ASCP CASESET
Laboratory Medicine

Publishing Team

Tae W Moon (design/production)
Joshua Weikersheimer (publishing direction)

Notice

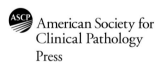

American Society for
Clinical Pathology
Press

Printed in China

16 15 14 13 12 11

ASCP CASESET
Laboratory Medicine

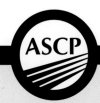

Edited by

Monte S. Willis, MD, PhD
Assistant Professor, Department of Pathology & Laboratory Medicine
University of North Carolina, Chapel Hill
Assistant Editor, *LABMEDICINE*

Frank H. Wians, Jr., PhD, MT(ASCP)
Technical Director, Core Laboratory
Baylor University Medical Center, Dallas, TX
Professor of Pathology (Ret), Department of Pathology,
University of Texas Southwestern Medical Center at Dallas
Lt Col (Ret), USAF, BSC
Editor-in-Chief, *LABMEDICINE*

Contributors (by last name)

A

Robert F. Aarstad
Fleurette Abreo
Syed A. Abutalib
Amy L. Adams
Julius Aitsebaomo
R. Scott Akins
Lisa Dunn-Albanasse
Jaffar Alfardan
M. Qasim Ansari
Rachna Arora
Mahnaz Shahidi-Asl
Vijay Aswani
Yara M. Audeh

B

Soon Bahrami
Jonathan Baker
Monette S. Baker
Jody A. Balko
Richard D. Barrera
Alice A. Basinger
Leland B. Baskin
Peter Bauer
Amanda Rivera-Begeman
Matthew L. Bell
Michael J. Bennett
Jason A Bennett
Mustafa Benekli
Roger L. Berkow
Seth M. Berney
Emmanuel C. Besa
Jill Zyrek-Betts
Parul Bhargava
Angelica Black
Diana L. Cochran-Black
Melissa M. Blann
Kenneth E. Blick
Michael B. Bober
Robert Booth
Barbara G. Border
Bradley Bryan
Charles Bradley
Beverly J. Brent
Chad F. Brouse
Michelle R. Brown
Sabrina Bryant
Christoph Buettner
Holly N. Burford
Linda K. Burnside
SF Bushor
Anthony W. Butch

Suleyman Buyukberber

C

Jeffrey A. Cadeddu
Patricia M. Canfield
Sharon E. Card
Elliot Carter
Dominick Cavuoti
Wendy Chamberlain
Wendy Chamberlain
Omer Chaudhry
Bai-Hsiun Chen
Hung-Jung Cheng
Yiqing Chi
Michael Cimo
Michael Constantinescu
James D. Cotelingam
Randy Coulter
Ugur Coskun

D

Michael D'Amarino
Jasbir Dhanoa
Asim Diab
Sandra Dietrich
Haig Donabedian
Robert F. Dons
Menka Doomra
Charles Dumontet
Dale M. Dunn
SL Dudley

E

Tze-Kiong Er
Tara N. Evans

F

Zheng Fan
Brent Farnesworth
Susan L. Fisher
Rachel B. Flamholz
Marjorie R. Fowler
Christine Lomas-Francis
J. Barry Freeman
Kristi Frenken
Karen Fritchie
Franklin S. Fuda
MK Fung

G

Rita Gander
Sujata Gaitonde
Seema Garg
Alde Carlo P. Gavino
Luc-Marie Gerland
Hossam Ghoneim

Peter Gilligan
Sandrine Kagialis-Girard
AJ Goodwin
Shweta Goyal
Debra Grant
Janice M. Matthews-Greer
Ratna Grewal
Luis A. Guarda

H

Ron G. Haas
Alexandra Harrington
Brian J. Harrington
Ibrahim A. Hashim
Emily Herndon
Elba A. Turbat-Herrera
Stephen Hill
Shu T. Huang
Jane Hudson
Sean M. Hussey

J

Majed Jeroudi
Mary John
Patricia M. Jones
Vivian Jones
Yuh-Jyh Jong
Cynthia Jumper

K

Andrea G. Kahn
Ali Osman Kaya
Ashraf M. Kahn
Eiad Kahwash
Samir Kahwash
Suthida Kankirawatana
Naveen Kakkar
Yuan S. Kao
Saliman A. Karsou
Anureet Kaur
Melanie S. Kennedy
Bryce Kerlin
Adil I. Khan
Eric Knudtson
Kathleen Kiefhaber
Karen C. Kirkley
Julie Kirkegaard
Marta L. Klein
Richard Komorowski
Ted Krafczyk
Steven Kroft
Karen K. Krisher
Dave Krugh
Ashwani Kumar

L

Meredith A. Lakey
Shahnila Latif
M. Jane Latimer
Jill Leonard
Valerie Lindgren
Cynthia Z. Liu
Alberto Locante
William Lockwood
Gifford Lum
Regina de Luna
Gillian Luxton
Andrew W. Lyon

M

Lisa Machor
Robert W. McKenna
B.R. MacPherson
Jonathan Marotti
Marisa B. Marques
Mary M. Mayo
Christopher R. McCudden
Qing H. Meng
Phylis Moder
Arshag D. Mooradian
Joseph Muenzer

N

Ranveer Nand
Meenakshi Nandedkar
Regina Y. Najera
Srinivas B. Narayan
Jason Nash
Michael F. Neerman
Jill Newstead
Kathleen Nicol
Frank Nizzi
Mary L. Nordberg

O

Richard O'Shaughnessy
Jeffrey W. Oliver
Yusra Othman
Banu Ozturk

P

Sangtae Park
K. Michael Parker
John R. Parker
Kara Partridge
Jigar S. Patel
Surekha Pendyal
Pete Pelletier
Kristin A. Pierce
Mary Plenzler
Matthew R. Plymyer

Judith O. Pretell
Kellous A. Price

Q

Reade Quinton

R

Dinesh Rakheja
Maria A. B. Reed
Stephanie D. Reilly
Paula Revell
Mark R. Rice
Mohammed Nabil Richi
Nada Rikabi
Danielle Treille-Ritouet
Dorothy Rivette
Damiano Rondelli
Melissa J. Rose
Karen Rossi
Michael Roth
Cynthia Rutherford

S

Steven J. Saccaro
Vishwas S. Sakhalkar
Yaseen Samman
Nancy L. Sapanara
Ravindra Sarode
Adam Seegmiller
Lisa Senzel
Corey J. Shamah
Deepti Shukla
Diane Snider
Guranjan Deep Singh
Sumi G. So
Satish K. Solanki
Paul M. Southern
Joseph Susa
Catherine Hammett-Stabler
Steffini Stalos
Mark R. Steciuk
Justin N. Steinert
Peggy Soung Sullivan
Martin I. Surks
Laurie J. Sutor
Lisa M Sutton
Vanlila Swami
Nawwar Swedan
Paula Szuflad

T

Louis Nova-Takara
Silvio S. Tanev
Reeta Thapa
John G. Thomas
Ronald Thomason

Marie W. Tortelli
Li-Yu Tsai
Rodney Tucay

U

Aytug Uner

V

Diana M. Veillon

W

Patrick C. J. Ward
Irfan Warraich
Arthur G. Weinberg
Michael D. White
Frank H. Wians, Jr.
JoAnna D. Williams
Monte S. Willis
Dennis C. Wooten
Jianhua Wu
Kathleen Wyne

X

Yin Xu

Y

Zhaohai Yang
Deniz Yamac
Emel Yaman
Manni Yeggapan
Ramazan Yildiz
Zhongxin Yu

Z

Fahim Zaman
Mandolin Ziadie

Preface

This ASCP CASESET provides case studies across the major subspecialties of clinical pathology:

- Chemistry
- Urinalysis
- Transfusion Medicine
- Microbiology
- Hematology
- Coagulation
- Immunology

The cases included within each subspecialty were selected from the library of case studies published in *LABMEDICINE*, a monthly, peer-reviewed publication of the American Society for Clinical Pathology (ASCP) dedicated to educating its readership on clinical pathology/laboratory medicine.

Cases are grouped within the major subspecialty areas of clinical pathology, recognizing that any attempt to strictly catalog many cases into a single subspecialty is fraught with difficulties because of the overlapping nature of the condition/disease between more than 1 subspecialty. For example, a case in which the final diagnosis is "multiple myeloma" could be categorized legitimately under Chemistry, Hematology, or Immunology subheadings. Therefore, the choice of subspecialties for categorizing cases was strictly the decision of the Editors. We also recognize that many of the major subspecialties of clinical pathology have sub-subspecialties (eg, Microbiology typically includes mycology, parasitology, and virology) within them; however, for simplicity we have chosen a hierarchical categorization of cases based on the 5 major subspecialties indicated above, with Urinalysis included with Chemistry.

The purpose of this ASCP CASESET is to provide allied health professionals and post-doctoral trainees in pathology and laboratory medicine involved in the teaching and training of clinical pathology with an extensive library of case studies covering a broad range of topics within each subspecialty of clinical pathology. Given the current emphasis on the "case study-based" approach to teaching medicine, including laboratory medicine, we believe that the case studies we have selected for inclusion in this ASCP CASESET will benefit both instructors and students. Moreover, to improve the teaching value of each case study, all cases use a standardized format involving the student's responses to the following questions, whenever applicable:

1. What are this patient's most striking clinical and laboratory findings?

2. What is (are) the most likely cause(s) of this patient's most striking laboratory findings?

3. What additional laboratory test(s) should be performed on this patient and why?

4. What is the principle of the critical laboratory test used to establish this patient's final diagnosis?

5. What condition does this patient's clinical, diagnostic, and laboratory findings suggest?

6. What is the pathophysiology of this patient's condition?

7. How should this patient's condition be treated?

Moreover, the answers to all questions, including detailed information, are provided for all of the above questions.

The principal advantages of the case studies are:

- The cases represent a broad spectrum of relatively rare, commonly occurring, and unusual conditions/diseases and the screening and confirmatory tests used typically to arrive at a definitive diagnosis

- The use of a standardized format to promote critical thinking and analysis of the clinical and laboratory information provided to arrive at a *differential diagnosis*, followed by synthesis of all patient-specific information necessary to arrive at a *definitive diagnosis*

- Case studies within each subspecialty Section are organized alphabetically by general "Topic Area," followed by a more specific "Topic" identifier to aid the reader in finding case studies pertinent to their teaching needs

- Each subspecialty Section contains an "Overview," written by an expert in the field, that provides useful information on the cases selected for inclusion

- Although the principal focus of the cases is topics in clinical pathology, some of the cases incorporate anatomic pathology (eg, histology) findings to strengthen further an understanding of the pathophysiology of the disease process associated with a particular condition/disease

- The content of the case studies can be easily translated into useful, colorful, and animated PowerPoint slides for student lecture presentations [**Note:** when using these case studies for teaching purposes, please be sure to provide appropriate attribution to the authors (not the Editors/Associate Editors of this ASCP CASESET) of each case]

- The answers are provided for all questions posed in each case study

- Each subspecialty section contains "Suggested Reading," including many books, and other educational resources, pertinent to the case studies within a chapter and available from ASCP Press via its online website: http://www.ascp.org/books

Last, the Introduction, "**Clinical Laboratory Tests: Which, Why, and What Do the Results Mean?**" provides useful information on the principal focus of all case studies – how clinical laboratory test results can and should be combined with other patient-specific information to arrive at a definitive diagnosis that improves patient care.

The Editors thank all authors of the cases selected for inclusion in this ASCP CASESET for providing what we believe is a "treasure-trove" of informative and useful cases with significant teaching value for instructors and students alike in all of the medical and allied health professions.

Monte S. Willis, MD, PhD

Frank H. Wians, Jr., PhD, MT(ASCP)

Table of Contents

vi   Preface

1   Chemistry Overview

Adrenal Gland

Blood Gases

Carbon Monoxide Intoxication

Calcium

CSF Beta-2-Transferrin

Diabetes

Electrolytes

Heart Disease

Hereditary Disease

Clinical Laboratory Tests: Which, Why, and What Do the Results Mean?

Frank H. Wians, Jr.

Department of Pathology, University of Texas Southwestern Medical Center, Dallas, TX

The purpose of this CE Update is to discuss the laboratory testing cycle and its importance in diagnostic decision making. This discussion will begin with some general comments about approaches to ordering clinical laboratory tests, followed by "real-world" examples to illustrate these approaches. We will then review the important diagnostic performance characteristics of laboratory tests, how they are calculated, and a principal tool (ie, receiver-operator characteristic [ROC] curves) used to assess the diagnostic accuracy of a laboratory test at specific cutoff values for the test. We will then discuss how laboratory tests are interpreted using a reference interval and its limitations, followed by some brief remarks about the concepts critical difference and neural network.

The "Laboratory Testing Cycle"

The "laboratory testing cycle" (**Figure 1**) consists of all steps between the time when a clinician thinks about and orders a laboratory test and the time the appropriate patient's sample for testing is obtained (eg, a blood specimen taken from an antecubital vein) and the results of the testing are returned to the clinician (often called the "vein-to-brain" turnaround time [TAT] of test results). This cycle consists of 3 phases: *preanalytical*, *analytical*, and *postanalytical* (**Figure 1**).

Common causes of *preanalytical* errors include a variety of factors, many of which are summarized in **T1**.

Analytical errors are of 2 types: random or systematic, and systematic errors can be subdivided further into constant or proportional error. Random errors can be caused by timing, temperature, or pipetting variations that occur randomly during the measurement process and are independent of the operator performing the measurement. Systematic error is caused frequently by a time-dependent change in instrument calibration that causes the calibration curve to shift its position and

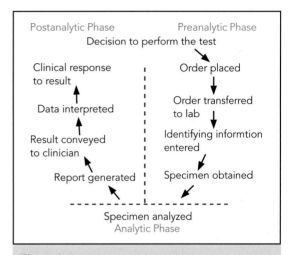

Figure 1_The "Laboratory Testing Cycle."

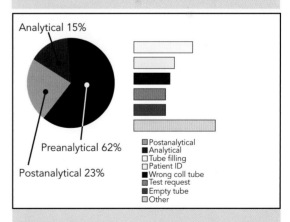

Figure 1A_Laboratory errors in stat testing. *Adapted from Ref 1.*

alter the accuracy and/or precision (reproducibility) of the quantitative results obtained using this curve.

Postanalytical errors include such mistakes as transcription errors (eg, an accurate and reliable result reported on the wrong patient, using the wrong value,

T1. Examples of Common Causes of Preanalytical Error

Biological
Age
Sex
Race (Blacks vs. Caucasians)
Behavioral
Diet
Obesity
Smoking
Alcohol intake
Caffeine intake
Exercise
Stress
Clinical (2⁰ Alterations)
Diseases:
Hypothyroidism
Insulin-dependent diabetes mellitus
Nephrotic syndrome/chronic renal failure
Biliary tract obstruction
Acute myocardial infarction
Drug Therapy:
Diuretics
Propanolol
Oral contraceptives with high [progestin]
Oral contraceptives with high [estrogen]
Prednisolone
Cyclosporine
Pregnancy
Specimen Collection & Handling
Specimen obtained from wrong patient*
Specimen mix-up*
Nonfasting vs. fasting (12 h)
Anticoagulant:
EDTA
Heparin
Capillary vs. venous blood
Hemoconcentration (eg, use of a tourniquet)
Specimen storage (@ 0–4 °C for up to 4 days)

Common sources of preanalytical error; however, frequency decreasing with advent of better quality assurance (QA) procedures to ensure positive patient ID and labeling of specimen tubes.

and/or with the wrong units [eg, mg/L instead of mg/day]).

The results of a relatively recent article on the sources of laboratory errors in stat testing, which should be very gratifying to laboratorians, has shown that analytical sources of error occurred least frequently (15%) while preanalytical errors occurred most frequently (62%) (**Figure 1A**).[1]

The top 5 causes of preanalytical errors were:[1]

- Specimen collection tube not filled properly.

- Patient ID error.

- Inappropriate specimen collection tube/container.

- Test request error.

- Empty collection tube.

Although 75.6% of all sources (preanalytical, analytical, or postanalytical) of laboratory errors had no effect on patient outcomes, ~25% had a negative impact, indicating much opportunity to reduce laboratory errors to Six Sigma levels (ie, < 3.4 errors/1 million opportunities) or near perfection.[1,2]

Diagnostic Decision Making

The use of clinical laboratory test results in diagnostic decision making is an integral part of clinical medicine. The menu of laboratory tests available to clinicians constitutes an impressive array that has expanded exponentially since 1920 when Folin and Wu devised the first useful test for the quantification of serum glucose concentration.[3] The current list of tests offered by 1 major reference laboratory includes nearly 3,000 analytes, which does not include the additional array of more commonly ordered tests (eg, complete blood count [CBC], electrolytes [sodium, potassium, chloride, carbon dioxide], thyroid stimulating hormone [TSH], glucose, etc.) routinely performed on site by most hospital-based clinical laboratories. Despite this ever-expanding plethora of useful and reliable clinical laboratory tests for diagnosing and monitoring the myriad of diseases effecting mankind, the recent emphasis on reducing health care costs and the emergence of managed care organizations led to efforts to reduce the abuse (over-ordering) and misuse (eg, ordering the right test for the wrong purpose or vice versa) of these tests.

Medical Necessity

As private health maintenance organizations (HMOs) and government-sponsored agencies (eg, Department of Health and Human Services [DHHS] and the Centers for Medicare and Medicaid Services [CMS]) seek to provide quality medicine cost effectively, reduction in the ordering of "unnecessary" laboratory tests has become a favorite target of these efforts. The critical question facing physicians, however, is: What constitutes an unnecessary laboratory test? In the current climate of business-oriented medicine, the answer should not be: Any test for which reimbursement by a payer (eg, Medicare) is likely to be denied. The correct answer is: Any test for which the results are *not* likely to be "medically necessary" in the appropriate management of the patient's medical condition. Thus, it is incumbent upon physicians and laboratorians to understand which laboratory tests are appropriate to order in the diagnosis and follow up of a patient's medical condition.

Questions to Ask Before Ordering a Laboratory Test

An understanding of which laboratory tests are appropriate to order in the diagnosis and follow up of a patient's medical condition should include prior consideration of the answers to the following questions:[4]

- Why is the test being ordered?

- What are the consequences of not ordering the test?

- How good is the test in discriminating between health versus disease?

- How are the test results interpreted?

- How will the test results influence patient management and outcome?

The answers to these questions are critical to the optimal selection and cost-effective use of laboratory tests likely to benefit patient management. A major misconception among clinicians is the feeling that a laboratory test is more objective than a patient's history and physical examination. Nevertheless, it is widely accepted that the judicious use of laboratory tests, coupled with thoughtful interpretation of the results of these tests, can contribute significantly to diagnostic decision making and patient management.

Reasons for Ordering a Laboratory Test

There are 4 major legitimate reasons for ordering a laboratory test:[4]

1. Diagnosis (to rule in or rule out a diagnosis).

2. Monitoring (eg, the effect of drug therapy).

3. Screening (eg, for congenital hypothyroidism via neonatal thyroxine testing).

4. Research (to understand the pathophysiology of a particular disease process).

Approaches for Establishing a Diagnosis Based on Laboratory Test Results

The principal approaches for establishing a diagnosis based on laboratory test results include:[4]

- Hypothesis deduction.

- Pattern recognition.

- Medical algorithms.

- Rifle versus shotgun approach.

Hypothesis deduction involves establishing a differential diagnosis based on the patient's history, including family, social, and drug history, and physical exam findings, followed by the selection of laboratory tests that are the most likely to confirm (ie, allow the clinician to deduce) a diagnosis on the list of differential diagnoses.

Example 1_*Hypothesis deduction* approach to laboratory test ordering: A 4-year-old child presents to the emergency room (ER) with an upper respiratory tract infection (URI), fever (102.2°F), and generalized seizures lasting 2 min. The clinician establishes a differential diagnosis of meningitis versus febrile seizures and deduces that the most appropriate

T2. Example of Pattern Recognition Approach to Diagnosis

Laboratory Test	Type of Pregnancy-Associated Thrombocytopenia						Patient
	ITP	GTP	TTP	HUS	DIC	HELLP	
Platelet count (×10³/uL)	<100	70-150	<50	LN to ↓	↓	<100	<50
Platelet antibody	+/–	+/–	–	–	–	–	–
PT and APTT	N	N	N	N	↑	N	N
D-dimer, µg/mL	<0.5	<0.5	<0.5	>0.5	>0.5	>0.5	<0.5
AST and ALT	N	N	N	N	N	↑	N
LD	N	N	↑↑↑	↑↑↑	↑	↑	N
BUN and creatinine	N	N	N or ↑	↑↑↑	↑	↑	N
RBC morphology	N	N	schistocytes	schistocytes spherocytes helmet cells	schistocytes	schistocytes	N

PT, prothrombin time; APTT, activated partial thromboplastin time; AST, aspartate aminotransferase; ALT, alanine aminotransferase; LD, lactate dehydrogenase; BUN, blood urea nitrogen; RBC, red blood cell; N, normal; LN, low-normal; ↓, decreased; ↑, increased, ↑↑↑, markedly increased; +/–, may be positive or negative; –, negative

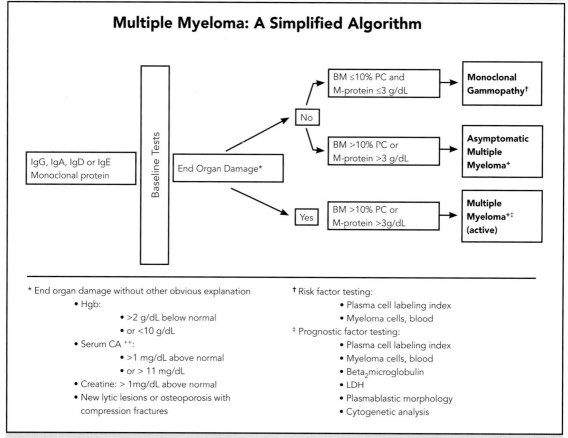

Multiple Myeloma: A Simplified Algorithm

IgG, IgA, IgD or IgE Monoclonal protein → Baseline Tests → End Organ Damage*

End Organ Damage* → No → BM ≤10% PC and M-protein ≤3 g/dL → **Monoclonal Gammopathy†**

No → BM >10% PC or M-protein >3 g/dL → **Asymptomatic Multiple Myeloma+**

End Organ Damage* → Yes → BM >10% PC or M-protein >3g/dL → **Multiple Myeloma+‡ (active)**

* End organ damage without other obvious explanation
- Hgb:
  - >2 g/dL below normal
  - or <10 g/dL
- Serum CA ++:
  - >1 mg/dL above normal
  - or > 11 mg/dL
- Creatine: > 1mg/dL above normal
- New lytic lesions or osteoporosis with compression fractures

† Risk factor testing:
- Plasma cell labeling index
- Myeloma cells, blood

‡ Prognostic factor testing:
- Plasma cell labeling index
- Myeloma cells, blood
- Beta₂microglobulin
- LDH
- Plasmablastic morphology
- Cytogenetic analysis

Figure 2_Simplified algorithm for the diagnosis of a monoclonal gammopthy versus asymptomatic multiple myeloma versus active multiple myeloma (Source: *Mayo Communique*. 2002;27:2).

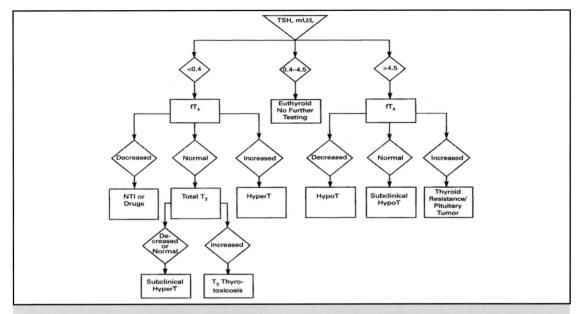

Figure 2.1_Algorithm for identifying individuals with thyroid disorders based on TSH level. TSH, thyroid-stimulating hormone; fT$_4$, free thyroxine; NTI, nonthyroid illness; T$_3$, triiodothyronine; HyperT, hyperthyroidism; HypoT, hypothyroidism.

laboratory tests to discriminate between these possibilities are the following tests performed on cerebrospinal fluid (CSF) from a spinal tap:

- White blood cell (WBC) and red blood cell (RBC) counts.

- Total protein.

- Glucose.

- Gram stain.

- Bacterial, viral, and/or fungal cultures.

- Rapid polymerase chain reaction (PCR) assay for a meningococcus-specific insertion sequence (IS).

All results for these tests were either "normal," "negative," or "no growth" (cultures), supporting a diagnosis of febrile seizure over bacterial, viral, or fungal meningitis.

Pattern recognition involves comparing the patient's pattern of results for several laboratory tests that have been determined previously to provide excellent power in discriminating between various competing and/or closely related diagnoses (**T2**). The pattern of laboratory test results shown for the pregnant "Patient" in **T2** most closely match those consistent with a diagnosis of idiopathic thrombocytopenic purpura (ITP), rather than other possible causes of pregnancy-associated thrombocytopenia: gestational thrombocytopenic (GTP); thrombotic thrombocytopenia (TTP); hemolytic uremic syndrome (HUS); disseminated intravascular coagulation (DIC); or, (syndrome of) hemolysis, elevated liver enzymes, and low platelet count (HELLP).

Medical algorithms (or "decision trees") are particularly useful in establishing a diagnosis based, in part, on information obtained from ordering the most appropriate (ie, necessary) laboratory tests. Such algorithms (cf., **Figures 2** and **2.1**) are advantageous because they:

- are logical and sequential;

- can be automated using a computer to achieve rapid turnaround time of results for tests included in the algorithm;

- *maximize* a clinician's efficiency;

- *minimize* the ordering of unnecessary laboratory tests;

- can be used by ancillary medical personnel (eg, physician assistants and nurse practitioners) and assisting physicians;

- can be easily updated with improved strategies for diagnostic decision making as new and better tests become available; and

- are incorporated into software programs that are relatively inexpensive to purchase and use.

The *rifle versus shotgun approach* to laboratory test ordering relates to ordering specific laboratory tests based on an assessment of their diagnostic accuracy and predictive value in identifying a particular disease (ie, using a "rifle" to hit the bulls-eye representing the correct diagnosis) versus indiscriminate ordering of a large number of laboratory tests that may or may not have adequate diagnostic accuracy and predictive value in identifying a particular disease (ie, using a "shotgun" to hit the target, which is likely to create a pattern of shots on the target, none of which may hit the bulls-eye). Ordering the following 20 laboratory (and other) tests on a 4-year-old child with signs and symptoms of an upper respiratory tract infection, fever (102.2 °F), and generalized seizure lasting 2 min represents a *shotgun*—and very expensive—approach to arriving at a diagnosis:

WBC count w/differential

Quantitative immunoglobulins (IgG, IgA, IgM)

Erythrocyte sedimentation rate (ESR)

Quantitative alpha-1-antitrypsin (AAT) level

Retic count

Arterial blood gasses (ABGs)

Throat culture

Sweat chloride

Nasal smear for eosinophils

Nasopharyngeal culture for pertussis infection

Viral cultures

Stool exam for ova and parasites (O & P)

Example 2			
	No. of Men With PCa	No. of Men Without PCa	Total
No. of men with positive[a]	160 (TP)	6,860 (FP)	7,020 PSA test
No. of men with negative[b] PSA test	40 (FN)	2,940 (TN)	2,980
Total	200	9,800	10,000

[a]Positive PSA test = men with a serum PSA concentration ≥4.0 ng/mL
[b]Negative PSA test = men with a serum PSA concentration <4.0 ng/mL

Urinalysis

Purified protein derivative (tuberculin) (PPD)/trichophyton/cocci skin tests

Electrolytes

Glucose

Total bilirubin

Aspartate aminotransferase (AST)
Alanine aminotransferase (ALT)

Chest X-ray (×3)

Electrocardiogram (ECG)

A rifle approach would involve ordering only those laboratory tests useful in discriminating between the diseases constituting the differential diagnosis (ie, meningitis or febrile seizure) as indicated in **Example 1** above (ie, the 7 to 9 "targeted" tests on CSF).

Clinical Performance Characteristics of Laboratory Tests

Because the clinical performance characteristics of all laboratory tests differ with respect to their diagnostic accuracy (ie, sensitivity and specificity), the selection of the appropriate laboratory test to order will vary depending on the purpose for which the test is to be used. Before considering this aspect of the selection of laboratory tests, we must first understand the terms that describe their diagnostic performance. These terms include prevalence, sensitivity, specificity, efficiency, and predictive value. To illustrate the mathematical calculation of values for each of these parameters, consider the example given below:[4,5]

Example 2_The laboratory test, prostate-specific antigen (PSA), was studied with regard to its ability to discriminate patients with prostate cancer (PCa) from those without PCa. This test was performed on 10,000 men, 200 of whom have biopsy-proven prostate cancer. Using this information, a *2 x 2 table* can be constructed as shown.

From this data, the values for prevalence, sensitivity, specificity, efficiency, positive predictive value (PPV), and negative predictive value (NPV) can be determined:

- *Prevalence* (p) = No. of individuals with disease/ No. of individuals in population to be tested

- = 200/10,000 = 0.020 = 2.0%

- *Sensitivity* = percentage of individuals *with* disease who have a *positive* test result = No. of true-positives/(No. of true-positives + No. of false-negatives) or $TP/(TP + FN) = 160/(160 + 40) = 160/200 = 0.800 = 80\%$

- *Specificity* = percentage of individuals *without* disease who have a *negative* test result = No. of true-negatives/(No. of true-negatives + No. of false-positives) or $TN/(TN + FP) = 2,940/ (2,940 + 6,860) = 2,940/9,800 = 0.30 = 30\%$

T2. The Effect of Disease Prevalence on the Positive (PPV) and Negative Predictive Value (NPV) of a Laboratory Test[a]

Disease Prevalence, %	PPV, %	NPV, %
0.1	1.9	99.9
1	16.1	99.9
10	67.9	99.4
50	95.0	95.0
100	100.0	n.a.

[a] In this example, the test is assigned 95% diagnostic specificity and 95% diagnostic sensitivity. n.a., not applicable.

- *Efficiency* =percentage of individuals correctly classified by test results as being either positive or negative for the disease = $(TP + TN)/(TP + FP + FN + TN) = (160 + 2,940)/10,000 = 3,100/10,000 = 0.31 = 31\%$

- *Positive Predictive Value (PPV)* = percentage of individuals with a *positive* test result who truly *have* the disease = $TP/(TP + FP) = 160/(160 + 6,860) = 160/7,020 = 0.023 = 2.3\%$, or

- $PPV = (\text{sensitivity})(p)/[(\text{sensitivity})(p) + (1 - \text{specificity})(1 - p) = (0.8)(0.02/[(0.8)(0.02) + (1 - 0.3)(1 - 0.02)] = 0.016/[0.016 + (0.7)(0.98)] = 0.016/[0.016 + 0.686] = 0.016/0.702 = 0.023 = 2.3\%$

- *Negative Predictive Value (NPV)* = percentage of individuals with a *negative* test result who do *not* have the disease = $TN/(TN + FN) = 2,940/ (2,940 + 40) = 2,940/2,980 = 0.987 = 98.7\%$, or $NPV = (\text{specificity})(1 - p)/[(\text{specificity})(1 - p) + (1 - \text{sensitivity})(p)] = (0.3)(1 - 0.02)/[(0.3)(1 - 0.02) + (1 - 0.8)(0.02)] = 0.294/0.298 = 0.987 = 98.7\%$

- *Sum of Sensitivity and Specificity* = 80 + 30 = 110 (*Note:* In general, a useful laboratory test will have a sum >170)

It is important to note that any test with a sensitivity = 50% and a specificity = 50% is no better than a coin toss in deciding whether or not a disease may be present. Tests with a combined sensitivity and specificity total = 170 or greater are likely to prove clinically useful. Most clinicians can achieve this total with a good history and physical examination! Thus, a laboratory test with 95% sensitivity and 95% specificity (sum = 190) is an excellent test.

The poor PPV (2.3%) in the example above makes it appear as if even good laboratory tests (which PSA is) are relatively useless. If the test is used selectively, however, for example on a population of individuals likely to have a disease (eg, a population in which the prevalence of disease is high), many laboratory tests have excellent PPVs. The effect of prevalence on predictive value is demonstrated in **T2**.

How do physicians increase the predictive value of laboratory tests? By appropriately selecting patients on whom the test is performed (ie, by maximizing the prevalence of disease in the population sampled). In the example cited above, performing PSA testing on men over age 50 years improves the PPV of PSA since the prevalence of prostate cancer increases from <1% in Caucasian men aged less than 50 years to 16% in men aged 50 to 64 years and to 83% in men over 64 years of age.

In some cases, it may be desirable to use a laboratory test with high sensitivity while sacrificing "some" specificity or vice versa. For example, if the risk associated with failure to diagnose a particular disease is high (eg, acquired immunodeficiency syndrome [AIDS]), false-negatives are unacceptable and only a laboratory test with high sensitivity is acceptable. On the other hand, if a disease is potentially fatal and no therapy, other than supportive care, is available (eg, cystic fibrosis), false-positives would be unacceptable. Thus, in this situation, a laboratory test with high specificity is desirable. In general, laboratory tests with both high sensitivity and high specificity are desirable since both false-negatives and false-positives are equally unacceptable under most clinical circumstances.

Diagnostic *sensitivity* refers to the proportion of individuals *with disease* who yield a *positive* test for an analyte (eg, PSA) associated with a particular disease. Diagnostic *specificity* refers to the proportion of individuals *without disease* who yield a *negative* test for the analyte. A "perfect" test would have both 100% diagnostic sensitivity and specificity, which seldom occurs in practice and if it does, the population of diseased and non-diseased patients studied was probably not large and varied enough to demonstrate that the test was not perfect. For any given test, there is always a trade-off between sensitivity and specificity, such that choosing a cutoff value (decision threshold) for a particular test that maximizes sensitivity occurs at the expense of specificity. This situation is illustrated in **Figure 2.2**.

Visual inspection of **Figure 2.2** reveals that, if the cutoff value, denoted by the dotted line at 4.0 ng/mL, is lowered to 2.0 ng/mL, the sensitivity of the PSA test improves from 80% at a cutoff of 4.0 ng/mL to 100% at a cutoff of 2.0 ng/mL since there are no false-negatives (ie, in this example, all individuals with prostate cancer have PSA values greater than 2.0 ng/mL). In addition, however, the number of false-positives increases, which causes the specificity of this test to worsen since specificity = $TN/(TN + FP)$, because any increase in the number of false-positives, a term in

the denominator of this equation, results in a decrease in the value given by this equation. Alternatively, if the cutoff value is increased to 10.0 ng/mL, the specificity of the PSA test improves from 30% at a cutoff of 4.0 ng/mL to 100% at a cutoff of 10.0 ng/mL since there are no false-positives (ie, in this example, all individuals without prostate cancer have PSA values less than 10.0 ng/mL). In addition, however, the number of false-negatives increases which causes the sensitivity of this test to worsen since sensitivity = $TP/(TP + FN)$.

Lastly, it is important to remember that knowing the sensitivity (ie, positivity in disease) and specificity (ie, negativity in health or non-disease) of a test is of limited value because these parameters represent the answer to the question: What is the probability of a patient having a positive test result if this patient has disease X? The more challenging question facing clinicians, however, is: What is the probability of this patient having disease X if the test result is positive (or negative)?[5] The reader is referred to reference 5 for a statistical briefing on how to estimate the probability of disease using likelihood ratios.

Receiver-Operator Characteristic (ROC) Curves

Receiver- (or relative-) operator characteristic (ROC) curves provide another useful tool in assessing the diagnostic accuracy of a laboratory test, because all (specificity, sensitivity) pairs for a test are plotted. The principal advantage of ROC curves is their ability to provide information on test performance at all decision thresholds.[3,6]

Typically, a ROC curve plots the false-positive rate (FPR = 1 - specificity) versus the true-positive rate (TPR = sensitivity). The clinical usefulness or practical value of the information provided by ROC curves in patient care may vary, however, even for tests that have good discriminating ability (ie, high sensitivity and specificity at a particular decision threshold). This may occur for several reasons:

- False-negative results may be so costly that there is no cutoff value for the test that provides acceptable sensitivity and specificity.

- The cost of the test and/or the technical difficulty in performing the test may be so high that its availability is limited.

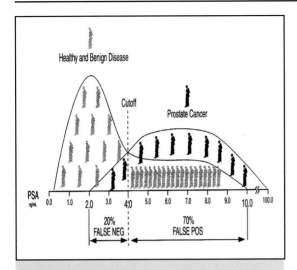

Figure 2.2_Dramatic representation of diagnostic sensitivity and specificity using the analyte PSA as an example.

- Less invasive or less expensive tests may provide similar information.

- The hardship (eg, financial and/or physical) associated with the test may cause patients to be unwilling to submit to the test.

A test with 100% sensitivity and 100% specificity in discriminating prostatic cancer from benign prostatic hyperplasia (BPH) and prostatitis at all decision thresholds would be represented by the y-axis and the line perpendicular to the y-axis at a sensitivity of 1.0 = 100% in a square plot of FPR versus TPR (**Figure 2.3A**).

A test for which the specificity and sensitivity pairs sum to exactly 100% at all decision thresholds would be represented by the diagonal of the square (**Figure 2.3A**) and represents a test with no clinical value.

Thus, in *qualitatively* comparing 2 or more tests in their ability to discriminate between 2 alternative states of health using ROC curves, the test associated with the curve that is displaced further toward the upper left-hand corner of the ROC curve has better discriminating ability (ie, a cutoff value for the test can be chosen that yields higher sensitivity and/or specificity) than tests associated with curves that lie below this curve. A more precise *quantitative* estimate of the superiority of 1 test over another can be obtained by comparing the area-under-the-curve (AUC) for each test and applying

statistics to determine the significance of the difference between AUC values.

The AUC (range: 0.5 to 1.0) is a quantitative representation of overall test accuracy, where values from 0.5 to 0.7 represent low accuracy, values from 0.7 to 0.9 represent tests that are useful for some purposes, and values >0.9 represent tests with high accuracy. The ROC curve (AUC = 0.66; 95% confidence interval: 0.60–0.72) in **Figure 2.3A** demonstrates that PSA has only modest ability in discriminating BPH from organ-confined prostate cancer.

However, other data using ROC curves to assess the ability of the tumor markers, prostatic acid phosphatase (PAP) and PSA, to differentiate prostate cancer from BPH and prostatitis at various cutoff values is illustrated in **Figure 2.3B**. Qualitatively, the ROC curve corresponding to PSA is displaced further toward the upper left-hand corner of the box than the curve for PAP. Quantitatively, the AUC values for PSA and PAP are 0.86 and 0.67, respectively. Thus, both qualitative and quantitative ROC analysis demonstrates that PSA provides better discrimination than PAP in distinguishing men with prostate cancer from those with BPH or prostatitis. Moreover, the diagnostic accuracy (ie, sensitivity *and* specificity) of PSA in providing this discrimination is higher (AUC = 0.86) in **Figure 2.3B** than in **Figure 2.3A** (AUC = 0.66), probably due to differences in the study designs represented by the data shown in each panel of **Figure 2.3**.

Reference Interval for Interpreting Laboratory Test Results

Once a clinical laboratory test with the appropriate diagnostic accuracy has been ordered, how are the results of the test interpreted? Typically, a *reference interval* or a *decision level* is used, against which the patient's test value is compared. *Decision level* refers to a particular cutoff value for an analyte or test that enables individuals with a disorder or disease to be distinguished from those without the disorder or disease. Moreover, if the diagnostic accuracy of the test and the prevalence of the disease in a reference population are known, then the predictive value of the decision level for the disorder or disease can be determined.

Reference interval relates to the values for an analyte (eg, PSA, glucose, etc.), determined on a defined population

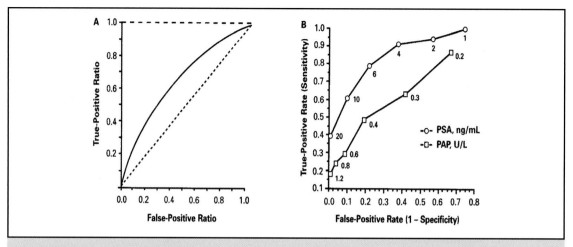

Figure 2.3_ROC curves for (**A**) perfect test (– – –), AUC=1.0; log PSA concentration in discriminating organ-confined prostate cancer from benign prostatic hyperplasia (———), AUC=0.66 (95% confidence interval, 0.60–0.72); test with no clinical value (-----), AUC=0.50. (**B**) Prostatic acid phosphatase (PAP) and PSA in differentiating prostate cancer from benign prostatic hyperplasia and prostatitis at various cutoff values (indicated adjacent to points on each of the curves). Reproduced with permission from Nicoll CD, Jeffrey JG, Dreyer J. *Clin Chem.* 1993;39:2540–2541.

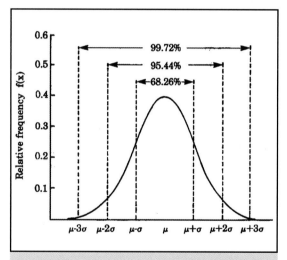

Figure 2.4_Example of a Gaussian (or bell-shaped) distribution of test values in which ~68% of the values are between the mean (μ) ± 1 standard deviation (σ); ~95% are between μ ± 2σ; and, ~99% are between μ ± 3σ.

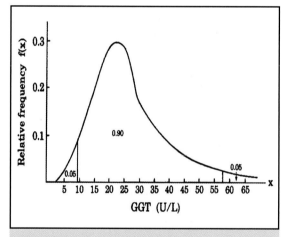

Figure 2.5_Example of a distribution of laboratory test values for an analyte (ie, the liver enzyme, gamma-glutamyl transferase [GGT]) for which the data are *not* Gaussian distributed.

of "healthy" individuals, that lie between the lower and the upper limits that constitute 95% of all values. Thus, an analyte value less than the lower limit of the reference interval would be classified as abnormally low, while any value greater than the upper limit of the reference interval would be classified as abnormally high, and values in between these limits would be classified as "normal." For example, after establishing the status of a population of individuals as "healthy," using such methods as history, physical exam, and findings other than the test being

evaluated, the reference interval for PSA, using many different assays, is typically stated as 0.0 ng/mL to 4.0 ng/mL. Thus, 95% of healthy men have a serum PSA concentration between these limits.

Although many laboratories publish the lower limit of a reference interval as "0," no analytical assay is capable of measuring a concentration precisely equal to 0 with high reproducibility. All quantitative assays have a finite lower limit of detection (LLD), distinct from 0, that more precisely constitutes the lower limit of the reference interval when this lower limit encompasses 0. For many PSA assays, the LLD is typically 0.05 ng/mL. Therefore, any PSA value less than 0.05 ng/mL would be reported appropriately as "less than 0.05 ng/mL" and not as 0.0 ng/mL. In addition, it is important to remember that reference intervals for an analyte are method dependent (ie, the reference interval established using 1 method cannot automatically be substituted for that of a different assay that measures the same analyte).

Since reference intervals for all analytes are based typically on the limits for the analyte that include 95% of all values obtained on healthy individuals with the assumption that the distribution of these values is Gaussian (or "bell-shaped"), it is important to recognize that 5% (or 1 out of 20; ie, the 2.5% of healthy individuals with analyte values in the left tail of the data distribution and the 2.5% of healthy individuals with analyte values in the right tail of the distribution when the reference interval is defined as the limits of the 2.5th and 97.5th percentiles of the distribution of all analyte values obtained on healthy individuals) of healthy individuals will have values outside these limits, either low or high (**Figure 2.4**).

Thus, reference intervals are intended to serve as a guideline for evaluating individual values and, for many analytes, information on the limits of an analyte for a population of individuals with the disease or diseases the test was designed to detect is even more informative. Also, it is important to recognize that values for some analytes in a population of healthy individuals may not be Gaussian distributed.

Figure 2.5 provides an illustration of this point applicable to the analyte, gamma-glutamyl transferase (GGT), in which the data is positively skewed. The reference interval for this data must be determined using a non-parametric statistical approach that does not make the assumption that the data is Gaussian distributed.

Lastly, to accurately interpret test results, it may be necessary to know gender-specific and/or age-stratified reference intervals since the values for many analytes vary with developmental stage or age. For example, alkaline phosphatase, an enzyme produced by osteoblasts (bone-forming cells), would be expected to be higher in a healthy 10- to 12-year-old during puberty and the growth spurt (ie, increased bone

formation during lengthening of the long bones) that normally accompanies puberty in adolescent males and females than those observed in a prepubertal or elderly individual.

Ideally, the best reference interval for an analyte would be *individual-specific* such that the value for the analyte, determined when the individual is ill, could be compared with the limits for this analyte, established on this same individual, when he or she was healthy or without the illness. For obvious reasons, it is difficult, if not impossible, to obtain such reference intervals. Thus, *population-based* reference intervals offer the most cost-effective and rational alternative. When using population-based reference intervals, however, it is critical that members of the reference population be free of any obvious or overt disease, especially diseases likely to affect the analyte for which the reference interval is being determined. For example, when determining a reference interval for TSH (also known as thyrotropin), it is critically important that the population of individuals tested be free of any pituitary or thyroid disease likely to affect the pituitary-hypothalamic-thyroid axis, which, under the action of the thyroid hormones tri- (T3) and tetraiodothyronine (T4), exert regulatory control over circulating levels of TSH.

Critical Difference Between Consecutive Laboratory Test Results

Since physicians frequently order the same test at multiple time points during the course of the patients' management, they are faced with the challenge of interpreting when the magnitude of the change in values for an analyte constitutes a significant change (or *critical difference* [CD]) that may (or should) affect medical decision making (eg, trigger a change in therapy, such as increasing or decreasing a drug dosage). Quantitative values for all analytes are affected by both imprecision (ie, lack of reproducibility) in the measurement of the analyte and *intra-individual variation* over time in the concentration of the analyte due to normal physiologic mechanisms (ie, biological variation) that are independent of any disease process. For example, the analyte cortisol, a glucocorticoid produced by the adrenal cortex that is important in glucose homeostasis, normally displays diurnal variation. Blood cortisol levels begin to rise during the early morning hours, peak at mid-morning, and then decline throughout the day to their lowest level between 8 PM and midnight. In patients with Cushing syndrome, this diurnal variation is lost and blood cortisol levels remain elevated throughout the day.

The degree of imprecision (ie, lack of reproducibility) in the quantitative measurement of any analyte is given by the magnitude of the coefficient of variation (CV), expressed usually as a percent, obtained from multiple measurements of the analyte using the formula: $\%CV = (SD/mean) \times 100$; where mean and SD are the mean and standard deviation of the values obtained from the multiple measurements of an analyte. There is a direct relationship between the magnitude of the CV and the degree of imprecision (ie, the lower the CV, the lower the imprecision [or the higher the degree of precision]). The magnitude of analytical variation is given by CV_a, while biological variability is defined by CV_b. Approaches to determining *assay-specific* values for CV_a, CV_b, and CD are beyond the scope of this CE Update.

Fortunately, most assays for a wide variety of analytes have excellent precision (ie, <5% to 10% CV_a), such that the principal component among these 2 sources of variation (ie, analytical or biological) is biological variation (CV_b). In addition, a change in values for an analyte that exceeds the change (ie, reference change value [RCV]) expected due to the combined effects of analytical and biological variation alone is due most likely to a disease process or to the affect of any therapy on the disease.

Neural Networks

More recently, neural networks, a branch of artificial intelligence, have been used to evaluate and interpret laboratory data.[7,8] These computerized networks mimic the processes performed by the human brain and can learn by example and generalize. Neural networks have been applied to such diverse areas as screening cervical smears (Pap smears) for the presence of abnormal cells and the identification of men at increased risk of prostate cancer by combining values for PSA, prostatic acid phosphatase (PAP), and total creatine kinase (CK). The use of neural networks in clinical and anatomic pathology is likely to expand because of their ability to achieve a higher level of accuracy than that attained by manual processes.

Laboratory Testing Paradox

Laboratory test results may influence up to 70 percent of medical decision making.[9] However, one must wonder whether the test results are being interpreted

correctly, and—if not—what the impact is of incorrect or inappropriate interpretation on the accuracy of diagnostic decision making based, in part, on laboratory test results. In a 2008 survey of junior physicians in the United Kingdom, only 18% of respondents were confident about requesting 12 common chemistry tests while more than half considered themselves usually confident or not confident in interpreting the results.[10] The lack of confidence in interpreting laboratory test results may be directly related, as suggested by Dr. Lopasata, to the sparse training in laboratory medicine provided in most United States medical schools.

Conclusion

In the final analysis, it is important for clinicians and laboratorians to recognize that laboratory data, although potentially extremely useful in diagnostic decision making, should be used as an aid and adjunct to the constellation of findings (eg, history, physical exam, etc.) relevant to the patient. *Laboratory data is never a substitute for a good physical exam and patient history (clinicians should treat the patient, not the laboratory results).*

1. Carraro P, Plebani M. Errors in a stat laboratory: Types and frequencies 10 years later. *Clin Chem*. 2007;53:1338–1342.

2. Gras JM, Philippe M. Application of Six Sigma concept in clinical laboratories: A review. *Clin Chem Lab Med*. 2007;45:789–796.

3. Wians FH Jr. Luminaries in laboratory medicine: Otto Folin. *Lab Med*. 2009;40:1–2.

4. Wians FH Jr, Baskin LB. Chapter 2: The Use of Clinical Laboratory Tests in Diagnostic Decision-Making. In: *Handbook of Clinical Pathology*, ASCP Press: Chicago; 2000: 9–24.

5. Lamb CR. Statistical briefing: Estimating the probability of disease. *Vet Radiol Ultrasound*. 2007;48:297–298.

6. Obuchowski NA, Lieber ML, Wians FH Jr. ROC curves in clinical chemistry: Uses, misuses, and possible solutions. *Clin Chem*. 2004;50:1118–1125.

7. Schweiger CR, Soeregi G, Spitzauer S, et al. Evaluation of laboratory data by conventional statistics and by 3 types of neural networks. *Clin Chem*. 1993;39:1966–1971.

8. Veltri RW, Chaudhari M, Miller MC, et al. Comparison of logistic regression and neural net modeling for prediction of prostate cancer pathologic stage. *Clin Chem*. 2002;48:1828–1834.

9. Forsman RW. Why is the laboratory an afterthought for managed care organizations? *Clin Chem*. 1996;42:813–816.

10. Khromova V, Gray TA. Learning needs in clinical biochemistry for doctors in foundation. *Ann Clin Biochem*. 2008;45:33–38.

Chemistry Overview

Frank H. Wians, Jr.

The case studies incorporated into this section represent a broad spectrum of organ systems, hereditary and acquired conditions/diseases, and subspecialties of Chemistry, including protein chemistry, liver function testing, and tests/hormones associated with the pituitary, parathyroid, and adrenal glands. The cases are arranged in alphabetical order by general "Topic Area," followed by a more specific "Topic" to aid the reader in quickly identifying the case studies of interest to their needs.

Representative hereditary and acquired conditions/diseases covered in this Section include:

- Analbuminemia

- Waldenström macroglobulinemia

- Congenital adrenal hyperplasia (CAH)

- Addison disease

- Hypercalcemia of malignancy

- Primary hyperparathyroidism

- Diabetic ketoacidosis (DKA)

- Hyperammonemia

- Pseudohyponatremia

- Syndrome of inappropriate anti-diuretic hormone (SIADH) secretion

- Chronic heart failure

- Inborn errors of metabolism

- Liver failure

- Renal failure

- Rhabdomyolysis

- Sarcoidosis

- Acute ethanol and ethylene glycol intoxication

- Hyperzincuria

- Benign prostatic hyperplasia and prostate cancer [ie, the role of the tumor marker, prostate-specific antigen (PSA), in discriminating between these 2 conditions]

Although only 2 tumor markers (CA 19-9 and PSA) are represented by case studies included in this Section, the following information is provided to expand the discussion of this important topic.

Tumor markers are substances that are either produced by tumor (or cancer) cells arising in certain tissues or are produced by the host in response to the tumor. They are produced often ectopically (ie, at tissue sites where the substance is not normally produced) and may differ, either quantitatively or qualitatively, from substances produced normally by the adult, differentiated tissue from which the tumor arises. Frequently, these substances are related to tissue antigens produced during fetal development (oncofetal antigens) that are lost usually during the normal tissue maturation process. The failure of several different kinds of cancer cells to lose their fetal antigens results in tumor markers that are not tumor specific and a reduction in their clinical usefulness in the diagnosis of a specific type of cancer. In addition, many of the commercially available assays for tumor markers are not approved by the Food and Drug Administration (FDA) for routine clinical use and are for "investigational use only" (IUO).

Pathophysiology of Cancer

Cancer is thought to be a disease of cell structure in which the normal scaffolding of cellular proteins with other intracellular components [eg, intermediate filaments of the cytoskeleton, ribonucleic (RNA) and dexoyribonucleic (DNA) acids] becomes deranged. Deregulation and uncoupling of the mechanisms that maintain normal nuclear and cellular structure, integrity, and function leads to *apoptosis* (ie, self-induced cell death).

Our understanding of the pathogenesis of cancer has progressed rapidly in the nearly 150 years since the report in 1848, of what may be considered the first tumor marker, Bence Jones protein in urine. The advent in the mid-1970s of hybridoma technology revolutionized the field of tumor biomarkers by providing a dependable means for preparing large quantities of high quality monoclonal antibodies capable of recognizing tumor-associated antigens in situ and in quantifying their concentration in body fluids (eg, serum, urine, and cerebrospinal fluid) with a high degree of analytical sensitivity and specificity. In addition, the clinical (or diagnostic) sensitivity and specificity of many of these markers has proved sufficient to use them clinically in:

- screening for cancer

- diagnosing cancer

- evaluating cancer prognosis

- tumor staging

- detecting tumor recurrence or remission

- localizing tumor and directing chemo- or radio-therapuetic agents

- monitoring the effectiveness of cancer therapy

The list of markers associated currently with a variety of human cancers has grown to well over 50 substances. These substances include proteins, glycoproteins, hormones, enzymes, and metabolic breakdown products. Moreover, they are associated with a wide range of different types of cancers involving many of the major human organ systems and/or tissues.

Advances in the laboratory techniques and methods used in molecular pathology, including hybridoma technology for the production of monoclonal antibodies, flow cytometry, DNA ploidy and cell cycle analysis, polymerase chain reaction (PCR) analysis, immunoblotting, immunophenyotyping, gene rearrangement analysis, digital imaging, immunohistoctyochemistry, and histopatholological staging of neoplastic disease have led to quantum leaps in our understanding of the pathogenesis and severity of a variety of cancers. In addition, application of these techniques has led to earlier diagnosis, treatment, and monitoring of many cancers.

Although tumor markers are not a panacea in the detection and surveillance of all cancers, they have become increasingly important in the clinical management of many of the malignancies that cause ~500,000 cancer-related deaths annually in the U.S. alone. It is likely that this trend will not only continue but will expand as new techniques and new markers become available in the fight against cancer.

The current list of tumor markers recognized by the National Academy of Clinical Biochemistry as useful for various purposes in certain cancers is summarized in the Table below:

Summary of NACB Recommendations/Guidelines on the Use of Various Tumor Markers

Type of Cancer	Tumor Marker	SCR	Dx/CF	STG/Px	DRC	M/S Rx
Breast	ER & PR	●	-	-	-	●
	CA 15-3	O	O	O	-	●
	BR 27.29	O	O	O	-	●
	CEA	O	●	●	-	●
Ovarian	CA 125	O	O	●	●	●
Colorectal	CEA	O	O	●	●	●
Lung	NSE	-	●	-	-	●
	CYFRA 21-1	-	-	-	-	●
	CEA	-	-	-	-	●
Germ cell	AFP & hCG	O	●	●	●	●
	LD	-	●	●	●	●
Thyroid	Tg	●	-	-	-	●
	CCT	-	-	-	-	●
Prostate	PSA	●	●	-	-	-
	%F/T	-	●	-	-	-
Neuroendocrine	VMA	-	●	-	-	-
	HVA	-	●	-	-	-

●, recommended for use; O, not recommended for use; -, no recommendation provided; ER, estrogen receptor; PR, progesterone receptor; CA, cancer antigen; BR, breast antigen; CEA, carcinoembryonic antigen; NSE, neuron-specific enolase; CYFRA, cytokeratin fragment; AFP, alpha-fetoprotein; hCG, human chorionic gonadotropin; LD, lactate dehydrogenase; Tg, thyroglobulin; CCT, calcitonin; PSA, prostate-specific antigen; F/T, free:total PSA ratio; VMA, vanillylmandelic acid; HVA, homovanillic acid; SCR, screening; Dx/CF, diagnosis/case finding; STG/Px, staging/prognosis; DRC, detecting tumor recurrence; M/S Rx, monitoring/selection of therapy

To supplement the information provided in the case studies included in this section, readers are referred to the "Suggested Reading" section below for books and additional articles related to the to the case study topics selected for inclusion in this section.

Suggested Reading

1. Mais DD. *Quick Compendium of Clinical Pathology*. Chicago: ASCP Press, 2009.

2. Leonard G, Mais DD. *Quick Compendium Companion for Clinical Pathology*. Chicago, ASCP Press, 2009.

3. McKenna R, Keffer J. *The Handbook of Clinical Pathology*, 2nd ed. Chicago: ASCP Press, 1999.

4. Dons RF, Wians FH Jr. *Endocrine and Metabolic Disorders: Clinical Lab Testing Manual.* Boca Raton, FL: CRC Press, 2009.

5. Wians FH Jr, Baskin LB. Chapter 2: The Use of Clinical Laboratory Tests in Diagnostic Decision-Making. In: *Handbook of Clinical Pathology,* ASCP Press: Chicago, IL, 2000, pp 9-24.

6. Wians, FH Jr. Chapter 20: Tumor Markers. In: *Handbook of Clinical Pathology,* ASCP Press: Chicago, IL, 2000, pp. 261-279.

7. Foster SV, Wians FH Jr, Chapter 5: Renal Function Tests. In: *Handbook of Clinical Pathology*, ASCP Press: Chicago, IL, 2000, pp 55-65.

8. Baskin LB, Wians FH Jr. Chapter 9: Serum Proteins. In: *Handbook of Clinical Pathology*, ASCP Press: Chicago, IL, 2000, pp 121-137.

9. Foster SV, Wians FH Jr. Chapter 16: Liver Function Tests. In: *Handbook of Clinical Pathology,* ASCP Press: Chicago, IL, 2000, pp 219-234.

10. Meny G, Jialal I, Wians FH Jr. Chapter 4: Calcium and Phosphorus. In: *Handbook of Clinical Pathology,* ASCP Press: Chicago, IL, 2000, pp 41-54.

11. Maxwell A, McCudden CR, Wians FH Jr, Willis MS. Recent advances in the detection of prostate cancer using epigenetic markers in commonly collected laboratory samples. *Lab Med* 2009;40:171-178.

12. Wians FH Jr. Clinical laboratory tests: which, why, and what do the results mean? *Lab Med* 2009;40;105-114.

13. Wians FH Jr. Use of Excel spreadsheets to create interpretive reports for laboratory tests requiring complex calculations. *Lab Med* 2009;40:5-12.

14. Valasek MA, Hopley RT, Wians FH Jr. Resolving the baneful and banal: bisalbuminemia in an adult with Waldenström macroglobulinemia. *Lab Med* 2008;39:723-726.

15. Terrell JD, Roehrborn CG, Wians FH Jr, Karakiewicz PI, Shariat SF. Update on prostate-specific antigen testing for the early detection of prostate cancer. *Lab Med* 2008;39:613-621.

16. Reddy V, Khan AI, Remaley AT, Wians FH Jr. Update on point-of-surgery testing. *Lab Med* 2006;37:754-756.

17. Park S, Cadeddu JA, Balko JA, Tortelli MW, Wians FH Jr. Persistently elevated prostate-specific antigen (PSA) level 4 months after successful laparoscopic radical prostatectomy in a 67-year-old man. *Lab Med* 2006;37:474-477.

18. Rutherford C, Wians FH Jr. A large skull mass in a 67-year-old woman. *Lab Med* 2006;37:417-421.

19. Khan AI, Cimo M, Hashim IA, Wians FH Jr. Hyperammonemia in a 20-year-old woman. *Lab Med* 2006;37:226-228.

20. Alfardan J, Wians FH Jr, Dons RF, Wyne K. The "perfect storm." *Lab Med* 2005;36:700-704

21. Ziadie M, Wians FH Jr. "CRAB" findings in a patient with fatigue and a history of poor apetite. *Lab Med* 2005;36:482-485.

22. Ziadie M, Wians FH Jr. A guide to the interpretation of CSF indices. *Lab Med* 2005;36:558-562 [CE Update].

23. Wians FH Jr. Lab methods/instruments – then and now: flame photometers and ion-selective electrodes. *Lab Med* 2004;35:599-600.

24. Hussey SM, Wians FH Jr. Shortness of breath in a 74 year-old woman. *Lab Med* 2004;35:408-412.

25. Chamberlain W, White MD, Wians FH Jr, Willis MS. Nasal discharge in a 50 year-old woman. *Lab Med* 2004;35:279-283.

26. Shariat SF, Roehrborn CG, Wians FH Jr. Update on prostate-specific antigen testing for the early diagnosis of prostate cancer. ASCP *Check Sample*, Clinical Chemistry 2003;43:67-89.

27. Willis MS, Wians FH Jr, Baskin LB. Abdominal tenderness in a male. *Lab Med* 2002;923-926.

28. Willis MS, Wians FH Jr, Kroft S, Baskin LB. The case of the needle-shaped urine crystals. *Lab Med* 2002;33:637-640.

29. Willis MS, Wians FH Jr. Marked proteinuria in a young male. *Lab Med* 2002;33:463-466.

30. Willis MS, Baskin LB, Wians FH Jr. Bone pain in a middle-age woman. *Lab Med* 2002;33:854-860.

31. Wians FH Jr. Tumor markers. *Lab Med* 2001;32:619-620.

32. Othman YH, Wians FH Jr. Tumor Markers. *Lab Med* 2001;32:621-622.

33. Wians FH Jr, Balko JA, Hsu RM, Byrd W, Snyder WH III. Intraoperative versus central laboratory Turbo PTH testing during parathyroidectomy surgery. *Lab Med* 2000;31:616-621.

34. Wians FH Jr. The Role of Prostate-Specific Antigen Testing in the Diagnosis, Treatment, and Follow-Up of Patients With Adenocarcinoma of the Prostate. ASCP *Check Sample,* Clinical Chemistry 1997;37:77-103.

A Newborn With Ambiguous Genitalia

Qing H. Meng, Stephen Hill, Gillian Luxton

Department of Pathology and Molecular Medicine, McMaster University, Ontario, Canada

Patient: 1-day-old baby.

Chief Complaint: Neonate was noted to have ambiguous genitalia.

Medical History: Neonate delivered by Cesarean section under spinal anesthesia at 39 weeks of gestation. After delivery, the baby was assigned as a male by the obstetrician.

Family History: The father is healthy. The mother (para 1, gravida 2) had a Cesarean section for her first baby girl 3 years ago at 40 weeks gestation due to failure to progress following 3 days of labor. The girl has been fine. The mother had no history of diabetes or hypertension.

Drug History: The mother did not take any medication during her most recent pregnancy. She had no history of drug abuse or contact with any toxic chemicals.

Physical Examination: The baby weighed 3,925 grams with APGAR scores of 9 at both 1 minute and 5 minutes after birth. Ambiguous genitalia (clitoromegaly and partial fusion of the labioscrotal folds) were equally observed. Cardiovascular and respiratory systems were normal.

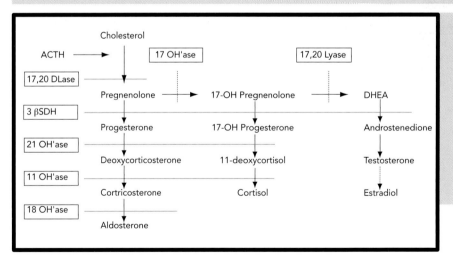

Figure 1_Pathway of adrenal steroid synthesis. 21 OH'ase, 21-hydroxylase; 11 OH'ase, 11β-hydroxylase; 18 OH'ase, 18-hydroxylase; 3 βSDH, 3 β-hydroxysteroid dehydrogenase; 17 OH'ase, 17α-hydroxylase; 17,20 DLase, 17,20-cholesterol-desmolase.

Questions

1. What is(are) this patient's most striking laboratory result(s)?

2. How do you explain this patient's most striking laboratory test results?

3. What is the most likely diagnosis relevant to this patient?

T1. Principal Laboratory Findings

Test	Patient's Result	"Normal" Reference Range
Hematology		
WBC count	14.8	$5.5-15.5 \times 10^3$/mL
RBC count	4.16	$3.25-5.50 \times 10^6$/mL
Hemoglobin	11.1	10.5-14.0 g/dL
Hematocrit	39.9	40-60%
MCV	78.3	70-95 fL
Differential: neutrophils	9.0	$1.5-7.0 \times 10^3$/mL
lymphocytes	4.1	$2.0-8.0 \times 10^3$/mL
monocytes	1.3	$0.0-1.1 \times 10^3$/mL
Chemistry		
Glucose	79	50-80 mg/dL
BUN	5	4-12 mg/dL
Sodium	130	135-145 mEq/L
Potassium	5.8	3.5-5.5 mEq/L
Chloride	100	95-105 mEq/L
Bicarbonate	18	22-30 mEq/L
Anion gap	12	5-14 mEq/L
TSH	1.8	0.5-5.5 mU/mL
Free T4	2.6	0.8-2.7 ng/dL
Cortisol (0800 h)	1.0	5-23 mg/dL
17-OH-progesterone	34,500	20-140 ng/dL
DHEA-S	822	26-444 mg/dL

WBC, white blood cell; RBC, red blood cell; MCV, mean corpuscular volume; BUN, blood urea nitrogen; TSH, thyroid stimulating hormone; T4, thyroxine; DHEA-S, dehydroepiandrosterone-sulfate

4. Which additional laboratory test(s) are appropriate to order on this patient and why?

5. What is the etiology of this patient's condition?

6. How is this patient's condition typically diagnosed?

7. How should this patient be treated?

Possible Answers _____

1. The most striking laboratory results are markedly elevated 17-OH-progesterone, and dehydroepiandrosterone-sulfate (DHEA-S) concentrations; elevated potassium; reduced sodium, cortisol, and urea levels; low osmolality; and a normal anion gap.

2. The reduced cortisol level and accumulation of its precursor, 17-OH-progesterone, suggest 21-hydroxylase deficiency, which is the most commonly seen enzyme deficiency in newborns with congenital adrenal hyperplasia (CAH). The accumulation of 17-OH progesterone may lead to the increased formation of dehydroepiandrosterone (DHEA) and its metabolite, DHEA-S, by an alternate pathway. The increased DHEA and DHEA-S concentrations lead to the peripheral synthesis in the liver of androstenedione and testosterone, which, together, are responsible for ambiguous genitalia, hirsutism, and virilization in females. Lack of the 21-hydroxylase enzyme blocks the pathways for both cortisol and aldosterone production, the principal glucocorticoids and mineralocorticoids produced by the adrenal cortex. Aldosterone causes increased sodium ion reabsorption and potassium and hydrogen ion excretion ($Na^+ \leftrightarrow K^+$ and $Na^+ \leftrightarrow H^+$ exchange) by the distal convoluted tubules and collecting duct of the kidney. Aldosterone is essential for the homeostasis of plasma water, sodium, and potassium ion concentrations. Aldosterone deficiency leads to hypovolemia, hyponatremia, hyperkalemia, and metabolic acidosis. In early or mild aldosterone and cortisol deficiency, these biochemical changes may not be evident. Severe cortisol deficiency may cause hypoglycemia.

3. ***Most likely diagnosis:*** *Congenital adrenal hyperplasia.* Congenital adrenal hyperplasia is an inherited autosomal recessive disorder that occurs with a population frequency of 1:1,000. It is classified in 2 forms based on different clinical presentations: classical and non-classical. The non-classical form of CAH due to partial 21-hydroxylase deficiency is the most common of all autosomal recessive diseases. The classical form of CAH due to hydroxylase deficiency occurs as a result of the imbalance in the production of cortisol, aldosterone, and androgens.[1] Too little cortisol during physical stress can lead to low blood pressure and even death. The lack of aldosterone production results in salt wasting. Excess androgen production causes abnormal physical development. The non-classical form

of CAH is a milder version of the classical form of this disease. Patients with non-classical CAH are not deficient in cortisol and aldosterone; however, they do produce excess androgens. Salt wasting forms of adrenal hyperplasia are accompanied by low serum aldosterone concentrations, hyponatremia, hyperkalemia, elevated plasma renin activity, hypovolemia, and hypotension. In contrast, hypertensive forms of adrenal hyperplasia (eg, 11-beta-hydroxylase deficiency and 17-alpha-hydroxylase deficiency) are associated with suppressed plasma renin activity and often hypokalemia. The diagnosis of CAH depends upon the demonstration of inadequate production of cortisol and/or aldosterone in the presence of accumulation of excess concentrations of precursor hormones. For example, the distinguishing characteristic of 21-hydroxylase deficiency is a very high (usually exceeding 1,000 ng/dL) serum 17-OH-progesterone and urinary pregnanetriol (a metabolite of 17-OH-progesterone) concentrations in the presence of clinical features suggestive of the disease (eg, a female with ambiguous genitalia, evidence of salt wasting, clitoromegaly, precocious pubic hair development, excessive growth, premature phallic enlargement in the absence of testicular enlargement, hirsutism, oligomenorrhea, and/or female infertility).

4. Serum aldosterone, plasma renin activity, serum testosterone, plasma ACTH, and urinary pregnanetriol levels. Low serum aldosterone concentration is expected in patients with CAH, while plasma renin may be increased or decreased depending on the type of enzyme deficiency present and the degree of mineralocorticoid deficiency. In addition, serum testosterone concentration is increased due to the decreased cortisol and aldosterone levels in such patients and shunting of cortisol precursors toward adrenal androgen production. Moreover, cortisol deficiency leads to an elevated ACTH concentration, which increases further the levels of cortisol and aldosterone precursor substances and results in bilateral adrenal hyperplasia (BAH). Measurement of urinary pregnanetriol (a metabolite of 17-OH-progesterone) concentration is also useful in the diagnosis of CAH. Genetic testing for mutations in the gene for the 21-hydroxylase enzyme is rarely necessary for the diagnosis of classical forms of adrenal

hyperplasia, but is essential in the prenatal diagnosis of adrenal hyperplasia. Subtle forms of adrenal hyperplasia associated with non-classical forms of 21-hydroxylase deficiency and 3-beta-hydroxysteroid dehydrogenase deficiency often require a Cortrosyn (synthetic ACTH) stimulation test to demonstrate the abnormal accumulation of precursor steroids.

5. Several enzyme deficiencies can cause CAH [**Figure 1**] and principal among these are: 21-hydroxylase, 11-beta-hydroxylase, 3-beta-hydroxysteroid dehydrogenase, 17-alpha-hydroxylase, 17,20-cholesterol-desmolase, and corticosterone 18-methyloxidase type II. Deficiency of the **21-hydroxylase enzyme** accounts for more than 90% of CAH cases.[1] In this type of CAH, there is increased production of progesterone, 17-OH-progesterone, DHEA, and androstenedione. Moreover, urinary concentrations of the metabolites of these substances (eg, 17-ketosteroids and pregnanetriol) are increased, while serum cortisol levels are decreased. The clinical symptoms of CAH are exacerbated by the stress (and demand for cortisol) of increased physical activity. The gene (CYP21) for the 21-hydroxylase enzyme is located on chromosome 6p21, adjacent to the human leukocyte antigen (HLA) genes. This gene is about 30 kilobases (kb) away from a pseudogene (CYP21P), which is 98% homologous in structure with the CYP21 gene; therefore, the minor differences between these genes are sufficient to render the pseudogene inactive in the production of functional 21-hydroxylase enzyme. Deficiency of the **11-beta-hydroxylase enzyme** causes 3% to 5% of all cases of CAH and is associated with a characteristic elevation of serum 11-deoxycortisol and deoxycorticosterone concentrations. In addition, urinary levels of 17-OH-corticosteroids are also usually high. Because of the mineralocorticoid activity of deoxycorticosterone, patients with 11-beta-hydroxylase enzyme deficiency exhibit salt retention, decreased plasma renin activity, and hypertension with hypokalemic alkalosis. The 11-beta-hydroxylase gene (CYP11B1) resides on chromosome 8q21. A neighboring gene (CYP11B2) codes for aldosterone synthetase, which catalyzes the conversion of corticosterone to aldosterone in the zona glomerulosa of the adrenal cortex. Mutations and deletions in the

CYP11B2 gene result in diminished aldosterone synthesis. Therefore individuals with a mutated CYP11B2 gene develop hyponatremia, hyperkalemia, and dehydration. Deficiency of the **3-beta-hydroxysteroid dehydrogenase enzyme** is indicated by an abnormal ratio of 17-hydroxypregnenolone to 17-hydroxyprogesterone and dehydroepiandrosterone to androstenedione concentration. The gene for 3-beta-hydroxysteroid dehydrogenase resides on chromosome 1p13. Deficiency of the **17-alpha-hydroxylase, 17,20-lyase,** and **17,20-cholesterol-desmolase enzymes** result in virilization of affected female infants and undervirilization of affected male infants. A single gene (CYP17) mutation causes the deficiency in the activity of these enzymes. Moreover, steroidogenic acute regulatory protein (StAR) appears to be involved in the transport of cholesterol across the mitochondrial membrane where it can be acted upon by the CYP450 system in the synthesis of pregnenolone which then is converted in various steroidogenic tissues into cortisol, aldosterone, or sex steroids. A deficiency of StAR results in a global steroid deficiency state. Lastly, deficiency of **corticosterone 18-methyloxidase type II** is characterized by aldosterone deficiency (low plasma aldosterone concentration) with chronic hyperkalemia and no abnormalities of sexual differentiation.

6. Prenatal diagnosis for 21-hydroxylase deficiency can be performed using DNA analysis on fetal cells obtained from amniotic fluid following amniocentesis or from chorionic villus samples (CVS).[2] This technique will detect 95% of all abnormal genes for CAH. Neonatal screening for 21-hydroxylase deficiency is sufficiently specific and sensitive to detect almost all infants with classical CAH and some infants with non-classical CAH. Analysis of 17-OH-progesterone levels in dried blood spot samples obtained from newborns between 48 to 72 hours of age is the typical method for screening newborns for CAH. A positive screening result must be confirmed by quantitative analysis of 17-OH-progesterone concentration, using a sensitive and specific method, in a second serum/plasma sample, urine steroid analysis, or mutation analysis of the CYP21 gene.

7. Early (less than 9 weeks after last menstrual period) treatment of a pregnant woman carrying a CAH-affected fetus appears to be somewhat successful in preventing the virilization of a female fetus with 21-hydroxylase enzyme deficiency. However, more detailed guidelines for the use of this treatment are needed. Infants with ambiguous genitalia should be observed closely for any signs or symptoms of salt wasting while the diagnosis of CAH is being established. Such infants should undergo surgical evaluation in case corrective surgery is indicated.[3] Moreover, newborns with dehydration, hyponatremia, hyperkalemia, or hypoglycemia must be treated immediately to correct these symptoms. Glucocorticoid and/or aldosterone replacement therapy may be necessary depending upon what enzyme deficiency is involved and whether cortisol and/or aldosterone synthesis is affected. A new therapy using the combination of a glucocorticoid, a mineralocorticoid, an aromatase inhibitor, and flutamide is currently under investigation.[2] A clitoroplasty was done on this patient and her external genitalia progresses well. Our patient has been on corticosteroid therapy and followed regularly by pediatric endocrinologists by monitoring 17-hydroxyprogesterone, renin, and electrolytes.

Keywords

congenital adrenal hyperplasia, 21-hydroxylase enzyme deficiency, cortisol, aldosterone, 17-hydroxyprogesterone

References

1. New MI, Carlson A, Obeid J, et al. Prenatal diagnosis for congenital adrenal hyperplasia in 532 pregnancies. *J Clin Endocrinoal Metab.* 2001;86:5651-5657.

2. Joint LWPES/ESPE CAH working group. Consensus statement on 21-hydroxylase deficiency from The Lawson Wilkins Pediatric Endocrine Society and The European Society for Paediatric Endocrinology. *J Clin Endocrinol Metab.* 2002;87:4048-4053.

3. Lee PA. Genital surgery among females with congenital adrenal hyperplasia: Changes over the past 5 decades. *J Pediatr Endocrinol Metab.* 2002;15:1473-1477.

Marked Hyponatremia in a 74-Year-Old Man

Matthew R. Plymyer

Department of Pathology, Easton Hospital, Easton, PA

Patient: 74-year-old man.

Chief Complaint: Weakness for several weeks with nausea, constipation, and cough.

History of Present Illness: The patient presented to the emergency department after experiencing generalized weakness, nausea, constipation, and an intermittent cough for about 3 weeks. He subsequently admitted anorexia and weight loss (approximately 15 pounds) over the past month. The patient denied fever, chills, chest pain, abdominal pain, diarrhea, and dysuria. He had begun treatment with antibiotics 1 week prior to presentation for a sinus infection.

Past Medical/Surgical History and Current Medications: The patient had a history of atrial fibrillation, hypothyroidism, and gastroesophageal reflux disease (GERD), and had had a hemorrhoidectomy. He reported no allergies. He had been treated with radioactive iodine about 40 years earlier for hyperthyroidism. Current medications included Synthroid (for hypothyroidism), Nexium (for GERD), and Tequin (for sinus infection).

Family/Social History: The patient is a widower who previously smoked 1.5 packs of cigarettes per day for 50 years (although he quit smoking 5 years ago) and reported drinking 1 to 2 beers per week. His mother had died of ovarian cancer and a sister also has thyroid dysfunction. There was no family history of neoplasms of the endocrine glands.

Physical Examination: Vital signs: temperature, 97.2°F; pulse, 106 beats per minute, irregularly irregular; respiratory rate, 20 per minute; blood pressure, 138/84 mmHg. The patient was thin with no palpable lymphadenopathy or organomegaly, and no edema or cyanosis.

Results of Other Diagnostic Tests: Electrocardiogram (ECG) showed atrial fibrillation with a heart rate of 106 beats per minute. Conventional radiographs of the abdomen showed no specific abnormalities. Computed tomography (CT) scan of the chest incidentally noted bilaterally enlarged adrenal glands, and follow-up CT of the abdomen and pelvis confirmed bulky masses involving both adrenal glands [**Image 1**]. The right and left adrenal glands measured 9.8 cm and 9.0 cm in greatest dimension, respectively; the adrenal masses were a new finding not present in an abdominal CT scan from 2 years earlier. Importantly, no other masses or evidence of lymphadenopathy were identified radiographically in the chest, abdomen, or pelvis.

T1. Principal Laboratory Findings

Test	Patient's Result	"Normal" Reference Range
Hematology		
WBC count	2.0	4.8-10.8 × 10³/μL
Hemoglobin	11.9	14.0-18.0 g/dL
Platelet count	178	130-400 × 10³/μL
Chemistry		
Sodium	108	133-145 mEq/L
Potassium	5.1	3.5-5.0 mEq/L
Chloride	76	96-108 mEq/L
CO_2	21	21-31 mEq/L
Glucose	91	70-105 mg/dL
BUN	13	6-20 mg/dL
Creatinine	0.9	0.5-1.2 mg/dL
Osmolality		
Serum	216	280-295 mOsm/kg H_2O
Urine	525	500-800 mOsm/kg H_2O
ACH (plasma, morning)	224	9-52 pg/mL (adult, morning)
ACH Stimulation Test		
Cortisol: Baseline	7.6	6.0-28.0 μg/dL (morning)
30-min	7.9	
60-min	8.6	>20 μg/dL

WBC, white blood cell; BUN, blood urea nitrogen; ACH, adrenocorticotropic hormone.

Fine needle aspiration (FNA) biopsy and thin needle core biopsy of the right adrenal gland were performed with ultrasound guidance, which showed a malignant neoplasm with significant necrosis. The neoplastic cells had little cytoplasm and large, irregular nuclei [**Image 2A**]. Flow cytometry evaluation of material obtained by FNA biopsy was unable to be completed secondary to low cell viability (probably a reflection of the necrosis). The neoplastic cells were immunoreactive (positive) by immunohistochemical evaluation for several markers, including leukocyte common antigen (LCA) [**Image 2B**] and CD20 and were non-immunoreactive for multiple additional markers (including carcinoma markers). Bone marrow aspiration and core biopsy were also performed, with no evidence of involvement by malignancy.

Questions

1. What is (are) this patient's most striking clinical, imaging, and laboratory findings?

2. How do you explain this patient's most striking laboratory findings?

3. Based on this patient's clinical, imaging, and laboratory findings, what is this patient's most likely diagnosis?

4. What are the most common causes of this patient's condition?

5. What are the most common signs, symptoms, and laboratory findings associated with this patient's condition?

6. Based on the FNA biopsy, immunohistochemical, and flow cytometry findings on adrenal gland tissue from this patient, what is the most likely cause of this patient's condition?

7. What are the most appropriate treatment and follow-up for this patient?

Possible Answers

1. Weakness, anorexia, gastrointestinal symptoms; bilaterally enlarged adrenal glands due to bulky masses involving both adrenal glands; markedly decreased serum sodium, decreased serum chloride, slightly increased serum potassium, elevated plasma adrenocorticotropic hormone (ACTH), abnormal ACTH stimulation test, and anemia.

2. The most common causes of hyponatremia are: overhydration, diuretic use/abuse, syndrome of inappropriate antidiuretic hormone (SIADH) secretion, adrenal failure, diabetic hyperosmolar state, and Bartter syndrome (a rare condition of unknown cause); chloride is generally low with hyponatremia, since chloride is the main counter-ion for sodium.[1] **Overhydration** should be apparent by a clinical history of consumption of a large volume of hypotonic fluids such as water and is usually associated with a low urine osmolality and blood urea nitrogen (BUN) concentration. **Diuretic use/abuse** should be

T2. Common Causes of Hyponatremia and Typical Clinical and Laboratory Findings

| | | "Typical" Clinical and Laboratory Findings | | | | | |
| | Clinical Findings, Hx of | Osmolality | | Serum | | | |
Cause		Serum	Urine	Na+	K+	BUN	Glu
Overhydration	Consumption of large volumes of a hypotonic fluid	↓				↓	
Diuretic use/abuse	Appropriate drug use	↓		↓*			
SIADH	Head trauma, CNS diseases, certain cancers	↓	>300				
Adrenal failure			>300		↑		
Diabetic hyperosmolarity	DM						↑↑↑↑
Bartter syndrome		↓		↓**			
Patient presented in this case study	None of the above clinical findings	↓	>300	↓↓↓	slt↑	↔	↔

*Fluid restriction corrects the hyponatremia. **Fluid restriction does not correct the hyponatremia. Hx, history; BUN, blood urea nitrogen; K+, potassium; Glu, glucose; SIADH, syndrome of inappropriate antidiuretic hormone; CNS, central nervous system; DM, diabetes mellitus; slt, slightly; ↓, decreased; ↑, increased; ↔, within normal limits.*

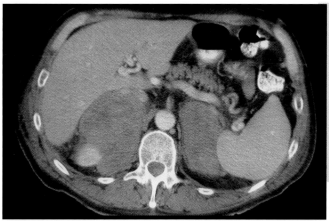

Image 1_Computed tomography scan of the patient's abdomen demonstrating large masses (arrows) involving both adrenal glands.

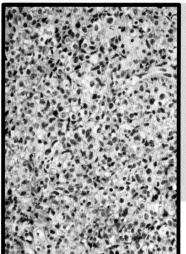 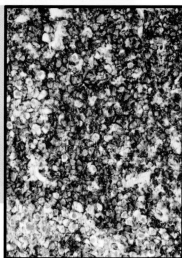

A   **B**

Image 2_Needle biopsy of the right adrenal gland mass illustrating **A**) neoplastic cells with little cytoplasm and large, irregular nuclei (hematoxylin and eosin stain, 400× magnification) and **B**) strong and uniform positive staining for leukocyte common antigen (immunoperoxidase stain for LCA, 400× magnification).

associated with the appropriate clinical drug history, low urine osmolality, and hypokalemia. **SIADH** is usually associated with a clinical history of head trauma, central nervous system (CNS) diseases, and certain cancers, and a urine osmolality greater than 300 mOsm but low serum osmolality. **Adrenal failure** is associated with increased serum potassium concentration (hyperkalemia) and a urine osmolality greater than 300 mOsm. **Diabetic hyperosmolarity** is associated with a clinical history of diabetes mellitus and a very high blood glucose level.[1] **Bartter syndrome** is characterized by laboratory findings similar to those of diuretic use/abuse except that fluid restriction does not correct the hyponatremia. Since ACTH is produced in the pituitary gland and stimulates the adrenal cortex to secrete glucocorticoids, principally cortisol, failure of the adrenal cortex leads to insufficient cortisol levels and elevated ACTH levels in a futile attempt to restore cortisol levels to their appropriate concentration.[2] Therefore, unlike individuals with normally functioning adrenal glands, in patients with primary adrenal insufficiency, intravenous administration of a synthetic ACTH analogue and measurement of baseline, 30-, and 60-minute serum cortisol levels results in no significant increase in cortisol levels at either of these time points.[1] The cortisol values on serum from the patient presented in this case study remained essentially unchanged from baseline at both 30- and 60-minutes after the administration of the ACTH analogue [**T1**].

3. *Most likely diagnosis: primary adrenal failure or primary adrenal insufficiency (Addison disease).*

4. In our patient, there was no history of excessive fluid intake, use of diuretic medications, head trauma, CNS diseases, known cancer, or diabetes mellitus. In addition, urine osmolality was greater than 300 mOsm/kg H_2O and serum glucose was not elevated; however, the potassium concentration was slightly increased [**T1** and **T2**]. The finding of bilateral adrenal gland masses on the CT scan suggests that there may be adrenal failure secondary to an anatomic abnormality of the adrenal glands. Primary adrenal failure is supported further by the elevated plasma ACTH level and the results of the ACTH stimulation test (ie, failure to increase the cortisol level above 20 μg/dL at 60 minutes following

the administration of the ACTH analogue, Cortrosyn).

5. Primary adrenal (adrenocortical) insufficiency is known as Addison disease, named for Thomas Addison who in 1855 determined that destruction of the adrenal glands was fatal in humans.[3] Specifically, the term Addison disease refers to *chronic* primary adrenal insufficiency and not *acute* primary adrenocortical insufficiency, which occurs in settings such as massive hemorrhage within the adrenal glands and rapid discontinuation of steroid medications.[4] Addison disease generally manifests after circulating levels of the glucocorticoids (mainly cortisol) and mineralocorticoids (mainly aldosterone) produced by the adrenal cortex are significantly decreased, which does not occur until at least 90% of both glands are destroyed.[4] At the time of Addison original description of this disease, most cases were caused by bilateral adrenal gland destruction in patients with tuberculosis.[2] In industrialized countries today, tuberculosis remains the second most common cause of Addison disease. The majority of cases are now caused by an autoimmune disorder known as autoimmune adrenal insufficiency which sometimes includes other autoimmune endocrine abnormalities (ie, polyendocrine deficiency syndrome).[3] The remaining cases are caused by a wide variety of conditions which can destroy the adrenal glands, including neoplasms (eg, metastatic carcinomas and lymphomas), other infections (eg, fungal infections), sarcoidosis, and amyloidosis.[4]

6. The most commonly observed signs in patients with Addison disease are weight loss (100%), skin hyperpigmentation (94%) due to melanocyte stimulation by increased ACTH precursors, and hypotension (88% to 94%), which sometimes is only orthostatic [ie, occurs only with a change in position (eg, going from a sitting to a standing position)].[2] Our patient noted weight loss; however, skin hyperpigmentation and hypotension were not noted. The most frequently reported symptoms of primary adrenal insufficiency include weakness/tiredness/fatigue (100%), anorexia (100%), and various gastrointestinal symptoms (92%), including nausea, vomiting, constipation, abdominal pain, and/or diarrhea.[2] The patient presented in this case study experienced the majority of these

classic symptoms. Lastly, a variety of laboratory abnormalities can be seen in patients with Addison disease, including hyponatremia (88%), hyperkalemia (64%), and anemia (40%).[2] All of these laboratory abnormalities were observed in our patient.

7. Based upon the right adrenal gland biopsy findings, a large B-cell lymphoma was diagnosed. Based on the CT findings and because there was no clinical or radiologic evidence of involvement of lymph nodes or other organs, the lymphoma was presumed to involve both adrenal glands and to be a primary adrenal gland lymphoma. Moreover, the microscopic appearance of hematoxylin and eosin-stained tissue sections from this patient's adrenal glands and the cytology preparations were consistent with lymphoma. The positive immunohistochemical stains for LCA (a marker present on most leukocytes, including most benign and malignant lymphocytes) and CD20 (a marker found on many B lymphocytes) also support the diagnosis of lymphoma, as do the negative stains for other markers that might indicate another type of malignancy such as metastatic carcinoma.

8. Metastasis is common among adrenal gland neoplasms. In addition, it is relatively common for carcinomas to metastasize to the adrenal glands, with the most common primary sites being breast, lung, kidney, stomach, pancreas, ovary, and colon.[5] Moreover, when carcinomas metastasize to the adrenal glands, they often do so bilaterally.[5] Lymphomas may involve 1 or both adrenal glands; however, both glands are usually affected only with disseminated disease involving many lymph nodes and organs.[5] In the case presented here, there was no evidence of lymphoma in sites other than the adrenal glands. About 25% of lymphomas in the United States are extranodal in origin (ie, they involve primarily organs other than lymph nodes),[6] although few cases of primary adrenal gland lymphoma have been reported.[7] According to a literature review by Mermershtain and colleagues in 2001, only 75 cases of primary adrenal gland lymphoma had been reported.[8] A variety of subtypes of lymphoma have been reported to involve primarily the adrenal glands; however, most have been B-cell lymphomas (as in our case), although T-cell lymphomas have also been reported.[9]

Lastly, only a minority of all cases of primary adrenal gland lymphoma present with Addison disease,[10] as was the case in our patient.

9. There are 2 important aspects to this patient's therapy, namely treatment of the adrenal insufficiency and treatment of the lymphoma, the underlying reason for the insufficiency. In primary adrenal insufficiency, both glucocorticoid (mainly cortisol) and mineralocorticoid (mainly aldosterone) production are deficient, so both must be replaced. Oral hydrocortisone and oral fludrocortisone can be used to replace the cortisol and aldosterone, respectively.[3] In addition, the patient needs to be educated regarding his/her condition, and liberal salt intake is encouraged.[2] Any stress on the body (such as illness or surgery) requires additional supplementation of the glucocorticoid replacement, and patients should have dexamethasone available for injection in times of emergency stress or trauma.[2] The adequacy of steroid hormone replacement therapy is determined by monitoring clinical signs and symptoms as well as monitoring serum sodium and morning plasma ACTH levels (for glucocorticoid replacement) and serum potassium and plasma renin activity (for mineralocorticoid replacement).[2,3]

10. In general, similar therapeutic principles are used to treat extranodal lymphomas as are used for localized nodal lymphomas and chemotherapy, with or without radiation therapy is most commonly used.[7] Radiation therapy can be used for cure only when the lymphoma is confined to a relatively small area. The chemotherapy used for large B-cell lymphoma usually consists of a doxorubicin (Adriamycin) combination.[7] Follow-up to monitor the efficacy of the treatment involves evaluation of the organ involved (in this case, monitoring the status of the adrenal insufficiency clinically and by laboratory tests as well as with follow-up radiographic studies) and general evaluation to assess disease progression (such as checking for evidence of lymphoma outside the adrenal glands and monitoring blood counts for evidence of subsequent bone marrow involvement).[7] Unfortunately, limited data exist for evaluating prognosis and guiding treatment of extranodal lymphomas in uncommon sites such as the adrenal glands.[7]

Treatment and Course

The patient was treated intravenously with 3% NaCl (higher sodium concentration than the normal physiologic amount) and steroid hormone replacement therapy. He was discharged on hospital day 20 with values for serum sodium, potassium, chloride, and carbon dioxide all within the normal reference limits for these analytes. As an outpatient, he was continued on oral hydrocortisone and fludrocortisone therapy and chemotherapy with CHOP (cyclophosphamide, hydroxydaunomycin, Oncovin, prednisone) was initiated several days later. The patient is alive and tolerating his treatment well 5 months later.

Keywords

hyponatremia, Addison disease, adrenal insufficiency, lymphoma

References

1. Henry JB. *Clinical diagnosis and management by laboratory methods*, 20th ed. Philadelphia: W.B. Saunders; 2001:98-99,321-322.

2. Wilson JD, Foster DW, Kronenberg HM, et al. *Williams textbook of endocrinology*, 9th ed. Philadelphia: W.B. Saunders; 1998:547-565.

3. DeGroot LJ, Jameson JL, Burger HG, et al. *Endocrinology*, 4th ed. Philadelphia: W.B. Saunders; 2001:1683-1690.

4. Cotran RS, Kumar V, Collins T. *Robbins pathologic basis of disease*, 6th ed. Philadelphia: W.B. Saunders; 1999:1159-1161.

5. Lack EE. *Tumors of the adrenal gland and extra-adrenal paraganglia*. Washington, DC: Armed Forces Institute of Pathology; 1997:199-212. Atlas of tumor pathology third series; fascicle 19.

6. Haskell CM. *Cancer treatment*, 5th ed. Philadelphia: W.B. Saunders; 2001:1426-1438.

7. Canellos GP, Lister TA, Sklar JL. *The lymphomas*. Philadelphia: W.B. Saunders; 1998:449-479.

8. Mermershtain W, Liel Y, Zirkin HJ, et al. Primary bilateral adrenal lymphoma relapsing as a solid cerebral mass after complete clinical remission. *Am J Clin Oncol.* 2001;24:583-585.

9. Schnitzer B, Smid D, Lloyd L. Primary T-cell lymphoma of the adrenal glands with adrenal insufficiency. *Hum Pathol.* 1986;17:634-636.

10. Serrano S, Tejedor L, Garcia B, et al. Addisonian crisis as the presenting feature of bilateral primary adrenal lymphoma. *Cancer.* 1993;71:4030-4033.

Hyperammonemia in a 20-Year-Old Woman

Adil I. Khan, Michael Cimo, Ibrahim A. Hashim, Frank H. Wians, Jr.

Department of Pathology, University of Texas Southwestern Medical Center, Dallas, TX

Patient: 20-year-old African American woman.

Chief Complaint: Fever (102°F) and cough that were not responding to amoxicillin treatment. Patient was lethargic and wheel chair bound.

History of Present Illness: Four days prior to presentation at the emergency department, the patient's mother noticed her daughter's cough and fever. The patient was seen by a primary care physician who prescribed amoxicillin. However, despite 4 days of treatment with amoxicillin, the patient showed no signs of improvement.

Past Medical History: She has static encephalopathy with a double spastic hemiparesis that was worse on the left than right side. Her neurological problems arose from meningitis at 3 months of age. She also had a ventriculoperitoneal shunt and global developmental delay.

Family/Social History: Non-contributory; no history of illicit drug, ethanol, or tobacco use.

Current Medications: Depakene/Depakote (valproic acid [VPA]; 250 mg bid) for seizures.

Physical Examination Findings: Non-ambulatory (wheel chair bound), resists manipulation, was non-verbal, and has scoliosis.

Questions _____

1. What is (are) this patient's most striking clinical and laboratory findings?

2. What are the causes of hyperammonemia?

3. What is this patient's most likely diagnosis?

4. What is the mechanism of ammonia production?

5. What is the mechanism of VPA-induced hyperammonemia?

6. What other drugs can induce hyperammonemia?

7. What are the effects of chronic hyperammonemia?

8. Is the magnitude of the VPA-induced hyperammonemia in our patient "clinically" significant?

9. What is the usual treatment for hyperammonemia?

10. What are the appropriate specimen collection and handling procedures for ammonia testing?

T1. Principal Laboratory Findings

Test	Patient's Result	Reference Interval
Chemistry		
Sodium	143	135-145 mg/dL
Potassium	4.0	3.6-5.0 mmol/L
Bicarbonate	31	22-31 mmol/L
Chloride	101	98-109 mmol/L
Calcium	8.8	8.4-10.2 mmol/L
Magnesium	2.5	1.4-1.8 mEq/L
Phosphorus	2.5	2.4-4.5 mg/dL
Glucose	97	65-110 mg/dL
BUN	31	7-21 mg/dL
Creatinine	0.6	0.6-1.2 mg/dL
Total protein	7.5	6.3-8.2 g/dL
Albumin	3.1	3.5-5.2 g/dL
Bilirubin, total	0.3	0.2-1.3 mg/dL
Bilirubin, direct	0.1	0.0-0.3 mg/dL
AST	14	13-40 U/L
ALT	5	10-40 U/L
ALP	65	38-126 U/L
GGT	12	8-78 U/L
Ammonia	46	9-33 mmol/L
VPA	140.5	50-100 mg/mL
Urinalysis		
Specific gravity	1.025	1.002-1.030
pH	6.0	5.0-7.0
Macroscopic findings	Negative	All dipsticks negative
Microscopic findings	Negative	

BUN, blood urea nitrogen; AST, aspartate aminotransferase; ALT, alanine aminotransferase; ALP, alkaline phosphatase; GGT, gammaglutamyl transferase.

T2. Principal Causes of Hyperammonemia[11]

Liver disease
Urinary tract infection with distension and stasis
Reye syndrome
Deficiency of enzymes in the urea cycle due to an inborn error of metabolism
HHH syndrome
Total parenteral nutrition
Ureterosigmoidostomy[a]
Sodium valproate therapy

[a]*Surgical implantation of a ureter into the sigmoid colon.*
HHH, hyperornithinemia-hyperammonemia-homocitrullinuria.

Possible Answers

1. Fever, lethargy, and cough unresponsive to treatment with amoxicillin; increased magnesium, BUN, ammonia, and VPA levels; and decreased ALT activity (**T1**). The most striking of the laboratory findings are the increased ammonia and VPA levels.

2. The principal causes of hyperammonemia are shown in (**T2**).

3. ***Most likely diagnosis:*** *VPA-induced hyperammonemia.* Among the principal causes of hyperammonemia, the most likely cause of our patient's hyperammonemia is valproic acid therapy, especially given the fact that she demonstrated no clinical or laboratory evidence of liver disease. Moreover, several studies have shown a link between VPA therapy and hyperammonemia.[1-8]

4. In healthy individuals, the gastrointestinal tract is the major source of ammonia, produced as a result of the action of bacterial proteases, ureases, and amine oxidases on the colon's contents and from the breakdown and metabolism of protein in food. As a result of these processes and the enterohepatic circulation, the ammonia concentration in the portal vein is 5 to 10 times higher than in the systemic circulation.[9] Upon entering the hepatic circulation, ammonia is detoxified by the urea cycle (**Figure 1**) in hepatocytes via its reaction with bicarbonate to produce urea, which then passes into the general circulation before being excreted by the kidneys into the urine. It should be noted that blood ammonia concentration is higher in infants than adults because the development of the hepatic circulation is fully completed only after birth.[10] The reference interval for ammonia in healthy adults is 9 to 33 μmol/L, while in neonates, the reference interval is much higher (64 to 107 μmol/L).[11] Thus, hyperammonemia arises from an abnor-

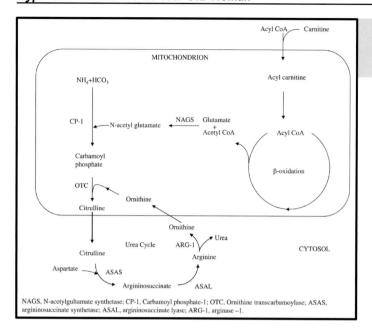

Figure 1_The urea cycle.

NAGS, N-acetylgultamate synthetase; CP-1, Carbamoyl phosphate-1; OTC, Ornithine transcarbamoylase; ASAS, argininosuccinate synthetase; ASAL, argininosuccinate lyase; ARG-1, arginase –1.

mality in ammonia metabolism, which can be either inherited or induced.

In children, hyperammonemia is largely due to an inborn error of metabolism associated with the enzymes of the urea cycle.[12] Urea cycle enzyme defects are usually autosomal genetic disorders with an overall prevalence of 1 in 30,000 births, with 84% of the cases associated with symptoms that present in the first year of life.[13,14] However, in individuals with partial enzyme deficiencies, symptoms of hyperammonemia may not occur until late adolescence or adulthood when these individuals demonstrate episodic hyperammonemia.[13] In adults, however, hyperammonemia often arises as a result of liver cirrhosis, liver failure, subacute liver necrosis, and less frequently, from the toxic ingestion of specific drugs, such as VPA.[10,12]

5. VPA-induced hyperammonemia occurs as a result of disruptions in the urea cycle in hepatocytes. Although it is not completely understood how VPA causes hyperammonemia in the absence of abnormally elevated liver-associated enzymes, 3 mechanisms have been proposed:

    (1) A metabolite (4-en-VPA) of VPA indirectly inhibits fatty acid oxidation resulting in the reduction of free coenzyme A (CoA) and acetyl CoA. Low acetyl CoA levels inhibit mitochondrial production of N-acetyl-glutamate

synthetase, which is a required activator of carbamoyl phosphate synthetase I, the first enzyme in the urea cycle, and thereby leads to an accumulation of ammonia in the blood.[15]

(2) Valproic acid inhibits intramitochondrial β-oxidation of long chain fatty acids leading to activation of the cytosolic w-oxidation pathway and increased utilization of free CoA, acetyl-CoA synthase, and acetyl CoA by this pathway that makes these substances less available for use in the urea cycle, which becomes less efficient in converting ammonia to urea.[1]

(3) Valproic acid causes a deficit in free carnitine, with subsequent reduction in mitochondrial transmembrane transportation of long chain fatty acids, and thus, a less active second pathway for acetyl CoA synthesis in supplying adequate levels of acetyl CoA required by the urea cycle.[1]

6. Topiramate (TPA) can induce hyperammonemia in patients being treated with VPA. It has been suggested that in the liver, TPA inhibits type V mitochondrial carbonic anhydrase.[1,16] Inhibition of this enzyme blocks the urea cycle by decreasing synthesis of bicarbonate necessary for the synthesis of carbamyl phosphate from free ammonia as a prelude to the detoxification of ammonia by the urea cycle.[1,17] Thus, the effects of TPA and VPA on the urea cycle are additive and facilitate the development of hyperammonemia.[1]

7. Cerebral edema and ischemia and death due to herniation of the brain. Hyperammonemia appears to be better tolerated in infants and young children than in adults since ammonia levels that cause minimal residual damage in infants can be fatal in adults. Animal and human studies have both shown that ammonia and glutamine, an amino acid in equilibrium with ammonia, appear to be the metabolites toxic to the central nervous system (CNS).[12] The primary toxic effect appears to be the uptake of fluid into astrocytes causing cerebral edema and resulting in cerebral ischemia and death due to herniation of the brain through the foramen magnum.[12]

8. No, because our patient's ammonia level was only modestly (1.4 × upper limit of normal) elevated and most patients do not "typically" exhibit signs and symptoms (eg, confusion, incoherent speech, and violent behavior) of hyperammonemia until plasma ammonia levels reach much higher levels (eg, ~74 to 99 μmol/L) and levels as high as 124 μmol/L have been reported.[15,18] If a patient on VPA or VPA+TPA does not exhibit any signs or symptoms of hyperammonemia and the blood levels of these drugs are in the therapeutic range, it is unlikely that the patient will become hyperammonemic due to VPA-induced hyperammonemia. Nevertheless, this case illustrates the importance of explaining an abnormal laboratory result for an analyte (ammonia) that, when elevated, can have serious clinical consequences. Also, it is important to remember that reference intervals for ammonia can vary significantly between laboratories and this finding may explain, in part, the wide range in ammonia concentrations associated with signs and symptoms of hyperammonemia.

9. Administration of lactulose (30 to 45 mL q2h with daily dose adjustments to produce 2 to 3 soft stools per day) is used to reduce the dietary and endogenous nitrogen load from the intestinal lumen.[5,15,19] Of course, if the patient is taking VPA, its use should be discontinued in favor of an anti-seizure medication not known to cause or exacerbate hyperammonemia.[15]

Blood should be collected by venipuncture into, preferably, a sodium (or lithium) heparin (or EDTA) tube and the sample tube completely filled and stoppered at all times to prevent contamination by ammonia in the air. Specimens must be placed on ice immediately, rotated periodically, and centrifuged promptly at 4°C to remove the plasma from the cells. If testing for ammonia will not be performed within 20 minutes of the venipuncture, the plasma should be frozen immediately. Plasma ammonia is stable for several days at -70°C. Potential causes for rejecting specimens for ammonia testing include improper collection tube, tube not stoppered, delayed delivery to the laboratory, and hemolysis (increases plasma ammonia concentration).[11]

Keywords

hyperammonemia, valproic acid, urea cycle, acetyl CoA

References

1. Latour P, Biraben A, Polard E, et al. Drug induced encephalopathy in 6 epileptic patients: Topiramate? Valproate? or both? *Hum Psychopharmacol*. 2004;19:193-203.

2. Mallet L, Babin S, Morais JA. Valproic acid-induced hyperammonemia and thrombocytopenia in an elderly woman. *Ann Pharmacother*. 2004;38:1643-1647.

3. Feil D, Chuang K, Sultzer DL. Valproate-induced hyperammonemia as a cause of altered mental status. *Am J Geriatr Psychiatry*. 2002;10:476-478.

4. Panikkar GP, Gilman SM. Valproate-induced hyperammonemia in the psychiatric setting: 2 cases. *J Clin Psychiatry*. 1999;60:557-559.

5. Eze E, Workman M, Donley B. Hyperammonemia and coma developed by a woman treated with valproic acid for affective disorder. *Psychiatr Serv*. 1998;49:1358-1359.

6. Duarte J, Macias S, Coria F, et al. Valproate-induced coma: Case report and literature review. *Ann Pharmacother*. 1993;27:582-583.

7. Gaskins JD, Holt RJ, Postelnick M. Nondosage-dependent valproic acid-induced hyperammonemia and coma. *Clin Pharm*. 1984;3:313-316.

8. Rawat S, Borkowski WJ, Jr., Swick HM. Valproic acid and secondary hyperammonemia. *Neurology*. 1981;31:1173-1174.

9. Tolman KG, Rej R. Liver function. In: Burtis CA and Ashwood ER *Tietz Textbook of Clinical Chemistry*. Philadelphia: W.B. Saunders Company, 1999:1125-1177.

10. Sherwin, JE. Liver function. In: Kaplan, LA, Amadeo JP, and Kazmierczak SC. *Clinical Chemistry: Theory, Analysis, Correlation*. St. Louis: Mosby, 2003:492-506.

11. Jacobs DS, DeMott WR, Strobel SL, et al. Chemistry. In: Jacobs DS and Wolfson WL. *Laboratory Test Handbook.* Stow: Lexi-Comp, 1990:84-85.

12. Cederbaum SD. Diseases of the urea cycle. In: Goldman L and Ausiello D. *Cecil Textbook of Medicine* 22nd Edition. Philadelphia: Elsevier, 2004:1286-1288.

13. Treem WR. Inherited and acquired syndromes of hyperammonemia and encephalopathy in children. *Semin Liver Dis.* 1994;14:236-258.

14. Rudolph CD, Rudolph AM, Hostetter MK. Inherited urea cycle and related disorders. In: *Rudolph's Pediatrics.* New York: Mc Graw Hill Medical Publishing Division, 2003:618-631.

15. McCall M, Bourgeois JA. Valproic acid-induced hyperammonemia: a case report. *J Clin Psychopharmacol.* 2004;24:521-526.

16. Dodgson SJ, Shank RP, Maryanoff BE. Topiramate as an inhibitor of carbonic anhydrase isoenzymes. *Epilepsia.* 2000;41 Suppl 1:35-S39.

17. Haussinger D, Kaiser S, Stehle T, et al. Liver carbonic anhydrase and urea synthesis. The effect of diuretics. *Biochem Pharmacol.* 1986;35:3317-3322.

18. Yehya N, Saldarini CT, Koski ME, et al. Valproate-induced hyperammonemic encephalopathy. *J Am Acad Child Adolesc Psychiatry.* 2004;43:926-927.

19. Hawkes ND, Thomas GA, Jurewicz A, et al. Non-hepatic hyperammonaemia: an important, potentially reversible cause of encephalopathy. *Postgrad Med J.* 2001;77:717-722.

Adventures in CO-Oximetry: Apparent Methemoglobinemia

Ron G. Haas,[1] Vijay Aswani,[2]

[1]*Laboratory and* [2]*Pediatrics, Marshfield Clinic, Marshfield, WI*

Patient: A 12-year-old female patient of Southeast Asian origin collapsed while watching a soccer game and was brought to the emergency room of a local hospital by her father.

Chief Complaint: Weakness, syncope, loss of appetite, cough.

History of Present Illness: Prior to hospital admission, the patient was seen as an outpatient at the request of her parents for fatigue, pallor, and lethargy. First menses started 2 months prior. The patient's family characterized the patient as quiet, a loner, tired, and sleeps as much as possible. Sibling noted the "patient never runs." The family also noted the patient urinates only twice daily and wets the bed 1 to 2×/week. Urine was foul smelling and turbid. History of constipation with bowel movements 1 to 2×/week.

Past Medical History: Tonsillectomy in 1997; hospitalized for pneumonia in 1995. Patient is reported to be full term vaginal birth with no significant prenatal, perinatal, or postnatal complications. No medication or food allergies are reported. The patient was not on any medications and denied the use of any herbal or natural products as health adjuncts or supplements.

Family History: The family history is negative for diabetes mellitus type 2, coronary artery disease, hypertension, cancers, bleeding disorders, cystic fibrosis, mental retardation, cerebral palsy, sudden infant death syndrome (SIDS), metabolic disorders, glucose-6-phosphate dehydrogenase (G6PD) deficiency, or any other hemoglobinopathies by report.

Social History: The family lives on a farm shared by 3 families who obtain drinking water from a common well. Nonsmoking parents and siblings are healthy with no chronic disorders. The family denied the use of any nitrogen fertilizers or pesticide products at their farm. The patient was in the sixth grade and helped out on the farm. The patient eats a little meat, a hot lunch at school, and dinner cooked by her parents at home.

Physical Examination: Based on an elevated methemoglobin (metHb) result, the patient was referred from Hospital A to Hospital B for treatment. The patient appeared pale and tired with some cyanosis around the lips. Vital signs were within normal limits for her age and gender. Respiration rate was 16 breaths per minute and pulse oximetry gave an O_2 saturation of 92% on 1.5 L/min oxygen via nasal cannula (about 23% oxygen).

Additional Diagnostic Procedures: An outpatient TSH performed a month prior was normal. An echocardiogram was performed and was unremarkable. An ultrasound of the urinary tract revealed a thickened bladder wall with significant bilateral hydroureteronephrosis. A cystometrogram demonstrated adequate overall bladder capacity.

Hospital Course: Following treatment for urinary tract infection, neurogenic bladder, and constipation, the patient was discharged 3 days after admission.

T1. Principal Laboratory Findings

Test	Patient's Result	"Normal" Reference Range
Urinalysis		
Color	Brown	
Turbidity	3+	None
Specific gravity	1.015	1.002–1.030
pH	8.0	4.6–8.0
Protein	>100 mg/dL	NEG
Glucose	NEG	NEG
Ketone	NEG	NEG
Bilirubin	NEG	NEG
Blood	3+	NEG
Urobilinogen	NEG	NEG
WBC	>100 Cells	NEG
RBC	>100 Cells	0–2/hpf
Bacti	4+	None seen
Esterase	2+	NEG
Nitrite	NEG	NEG
Clumps of WBCs seen per hpf		
Urine culture: *Escherichia coli* >100,000 org/mL		
Hematology		
WBC	12.1	4.5–13.5 × 10^3/µL
RBC	3.96	4.10–5.30 × 10^6/µL
Hgb	11.1	12.0–15.0 g/dL
Plt	416	150–450 × 10^3/µL
MPV	7.6	6.0–9.5 fL
Neut	71	32–65%
ANC#	8.6	1.8–8.0 × 10^3/µL
Lymph	15	28–48%
Lymph#	1.9	1.2–6.0 × 10^3/µL
Mono	12	1–12%

T1. Principal Laboratory Findings

Chemistry		
BNP	9	5–100 pg/mL
D-dimer	0.68	0.10–0.69 µg/mL(DDU)
Na	140	133–144 mmol/L
K	3.5	3.4–5.1 mmol/L
Urea N	13	5–20 mg/dL
Creat	0.8	0.5–0.9 mg/dL
Ca	9.1	8.5–10.3 mg/dL
G6PDH	278	146–376 nU/RBC
C-reactive protein	7.4	0.0–1.0 mg/dL
Drug screen, urine:	none detected	
Lead, blood:	1	0–10 µg/dL
Heavy metals screen, blood		
(As, Hg, Cd):	normal	
Arterial blood gas		
pH	7.45	7.35–7.45
pCO$_2$	36	5–45 mm Hg
pO$_2$ (room air)	96	80–105 mm Hg
HCO$_3$- calc.	25	22–28 mmol/L
BE calc.	1.2	-3.0–3.0 mmol/L
CO-oximetry Hospital Lab A		
FiO$_2$	Room Air	
Fractional OxyHgb	78.1	94.0–99.0%-Sat
Carboxy-Hgb	<5.0	0.0-7.0% (nonsmokers <5%)
Methemoglobin	20.6	0.1–1.9%
CO-oximetry: Hospital Lab B		
Methemoglobin: "interferences present"		
(Also carboxyhemoglobin, fractional oxyhemoglobin)		
CO-oximetry: Hospital Lab C		
Methemoglobin	>10%	0–2%

WBC: white blood cell; RBC: red blood cell; Hgb: hemoglobin; Plt: platelet; MPV: mean cell volume; Neut: neutrophils; ANC: absolute neutrophil count; Lymph: lymphocytes; Mono: monocytes; BNP: brain natriuretic peptide; Urea N: urea nitrogen; Creat: creatinine; G6PDH: glucose-6-phosphate dehydrogenase

T2. Methemoglobin Evaluation Panel		
Test	Patient's Result	"Normal" Reference Range
Day of discharge:		
Hemoglobin A2	3.1	2.0–3.3%
Hemoglobin F	2.2	0.0–2.0%
Variants:		none
Methemoglobin	0.0	0.0–1.5%
Sulfhemoglobin	5.3	0.0–1.0%
Methemoglobin M 630/600 nm ratio	1.43	≥1.25
Methemoglobin M 500/600 nm ratio	3.25	≥2.80
Methemoglobin reductase	14.1	8.2–19.2 IU/g Hb
Small abnormal peaks on HPLC and spectral scan consistent with sulfhemoglobin. Slight increase of Hgb F of uncertain significance.		
3 weeks later:		
Sulfhemoglobin	2.5	0.0–1.0%

Questions

1. What are the patient's most striking clinical and laboratory findings?

2. What is the patient's most likely diagnosis?

3. What is methemoglobinemia (metHb-emia) and its clinical features?

4. What simple observational tests are available to distinguish metHb?

5. What is the treatment for significantly-elevated levels of metHb, and what considerations arise with treatment?

6. What are the causes of acquired metHb-emia?

7. What is the physiologic basis of inherited metHb-emia?

8. What confirmatory tests are available for metHb-emia and dyshemoglobins given positive results by CO-oximetry?

9. What is sulfhemoglobin (sulfHb) and documented causes of increased levels?

10. How do metHb-emia and sulfhemoglobinemia (sulfHb-emia) differ in their clinical effects?

11. What is the significance of the dyshemoglobin abnormality in this patient and outcome?

12. What are the lessons learned?

Possible Answers

1. The patient had a pale cyanotic appearance and a markedly elevated metHb (**T1**) upon admission. C-reactive protein levels suggested an inflammatory process. Urinalysis and urine culture indicated pyelonephritis and treatment was initiated for a urinary tract infection. The most notable finding is the significantly elevated metHb level observed at Hospital Laboratory A as measured by CO-oximetry (Instrumentation Laboratory, GEM OPL, Lexington, MA) prior to transfer of the patient to Hospital B for further treatment. Following transfer, Hospital B's laboratory was unable to confirm the elevated metHb levels on an integrated blood gas/CO-oximeter instrument (AVL/Roche, Omni 6, Indianapolis, IN) as identical analyzers gave an "interferences present" printout upon analysis of 3 serial blood samples over a 2-day period for all of the hemoglobin fractions (oxy-, carboxy- and met-hemoglobin). One of the serial samples was transported to a sister hospital 35 miles away (Hospital C) with a standalone CO-oximeter (Instrumentation Laboratory, Model 682, Lexington, MA) that did confirm the original elevated metHb report, giving a level >10%.

2. ***Most likely diagnosis?*** *Methemoglobinemia.* The urinalysis data clearly indicated a urinary tract infection, and the patient was started on an antibiotic, cefixime. Although there were inconsistencies across CO-oximeters, the presence of high levels of methemoglobin on 2 different analyzers plus the patient's cyanotic appearance supported a diagnosis of metHb-emia.

3. Adult hemoglobin contains 4 polypeptide chains each of which has a heme group with an atom of iron in the ferrous (+2) state which facilitates the binding of oxygen. In metHb-emia, 1 or more of the iron atoms is in the ferric (+3) oxidation state and these heme groups are incapable of binding oxygen. Additionally, the conversion of 1 or more of the iron atoms to the ferric state compromises the overall release of oxygen by the remaining heme groups containing ferrous iron. This causes a functional anemia disproportionate to the metHb level and decreased oxygen release (ie, a leftward shift in the oxyhemoglobin dissociation curve). Normal levels of metHb are generally considered to be <1.5% to 2% with levels of 15% producing an asymptomatic cyanosis. At levels of 20% or more, symptoms include dyspnea, fatigue, nausea, dizziness, headache, and syncope. As levels increase, symptoms worsen, with levels of 70% or more having a high mortality.

4. Deoxyhemoglobin has a dull red appearance, whereas blood containing significant amounts of metHb (and sulfhemoglobin) will have more of a chocolate brown appearance due to significant absorbance at longer wavelengths. Arterial blood from this patient had a brownish appearance consistent with metHb. A convenient bedside test that has been reported is to add several drops of blood to white filter paper. The chocolate brown appearance due to metHb does not change with time, whereas deoxyhemoglobin, which is initially dark red, brightens to a vivid red upon exposure to oxygen due to the formation of oxyhemoglobin.[2]

5. *Treatment.* The treatment of choice for acutely elevated levels of metHb is methylene blue that is infused intravenously. The dose is usually 1 to 2 mg/kg administered over 3 to 5 minutes and is recommended for metHb levels >20%. Typically, metHb levels will be lowered significantly within an hour. Methylene blue is actually an oxidant, however, and it is the reduced leucomethylene blue form produced in vivo which is the active agent involved in reducing the metHb ferric iron to the ferrous state. This reduced form is generated by a reaction involving the enzyme nicotinamide adenine dinucleotide phosphate (NADPH)-dependent methemoglobin reductase. The NADPH enzyme is produced by the hexose monophosphate shunt pathway and requires adequate levels of G6PDH. Additionally, dextrose infusion is desirable to provide adequate substrate for metabolic conversion of methylene blue to the reduced form. Patients with genetic deficiencies of G6PDH may not produce sufficient NADPH to convert methylene blue to the active reduced form. In this scenario, methylene blue (being an oxidant) will actually increase metHb levels, and therapy will be ineffective. Exchange transfusion should then be considered as an alternative.[2] A predose G6PDH level in this patient indicated normal enzyme activity (**T1**). Additionally, methylene blue may interfere with CO-oximetry measurements by virtue of its significant absorption in the 600 nm region and weaker absorption at shorter wavelenths. Methylene blue is fairly rapid acting and has a reported half-life of 55 min at normal G6PDH levels.[1] Two doses were administered to the patient during hospitalization with blood metHb levels being sampled 4.5 hours prior to the initial dose and 6.5 hours subsequent to the final dose. Spectral interference by methylene blue in the CO-oximeter measurements was not thought to be contributory to the discordant results among instruments. The metHb level at discharge following 2 cycles of methylene blue treatment and measured at Hospital A's laboratory was 18.5%.

6. *Acquired metHb-emia.* Increased metHb levels are frequently a consequence of oxidant exposure. The reader is referred to several recent reviews for a complete listing of drugs and precipitating agents.[1,2] High nitrate levels in drinking water and certain vegetables has been commonly implicated due to the formation of nitrites produced by endogenous bacteria in the gastrointestinal tract. A number of case studies have also documented the overuse of local anesthetics such as benzocaine. In the case of this patient, none of these agents or common causes appeared reasonable, given that other family members and other families sharing water or food were unaffected. Subsequent water testing also demonstrated insignificant levels of nitrate. Additionally, no oxidant drugs were detected during the course of a comprehensive drug screen.

7. *Inherited metHb-emia.* Roughly 3 percent of hemoglobin is converted to metHb on a daily basis. Yet, metHb does not accumulate due largely to the protective effect of cytochrome b5 reductase which facilitates conversion of metHb formed by everyday oxidative processes to functional ferrous-containing hemoglobin. Genetic abnormalities have been reported related to decreased cytochrome b5 reductase (NADH-dependent methemoglobin reductase) activity, which are inherited in an autosomal recessive fashion. A particularly interesting case study of inherited cytochrome b5 reductase deficiency involving several generations of a family from Appalachia has been documented.[4,5] Additionally, newborns have activities only 50% to 60% of adult levels and are more susceptible to oxidant exposure (eg, with nitrate-contaminated drinking water). Of note is that this red cell enzyme maintains sufficient activity even at refrigerated temperatures and, thus, significantly contributes to the labile nature of metHb in stored samples, resulting in a relatively rapid disappearance of metHb and necessitating its assay in a timely manner. An additional genetic cause of metHb-emia is the presence of hemoglobin M variants. These abnormal hemoglobins have mutations in the globin chain that stabilize heme iron in the ferric state and may also give rise to misleading CO-oximetry results. They can be detected by spectrophotometric scanning of hemolysates, examining absorbances at 500, 600, and 630 nm and calculating absorbance ratios, or by performing hemoglobin electrophoresis.[1]

8. The lack of an apparent causative agent for metHb in the patient, the lack of agreement across CO-oximeters, and the minimal change in metHb results following 2 doses of methylene blue were problematic in this case. Particularly frustrating was the inability to provide timely data to the clinician following treatment with methylene blue as a consequence of an "interferences present" CO-oximeter response at Hospital B where treatment occurred. This was compounded by the observation that the Hospital B instrument was perceived to have more wavelengths available than the 2 other CO-oximeters and ostensibly capable of providing more information. Inquiries to the vendor (Roche) for the AVL/Roche Omni 6 analyzer used at Hospital B indicated that information

on the number of wavelengths was considered proprietary, but after further inquiries a service representative indicated that >100 wavelengths are available for resolving hemoglobin fractions in contrast to only 7 wavelengths for the instruments used at Hospitals A and C. Because of these inconsistencies, consideration was given to other means for assessing the presence of metHb. In particular, a relatively simple manual method for metHb is available in standard textbooks.[6] This assay involves measuring metHb at its peak absorbance of 630 nm and involves the addition of cyanide to convert metHb to cyan-metHb, which absorbs at shorter wavelengths resulting in an absorbance decrease at 630 nm due to disappearance of metHb. Given the additional availability of a scanning spectrophotometer, such a procedure was initiated as an ad hoc confirmatory test. Results from this experiment were remarkable in that no reactivity or absorbance change was observed at 630 nm upon addition of cyanide. Additionally, upon scanning, an absorbance peak was observed at 620 nm rather than at the stated metHb peak of 630 nm. This 620 nm absorption peak is consistent with the presence of sulfHb rather than metHb.[6] Reanalysis of the same sample 24 hours later after overnight refrigeration again showed a 620 nm peak with a comparable absorbance, a finding also inconsistent with the labile nature of metHb. Based on these observations, blood was referred on the final day of discharge for a "methemoglobinemia evaluation" (Mayo Medical Laboratories) for a reflexive panel of tests involving hemoglobin electrophoresis, metHb, and sulfHb quantitation, methemoglobin (cytochrome b5) reductase activity, and a hemoglobin spectral scan providing the absorbance ratios A_{630}/A_{600} and A_{500}/A_{600} for detection of hemoglobin M variants. Results received several days later are summarized in **T2** and confirmed the qualitative observations in the authors' laboratory obtained during admission regarding the presence of sulfHb rather than metHb.

9. SulfHb is a green-pigmented molecule with a sulfur atom incorporated into the porphyrin ring of heme. SulfHb is thought to be derived from hydrogen sulfide produced by intestinal bacteria. Increases have been associated with drug exposure, occupational exposure to sulfur compounds, and environmental exposure to polluted air. A

common, although not universal, finding has been a history of chronic constipation. A 1950s study of 62 cases of sulfhemoglobinemia at the Mayo Clinic noted this symptom in 26 patients.

10. Sulf Hb also causes a functional anemia in that the altered heme-like metHb is incapable of transporting oxygen. Whereas metHb causes a leftward shift in the oxyhemoglobin dissociation curve resulting in a decreased oxygen release at the tissue level, sulf Hb causes a rightward shift. Thus, while the patient with sulf Hb-emia would appear bluer than the patient with a comparable level of metHb due to spectral differences between the pigments, the patient with sulf Hb would have less of a tissue oxygenation deficit because oxygen delivery is facilitated rather than impaired.[7] Sulf Hb is also resistant to treatment with methylene blue and is eliminated with normal red blood cell turnover.

11. A sulfhemoglobin result of 5.3% was obtained, which, based on the admission hemoglobin of 11.1 g/dL, would give a sulf Hb concentration of 0.6 g/dL. Levels of 0.5 g/dL or more are reported to produce a skin discoloration equivalent to that for deoxyhemoglobin levels of 5 g/dL or more (ie, a discernible cyanosis).[9] This level of sulf Hb, however, would not likely be expected to cause chronic fatigue and dizziness. Thus, the patient's fatigue is more likely a consequence of her urinary tract infection. The cause of the increased sulf Hb level is also unclear, although there is a strong association with chronic constipation.[8] With counseling by medical staff, patient bowel habits were improved, and the quantitative sulf Hb level decreased about half-fold to 2.5% (**T2**) several weeks later.

12. *Lessons learned.* Three current-generation CO-oximeters failed to identify the hemoglobin abnormality present in this case with 2 of the instruments giving erroneous levels for metHb. Documentation for 2 of the 3 instruments specifies the ability to detect sulf Hb, but neither instrument provided any indication in this case. A false elevation of metHb in the presence of sulf Hb had been reported previously using an earlier-generation CO-oximeter. Identification of sulf Hb was likewise confirmed by manually scanning both before and after the addition of neutralized cyanide solution. In vitro production

of metHb was also noted following freezing of samples and use of fluoride-oxalate collection tubes.[10] Seemingly, identification of dyshemoglobins such as sulf Hb in the presence of other blood pigments (eg, lipemia and bilirubin) still remains a challenging task even with current-generation analyzers and appropriate sample collections. Instruments which incorporate diode array technology and which enable sampling at 100 or more wavelengths would appear to have advantages, but this is also dependent on robust computer algorithms for identifying dyshemoglobins and discriminating against other artifacts and interferences. The availability of a recording spectrophotometer for scanning a hemolysate was particularly valuable in this situation and provided an important clue. Additionally, rapid transport of samples to laboratories over a distance of 35 to 50 miles, and the cooperation of staff in providing results using different analyzers was helpful in creating awareness of a problem. Fortunately, the treatment for metHb-emia is relatively innocuous (given normal G6PDH activity) and did not exacerbate clinical outcome. Use of a manual metHb method and, in particular, reactivity (or lack of reactivity) of the hemolysate with cyanide was useful in resolving this case, although recognition was not timely enough to prevent treatment for metHb-emia.

Keywords _____

CO-oximetry, methemoglobin, sulfhemoglobin, dyshemoglobins

References _____

1. Haymond S, Cariappa R, Eby CS, et al. Laboratory assessment of oxygenation: Methemoglobinemia. *Clin Chem.* 2005;51:434–444.

2. Wright RO, Lewander WJ, Woolf AD. Methemoglobinemia: Etiology, pharmacology, and clinical management. *Ann Emer Med.* 1999;34:646–656.

3. Gourlain H. Interference of methylene blue with CO-oximetry of hemoglobin derivatives. *Clin Chem.* 1997;43:1078–1080.

4. Trost C. Blue People of Troublesome Creek. Science. 82 Nov, 1982. Available at: www.nclark.net/BluePeopleofTroubleCreek.html.

5. Cawein M, Behlen CH 2nd, Lappat EJ. Hereditary diaphorase deficiency and methemoglobinemia. *Arch Int Med*. 1964;113:578–585.

6. Fairbanks VF, Klee GG. Biochemical aspects of hematology. In: Burtis CA, Ashwood ER, eds. *Tietz Textbook of Clinical Chemistry*. 2nd ed. Philadelphia: WB Saunders; 1994: 2025–2027.

7. Park CM, Nagel RL. Sulfhemoglobinemia—Clincal and molecular aspects. *New Eng J Med*. 1984;310:1579–1584.

8. Brandenburg RO, Smith HL. Sulfhemoglobinemia: A study of 62 clinical cases. *Am Heart J*. 1951;42:582–588.

9. Wu C, Kenny MA. A case of sulfhemoglobinemia and emergency measurement of sulfhemoglobin with an OSM3 CO-oximeter. *Clin Chem*. 1997;43:162–166.

10. Kellner MJ, Bailey DN. Mismeasurement of methemoglobin ("methemoglobin revisited"). *Clin Chem*. 1985;31:168–169.

Severe Crushing Headaches, Nausea, and Weakness in a 30-Year-Old Man

Leland B. Baskin

General Laboratory, Calgary Laboratory Services and Department of Pathology and Laboratory Medicine, University of Calgary, Calgary, AB, Canada

Patient: 30-year-old man, non-smoker.

Drug History: Nortriptyline for migraine headaches.

Chief Complaint: The patient was found unresponsive and apneic by a relative at home, brought to the emergency department (ED), and admitted to the hospital.

History of Present Illness: Two months prior to admission, the patient experienced severe, crushing headaches associated with nausea and weakness that awakened him at 2:00 AM. He continued to awaken with increasingly severe headaches over the following 2 months and was seen 6 times in the local ED during the early morning hours. A magnetic resonance imaging (MRI) scan of his head and an electroencephalogram (EEG) were unremarkable. He was told that the headaches were probably migraines and was treated with nortriptyline. Immediately prior to admission, he had taken a 1-week ski trip during which he did not experience any of his previous symptoms. During his most recent hospital admission, he was treated with 100% O_2 by facemask.

Past Medical History: Eight years earlier, the patient had been found in a hypotensive state after chain smoking a carton of cigarettes and drinking 2 to 3 liters of high caffeine content cola. He was diagnosed with Wolf-Parkinson-White syndrome (or anomalous atrioventricular excitation) and underwent radiocatheter ablation.

Family History: Noncontributory.

Physical Examination: Unremarkable.

Social History: The patient is an unmarried medical resident.

Questions

1. What is (are) this patient's most striking laboratory result(s)?

2. How do you explain this patient's most striking laboratory results?

3. What is the pathogenesis of carbon monoxide toxicity?

4. What are the short- and long-term sequelae of carbon monoxide intoxication?

5. How is carbon monoxide concentration measured?

6. What is the optimal sample for quantifying carboxyhemoglobin concentration?

7. What is the treatment for carbon monoxide intoxication?

T1. Principal Laboratory Findings

Test	Patient's Result	"Normal" Reference Range	
Arterial Blood Gases			
pH	7.48	7.37 – 7.43	
pCO_2	33	38-42 mm Hg	
pO_2	297	90-100 mm Hg	
HCO_3	35	22-26 mmol/L	
O_2 saturation (on 100% O_2 for 2 h)	98	95-98%	
Carboxyhemoglobin level	23	<0.5%	Rural non-smoker
		1-2%	Urban non-smoker
		5-6%	Smoker
		>3%	Hemolytic anemia
Hematology			
Hemoglobin	14.8	13.2-16.2 g/dL	
Hematocrit	42.6	40-52%	
Chemistry			
Ethanol, blood	<10	<10 mg/dL	
Urine Drug Screen:			
Phencyclidine	Negative	Negative	
Barbiturates	Negative	Negative	
Cannabinoids	Negative	Negative	
Cocaine	Negative	Negative	
Opiates	Negative	Negative	

T2. Typical Signs and Symptoms of CO-Intoxication

CO-Hb Conc, %	Signs and Symptoms
10	Frontal headache Unable to perform complex tasks or strenuous labor Aggravation of existing heart disease Gastroenteritis misdiagnosed as food poisoning or as due to a viral syndrome
20	Throbbing headache Dyspnea with exertion
30	Dizziness Nausea
40	Confusion Syncope
50	Coma Seizures
60	Hypotension Respiratory failure
70	Death

Possible Answers

1. Markedly elevated arterial pO_2 and carboxyhemoglobin (CO-Hb) levels, increased arterial pH and HCO_3, and decreased pCO_2.

2. Carbon monoxide intoxication. The patient was on 100% O_2 by facemask; therefore, his pO_2 is expected to be markedly elevated. The combination of increased pH and HCO_3 and decreased pCO_2 define metabolic alkalosis that may have resulted from vomiting secondary to nausea.

3. **Carbon Monoxide.**[1-5] *Biochemistry:* Carbon monoxide (CO) is a clear, colorless, odorless gas, with a specific gravity of 0.97 (slightly lighter than air), and a molecular weight of 28 Daltons. It is produced by incomplete combustion of organic fuels and is the most abundant air pollutant in the world. It is also the leading cause of death from poisoning in the United States, accounting for up to 5,000 deaths per year. Cigarette smoke contains approximately 4% CO,

while automobile exhaust contains 0.5 to 10% CO. The threshold limit value (TLV) for CO is 50 ppm (ie, 0.05 mL of CO/L of air). Being in a smoke-filled room for 1.5 hours causes a 38% increase in blood CO levels in non-smokers. *Physiology:* Under normal physiological circumstances, metabolism of heme to biliverdin by heme oxidase generates CO as a by-product at a rate of 0.4 mL/hour, producing a background concentration of CO-Hb of 0.4% to 0.7%. Thus, increased heme metabolism caused by hemolysis increases CO production. Metabolism of methylene chloride (dichloromethane, CH_2Cl_2) also generates CO. As a gas, CO is excreted via pulmonary expiration and less than 1% is metabolized. The half-life ($t_{1/2}$) of CO in resting adults at sea level is 4 to 6 hours. With administration of pure O_2, $t_{1/2}$ is decreased to approximately 1.5 hours. At 2 to 3 atmospheres on pure O_2, $t_{1/2}$ is approximately 25 minutes. *Toxicology:* Four mechanisms of CO toxicity have been proposed: 1) displacement of O_2 from Hb, 2) increased O_2 affinity of Hb, 3) limiting O_2 utilization, and 4) increased production of superoxide (O_2^-) radicals. Due to the high affinity of Hb for CO (approximately 200 to 250 times greater than that for O_2), CO displaces O_2 from Hb to form CO-Hb. Carbon monoxide binding to Hb causes a shift in the Hb-O_2 dissociation curve to the left, which increases the O_2 affinity of the remaining 3 units of the Hb tetramer. Thus, less O_2 is available to the tissues. In addition, CO binding to other heme proteins such as myoglobin, cytochrome P_{450}, and cytochrome oxidase a_3 may limit O_2 utilization by the tissues. Increased carboxymyoglobin concentration causes cardiac hypoxia and depression. Lastly, CO converts xanthine dehydrogenase to xanthine oxidase that oxidizes xanthine to uric acid and produces O_2^- as a by-product. Superoxide production causes peroxidation of lipids in the brain, resulting in neuronal injury. Tissue hypoxia is the primary toxic mechanism of CO and the organ systems most sensitive to hypoxia are the neurologic, cardiovascular, pulmonary, and renal systems. This hypoxia is not due simply to binding of CO to Hb but due to binding with other heme proteins as well. Acute mortality due to CO intoxication is attributed to cardiac dysrhythmia due to hypoxia. Acute effects correlate roughly with CO-Hb concentration. Toxicity increases with length of exposure, decreased metabolic

activity, and the presence of underlying cardiac or cerebrovascular disease. Metabolic acidosis is common in severe CO intoxication due to the accumulation of lactic acid, while respiratory acidosis occurs less commonly but may be severe.

4. Typical signs and symptoms associated with acute CO intoxication are indicated in **T2**. Chronic signs and symptoms may be due to delayed toxicity secondary to hemorrhagic necrosis in perivascular areas. Delayed effects of CO intoxication include neuropsychiatric changes such as personality alterations, memory impairment, and motor disturbances. Moreover, injury to the hippocampus and globus pallidus regions of the brain can result in Parkinson syndrome and dementia. These consequences are more likely in patients experiencing deep coma regardless of length of exposure to CO or maximum CO-Hb level. Because various factors affect the degree of toxicity experienced by individuals suffering from CO intoxication, the CO-Hb concentration alone is not a reliable indicator of intoxication or prognosis. It must be correlated with the patient's history and presentation, particularly mental status.

Gas chromatography and spectrophotometry are the principal methods for quantifying CO-Hb concentration. Pulse oximetry and other methods are less precise and accurate. The reference method is gas chromatography (GC). It is the most accurate and precise, especially at low concentrations, of all methods for quantifying CO-Hb concentration. Using this method, ferric cyanide [$Fe(CN)_3$] is added to a whole blood sample to release CO for quantification. A molecular sieve column and a thermal conductivity detector are used to isolate and detect CO. The analytical sensitivity of the GC method may be increased by reducing CO to methane (CH_4) with a catalyst, such as nickel, after its emergence from the column and measuring CH_4 using a flame ionization detector. Prior to calculating the CO-Hb concentration, the CO binding capacity of hemoglobin is determined by measuring the CO content after saturation of an aliquot of the patient's blood sample with CO. CO-Hb concentration is then calculated using the formula: CO-Hb, % = ($CO_{content}/CO_{binding\ capacity}$) × 100. Because it is both rapid and convenient, the most commonly used method for quantifying CO-Hb concentration is automated visible spectrophotometry at 4 to 7 wavelengths ("co-oximetry"). The CO-Hb concentration is then determined along with the concentrations of deoxy-Hb, O_2-Hb, CO-Hb, methemoglobin [met-Hb; ie, deoxy-Hb whose ferrous iron (Fe^{2+}) has been oxidized to the ferric form (Fe^{3+})] and sometimes sulfhemoglobin (S-Hb; Hb with sulfur inserted into the Hb porphyrin ring structure), and cyanmethemoglobin (cyanmet-Hb; Hb bound to cyanide) by a formula based on a series of matrix coefficients. This method correlates well with GC at CO-Hb levels greater than 3%. Hemoglobin F (Hb F) has different spectral properties from Hb A that causes CO-Hb concentration to be overestimated by 4% to 7% in neonates. A simpler, manual spectrophotometric method for the quantification of CO-Hb concentration uses only the absorbance at 541 nm and 555 nm. Blood is treated with sodium hydrosulfite ($Na_2S_2O_4$) to convert O_2-Hb and met-Hb to deoxy-Hb with no effect on CO-Hb. Then the ratio of the absorbance at 541 nm (CO-Hb) and 555 nm (deoxy-Hb) is used to determine the %CO-Hb concentration. Pulse oximetry falsely measures CO-Hb as O_2-Hb leading to a falsely high %O_2 saturation. The difference between %O_2 saturation by pulse oximetry and spectrophotometry is called the "saturation gap" and usually represents CO-Hb.

5. The optimal sample for quantification of CO-Hb concentration is a fresh whole blood sample preserved with sodium fluoride and stored at 4°C or frozen. Bacterial contamination must be avoided because bacteria can produce CO and denature Hb. Fresh whole blood is essential because as red blood cells age more methemoglobin is produced which may be falsely measured as CO-Hb by some laboratory methods. In addition, other potentially interfering forms of Hb in the quantitation of CO-Hb concentration include cyanmet-Hb and S-Hb. Some spectrophotometric methods will allow the use of capillary blood.

6. The mainstay of treatment for CO intoxication is 100% O_2 replacement. This accelerates the elimination of CO. If the CO-Hb concentration is greater than 25%, or if the patient is comatose, the use of hyperbaric oxygen (HBO) therapy may be beneficial. Institution of HBO therapy, however, should occur within 6 hours

of exposure. In the case of CO intoxication in a pregnant woman, HBO therapy has not been shown to benefit or harm the fetus. In this case, the patient recovered completely and continued in his residency training program.

Keywords

carbon monoxide intoxication, carboxyhemoglobin, gas chromatography, hyperbaric oxygen therapy

References

1. Baselt RC, Cravey RH. *Disposition of Toxic Drugs and Chemicals in Man.* 3rd ed. Chicago, IL: Yearbook Medical Publishers. 1989:133-136.

2. Porter WH. Chapter 27: Clinical toxicology. In Burtis CA, Ashwood ER, eds. *Tietz' Textbook of Clinical Chemistry.* 3rd ed. Philadelphia: W.B. Saunders. 1999:917-920.

3. Tomaszewski C. Chapter 86: Carbon monoxide. In Goldfrank LR, Flomenbaum NE, Lewin NA, et al. *Goldfrank's Toxicologic Emergencies.* 5th ed. Norwalk, CT: Appleton & Lange. 1994:1199-1214.

4. Ellenhorn MJ. Chapter 66: Respiratory toxicology. In: *Ellenhorn's Medical Toxicology. Diagnosis and Treatment of Human poisoning.* 2nd ed. New York: Elsevier Science Publishing. 1997:1465-1476.

5. Reisdorff EJ, Shah SM. Carbon monoxide poisoning: from crib death to pickup trucks. *Emerg Med Reports.*

Polyuria and Abdominal Pain in a Young Jamaican Woman

Lisa Senzel,[1] Martin I. Surks,[2] Christoph Buettner[2]

[1]*Departments of Pathology and* [2]*Medicine, Montefiore Medical Center and Albert Einstein College of Medicine, Bronx, NY*

Patient: 25-year-old female.

Past Medical History: Unremarkable.

Chief Complaint: Polyuria and abdominal pain with nausea and vomiting.

History of Present Illness: The patient had come to the United States from Jamaica and developed polyuria with abdominal discomfort. During a 2-week period, her symptoms did not improve and after developing nausea and vomiting, she presented to our emergency department (ED). She reported that eating did not appear to make her abdominal pain worse. She denied melena (black stools or vomit), hematochezia (passage of bloody stools), diarrhea, fever, chills or night sweats, weight loss, and alcohol or drug use.

Physical Examination: Vital signs were: temperature, 99.9°F; BP, 139/95 mm Hg; pulse, 111 bpm; respirations, 22 per min. Physical exam findings were normal except for moderate abdominal tenderness and II/VI systolic murmur.

Results of Additional Diagnostic Procedures: A skeletal survey, bone scan, chest X-ray, and computed tomography (CT) scan of the soft tissues of the neck were unremarkable. The purified protein derivative (PPD) test was negative. Bone marrow biopsy was normal except for evidence of increased bone resorption.

Questions

1. What is (are) this patient's most striking laboratory result(s)?

2. How do you explain this patient's most striking laboratory result(s)?

3. What condition(s) does this patient's clinical and laboratory findings suggest?

4. Which additional laboratory test(s) are appropriate to order on this patient and why?

5. What is this patient's most likely diagnosis?

6. What are the principal complications found in this patient's condition?

7. What is the most appropriate treatment for this patient?

Possible Answers

1. Markedly increased total calcium and alkaline phosphatase; increased urine calcium excretion rate, WBC count, total protein, and creatinine.

2. Hypercalcemia is due to either: excessive skeletal calcium release, increased intestinal calcium absorption, or inadequate renal calcium excretion. Excessive skeletal calcium release is the most likely cause of this patient's hypercalcemia,

T1. Principal Laboratory Findings

Test	Patient's Result	"Normal" Reference Range
Hematology		
WBC count	20	$4.1-10.9 \times 10^3$/mL
Hemoglobin	11	12.0-15.2 g/dL
Hematocrit	35	37-46%
Platelet count	278	$150-450 \times 10^3$/mL
Chemistry		
Sodium	137	135-145 mEq/L
Potassium	3.6	3.5-5.0 mEq/L
BUN	17	7-21 mg/dL
Total protein	9.5	6.3-8.2 g/dL
Albumin	4.9	3.5-4.8 g/dL
Creatinine	2.1	0.6-1.2 mg/dL
Calcium, total	19.2	8.4-10.2 mg/dL
Urine calcium excretion	2,066	0-300 mg/24 h
Phosphorous	2.7	2.4-4.5 mg/dL
Alkaline phosphatase	782	38-126 IU/L
TSH	0.3	0.4-4.5 µIU/mL
Free T4	0.8	0.8-1.8 µg/dL

WBC, white blood cell; BUN, blood urea nitrogen; TSH, thyroid stimulating hormone; T4, thyroxine

since the dietary history as well as the increased urinary calcium excretion make the latter 2 causes less likely. The elevated alkaline phosphatase suggested increased new bone formation by osteoblasts, most likely in response to osteoclast stimulation that leads to calcium release from the bone.

3. In general, causes of hypercalcemia include primary hyperparathyroidism, due to a parathyroid gland adenoma, or, less commonly, hyperplasia, humoral hypercalcemia of malignancy (HHM), malignancies metastatic to bone causing lytic lesions leading to local release of calcium, granulomatous diseases such as sarcoidosis, the milk-alkali syndrome, vitamin D intoxication, and familial hypocalciuric hypercalcemia. Primary hyperparathyroidism presents with hypercalcemia, an elevated alkaline phosphatase, and rarely, also with renal failure. In primary hyperparathyroidism the phosphaturic effect of parathyroid

hormone (PTH) usually leads to a low serum phosphorous; however, the serum phosphorous concentration was normal in this patient. Our patient's markedly increased serum calcium level strongly suggested humoral hypercalcemia of malignancy because such a marked increase is rare in primary hyperparathyroidism and is essentially never observed with other causes of hypercalcemia.

4. Parathyroid hormone (PTH) and parathyroid hormone related peptide (PTHrP). To differentiate between primary hyperparathyroidism and HHM, it is helpful to determine whether the hypercalcemia is PTH driven. In our patient, the PTH level was appropriately suppressed at 3 pg/mL (normal reference interval: 7-53 pg/mL). Primary hyperparathyroidism was therefore ruled out. Parathyroid hormone-related protein (PTHrP) is most commonly elevated in HHM. It was therefore somewhat unexpected to find it normal (<1.3 pmol/L) in this patient. However, PTHrP may not be increased in some malignancies associated with HHM. Further workup was aimed at ruling out malignancies. Bone marrow examination showed no evidence of malignancy and the lack of lymphadenopathy precluded nodal biopsy. Both urine and serum protein electrophoresis patterns did not reveal any evidence of paraproteinemia. Mammography and CT of the thorax, abdomen, and pelvis were unremarkable. Thus, common causes of HHM, such as a solid tumor, multiple myeloma, or lymphoma, were less likely causes of our patient's hypercalcemia. In this woman of Caribbean descent, an important consideration was adult T-cell leukemia/lymphoma (ATLL), which is associated with human T-cell lymphotropic virus-1 (HTLV-1) infection. HTLV-1 infection is endemic to the Caribbean and Japan. In the United States, Brooklyn, New York is considered an endemic area because of the large number of immigrants from HTLV-1 endemic countries of the world who have settled in Brooklyn. Diagnosis of ATLL depends on HTLV seropositivity and on morphologic or other evidence of abnormal cells in lymph nodes, bone marrow, and/or peripheral blood. Our patient's serum was positive for antibodies to both HTLV types 1 and 2. Flow cytometry was performed on peripheral blood from our patient and revealed a typical pattern for ATLL—a high CD4/CD8 ratio (17.8:1 for

our patient) and loss of the T-cell cluster of differentiation (CD) marker, CD7. Finally, extraction of DNA from our patient's peripheral blood lymphocytes, followed by polymerase chain reaction (PCR) testing using primers to the V1-8/J1 regions of the T-cell receptor gene, revealed a single band on gel electrophoresis, consistent with a monoclonal T-cell population.

5. ***Most likely diagnosis:*** *hypercalcemia of malignancy associated with adult T-cell leukemia/lymphoma (ATLL).*

   This patient's HTLV seropositivity, high CD4/CD8 ratio, loss of the CD7 T-cell marker, and PCR findings consistent with a monoclonal T-cell population strongly support the diagnosis of ATLL.

6. Overall, up to 10% to 20% of patients with malignancies experience hypercalcemia, usually in advanced stages of the disease. In most cases, it is not difficult to make the diagnosis of HHM if the patient already has a diagnosis of malignancy. Adult T-cell leukemia/lymphoma is a notable exception in that hypercalcemia is commonly the presenting feature of this disease before any other organ system, including the bone marrow, is detectably involved. Hypercalcemia is seen in as many as 70% of patients with ATLL and is often severe, with calcium levels as high as 20 mg/dL, sometimes causing obtundation. The majority of patients with HHM die within several months after the hypercalcemia is discovered. Both solid tumors and hematological malignancies can lead to hypercalcemia, most commonly breast and lung cancer and multiple myeloma. Hypercalcemia of malignancy is mostly due to increased bone resorption with consequent release of calcium from bone. This can occur by 3 possible mechanisms of action: 1) tumor secretion of PTHrP, 2) tumor production of calcitriol (1,25-dihydroxyvitamin D), or 3) the release of cytokines by the tumor.[1-3] PTHrP is the most common cause of hypercalcemia in patients with nonmetastatic solid tumors, ATLL, or non-Hodgkin lymphoma. PTHrP has important physiological functions during development where it is expressed in many different tissues. Its functions include cartilage, tooth, and mammary gland development.[4]

In a knock-out model of PTHrP in mice, one finds a severe defect in cartilage development that leads to early death within several days after birth.[5] Transgenic over-expression of PTHrP delays chondrocyte cell maturation.[6] PTHrP shows amino acid sequence homology with PTH in its amino terminus—the portion of the molecule associated with binding to the PTH receptor. The first 13 amino acids in the amino terminus are almost identical in both PTH and PTHrP.[4] This sequence homology confers on PTHrP the ability to bind and activate the PTH receptor. PTHrP can elicit all of the biologic effects of PTH. In contrast to primary hyperparathyroidism, where the calcitriol levels are typically elevated, serum calcitriol concentrations, for reasons that are not fully understood, are normal or low in PTHrP-mediated HHM.[7] Increased production of calcitriol is found in about 50% of all cases of HHM caused by lymphomas, and it is the main cause of hypercalcemia in Hodgkin disease.[2,8] The hypercalcemia is believed to be due to an increased production of 1,25-dihydroxyvitamin D from 25-hydroxyvitamin D by tumor cells and in this respect, resembles the hypercalcemia of granulomatous disease, which is also due to enhanced extrarenal production of 1,25-dihydroxy-vitamin D.[9,10]

Hypercalcemia induced by calcitriol usually responds to glucocorticoid therapy. In patients with ATLL, multiple myeloma, and in some patients with breast cancer, however, cytokine release, and not invasion of tumor cells into bone, is most commonly the cause of the hypercalcemia observed in these patients. Cytokines stimulate active osteoclasts, the likely proximate mediators of bone resorption, found near the tumor cells. Cytokines that stimulate bone resorption include interleukin-1 beta (IL-1β), IL-6, and tumor necrosis factor-beta.[10] In the case of ATLL, recent evidence points to an increased expression of the receptor activator of nuclear factor kappaB ligand (RANKL) gene, and this over-expression correlates with hypercalcemia.[11] RANKL is part of the OPG/RANKL/RANK system, which was recently identified as the dominant, final mediator of osteoclastogenesis.[12] This finding could explain the hypercalcemia seen in these patients with ATLL in which PTHrP is not elevated.

7. The mainstay of treatment in marked hypercalcemia is to reverse dehydration caused by the hypercalcemia-induced diuresis, loss of renal concentrating ability, and vomiting. Once rehydration has been achieved, inducing diuresis via saline plus furosemide administration will decrease the tubular reabsorption of calcium. With this approach, the serum calcium may decrease by up to 4 mg/dL within 24 hours. One needs to be careful to avoid potassium and magnesium depletion as well as pulmonary edema. Forced diuresis should be supplemented with the use of agents that block bone resorption. The most popular agents are bisphosphonates, either alone or in combination with calcitonin because of its earlier onset of action. In patients with malignancies, mithramycin and gallium nitrate may be used because of their potent osteoclast inhibitory effects. Especially in hematologic malignancies, glucocorticoids have been proven to be efficient agents in inhibiting calcium release.

In our patient, the use of bisphosphonates plus calcitonin for the first 48 hours led to a drop in her serum calcium to 12 mg/dL, which lasted for only a few days and was followed by a rise in serum calcium concentration. Repeated bisphosphonate administration led to a decreased efficiency in lowering the serum calcium concentration because the inhibition of osteoclasts by bisphosphonates was exhausted. Therefore, prednisone therapy was initiated and the serum calcium concentration decreased to a level within the normal reference range. After tapering the prednisone therapy, the patient was maintained on a dose of 5 mg of prednisone for several months with no recurrence of hypercalcemia. Treatment of ATLL can be undertaken with several cycles of combination chemotherapy, although complete response rates are typically 20% to 45%, with responses usually lasting only a few months. Current experimental protocols at the National Institutes of Health (NIH) for the treatment of patients with ATLL are examining the effectiveness of combination antiretroviral drug (ie, interferon-γ and zidovudine) therapy in patients with ATLL and of monoclonal antibodies directed against CD25—the IL-2 receptor alpha subunit that is activated on ATLL cells but not on normal lymphocytes. Our patient was referred to the NIH for participation in such an experimental protocol.

Keywords

hypercalcemia, humoral hypercalcemia of malignancy, parathyroid hormone, parathyroid hormone related peptide, adult T-cell leukemia/lymphoma, bisphosphonates, calcitriol

References

1. Rosol TJ, Capen CC. Mechanisms of cancer-induced hypercalcemia. *Lab Invest*. 1992;67:680-702.

2. Seymour JF, Gagel RF. Calcitriol: The major humoral mediator of hypercalcemia in Hodgkin's disease and non-Hodgkin's lymphomas. *Blood*. 1993;82:1383-1394.

3. Francini G, Petrioli R, Maioli E, et al. Hypercalcemia in breast cancer. *Clin Exp Metastasis*. 1993;11:359-367.

4. Strewler, GJ. The physiology of parathyroid hormone-related protein. *N Engl J Med*. 2000;342:177-185.

5. Karaplis AC, Luz A, Glowacki J, et al. Lethal skeletal dysplasia from targeted disruption of the parathyroid hormone-related peptide gene. *Genes Dev*. 1994;8:277287.

6. Weir EC, Philbrick WM, Amling M, et al. Targeted overexpression of parathyroid hormone-related peptide in chondrocytes causes chondrodysplasia and delayed endochondral bone formation. *Proc Natl Acad Sci USA*. 1996;93:10240-102405.

7. Schilling T, Pecherstorfer M, Blind E, et al. Parathyroid hormone-related protein (PTH-rP) does not regulate serum 1,25-dihydroxyvitamin D levels in hypercalcemia of malignancy. *J Clin Endocrinol Metab*. 1993;76:801-803.

8. Roodman GD. Mechanisms of bone lesions in multiple myeloma and lymphoma. *Cancer*. 1997;80:1557-1563.

9. Barbour GL, Coburn JW, Slatopolsky E, et al. Hypercalcemia in an anephric patient with sarcoidosis: evidence for extrarenal generation of 1,25-dihydroxyvitamin D. *N Engl J Med*. 1981;305:440-443.

10. Stern PH, De Olazabal J, Bell NH. Evidence for abnormal regulation of circulating 1 alpha, 25-dihydroxyvitamin D in patients with sarcoidosis and normal calcium metabolism. *J Clin Invest*. 1980;66:852-855.

11. Nosaka K, Miyamoto T, Sakai T, et al. Mechanism of hypercalcemia in adult T-cell leukemia: Overexpression of receptor activator of nuclear factor kB ligand on adult T-cell leukemia cells. *Blood*. 2002;99:634-640.

12. Khoshla S. Minireview. The OPG/RANKL/RANK system. *Endocrinology*. 2001;142:5050-5055.

Nasal Discharge in a 50-Year-Old Woman

Wendy Chamberlain, Michael D. White, Frank H. Wians, Jr., Monte S. Willis

Department of Pathology, The University of Texas Southwestern Medical Center, Dallas, TX

Patient: 50-year-old G3P3 African-American woman.

Chief Complaint: Fluid leaking from her nose.

History of Present Illness: The patient indicated that fluid had been leaking from her nose for approximately 6 weeks, which worsened when she leaned over. No history of recent infection, excessive sneezing, coughing, or trauma was elicited.

Past Medical History: The patient was currently being treated for hypertension, chronic microcytic anemia, asthma, and epilepsy. The patient reported a single episode of tonic-clonic seizures approximately 20 months prior to presentation, for which she was being treated with Tegretol. Her previous surgeries included a cholescystectomy approximately 10 years ago and fallopian tube ligation approximately 20 years earlier.

Drug History: Tegretol (carbamazepine), 400 mg every 12 hours; aspirin, 81 mg/day; Zyrtec, 10 mg/day; diovan hydrochlorothiazide, 18.75 mg (12.5 mg/tab, 1.5 tab/day); Niferex (cyanocobalamin; folic acid; iron polysaccharide complex), 50 mg/day.

Family/Social History: The patient's brother, sister, and mother had a history of hypertension. Her mother suffered a "mild" stroke several years ago (in her 70s) and her father died at age 78 of colon cancer. The patient admitted frequent use of snuff and smoking 4 cigarettes/day for approximately the last 10 years. She denied alcohol or illicit drug use.

Physical Examination: The patient was alert, well-hydrated, appeared healthy, and was in no apparent distress. Clinically, she was determined to be obese [body mass index (BMI) >35]. Her physical examination was remarkable only for left-sided clear nasal discharge.

Additional Diagnostic Procedures: A magnetic resonance imaging (MRI) of the patient's head was performed 20 months earlier at the time of her initial (and only) seizure. It demonstrated what appeared to be a left choroidal arachnoid cyst impressing on the body and tail of the hippocampus, which was the presumed etiology of her seizure. No other defects were detected at that time.

T1. Principal Laboratory Findings

Test	Patient's Result	"Normal" Reference Range
Hematology		
WBC count Differential, % (absolute number)	12.7	4.1-11.1 × 10³/µL
Neutrophils	78.3 (10)	48.8-68.8% (2-7.5 × 10³/µL)
Lymphocytes	15.8 (2)	20.0-51.0% (0.9-4.7 × 10³/µL)
Monocytes	3.9 (0.5)	4.0-11.0% (0.1-0.9 × 10³/µL)
Eosinophils	1.5 (0.2)	1.0-7.0% (0.0-0.5 × 10³/µL)
Basophils	0.5 (0.1)	0.0-1.0% (0.0-0.2 × 10³/µL)
RBC count	5.08	4.01-5.31 × 10⁶/µL
Hemoglobin	11.2	12.1-16.1 g/dL
Hematocrit	36.6	36.8-48.7%
MCV	72	79-101 fL
MCH	22	27-38 pg
MCHC	30.6	31.6-35.4 g/dL
RDW	9.1	<14.5%
Platelet count	436	174-404 × 10³/µL
Chemistry		
BUN	18	7-21 mg/dL
Creatinine	0.8	0.6-1.2 mg/dL
Bilirubin, total	0.3	0.2-1.3 mg/dL
Uric acid	4.5	2.6-6.0 mg/dL
AST	32	13-40 U/L
ALT	40	10-40 U/L
ALP	112	38-126 U/L
GGT	196	8-78 U/L

ALT, alanine aminotransferase; ALP, alkaline phosphatase; AST, aspartate aminotransferase; BUN, blood urea nitrogen; GGT, g-glutamyltranspeptidase; MCH, mean corpuscular hemoglobin; MCHC, mean corpuscular hemoglobin concentration; MCV, mean corpuscular volume; RBC, red blood cell; RDW, red blood cell distribution width; WBC, white blood cell.

Questions

1. What are this patient's most striking clinical and laboratory findings?

2. What is (are) the most likely cause(s) of this patient's most striking laboratory findings?

3. What additional laboratory test(s) should be performed on this patient and why?

4. What is the principle of the test used to determine if ear or nasal fluid contains cerebrospinal fluid (CSF)?

5. What are some of the conditions in which CSF can be found in ear or nasal fluid?

6. What condition does this patient's clinical, diagnostic, and laboratory findings suggest?

7. What is the pathophysiology of CSF leaks?

8. How should this patient's condition be treated?

Possible Answers

1. Striking *clinical* findings include a history of a single seizure 20 months prior to presentation that was completely controlled with carbamazepine; a normal head MRI post-seizure, except for a minimal defect thought to be an arachnoid cyst; clear rhinorrhea (nasal discharge), worsening when she leaned over; no clinical (eg, coughing, sore throat, swollen lymph nodes, colored mucous drainage) or laboratory (eg, normal WBC) evidence of infection; and no history of trauma. Striking *laboratory* findings include a low hemoglobin, hematocrit, and MCV consistent with mild microcytic anemia, and a significantly elevated GGT with normal AST, ALT, and ALP values [**T1**].

2. **Microcytic anemia.** The most likely cause of this patient's microcytic anemia is decreased body iron stores, which is why she was taking iron supplementation, and explains why her anemia was relatively mild when she presented to the emergency department. **Elevated GGT.** Some of the more common causes of an elevated GGT include bile duct obstruction and liver damage from acute hepatitis or acetaminophen overdose.[1] In addition, an elevated GGT has been described in patients with epilepsy, both unrelated and related to therapy with anti-seizure medications (eg, phenobarbitol and dilantin).[1]

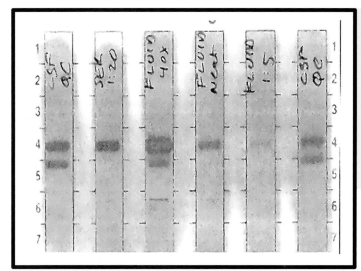

Image 1_Immunoelectrophoresis of patient's nasal fluid. Lane: **1**, CSF QC sample (positive control); **2**, patient's serum diluted 1:20; **3**, patient's nasal fluid concentrated 40-fold (40×); **4**, patient's nasal fluid, unconcentrated and undiluted (neat); **5**, patient's nasal fluid diluted 1:5; **6**, repeat of CSF QC sample. Arrows indicate position of parent transferrin (Trf) and its less negatively charged isoform, β2-transferrin (β2-Trf).

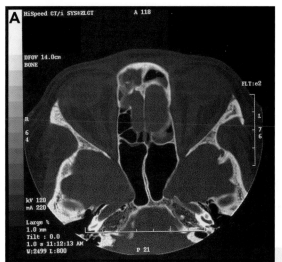
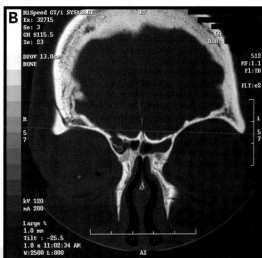

Image 2_Head and sinus CT without contrast. **A**. Axial section demonstrating defects involving the posterior aspect of the frontal sinuses bilaterally and the cribriform plate that are more prominent on the left side with adjacent soft tissue or fluid in the frontal sinuses and nasal vault. **B**. Coronal section further demonstrating the defect in the right frontal sinus. Upon surgical repair, a meningocele was found to be the cause of this defect, although a mass could not be excluded based on the CT findings alone. F, frontal sinuses; CP, cribriform plate; NV, nasal vault; RF, right frontal sinus; LF, left frontal sinus.

The patient presented in this case study was currently being treated for epilepsy.

3. Simultaneous immunofixation electrophoresis (IFE) of both the fluid leaking from the patient's nose and serum using transferrin antiserum. The rationale for this testing is based on the patient's symptoms of clear rhinorrhea suggestive of a cerebrospinal fluid (CSF) leak and the ability of IFE with transferrin antiserum to detect

β_2-transferrin, an isoform of transferrin found only in fluids containing CSF. Based on a retrospective analysis of patients from our institution, a diagnostic algorithm has been developed recently for evaluating patients with suspected CSF leakage into the nasal or auditory canals.[5] Initially, the presence of CSF in nasal or ear fluid in patients with rhinorrhea or otorrhea is confirmed by simultaneous IFE of the fluid and the patient's serum using transferrin antiserum that detects both parent transferrin and its less negatively charged isoform, β_2-transferrin.[2-4] The fluid is interpreted as containing CSF if both parent and β_2-transferrin bands are detected in the IFE pattern of the fluid and only the parent transferrin band is observed in the patient's serum sample. Immunofixation electrophoresis is the method of choice for the detection of CSF in nasal or ear fluid because of its high specificity and sensitivity (95% to 100%).[6,7] If the fluid is determined to contain CSF, follow-up should include localization of the defect by high resolution CT.[5] The complete diagnostic algorithm is based on the most cost effective and efficacious approach to the diagnosis and treatment of suspected CSF leaks and includes the use of imaging modalities such as radionuclide cisternography, magnetic resonance cisternography, and intrathecal administration of fluorescein.

Cerebrospinal fluid results from the ultrafiltration of plasma containing low molecular weight serum proteins such as albumin, pre-albumin, and transferrin. When transferrin, a protein responsible for the transport of iron, is filtered into the CSF, it is acted upon by intrathecal cerebral neuraminidases. These neuraminidases cleave sialic acid moieties from transferrin (the β_1 form, also called the intact or parent form) resulting in a less negatively charged isoform referred to as β_2-transferrin, t-protein, or CSF transferrin. Using transferrin-specific antiserum, immunofixation electrophoresis (IFE) can be used to identify parent transferrin and β_2-transferrin in fluids suspected of containing CSF. The agarose gel IFE pattern of this patient's nasal fluid is shown in **Image 1**. Because the less negatively charged β_2-transferrin does not migrate toward the anode (positively-charged electrode) as fast as β_1-transferrin, 2 distinct bands can be observed in the IFE pattern of nasal or ear fluid containing CSF [**Image 1**], the more anodally migrating β_1-transferrin followed by the slower migrating β_2-transferrin isoform.[8] Whenever IFE is performed on fluids suspected of containing CSF, a patient's serum control, a positive CSF control, and various concentrations of the ear or nasal fluid [ie, concentrated, neat (not diluted or concentrated), and diluted] must be run with each fluid sample to correctly interpret the results.[9] Intact, β_1-transferrin is found predominantly in the plasma; however,

it can also be found in CSF, nasal secretions, tears, saliva, lymph fluid, and aqueous humor.[10,11] The β_2-transferrin isoform is found in the CSF; however, it can also be present in various clinical scenarios, including in the serum of patients with liver disease secondary to alcohol consumption[10] and in individuals with a rare genetic variant of transferrin, in which sialic-acid is depleted, giving rise to multiple transferrin bands on IFE, and mimicking what occurs in CSF.[12] Thus, it is necessary to run the patient's serum as a control as described above in order to prevent false positive interpretations of fluids as containing CSF.[9]

The most common cause of CSF drainage into ear or nasal fluid is accidental trauma from a closed head injury.[13] In such cases, leakage of CSF into ear or nasal discharge begins typically within approximately 48 hours after the trauma and in nearly all cases within 3 months of the traumatic episode.[14] Moreover, endoscopic sinus and neurologic surgery are leading causes of iatrogenic skull base fractures.[13] Other causes of CSF discharge from the nose or ear include central nervous system neoplasms, congenital skull defects (eg, hydrocephalus), and individuals with spontaneous CSF encephalocele. Individuals with spontaneous CSF encephalocele may represent a distinct group. They do not have the other etiologies that characterize the other aforementioned groups. Lastly, some studies have demonstrated that some spontaneous CSF leaks can occur in patients with Marfan syndrome, in patients with Marfanoid features, or in patients with other connective tissue diseases.[15,16]

4. **Spontaneous CSF leak.** The patient's history of positional heachaches in the absence of any trauma, CT findings consistent with frontal sinus defects [**Image 2**], and the presence of β_2-transferrin in her nasal fluid but not in her serum support the diagnosis of spontaneous CSF leak.

5. Normal CSF physiology involves a balance between the production of CSF, mainly by the choroid plexus found in the ventricles (the open areas in the center of the brain) and the absorption of CSF by the arachnoid villi. Cerebrospinal fluid is produced at a rate of about 0.35 mL/minute, or approximately 350 to 500 mL/day, although no more than 90 to 150 mL are present in the CNS at any 1 time.[13] The balance between

this production and absorption of CSF results in a turnover of 3 to 5 volumes of CSF per day. Moreover, normal intracranial pressure (ICP) lying down is 5 to 15 cm H_2O and increases up to 40 cm H_2O upon sitting. Sneezing, laughing, and Valsalva maneuvers (that increase intra-abdominal pressure) may increase ICP significantly. There are several etiologies of CSF leakage which are categorized according to the bony defect, degree and nature of the dural disruption, and the associated ICP. These common etiologies include accidental trauma, surgical trauma, CSF tumors, congenital defects (ie, Marfan syndrome and embryogenic defects), spontaneous CSF leaks, and fistulas.[13,15-17]

Fistulas of the CSF occur when the subarachnoid space communicates with a portion of the skull base which can then manifest itself as a sinonasal tract or temporal bone defect (ie, encephalocele).[5] Repair by surgical means is indicated if leaks do not stop by conservative means or if they were created iatrogenically (eg, during surgery), discovered during surgery, or resulted from trauma or other intracranial injuries.[5] The incidence of encephaloceles is reported to be between 1:10,000 and 1:100,000, with 10% to 25% occurring in the anterior base of the skull.[18,19] Rarely, do multiple defects in the skull base occur and only 6 reports have been published previously.[17] The recognition of spontaneous CSF leaks has increased, leading to a more complete description of this disorder. Headaches are commonly associated with CSF leaks, are orthostatic, and range from transient to more chronic daily headaches.[15] Reports of Valsalva-induced transient headaches have also been published.[15]

Spontaneous CSF leaks occur in patients for which no etiology is clear, as occurred in this case.[13] The cause of spontaneous CSF leaks has been attributed to a variety of causes such as tumors, delayed trauma, and congenital causes,[20,21] and their description as a distinct clinical entity has been proposed by Schlosser and colleagues.[13] These authors propose that the development of CSF leaks may be due to impaired absorption of CSF leading to elevated ICP that in turn exerts forces throughout the skull base.[13] This may result in dura and brain pressure exerted in all directions that moves

through anatomically weakened sites resulting in a small herniation and encephalocele that leaks CSF.[13] Spontaneous CSF leaks occur predominantly in middle-aged obese women (as in this case). Interestingly, this group of women also have an increased prevalence of benign intracranial hypertension (BIH) or pseudotumor cerebri. Patients with BIH have CSF pressures ranging from 25 to 60 cm of H_2O, and therapy is aimed at reducing ICP using diuretics, oral steroids, ongoing lumbar punctures, or shunts.[22] Elevated ICP is associated with both spontaneous CSF leaks and BIH.[23,24]

6. The treatment of choice for spontaneous or iatrogenic CSF rhinorrhea is endoscopic repair, unless the defect is in the posterior wall of the frontal sinus or larger than 5 cm.[25] In the last 10 years, success rates of repair after an initial repair attempt have ranged from 76% to 97%, while success after a second attempt ranges from 86% to 100%.[26-32] Otolaryngologists use many different approaches to repair skull base defects where CSF leaks are occurring. With endoscopic techniques, a greater than 90% success rate may be achieved allowing most individuals to avoid a craniotomy.[13] The success rate by craniotomy has been estimated at 70% to 80%.[27,33] The basic concepts in endoscopic repair are determining the leak site accurately, adequately preparing the area that is leaking, and placing the graft material appropriately.[13] Depending on the site of the defect, various approaches are taken. For example, to repair the ethmoid roof and cribriform area (as in this patient), a transnasal endoscopic approach is used.[13] An ethmoidectomy and maxillary antrostomy are generally needed to approach the area where the leak is located. Positive identification of the leak can be accomplished by direct inspection or intrathecal fluorescein injection.[13] Using different approaches, the entire anterior and central areas of the skull base can be reached endoscopically. The size, anatomic character, location, and presence of elevated CSF pressures all play a role in determining the type of graft that is used in repairing each defect.[13] Perioperatively, it is important to have lumbar access to inject flourescein and decrease CSF pressure if necessary to aid in the reduction of an encephalocele.[13] A lumbar drain is important post-operatively for 24 to 36 hours to avoid spikes in ICP.[13] Acetazolamide

(Diamox), a diuretic that decreases CSF production up to 48%,[34] is used in some cases in which ICP is elevated.[13] Positive pressure ventilation is avoided as much as possible to avoid the risk of pneumocephalus after the patient is extubated. Bed positioning post-operatively is also important to avoid increased CSF pressures while the repaired area is healing. Conservative debridement is generally performed for 1 to 2 weeks after surgery to keep the sinus areas open, and by 6 weeks after the surgery most patients are back to "normal."

Follow-up and Treatment

A head and sinus computed tomography (CT) scan was performed [**Image 2**] after her nasal discharge was reported as positive for β_2-transferrin [**Image 1**]. Her head CT indicated bilateral anterior fossa defects in the base of the skull with a left-sided ethmoidal sinus defect and encephalocele. Additionally, bilateral cribriform plate and left- and right-frontal sinus defects were noted, several of which were leaking CSF. Endoscopic repair of the left meningoencephalocele was performed a month after her initial presentation. Six months after her surgery, the patient no longer suffered from chronic headaches; however, she had a mild rhinorrhea of significantly less intensity than before her surgery.

Keywords

rhinorrhea, otorrhea, cerebrospinal fluid, beta-2-transferrin, sialic acid, neuraminidase, immunofixation electrophoresis, intracranial pressure

References

1. Ravel R. Liver and biliary tract tests. In: *Clinical laboratory medicine: Clinical application of laboratory data.* St. Louis: Mosby, 1995:309-330.

2. Nandapalan V, Watson ID, Swift AC. Beta-2-transferrin and cerebrospinal fluid rhinorrhoea. *Clin Otolaryngol.* 1996; 21:259-264.

3. Marshall AH, Jones NS, Robertson IJ. An algorithm for the management of CSF rhinorrhoea illustrated by 36 cases. *Rhinology.* 1999;37:182-185.

4. Bateman N, Jones NS. Rhinorrhoea feigning cerebrospinal fluid leak: Nine illustrative cases. *J Laryngol Otol.* 2000;114:462-464.

5. Zapalac JS, Marple BF, Schwade ND. Skull base cerebrospinal fluid fistulas: a comprehensive diagnostic algorithm. *Otolaryngol Head Neck Surg.* 2002;126:669-676.

6. Oberascher G, Arrer E. Efficiency of various methods of identifying cerebrospinal fluid in oto- and rhinorrhea. *ORL J Otorhinolaryngol Relat Spec.* 1986;48:320-325.

7. Skedros DG, Cass SP, Hirsch BE, et al. Sources of error in use of beta-2 transferrin analysis for diagnosing perilymphatic and cerebral spinal fluid leaks. *Otolaryngol Head Neck Surg.* 1993;109:861-864.

8. Wians FH, Baskin LB. Electrophoretic methods for the evaluation of proteins in human body fluids. *Diag Endo Metab.* 1998;16:371-383.

9. Normansell DE, Stacy EK, Booker CF, et al. Detection of beta-2 transferrin in otorrhea and rhinorrhea in a routine clinical laboratory setting. *Clin Diagn Lab Immunol.* 1994;1:68-70.

10. Storey EL, Anderson GJ, Mack U, et al. Desialylated transferrin as a serological marker of chronic excessive alcohol ingestion. *Lancet.* 1987;1:1292-1294.

11. Tripathi RC, Millard CB, Tripathi BJ, et al. Tau fraction of transferrin is present in human aqueous humor and is not unique to cerebrospinal fluid. *Exp Eye Res.* 1990;50:541-547.

12. Jaeken J, van Eijk HG, van der Heul C, et al. Sialic acid-deficient serum and cerebrospinal fluid transferrin in a newly recognized genetic syndrome. *Clin Chim Acta.* 1984;144:245-247.

13. Schlosser RJ, Bolger WE. Nasal cerebrospinal fluid leaks. *J Otolaryngol.* 2002;31:S28-37.

14. Zlab MK, Moore GF, Daly DT, et al. Cerebrospinal fluid rhinorrhea: A review of the literature. *Ear Nose Throat J.* 1992;71:314-317.

15. Mokri B. Spontaneous CSF leaks mimicking benign exertional headaches. *Cephalalgia.* 2002;22:780-783.

16. Mokri B, Maher CO, Sencakova D. Spontaneous CSF leaks: Underlying disorder of connective tissue. *Neurology.* 2002;58:814-816.

17. Raghavan U, Majumdar S, Jones NS. Spontaneous CSF rhinorrhoea from separate defects of the anterior and middle cranial fossa. *J Laryngol Otol.* 2002;116:546-547.

18. Orkin M, Fisher I. Heterotopic brain tissue (heterotopic neural rest). Case report with review of related anomalies. *Arch Dermatol.* 1966;94:699-708.

19. Nager GT. Cephaloceles. *Laryngoscope.* 1987;97:77-84.

20. Hubbard JL, McDonald TJ, Pearson BW, et al. Spontaneous cerebrospinal fluid rhinorrhea: Evolving concepts in diagnosis and surgical management based on the Mayo Clinic experience from 1970 through 1981. *Neurosurgery.* 1985;16:314-321.

21. Ommaya AK, Di Chiro G, Baldwin M, et al. Non-traumatic cerebrospinal fluid rhinorrhoea. *J Neurol Neurosurg Psychiatry.* 1968;31:214-225.

22. Corbett JJ, Thompson HS. The rational management of idiopathic intracranial hypertension. *Arch Neurol.* 1989;46:1049-1051.

23. Zagardo MT, Cail WS, Kelman SE, et al. Reversible empty sella in idiopathic intracranial hypertension: an indicator of successful therapy? *AJNR Am J Neuroradiol.* 1996;17:1953-1956.

24. Shetty PG, Shroff MM, Fatterpekar GM, et al. A retrospective analysis of spontaneous sphenoid sinus fistula: MR and CT findings. *AJNR Am J Neuroradiol.* 2000;21:337-342.

25. Hughes RG, Jones NS, Robertson IJ. The endoscopic treatment of cerebrospinal fluid rhinorrhoea: The Nottingham experience. *J Laryngol Otol.* 1997;111:125-128.

26. Zweig JL, Carrau RL, Celin SE, et al. Endoscopic repair of cerebrospinal fluid leaks to the sinonasal tract: predictors of success. *Otolaryngol Head Neck Surg.* 2000;123:195-201.

27. Lanza DC, O'Brien DA, Kennedy DW. Endoscopic repair of cerebrospinal fluid fistulae and encephaloceles. *Laryngoscope.* 1996;106:1119-1125.

28. Dodson EE, Gross CW, Swerdloff JL, et al. Transnasal endoscopic repair of cerebrospinal fluid rhinorrhea and skull base defects: A review of 29 cases. *Otolaryngol Head Neck Surg.* 1994;111:600-605.

29. Mattox DE, Kennedy DW. Endoscopic management of cerebrospinal fluid leaks and cephaloceles. *Laryngoscope.* 1990;100:857-862.

30. Casiano RR, Jassir D. Endoscopic cerebrospinal fluid rhinorrhea repair: Is a lumbar drain necessary? *Otolaryngol Head Neck Surg.* 1999;121:745-750.

31. Mao VH, Keane WM, Atkins JP, et al. Endoscopic repair of cerebrospinal fluid rhinorrhea. *Otolaryngol Head Neck Surg.* 2000;122:56-60.

32. Wax MK, Ramadan HH, Ortiz O, et al. Contemporary management of cerebrospinal fluid rhinorrhea. *Otolaryngol Head Neck Surg.* 1997;116:442-449.

33. Schick B, Ibing R, Brors D, et al. Long-term study of endonasal duraplasty and review of the literature. *Ann Otol Rhinol Laryngol.* 2001;110:142-147.

34. Carrion E, Hertzog JH, Medlock MD, et al. Use of acetazolamide to decrease cerebrospinal fluid production in chronically ventilated patients with ventriculopleural shunts. *Arch Dis Child.* 2001;84:68-71.

Recurrent Confusion and Seizures in an Adult Male

Qing Meng,[1] Gillian Luxton[2]

[1]*Department of Pathology, Royal University Hospital, University of Saskatchewan, Saskatoon, Canada*

[2]*Department of Pathology and Molecular Medicine, McMaster University, Ontario, Canada*

Patient: 49-year-old male.

Chief Complaint: Recurrent confusion and seizures with violent behavior.

History of Present Illness: For the last 10 years, the patient had recurrent difficulty with early morning spells of confusion. Recently, this symptom became worse, with violent behavior and seizures, and he was sometimes incontinent of stool and urine. He indicated, however, that he felt better after eating snacks or breakfast, particularly if they included orange juice. He denied any problems with palpitations, diaphoresis, tremor, or paralysis. He had no nausea, vomiting, headache, or vision change.

Medical History: Six months previously, he presented with low back pain and was diagnosed with seminoma and a large retroperitoneal/periaortic encasing mass with residual tumor and received chemotherapy. He had no history of diabetes mellitus, alcoholism, drug addiction, heart disease, hypertension, or epilepsy.

Family History: No family history of diabetes mellitus, stroke, seizure, or alcoholism.

Drug History: The patient denied drug abuse and taking any medications.

Physical Examination: Vital signs were: BP, 120/70 mm Hg; HR, 86/min. He was conscious but appeared anxious. There were no remarkable findings on review of cardiovascular and respiratory systems. Liver and spleen were not palpable. The movement and strength were normal for both arms and legs.

Questions _____

1. What are this patient's most striking clinical and laboratory findings?

2. How do you explain this patient's most striking clinical and laboratory findings?

3. What are the causes of hypoglycemia?

4. What is the most likely source of this patient's increased insulin level?

5. What is this patient's differential diagnosis?

6. What is this patient's most likely diagnosis?

7. How should this patient be treated?

T1. Principal Laboratory Findings

Test	Patient's Result	"Normal" Reference Range
Hematology		
WBC count	5.4	4.0-11.0 × 10³/mL
RBC count	3.38	4.5-6.5 × 10⁶/mL
Hemoglobin (Hb)	7.8	13.0-18.0 g/dL
Hematocrit (Hct)	24.1	40.0-54.0%
MCV	71.1	82-99 fL
MCH	23	27-32 pg
MCHC	30	30-35 g/dL
RDW	30.3	11.5-15.0%
Platelet count	136	150-400 × 10³/mL
Chemistry		
BUN	13	8-18 mg/dL
Creatinine	1.1	0.6-1.2 mg/dL
Sodium	138	135-145 mEq/L
Potassium	4.5	3.5-5.5 mEq/L
Chloride	102	98-107 mEq/L
Total CO$_2$	26	22-30 mEq/L
Calcium	9.76	8.6-10.2 mg/dL
Phosphorus	4.4	2.5-4.5 mg/dL
Magnesium	0.8	0.6-1.1 mEq/L
CK, total	37	<225 U/L
Total protein	6.8	6.0-8.0 g/dL
Albumin	3.2	3.5-5.5 g/dL
A/G ratio	0.9	1.4-1.6
INR-PT	1.5	0.9-1.2
Urate	4.0	3.6-7.6 mg/dL
Bilirubin, total	0.5	0.1-1.1 mg/dL
ALP	164	40-120 U/L
GGT	82	0-50 U/L
LD	457	100-220 U/L
AST	46	<35 U/L
ALT	37	0-40 U/L
PTH	17	10-65 pg/mL
Iron	45	67-178 mg/dL
TIBC	270	250-447 mg/dL
%TS	17	20-50%
Ferritin	73	18-300 ng/mL
AFP	2	<10 mg/L
hsCRP	9,320	<20 mg/dL
Troponin I	<0.3	£0.5 mg/L

WBC, white blood cell; RBC, red blood cell; MCV, mean corpuscular volume; MCH, mean corpuscular hemoglobin; MCHC, mean corpuscular hemoglobin concentration; RDW, red cell distribution width; BUN, blood urea nitrogen; CK, creatine kinase; A/G, albumin/globulin; INR-PT, international normalized ratio of prothrombin time; ALP, alkaline phosphatase; GGT, gamma glutamyl transferase; LD, lactate dehydrogenase; AST, aspartate aminotransferase; ALT, alanine aminotransferase; PTH, parathyroid hormone; TIBC, total iron binding capacity; %TS, percent transferrin saturation; AFP, alpha fetoprotein; hsCRP, high sensitivity C-reactive protein

T2. Hormones

Test	Patient's Result	"Normal" Reference Range
Chemistry		
Glucose (random)	46	70-100 mg/dL
Glucose (fasting)	32	70-110 mg/dL
Ketones	Negative	Negative
Proinsulin	133.2	6.4-9.4 pmol/L
C-peptide	10.0	0.78-1.89 ng/mL
Insulin	65.1	6.19-27.93 µU/mL
Insulin: glucose ratio: Random	1.4	<0.3
Fasting	2.0	<0.3
IGF I	89	94-252 µg/L
Cortisol (0800 h)	13	7-24 mg/dL
ACTH	27	9-50 pg/mL
hCG	2	<2 mIU/mL
Prolactin	20	<18 µg/L
TSH	2.0	0.4-5.0 µU/mL
LH	32.0	2.0-12.0 U/L
FSH	51.6	1.0-12.0 U/L
Testosterone, total	202	288-865 ng/dL

IGF I, insulin-like growth factor I; ACTH, adrenocorticotropic hormone; hCG, human chorionic gonadotropin; TSH, thyroid stimulating hormone; LH, luteinizing hormone; FSH, follicle-stimulating hormone

Possible Answers

1. Neurological symptoms, including confusion and seizures; markedly decreased random and fasting glucose; markedly increased insulin, C-peptide, proinsulin, and high sensitivity C-reactive protein (hsCRP); decreased RBC count, Hb, Hct, platelet count, MCV and MCH, with an increased RDW; prolonged INR; decreased iron, albumin, and A/G ratio; increased ALP and LD; slightly increased LH and FSH levels; decreased testosterone [**T1**] and [**T2**].

2. The explanation of this patient's most striking clinical and laboratory findings are complicated by his cancer. Neurological symptoms such as confusion and seizures, coupled with markedly decreased random and fasting glucose concentrations and markedly increased insulin, C-peptide, and proinsulin values, indicate that this patient has hypoglycemia. The low RBC, Hb, Hct, MCV, MCH, increased RDW, and low serum iron indicate iron deficiency anemia (IDA). Iron deficiency anemia may be related to the patient's poor nutrition, glucose malabsorption, or chemotherapy. Serum ferritin is a sensitive, but less specific, early marker for IDA because it can be increased in clinical conditions such as acute phase reaction and inflammation. When these conditions are present, a normal serum ferritin concentration can occur in individuals with severe IDA. An acute phase reaction in our patient is supported by the markedly increased hsCRP concentration. C-reactive protein is a *positive* acute phase reactant whose concentration is increased in individuals with an acute phase reaction. A total iron binding capacity (TIBC) within the limits of the (normal) reference interval does not eliminate the diagnosis of IDA because TIBC is a surrogate marker of transferrin, a *negative* acute phase reactant (ie, transferrin concentration decreases in individuals with an acute phase reaction). High transferrin saturation (>15%) may suggest coexistence of anemia of chronic disease (ACD) with IDA; however, IDA alone is not excluded because TIBC can be influenced by many physiological and pathophysiological conditions.[1] Low platelet count, prolonged INR, decreased albumin and A/G ratio, high ALP, LD, and AST suggest that the patient has chronic liver disease. Testicular tissue damage from tumor (seminoma) infiltration or chemotherapy could be the cause of the patient's low testosterone concentration. A low testosterone concentration stimulates the hypothalamus to secrete gonadotropin releasing hormone (GnRH) which acts on the anterior pituitary to increase the release of LH and FSH.

3. Hypoglycemia (ie, a serum glucose concentration <50 mg/dL) can arise due to alimentary and endocrine problems, idiopathic, extrapancreatic, and pancreatic (eg, insulinomas) tumors, and miscellaneous causes, including fasting and malnutrition, hepatic and other diseases, as a side effect of diabetes treatment, treatment with various medications (eg, sulfonylureas and chemotherapeutic agents), and hormone or enzyme deficiencies. Malnutrition was not a severe problem for the patient because his serum albumin concentration was close to the lower limit of the reference interval and he denied any vomiting and diarrhea. Based on his increased liver function test values, he appeared to have a chronic hepatic injury, which could impair gluconeogenesis, increase depletion of glycogen stores, and cause hypoglycemia. Cancer chemotherapy is known to be associated with development of hypoglycemia. The findings of a low blood glucose concentration, coupled with markedly increased insulin, C-peptide, and proinsulin values, are consistent with insulin-induced hypoglycemia, which is usually due to an insulin-producing tumor.[2]

4. Because the patient had a testicular tumor (seminoma) with metastases to the retroperitoneal and mesenteric areas, the pancreas might contain an insulin-secreting tumor or the testicular tumor itself might be secreting insulin. Rarely do non-pancreatic tumors secrete insulin, and there has been only 1 report of such a case involving an insulin-secreting small-cell carcinoma of the cervix.[3] Moreover, a tissue specimen resected from the patient's tumor was negative for insulin staining. In addition, the patient's markedly increased proinsulin and C-peptide values eliminated exogenous insulin as the cause of his hypoglycemia, while the patient's negative drug history, including lack of treatment with a sulfonylurea, ruled out the possibility of medication-induced insulin secretion. Based on the collection of

these findings, the most likely source of this patient's markedly increased insulin concentration is a pancreatic insulinoma.

5. Specific causes of a markedly decreased glucose concentration include: factitious, fasting, or reactive hypoglycemia, nesidioblastosis, or drug-, alcohol-, critical illness-, hormone deficiency-, autoimmune-, and tumor-induced hypoglycemia. **Factitious hypoglycemia** can occur in patients with psychiatric disturbances, a need for attention, and access to insulin. The triad of hypoglycemia, high immunoreactive insulin levels, and suppressed plasma C-peptide levels is pathognomonic of exogenous insulin administration. Exogenous insulin-induced hypoglycemia can be detected by an insulin:C-peptide ratio greater than 1.0. **Fasting hypoglycemia** is diagnosed from a blood sample that shows a blood glucose level of less than 50 mg/dL after an overnight fast, between meals, or after exercise. In **reactive hypoglycemia** (postprandial) symptoms appear within 4 hours after a meal. The cause(s) of reactive hypoglycemia are controversial. Some investigators have suggested that certain individuals may be more sensitive than others to the effects of epinephrine, which cause many of the symptoms of hypoglycemia.[4] Others believe that a deficiency in glucagon secretion leads to hypoglycemia.[5] Causes of reactive hypoglycemia include gastric surgery, because of the rapid passage of food into the small intestine, drugs, antibodies to insulin or the insulin receptor, and hereditary fructose-1,6-diphosphatase deficiency. **Nesidioblastosis**, or hyperplasia of the pancreatic islet cells, causes hyperinsulinemic hypoglycemia. It is predominantly a neonatal disorder, although cases in adults have been reported.[6] **Drug-induced hypoglycemia** can occur in diabetics taking certain drugs (eg, insulin) to control blood glucose levels, including inadvertent ingestion of sulfonylurea due to patient or pharmacist error. Other drugs associated with drug-induced hypoglycemia include haloperidol, salicylates, quinine, pentamidine, and sulfonamides. The patient was not an insulin-dependent diabetic, and he was not taking any drugs or medications. **Alcohol-induced hypoglycemia** results from chronic alcohol ingestion that can impair hepatic gluconeogenesis and glycogen storage that is aggravated further by the malnutrition that frequently accompanies chronic alcoholism. **Critical illness-induced hypoglycemia** can occur in individuals with renal failure or severe liver disease, such as drug-induced hepatitis and liver failure. Long-term starvation, as may occur in the eating disorder anorexia nervosa, can result in the depletion of substances needed in gluconeogenesis, resulting in hypoglycemia. **Hormone deficiency-induced hypoglycemia** can occur in certain disorders of the adrenal (eg, Addison disease) and pituitary glands (eg, hypopituitarism) that result in a deficiency of key hormones that regulate glucose homeostasis. Hormone deficiencies cause hypoglycemia in children more frequently than in adults. Decreased blood levels of cortisol, growth hormone, glucagon, thyroxine, or epinephrine can lead to fasting hypoglycemia. Moreover, hypoglycemia with adrenal insufficiency should be accompanied by suppressed insulin levels. Laboratory tests for hormone levels establish the diagnosis. In this patient, cortisol, ACTH, and TSH levels were within the limits of the (normal) reference interval for these hormones. **Autoimmune-induced hypoglycemia** is a rare disorder caused by the interaction of endogenous antibodies with insulin or the insulin receptor. When this disorder occurs, laboratory testing demonstrates low plasma C-peptide and high plasma insulin concentrations. **Tumor-induced hypoglycemia** occurs in individuals with pancreatic (insulinomas) and extrapancreatic insulin-producing tumors that cause hypoglycemia by disproportionately raising the serum insulin level in relation to the blood glucose level. Insulinomas do not normally metastasize to other parts of the body. Nonpancreatic, non-insulin producing neoplasms can also cause hypoglycemia; however, in such cases, the tumor secretes factors [eg, insulin-like growth factors I (IGF I) and II (IGF II)] other than insulin, which, when elevated, cause hypoglycemia. The patient had an increased plasma insulin level and a low IGF I level, suggesting that his insulin-secreting tumor was of pancreatic origin.

6. ***Most likely diagnosis:*** *hypoglycemia due to a pancreatic insulinoma.*

Hypoglycemia with highly elevated insulin, C-peptide, and proinsulin strongly suggests that this patient had hyperinsulinemia due to an insulin-secreting pancreatic insulinoma.

This diagnosis was confirmed by ultrasound, octreotide scan, and surgical findings, which indicated the presence of an insulinoma in the head of the pancreas. The patient was unusual in that he presented with only neuroglycopenic symptoms of hypoglycemia.[7] An insulinoma is a neuroendocrine tumor, derived mainly from pancreatic islet cells, that produces excessive amounts of insulin and is the most common type of tumor causing hypoglycemia. In healthy individuals, insulin and C-peptide are secreted in equimolar amounts because they are both derived from the same inactive precursor molecule, proinsulin. Some insulinomas secrete additional hormones, such as gastrin, 5-hydroxy-indole acetic acid (5-HIAA), ACTH, glucagon, hCG, and somatostatin. Insulinomas are the most common pancreatic endocrine tumor. The incidence of insulinomas in the United States population is about 1 to 4 per million people, and women are slightly more affected than men (male:female ratio = 2:3). Moreover, these tumors may secrete insulin in short bursts, causing wide fluctuations in blood glucose levels. About 90% of insulinomas are benign, while malignant insulinomas are often seen in patients with multiple endocrine neoplasia (MEN).[1] The pathogenesis of, and particularly the genetic changes that occur in, neuroendocrine tumors is not fully understood. In individuals with an insulinoma, symptoms vary widely; however, in general, they are characterized by central nervous system (headache, confusion, blurred vision, personality changes, seizures), cardiovascular (tachycardia, palpitations), GI (hunger, nausea, belching), and adrenergic effects (weakness, sweating, anxiety, tremulousness, nervousness). A diagnosis of hypoglycemia should not be made unless a patient meets the criteria of Whipple triad: (1) low blood glucose concentration with (2) typical symptoms of hypoglycemia that are (3) alleviated by glucose administration.[8] The diagnosis of insulinoma is normally established by the laboratory findings of low plasma glucose, inappropriately elevated levels of insulin and C-peptide, and to a lesser degree, high levels of proinsulin.[2] The biochemical diagnosis of insulinoma is established in 95% of patients during prolonged fasting (up to 72 h) when the following laboratory test results are found in patients not on sulfonylurea therapy: serum insulin levels of 10 mU/mL or more [(normal)

reference interval: <6 mU/mL], glucose levels of less than 40 mg/dL [(normal) reference interval: 70-110 mg/dL], C-peptide levels exceeding 2.5 ng/mL [(normal) reference interval: <2 ng/mL), and proinsulin levels greater than 25% (or up to 90%) that of the immunoreactive insulin level. Moreover, an insulin (mU/mL) to plasma glucose (mg/dL) ratio of >0.3 is diagnostic of an insulinoma. In patients with an insulinoma, this ratio rises during fasting as seen in this patient whose insulin to glucose ratio was 1.4 [**T2**]. Stimulation tests are no longer recommended in the diagnostic workup of patients suspected of having an insulinoma. The intravenous administration of tolbutamide, glucagon, or calcium can be hazardous to the patient by inducing prolonged and refractory hypoglycemia. Moreover, an oral glucose tolerance test (OGTT) should not be used for evaluating a patient suspected of having hypoglycemia. Imaging studies, including computed tomography (CT) scan, magnetic resonance imaging (MRI), transabdominal ultrasonography, or arteriography is performed only after the diagnosis of insulinoma has been established biochemically. The sensitivity of these imaging techniques is low particularly when the insulinomas are small (< 2 cm).

7. The initial treatment of hypoglycemia depends on the patient's symptoms. It may be helpful for patients to eat snacks, drink orange juice, swallow glucose tablets, or eat candy to raise their blood sugar level. If the symptoms are more severe, intravenous glucose administration or an injection of glucagon may be needed. In any event, treatment of a patient with signs and symptoms of hypoglycemia should not be withheld while waiting for a laboratory glucose values. For the long term, treatment of hypoglycemia may involve the use of an insulin inhibitory drug and surgical removal of the tumor (insulinoma). Diazoxide, a direct inhibitor of insulin secretion, which can increase hepatic glucose output and decrease cellular glucose uptake, may be indicated in patients with an insulinoma. Because insulinoma resection is curative in approximately 90% of patients with hypoglycemia due to an insulinoma, such surgery is currently the therapy of choice. After starting diazoxide therapy, the patient had no further episodes of severe hypoglycemic reactions, such as loss of consciousness or seizures. His blood glucose levels improved;

however, they were still lower than normal. Subsequently, the patient underwent surgery and recovered well. Following surgery, he had no symptoms of hypoglycemia and all previously abnormal laboratory test values returned to values within the normal reference interval for each test.

Keywords

hypoglycemia, insulinoma, nesidioblastosis

References

1. Wians FH Jr, Urban JE, Keffer JH, et al. Discriminating between iron deficiency anemia and anemia of chronic disease using traditional indices of iron status vs transferrin receptor concentration. *Am J Clin Pathol.* 2001;115:112-118.

2. Roith DL. Tumor-induced hypoglycemia. *N Engl J Med.* 1999;341:757-758.

3. Seckl MJ, Mulholland PJ, Bishop AN, et al. Brief report: Hypoglycemia due to an insulin-secreting small-cell carcinoma of the cervix. *N Engl J Med.* 1999;341:733-736.

4. Service FJ. Hypoglycemic disorders. *N Engl J Med.*1995;332:1144-1152.

5. Brun JF, Fedou C, Mercier J. Postprandial reactive hypoglycemia. *Diabetes Metab.* 2000;26:337-351.

6. Kaczirek K, Soleiman A, Schindl M, et al. Nesidioblastosis in adults: A challenging cause of organic hyperinsulinism. *Eur J Clin Investigat.* 2003;33:488-492.

7. Dizon AM, Kowalyk S, Hoogwerf BJ. Neuroglycopenic and other symptoms in patients with insulinomas. *Am J Med.* 1999;106:307-310.

8. Burtis CA, Ashwood ER. *Tietz Textbook of Clinical Chemistry.* 3rd ed. Philadelphia: W.B. Saunders Company.

Severe Head Trauma During a Motor Vehicle Accident

Barbara G. Border

Department of Diagnostic and Primary Care, Texas Tech University Health Sciences Center, Lubbock TX

Patient: 31-year-old male.

Surgical History: None.

Family History: Unremarkable.

Chief Complaint: Patient presented to the emergency room of a large urban hospital with severe scalp abrasions and head trauma following a motor vehicle accident (MVA). A cranial computed tomography (CT) scan was performed to determine the extent of neural damage, and massive hemorrhage was noted below and around the hypothalamic area. Craniectomy and craniotomy of right frontal lobe tissue was performed to relieve the excess intracranial pressure. The patient was admitted to the surgical intensive care unit (SICU) in critical condition.

Drug History: Family claimed no knowledge of patient's drug history.

Laboratory Findings: All results for the initial chemistry tests performed on this patient prior to admission to the SICU were within the normal reference limits for these tests. A CBC count revealed a moderately low RBC count and decreased hemoglobin and hematocrit values. Analysis of cerebrospinal fluid (CSF) indicated 1,300 RBCs/mm^3 (normal reference limits: 0 to 100) and 400 WBCs/mm^3 (normal reference limits: 0 to 5). One week after admission to the SICU, all results for chemistry tests were still within the normal reference limits for these tests; urinalysis results were unremarkable, except for a trace of blood and a few (3 to 5) epithelial cells; and, analysis of CSF following a second lumbar spinal tap continued to demonstrate the presence of increased numbers of RBCs (mostly crenated) and WBCs. Subsequently, the patient was moved from the SICU to the neurological rehabilitation unit (NRU), and his status was downgraded to serious.

Results of Additional Diagnostic Procedures: A second cranial CT was performed approximately 1 week after admission and demonstrated typical postoperative changes indicative of craniectomy, craniotomy, and cranioplasty. Evidence of hemorrhage was noted; however, the size and extent of the hemorrhage and subdural hematoma were reduced. Noninfusion cranial CTs were performed at 2 and 3 weeks postcraniotomy. The CT findings included mild dilatation of the ventricular system and encephalomalacia. As before, there was no radiographic evidence of the presence of a brain mass.

Results of Additional Laboratory Procedures: Approximately 2 weeks following admission and 1 week after moving into the NRU, the patient's serum glucose concentration was increased, and the results of laboratory tests for a wide variety of chemistry analytes were closely monitored during the next 2.5-week period [**T1**]. In addition, several endocrine laboratory tests were ordered with results shown in **T2**.

T1. Patient's Principal Laboratory Findings

Analyte	Day Postadmission to NRU[a]										Reference Limits		Units
	1	4	5	6	8	11	12	13	15	17	LLN	ULN	
Total Protein		6.7	7.9	6.3	7.3	7.5	6.7	6.7	6.9	7.1	6.0	8.5	g/dL
Albumin		3.9	4.5	3.5	4.2	4.3	3.8	3.7	3.7	3.8	3.0	5.5	g/dL
Globulin		2.8	3.0	3.3	3.1	2.8	3.4	3.9	3.5	3.3	1.5	3.5	g/dL
Sodium	138	148	150	144	146	160	152	151	146	145	135	145	mmol/L
Potassium	4.0	4.0	4.1	3.7	4.1	3.9	3.9	3.9	4.0	3.9	3.5	5.0	mmol/L
Chloride	101	109	108	107	108	118	116	113	106	107	96	106	mmol/L
CO_2	25	26	25	27	24	27	26	29	26	24	22	32	mmol/L
Anion gap	12	13	11	12	15	16	16	16	15	14	8	16	
Calcium		9.4	9.4	9.9	8.7	9.8	10.1	9.0	9.3	8.8	8.5	10.5	mg/dL
Phosphorus		4.5	4.0	3.0	6.0	4.5	4.4	3.7	3.6	3.7	2.5	4.5	mg/dL
Creatinine		1.2	1.2	1.0	1.1	1.1	1.2	1.2	1.3	1.1	0.7	1.5	mg/dL
BUN	14	17	16	13	15	14	17	17	20	23	10	20	mg/dL
Iron		57	129	63	91	85	66	65	60	62	49	181	µg/dL
Total bilirubin		0.5	0.7	0.5	0.4	0.5	0.5	0.5	0.5	0.5	0.2	1.2	mg/dL
Direct bilirubin		0.0	0.0	0.0	0.0	0.0	0.0	0.0	0.0	0.0	0.0	0.2	mg/dL
Uric Acid		9.8	9.9	8.4	7.9	11.6	10.6	10.1	9.6	8.3	2.5	8.5	mg/dL
Glucose	143	198	129	149	332	165	297	219	170	375	70	125	mg/dL
Cholesterol		276	308	239	325	339	345	325	289	327	0	200	mg/dL
Triglycerides		1141	974	752	1284	931	2000	1251	1034	3476	0	250	mg/dL
$Osmo_{meas}$	300										270	300	mOsm/kg
$Osmo_{calc}$[b]	289												mOsm/kg
Osmolal gap	11										10		

Enzymes

										LLN	ULN	Units
ALP	158	166	147	178	149	144	141	142	165	30	115	U/L
ALT	523	524	329	243	212	189	160	108	89	8	40	U/L
AST	242	183	98	56	88	97	57	33	35	5	50	U/L
AST/ALT ratio	0.46	0.35	0.30	0.23	0.42	0.51	0.36	0.31	0.39	0.7	1.4	
CK	33	49	43	65	40	47	56	76	51	15	105	U/L
GGT	523	538	445	543	695	623	570	473	518	8	78	U/L
LD	378	340	277	316	283	295	233	199	240	100	190	U/L

aBolded values are outside the analyte-specific reference limits. bOsmo_calc = 2[Sodium] + ([Glucose]/18) + ([BUN]/2.8); [Sodium] = 138 mmol/L; [Glucose] = 143 mg/dL; [BUN] = 14 mg/dL. NRU, neurological rehabilitation unit; LLN, lower limit of normal; ULN, upper limit of normal; Osmo_calc, calculated osmolality; Osmo_meas, measured osmolality; ALP, alkaline phosphatase; ALT, alanine aminotransferase; AST, aspartate aminotransferase; BUN, blood urea nitrogen; CK, creatine kinase; GGT, gamma-glutamyl transferase; LD, lactate dehydrogenase

T2. Results of Additional (Endocrine) Laboratory Tests

Analyte	Patient's Result^a	Reference Limits LLN	ULN	Units
FT4	**0.1**	0.8	2.3	ng/dL
TT3	**10**	100	200	ng/dL
TSH	**Und**	0.4	4.2	μIU/mL
LH	**Und**	1.0	8.0	mIU/mL
Total testosterone	**25**	280	2200	ng/dL
ACTH (supine)	Und	10		pg/mL
Cortisol:				
8:00 AM	**1.0**	5	23	μg/dL
8:00 PM	0.4			<½ of 8:00 AM value
ADH	**1.0**	4	14	pg/mL

aBolded values are outside the analyte-specific reference limits defined by the lower (LLN) and upper (ULN) limits of the normal reference interval. FT4, free thyroxine; TT3, total triiodothyronine; TSH, thyroid stimulating hormone; Und, undetectable; LH, luteinizing hormone; ACTH, adrenocorticotropic hormone; ADH, anti-diuretic hormone.

Questions

1. What are this patient's most striking laboratory results?

2. How do you explain this patient's most striking laboratory results?

3. What condition(s) does this patient's laboratory and other findings suggest?

4. Which additional laboratory test(s) are appropriate to order on this patient and why?

5. What is the most likely diagnosis (diagnoses) relevant to this patient?

Possible Answers

1. Abnormal initial and follow-up CSF findings (ie, increased RBCs and WBCs); markedly increased serum glucose, cholesterol, triglycerides, ALP, ALT, AST, GGT, LD values, and slightly increased osmolal gap ([**T1**] and [**Figure 1**]); markedly decreased serum FT4, TT3, TSH, LH, total testosterone, ACTH, cortisol, and ADH

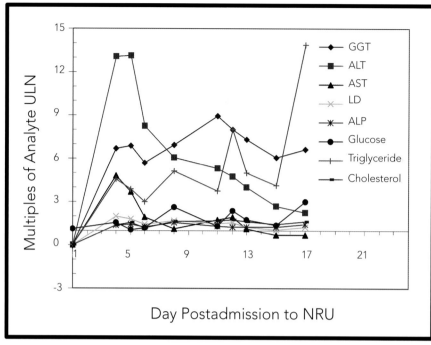

Figure 1_Changes in serum levels, expressed as a multiple of the analyte-specific upper limit of normal (ULN), of various analytes during the patient's stay in a neurological rehabilitation unit (NRU). The x-axis line that crosses the y-axis at a value of 1 multiple of the ULN represents the ULN for each analyte shown.

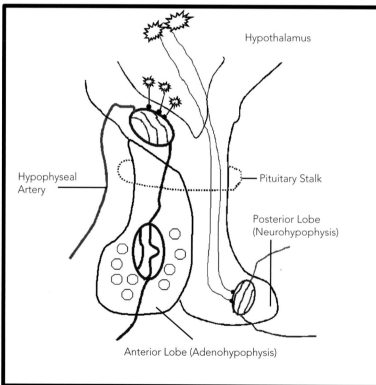

Figure 2_Routes by which the hypothalamus influences the pituitary gland. Anti-diuretic hormone (ADH; vasopressin) and oxytocin are synthesized by neurons in the supraoptic and paraventricular nuclei of the hypothalamus and transported down axons in the pituitary stalk to capillaries of the posterior pituitary lobe (neurohypophysis). Neurons in the arcuate and periventricular nuclei of the hypothalamus secrete releasing hormones into hypothalamic capillaries where they gain access to the hypophyseal portal system to reach the cells of the anterior lobe of the pituitary (adenohypophysis). These cells, when stimulated by the releasing hormones secreted by the hypothalamus, synthesize various hormones (eg, TSH, LH, FSH, prolactin, ACTH, etc) that are released into the general circulation.

values [**T2**]; and, increased serum sodium concentration [**T1**].

2. The patient's most striking laboratory results might be explained as follows:

Abnormal CSF findings: Most likely caused by the head trauma sustained during the MVA.

Markedly increased serum glucose: The primary cause of an elevated *glucose* value is uncontrolled diabetes mellitus (DM); however, the patient had no known history of diabetes, and the initial urinalysis did not indicate the presence of glucose or ketones. The patient's glucose value began to rise 2 weeks after admission and reached its highest value approximately 4 weeks postadmission. Further urine studies (*results not shown*) indicated elevated glucose and ketones. Because of the acute nature of the rise in glucose values, idiopathic type 1 DM is the most likely cause. The cause of this patient's sudden onset of DM is unclear; however, it might be stress-induced due to the trauma of the MVA. Stress-induced DM is often overlooked in patients who undergo a stressful surgical procedure and demonstrate postsurgery elevated serum glucose and lipid values.

Markedly increased serum cholesterol and triglycerides: The patient's serum samples were grossly lipemic. Elevated lipid (*cholesterol and triglycerides*) values in a diabetic indicate an abnormality in the citric acid cycle, which occurs commonly in individuals with uncontrolled DM and Fredrickson Type IV hyperlipoproteinemia. Elevated triglycerides also occur in patients with hypothyroidism (see below). On day 17 of this patient's stay in the NRU, his triglycerides concentration increased dramatically during an episode of diabetic hyperglycemia that precipitated the mobilization and breakdown of adipose tissue triglycerides to fatty acids as a cellular source of energy in the absence of glucose.

Markedly increased serum ALP, ALT, AST, GGT, and LD values: The increased levels of liver tissue-specific (*ALT, AST*, and *GGT*) and nonspecific (*ALP* and *LD*) enzymes are typical of acute hepatic injury, which could have been sustained by the patient as a result of the MVA. The activity of ALT is much higher than AST and therefore, the AST/ALT ratio <1.0, indicating a possible inflammatory condition of the liver (eg, acute viral hepatitis). However, the patient's total protein and albumin concentrations were within reference interval limits, suggesting normal hepatic synthetic function. Additionally, hepatocytic excretory function was normal because the total and direct bilirubin values were within normal reference limits for these analytes. Lastly, evidence of the patient's liver recovering from acute liver injury was provided by the marked decrease in ALT and AST values over a 2.5-week period in the NRU (**Figure 1**).

Markedly decreased serum FT4, TT3, TSH, LH, total testosterone, ACTH, cortisol, and ADH values: Massive hemorrhage in the area of the hypothalamus and pituitary stalk made it likely that the hormones associated with the hypothalamic-pituitary-thyroid (HPT) and -adrenal (HPA) axes were affected. The hypothalamic-pituitary portion of these axes constitute a group of structures (eg, hypothalamus, anterior, and posterior pituitary glands) with a complex interrelationship that utilizes negative feedback control mechanisms to maintain normal homeostasis of the analytes whose plasma concentration is governed by the hormones produced within these structures [**Figure 2**]. Loss of function by any of the components of these axes will lead to insufficiency of 1 or more hormones or analytes produced by a target organ. By examining which values are decreased and which are elevated, it can be determined which component of the axis has been affected. Protein hormones synthesized in the adenohypophysis (anterior pituitary gland) include TSH, LH, follicle stimulating hormone (FSH), ACTH, growth hormone, β-endorphin, and prolactin. Thus, damage to both the hypothalamus and pituitary glands would be expected to have a profound downstream effect on the target tissues and organs of the hormones produced by these glands. For example, a decrease in the availability of the hypothalamic hormones, thyrotropin-releasing hormone (TRH), corticotrophin-releasing hormone (CRH), and gonadotropin-releasing hormone (GnRH), would lead to decreased production and release of *TSH, ACTH, LH*, and *FSH* from the anterior pituitary and decreased production and release of *T4* and *T3* by the thyroid gland, *cortisol* by the adrenal cortex, and *testosterone* by Leydig cells of the testes. Although decreased T4 (and free T4) and T3 values are typical of patients with primary hypothyroidism, such patients, with a normal functioning HPT axis, would be expected to have an increased TSH concentration as the hypothalamus and anterior pituitary glands responded to low free T4 and T3 concentrations by producing and secreting more TRH and TSH, respectively. The undetectable TSH value in our patient's serum suggests secondary hypothyroidism due to pituitary loss or tertiary hypothyroidism due to hypothalamic damage. Similarly, although a decreased testosterone concentration is consistent with primary hypogonadism, such patients, with normal functioning hypothalamus and pituitary glands, would be expected to have an increased LH concentration. The profoundly decreased total testosterone concentration in our patient suggests either secondary hypogonadism due to pituitary damage or tertiary hypogonadism due to loss of hypothalamic function. Lastly, although a decreased cortisol concentration may indicate primary hypoadrenalism, such a decrease should trigger increased release of CRH from the hypothalamus, increased release of ACTH from the anterior pituitary, and increased production and secretion of cortisol by the adrenal cortex in an effort to restore the cortisol level to normal. Because our patient's plasma ACTH was undetectable, this finding suggests a loss of pituitary and/or hypothalamic function. Potential causes of decreased pituitary hormones include primary and secondary hypopituitarism. Destruction of the anterior pituitary, either by an adenoma or by trauma, is a primary cause of decreased pituitary hormone concentrations as many of these hormones are synthesized by cells of the adenohypophysis. Secondary hypopituitarism is caused by damage to the hypothalamus, particularly the arcuate and periventricular regions, which contain parvocellular neurons that stimulate production of TRH, CRH, and GnRH. Shearing of the delicate blood vessels in the pituitary stalk that transport these hormones to the anterior pituitary will also lead to hypopituitarism. With the severe head trauma suffered by this patient, and the visualization of hemorrhage below and including the hypothalamus on the initial head CT, it is highly likely that damage to the hypothalamus, pituitary stalk, and anterior pituitary gland all played a role in the hypopituitarism demonstrated by this patient.

Increased serum sodium concentration and osmolal gap: Hypernatremia has a myriad of causes; however, the combination of grossly lipemic serum, hyperlipidemia, and an osmolal gap >10, suggests that decreased serum water content is the most likely cause. Moreover, this patient's markedly decreased ADH (or vasopressin) concentration is consistent with this suggestion. Magnocellular neurons in the supraoptic and paraventricular regions of the hypothalamus synthesize ADH (and oxytocin) and transport these substances down axons in the pituitary stalk to the neurohypophysis (posterior pituitary gland). Here ADH is stored in cells or directly released into capillaries when the hypothalamus receives signals from the blood or higher brain centers indicating a need for water retention. Anti-diuretic hormone acts on the cells of the distal convoluted tubule of the kidney to decrease urine volume. If ADH concentration is low, urine volume increases, and sodium levels in the blood rise due to hemoconcentration resulting from the increased loss of plasma water in the urine. Clinically, reduced production of ADH is referred to as diabetes insipidus, a disorder that includes symptoms of polyuria, polydipsia, and hypernatremia.

3. Diabetes mellitus, diabetes insipidus, and panhypopituitarism.

4. In the short term, no additional laboratory tests are needed because all of the patient's laboratory findings could be explained as a consequence of the head trauma and other injuries sustained by the patient during the MVA. After successful recovery and convalescence from his injuries, if a fasting glucose was still elevated (ie, >126 mg/dL) and/or hypopituitarism was still present, additional laboratory tests would include a serum insulin level to determine whether or not he had type 1 (insulin-dependent) or type 2 (noninsulin-dependent) DM. Also, various stimulation tests (eg, ACTH, insulin, or metyrapone stimulation tests), in conjunction with serum aldosterone determinations, could be used to distinguish between primary and secondary (ie, resulting from pituitary or hypothalamic dysfunction) adrenal insufficiency.

5. ***Most likely diagnosis:*** idiopathic DM and
panhypopituitarism caused by injury to the
hypothalamus and pituitary glands from head
trauma sustained during a MVA. In patients
with confirmed type 1 diabetes, therapy would
include conformity with a diet meeting the
guidelines of the American Diabetes Association
and insulin injection. Treatment modalities for
thyroid hormone, cortisol, testosterone, and
ADH deficiencies would include oral thyroxine,
hydrocortisone (dexamethasone injection if
the patient was unable to take oral cortisone),
testosterone patch, and DDAVP nasal spray,
respectively.

Pseudohyponatremia in a Myeloma Patient: Direct Electrode Potentiometry Is a Method Worth its Salt

Andrew W. Lyon, Leland B. Baskin

Department of Pathology and Laboratory Medicine, University of Calgary and Calgary Laboratory Services, Calgary, Alberta, Canada

Patient: 49-year-old Caucasian male.

Chief Complaint: He presented to our cancer clinic complaining of malaise, tiredness, and bone pain.

Prior Medical History: The patient had a 4-year history of progressive multiple myeloma (IgG-lambda immunophenotype) with gradually increasing bone pain that was refractory to high dose chemotherapy and autologous stem cell transplantation. He had been treated recently with morphine, a bisphosphonate (pamidronate disodium), and radiation to the shoulders. During his recent visit, he received 2 units of packed red blood cells and 40 grams of intravenous immune globulin.

Recent Drug History: Morphine sulfate [MS Contin®], 220 mg bid; testosterone enanthate (Delatestryl®, to boost energy), 300 mg intramuscularly; pamidronate disodium, 90 mg intravenously; dexamethasone, 4 mg bid.

Results of Additional Diagnostic Procedure and Laboratory Tests: At the request of the laboratory director, the initial electrolyte measurements (sodium, potassium, and chloride) by an indirect ion-specific electrode (ISE) method were repeated using an alternate method/instrument (direct potentiometry/blood gas analyzer) [**T2**].

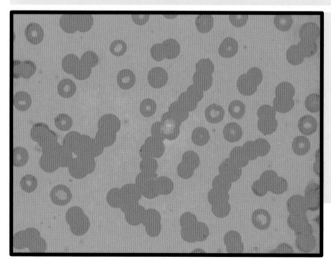

Image 1_Rouleaux in a stained peripheral blood smear from our patient with multiple myeloma. The background is a consequence of the markedly increased protein concentration in this patient's serum.

Pseudohyponatremia in a Myeloma Patient: Direct Electrode Potentiometry Is a Method Worth its Salt

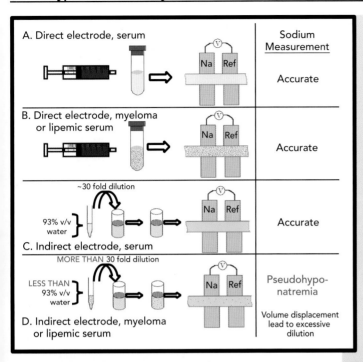

A. Direct electrode, serum — Sodium Measurement — Accurate

B. Direct electrode, myeloma or lipemic serum — Accurate

~30 fold dilution
93% v/v water
C. Indirect electrode, serum — Accurate

MORE THAN 30 fold dilution
LESS THAN 93% v/v water
D. Indirect electrode, myeloma or lipemic serum — Pseudohypo-natremia — Volume displacement lead to excessive dilution

Figure 1_Schematic view of indirect and direct sodium electrodes depicting the susceptibility of serum samples from myeloma patients or lipemic serum samples to pseudohyponatremia when sodium is quantified by indirect electrode methods. The potentiometric measurement of sodium by direct electrode methods occurs on undiluted specimens (directly) using either anticoagulated whole blood, plasma, or serum, and the accuracy of these methods is not influenced by the "volume exclusion effect" (Panels **A** and **B**). Indirect electrode methods require an approximately 30-fold dilution of the specimen prior to the potentiometric measurement of sodium by an ion selective electrode, which renders sodium values by this method susceptible to a dilution error commonly referred to as pseudohyponatremia (Panels **C** and **D**).[6]

T1. Principal Laboratory Findings

Test	Patient's Result	"Normal" Reference Interval
Hematology		
WBC count	4.1	$4.0\text{-}11.0 \times 10^3/\text{mL}$
Neutrophils	2.2	$2.0\text{-}8.0 \times 10^3/\text{mL}$
Bands	0.1	$0.0\text{-}1.3 \times 10^3/\text{mL}$
Lymphocytes	0.7	$0.7\text{-}3.5 \times 10^3/\text{mL}$
Monocytes	1.1	$0.0\text{-}1.0 \times 10^3/\text{mL}$
Eosinophils	0.0	$0.0\text{-}0.7 \times 10^3/\text{mL}$
Polychromasia	1+	Negative
Rouleaux	3+	Negative
Nucleated RBCs/100 WBCs	1	0
Hemoglobin	8.6	13.7-18.0 g/dL
Hematocrit	25	40-54%
RBC count	2.4	$4.5\text{-}6.0 \times 10^6/\text{mL}$
MCV	102	82-100 fL
MCHC	34.6	32.0-36.0 g/dL
Platelet count	181,000	150,000-400,000/mL

T1. Principal Laboratory Findings

Chemistry		
Sodium	128	133-145 mmol/L
Potassium	4.4	3.5-5.0 mmol/L
Chloride	95	98-111 mmol/L
CO_2	28	21-31 mmol/L
Anion gap*	5	7-16 mmol/L
Creatinine	1.3	0.7-1.4 mg/dL
Calcium	10.9	8.4-10.2 mg/dL
Triglycerides	60	55- 327 mg/dL
Total protein†	17.1	6.3-8.0 g/dL

*Anion gap = [sodium] – [chloride + CO_2].
†Using a diluted serum sample and correcting the result for the dilution factor. WBC, white blood cell; RBC, red blood cell; MCV, mean corpuscular volume; MCHC, mean corpuscular hemoglobin concentration

T2. Repeat Electrolyte Results by Direct Potentiometry Method

Test	Patient's Result, mmol/L
Sodium	137
Potassium	4.8
Chloride	99
Anion gap*	10

*Calculated using the equation and CO_2 value from **T1**.

Questions

1. What (is)are this patient's most striking laboratory result(s)?

2. How do you explain this patient's most striking laboratory result(s)?

3. Which additional test(s) should be performed? Why?

4. What is the most likely cause of the disparity between sodium values by indirect ISE versus direct potentiometry methods?

5. What is the most appropriate treatment for this patient and the most appropriate actions for the laboratory?

Possible Answers

1. Markedly elevated serum total protein, hyponatremia, hypochloremia, Rouleaux formation (3+), and macrocytic anemia (increased MCV and decreased hemoglobin, hematocrit, and RBC count) with polychromasia and the presence of nucleated red blood cells (1 NRBC/100 WBCs) [**Image 1**].

2. The markedly elevated serum total protein concentration was caused by unregulated synthesis of a monoclonal immunoglobulin as occurs typically in patients with a plasma cell dyscrasia such as multiple myeloma or Waldenström macroglobulinemia. The patient was known to have multiple myeloma and an IgG-lambda monoclonal serum component. The patient's hyponatremia and hypochloremia were not clinically anticipated. Rouleaux formation, the linear alignment of at least 4 RBCs in a thin area of a blood smear resembling a stack of coins, is caused by changes in the surface charge of the erythrocyte membrane when this membrane is coated with excessive amounts of protein such as globulins and fibrinogen. Other causes of Rouleaux formation include plasma expanders (dextran and hydroxyethyl starch) and radiographic contrast materials. The most common cause of Rouleaux formation, however, is paraproteinemia due to a monoclonal gammopathy. Rouleaux formation

often increases the erythrocyte sedimentation rate as well. Moreover, hyperproteinemia may cause RBC aggregation leading to a spuriously high mean corpuscular volume (MCV). Another mechanism for an increased MCV in neoplastic diseases such as multiple myeloma is folate deficiency caused by increased folate utilization by the neoplasm leading to a macrocytic anemia. Elevated protein concentration may expand the plasma volume and displace some of the RBCs, thereby reducing the hemoglobin concentration disproportionately to the total RBC mass and exaggerating the anemia. It also may render a bluish background to a stained peripheral blood smear as in this case [**Image 1**].[1-5] Accelerated bone marrow release of reticulocytes in response to the marked anemia is the most likely explanation of the macrocytosis, polychromasia, and nucleated RBCs observed on this patient's stained peripheral blood smear.[1-2]

3. Repeat sodium and chloride testing using an alternate method/instrument. Our patient's decreased sodium, chloride, and anion gap results, in conjunction with a markedly elevated serum total protein value, were brought to the attention of the laboratory director. We considered the possibility that protein precipitation during the quantitative measurement of total protein in our patient's serum sample may have resulted in a falsely increased total protein value; however, our patient was not prone to cryoglobulinemia and the total protein result was obtained using a diluted specimen. Once the serum total protein result was considered valid, we suspected that the sodium and chloride values might be falsely decreased due to protein interference with the indirect ISE method used in our chemistry analyzer (Hitachi 917, Roche Diagnostics , Indianapolis, IN). Therefore, sodium and chloride (and potassium) testing on our patient's serum sample was repeated using the direct potentiometry method in a blood gas analyzer (ABL 725, Radiometer America, Westlake, OH) with the results shown in **T2**.

4. The "volume exclusion effect" that occurs in sera with high protein concentrations. The initial low sodium concentration in our patient's serum sample by an indirect electrode method that corrected to a value within the reference range for sodium when this sample was re-tested for

sodium using a direct electrode method is indicative of *pseudohyponatremia*. Pseudohyponatremia is associated with the "volume exclusion effect" that occurs in lipemic serum samples and in sera with high concentrations of protein when these sera are assayed for sodium concentration using indirect electrode methods.[6] Direct and indirect ion-specific electrodes are both widely used in clinical laboratory instrumentation. As the name suggests, a direct ion-specific electrode method detects the activity of a specific ion in an undiluted specimen (ie, the specimen is analyzed "directly" with no intermediate specimen dilution step). Indirect ion-specific electrodes measure the activity of specific ions in a specimen following dilution of the specimen with a diluent of fixed composition [**Figure 1**]. The advantages and disadvantages of each design have been reviewed elsewhere.[6] The typical water content of plasma is approximately 93% and indirect electrode methods for quantifying electrolyte concentrations assume that this proportion is constant. When plasma contains large concentrations of lipid or paraprotein, these extra components occupy volume and displace water, so that plasma contains less water per unit volume and less electrolytes per unit volume. Automated instruments with indirect electrodes pipette aliquots of plasma (eg, 10 μL of plasma contains 9.3 μL water) and add diluent (eg, 300 μL buffer) before determining the electrolyte concentration with an ion selective electrode. Lipemia and hyperproteinemia cause predictable decreases in the amount of water per unit volume of plasma (W_p) which can be estimated using Waugh's empirical equation [values for serum total protein concentrations (P_s) and serum triglyceride concentration (L_s) below were taken from **T2**][7]:

$$W_p \, (g/dL) = 99.1 - 0.73 \times P_s \, (g/dL) - 1.03 \times L_s \, (g/dL)$$

$$= 99.1 - 0.73 \times 17.1 - 1.03 \times 0.06$$

$$= 99.1 - 12.5 - 0.06$$

$$= 86.6 \, (or \sim 87\%; \% = g/100 \, mL = g/dL)$$

Therefore, the decrease in plasma water content = 100 - 86.6 = 13.4%.

Thus, a 10 μL aliquot of our patient's plasma contains 8.7 μL (ie, 87% of 10 μL) of water

and the addition of a fixed volume of diluent (eg, 300 μL) will cause excess dilution (overdilution) of the water-phase of the aliquot and falsely low concentrations of electrolytes. Moreover, this effect will be directly proportional to the volume of water displaced by the lipid or paraprotein. Therefore, our patient's expected sodium concentration by an indirect electrode method can be estimated as follows:

$$\frac{8.7 \, mL}{9.3 \, mL} \times 137 \, mmol/L \, Na^+_{Direct \, Electrode} = 128 \, mmol/L \, Na^+_{Indirect \, Electrode}$$

Our patient's observed Na^+ concentration by an indirect electrode method was 128 mmol/L [**T1**].

Moreover, blood specimens from patients with multiple myeloma are prone to generating erroneous laboratory results through a variety of other mechanisms, including turbidity from precipitation of the paraprotein in cuvettes during the analysis, inaccurate pipetting due to the high viscosity of serum samples from patients with myeloma, and the inactivation of reagents by binding to the paraprotein. Monoclonal protein precipitates are responsible for the most obvious forms of cryoglobulins (type I and type II) that can erroneously lower measured values for the serum total protein concentration by creating flocculent precipitates that cause turbidity and optically interfere with many methods. Numerous examples of such interference have appeared as case reports and reviews, and monoclonal IgM is often responsible.[8-17] Due to the intermittent nature of the interference and the frequent reformulation of reagents by manufacturers, this type of laboratory error is difficult to anticipate, but it can be recognized within the laboratory by alert staff and brought to the attention of clinical colleagues to avoid misinterpretation. Some of the laboratory tests prone to interference by hyperparaproteinemia include: albumin, creatinine (Jaffe method), C-reactive protein, hemoglobin, MCH, MCHC, inorganic phosphate, thyroxine, urea nitrogen, uric acid, and sodium.

5. The patient should not be treated for hyponatremia. It is difficult for laboratory professionals to identify potentially erroneous laboratory test results due to hyperproteinemia; however, when marked hyperproteinemia is observed

on any serum specimen, the results of the tests identified above should be reviewed and electrolyte measurements repeated by a direct ISE method. Moreover, when pseudohyponatremia is confirmed, it is prudent to alert clinicians of this finding by providing this information on the laboratory report. Laboratories that serve cancer treatment clinics with large numbers of multiple myeloma patients may consider conducting all electrolyte tests on instruments with direct electrodes to avoid the repetitive uncertainty in the validity of the results.

Treatment and Course

The patient received 2 units of packed red cells and 40 grams of intravenous immune globulin. The laboratory report contained an interpretive comment about the likelihood of pseudohyponatremia, along with the serum sodium result from the direct electrode method. Treatment for hyponatremia was not initiated. The patient returned to the clinic 4 weeks later with hyperproteinemia, Rouleaux, and persistent pseudohyponatremia. "Any man is liable to err, only a fool persists in error." Marcus Tullius Cicero (106-43 B.C.), Roman orator.

Keywords

pseudohyponatremia, ion-specific electrode, multiple myeloma, hyperproteinemia, paraproteinemia

References

1. Williams WJ, Beutler E, Erslev AJ, Lichtman MA. *Hematology*, 4th ed. New York: McGraw-Hill Publishing. 1990:307-309, 1588.

2. Morris MW, Davey FR. Chapter 24: Basic examination of blood. Henry JB. *Clinical Diagnosis and Management by Laboratory Methods*. 19th ed. Philadelphia: WB Saunders. 1996:581-582.

3. Henry JB, Beadling WV. Chapter 30: Immunohematology. Henry JB. *Clinical Diagnosis and Management by Laboratory Methods*. 19th ed. Philadelphia: WB Saunders. 1996:777.

4. Pincus MR, Preuss HG, Henry JB. Chapter 7: Evaluation of renal function, water, electrolytes, acid-base balance, and blood gases. Henry JB. *Clinical Diagnosis and Management by Laboratory Methods*. 19th ed. Philadelphia: WB Saunders. 1996:139-161.

5. CAP Surveys Manual. Section 2: *Hematology, coagulation, clinical microscopy*. Chicago, IL, 1994:44.

6. Scott MG, Heusel JW, LeGrys VA, et al. Chapter 31: Electrolytes and blood gases. Burtis CA, Ashwood EA, eds. *Tietz Textbook of Clinical Chemistry*. 3rd ed. Philadelphia: WB Saunders. 1999:1061-1063.

7. Waugh, WH. Utility of expressing serum sodium per unit of water in assessing hyponatremia. *Metabolism*. 1969;18:706-712.

8. Reed RG. Interference by an IgM paraprotein in the bromcresol green method for determination of serum albumin. *Clin Chem*. 1987;33:1075-1076.

9. Datta P, Graham GA, Schoen I. Interference by IgG paraproteins in the Jaffe method for creatinine determination. *Am J Clin Pathol*. 1986;85:463-468.

10. Yu, A. Pira U. False increase in serum C-reactive protein caused by monoclonal IgM-lambda : A case report. *Clin Chem Lab Med*. 2001;39:983-987.

11. Linz LJ. Elevation of hemoglobin, MCH, MCHC by paraprotein: How to recognize and correct the interference. *Clin Lab Sci*. 1994;7:211-212.

12. Zaman Z, Sneyers L, Van Orshoven A, et al. Elimination of paraprotein interference in determination of plasma inorganic phosphate by ammonium molybdate method. *Clin Chem*. 1995;41:609-614.

13. Larner AJ. Pseudohyperphosphatemia. *Clin Biochem*. 1995;28:391-393.

14. Alexander NM, Gattra R, Nashimoto M. Myeloma immunoglobulin interferes with serum thyroxine analysis by homogeneous enzyme immunoassay. *Clin Chim Acta*. 1980;100:301-305.

15. Pierce GF, Garrett NC, Koenig J, et al. Interference by monoclonal proteins in the o-phthalaldehyde method for blood urea nitrogen. *Clin Chim Acta*. 1986;154:233-236.

16. Langman LJ, Allen LC, Romaschin AD. Interference of IgM paraproteins in the Olympus AU800 urine acid assay. *Clin Biochem*. 1998;31:517-521.

17. Kroll MH, Elin RJ. Interference with clinical laboratory analyses. *Clin Chem*. 1994;40:1996-2005.

Shortness of Breath in a 74-Year-Old Woman

Sean M. Hussey, Frank H. Wians, Jr.

Department of Pathology, University of Texas Southwestern Medical Center, Dallas, TX

Patient: 74-year-old Caucasian woman.

Chief Complaint: Progressive increase in episodic shortness of breath for the past 2 weeks.

History of Present Illness: The patient had been in her normal state of health until 2 weeks ago when she noticed that she had difficulty catching her breath while walking. She was used to walking 2 miles without difficulty, but was now becoming short of breath after just 100 yards. The symptoms were progressing and over the past 3 days the patient stated that she was short of breath lying down. She had always slept with only 1 pillow, but was now requiring 2 pillows. The patient also reported an 8 to 10 pound weight gain over the past 6 weeks.

Past Medical History: Moderately controlled hypertension for the past 50 years.

Past Surgical History: Benign parotid gland tumor removed in 1963.

Drug History: Diovan HCT, once a day; aspirin, 325 mg tablet, prn.

Family/Social History: The patient's father died at age 56 from a heart attack secondary to coronary artery disease. Her mother died at age 77 secondary to colon cancer. Her brother died at age 49 from an unknown cancer, and her sister died at age 68 from acute renal failure secondary to diabetes mellitus. The patient has 4 children, all of whom are alive and healthy. She had no history of smoking, alcohol abuse, or blood transfusion.

Physical Examination: Vital signs: temperature, 35.8°C; heart rate, 82 beats per minute; respiratory rate, 18 breaths per minute; blood pressure, 157/64 mm Hg. The patient was well-nourished and in no acute respiratory distress (oxygen saturation of 95% on room air). Her current weight was 126 pounds. The patient's physical exam was normal with clear respiratory sounds and no lower extremity edema.

Results of Additional Diagnostic Procedures and Tests: A chest X-ray revealed bilateral pleural effusions. An electrocardiogram showed normal sinus rhythm. A transthoracic echocardiogram revealed a dilated left atrium, an increase in right-sided filling pressure, and mild to moderate mitral regurgitation. The left ventricular ejection fraction (LVEF) was within normal limits.

T1. Principal Laboratory Findings

Test	Patient's Result	"Normal" Reference Range
Hematology		
WBC count	9.7	$4.1-11.1 \times 10^3$/mL
RBC count	4.19	$4.01-5.31 \times 10^3$/mL
Hemoglobin	12.0	12.1-16.1 g/dL
Hematocrit	38.3	36.8-48.7%
Platelet count	244	$174-404 \times 10^3$/mL
Differential:		
Neutrophils	62	35-80%
Lymphocytes	33	20-50%
Monocytes	4	2-12%
Eosinophils	1	0-7%
Basophils	0	0-2%
Coagulation		
PT	10.3	9.8-11.9 sec
INR	0.9	
PTT	31.8	23.0-32.5 sec
D-Dimer	0.7	0-3 mg/L
Chemistry		
Sodium	136	135-145 mEq/L
Potassium	3.6	3.6-4.0 mEq/L
Chloride	101	98-109 mEq/L
CO_2	25	22-31 mEq/L
BUN	11	7-21 mg/dL
Creatinine	0.5	0.6-1.2 mg/dL
AS	34	13-40 U/L
AL	28	10-40 U/L
Total protein	7.1	6.3-8.2 g/dL
Albumin	4.2	3.5-5.2 g/dL
Total bilirubin	0.7	0.2-1.3 mg/dL
Direct bilirubin	0.1	0.0-0.3 mg/dL
BNP	827	<100 pg/mL*

*A BNP value <100 pg/mL is generally not consistent with a diagnosis of decompensated heart failure; a BNP value >400 pg/mL is often seen in patients with advanced or decompensated heart failure due to left ventricular systolic or diastolic dysfunction; a BNP value between 100 pg/mL and 400 pg/mL may be difficult to interpret in patients with concomitant diseases that can affect BNP levels, such as COPD and PE; and, BNP results must always be evaluated in concert with other patient-specific clinical and laboratory findings.

WBC, white blood cell; RBC, red blood cell; P, prothrombin time; INR, International Normalized Ratio; P, partial thromboplastin time; BUN, blood urea nitrogen; AS, aspartate aminotransferase; AL, alanine aminotransferase; BNP, B-type natriuretic peptide.

T2. Characteristics of Pleural Fluid

PF Characteristic	Transudate	Exudates
Protein, g/dL	<3	
LD, U/L	<200	>200
Glucose, mg/dL	>60	
WBC count/mm^3	<1,000	
Cholesterol, mg/dL	<45	>45
[Protein]$_{PF}$:[Protein]$_S$	<0.5	>0.5
[LD]$_{PF}$:[LD]$_S$	<0.6	>0.6
[Glucose]$_{PF}$:[Glucose]$_S$	1.0	
Associated diseases	Biventricular HF with venous HF Nephrotic syndrome Peritoneal dialysis Atelectasis Urinothorax	Pneumonia Lung abscess Pancreatitis Pancreatic pseudocyst TB Actinomycosis Pleurisy Asbestosis Malignant mesothelioma Lymphoma Meigs syndrome* Lung cancer Pneumothorax

*Triad of benign fibroma (or other ovarian tumors) with ascites and large pleural effusions. PF, pleural fluid; LD, lactate dehydrogenase; WBC, white blood cell; S, serum; HF, heart failure; HTN, hypertension; TB, tuberculosis.

T3. Diagnostic Performance of BNP as a Screening Test for Heart Failure*

Diagnostic Parameter	Type of Patient Population	
	General	Symptomatic PC
Sensitivity	76[a]	97[b]
Specificity	87[a]	84[b]
PPV	16	70
NPV	98	98

*Modified from Reference #8. [a]At a BNP cutoff value of 17.9 pg/mL. [b]At a BNP cutoff value of 76.8 pg/mL. BNP, B-type natriuretic peptide; PC, primary care; PPV, positive predictive value; NPV, negative predictive value.

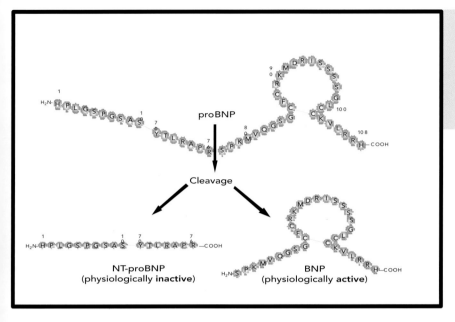

Figure 1_Formation of BNP (32 amino acids) and NT-proBNP (76 amino acids) from cleavage of the proBNP (108 amino acids) precursor molecule.

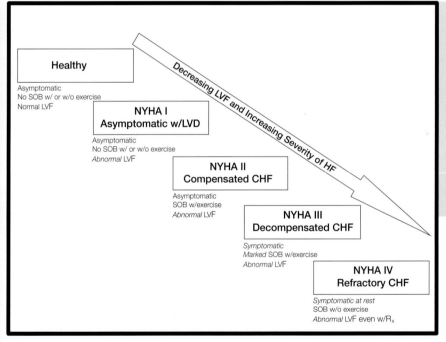

Figure 2_The evolution of the clinical stages of congestive heart failure (CHF) according to the classification scheme developed by the New York Heart Association (NYHA). SOB, shortness of breath; LVD, left ventricular dysfunction; LVF, left ventricular function; Rx, therapy.

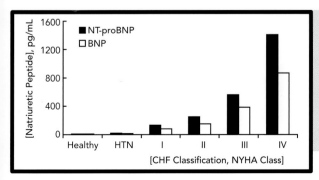

Figure 3_Relative concentrations of BNP and N-terminal pro-BNP (NT-proBNP) in healthy patients, patients with hyptertension (HTN), or congestive heart failure (CHF) of variable severity (Class I, least severe to Class IV, most severe) according to the CHF classification scheme developed by the New York Heart Association (NYHA)

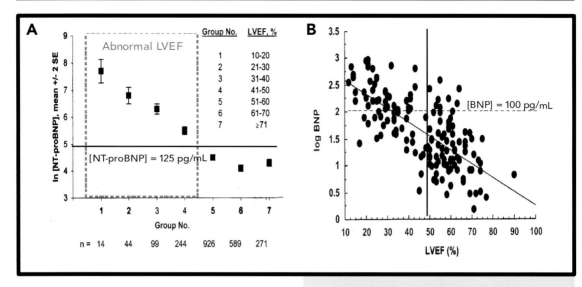

Figure 4_A Inverse relationship between NT-proBNP and left ventricular injection fraction (LVEF) (modified from Reference 3; solid line corresponds to an NT-proBNP concentration of 125 pg/ml; dotted lines encompass patient groups with an abnormal LVEF (ie, <50%). **B** Inverse relationship between BNP concentration and LVEF (modified from Reference 4; solid line corresponds to an LVEF of 50%; dotted line corresponds to a BNP concentration of 100 pg/mL). Note that some patients with an abnormal LVEF (ie, <50%) have a BNP concentration less than a cutoff value of 100 pg/ml.

Questions

1. What is (are) this patient's most striking clinical and laboratory result(s)?

2. How do you explain the patient's most striking clinical and laboratory result(s)?

3. What condition(s) does this patient's laboratory and other findings suggest?

4. What is the pathophysiology of this patient's disease?

5. What are the clinical manifestations of this patient's disease?

6. What is the prognosis for this patient?

7. What is the most appropriate treatment for this patient?

Possible Answers

1. A progressive dyspnea on exertion (the patient was unable to walk 100 yards without getting short of breath); orthopnea; a chest X-ray with bilateral pleural effusions; an increased right-sided filling pressure on echocardiogram; and a markedly increased EDTA-plasma B-type natriuretic peptide (BNP) level.

2. Dyspnea on exertion. The causes of shortness of breath during physical exertion include: 1) pulmonary disease [eg, malignancy, asthma, chronic obstructive pulmonary disease (COPD), pulmonary embolus (PE)]; 2) cardiac disease [eg, congestive heart failure (CHF), mitral valve prolapse]; 3) deformity of the chest wall; and 4) diseases associated with weakness of the respiratory muscles. **Orthopnea.** Orthopnea, or shortness of breath while lying down that is relieved with elevating the head, is most often secondary to left ventricular cardiac failure. Other etiologies include pulmonary congestion, asthma, COPD, pulmonary infection, chronic cough, obesity, and abdominal distension. **Pleural effusions on X-ray.** The differential diagnosis of a pleural effusion is extensive; however, thoracentesis to obtain pleural fluid and analysis of the fluid for certain constituents allows the fluid to be categorized as a transudate or an exudate [**T2**]. Transudates occur when there is an imbalance between hydrostatic and

oncotic pressures (eg, in patients with heart failure in whom the hydrostatic pressure of the fluid in the peritoneal tissue becomes higher than the oncotic pressure of the fluid in the pleural space causing the movement of fluid from the peritoneum into the pleural space), while exudates are defined by the presence of at least 1 of the following criteria: 1) [protein]$_{pleural\ fluid}$:[protein]$_{serum}$ ratio > 0.5; 2) [LD]$_{pleural\ fluid}$:[LD]$_{serum}$ ratio > 0.6; 3) [LD]$_{pleural\ fluid}$ >200 U/L.[1] The classification of a pleural fluid as a transudate or exudate can be useful in suggesting additional testing for differentiating between various diagnoses. In the case of this patient, the effusions were too small to warrant a thoracentesis. Therefore, the differential diagnosis must include conditions associated potentially with either a transudative or an exudative pleural fluid, including CHF, liver cirrhosis, nephrotic syndrome, infection (bacterial, viral, mycobacterial), drug-induced (the most common being treatment with amiodarone or nitrofurantoin), sarcoidosis, systemic lupus erythematosis (SLE), rheumatoid arthritis, pancreatitis, and PE. **Elevated BNP.** B-type (or brain, the tissue in which it was first discovered) natriuretic peptide (BNP) is a small protein (32 amino acids) produced following the cleavage of a larger precursor protein (proBNP) that yields the physiologically inactive N-terminal proBNP molecule (NT-proBNP) and the physiologically active hormone, BNP [**Figure 1**]. The family of natriuretic peptides includes atrial natriuretic peptide (ANP), BNP, and C-type natriuretic peptide (CNP), all of which are involved in the regulation of blood pressure and fluid homeostasis.[2] The basic functions of the natriuretic peptide hormones are: natriuresis, diuresis, and vasodilation. Among the natriuretic peptides however, BNP has been shown to be the most stable to degradation, and the most diagnostically specific for identifying patients with CHF and abnormal left ventricular function.[3,4] The right ventricle of the heart pumps blood directly to the lungs against a much lower resistance to blood flow compared to the left ventricle which must pump blood to all other parts of the body against a much greater resistance to blood flow. Thus, patients with CHF can have abnormal left ventricular function or mitral regurgitation [ie, failure of the mitral (or bicuspid) valve to prevent blood from flowing back into the left atrium from the left ventricle]. The principal

hemodynamic measure of left ventricular function is the left ventricular ejection fraction (LVEF). The LVEF is determined by M-mode or 2D echocardiography and a normal functioning left ventricle ejects through the aorta >50% of its end diastolic blood volume. Both BNP and NT-proBNP are elevated in patients with signs and symptoms of HF and abnormal left ventricular function (LVF) [**Figure 2** and **Figure 3**] or LVEF [**Figure 4A** and **Figure 4B**] according to the scheme for evaluating the severity of CHF developed by the New York Heart Association (NYHA).[3-5] However, mitral regurgitation, trauma, abdominal or thoracic surgery, subarachnoid hemorrhage, certain brain disorders, and diabetic nephropathy have all been shown to raise natriuretic peptide levels.[6] Moreover, elevated BNP levels (>80 pg/mL) in patients with an acute coronary syndrome are associated with a higher incidence of death, new or progressive CHF, and new or recurrent myocardial infarction.[7] Our patient had a normal LVEF, but mild to moderate mitral regurgitation, thus accounting for her markedly elevated EDTA-plasma BNP level. The diagnostic accuracy of BNP as a screening test for CHF depends on the nature of the population being screened. As expected, the diagnostic accuracy (ie, sensitivity and specificity) of BNP in identifying patients with heart failure or LV systolic dysfunction is higher in symptomatic primary care patients than in individuals selected from a cross-section of a community or general population [**T3**].[8]

3. ***Most likely diagnosis:*** *congestive heart failure (CHF).* The constellation of our patient's clinical and laboratory findings, including dyspnea on exertion, orthopnea, bilateral pleural effusions, increased right-sided cardiac filling pressure, mild to moderate mitral regurgitation, and an elevated plasma BNP level makes CHF the most likely diagnosis.

4. **Pathophysiology of CHF.** Congestive heart failure is the result of an alteration of Starling forces in the cardiac contractile myocytes. This alteration is most often related to an index event. That event could be acute, as occurs with an acute myocardial infarction, or chronic, such as long-standing hypertension or mitral valve disease. The patient had both chronic hypertension and mitral regurgitation. With

mitral valve insufficiency, increased loading conditions (ie, increased blood requirements by the tissues brought on by increased exercise resulting in a higher heart rate as the heart works harder to keep up with the demand for blood) lead to abnormal chemical signals being sent to the cardiac myocytes and fibroblasts that cause myocyte hypertrophy and an increase in collagen deposition in the heart wall, a process known as "remodeling."[9] Myocytes elongate eccentrically and consequently the cardiac chamber dilates. This leads to alterations in the anatomical relationship between the papillary heart muscles and the valve leaflets, which worsens both the valve abnormality and volume overload (dilation) of the heart chambers. Over time, the chamber dilation exceeds the myocyte hypertrophy and leads to increased cardiac wall tension and systolic dysfunction. Long-standing hypertension, on the other hand, results as an increase in the cross-sectional thickness of individual myocytes. Thus, CHF occurs when the heart is incapable of maintaining a cardiac output sufficient to accommodate metabolic requirements for oxygenated blood. When this occurs, heart rate, pulse rate, blood pressure, and the release of natriuretic peptides increase to compensate for these changes. Over time, however, these mechanisms may fail to relieve the stress on the heart and when this occurs, decompensated CHF of variable severity results in a medical emergency requiring prompt medical intervention. The severity of CHF is gauged typically using the classification scheme developed by the New York Heart Association (NYHA) [**Figure 2**].

5. **Clinical manifestations of CHF**. Congestive heart failure can manifest itself clinically by a number of non-specific symptoms including fatigue, decreased appetite, and increased heart rate. The principal clinical hallmarks of CHF include pulmonary and peripheral edema from sodium and water retention. In addition, because of the inadequate supply of blood to perfuse all vital organs, blood is shunted away from the periphery to compensate for this deficiency. The decreased blood flow to the muscles and limbs leads to fatigue and peripheral edema. Moreover, the stomach also receives less blood, which can lead to digestive problems. Symptoms more specific for cardiac disease that are frequently seen in patients with CHF are shortness of breath, peripheral edema (most often in the lower extremities), wheezing, and persistent cough. As heart muscle function declines in patients with CHF, pulmonary pressures increase, ultimately progressing to fluid accumulating in the air spaces (alveoli) of the lung. Once this happens, breathlessness, cough, and wheezing soon follow. Eventually, right-sided heart failure develops followed by leakage of fluid into the peripheral soft tissues. In addition, decreased renal function secondary to the lack of adequate renal blood perfusion leads to sodium and water retention by the kidneys and a worsening of the pre-existing peripheral edema.

6. **The prognosis** for patients with CHF is variable depending on several factors, including age, severity of the heart failure, and the overall health of the patient. Two-thirds of patients with CHF die within 5 years, while 20% of patients with CHF die within 12 months of diagnosis. Moreover, the prognosis is slightly worse in men than in women. The biggest medical concern in patients with CHF is lethal cardiac arrhythmia, which occurs at a rate 9 times higher than that of the general population. Despite advances in the treatment of hypertension and myocardial infarction, the survival rate for patients with CHF has not improved dramatically. Patients can improve their survival by closely monitoring their diet, controlling their weight, and not smoking or consuming large amounts of alcohol.

7. **The appropriate treatment** for patients with CHF usually consists of a combination of prescription medications and lifestyle changes. Controlling dietary intake of fats, limiting alcohol intake, and smoking cessation can increase the effectiveness of any pharmacologic treatment regimen. Multiple medications have been shown to improve both cardiac function and CHF symptoms. Angiotensin converting enzyme (ACE)-inhibitors are considered by many to be the first-line of CHF therapy and act by blocking the production of angiotensin, a hormone with significant vasoconstrictor activity, thus lowering the heart's workload by causing vasodilation. Diuretics are often prescribed to increase the amount of sodium and water excreted by the kidneys. This will help decrease the total body fluid volume and decrease cardiac workload. Digoxin, an inotropic agent that increases the

force of the heart's contractions, is used to improve cardiac contractility and decrease atrial fibrillation. Other medications used in the treatment of patients with CHF include vasodilators, beta blockers, calcium channel blockers, and anticoagulants. In some patients, insertion of an automated implantable cardioverter defibrillator (AICD), or pacemaker, under the skin below the left or right collar bone may be beneficial in reducing mortality due to cardiac arrhythmias.

Treatment and Course

The patient was continued on Diovan HCT and started on Lasix, Toprol, and daily aspirin therapy. She was referred for follow-up to the cardiology service. She had several follow-up BNP measurements and 6 months following the initiation of her therapy, her plasma BNP level was 178 pg/mL.

Keywords

congestive heart failure, dyspnea, orthopnea, B-type natriuretic peptide, pleural fluid, transudate, exudate

References

1. Celli BR. Diseases of the diaphragm, chest wall, pleura, and mediastinum. In: *Cecil Textbook of Medicine,* 22nd ed, Goldman L, Ausiello D, eds. Philadelphia: Saunders. 568-576.

2. Ruskoaho H, Leskinen H, Magga J, et al. Mechanisms of mechanical load-induced atrial natriuretic peptide secretion: Role of endothelin, nitric oxide, and angiotensin II. *J Mol Med.* 1997;75:876-885.

3. Bay M, Kirk V, Parner J, et al. NT-proBNP: A new diagnostic screening tool to differentiate between patients with normal and reduced left ventricular systolic function. *Heart.* 2003;89:150-154.

4. Valli N, Georges A, Corcuff JB, et al. Assessment of brain natriuretic peptide in patients with suspected heart failure: Comparison with radionuclide ventriculography data. *Clinica Chimica Acta.* 2001;306:19-26.

5. Maisel AS, Koon J, Krishnaswamy P, et al. Utility of B-natriuretic peptide as a rapid, point-of-care test for screening patients undergoing echocardiography to determine left ventricular dysfunction. *Am Heart J.* 2001;141:367-374.

6. Cowe MR, Mendez GF. BNP and congestive heart failure. *Prog Cardiovasc Dis.* 2002;44:293-321.

7. DeLemos JA, Morrow DA, Bentley JH, et al. The prognostic value of B-type natriuretic peptide in patients with acute coronary syndromes. *N Engl J Med.* 2001;345:1014-1021.

8. Struthers AD. Heart failure: The diagnosis of heart failure. *Heart.* 2000;84:334-338.

9. Gould BE. *Pathophysiology for the health professions,* 2nd ed. Philadelphia: WB Saunders Company, 2002, 284-288.

Lethargy and Hyperammonemia in a Neonate

Emily Herndon,[1] Vivian Jones, [2] Michael J. Bennett[1,2]

Departments of Pathology, [1]University of Texas Southwestern Medical Center and [2]Children's Medical Center, Dallas, TX

Patient: 3-day-old female.

Chief Complaint: Lethargy.

Past Surgical History: None.

History of Present Illness: The infant was delivered at 39 weeks gestational age following the uneventful pregnancy of her mother (G2P2). She began breast-feeding without difficulty and went home 2 days after delivery. That evening, approximately 24 hours prior to presentation at our tertiary care pediatric medical center, she became lethargic and would not awaken for feeding. She was taken first to her primary care physician (PCP), where she was found to be breathing deeply. She was subsequently transferred to a local hospital. While at this hospital, plasma ammonia testing was performed, and the level was 700 mmol/L (normal reference range: 64-107 mmol/L). She was subsequently intubated and given D10 fluid intravenously; after blood, urine, and cerebrospinal fluid (CSF) samples were obtained for culture, she was given ampicillin and claforan antibiotics. She was then transferred to our tertiary care pediatric medical center for further treatment.

Past Medical History: The infant was delivered by spontaneous vaginal delivery and had APGAR [Appearance (color); Pulse (heart rate); Grimace (reflex irritability); Activity (muscle tone), and Respirations] scores of 8 and 9 (maximum score = 10) immediately after birth.

Family History: The patient's sibling is a healthy 2-year-old sister.

Social History: The patient lives at home with her mother and sister.

Physical Examination: The infant was lethargic (but arousable), afebrile, and tachycardic with slightly cool extremities, equal, round, and sluggishly reactive pupils, and normal bowel sounds. The chest was clear to auscultation bilaterally and the neck was supple with a full range of motion.

Questions

1. What are this patient's most striking clinical and laboratory findings?

2. How do you explain this patient's most striking clinical and laboratory findings?

3. What additional test(s) should be performed on this infant and why?

4. What is this patient's most likely diagnosis?

5. How is this patient's disorder "definitively" diagnosed?

6. How should this patient be treated?

T1. Principal Laboratory Findings

Test	Patient's Result	"Normal" Reference Interval
Arterial Blood Gases		
pH	7.52	7.35-7.45
pCO_2	21	27-41 mm Hg
pO_2	62	83-108 mm Hg
Bicarbonate	17	17-24 mEq/L
Chemistry		
Sodium	147	134-146 mEq/L
Potassium	3.4	4.5-7.2 mEq/L
Chloride	108	95-110 mEq/L
Bicarbonate	18	18-31 mmol/L
BUN	5	2-19 mg/dL
Creatinine	0.8	0.1-0.6 mg/dL
Glucose	139	45-100 mg/dL
Ammonia, plasma	490	64-107 mmol/L
Lactic acid	7.8	0.7-2.3 mmol/L
AST	68	47-150 U/L
ALT	41	5-45 U/L
GGT	345	34-263 U/L
Total bilirubin	11.9	0.1-13.3 mg/dL

BUN, blood urea nitrogen; AST, aspartate aminotransferase; ALT, alanine aminotransferase; GGT, gamma-glutamyltransferase

T2. Plasma and Urine Testing for Urea Cycle Intermediates by High Performance Liquid Chromatography

Test	Patient's Result	"Normal" Reference Interval
Glutamine	1,553	200-1,200 µmol/L
Asparagine	70	15-132 µmol/L
Citrulline	2,098	3-55 µmol/L
Argininiosuccinic acid	<1.0	0 µmol/L
Arginine	206	6–140 µmol/L
Ornithine	166	10-211 µmol/L
Orotic acid, urine	Elevated	None detectable

Possible Answers

1. Difficulty breathing and lethargy after feeding; increased *blood* pH with decreased pCO_2 and pO_2; markedly decreased *serum* potassium and increased glucose concentration and GGT activity; markedly increased *plasma* ammonia concentration.

2. The constellation of these abnormal clinical and laboratory findings in a newborn is highly suggestive of an inherited metabolic disease. Moreover, the combination of an increased blood pH (most likely in this case from a metabolic alkalosis), normal serum bicarbonate concentration, and increased plasma ammonia concentration is more consistent with a urea cycle disorder than an aminoacidopathy, galactosemia, or an organic acidemia.

3. To "presumptively" identify a urea cycle disorder, plasma, and urine levels of intermediates in the urea cycle should be quantified by an analytically sensitive and specific method such as high performance liquid chromatography (HPLC). The results of testing our patient's plasma and urine by HPLC for a variety of urea cycle intermediates are shown in **T2**. Most notably, plasma glutamine and arginine concentrations were increased; however, citrulline concentration was markedly increased to approximately 40 times the upper limit of the normal reference interval and urinary orotic acid concentration was elevated.

4. **Most likely diagnosis:** *argininosuccinate synthase deficiency.*

5. Dietary protein is first degraded to its constituent amino acids by extracellular proteases found in the stomach and small intestine and then by intracellular proteases. Free amino acids can be used by cells to synthesize new proteins and other macromolecules or they can be catabolized to their carbon chain backbone by removal of their amino group in a process that converts this group to ammonia. Because ammonia is toxic to cells, it must be removed before levels accumulate. In 1932, Krebs and Henseleit identified the enzymes and intermediates in a cyclic series of reactions for detoxifying ammonia by converting

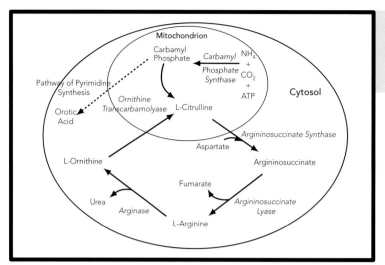

Figure 1_The urea cycle.

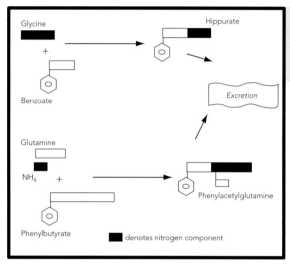

Figure 2_Alternative modes of nitrogen excretion.

it to a neutral, non-toxic, water-soluble end product (ie, urea) that can be easily eliminated in the urine by healthy kidneys. This cyclic series of reactions occur exclusively in hepatocytes and are referred to as the Krebs-Henseleit cycle, or more commonly, the urea cycle. The enzymes involved in this cyclic series of reactions are shown in [**Figure 1**] and include the mitochondrial enzymes, cabamyl phosphate synthase (CPS) and ornithine transcarbamylase (OTC); and the cytosolic enzymes, argininosuccinate synthase (AS), argininosuccinate lyase (AL), and arginase.[1] Moreover, these enzymes are induced in the perinatal period by the presence of protein in the gastrointestinal (GI) tract and by hormones such as glucagon and cortisol.[2] Inherited deficiencies in 1 or more enzymes of the urea cycle occur both in neonates and in older

patients. In older individuals, OTC deficiency occurs most commonly in female carriers due to a mutation in the OTC gene on 1 of their X chromosomes. The overall incidence of all urea cycle disorders is approximately 1 in 8,000, and in Japan, these disorders represent the most important inborn error of metabolism.[2,3] Clinically, individuals with a urea cycle disorder typically present with hyperammonemia, encephalopathy, and respiratory alkalosis; however, signs and symptoms vary depending on the specific enzyme defect and the increased concentration of metabolites associated with each defect.[3] Moreover, symptoms such as lethargy can occur within 24 hours to 72 hours of birth, requiring arousal of the infant for feeding, as occurred in our patient. As toxic intermediates accumulate, adverse neurologic changes progress and include cerebral edema and herniation of the cerebellar tonsils.[2] If a bulging fontanel is noted, an intracranial hemorrhage may be present; however, this possibility can be easily confirmed or rejected by imaging studies.[3] In addition, sepsis, a condition often among the differential diagnoses in patients with a urea cycle disorder, can be ruled in or out on the basis of the presence or absence of fever and positive or negative cultures for a causative organism. Therefore, the "presumptive" identification of the specific enzyme defect in patients suspected of having a urea cycle disorder is based principally on plasma and urine levels of urea cycle intermediates. The increased glutamine, orotic acid, and citrulline levels in our patient are highly indicative of AS deficiency. Orotic acid is formed from the combination of carbamyl phosphate and aspartic acid such that increased concentrations of both of these substrates would promote increased urinary excretion of orotic acid. Carbamyl phosphate, citrulline, and aspartic acid are all intermediates that occur upstream from the AS step in the urea cycle [**Figure 1**]. Thus, a deficiency of AS explains the increased plasma concentrations of glutamine (a precursor of glutamate) and citrulline and the increased urine concentration of orotic acid; however, it is not consistent with our patient's increased plasma concentration of arginine, a downstream intermediate from the AS step in the urea cycle. This finding is explained by the fact that our patient was given exogenous arginine prior to the collection of plasma and urine samples for testing.

6. Although serum and urine screening for the presence of increased concentrations of substances characteristic of argininosuccinate synthetase deficiency provides "presumptive" evidence of this disorder, "definitive" diagnosis is made by assessing the enzymatic activity of this enzyme using cultured leukocytes or fibroblasts or, prenatally, using cells cultured from specimens obtained by chorionic villus sampling or by amniocentesis.[4,5]

7. The treatment of patients with urea cycle disorders involves restriction of dietary protein content, re-introduction of essential amino acids (eg, arginine), and the activation of alternative pathways for the elimination of ammonia [**Figure 2**]. Because most patients with AS deficiency are diagnosed at a young age and require adequate protein and essential amino acids in their diet for normal growth and development, achieving the right balance between dietary restriction of protein content and normal growth and development is challenging for the neonatologist. Patients with AS deficiency should be monitored closely for symptoms of neurologic damage, and both ammonia and glutamine levels should be monitored when the evidence for such damage is inconclusive. Monitoring glutamine levels is useful because studies have shown that it typically rises before ammonia.[6] In addition, administration of phenylbutyrate is useful in reducing the formation of ammonia by promoting the excretion of glutamine as phenylacetylglutamine, the adduct formed when glutamine combines with phenylbutyrate [**Figure 2**]. Last, if ammonia levels must be lowered in an emergency, hemodialysis is an option.[2,3] Despite these treatments, however, the prognosis is bleak for most patients with a urea cycle disorder. For example, about half of all patients with OTC deficiency die by 4 years of age, while the half that survive typically have a mean IQ of less than 50.[3]

Keywords

argininosuccinate synthase deficiency, citrullinemia, urea cycle, hyperammonemia

References

1. Zubay G. *Biochemistry*. New York: Macmillan, 1988:615-645.

2. Gilbert-Barness E. *Metabolic Diseases: Foundations of Clinical Management, Genetics, and Pathology*. Natick, MA: Eaton Publishing, 2000:95-111.

3. Brusilow SW, Horwich ER. Urea cycle enzymes. In: Scriver CR, Beaudet AL, Valle D, Sly WS, eds. *The Metabolic and Molecular Basis of Inherited Disease*, 8th ed. New York: McGraw-Hill, 2001:1909-1963.

4. Nyhan LN, Ozamd PT. *Atlas of Metabolic Diseases*. New York: Chapman and Hall Medical, 1998:1-12.

5. Rezvani I, Rosenblatt DS, Matalon RK. Defects in metabolism of amino acids. In: Behrman RE, Kleigman RM, Jenson HB. *Nelson Textbook of Pediatrics*. 16th ed. Philadelphia, PA: WB Saunders, 2000:345-377.

6. Wilson CJ, Lee PJ, Leonard JV. Plasma glutamine and ammonia concentrations in ornithine carbamoyltransferase deficiency and citrullinemia. *J Inher Metab Dis*. 2001;24:691-695.

Fatigue, Bronze-Colored Skin, and Skin Ulcerations in a 51-Year-Old Alcoholic Woman

Amanda Rivera-Begeman, Manni Yeggapan

Department of Pathology, University of Texas Southwestern Medical Center, Dallas, TX

Patient: 51-year-old Caucasian woman.

Family History: Unremarkable.

Chief Complaint: Fatigue, "bronze-colored" skin, and ulcerations on the dorsum of both hands.

Past Medical History: The patient's medical history included hepatitis C and porphyria cutanea tarda diagnoses 10 and 8 years ago, respectively, bipolar disorder, cholelithiasis, and ascites 1 month prior to presentation that resolved after decreased alcohol consumption. She indicated that she had undergone multiple therapeutic phlebotomies and a liver biopsy; however, records of these events were not available.

Drug History: Lithium (antimanic), Loxapine (antipsychotic), and Wellbutrin (antidepressant).

Past Surgical History: Bilateral tubal ligation 8 years ago.

Past Social History: Tobacco abuse (2.5 packs per day for 39 years), alcohol abuse (up to 1 case of beer/day), and intravenous (IV) drug abuse 15 years ago.

Physical Examination: The patient was afebrile with signs and symptoms of a peripheral neuropathy, normal vital signs, and hepatomegaly without signs of portal hypertension, ascites, or jaundice.

Results of Additional Diagnostic Procedures: Liver ultrasound and biopsy results demonstrated severe hepatocellular iron deposition and cirrhosis (**Image 1**). HFE gene mutation analysis demonstrated that our patient was homozygous-affected for the cytosine (C) to guanine (G) transversion at nucleotide position 187 (C187G) that results in a cysteine (C) to tyrosine (Y) substitution at amino acid position 282 (C282Y) in the HFE protein (**Image 2**).

Questions _____

1. What are this patient's most striking clinical and laboratory findings?

2. How do you explain this patient's most striking clinical and laboratory findings?

3. What additional test(s) should be ordered on this patient and why?

4. What condition(s) is(are) suggested by this patient's most striking clinical and laboratory findings?

5. What is this patient's most likely diagnosis?

T1. Principal Laboratory Findings

Test	Patient's Result	"Normal" Reference Interval
Hematology		
WBC count	14.5	4.1-10.9 × 10³/μL
Hemoglobin	16.2	12.0-15.2 g/dL
Hematocrit	49.3	37.0-46.0%
Platelet count	225	150-450 × 10³/μL
Chemistry		
Sodium	135	137-145 mEq/L
Potassium	4.3	3.6-5.0 mEq/L
Chloride	100	101-111 mEq/L
Calcium	9.7	8.9-10.6 mg/dL
Magnesium	1.5	1.4-1.8 mEq/L
Glucose	122	65-110 mg/dL
Phosphorous	4.2	2.3-4.5 mg/dL
BUN	8	7-21 mg/dL
Creatinine	0.8	0.5-1.4 mg/dL
Bilirubin, total	0.5	0.0-1.3 mg/dL
Total protein	7.4	6.3-8.2 g/dL
Albumin	3.8	3.5-4.8 g/dL
AST	44	5-35 U/L
ALT	23	10-40 U/L
ALP	126	38-126 U/L
GGT	90	8-78 U/L
Iron, total	137	48-180 μg/dL
TIBC	246	262-474 μg/dL
Ferritin	438	7-282 ng/mL
Transferrin	192	212-360 mg/dL
Transferrin saturation*	51	15-45%
Immunology		
Anti-HCV antibody	Reactive	Non-reactive

*Transferrin saturation, % = ([SIC, μg/dL] × 100)/([transferrin, mg/dL] × 1.42); 1.42 represents a multiplication factor based on the molecular weight, in Daltons (Da), of iron (56 Da) and apotransferrin (79570 Da) and a factor of 1000 to convert mg to μg [ie, (56 × 1000)/79570 = 0.704 and 1/0.704 = 1.42]. WBC, white blood cell; BUN, blood urea nitrogen; TIBC, total iron binding capacity; AST, aspartate aminotransferase; ALT, alanine aminotransferase; ALP, alkaline phosphatase; GGT, gamma-glutamyl transferase; HCV, hepatitis C virus.

6. How is this patient's condition typically treated?

Possible Answers

1. "Bronze-colored" skin and ulcerated skin lesions on the hands; increased hemoglobin, hematocrit, ferritin, and % transferrin saturation with decreased transferrin and TIBC values and a normal serum total iron concentration; and modestly increased AST and GGT values (**T1**).

2. The increased ferritin and % transferrin saturation, coupled with decreased transferrin and TIBC values and a normal serum total iron concentration suggests compensated iron overload. The TIBC is the quantity of iron that can be bound by transferrin in a specified volume of serum and represents an indirect measure of the serum transferrin concentration, thus explaining our patient's decreased values for both of these parameters. Typically, in patients with iron overload, the serum total iron concentration is increased; however, it can be within normal limits, especially in a patient who has recently undergone a therapeutic phlebotomy to reduce their iron stores. Moreover, iron overload is categorized as "representative" (ferritin concentration >400 ng/mL) or "non-representative" (ferritin concentration <400 ng/mL) based on the serum ferritin concentration.[1] Iron storage diseases associated with a representative ferritin increase can be divided into 2 forms: primary and secondary. The primary and secondary causes of representative iron overload include hereditary hemochromatosis and acquired hemochromatoses (also known as hemosideroses), respectively. Moreover, values for transferrin saturation are >50% in conditions associated with a representative increase in ferritin concentration and are decreased in conditions associated with a non-representative increase in ferritin concentration. Increased transferrin saturation results in a compensatory decrease in serum transferrin concentration and its surrogate marker, TIBC. The effect of phlebotomy is a stimulation of bone marrow erythropoiesis with increased production of and incorporation of iron from storage depots (ie, ferritin and hemosiderin) into hemoglobin of newly formed red blood cells, thus accounting for this patient's increased hemoglobin and hematocrit values.

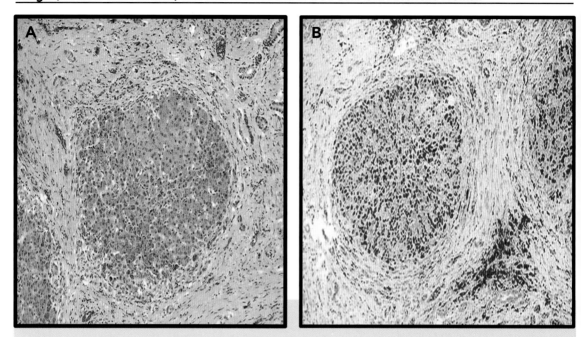

Image 1_Histopathology results of liver biopsy tissue demonstrating **A**) extensive fibrosis and small nodules of hepatocytes without fatty changes (H&E stain; 200× magnification) and **B**) abundant hemosiderin granules (Prussian Blue iron stain; 200× magnification).

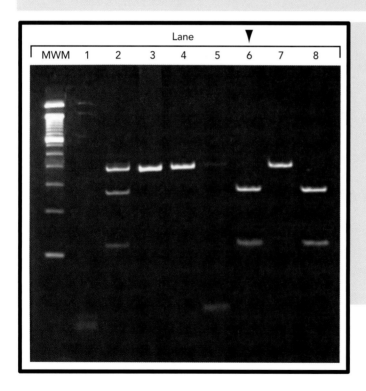

Image 2_Polyacrylamide gel (10%) electrophoresis pattern for PCR testing for the C282Y HFE protein mutation: *lane MWM*, various molecular weight markers; *lane 1*, negative control (no DNA); *lane 2*, positive (heterozygote for the C282Y HFE mutation) patient control; *lanes 3, 4, 5, and 7*, negative (homozygous-normal) patient controls; *lane 6 (arrowhead)* - our patient who is homozygous-affected for the C282Y HFE mutation; *lane 8*, homozygous-affected patient for the C282Y HFE mutation. *PCR, polymerase chain reaction.*

Depot iron refers to the approximately 20% of the total iron content in the body stored in ferritin and hemosiderin in cells of the recticuloendothelial system (liver, spleen, and bone marrow). The human body is not capable of actively excreting excess iron. Therefore, when the concentration of free iron in the plasma exceeds the iron-binding capacity of transferrin and the iron storage capacity of ferritin and hemosiderin, iron can become deposited in the skin (and other parenchymatous tissues) and produce a "bronze" discoloration and ulcerative lesions from the cell damage and death caused by the increased concentration of free iron ions within skin cells. This patient's modestly increased AST and GGT values are consistent with her prior history of alcohol and IV drug abuse and liver cirrhosis.

3. Polymerase chain reaction (PCR)-based DNA testing for the HFE gene mutation. Hereditary hemochromatosis (HH) is an HLA-associated autosomal recessive disorder of iron metabolism in which the genetic defect is a mutation in a gene closely linked with the human leukocyte antigen (HLA)-A locus on the short arm of chromosome 6. Because of the association between this defective gene, primary hemochromatosis (H), and a disorder of iron (FE) metabolism, this gene has been given the name "HFE gene." The protein product of the HFE gene is a transmembrane major histocompatibility (MHC) class 1-like glycoprotein, containing 343 amino acids, termed "HFE," that modulates iron transport.[2] Two mutations in the HFE gene [ie, guanine (G) to adenine (A) transition at nucleotide 845 (G845A) and a cytosine (C) to guanine (G) transversion at nucleotide position 187 (C187G)] result in HFE protein mutations [ie, cysteine (C) to tyrosine (Y) substitution at amino acid position 282 (C282Y) and a histidine (H) to aspartic acid (D) substitution at amino acid position 63 (H63D)] that cause the majority of cases of HH. Interestingly, however, hemochromatosis occurs in some populations (eg, China) due to mutations in genes other than the HFE gene (ie, non-HFE hemochromatosis).[2] When the mutation occurs in the HFE gene, it results in a defective HFE protein localized principally within cells of the gastrointestinal tract that is not capable of migrating outside of these cells, resulting in increased iron absorption in the small intestine and increased storage in affected organs (ie, parenchymal cells of the liver, the heart, pancreas, and adrenal glands). The accumulation of iron within these organs causes clinical complications including diabetes, liver cirrhosis, arthropathy, cardiomyopathy, and impotence.[1,2] The availability of genetic testing for HFE gene mutations has reduced substantially the need for liver biopsy and the histochemical identification of increased hepatic iron (**Image 1B**) to confirm iron overload.

Liver biopsy may be useful, however, to assess prognosis in some cases of iron overload in subclinical cases and in individuals with additional risk factors for liver disease.[3]

4. In patients with clinical and laboratory findings suggestive of iron overload, the differential diagnosis should include primary (hereditary) hemochromatosis, secondary (acquired) hemochromatosis, and dietary causes. Secondary, or acquired, causes of hemochromatosis include ineffective erythropoiesis, thalassemia major, sideroblastic and aplastic anemias, and blood transfusions. Dietary causes of iron overload include extreme ingestion of iron, African dietary iron overload (from alcoholic beverages brewed in vessels made of iron), and chronic alcoholism.[2] To determine the cause of our patient's iron overload, HFE genotyping, liver ultrasonography, and a liver biopsy to determine the existence or extent of liver damage were performed. These procedures indicated that our patient was homozygous for the C187G HFE gene mutation and C282Y protein mutation (**Image 2**), and had severe hepatic iron deposition and cirrhosis.

5. ***Most likely diagnosis:*** *iron overload due to hereditary hemochromatosis.*

Hereditary hemochromatosis is 1 of the most common genetic diseases in individuals of Northern European descent (prevalence = 1 in 200 to 300 individuals).[2] Approximately 1 in 10 of these individuals are carriers of, and about 1 in 200 to 300 are homozygous for, an HFE gene mutation. In individuals with a homozygous HFE gene mutation, iron absorption by the intestines is increased nearly 2-fold. Symptoms (eg, fatigue) of HH often occur after the age of 50 and occur more frequently in males (M) than females (F) (M:F = 3:1).[2] Excessive accumulation of iron causes iron storage in the parenchymal cells of a variety of organs, including liver, pancreas, heart, and pituitary gland. Moreover, the increased concentration of free iron ions in the tissues of these organs causes free radical-induced lipid peroxidation that damages these tissues and impairs organ function.[4,5] The increase in intracellular free iron ions is thought to occur because of defective HFE protein. Although the function of the HFE protein is still under investigation, it has been postulated that this protein affects iron homeostasis by competing with transferrin, the principal iron transport protein in the blood, for binding to the transferrin receptor, thus decreasing cellular iron absorption. Mutated HFE protein (eg, in individuals with a homozygous HFE gene mutation) is unable to fold correctly and is degraded before it can reach its usual location at the cell surface. Therefore, the decrease in the concentration of HFE protein to compete with transferrin for the transferrin receptor results in increased binding of transferrin to this receptor and an increase in intracellular iron concentration. Excess intracellular iron is stored in parenchymal cells in the form of ferritin and hemosiderin. Moreover, in the early stages of iron overload, iron deposition occurs predominantly in the periportal cells of the liver. When the iron storage capacity of these cells is exceeded during further iron accumulation by these cells, perilobular hepatic fibrosis occurs, followed by iron deposition in Kupffer cells, fibrous septa, and bile duct epithelium. In the later stages of iron overload, macronodular or mixed macro- and micronodular cirrhosis occurs.

6. If left untreated, hemochromatosis causes death due to cardiac or hepatocellular failure, portal hypertension, or hepatocellular cancer. Fortunately, hemochromatosis is a treatable disease and the prognosis depends on how early the diagnosis is made and treatment is initiated. If the patient is treated early enough, most if not all, of the manifestations of this disease can be prevented. If treated at a later stage, life expectancy is still improved with an increase in 5-year survival from 33% to 89%.[4,5] The mainstay of treatment for hemochromatosis consists of an initial therapeutic phlebotomy of 500 mL, followed by phlebotomy 1 to 2 times per week until iron levels normalize. Once normal iron levels are achieved, therapeutic phlebotomy is performed only as needed. Moreover, it is important to follow these patients' hematocrit and serum ferritin concentrations closely to prevent iron-deficiency anemia (IDA). If the patient is already anemic, phlebotomy is contraindicated and therapy with the iron-chelating agent, deferoxamine (Desferal) can be instituted. In addition, in patients with HH, screening for HFE gene mutations in family members should be done. Because HH is not an uncommon disease among Caucasians, the College of American

Pathologists (CAP) recommends population screening. Cost-effective screening of the general population is possible using percent transferrin saturation (%TS) or serum iron concentration (SIC) as an initial screening test, followed by confirmatory DNA testing of individuals with a %TS >60% (>50% in premenopausal women) or a SIC >150 μg/dL.[2,6] Nevertheless, this screening is not universally accepted because the natural history and burden of suffering of this disease are unknown.[7]

Keywords

iron overload, ferritin, hemosiderin, percent transferrin saturation, hereditary hemochromatosis, acquired hemochromatosis, genotyping, liver biopsy, HFE gene, HFE protein

References

1. Wick M, Pinggera W, Lehmann P. *Iron Metabolism, Anemias Diagnosis and Therapy*, 4th ed. New York: Springer Verlag, 2000.

2. Lyon E, Frank EL. Hereditary hemochromatosis since discovery of the HFE gene. *Clin Chem.* 2001;47:1147-1156.

3. Adams PC. Role of genetic testing testing and liver biopsy in the diagnosis of hemochromatosis. *Curr Gasteroenterol Rep.* 1999;1:27-29.

4. Bacon B, Tavill A. *Hemochromatosis.* National Digestive Diseases Information Clearinghouse (NDDIC). NIH publication No. 02-4621, August 2002. http://digestive.niddk.nih.gov/ddiseases/pubs/hemochromatosis/index.htm. Accessed July 12, 2004.

5. Powel L, Isselbacher K. Hemochromatosis. In: *Harrison's Principles of Internal Medicine,* 14th ed. Edited by Fauci AS, Braunwald E, Isselbacher KJ, et al. New York: McGraw-Hill, 1998, 2149-2152.

6. Bassett ML. Analysis of the cost of population screening for hemochromatosis using biochemical and genetic markers. *J Hepatol.* 1997;27:517-524.

7. Burke W, Thompson E, Knoury MJ, et al. Hereditary hemochromatosis gene discovery and its implication for population-based screening. *JAMA.* 1998;280:172-178.

Lethargy, Failure to Thrive, and Psychomotor Retardation in an Infant

Jaffar Alfardan, Michael J. Bennett

Department of Pathology, Children's Hospital and the University of Texas Southwestern Medical Center, Dallas, TX

Patient: 13-month-old female infant.

Chief Complaint: Loss of responsiveness, decreased appetite and energy level, and an inability to sit, crawl, or stand.

History of Present Illness: The infant was delivered at 39 weeks gestation to a 15-year-old mother who had received only 4 weeks of prenatal care. At birth, she weighed 7 pounds 5 ounces and was discharged with her mother. The mother indicated that the infant demonstrated normal developmental milestones and was healthy up until 5 days prior to being seen in the emergency department (ED). At that time, the baby spiked a fever of 103.3°F, and her mother took her to a local clinic, where she was treated with Omnicef for otitis media and a respiratory infection. Over the next 5 days, the infant demonstrated the signs and symptoms indicated above and her mother brought her to the ED. Subsequently, the infant was admitted to the intensive care unit (ICU).

Medical History: There was no history of the child having ingested honey.

Family History: The mother claimed no history of drug abuse or hereditary disease, and she knew very little about the biological father's family history.

Physical Examination Findings: Altered mental status, mild tachypnea, warm dry skin, marked generalized hypotonia, 4/5 and 1-2/5 power in upper and lower limbs, respectively, and normal reflexes.

Additional Diagnostic Testing: An electrocardiogram (EKG) and an echocardiogram (ECG) were obtained to rule out heart disease, and both were normal. An electroencephalogram (EEG) demonstrated no specific abnormalities; a computed tomography (CT) scan showed low density within the globus pallidi; and a magnetic resonance imaging (MRI) scan showed symmetric foci of T1 and T2 prolongation involving the globus pallidi portion of the brain. Proton magnetic resonance spectroscopy (1HMRS) was cancelled because the patient woke up in the MRI room. Since the results of the imaging studies suggested the presence of a metabolic disorder [eg, methylmalonic acidemia, glutaric acidemia type 1], serum amino acid and acylcarnitine levels were measured and a urine organic acid screen was performed by gas chromatography/mass spectrometry (GC/MS) (**T1**).

T1. Principal Laboratory Findings

Test	Patient's Result	"Normal" Reference Range
Hematology		
WBC count	5.8	$5.0\text{-}14.5 \times 10^3/\mu L$
Hemoglobin	12.6	4.2-11.1 g/dL
Hematocrit	37.6	30.0-42.0%
Platelet count	501	$150\text{-}550 \times 10^3/\mu L$
Chemistry		
Sodium (Na^+)	144	139-146 mEq/L
Potassium	4.7	3.5-5.0 mEq/L
Chloride (Cl^-)	110	98-106 mEq/L
CO_2	21	18-31 mmol/L
Anion gap[a]	13	5-14 mEq/L
Glucose	86	74-127 mg/dL
Calcium	10	8.4-10.7 mg/dL
Phosphorus	5.6	3.8-6.5 mg/dL
Magnesium	2.1	1.6-2.6 mEq/L
Ammonia	21	21-50 umol/L
Lactate	1.2	0.7-2.3 mmol/L
Amino acid screen	No abnormally increased amino acid present	No abnormally increased amino acid present
Carnitine screen	No abnormal acylcarnitine present	No abnormal acylcarnitine present

T1. Principal Laboratory Findings

Organic acid screen	Positive for increased concentrations of 4-HBA and 3,4-DHBA	Negative for an increased concentration of an organic acid
Venous blood gases		
pH	7.40	7.35-7.45
pO_2	40	30-50 mm Hg
pCO_2	34	31-54 mm Hg
Base excess	-3.2	-4.0 to -2.0 mEq/L
DAU testing		
Phencyclidine	Negative	Negative
Benzodiazepines	Negative	Negative
Cocaine metabolite	Negative	Negative
Amphetamines	Negative	Negative
Cannabinoids	Negative	Negative
Opiates	Negative	Negative
Barbiturates	Negative	Negative
Microbiology		
Blood culture	Negative	Negative
CSF culture	Negative	Negative
Viral PCR testing	Negative	Negative

[a]$Na^+ - (Cl^- + CO_2)$.
WBC, white blood cell; 4-HBA, 4-hydroxybutyric acid; 3,4-DHBA, 3,4-dihydroxybutyric acid; DAU, drugs of abuse in urine; CSF, cerebrospinal fluid; PCR, polymerase chain reaction

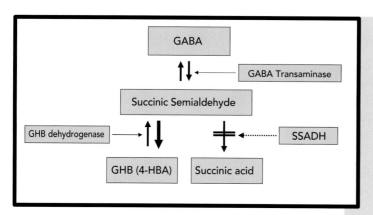

Figure 1_Metabolic pathway of GABA illustrating the block in the conversion of succinic semialdehyde to succinic acid that occurs in patients with SSADH deficiency and results in the accumulation of 4-HBA in the plasma, urine, and CSF of affected individuals.

GHB, gamma-hydroxybutyrate; 4-HBA, 4-hydroxybutyric acid; SSADH, succinic semialdehyde dehydrogenase.

Questions _____

1. What are this patient's most striking clinical and laboratory findings?

2. How do you explain this patient's most striking clinical and laboratory findings?

3. What is this patient's most likely diagnosis?

4. What condition could be confused with this patient's disease?

5. What is the pathophysiology of this patient's disease?

6. What are the principal signs and symptoms associated with this patient's disease?

7. What are the principal laboratory findings associated with this patient's disease?

8. What imaging studies are useful in establishing the diagnosis of this patient's disease?

9. What additional test should be performed to confirm the diagnosis of this patient's disease?

10. What are the genetics of this patient's disease?

11. How should this patient's disease be treated?

Possible Answers _____

1. Lethargy, altered mental status, failure to thrive, hypotonia, and psychomotor retardation; prolonged T1- and T2-weighted MRI images involving the globus pallidi bilaterally; and a large amount of 4-HBA and 3,4-DHBA in the urine in the absence of an increased anion gap or a metabolic acidosis [ie, anion gap, blood pH, and venous blood gas values were within the normal reference range for these parameters (**T1**)].

2. The constellation of this infant's signs and symptoms are consistent with several conditions, especially CNS infection, a cardiovascular anomaly, botulism, and an inborn error of metabolism. However, follow-up diagnostic and laboratory testing, including negative

ECG, echocardiography, viral PCR, and blood and CSF culture findings, when coupled with positive MRI and urine GC/MS findings for increased concentrations of unexpected metabolites [ie, 4-HBA and 3,4-DHBA (**T1**)], were highly suggestive of an inborn error of metabolism as the most likely explanation for this infant's most striking clinical and laboratory findings.

3. ***Most likely diagnosis:*** *succinic semialdehyde dehydrogenase (SSADH) deficiency (or 4-hydroxybutyric aciduria).* The presence of 4-hydroxybutyric acid (4-HBA) and 3-4 dihydroxybutyrate (3,4-DHBA) peaks on the GC/MS chromatogram of our patient's urine is consistent with SSADH deficiency or ingestion of gamma-hydroxybutyrate (GHB or 4-HBA), a drug of abuse. Because the infant was being closely monitored in the hospital for almost 3 days without the disappearance of the metabolites, 4-HBA and 3,4-DHBA, it was assumed that SSADH deficiency was the most likely cause of the increased concentrations of these metabolites in her urine.

4. Gamma-hydroxybutyrate drug abuse. Gamma-hydroxybutyrate is a naturally occurring short-chain fatty acid found in mammalian tissues. It has sedative-hypnotic effects similar to those of barbiturates and benzodiazepines. High doses of GHB have been used as an anesthetic agent in Europe and also for drug and alcohol addiction treatment and narcolepsy.[1] Gamma-hydroxybutyrate also has purported euphoric and "fat-burning" effects. It has been abused as a recreational drug with properties of addiction, tolerance, withdrawal, and intoxication.[2] It has also been used as a date-rape drug, often in combination with alcohol.[3] Prior to 1990, GHB was available over-the-counter (OTC) in the United States as a dietary supplement and for bodybuilding. After reports of its toxicity and illicit use as a "club drug" and date-rape drug, the Food and Drug Administration (FDA) banned GHB for non-medical uses in 1991. Unfortunately, this ban was not effective, and GHB is still widely and easily available online, from street sources, and from certain stores under street drug names like Liquid X, Liquid Ecstasy, Scoop, Blue Nitro, and Grievous Bodily Harm. In addition, the ban has been circumvented by the sale of "chemistry kits" which contain precursors of GHB and

instructions on how to make GHB.[4] Gamma-hydroxybutyrate can also be given as a precursor substance, gamma-hydroxybutyrolactone, which is converted to GHB in the body. Gamma-hydroxybutyrate abuse has reached "mini-epidemic" proportions in the United States, especially in metropolitan areas, where 68 GHB-related deaths have been reported in a period of 4 years.[5] Therefore, physicians should be aware of its potential for abuse and the signs, symptoms, and laboratory testing associated with recognizing and managing patients with GHB intoxication or withdrawal. Because the GC/MS chromatogram of our patient's urine demonstrated a peak consistent with an increased concentration of 4-HBA, GHB abuse was considered possible in this case. However, GHB disappears completely from plasma within 2 to 4 hours and from urine within 8 hours after ingestion.[6] Repeat testing of our patient's urine 3 days after the initial test demonstrated a persistent 4-HBA level, thus ruling out GHB abuse and ruling in SSADH deficiency as the most likely cause of our patient's increased urine 4-HBA level.

5. Succinic semialdehyde dehydrogenase deficiency causes decreased succinic acid production from gamma-aminobutyric acid (GABA) with shunting of the accumulated succinic semialdehyde intermediate to 4-HBA (**Figure 1**) and subsequently, 3,4-DHBA. Gamma-aminobutyric acid functions as both a metabolic intermediate in neuronal and extra-neuronal tissues and as a neurotransmitter in neural tissue. Gamma-aminobutyric acid is found predominantly in brain cells; however, it also occurs in kidney and B-cells of the pancreas. Gamma-aminobutyric acid is converted to succinic semialdehyde by GABA transaminase. Succinic semialdehyde is either metabolized to GHB by GHB dehydrogenase or to succinate by SSADH. Deficiency of SSADH causes the accumulation of GHB in body fluids, which causes the clinical manifestations of SSADH deficiency, also known as 4-hydroxybutyric aciduria. Interestingly, despite the presence of increased serum concentrations of the organic acids, 4-HBA and 3,4-DHBA, SSADH deficiency is not associated with an increased anion gap or a metabolic acidosis because the molar concentrations of these acids

in the blood are not sufficiently high enough to cause these abnormalities.

6. The disorder usually presents in childhood, and the most common symptoms are mild to severe psychomotor retardation, expressive language impairment, and behavioral abnormalities, including aggressiveness and hallucinations. Other symptoms include hypotonia, non-progressive ataxia, oculomotor apraxia, and autistic features. Seizures occur in about 50% of patients.[7,8]

7. The biochemical hallmark of SSADH deficiency is accumulation of 4-HBA in physiological fluids without accompanying metabolic acidosis. Levels of 4-HBA range from 2- to 800-fold higher in urine, 4- to 200-fold higher in plasma, and 100- to 1,200-fold higher in CSF, compared to the levels found in these fluids from healthy children.[9] Other compounds that can be elevated in patients with SSADH deficiency include 3,4-DHBA, 3-oxo-4-hydroxybutyric acid, and glycolic acid. 4-HBA is highly volatile and its presence may be obscured on routine total ion GC/MS by a high urea peak; however, it can be readily detected by selective ion monitoring (SIM) GC/MS. Selective ion monitoring GC/MS is both specific and sensitive for 4-HBA with a lower limit of detection (LLD) of 1 μg/mL. Isotope dilution gas chromatography-mass spectrometry, using ^{2}H- and ^{13}C-labeled internal standards, remains the gold standard method for detecting increased concentrations of GHB in physiological fluids.[7,8]

8. Neuro-imaging studies for SSADH deficiency include cranial CT, MRI, fluorodeoxyglucose positron emission tomography (PET), and proton magnetic resonance spectroscopy (^{1}H-MRS). The most consistent MRI abnormality in patients with SSADH deficiency is increased T2-weighted signal bilaterally and symmetrically in the globus pallidus and subcortical white matter areas of the brain. Other areas of the brain that can be affected include the brainstem and cerebellar dentate nucleus.[7] Proton MR spectroscopy is increasingly being used to aid in the diagnosis and may be helpful in disease follow-up. A characteristic ^{1}H-MRS pattern with clearly elevated GABA levels and traces of GHB

was found in both the white and gray matter of the brain of 1 patient with SSADH deficiency.[10]

9. Once an elevation of 4-HBA is observed by GC/MS of a patient's urine, plasma, and/or CSF, the diagnosis of SSADH deficiency is confirmed by measurement of SSADH activity in peripheral lymphocytes or cultured lymphoblasts. In patients with SSADH deficiency, the level of SSADH activity is about 10% of normal in a proband.[11] Intermediate levels between probands and normals is noted in cells from the parents of probands, thus supporting the autosomal recessive inheritance of this disease. This testing on our patient demonstrated minimal residual SSADH activity, thus confirming the diagnosis of SSADH deficiency. In addition, SSADH activity can be measured in cultured amniocytes and biopsied chorionic villus tissue, and 4-HBA levels can be measured in amniotic fluid.[12] Moreover, if the results of enzyme and metabolic studies are not concordant, gene sequencing and mutation analysis using DNA from chorionic villus cells and reverse transcriptase-polymerase chain reaction (RT-PCR) testing can be performed.[13] In addition, prenatal testing is feasible using metabolic, enzyme, and DNA analysis.

10. The index case of gamma-hydroxybutyric aciduria was described in 1981 by Jakobs and coworkers.[14] Succinic semialdehyde dehydrogenase deficiency is a rare autosomal recessive disorder of GABA metabolism. The disorder has been identified in approximately 350 individuals worldwide.[7] The SSADH gene has been mapped to chromosome 6p22.[15] The mutations thus far described in this gene are private mutations within families and no clear phenotype/genotype correlation has been documented. In 1 study, a total of 33 mutations were identified including 25 point mutations, 4 small insertions, and 5 small deletions.[16] Twenty of these mutations were unique to individual families.[16] Until recently, there has been no clinical phenotype described with heterozygosity for SSADH deficiency. In a single case report from Turkey, a heterozygous sibling of a patient with SSADH deficiency presented with photosensitive absence epilepsy and myoclonic seizures.[17] The heterozygous patient and parents did not manifest 4-OH-butyric aciduria, but SSADH activity levels were low, and a splice site mutation

in the SSADH gene was identified in each of these individuals.[17]

11. Vigabatrin, an irreversible GABA transaminase inhibitor, remains the sole treatment for SSADH deficiency. However, Vigabatrin is not available in the United States and its long-term efficacy is questionable. It has not shown consistent results, which may be due to its inability to decrease brain GHB concentrations. It is also associated with irreversible visual-field changes and has not been approved by the FDA.[18] With the development of the Aldh5a1 mice model of SSADH deficiency, preclinical agents like taurine and NCS-382 are being investigated for use in clinical trials.[18]

Treatment and Course

The patient was started on acyclovir, ceftriaxone, and vancomycin; however, these medications were discontinued when blood and CSF cultures and viral PCR test results came back negative. The patient developed seizures during her ICU stay and was started on phenytoin and later switched to phenobarbital before discharge. The mother was informed about the diagnosis, the variability of symptoms among affected individuals, and the absence of any dietary modifications or effective treatment for SSADH deficiency. In addition, she was informed that because SSADH deficiency is a rare, autosomal recessive disorder and she was no longer involved with the father of this child, she had little chance of having another SSADH-affected baby. She was also advised of the need for good follow-up with her primary care physician. We arranged follow-up for her and her child with the metabolic/genetic, neurology, and physical therapy clinics and she was enrolled in an early childhood intervention program.

Keywords

inborn error of metabolism, succinic acid semialdehyde deficiency, gamma-aminohydroxy butyric acid, gas chromatography-mass spectrometry

References

1. Wong GT, Bottiglieri T, Carter SO. GABA, gamma-hydroxybutyric acid, and neurological disease. *Ann Neurol.* 2003;54:3-12.

2. Li J, Stokes AS, Woeckener A. A tale of novel intoxication: A review of the effects of G-hydroxybutyric acid with recommendations for management. *Ann Emerg Med.* 1998;31:729-36.

3. Wong CG, Gibson KM, Snead OC. From the street to the brain: Neurobiology of the recreational drug gamma-hydroxybutyric acid. *Trends Pharmacol Sci.* 2004;25:29-34.

4. Nicholson KL, Balster RL. GHB: A new and novel drug of abuse. *Drug and Alcohol Dependence* 2001;63:1-22

5. McDaniel CH, Miotto KA. Gamma hydroxybutyrate and gamma butyrolactone withdrawal: Five case studies. *J Psychoactive Drugs.* 2001;33:143-149.

6. Ferrara SD, Zotti S, Tedeschi L, et al. Pharmacokinetics of gamma-hydroxybutyric acid in alcohol dependent patients after single and repeated oral doses. *Br J Clin Pharmacol.* 1992;34:231-5.

7. Pearl PL, Novotny EJ, Acosta MT, et al. Succinic semialdehyde dehydrogenase deficiency in children and adults. *Ann Neurol.* 2003;54:S73-S80.

8. Pearl PL, Gibson KM, Acosta MT, et al. Clinical spectrum of succinic semialdehyde dehydrogenase deficiency. *Neurology.* 2003;60:1413-1417.

9. Gibson KM, Aramaki S, Sweetman L, et al. Stable isotope dilution analysis of 4-hydroxybutyric acid: An accurate method for quantification in physiological fluids and the prenatal diagnosis of 4-hydroxybutyric aciduria. *Biomed Environ Mass Spectrom.* 1990;19:89-93.

10. Ethofer T, Seeger U, Klose U, et al. Proton MR spectroscopy in succinic semialdehyde dehydrogenase deficiency. *Neurology.* 2004;62:1016-1018.

11. Pattarelli PP, Nyhan WL, Gibson KM. Oxidation of [U-^{14}C] succinic semialdehyde in cultured human lymphoblasts: Measurement of residual succinic semialdehyde dehydrogenase activity in 11 patients with 4-hydroxybutyric aciduria. *Pediatr Res.* 1988;24:455-60.

12. Gibson KM, Baumann C, Ogier H, et al. Pre- and postnatal diagnosis of succinic semialdehyde dehydrogenase deficiency using enzyme and metabolite assays. *J Inherit Metab Dis.* 1994;17:732-737.

13. Hogema BM, Akaboshi S, Taylor M, et al. Prenatal diagnosis of succinic semialdehyde dehydrogenase deficiency: Increased accuracy employing DNA, enzyme, and metabolite analyses. *Mol Genet Metab.* 2001;72:218-222.

14. Jakobs C, Bojasch M, Monch E, et al. Urinary excretion of gamma-hydroxybutyric acid in a patient with neurological abnormalities: The probability of a new inborn error of metabolism. *Clin Chim Acta.* 1981;111:169-178.

15. Trettel F, Malaspina P, Jodice C, et al. Human succinic semialdehyde dehydrogenase: Molecular cloning and chromosomal localization. *Adv Exp Med Biol.* 1997;414:253-260.

16. Akaboshi S, Hogema BM, Novelletto A, et al. Mutational spectrum of the succinate semialdehyde dehydrogenase (ALDH5A1) gene and functional analysis of 27 novel disease-causing mutations in patients with SSADH deficiency. *Hum Mutat.* 2003;22:442-450.

17. Dervent A, Gibson KM, Pearl PL, et al. Photosensitive absence epilepsy with myoclonias and heterozygosity for succinic semialdehyde dehydrogenase (SSADH) deficiency. *Clin Neurophysiol.* 2004;115:1417-1422.

18. Gropman A. Vigabatrin and newer interventions in succinic semialdehyde dehydrogenase deficiency. *Ann Neurol.* 2003;54:S66-S72.

Recurrent Nephrolithiasis in a 9-Year-Old Child

Monte S. Willis

University of North Carolina, Chapel Hill, NC

Patient: 9 ½ year-old female.

Chief Complaint: Recurrent kidney stones.

History of Present Illness: The child's parents reported she had experienced 2 previous episodes of kidney stones (nephrolithiasis) within the last 10 months. These episodes were associated with fever, intense abdominal pain, back pain, and vomiting. Kidney stones were identified by computed tomography (CT) scan as the cause of these symptoms.

Past Medical History: Non-contributory.

Family History: Non-contributory.

Physical Examination: Vital signs: blood pressure, 107/70 mm Hg; temperature, 37.4°C; pulse, 112 bpm. Height: 134 cm (approximately 50th percentile for age/gender); weight, 28.7 kg (approximately 50th percentile for age/gender); body mass index (BMI), 15.8.

Additional Diagnostic Procedures: Renal ultrasonography demonstrated kidneys that were normal in size and echotexture with no evidence of hydronephrosis or masses. However, 2 areas of echogenic foci representing renal calculi were identified in the right kidney (**Image 1**). No distinct renal calculi were identified in the left kidney.

T1. Principal Laboratory Findings

Test	Patient's Result	Reference Interval
Chemistry		
Creatinine, serum	0.6	0.4-0.9 mg/dL
Creainine, urine (24 h)	486	800-2,800 mg/dL
Urinalysis		
Macroscopic: Leuckocyte esterase	1+	Negative
Blood/hemoglobin	1+	Negative
Microscopic: RBCs/hpf	3-5	Negative
Crystals	Clear, hexagonal plates	Negative

T1. Principal Laboratory Findings

Special Chemistry		
Urine amino acid analysis:	(Ages 3-15 years)	
Cystine	796	11-53 µmol/24 h
Lysine	3,665	19-140 µmol/24 h
Ornithine	966	3-16 µmol/24 h
Arginine	2,116	10-25 µmol/24 h

RBCs, red blood cells; hpf, high power field.

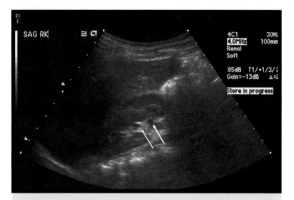

Image 1_Ultrasound of the right kidney illustrating at least 2 echogenic foci with posterior acoustic shadowing which were consistent with renal calculi (arrows).

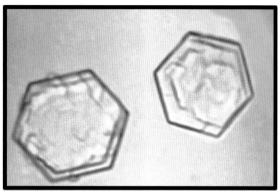

Image 2_Example of the clear, hexagonal crystals found in our patient's urine.

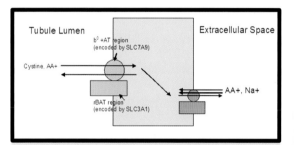

Figure 1_The heterodimeric amino acid transporter protein, consisting of bo+AT and rBAT regions, transports cystine in the proximal renal tubule. Mutations in the SLC3A1 (rBAT) gene are detected in most cases of Type A cystinuria. Adapted from Verrey, et al.[33]

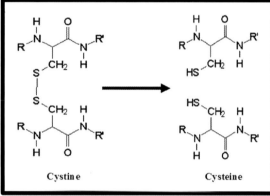

Figure 2_Cleavage of the cystine disulfide bond by D-penicillamine, a-mercaptopropionylglycine (MPG), or ascorbic acid converts cystine to cysteine, a form 50-fold more water soluble than cystine.

Questions _____

1. What are this patient's most striking clinical and laboratory findings?

2. How do you explain these findings?

3. What is the differential diagnosis and how can this patient's clinical and laboratory findings be used to differentiate between these diagnoses?

4. What is this patient's most likely diagnosis?

5. Under what conditions should this patient's diagnosis be suspected?

6. What is the epidemiology and basic defect in this patient's disease?

7. What is the molecular pathogenesis of this patient's disease?

8. What is the medical therapy used in the treatment of this patient's condition?

9. What other treatment modalities have been used in the treatment of this patient's condition?

Possible Answers

1. The most striking clinical finding is a history of recurrent kidney stones in a child. Significant laboratory findings include: a normal urine (random and 24-hour) creatinine concentration; a urinalysis positive for leukocyte esterase, hemoglobin, and red blood cells (RBCs); the presence of clear hexagonal crystals on urine microscopic analysis (**Image 2**); and abnormally elevated urinary concentrations of cystine, ornithine, lysine, and arginine (**T1**).

2. Leukocyte esterase activity in a urine specimen indicates the presence of neutrophil esterolytic activity. Therefore, a positive urine leukocyte esterase test indicates the presence of a significant number of intact or lysed neutrophils associated typically with a urinary tract infection. In a patient with recurrent kidney stones, this may be due to stasis-associated ascending infection or to a localized mucosal inflammatory response secondary to calculous formation.[1] Under high power microscopy, unstained RBCs in the urine are normally found in small numbers [0-2 cells/high power field (hpf)]. More than 3 cells/hpf, as found in this case, is considered abnormal and can be the result of calculi formation.[1] Urine amino acid testing is often performed to screen for congenital abnormalities of amino acid metabolism.

3. Four disease entities that exhibit abnormal transport of the cationic amino acids (ie, cystine, ornithine, lysine, and arginine) found in our patient's urine include: (1) classic cystinuria, (2) lysinuric protein intolerance (LPI), (3) hyperdibasic aminoaciduria type 1, and (4) isolated lysinuria (lysine malabsorption syndrome).[2,3] The symptoms of LPI and hyperdibasic aminoaciduria type 1 include vomiting and diarrhea after weaning.[4,5] The hyperammonemia associated with protein ingestion leads to avoidance of high protein foods after which a host of medical problems ensue including poor growth, enlarged liver and spleen, osteoporosis, muscle hypotonia, and mental retardation.[5] The single patient with isolated lysinuria identified to date suffered from growth failure, seizures, and mental retardation. Therefore, our patient's clinical (normal mental status and growth) and laboratory findings rule out LPI, hyperdibasic aminoaciduria type 1, and isolated lysinuria as the cause of her recurrent nephrolithiasis, leaving cystinuria as the most likely cause of our patient's disease.

4. *Most likely diagnosis: cystinuria.* The patient's history of recurrent nephrolithiasis, the presence of hexagonal crystals in the urine, and significantly elevated concentrations of cystine, ornithine, lysine, and arginine in a 24-hour urine specimen support the diagnosis of cystinuria.

5. The diagnosis of cystinuria should be suspected in patients with cystine stones, especially if they have a family history of cystine nephrolithiasis. Up to 10% of urinary stones that occur in children are caused by cystinuria.[6] More than 50% of patients with cystinuria develop cystine stones in their lifetime, most of which form stones recurrently and require the need for repeated interventions.[7] Cystine stones can be detected by ultrasound and are difficult to visualize by x-ray imaging. Hexagonal crystals detected by urinalysis can confirm the diagnosis; however, only 20% to 25% of patients with cystinuria have detectable crystals.[8] Due to this fact, definitive diagnosis of cystinuria is made by quantifying urine amino acids in a 24-hour urine specimen using ion-exchange chromatography, high performance liquid chromatography (HPLC), or tandem mass spectrometry (MS/MS).[9-11] Simpler methods utilizing colorimetric assays have been described as an economical method for population screening for this disease.[12,13]

6. Cystinuria is an autosomal recessive disease with a prevalence estimated between 1:1,000 to 1:17,000 in the United States and Europe.[14,15] The basic defect in cystinuria is impaired transport of dibasic amino acids in the proximal renal tubule. While this defect results in elevated urine concentrations of cystine, ornithine, lysine, and arginine, only cystine is insoluble enough in urine to form stones, particularly at pH 5-7. A 3-fold increase in solubility occurs when the pH is >8, which is why this disease has been treated by urine alkalinization for nearly 5 decades.[16] In addition, to more accurately quantify urine cystine concentration, the solubility of cystine can be enhanced by adding sodium bicarbonate to urine samples until the pH is greater than 7.5.[17] While a 24-hour urine collection is optimal to

determine cystine levels, the cystine/creatinine ratio on a random urine sample may distinguish individuals with homozygous disease from heterozygous carriers. A random urine cystine/creatine ratio can also be used to monitor therapy. It should be noted, however, that the urinary excretion level of cystine (and other dibasic amino acids such as ornithine, lysine, arginine) does not correlate with the frequency of cystine stone formation. Therefore, whenever possible, it is important to analyze kidney stone content, as renal stones composed of complex mixtures of amino acids and other substances can occur, requiring further, or different, interventions than might occur in the presence of pure cystine stones.

7. There is growing evidence that kidney stone formation is associated with specific mutations in calcium, oxalate, uric acid, and cystine transporters in the kidney.[18] The molecular basis of cystinuria involves 2 mutations in the renal dibasic amino acid transporter.[19,20] The mutation in the SLC3A1 gene, found on chromosome 2, encodes the rBAT subunit of this transporter (**Figure 1**). The second mutation in the SLC7A9 gene, found on chromosome 19, encodes the b⁰+AT region of the transporter. Cystinuria has recently been re-classified following the identification of these molecular defects into 3 types: Type A (SLC3A1 mutation only); Type B (SLC7A9 mutation only); or Type AB (having both SLC3A1/SLC7A9 mutations).[21] Abnormalities in 1 or both of these genes identifies 75% of all affected individuals with cystinuria, suggesting that there remain unidentified mutations in the renal dibasic amino acid transporter.[18] While progress has been made in identifying the mutations associated with cystinuria, it is not necessary clinically to detect these specific underlying mutations by molecular methods, as they can be accurately predicted based on the results of standard laboratory test values.[18] Patients with homozygous mutations in genes associated with cationic amino acid transport proteins have urine cystine concentrations exceeding 1,300 μmol/L.[8,22] Alternatively, healthy individuals excrete less than 100 μmol/L. Patients with heterozygous mutations may have urine cystine concentrations <100 μmol/L; however, they can be distributed in the normal range and extend up to, but typically do not exceed, 1,000 μmol/L.[8,22]

Recurrent kidney stones (nephrolithiasis) result from a diversity of mechanisms, many of which involve mutations in various transport proteins. In contrast to individuals that do not form calcium renal stones, patients that form stones made primarily of calcium have been shown to have specific mutations in genes (eg, CLCN5 and CLCNKB, WNK Kinases, ATPB61, and NPT2) that regulate renal chloride excretion and reabsorption.[18] Similarly, hyperoxaluria has been associated with mutations in the AGXT and GRHPR genes and defects in the glyoxalate metabolic pathway.[18] Moreover, distinct mutations in the cystine transport protein genes SLC3A1 and SLC7A9 have been shown to lead to cystine stones associated with cystinuria. In addition, hyperuricosuria, the underlying cause of uric acid stones, has been associated with familial clusters of gene mutations in uric acid transport proteins. Taken together, these findings explain the growing appreciation of the role of specific gene mutations in the pathogenesis of nephrolithiasis.[18]

8. Medical therapy in the treatment of cystinuria involves regular examinations, dietary methionine restriction, and pharmacological therapy. Since the metabolism of methionine results in cystine, dietary restriction of methionine, found in protein-rich foods, would be ideal. However, such strict restriction is not followed by most patients and not recommended in children, as in the present case. However, a low protein diet (<0.8 g protein/day) is recommended in concert with a reduction in salt intake, which has been shown to reduce cystine excretion.[23] Fluid intake of at least 4-5 L of water per day (3 L in children) will dilute urinary cystine concentrations and reduce precipitation. Intake should ensure diuresis throughout the night, including the post-micturation period.[24,25] Alkalinization of the urine increases the solubility of cystine, so administration of potassium citrate is recommended in patients with severe renal disease. To adequately alkalinize the urine, urinary pH determination should initially be made at least 3 times a day. High alkalinization of the urine carries the risk of calcium phosphate kidney stone formation. If these methods fail, agents that induce the conversion of cystine to cysteine can be used if cystine excretion is >3 mmol/day.[8] The most widely used agents for this purpose are D-penicillamine

and a-mercaptopropionylglycine (MPG), which effectively cleave the disulfide bond of cystine to form cysteine (**Figure 2**), resulting in a 50-fold increase in solubility.[26-28] High dose ascorbic acid acts similarly by cleaving the disulfide bond in cystine. Unfortunately, the treatment of patients with cystinuria by these various modalities has limited efficacy, major side effects, and high recurrence rates resulting in poor patient compliance and a high risk of renal impairment over time.

9. In addition to medical therapy to prevent kidney stones, shock wave lithotripsy, uteroscopy and laser lithotripsy, percutaneous nephrolithotome, open surgery, and renal transplantation can be utilized to remove kidney stones once they are formed. Shock wave lithotripsy is a non-invasive method to disrupt upper urinary tract stones <1.5 cm in size. Uteroscopy and laser lithotripsy can be used on larger stones (1.5 to 2 cm), while percutaneous nephrolithotomy may be utilized when stones are >2 cm in diameter. For larger, complex stones, open surgery may be necessary. Renal transplantation has been performed on patients with renal failure precipitated by cystine renal stones. Interestingly, it appears that recurrent nephrolithiasis does not occur in transplanted kidneys as would be expected based on the pathophysiology of this disease.[29-32]

10. **Patient follow-up:** The patient's parents were instructed to increase the patient's fluid intake to 3 L/day, alkalinize the urine with Polycitra-K (potassium citrate, 7.5 mL b.i.d.), and monitor the child's urine pH. Two months later, no intervening abdominal, pelvic, or flank pain, or gross hematuria, was reported. Daily urine pH values were consistently in excess of 7, and the child had been compliant with her increased fluid intake. No crystals were found in her urine, and a renal ultrasound revealed only persistent small stones in the right kidney.

Keywords _____

cystinuria, cystine, nephrolithiasis, kidney stones, crystals, inborn errors of metabolism, rBAT, b^0+AT

References _____

1. Fuller CE, Threatte GA, Bernard JB. Basic examination of urine. In *Clinical Diagnosis and Management by Laboratory Methods.* Henry, JB, 3d. Philadelphia: W.B. Saunders Company; 2001:367-402.

2. Perheentupa J, Visakorpi JK. Protein intolerance with deficient transport of basic aminoacids. Another inborn error of metabolism. *Lancet.* 1965;2:813-816.

3. Kekomaki M, Visakorpi JK, Perheentupa J, et al. Familial protein intolerance with deficient transport of basic amino acids. An analysis of 10 patients. *Acta Paediatr Scand.* 1967;56:617-30.

4. Norio R, Perheentupa J, Kekomaki M, et al. Lysinuric protein intolerance, an autosomal recessive disease. A genetic study of 10 Finnish families. *Clin Genet.* 1971;2:214-22.

5. Simell O. Lysinuric Protein Intolerance and Other Cationic Aminoacidurias: In *The Online Metabolic & Molecular Bases of Inherited Disease.* Scriver, et al, eds. The McGraw-Hill Companies, 2001-2005.

6. Coward RJ, et al. Epidemiology of paediatric renal stone disease in the UK. *Arch Dis Child.* 2003;88: 962-965.

7. Pras E. Cystinuria at the turn of the millennium: clinical aspects and new molecular developments. *Mol Urol.* 2000;4:409-414.

8. Knoll T, Zollner A, Wendt-Nordahl G, et al. Cystinuria in childhood and adolescence: recommendations for diagnosis, treatment, and follow-up. *Pediatr Nephrol.* 2005;20:19-24.

9. Fekkes D. State-of-the-art of high-performance liquid chromatographic analysis of amino acids in physiological samples. *J Chromatogr B Biomed Appl.* 1996;682:3-22.

10. Holmgren G, Jeppson JO, Samuelson G. High-voltage electrophoresis in urinary amino acid screening. *Scand J Clin Lab Invest.* 1970;26;313-318.

11. Bayer E, Grom E, Kalteneger B, et al. Separation of amino acids by high performance liquid chromatography. *Anal Chem.* 1976;48:1106-1109.

12. Guerra A, et al. A simple quantitative test for screening cystinuria. *Lab Med.* 2002;33:214-217.

13. Trinchieri A, Dormia G, Montanari E, et al. Cystinuria: definition, epidemiology and clinical aspects. *Arch Ital Urol Androl.* 2004;76:129-134.

14. Schon R, Thalhammer O. [Routine screening for inborn errors using urine filterpaper specimens at age 4-5 weeks (author's transl)]. *Padiatr Padol.* 1976;11:319-325.

15. Cabello-Tomas ML, Garcia-Gomez AM, Guillen-Dominguez ML. Pilot screening programme for cystinuria in the Valencian community. *Eur J Epidemiol.* 1999;15:681-684.

16. Dent CE, Senior B. Studies on the treatment of cystinuria. *Br J Urol.* 1955;27:317-332.

17. Nakagawa Y, Asplin JR, Goldfarb DS, et al. Clinical use of cystine supersaturation measurements. *J Urol.* 2000;164:1481-5.

18. Langman CB. The molecular basis of kidney stones. *Curr Opin Pediatr.* 2004;16:188-193.

19. Chillaron J, et al. An intracellular trafficking defect in type I cystinuria rBAT mutants M467T and M467K. *J Biol Chem.* 1997;272:9543-9549.

20. Calonge MJ, et al. Cystinuria caused by mutations in rBAT, a gene involved in the transport of cystine. *Nat Genet.* 1994;6:420-425.

21. Dello Strologo L, et al. Comparison between SLC3A1 and SLC7A9 cystinuria patients and carriers: A need for a new classification. *J Am Soc Nephrol.* 2002;13:2547-53.

22. Guillen M, Corella D, Cabello ML, et al. Reference values of urinary excretion of cystine and dibasic aminoacids: Classification of patients with cystinuria in the Valencian Community, Spain. *Clin Biochem.* 1999;32:25-30.

23. Rodriguez LM, Santos F, Malaga S, et al. Effect of a low sodium diet on urinary elimination of cystine in cystinuric children. *Nephron.* 1995;71:416-418.

24. Monnens LA, Noordam K, Trijbels F. Necessary practical treatment of cystinuria at night. *Pediatr Nephrol.* 2000;14:1148-9.

25. Fjellstedt E, Denneberg T, Jeppsson JO, et al. A comparison of the effects of potassium citrate and sodium bicarbonate in the alkalinization of urine in homozygous cystinuria. *Urol Res.* 2001;29:295-302.

26. Chow GK, Streem SB. Medical treatment of cystinuria: Results of contemporary clinical practice. *J Urol.* 1996;156:1576-8.

27. Harbar JA, Cusworth DC, Lawes LC, et al. Comparison of 2-mercaptopropionylglycine and D-penicillamine in the treatment of cystinuria. *J Urol.* 1986;136:146-9.

28. Pak CY, Fuller C, Sakhaee K, et al. Management of cystine nephrolithiasis with alpha-mercaptopropionylglycine. *J Urol.* 1986;136:1003-8.

29. Tuso P, Barnett M, Yasunaga C, et al. Cystinuria and renal transplantation. *Nephron.* 1993;63:478.

30. Hayes JM, Streem SB, Graneto D, et al. Urolithiasis after renal transplantation. *Transplant Proc.* 1989;21:1960-1961.

31. Krizek V, Erben J, Lazne M, et al. Disappearance of cystinuria after kidney transplantation. *Br J Urol.* 1983;55:575.

32. Hoitsma AJ, Koene RA, Trijbels FJ, et al. Disappearance of cystinuria after renal transplantation. *JAMA.* 1983;250:615.

33. Verrey F, et al. Novel renal amino acid transporters. *Annu Rev Physiol.* 2005;67:557-72.

Hepatosplenomegaly in an 8-Month-Old Child

Monte S. Willis, Alice A. Basinger, Zheng Fan, Surekha Pendyal, Joseph Muenzer, Catherine Hammett-Stabler

Departments of Pathology & Laboratory Medicine and Pediatrics, University of North Carolina, Chapel Hill, NC

Patient: 8-month-old female.

Chief Complaint: Enlarged abdomen and leg weakness.

History of Present Illness: The mother reported that the child had a 3-month history of increasing abdominal girth and progressive loss of leg strength.

Past Medical History: The mother stated that during her full-term pregnancy with the child, there were no complications. Additionally, an expanded newborn screen by tandem mass spectrometry was negative for abnormal metabolites in a blood sample obtained at 36 hours post-delivery.

Family History: A sibling died at age 3 with an enlarged abdomen; however, the cause of death was undetermined.

Physical Examination Findings: The patient's abdomen was markedly distended and both the liver and spleen were palpable approximately 6 cm below the costal margin (**Image 1A**). While the patient's upper extremities had normal tone and strength, her lower extremities were weak bilaterally (**Image 1B**).

Additional Laboratory Studies: A urine organic acid profile revealed elevated tyrosine metabolites, specifically 4-hydroxy-phenylpyruvate (4-HPP), succinylacetoacetate (SAA) oxime derivative, and succinylacetone (SA). Plasma amino acid analysis detected an elevated tyrosine level (245 µmol/L; reference range: 26-110 µmol/L).

Additional Clinical Studies: Magnetic resonance imaging (MRI) studies revealed a fibrotic, cirrhotic-appearing liver with enumerable nodules (**Image 2A**). Gadolinium-contrast MRI did not detect lesions that became enhanced (ie, white on MRI) (**Image 2B**), which is a characteristic finding in patients with hepatocellular carcinoma. In addition, MRI detected portal vein dilation and splenomegaly consistent with portal hypertension.

Questions _____

1. What are this patient's most striking clinical and laboratory findings?

2. How do you explain this patient's most striking clinical and laboratory findings?

3. How is tyrosine catabolized in vivo?

4. Is the patient's increased plasma tyrosine level diagnostically specific in identifying the cause of this patient's signs and symptoms?

5. What is this patient's most likely diagnosis?

6. What is the pathophysiology of this patient's disease?

T1. Principal Laboratory Findings

Test	Patient's Result	"Normal" Reference Interval
Hematology		
WBC count	13.9	6.0-17.5 × 10³/μL
RBC count	4.0	3.7-5.3 × 10⁶/μL
Hemoglobin	12.1	10.5-13.5 g/dL
Hematocrit	36.3	33-39%
Platelet count	145	150-440 × 10³/μL
PBS findings	Anisopoikilocytosis; atypical lymphocytes	
Coagulation		
PT	17.7	11.0-14.0 sec
INR	1.5	
aPTT	54.7	22.0-32.4 sec
Chemistry		
Sodium	139	135-145 mEq/L
Potassium	4.7	4.1-5.3 mEq/L
Chloride	105	98-107 mEq/L
CO_2	23	23-30 mEq/L
Total protein	6.8	6.6-8.0 g/dL
Albumin	4.4	3.5-5.0 g/dL
AST	109	22-63 U/L
ALT	74	12-45 U/L
ALP	1051	145-320 U/L
GGT	384	11-48 U/L
α-Fetoprotein	8,862	<10 ng/mL
Phosphorus	2.9	4.8-8.1 mg/dL
Creatinine	0.3	0.3-0.6 mg/dL
BUN	5	4-19 mg/dL
Ammonia	<5	9-33 μmol/L
Amylase	33	0-79 U/L
Lipase	101	10-128 U/L

WBC, white blood cell; RBC, red blood cell; PBS, peripheral blood smear; PT, prothrombin time; INR, International Normalized Ratio; aPTT, activated partial thromboplastin time; AST, aspartate aminotransferase; ALT, alanine aminotransferase; GGT, gamma-glutamyltransferase; BUN, blood urea nitrogen.

7. What are the consequences of failing to identify and adequately treat this patient's disease?

8. How should individuals suspected of having this patient's disease be monitored?

9. How is this patient's condition typically treated?

10. What is the role of laboratory testing in this patient's condition?

11. How should this patient's disease be confirmed?

12. What is the patient's prognosis?

Possible Answers

1. The most striking clinical findings in this patient include: a 3-month history of abdominal distension and leg weakness; a dramatically enlarged liver and spleen on physical exam; and muscle weakness/hypotonia. Strikingly abnormal laboratory values included: elevated liver function tests (LFTs: AST, ALT, ALP, GGT); elevated a-fetoprotein (AFP); elevated direct and indirect bilirubin concentrations; prolonged PT and PTT; decreased phosphorous level; the presence of urinary SAA and SA; and an elevated serum tyrosine level.

2. From the infant's physical examination and imaging studies, the progressive abdominal distension observed by her mother is explained by the enlarged liver and spleen. Furthermore, the basic biochemical and hematological laboratory test results indicate that neither organ was functioning appropriately. When investigating hepatosplenomegaly and abnormal LFTs in a child of this age, one should include in the differential causes of physical obstruction, primary liver disease, toxic injury, infectious agents, as well as several inherited metabolic disorders. Although the imaging studies found evidence of hepatic fibrosis and portal hypertension, there was no evidence of a structural cause of obstruction such as a tumor. While primary liver diseases such as hemolytic uremic syndrome, primary biliary cirrhosis, and sclerosing cholangitis are possible, these diseases do not have an association with peripheral neuropathies. Since a sibling of this child had exhibited an extended abdomen

T2. Diseases Associated With Inborn Errors of Metabolism and Hepatosplenomegaly

Disease	Defect	Symptoms/Features
Glycogen storage diseases	Enzymes that form or release glycogen	General muscle symptoms, such as weakness and cramps; specific syndromes, such as hypoglycemic seizures or cardiomegaly, may be present
Lysosomal storage diseases	Lysosomal enzymes responsible for the turnover of cell constituents	Neurodegeneration
Galactosemia	Enzymes responsible for degrading galactose	Acute: Jaundice, vomiting, lethargy, irritability, and convulsions
		Chronic: Continued feeding of milk products leads to liver cirrhosis, cataract formation, and mental retardation
Peroxisomal storage diseases	Perioxisome metabolic pathway enzymes participating in β-oxidation of certain fatty acids and biosynthesis of phospholipids, bile acids, and isoprene compounds	Complex developmental and metabolic phenotypes
Tyrosinemia	Deficiency in the enzymes necessary for tyrosine degradation	Highly variable and include cirrhosis, acute liver failure, hepatocarcinoma, renal Fanconi syndrome, and peripheral neuropathy crises
Bile acid disorders	Enzymes in bile acid biosynthesis	Jaundice, hepatomegaly, pale stools, dark urine
Congenital glycosylation diseases	Defects in the synthesis of the glycan moiety of glycoproteins	Specific dysmorphy with moderate to severe neurologic involvement

T3. Diseases Associated With Defects in Enzymes of the Tyrosine Catabolic Pathway

Disease	Enzyme Defect	Symptoms/Features
Hereditary tyrosinemia type I[a]	Fumaryl-acetoacetate hydrolase	Severe neurological symptoms, acute liver failure, hepatocellular carcinoma
Hereditary tyrosinemia type II	Tyrosine aminotransferase	Corneal ulcers, dendritic keratitis, photophobia, pain, excessive lacrimation
Hereditary tyrosinemia type III	4-Hydroxyphenyl pyruvate dioxygenase	Neurologic dysfunction, ataxia, seizures, psychomotor retardation
Alkaptonuria	Homogentisate oxidase	Arthritis, alkylosis

[a]*Most severe form of hereditary tyrosinemia.*

before death, the focus of efforts to identify the cause of this infant's hepatosplenomegaly was a genetic disorder (**T2**) not detected by the newborn screen. The genetic disorders shown in **T2** are congenital inborn errors of metabolism associated with hepatosplenomegaly.

3. Tyrosine is an essential component of thyroid hormone, catecholamines, and melanin and is degraded through a series of enzymatic reactions (**Figure 1**). Impaired tyrosine catabolism is a feature of several genetic disorders, in which

enzymatic defects lead to an accumulation of metabolites [ie, fumarylacetoacetic acid (FAA), maleylacetoacetic acid (MAA), and SA] that precede the defect in the catabolic pathway. The specific diseases associated with these enzymatic defects are a result of the toxicity of these metabolites. Depending on the enzyme defect, the resulting phenotype can range from mild to extremely severe, resulting in death in infancy.

4. Unfortunately, the finding of an increased plasma tyrosine level is not diagnostically specific for

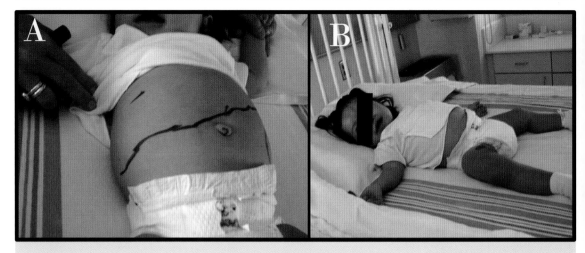

Image 1_At presentation, the patient's liver was 6 inches below (lower black marker line) the costal margin (**A**), while the patient's lower extremities demonstrated weakness/hypotonia bilaterally (**B**).

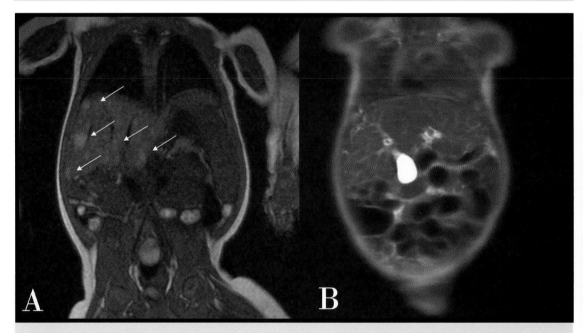

Image 2_MRI showing the patient's fibrotic, nodular, cirrhotic-appearing liver with numerous nodules (arrows) (**A**) that were not enhanced with contrast media (**B**), suggesting that hepatocarcinoma was not present.

an inborn error of metabolism. Mildly increased tyrosine concentrations are seen in scurvy, hyperthyroidism, in response to fasting, and following ingestion of tyrosine-rich foods. Mild to extremely elevated tyrosine concentrations are commonly encountered in patients with severe liver dysfunction or 1 of the several types of tyrosinemia. Laboratory testing plays a key role in the evaluation of these patients as pertinent findings can allow some disorders to be excluded and others to be investigated further. The most difficult differentiation to make in patients presenting with tyrosinemia is between inherited forms and liver disease of other etiologies. In addition to transient tyrosinemia of the newborn, 3 types of tyrosinemia have been described: type I, type II, and type III.[1-3] Transient tyrosinemia of the newborn occurs in up to 10% of premature infants and to a lesser degree in full-term infants.[1-3] It results from the

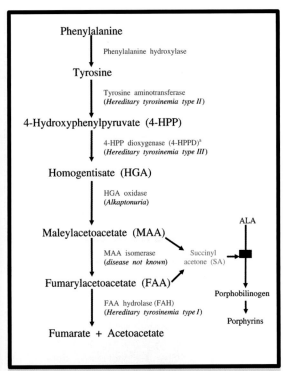

Figure 1_Tyrosine catabolic pathway found predominantly in hepatocytes and cells of the proximal renal tubules. The disease associated with an enzyme deficiency is shown in parentheses below the affected enzyme (modified from Endo, et al, 2003). Black box indicates site where SA blocks the conversion of delta-aminolevulinic acid (ALA) to porphobilinogen. Nitisinone inhibits 4-HPPD.

immaturity of the newborn hepatic microsomal enzymes, specifically 4-hydroxy-phenylpyruvate dioxygenase (4-HPPD) (**Figure 1**). As the name suggests, the infant's tyrosine concentrations return to normal as the liver matures in the weeks/months following birth. Typically, these infants do not exhibit neurological symptoms as were seen in our patient. Acute neurologic crises are associated with the inherited forms of tyrosinemia and can manifest as ataxia, seizures, psychomotor retardation, severe central nervous system (CNS) dysfunction, and peripheral neuropathies. Peripheral neuropathies are often found in cases of hereditary tyrosinemia type I (HTI) while patients with hereditary tyrosinemia type III (HTIII) tend to present with more severe CNS involvement. In determining the cause of an elevated serum tyrosine concentration, it is most important to look for other causes of liver disease as soon as possible, because HTI

requires immediate, aggressive therapy to reduce morbidity and mortality.[4]

5. **Most likely diagnosis**: *hereditary tyrosinemia type I.* The physical exam, most notably leg weakness and hepatosplenomegaly, and laboratory findings [eg, increased urine concentration of the tyrosine metabolite, SA] in our patient are most consistent with HTI.

Hereditary tyrosinemia type I (HTI) is a rare disorder estimated to occur at a rate of 1 case per 100,000-120,000 newborns.[5] The presence of urine SA is pathognomonic for HTI and reflects a defect in the tyrosine metabolic pathway. There are, however, a few cases of HTI in which SA was not increased, yet HTI was documented via genetic testing.[5] The gene mutations involved result in a deficiency in the enzyme fumarylacetoacetate hydrolase (FAH) (**Figure 1**) and lead to the accumulation of upstream metabolites (ie, SA). Since the tyrosine metabolic pathway is found predominantly in hepatocytes and cells of the proximal renal tubules, the liver and kidneys are the organs primarily affected by defects in tyrosine catabolism.[6] To date, 34 mutations in the FAH gene have been associated with HTI.[7] These mutations cluster between amino acids 230-250. These findings have led to the development of animal models for studying the effect of these mutations on the development and severity of HTI.[8]

6. The pathophysiology of HTI is a direct result of the accumulation of upstream metabolites. Both FAA and MAA are thought to act as alkylating agents and act as alkylating agents and disrupt sulfhydryl metabolism. These actions likely contribute to the increased incidence of hepatocellular carcinoma observed in affected patients. In addition, FAA is known to deplete glutathione, initiate premature cell apotosis, and induce chromosomal breakage.[9-11] Damage to the proximal renal tubules results in defective phosphorous uptake and mimics the defect found in Fanconi anemia.

7. Without treatment, HTI patients have a shortened lifespan. Many die of acute liver failure before age 2, while those who survive childhood often develop chronic liver failure or hepatocellular carcinoma by the age of 20.[4] Clinically,

untreated HTI manifests in hepatic, renal, and neurologic disease. Complications of liver failure that may occur include jaundice, ascites, and hemorrhage. In some HTI patients, a prominent coagulopathy due to liver failure is the main presenting feature.[12] Renal involvement, which may be irreversible, ranges from mild tubular dysfunction to renal failure.[13-15] Because of the defective phosphorous uptake, it is not unusual to find hypophosphatemic rickets in association with HTI. Neurologic involvement relates to the inhibition of aminolevulinate dehydratase by increased plasma levels of SA. Disruption of the heme pathway at this point leads to an accumulation of porphyrins and a secondary peripheral neuropathy and muscle weakness. Acute neurologic crises in HTI, presenting as sudden peripheral neuropathies, have 2 phases: (1) active painful parathesias; and (2) a reprieve followed by paralytic crisis. Porphyria-like neurologic symptoms manifesting as muscle weakness or paralysis, generally seen in patients not undergoing therapy, have been identified in 42% of HTI patients.[16] In our patient with HTI, hepatocyte and proximal renal tubule damage may have manifested in abnormal liver function tests and hypophosphatemia. Direct liver damage can be identified by the presence of abnormally elevated a-fetoprotein and LFTs (**T1**). The inability of the liver to synthesize clotting factors is likely responsible for the patient's prolonged PT and PTT results. Although porphyrins were not quantified, the patient's lower extremity weakness/hypotonia is likely related to an inhibition of heme synthesis by SA.

8. Therapy for HTI includes dietary management, oral administration of NTBC [2-(2-nitro-4-trifluoromethylbenzoyl)-1,3-cyclohexanedione], and liver transplantation. The goal of dietary management is to reduce tyrosine intake. This is achieved by limiting dietary intake of phenylalanine and tyrosine. Specifically, special metabolic formulas that lack tyrosine and phenylalanine, but which are otherwise nutritionally complete, are used in infants and older individuals to meet overall protein needs. High protein foods (eg, meats, poultry, dairy, nuts, and legumes) are eliminated from the diet. Additionally, fruits, vegetables, and starchy foods are used to make up the natural protein component of the diet and are used to supply the phenylalanine and

tyrosine necessary to maintain blood levels in the range required to support normal growth and development. The drug NTBC, originally developed as a herbicide, inhibits the second step of tyrosine degradation by inhibiting 4-HPPD (**Figure 1**). Inhibition of this enzyme prevents the accumulation of FAA, MAA, and SA and as a result leads to a milder clinical presentation that is biochemically similar to hereditary tyrosinemia type III (**T3**). The first trial of NTBC in HTI patients, performed over a decade ago, demonstrated a significant clinical improvement in 90% of treated patients.[17] The success of NTBC treatment is monitored by quantifying serum tyrosine and SA concentrations, and monitoring the patient clinically for the development of signs and symptoms of hepatic carcinoma and renal dysfunction. Neurologic crises, when they occur, may be managed by glucose infusion, which inhibits delta-aminolevulinic acid (ALA) synthetase and porphyrin accumulation.[18] For patients who have persistent liver dysfunction or develop hepatic carcinoma, liver transplantation is an option.[19-21]

9. Laboratory testing is important in both the diagnosis of HTI and its management. Although the patient underwent expanded newborn screening that included measurement of tyrosine concentrations using tandem mass spectrometry, the diagnosis of HTI was not made until later. Unfortunately in HTI, tyrosine concentrations do not typically exceed the cutoff value (500 μmol/L in this particular case) associated with HTI until after the time at which most newborn screening is performed. In this case, the patient's screen, obtained 36 hours after birth, demonstrated a tyrosine value of 120 μmol/L, well under the cutoff value of 300 μmol/L. Conversely, the defect in hereditary tyrosinemia type II occurs at the initial step of tyrosine degradation, resulting in higher tyrosine levels in the first few days after birth that are more likely to be detected if included in newborn screening. As mentioned above, elevated serum tyrosine levels in transient tyrosinemia of the newborn are also detected in the first few days after birth. Therefore, a serum tyrosine cutoff value of 300 μmol/L is used to reduce the number of false positives relating to transient tyrosinemia. Nevertheless, the distinction between HTI and transient tyrosinemia by tyrosine levels

alone is difficult. Some states have instituted multiple newborn screenings with a second sample collected several weeks after birth. In such protocols, the likelihood of detecting HTI by measuring serum tyrosine concentration is greatly increased. Measurement of SA in blood or urine, however, offers the greatest diagnostic specificity.[22,23] Due to the high incidence of HTI in some regions of Quebec, Canada, that province's newborn screening program includes evaluation of SA by GC-MS using dried blood spots from individuals with elevated tyrosine levels. A similar approach to identifying affected newborns is being considered by some states in the United States for inclusion in their newborn screening programs.

10. Since FAA's short half-life makes it difficult to detect, the longer-lived SA metabolite is monitored. Detection of urine SA using GC-MS as part of an organic acid profile is adequate for both the diagnosis and can be used in the management of HTI. Additionally, plasma tyrosine and phenylalanine levels are often monitored. Monitoring of urine organic acid and plasma tyrosine levels should be performed monthly for the first year after diagnosis and subsequently every 3 months. Since leukopenia and thrombocytopenia may occur in HTI, it is important that a routine CBC be performed. Additional testing should include an annual ophthalmologic exam and hepatic MRI with and without contrast media.[4]

11. Confirmation of HTI can be made by assaying cultured skin fibroblasts for FAH enzyme activity. Presently, at least 9 laboratories in the United States commercially perform FAH enzyme activity testing (www.GeneTests.com). These laboratories offer additional, although mainly research-oriented, FAH mutation analysis.

In an international study of 108 HTI patients receiving dietary treatment alone, survival correlated with the age of disease onset.[24] In this study, the most common causes of death included recurrent bleeding and liver failure (67%), hepatocellular carcinoma (17%), and a porphyria-like syndrome associated with respiratory failure (10%).[24] If the onset of symptoms occurred before 2 months of age, there was a 38% and 29% probability of 1- and 2-year survival, respectively.

If symptoms began between 2 and 6 months, the 1- and 2-year survival increased to 74%. Onset of symptoms after 6 months increased 1- and 2-year survival to 96%.[24] In general, chronic hepatic failure occurs by age 2 in patients presenting earlier, while those with later onset die in mid-childhood from hepatic carcinoma or liver failure. The international study of HTI indicated above did not include patients on NTBC therapy. Since NTBC therapy for HTI is relatively new and the disease is relatively rare, long-term outcome studies are needed to assess the impact of this treatment on patient outcome and survival. Based on initial studies, however, it is predicted that NTBC therapy will increase life expectancy and decrease the risk of hepatocellular carcinoma.[17] Despite this optimistic initial study, however, recent studies have reported the occurrence of hepatocellular carcinoma after NTBC treatment, demonstrating that it remains to be determined if NTBC therapy is sufficient to prevent the development of carcinoma if it is already present.[25]

Patient Follow-up

The patient was placed on a low tyrosine, low phenylalanine food formula, along with NTBC (4 mg BID mixed in formula). Within days of therapy initiation, marked improvement was seen in the patient's irritability. After 1 month of therapy, SA was undetectable in her urine, her lower extremity weakness resolved, and her liver enzyme levels decreased (ALP, 265 U/L; total bilirubin, 0.3 mg/dL; AFP, 2,537 ng/mL). Since the initial elevated (1.6-8–fold the upper limit of normal) liver enzyme levels (**T1**) reflected significant hepatocellular damage, an extended period of time for enzyme values to normalize is expected. Close monitoring for adequate NTBC therapy, hepatocellular carcinoma, and neurologic symptoms will be the focus of future follow-up of this patient. The patient's diet will be titrated to maintain plasma phenylalanine concentration in the normal range, tyrosine levels <400 μM, and to allow for normal growth and development.

Keywords

FAH deficiency, hepatorenal tyrosinemia, hereditary tyrosinemia type I

References

1. Neto EC, Schulte J, Anele E, et al. Persistent tyrosinemia detected by thin-layer chromatography. *Southeast Asian J Trop Med Public Health.* 1999;30(Suppl 2):151.

2. Levy HL, Shih VE, Madigan PM, et al. Transient tyrosinemia in full-term infants. *JAMA.* 1969;209:249-250.

3. Fernbach SA, Summons RE, Pereira WE, et al. Metabolic studies of transient tyrosinemia in premature infants. *Pediatr Res.* 1975;9:172-176.

4. Grompe M. Disorders of tyrosine metabolism. *Up-to-date.* 2005.

5. De Braekeleer M. Hereditary disorders in Saguenay-Lac-St-Jean (Quebec, Canada). *Hum Hered.* 1991;41:141-146.

6. Grompe M. The pathophysiology and treatment of hereditary tyrosinemia Type I. *Semin Liver Dis.* 2001;21:563-571.

7. St-Louis M, Tanguay RM. Mutations in the fumarylacetoacetate hydrolase gene causing hereditary tyrosinemia type I: Overview. *Hum Mutat.* 1997;9:291-299.

8. Endo F et al. Animal models reveal pathophysiologies of tyrosinemias. *J Nutr.* 2003;133:2063S-2067S.

9. Liang HC, Shertzer HG, Nebert DW. "Oxidative stress" response in liver of an untreated newborn mouse having a 1.2-centimorgan deletion on chromosome 7. *Biochem Biophys Res Commun.* 1992;182:1160-1165.

10. Jorquera R, Tanguay RM. The mutagenicity of the tyrosine metabolite, fumarylacetoacetate, is enhanced by glutathione depletion. *Biochem Biophys Res Commun.* 1997;232:42-48.

11. Manning K, Al-Dhalimy M, Finegold M, et al. In vivo suppressor mutations correct a murine model of hereditary tyrosinemia type I. *Proc Natl Acad Sci USA.* 1999;96:11928-33.

12. Nussinovitch M, Campino G, Shapira R, et al. Liver failure with coagulopathy in an infant with tyrosinemia. *Harefuah.* 2001;140:578-9, 680.

13. Suzuki Y, Konda M, Imai I, et al. Effect of dietary treatment on the renal tubular function in a patient with hereditary tyrosinemia. *Int J Pediatr Nephrol.* 1987;8:171-6.

14. McDiarmid SV. Renal function in pediatric liver transplant patients. *Kidney Int Suppl.* 1996;53:S77-84.

15. Kvittingen EA, Jellum E, Stokke O, et al. Liver transplantation in a 23-year-old tyrosinaemia patient: Effects on the renal tubular dysfunction. *J Inherit Metab Dis.* 1986;9:216-224.

16. Mitchell G et al. Neurologic crises in hereditary tyrosinemia. *N Engl J Med.* 1990;322:432-437.

17. Holme E, Lindstedt S. Tyrosinaemia type I and NTBC (2-(2-nitro-4-trifluoromethylbenzoyl)-1,3-cyclohexanedione). *J Inherit Metab Dis.* 1998;21:507-517.

18. Handschin J, Lin J, Rhee J, et al. Nutritional regulation of hepatic heme biosynthesis and porphyria through PGC-1alpha. *Cell.* 2005;122:505-15.

19. Mohan N, McKiernan P, Preece MA, et al. Indications and outcome of liver transplantation in tyrosinaemia Type I. *Eur J Pediatr.* 1999;158(Suppl 2):S49-54.

20. Esquivel CO, Mieles L, Marino IR, et al. Liver transplantation for hereditary tyrosinemia in the presence of hepatocellular carcinoma. *Transplant Proc.* 1989;21:2445-6.

21. Mieles LA, Esquivel CO, Van Thiel DH, et al. Liver transplantation for tyrosinemia. A review of 10 cases from the University of Pittsburgh. *Dig Dis Sci.* 1990;35:153-7.

22. Allard P, Grenier A, Korson MS, et al. Newborn screening for hepatorenal tyrosinemia by tandem mass spectrometry: Analysis of succinylacetone extracted from dried blood spots. *Clin Biochem.* 2004;37:1010-1015.

23. Rashed MS, Al-Ahaidib Ly, Al-Dirbashi OY, et al. Tandem mass spectrometric assay of succinylacetone in urine for the diagnosis of hepatorenal tyrosinemia. *Anal Biochem.* 2005;339:310-317.

24. van Spronsen FJ, Bijlveld CM, van Maldeger BI, et al. Hereditary tyrosinemia type I: A new clinical classification with difference in prognosis on dietary treatment. *Hepatology.* 1994;20:1187-1191.

25. van Spronsen FJ, Bijleveld CM, van Maldegem BT, et al. Hepatocellular carcinoma in hereditary tyrosinemia type I despite 2-(2 nitro-4-3 trifluoro- methylbenzoyl)-1, 3-cyclohexanedione treatment. *J Pediatr Gastroenterol Nutr.* 2005;40:90-93.

A Neonate With Hyperammonemia

Dinesh Rakheja,[1] Michael B. Bober,[2] Susan L. Fisher,[1] Patricia M. Jones[1]

[1]*Departments of Pathology and* [2]*Pediatrics, Children's Medical Center and The University of Texas Southwestern Medical Center, Dallas TX*

Patient: 12-day-old African-American male infant.

Chief Complaint: Failure to thrive, lethargy, feeding intolerance, and strong body odor.

History of Present Illness: The patient was the smaller of a pair of twins delivered by a 24-year-old primigravida at an outside institution. Because of this twin's intrauterine growth retardation, labor was induced at 36 weeks gestation. At birth, he weighed 3 pounds and 9 ounces. Over the first 9 days of life, he required intravenous (IV) glucose in addition to his Isomil feeds to maintain euglycemia. He was switched to breast milk on day 9 and subsequently developed feeding intolerance and emesis. On day 10, he became lethargic and developed a strong body odor. Laboratory tests revealed mildly elevated serum ammonia (206 mmol/L) with no acidosis. The next day he became progressively more lethargic and subsequently comatose; his serum ammonia was 1,396 mmol/L and there was no acidosis. At this time, he was transferred to our hospital.

Past Medical/Surgical History: The perinatal course had been apparently unremarkable.

Family/Social History: The twin sibling is apparently healthy.

Physical Examination: At the time of admission, the infant appeared dehydrated with dry, wrinkled skin and decreased subcutaneous fat stores. He was comatose with minimal spontaneous movements. Neurological examination showed generalized hypotonia with 4+ reflexes. There was ankle clonus with 9 beats.

Additional Diagnostic Procedures and Tests: Sonographic examination of the head showed symmetric increased echogenicity of the periventricular white matter and thalami. These were interpreted as nonspecific findings related either to a hypoxic event or to a metabolic disorder.

Questions _____

1. What are this patient's most striking clinical and laboratory findings?

2. How do you explain these findings?

3. What additional laboratory testing should be performed on this neonate and why?

4. What is the patient's most likely diagnosis?

5. What is the biochemical and pathophysiologic basis of this disease?

6. What is the genetic basis of this disease?

T1. Principal Laboratory Findings

Test	Patient's Result	"Normal" Reference Range
Hematology		
WBC count	1.7	5-19 × 10³/µL
RBC count	3.26	3.6-6.2 × 10³/µL
Hemoglobin	10.9	12.5-20.5 g/dL
Hematocrit	32.6	39-63%
MCV	100	86-124 fL
MCH	33.4	28-40 pg
MCHC	33.4	32-36 g/dL
RDW	17	11.5-15.0%
Platelet count	3	150-600 × 10³/µL
Absolute neutrophil count	0.14	1.00-9.00 × 10³/µL
Chemistry		
Sodium	138	139-146 mEq/L
Potassium	4.5	3.0-7.0 mEq/L
Chloride	103	98-106 mEq/L
CO_2	25	18-31 mEq/L
Anion gap	11	5-14
Glucose	275	74-127 mg/dL
Calcium, ionized	1.09	1.12-1.32 mmol/L
Phosphorus	4.6	5.0-8.0 mg/dL
Magnesium	1.8	1.6-2.4 mEq/L
BUN	12	2-19 mg/dL
Creatinine	1.1	0.2-0.6 mg/dL
Albumin	1.9	3.9-5.0 g/dL
Ammonia	1182	56-92 mmol/L
Lactic acid	2.5	0.7-2.3 mmol/L
Venous blood: pH	7.31	7.35-7.45
gases pCO_2	45	41-54 mm Hg
pO_2	30	30-50 mm Hg
HCO_3	23	17-24 mEq/L
Amino acid screen: Serum	2,606 (arginine)	6-140 µmol/L
Organic acid screen: Urine	Positive for increased concentrations of: lactic acid, 3-hydroxyisovaleric acid, methylsuccinic acid, methylfumaric acid, isovalerylglycine	Negative for increased concentration of an organic acid

WBC, white blood cell; RBC, red blood cell; MCV, mean corpuscular volume; MCH, mean corpuscular hemoglobin; MCHC, mean corpuscular hemoglobin concentration; RDW, red blood cell distribution width; BUN, blood urea nitrogen

T2. Possible Causes of Hyperammonemia in Infants

Urea cycle disorders
- N-acetylglutamate synthetase deficiency
- Carbamyl phosphate synthetase 1 deficiency
- Ornithine transcarbamylase deficiency
- Argininosuccinic acid synthetase deficiency
- Argininosuccinic lyase deficiency
- Arginase deficiency

Organic acidemias
- Isovaleric acidemia
- Propionic acidemia
- Methylmalonic acidemia
- Glutaric acidemia type II
- Multiple carboxylase deficiency
- Beta-ketothiolase deficiency

Congenital lactic acidosis
- Pyruvate dehydrogenase deficiency
- Pyruvate carboxylase deficiency
- Mitochondrial disorders

Disorders of dibasic amino acid transport
- Lysinuric protein intolerance
- Hyperammonemia-hyperornithemia-homocitrullinuria

Fatty acid oxidation disorders

Transient hyperammonemia of the newborn

Asphyxia

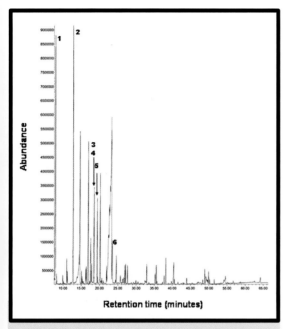

Figure 1_Gas chromatography/mass spectrometry results from the patient's initial urine specimen showed elevated levels of lactic acid (peak #1), 3-hydroxyisovaleric acid (peak #2), methylsuccinic acid (peak #3), methylfumaric acid (peak #5), and isovalerylglycine (peak #6). Peak #4 represents the internal standard (2-phenylbutyric acid).

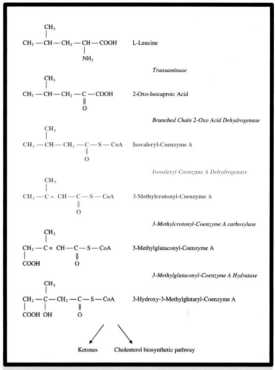

Figure 2_Isovaleryl-coenzyme A dehydrogenase catalyzes the oxidation of isovaleryl-coenzyme A to 3-methylcrotonyl-coenzyme A, a step in the catabolic pathway of the amino acid leucine.[1] Its deficiency leads to isovaleric acidemia.

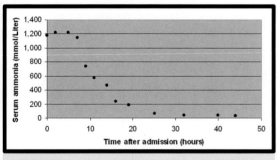

Figure 3_The markedly elevated levels of ammonia in the patient's serum responded rapidly to therapy with intravenous glucose, carnitine, and glycine.

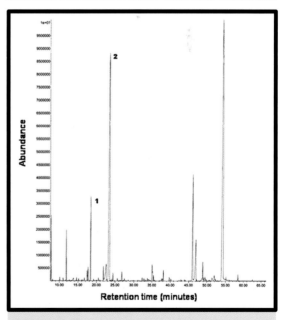

Figure 4_Three days after therapy, gas chromatography/mass spectrometry results from the patient's urine specimen showed only a large amount of isovalerylglycine (peak # 2). Peak #1 represents the internal standard (2-phenylbutyric acid).

7. How do patients with this disease usually present?

8. What is the appropriate management for patients with this disease?

Possible Answers _____

1. Low birth weight, failure to thrive, lethargy, feeding intolerance, strong body odor, dehydration, generalized hypotonia with brisk reflexes and ankle clonus; mild acidosis, hyperglycemia, hypoalbuminemia, hyperammonemia, hypocalcemia, pancytopenia, and hyperargininemia (**T1**); bilaterally symmetric increased periventricular and thalamic echogenicity; abnormal urine organic acid screen with increased levels of lactic acid, 3-hydroxyisovaleric acid, methylsuccinic acid, methylfumaric acid, and isovalerylglycine (**Figure 1**).

2. The patient's clinical signs and symptoms are suggestive of an inborn error of metabolism. The markedly elevated serum ammonia level suggests a urea cycle disorder; however, other metabolic causes of hyperammonemia including organic acidemias are in the differential diagnosis (**T2**).

3. Marked hyperammonemia in the absence of significant acidosis is suggestive of a urea cycle disorder, which should prompt serum amino acid analysis by high performance liquid chromatography (HPLC) and urine organic acid analysis by gas chromatography/mass spectrometry (GC/MS). Since a urea cycle disorder was considered the most likely possibility among the possible causes of hyperammonemia in infants (**T2**), the patient was started on parenteral arginine in an effort to reduce the ammonia levels. This led to the observed increase in serum arginine. In the absence of this history, the elevated arginine levels would have suggested a deficiency of arginase, a urea cycle disorder. However, arginase deficiency does not have this type of neonatal presentation. Moreover, the patient's acidosis and urine organic acid profile (**Figure 1**) are consistent with an organic acidemia.

4. ***Most likely diagnosis***: *isovaleric acidemia (or isovaleryl-coenzyme A dehydrogenase deficiency; OMIM #243500).*

5. The presence of 3-hydroxyisovaleric acid, isovalerylglycine, methylsuccinic acid, and methylfumaric acid in the patient's urine sample is characteristic for isovaleric acidemia. The diagnosis can be confirmed by an assay for isovaleryl-coenzyme A dehydrogenase in cultured fibroblasts of the patient. However, the enzyme assay is not readily available and the urine organic acid profile by GC/MS is virtually diagnostic for this disease.[1]

6. Isovaleryl-coenzyme A dehydrogenase (*EC 1.3.99.10*) is a mitochondrial enzyme that catalyzes a step in the catabolic pathway of the ketogenic branched chain amino acid leucine (**Figure 2**). More specifically, it catalyzes the oxidation of isovaleryl-coenzyme A to 3-methylcrotonyl-coenzyme A. Therefore, a deficiency of isovaleryl-coenzyme A dehydrogenase leads to an excessive accumulation of isovaleryl-coenzyme A. Isovaleryl-coenzyme A is converted to isovalerylglycine, which is non-toxic and readily excreted in the urine. Another non-toxic conjugate product is isovalerylcarnitine, which can be detected by liquid chromatography/tandem mass spectrometry (LC/MS/MS) in urine and blood. Other metabolites of isovaleric acid that are formed include 3-hydroxyisovaleric acid and 4-hydroxyvaleric acid; the latter is further oxidized to methylsuccinic acid, which is then dehydrogenated to methylfumaric acid. Some other minor metabolites that may be detected include 3-hydroxyisoheptanoic acid, isovalerylglutamic acid, isovalerylglucuronide, isovalerylalanine, and isovalerylsarcosine.[1] The pathophysiologic basis of the toxicity of isovaleric acid and its metabolites is yet to be completely elucidated. In high concentrations seen in symptomatic isovaleric acidemia patients, isovaleric acid inhibits succinate-coenzyme A ligase in the Krebs cycle and is also toxic to granulopoietic precursors in bone marrow cultures.[2-3] Inhibition of the urea cycle enzyme, N-acetylglutamate synthetase, by isovaleryl-coenzyme A may explain the occasional occurrence of hyperammonemia in patients with isovaleric acidemia.[4]

7. Isovaleric acidemia, first described in 1966, is an autosomal recessive disorder caused by a deficiency of the enzyme isovaleryl-coenzyme A dehydrogenase.[5] Isovaleryl-coenzyme A dehydrogenase is encoded by a gene that resides

on chromosome 15q14-q15.[6] The enzyme is synthesized in the cytoplasm as a 45 kDa precursor protein. During transport into the mitochondria, the precursor protein is processed to form the mature 43 kDa protein. Four of these 43 kDa peptides come together to form a homotetramer that has the dehydrogenase activity.[7-8] Six molecular variants have been identified in patients with isovaleric acidemia. Class I mutant alleles show point mutations in the gene encoding isovaleryl-coenzyme A dehydrogenase so that the molecular weights of the precursor and mature peptides are normal. Class II-IV mutant alleles produce smaller precursor and/or mature peptides and represent point mutations or small deletions. Class V and VI mutant alleles form no protein product. Class V mutants have an abnormality in mRNA translation, while class VI mutants have defective transcription with no mRNA being formed.[9-10] A genotype-phenotype correlation has been suggested with the identification of a common mutation [932Cytosine (C) Ō Thymidine (T)] in association with a mild phenotype.[11]

8. Patients with isovaleric acidemia may present in early neonatal life with a sudden onset, severe illness or may present later in infancy with a chronic intermittent form of the disease.[1] Patients with neonatal onset, if they survive the acute illness, go on to follow a chronic intermittent course. Usually, the illness begins within a few days of birth with increasing lethargy and difficulty in feeding leading to dehydration and weight loss. An "odor of sweaty feet" may be found and represents the accumulation in the body of isovaleric acid and related compounds. Laboratory investigation typically shows metabolic acidosis with mild lactic acidemia and ketosis. In addition, there is pancytopenia and hypocalcemia. Marked hyperammonemia has also been described but is not a common finding.[12-14] Many patients do not survive the acute illness and die of acidosis, cerebral edema, infections, and/or bleeding. Patients with the chronic intermittent form of the disease usually have their first illness before their first birthday, usually following a minor respiratory infection, or other type of stress, and sometimes following increased intake of protein-rich foods. The symptoms include lethargy, vomiting, and "sweaty feet odor," with laboratory investigations

revealing acidosis and pancytopenia. There may be hyperglycemia, which along with ketosis, may be mistaken for diabetic ketoacidosis.[14-15] The patient's signs and symptoms resolve with treatment including protein restriction and administration of carnitine and/or glycine. The diagnosis of isovaleric acidemia can be made on the basis of the characteristic urine organic acid profile for this disorder. Newborn screening with LC/MS/MS can detect isovalerylcarnitine in microliter quantities of blood.[16-18] In addition, LC/MS/MS can detect isovalerylcarnitine in amniotic fluid which can be used for prenatal diagnosis of isovaleric acidemia.[19-20] Newborn screening programs have established the prevalence of isovaleric acidemia to be 1 in 62,500 newborns in Germany.[17] A review of the literature suggests that this case report is the first description of isovaleric acidemia in an African-American neonate.

9. The principle behind the treatment of patients with isovaleric acidemia includes restriction of leucine in their diets and treatment with carnitine and/or glycine, both of which conjugate with isovaleric acid to form the non-toxic and easily excreted products—isovalerylcarnitine and isovalerylglycine.[21-23]

Treatment and Course _____

The patient underwent immediate intubation and peritoneal dialysis to rapidly decrease his serum ammonia concentration. In addition, intravenous glucose was administered at high infusion rates. Following diagnosis, the patient was started on carnitine (25 mg/kg every 6 hours) and glycine (45 mg/kg every 4 hours). The patient responded by rapid reduction in his ammonia levels (**Figure 3**). When he awakened and was able to feed, he was placed on a protein restricted diet. A combination of Enfamil and Ivalex was used to provide 3.7 g/kg/day of total protein and 150 g/kcal/day. Three days later, a follow-up urine organic acid analysis showed no 3-hydroxyisovaleric acid and a larger amount of isovalerylglycine (**Figure 4**). Clinically, the patient appeared to do well, but will need life-long dietary management.

Keywords

isovaleric acidemia, gas chromatography/mass spectrometry, hyperammonemia

References

1. Sweetman L, Williams JC. Branched chain organic acidemias. In Scriver CR, Beaudet AL, Sly WS, Valle D (Eds.). *The Metabolic and Molecular Bases of Inherited Disease*, 8th ed. New York: McGraw-Hill; 2002:2132-2135.

2. Bergen BJ, Stumpf DA, Haas R, et al. A mechanism of toxicity of isovaleric acid in rat liver mitochondria. *Biochem Med*. 1982;27:154-160.

3. Hutchinson RJ, Bunnell K, Thoene JG. Suppression of granulopoietic progenitor cell proliferation by metabolites of the branched-chain amino acids. *J Pediatr*. 1985;106:62-65.

4. Coude FX, Sweetman L, Nyhan WL. Inhibition by propionyl-coenzyme A of N-acetylglutamate synthetase in rat liver mitochondria. A possible explanation for hyperammonemia in propionic and methylmalonic acidemia. *J Clin Invest*. 1979;64:1544-1551.

5. Tanaka K, Budd MA, Efron ML, et al. Isovaleric acidemia: a new genetic defect of leucine metabolism. *Proc Natl Acad Sci USA*. 1966;56:236-242.

6. Kraus JP, Matsubara Y, Barton D, et al. Isolation of cDNA clones coding for rat isovaleryl-CoA dehydrogenase and assignment of the gene to human chromosome 15. *Genomics*. 1987;1.264-269.

7. Ikeda Y, Tanaka K. Purification and characterization of isovaleryl coenzyme A dehydrogenase from rat liver mitochondria. *J Biol Chem*. 1983;258:1077-1085.

8. Tanaka K, Ikeda Y, Matsubara Y, et al. Molecular basis of isovaleric acidemia and medium-chain acyl-CoA dehydrogenase deficiency. *Enzyme*. 1987;38:91-107.

9. Ikeda Y, Keese SM, Tanaka K. Molecular heterogeneity of variant isovaleryl-CoA dehydrogenase from cultured isovaleric acidemia fibroblasts. *Proc Natl Acad Sci USA*. 1985;82:7081-7085.

10. Vockley J, Parimoo B, Tanaka K. Molecular characterization of 4 different classes of mutations in the isovaleryl-CoA dehydrogenase gene responsible for isovaleric acidemia. *Am J Hum Genet*. 1991;49:147-157.

11. Ensenauer R, Vockley J, Willard JM, et al. A common mutation is associated with a mild, potentially asymptomatic phenotype in patients with isovaleric acidemia diagnosed by newborn screening. *Am J Hum Genet*. 2004;75:1136-1142.

12. Yoshino M, Yoshida I, Yamashita F, et al. Neonatal isovaleric acidemia associated with hyperammonemia. *Adv Exp Med Biol*. 1982;153:141-146.

13. Mendiola J Jr, Robotham JL, Liehr JG, et al. Neonatal lethargy due to isovaleric acidemia and hyperammonemia. *Tex Med*. 1984;80:52-54.

14. Hou JW, Wang TR. Isovaleric acidemia: report of one case. *Zhonghua Min Guo Xiao Er Ke Yi Xue Hui Za Zhi*. 1990;31:262-265.

15. Attia N, Sakati N, al Ashwal A, et al. Isovaleric acidemia appearing as diabetic ketoacidosis. *J Inherit Metab Dis*. 1996;19:85-86.

16. Zytkovicz TH, Fitzgerald EF, Marsden D, et al. Tandem mass spectrometric analysis for amino, organic, and fatty acid disorders in newborn dried blood spots: a 2-year summary from the New England Newborn Screening Program. *Clin Chem*. 2001;47:1945-1955.

17. Schulze A, Lindner M, Kohlmuller D, et al. Expanded newborn screening for inborn errors of metabolism by electrospray ionization-tandem mass spectrometry: results, outcome, and implications. *Pediatrics*. 2003;111:1399-1406.

18. Chace DH, Kalas TA, Naylor EW. Use of tandem mass spectrometry for multianalyte screening of dried blood specimens from newborns. *Clin Chem*. 2003;49:1797-1817.

19. Shigematsu Y, Kikawa Y, Sudo M, et al. Prenatal diagnosis of isovaleric acidemia by fast atom bombardment and tandem mass spectrometry. *Clin Chim Acta*. 1991;203:369-374.

20. Shigematsu Y, Hata I, Nakai A, et al. Prenatal diagnosis of organic acidemias based on amniotic fluid levels of acylcarnitines. *Pediatr Res*. 1996;39:680-684.

21. Roe CR, Millington DS, Maltby DA, et al. L-carnitine therapy in isovaleric acidemia. *J Clin Invest*. 1984;74:2290-2295.

22. Berry GT, Yudkoff M, Segal S. Isovaleric acidemia: medical and neurodevelopmental effects of long-term therapy. *J Pediatr*. 1988;113:58-64.

23. Fries MH, Rinaldo P, Schmidt-Sommerfeld E, et al. Isovaleric acidemia: response to a leucine load after 3 weeks of supplementation with glycine, L-carnitine, and combined glycine-carnitine therapy. *J Pediatr*. 1996;129:449-452.

Severe Acid-Base Imbalance in a 1-Day-Old Infant

Patricia M. Jones

Assistant Professor of Pathology, University of Texas Southwestern Medical Center, and Assistant Director of Chemistry, Children's Medical Center of Dallas

Patient: 4-day-old, Caucasian male.

Family History: Unremarkable.

Medical History: No medical history, 4 days old.

Drug History: None.

Chief Complaint: Infant presented with respiratory distress, vomiting, and refusal to feed.

Physical Examination: This infant was lethargic and hypotonic and appeared dehydrated.

T2. Principal Laboratory Findings

Test Reference	Abnormal Result	Normal Range
pH	7.10	7.35-7.45
pCO_2, mm Hg	21	41-54
HCO_3, mEq/L (mmol/L)	6 (6)	16-24 (16-24)
Base excess, mEq/L	−23.2	−7.0 to −1.0
Sodium mEq/L (mmol/L)	151 (151)	139-146 (139-146)
Chloride mEq/L (mmol/L)	116 (116)	96-106 (96-106)
Total CO_2, mEq/L (mmol/L)	6 (6)	18-31 (18-31)
AGAP mEq/L (mmol/L)	29 (29)	5-14 (5-14)
Ammonia (mmol/L)	(342)	(56-92)
UA ketones	>80	Negative
Glucose mg/dL (mmol/L)	56 (3.1)	<1 wk, 45-100 (2.5-5.6)
		>1 wk, 74-127 (4.1-7.0)

AGAP, anion gap; UA, urinalysis.

Questions

1. What condition(s) does this patient's signs and symptoms suggests?

2. What diagnosis do the laboratory test findings in **T2** suggest?

3. What additional tests would you order and why?

4. What is the most likely diagnosis for this infant?

Results of Additional Diagnostic Tests _____

Serum amino acid analysis: Elevations of leucine, isoleucine, lysine, valine, and tyrosine, with excessive elevation of glycine.

Urine organic acid analysis: Elevated excretion of methylcitrate, 3-hydroxypropionic, and 3-hydroxy-valeric acids.

Possible Answers _____

1. All these symptoms could be suggestive of an inborn error of metabolism. The respiratory distress, vomiting, and dehydration could also be signs of an infectious disease.

2. The laboratory tests show a profound metabolic acidemia with an elevated anion gap. The acidemia is accompanied by ketosis, hyperammonemia, and borderline hypoglycemia. Elevated sodium and chloride are probably related to the dehydration, as well as the metabolic acidosis.

3. A work-up for a metabolic disorder should be ordered, including a plasma amino acid and a urine organic acid. Cultures should probably be taken to rule out sepsis and because inborn errors of metabolism are often precipitated by intercurrent infections.

4. Diagnosis: Propionic acidemia. The excretion of 3-hydroxypropionic acid, 3-hydroxyvaleric acid and methylcitrate in the urine is consistent with a diagnosis of propionic acidemia. Marked elevations of serum glycine are often seen also. Treatment walks a fine line between supplying sufficient essential amino acids for growth and supplying enough to precipitate ketoacidotic crises. Fibroblast or leukocyte studies of propionyl-CoA carboxylase activity will confirm the diagnosis.

Seizures and Vertigo in a Young Infant

Srinivas B. Narayan,[1] Patricia M. Jones,[1,2] Michael J. Bennett,[1,2]

Department of Pathology, [1]University of Texas Southwestern Medical Center, [2]Children's Medical Center, Dallas, TX

Patient: 23-month-old male infant.

Past Surgical History: None.

Chief Complaint: Breathing problems, seizures, and walking off balance.

History of Present Illness: Epileptic attacks, ataxia, vertigo, and seizures requiring the care of a neurologist for the past 1.5 years.

Past Medical History: The patient had been hospitalized several times previously for seizures and vertigo. No significant abnormalities seen on magnetic resonance imaging (MRI) and computed tomography (CT) scans during those hospitalizations. The infant was treated with albuterol (Salbutamol, 2.5 mg) for breathing problems.

Drug History: A urine toxicology screen performed on the patient was negative.

Family/Social History: Mother with type I diabetes mellitus.

Physical Examination: Vital signs: temperature, 36.8°C; blood pressure, 131/84 mm Hg; heart rate, 87 bpm; respiratory rate, 27/minute. The physical examination was within normal limits.

Results of Additional Laboratory Diagnostic Procedures: Laboratory tests for disorders of amino acid metabolism were negative.

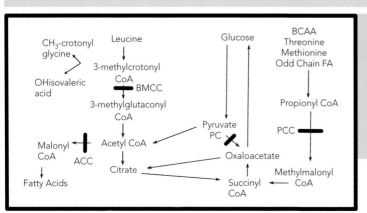

Figure 1_Metabolic pathways depicting the sites (carboxylase enzymes) blocked by the absence of biotin. BMCC, beta-methylcrotonyl coenzyme A (CoA) carboxylase; ACC, acetyl CoA carboxylase; PC, pyruvate CoA carboxylase; PCC, propionyl CoA carboxylase.

T1. Principal Laboratory Findings

Test	Patient's Result	"Normal" Reference Range
Whole Blood		
WBC Count	7.7	4.1-11.1 × 10³/
Differential: Neutrophils	32	0-11%
Lymphocytes	56	20-51%
Monocytes	8	4-11%
Eosinophils	4	1-7%
Hemoglobin	10.8	13.2-16.9 g/dL
Platelet Count	368	174-404 × 10³/ mL
MCV	71.1	72-86 fL
MCH	22.4	24-31 pg
MCHC	31.4	32.0-36.0 g/dL
pH	7.34	7.35-7.45
pCO$_2$	20	41-54 mm Hg
Serum/Plasma		
Ammonia	14	21-50 mmol/L
Lactate	4.5	0.7-2.3 mmol/L
Sodium	140	139-146 mEq/L
Potassium	4.7	3.7-5.6 mEq/L
Chloride	108	97-104 mEq/L
Anion Gap	19	5-14 mmol/L
BUN	10	5-17 mg/dL
Creatinine	0.4	0.1-0.6 mg/dL
Calcium	10.7	8.7-9.8 mg/dL
Ionic Calcium	1.35	1.12-1.32 mmol/L
Phosphorus	3.5	2.4-4.5 mg/dL
AST	27	9-80 U/L
ALT	13	5-45 U/L
(a) ALP	207	145-320 U/L
GGT	22	6-19 U/L
Biotinidase	None Detected	3.5-13.8 U/L
Urine		
Toxicology screen	Negative	Negative
Organic acid screen	Positive[a]	Negative

[a]*Markedly increased concentrations of methylcrotonyl glycine, 3-hydroxyisovaleric acid, and methylcitrate identified by GC-MS. WBC, white blood cell; MCV, mean corpuscular volume; MCH, mean corpuscular hemoglobin; MCHC, mean corpuscular hemoglobin concentration; BUN, blood urea nitrogen; AST, aspartate aminotransferase; ALT, alanine aminotransferase; ALP, alkaline phosphatase; GGT, gammaglutamyl transferase.*

Figure 2_Illustration of the amide linkage of the biotin cofactor to a carboxylase apoenzyme via an amino group of a lysine residue of the apoenzyme.

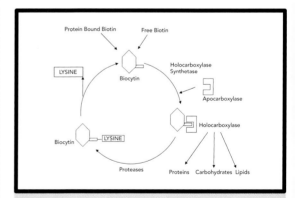

Figure 3_The role of biotinidase in the metabolism of biotin.

Questions

1. What is(are) this patient's most striking laboratory result(s)?

2. How do you explain this patient's most striking laboratory result(s)?

3. What condition(s) does this patient's clinical and laboratory findings suggest?

4. What is the biochemical basis of this patient's condition(s)?

5. What are the consequences of this patient's condition if left untreated?

6. What is the most appropriate treatment for this patient?

Possible Answers

1. Lactic acidemia, increased anion gap, decreased blood pH and pCO_2, undetectable biotinidase level, and positive urine organic acid screen with massive elevation of urinary levels of 3-hydroxy-isovaleric acid, 3-methylcrotonyl glycine, and methylcitric acid.

2. The metabolic acidosis caused by increased concentrations of organic acids (ie, lactic acid and those excreted in the urine) in the blood account for the increased anion gap and decreased pH and pCO_2 levels. Moreover, the absence of biotinidase activity, coupled with high urinary levels of 3-hydroxyisovaleric acid, 3-methyl-crotonyl glycine, and methylcitric acid, identified and quantified in this patient's urine by gas chromatography-mass spectrometry (GC-MS), are strongly suggestive of biotinidase deficiency.

3. ***Most likely diagnosis:*** *biotinidase deficiency.* The enzyme, biotinidase, was first characterized by Pispa in 1965.[1] The 56-kilodalton (kDa) native protein is produced from post-translational modification of a 70 to 76 kDa precursor in serum, and there are at least 4 major isoenzymes. Biotinidase activity can be seen in almost all tissues, with high activities in serum, liver, adrenal glands, and kidney. The enzyme has been purified to homogeneity from both plasma and serum.[2,3] Biotinidase deficiency is inherited as an autosomal recessive trait. Because testing for biotinidase deficiency meets many of the major criteria for inclusion in a newborn screening program, including the availability of an effective treatment, many states and countries perform population screening for this disorder.

4. Biotinidase is required for the conversion of the precursor, biocytin, to biotin, an essential vitamin cofactor for carboxylase enzymes, such as those found in the Krebs cycle. The absence of biotin blocks the conversion of 3-methylcrotonyl-CoA to 3-hydroxyisovaleric acid by 3-methylcrotonyl-CoA carboxylase and the conversion of 3-methylcrotonylglycine to propionyl-CoA by propionyl-CoA carboxylase,

resulting in urinary excretion of large amounts of 3-hydroxyisovaleric acid, 3-methylcrotonylg-lycine, and methylcitric acid [**Figure 1**]. High urinary levels of these organic acids are pathognomonic of biotinidase deficiency. These metabolites are formed only when inadequate amounts of biotin are available for the normal function of multiple carboxylases. Along with prominent organic aciduria, ketoacidosis and hyperammonemia may be seen as late manifestations of biotinidase deficiency in previously undiagnosed cases. The biotin-requiring apocarboxylases that are affected in these individuals are shown in **Figure 1**. Biotin is covalently bound to these apocarboxylases by the action of holocarboxylase synthetase.[4,5] These carboxylases play important roles in gluconeogenesis, fatty acid synthesis, and the catabolism of branched chain amino acids (BCAAs). Mammals cannot synthesize biotin and therefore, derive the vitamin from the diet or endogenous turnover of the biotin attached to carboxylases.[6] The side chain of the carboxy-terminus of biotin is linked to an epsilon amino group of a specific lysine residue of the apoenzyme through an amide linkage. The amide linkage connecting biotin and apoenzyme is long and flexible, which allows biotin to move from 1 active site to another [**Figure 2**]. On degradation of the holoenzyme, the protein bound biotin requires digestion by proteolytic enzymes to yield free biotin for recycling and conversion to biocytin (biotinyl-amino-lysine). Biotinidase acts as a hydrolase by cleaving biocytin and biotinyl peptides into free biotin and the amino acid, lysine. Biotinidase also hydrolyzes the undigested biocytin absorbed from the intestine into plasma in order to release free biotin that can readily enter cells to become incorporated into the apoenzyme. Unmetabolized biocytin is excreted in the urine. It remains unknown as to whether biotin recycling by biotinidase takes place intracellularly or in the extracellular compartment. The role of biotinidase in the recycling of biotin is depicted in **Figure 3**. Suggested additional functions of biotinidase include a role in the transportation and bioavailability of biotin, biotinylation of nuclear protein, and in neuronal uptake of biotin.[7]

5. If left untreated, the clinical consequences of profound biotinidase deficiency (ie, less than 10% residual serum biotinidase activity) include

seizures, hypotonia, skin rashes, alopecia, breathing abnormalities, hearing loss, eye problems, and cellular immunological abnormalities.[8] The neurosensory deafness and optic atrophy seen in biotinidase deficiency are not seen in holocarboxylase synthetase deficiency. The etiology of the neurological problems associated with biotinidase deficiency is not clearly understood.

6. Administration of pharmacologic doses of the vitamin, biotin. Currently the only known treatment for biotinidase deficiency is administering biotin. Anywhere from 5 to 10 mg of biotin daily for life in profoundly affected individuals effectively reverses the symptoms of biotinidase deficiency, especially if the treatment is started early before irreversible neurological damage has occurred. Neurologic damage cannot be completely reversed even with high doses of biotin. This characteristic of biotinidase deficiency strongly supports newborn screening for this disorder.[8] Inherited metabolic disorders which improve upon treatment with pharmacological doses of vitamins are described as vitamin-responsive disorders.[9] Biotinidase deficiency is a classical example of a vitamin-responsive disorder. The early onset or neonatal form of multiple carboxylase deficiency is usually due to biotin holocarboxylase synthetase deficiency and most children with the late onset or infantile form of multiple carboxylase deficiency have biotinidase deficiency.[10,11] Affected individuals with biotinidase deficiency often become asymptomatic when treated with pharmacologic doses of biotin.

Treatment and Course

After the infant was diagnosed with biotinidase deficiency, treatment was started with oral biotin supplementation. He was treated with 0.25 mL of 25 mg/mL biotin twice daily. The patient responded well to the treatment with obvious signs of vertigo disappearing within a few days. The patient continues to do well on this treatment.

Keywords

biotinidase deficiency, biotin, carboxylase

References

1. Pispa J. Animal biotinidase. *Ann Med Exp Biol.* 1963;43(Suppl):1-39.

2. Craft DV, Goss NH, Chandramouli N, et al. Purification of biotinidase from human plasma and its activity on biotinyl peptides. *Biochem.* 1985;24:2471-2476.

3. Chauhan J, Dakshinamurthy J. Purification and characterization of biotinidase from human serum. *J Biol Chem.* 1986;261:4268-4274.

4. Lane MD, Young DL, Lynen F. The enzymatic synthesis of holotranscarboxylase from apotranscarboxylase and (+)-biotin. I. Purification of apoenzyme and synthetase: characteristics of the reaction. *J Biol Chem.* 1964;239:2858-2864.

5. Achutamurthy PN, Mistry SP. Synthesis of biotin-dependent carboxylases from their apoproteins and biotin. *Biochem Rev (India).* 1972;43:1-12.

6. Heard GS, Wolf B, Reddy JK. Pancreatic biotinidase activity: the potential for intestinal processing of dietary protein bound biotin. *Pediatr Res.* 1984;18:198A-208A.

7. Hymes J, Wolf B. Biotinidase and its roles in biotin metabolism. *Clin Chim Acta.* 1996;255:1-11.

8. Wolf B. Disorders of biotin metabolism. In: Scriver CR, Beaudet AL, Valle D Sly WS eds. *The Metabolic and Molecular Bases of Inherited Diseases*, 8th ed. New York: McGraw Hill, 2001:3935-3964.

9. Wolf B. Vitamin-dependent metabolic diseases. In: Kelly VC, editor. *Practice of Pediatrics.* Philadelphia: Harper and Row, 1982;1-9.

10. Munnich A, Saudubray JM, Carre G et al. Defective biotin absorption in multiple carboxylase deficiency. *Lancet.* 1981;2:263-268

11. Wolf B, Grier RE, Allen RJ, et al. Biotinidase deficiency: The enzymatic defect in late onset multiple carboxylase deficiency. *Clin Chim Acta.* 1983;131;273-281.

Failure to Thrive in a 14-Month-Old Child

Monte S. Willis,[1] Michael J. Bennett,[2]

Departments of Pathology, [1]University of Texas Southwestern Medical Center and [2]The Children's Medical Center, Dallas, TX

Patient: 14-month-old Hispanic male.

Chief Complaint: Failure to thrive, ongoing emesis, and particularly foul-smelling stools.

History of Present Illness: The patient was born at term without any complications. Two days after going home, his parents noted daily emesis and progressively worsening diarrhea with foul-smelling stools. Additionally, his mother noted that he struggled to breathe at times and other times he would breathe rapidly, particularly at night. The child was hospitalized at the age of 4 months for fever, dehydration, and emesis. At that time, it was noted that he was very physically inactive. Medical records from this visit indicated the patient had good hearing bilaterally. At approximately 10 months of age, the patient had stool fecal fat testing because of his chronic foul-smelling "diarrhea." At that time his stool cultures were negative; however, microscopically, his stool was noted to have more than 100 fatty acid droplets per high power field (hpf) (normal <60 droplets/hpf). In addition, the child was noted to have gained only approximately 1 pound every 2 to 3 months since birth. Normally, children gain weight at the rate of approximately 1.25 pounds/month or 2.5 to 3.75 pounds in 2 to 3 months. The child had been on several different formulas in order to increase his body weight. He was currently on Neocate, which had decreased his episodes of emesis and stool volume, although his stools were still particularly foul-smelling.

Past Medical History: The patient had 2 previous episodes of otitis media and 1 hospitalization at an outside private hospital at 4 months of age.

Past Surgical History: None.

Drug History: The patient was currently being treated with nebulized albuterol (3 times daily) and Pulmicort (budesonide, an inhaled corticosteroid), once daily. He was recently given a course of amoxicillin for otitis media to which he did not respond.

Family/Social History: The patient has a cousin with asthma and an aunt that died at the age of 10 due to complications of spina bifida.

Physical Examination: Vital signs: T, 37.3°C; HR, 112; RR, 20; BP, 84/64 mm Hg. The child was noted to be a small male child in no acute distress with an occasional cough noted. Oxygen saturation was 98% on room air. His current weight and length (8.29 kg and 74.5 cm, respectively) were less than the fifth percentile for his age. The patient's physical examination was normal except for bilateral otitis media and congested nares with dried nasal crusting.

Procedures and Additional Tests: A chest X-ray revealed patchy areas of bronchial wall thickening as well as left lower lobe atelectasis. Sputum cultures identified moderate growth of oropharyngeal flora, light growth of non-fermenting gram-negative rods (not Pseudomonas spp.), moderate growth of Staphylcoccus aureus (oxacillin sensitive), and moderate growth of Hemophilus influenza (beta-lactamase negative). A sweat chloride test was performed and the result was 102 mEq/L (normal: <40 mEq Cl/L sweat). A second sweat test performed 2 weeks later gave a chloride result of 111 mEq/L. In addition, mutation analysis of DNA from nucleated cells obtained from an anticoagulated whole blood specimen from our patient revealed a single ΔF508 mutation in the cystic fibrosis transmembrane conductor regulator (CFTR) gene.

T1. Principal Laboratory Findings

Test	Patient's Result	"Normal" Reference Range
Hematology WBC count	19.8 5.0-14.	$5.0 \times 10^3/mL$
RBC count	5.02	$3.9-5.3 \times 10^6/mL$
Hemoglobin	13	11.1-14.2 g/dL
Hematocrit	41.1	30-42%
MCV	81.9	72-86 fL
MCH	25.9	24-31 pg
MCHC	31.7	32-36 g/dL
Platelet count	570	$150-550 \times 10^3/mL$
MPV	7.2	9.0-12.0 fL
Differential:		
neutrophils	50.3	20-40%
lymphocytes	43.2	46-76%
monocytes	5.3	0-10%
eosinophils	1.3	0-5%
basophils	0	0-2%
ANC	9.96	$1.5-8.0 \times 10^3/mL$
atypical lymphocytes	3	<0%
Chemistry Sodium	142	139-146 mEq/L
Potassium	4.2	3.5-5.0 mEq/L
Chloride	108	98-106 mEq/L
CO_2	22	18-31 mEq/L
Anion Gap	13	5-14 mEq/L
IgE	8	<60 IU/mL
Glucose	109	74-127 mg/dL
HbA1c	4.1	<6%
BUN	15	5-18 mg/dL
Creatinine	0.3	0.2-0.6 mg/dL
AST	56	15-55 U/L
ALT	59	5-45 U/L
GGT	17	2-22 U/L
Vitamin levels		
Vitamin A: retinol	0.29	0.2-0.5 mg/L
retinyl esters	0.08	0.0-0.10 mg/L
Vitamin D (25-OH)	26	20-59 ng/mL
Vitamin E: α-tocopherol	1.6	5.5-9.0 mg/L
γ-tocopherol	0.2	0.0-6.0 mg/L

WBC, white blood cell; RBC, red blood cell; MCV, mean corpuscular volume; MCH, mean corpuscular hemoglobin; MCHC, mean corpuscular hemoglobin concentration; MPV, mean platelet volume; ANC, absolute neutrophil count; HbA1c, hemoglobin A1c; BUN, blood urea nitrogen; AST, aspartate aminotransferase; ALT, alanine aminotransferase; GGT, gamma-glutamyltransferase.

Questions

1. What is(are) this patient's most striking clinical and laboratory result(s)?

2. How do you explain this patient's most striking laboratory result(s)?

T2. CF Mutations Constituting the 87-Mutation Panel*

ΔF508	G91R	R117C	S549R	1949del84	3849+4A>G
ΔDF311	I148T	R117H	T338I	2043delG	3876delA
ΔI507	K710X	R1283M	V520F	2143delT	3905insT
A455E	L206W	R334W	W1089X	2183delAA>G	394delTT
A559T	M1101K	R347H	W1282X	2184delA	405+1G>A
C524X	N1303K	R347P	Y1092X	2307insA	405+3A>C
D1152	H P574H	R352Q	Y563D	2789+5G>A	444delA
D127	0N Q1238X	R553X	1078delT	2869insG	574delA
E60X	Q359K/T360K	R560T	1161delC	3120+1G>A	621+1G>T
G178R	Q493X	S1196X	1609delCA	3120G>A	711+1G>T
G330X	Q552X	S1251N	1677delTA	3659delC	711+5G>A
G480C	Q890X	S1255X	1717-1G>A	3662delA	712-1G>T
G542X	R1066C	S364P	1812-1G>A	3791delC	
G551D	R1158X	S549I	1898+1G>A	3821delT	
G85E	R1162X	S549N	1898+5G>T	3849+10kbC>T	

*Genzyme General Genetics: www.genzymegenetics.com/clinicalinfo/molgen/cystic.htm.

T3. CF Carrier Risk and Detection Rate by Ethnic Background Using the 87-Mutation Screening Panel *

Ethnic Background	Carrier Risk	Detection Rate
Northern European Caucasian	1/25	90%
Southern European Caucasian	1/25	90%
Ashkenazi Jew	1/26	97%
African American	1/65	75%
Hispanic	1/46	58%[5]
Asian	1/90	38%[5]
Native American	1/52	81%[5]

*Genzyme General Genetics: www.genzymegenetics.com/clinicalinfo/molgen/cystic.htm.

3. What condition(s) does this patient's laboratory and other findings suggest ?

4. What is the pathophysiology of this patient's disease?

5. What are the clinical manifestations of this patient's disease?

6. What are typical complications associated with this patient's disease?

7. What is the long-term prognosis for this patient?

8. What is the most appropriate treatment for this patient?

Possible Answers

1. The most striking clinical and laboratory findings include: a marked failure to thrive (<fifth percentile for height and weight); ongoing diarrhea with particularly foul smelling stool and increased fat droplets in the stool; chronic cough; *S. aureus* and *H. influenza* growth from sputum cultures; a chest X-ray with patchy areas of bronchial wall thickening with left lower lobe atelectasis; increased WBC, ANC, AST, ALT values and decreased a-tocopherol levels; 2 positive sweat chloride tests; and a single copy of the ΔF508 mutation in the CFTR gene.

2. Each of our patient's most striking laboratory and clinical findings can be best explained as follows. **Failure to thrive.** A detailed dietary history determined that the child was receiving and ingesting adequate amounts of food indicating the child was not properly utilizing or retaining the calories provided by the food he ingested.

Ongoing diarrhea, particularly foul smelling feces, and increased fat droplets in the stool by qualitative fecal fat analysis. Steatorrhea (increased fecal fat content) can be the cause of ongoing diarrhea that is particularly foul smelling. The determination of increased fecal fat is performed by Sudan III staining of the feces. Increased stool fatty acids suggests pancreatic disease, although this qualitative method does not detect low levels of steatorrhea well.[1] The finding of increased quantities of fat in the stool is the principal manifestation of most malabsorption syndromes. In children, the main disease processes associated with steatorrhea and malabsorption syndrome are celiac disease and cystic fibrosis (CF). Cystic fibrosis screening should be performed if therapy for celiac disease does not improve symptoms or if other symptoms of CF are present (ie, chronic lung problems). Celiac disease is an inflammatory condition of the small intestine in which the initiating factor in certain individuals predisposed to this disease is the ingestion of gluten- and prolamin-containing foods such as wheat, rye, and barley. Screening tests for anti-gliadin and anti-endomysial antibodies, which are associated with celiac disease, can help diagnose this disease so that appropriate therapy can be initiated. **Positive sputum cultures for *S. aureus* and *H. influenza.*** Bacterial colonization of the airways in patients with CF occurs early in the disease process and becomes impossible to eliminate. Generally, *S. aureus* and *H. influenzae* colonize first (as in this case), but in time, growth of *Pseudomonas aeruginosa* and *Burkholderia cepacia* can also occur.[2] **Abnormal chest X-ray with patchy areas of bronchial wall thickening and left lower lobe atelectasis.** Bronchial wall thickening is a morphological finding that is observed in chronic airway diseases such as chronic bronchitis, cystic fibrosis, bronchiectasis, asthma, and bronchiolitis. It appears as a thickening of the bronchial wall causing ring shadows and parallel linear shadows (tubular shadows) on chest X-ray. Atelectasis (airless or collapsed lung) present in this case differs from a consolidation in that a consolidation is the replacement of lung space by fluid, whereas in atelectasis the air in the lung space is resorbed, not replaced. Bronchial obstruction (eg, mucous), compression by adjacent structures, or scarring from pneumonia are the major causes of atelectasis.[3]

Difficulty breathing, tachycardia, and chronic cough. These symptoms correlate with the chronic lung process indicated radiographically (ie, chronic airway disease due to cystic fibrosis, chronic bronchitis, etc). The moderate growth of beta-lactamase negative *H. influenza* and oxacillin-sensitive *S. aureus* from our patient's sputum culture indicates that an infection/colonization with these 2 bacteria has occurred. **Increased WBC count with increased absolute neutrophil count (ANC).** Leukocytosis is generally seen in patients with a bacterial infection, while viral infections tend to be associated with normal or low leukocyte counts. Our patient's leukocytosis is most likely related to his bacterial lung infection and/or his chronic bilateral bacterial otitis media.[1] **Increased liver function test (AST, ALT) results.** Increases in AST and ALT levels are most commonly seen in patients with liver damage (eg, viral and alcoholic hepatitis, alcoholic cirrhosis, fatty liver). The AST and ALT increases observed in serum from our patient were modest and not indicative of major liver damage. **Decreased a-tocopherol level**. In an individual with an adequate dietary intake of vitamin E (a-tocopherol), a decreased serum concentration of a-tocopherol indicates that this fat-soluble vitamin is not being adequately absorbed from the GI tract. Because the levels of other fat-soluble vitamins (A and D) in our patient were within the normal reference interval for these vitamins [**T1**], and his prothrombin time (PT) and partial thromboplastin time (PPT) results (ie, indirect tests of vitamin K-dependent clotting factor activity) were normal (*data not shown*), our patient's malabsorption syndrome was modest. **Abnormal sweat chloride tests.** Increased concentrations of sodium and chloride in sweat are a consistent finding in patients with CF as sweat glands (exocrine glands) are affected by this disease. The definitive sweat chloride test is performed by collecting sweat by pilocarpine iontophoresis. Pilocarpine is a cholinergic agonist which increases sweat production when applied to the skin via iontophoresis. Two electrodes create a small current that transports the sweat-stimulating drug into the sweat glands and the resulting sweat is collected.[1] This test is technically difficult to perform on neonates, so it is better, if possible, to wait until they are 4 weeks old. A sweat chloride result >60 mEq/L or a sweat sodium result >70 mEq/L is definitively abnormal. Levels of sweat chloride >60 mEq/L in a patient with major clinical manifestations of CF makes the diagnosis of CF virtually unequivocal. A small percentage of patients (2%) with CF will, however, have a normal sweat chloride test.[2] While the sweat chloride test may appear easy to perform, surveys have demonstrated that a majority of laboratories have low accuracy when performing this test. To avoid inaccurate diagnosis of CF, the diagnosis of CF should not be made or excluded on the basis of the results from a single sweat chloride test.[1] This is why multiple sweat chloride tests were performed on our patient. **ΔF508 mutation in the CFTR gene.** Mutations in the CFTR gene cause CF. There are more than 900 mutations in the CFTR gene that can cause CF. The most common mutation is ΔF508, accounting for 70% of CF cases in the Caucasian population. Moreover, the highest risk of CF with pancreatic disease exists when the ΔF508, G542X, G551D, N1303K, or W1282X mutations are combined with another CFTR mutation.[4]

3. **The patient's clinical and laboratory findings are most consistent with:** Cystic fibrosis with *S. aureus* and *H. influenza* lung infection and chronic otitis media. The constellation of our patient's findings, including failure to thrive, steatorrhea, a chronic lung process (sputum cultures positive for *S. aureus* and *H. influenza)*, along with 2 increased sweat chloride tests, and the detection of a single positive ΔF508 mutation by polymerase chain reaction (PCR)-based assays, makes CF the most likely diagnosis. Cystic fibrosis is an autosomal recessive genetic disease that is caused by an underlying mutation in the gene for the CFTR necessitating the presence of 2 mutations in the CFTR gene for the disease to be clinically present. Our patient had multiple positive sweat chloride tests, along with symptoms of CF, that allowed the definitive diagnosis of CF. Frequently, a 25-mutation screen is used to detect many of the more common CF mutations in the Caucasian population.[4] In addition, this screen detects 17 mutations found mainly in the Hispanic population. However, since our patient is Hispanic, a more complete screening, using the 87-mutation screen, was performed, which detects 28 mutations found mainly in the Hispanic population.[5] The CFTR

gene mutation analysis method performed on this patient's cells detects 87 CFTR mutations [**T2**], which account for 90% of the mutations found in Caucasians of northern European descent [**T3**]. However, since this patient is of Hispanic descent, and only 58% of CFTR mutations are detected by this method, this patient must have an additional, unrecognized mutation in addition to the single DF508 mutation that was detected. The findings of leukocytosis and an increased ANC are most likely related to this patient's lung and otitis media infections. While otitis media can be seen more frequently in younger children, several studies have shown that it is not more common in patients with CF. In a prospective prevalence survey, it was demonstrated that 10% of CF patients, ages 4 months to 17 years, presented with unilateral or bilateral otitis media, which is a low prevalence compared to the prevalence in children without CF.[6] Another study confirmed this prevalence using children with CF between the ages of 2 and 17 years.[7] It should be noted, however, that other ear, nose, and throat (ENT) complications (eg, sinusitis) are more prevalent in patients with CF. The incidence of CF in the United States is 1:2,000 to 1:3,000 in Caucasians and approximately 30,000 people have this disease. Moreover, CFTR gene mutations are found in 1:20 to 1:25 Caucasians who are carriers and have no symptoms of disease.

4. **Pathophysiology of CF.** The gene that encodes the CFTR was cloned in 1989, and encodes a 1,480 amino acid-containing protein. The CFTR forms a chloride permeable membrane which is regulated by phosphorylation and is found on a variety of tissues to varying degrees.[2] The testing of a patient's DNA for specific mutations in the CFTR gene may provide definitive evidence of CF. This testing is performed by commercial and academic/university laboratories and has the value of detecting carriers thereby allowing preconception genetic counseling and prenatal screening. In general, a swab of the inner cheek is collected and DNA isolated from the nuclei of buccal cells is tested for the presence of CFTR gene mutations. Testing is done for the most common mutations [**T2**], especially those found in 90% of Caucasians of northern European descent; however, other CFTR mutations are more common in descendants of other races,

and therefore the results of the 87-mutation screen cannot always be depended upon for the diagnosis of CF. What makes our patient's case most interesting is that he had only a single mutation in the CFTR gene among the 87 mutations that were screened for; however, when coupled with 2 positive sweat chloride tests by pilocarpine iontophoresis and the patient's characteristic clinical signs and symptoms, the diagnosis of CF was unequivocal.

5. **The clinical manifestations of CF** are varied and depend on the age of the patient. Newborns with CF may present with meconium ileus or failure to thrive (as in this case). In children or adults, ongoing respiratory tract infections may be the only presenting symptom. However, the course of CF is characterized by exacerbations of lung disease that increase in severity and frequency and improve with therapy, increases in sputum production (in which a change of color is often noted), a feeling of congestion in the chest, and a reduced appetite. Breathing rate increases, as does the use of the accessory muscles of respiration, and rales, rhonchi, and wheezes occur. Pulmonary function worsens and new infiltrates are observed on X-ray accompanied by a leukocytosis. Increased breathing, infiltrates on X-ray, and a leukocytosis were all seen in the present case. The earliest manifestation of lung involvement is a cough, generally worse at night and upon waking. Wheezing may also be present and the cough persists for longer periods than in a normal respiratory illness. Thick, purulent, green sputum eventually becomes apparent and symptoms of bronchitis persist for years to decades.[2] Shortness of breath and difficulty breathing progress as the severity of the disease and its symptoms worsen. Bacterial colonization of the airways starts with *S. aureus* and *H. influenzae* and over time, *P. aeroginosa* and *B. capacia* infections become a common finding. Sputum cultures are valuable in evaluating the antibiotic susceptibility pattern of the bacteria present. In the present case, the patient's sputum grew *H. influenza*, but not *P. aeroginosa* or *B. capacia*, which would not be expected until later in the disease process. Changes in pulmonary function occur with obstructive airway disease when the airways are obstructed with thick mucus.

6. **The complications of CF include**: pulmonary, pancreatic, gastrointestinal, genitourinary, and hepatobiliary disease. **Pulmonary disease.** The accumulation of air or gas in the pleural space may occur (pneumothorax) due to spontaneous disruption of lung function by changes in the internal pressure in the thorax. Without normal CFTR function in the epithelial cells of the intrapulmonary and upper airways, particularly the sinuses, the airways are adversely affected. While the sinuses are almost always involved, sinus infection (acute or chronic) is not a common finding among patients with CF. **Pancreatic disease.** The exocrine function of the pancreas fails in 85% of patients with CF. Exocrine pancreatic failure is universal in patients who are homozygous for the ΔF508 mutation. Apparently some of the mutations in the CFTR gene provide sufficient function to prevent the complete failure of the pancreas. **Gastrointestinal disease.** Gastrointestinal symptoms occur commonly with CF, but they do not commonly cause life-threatening consequences. Meconium ileus occurs in about 20% of newborns with CF and is practically diagnostic of CF in these individuals. Small bowel obstruction, intussusception, and rectal prolapse occur occasionally in children, but not in adults.[2] **Genitourinary disease.** Nearly all (95%) males with CF are sterile due to Wolffian duct atropy; however, spermatogenesis occurs and retrieval of sperm has been performed for in vitro fertilization. Females are less fertile due to nutritional deficits, lung disease, and thick cervical mucus plugs that can occur at the cervical opening. **Hepatobilliary disease.** Liver disease is subtle in patients with CF and manifests broadly from cholestasis to cirrhosis with increases in AST and ALT levels. In patients with pancreatic insufficiency, nearly 20% have an elevated ALT level and the next most commonly elevated liver enzyme is alkaline phosphatase (ALP). Our patient had both elevated ALT and a slightly elevated AST level [**T1**] in the absence of an elevated ALP level (*data not shown*), indicating some involvement of the liver.

7. Due to several factors, the prognosis for patients with CF has improved dramatically over the last several decades.[8] The strongest correlation with 8-year survival of patients with CF is aerobic fitness and an active lifestyle.[9] Moreover, treatment improves prognosis and early, aggressive,

CF-centered care is associated with better patient outcomes.[10-12] Improvement in nutrition in patients with CF has been associated with improved survival and pancreatic-sufficient patients have better outcomes when compared to those with pancreatic insufficiency. Low socio-economic status is associated with a worse outcome, probably due to the cost of aggressive treatment, frequent hospital visits, and the antibiotics that make such a difference in the long-term outcome of patients with CF. Interestingly, patients with CF that lack medical insurance or have Medicaid tend to have worse lung function than non-Medicaid patients.[13,14] Second-hand smoke exposure and viral respiratory infections are also associated with worse outcomes in patients with CF.[15,16] Other factors that influence survival in patients with CF include being female (protective)[17] and infection with *P. aeruginosa* or some strains of *B. cepacia* (detrimental).[8]

8. The most appropriate treatment for this patient is multi-faceted and includes antibiotics, chest physiotherapy, bronchodilators, DNase (deoxyribonuclease), anti-inflammatory agents, pancreatic enzymes, and nutritional support.[2] At times when the lung disease in patients with CF worsens acutely, antibiotics given intensely and parenterally over a 2- to 3- week period are recommended. The use of specific antibiotics is based on the results of susceptibility testing of the organisms isolated in sputum. Infection with the most common pathogen, *P. aeruginosa*, can generally be treated with an aminoglycoside and a beta-lactam antibiotic. Response to therapy is assessed by improvement in symptoms, pulmonary function testing, and sometimes by quantitative bacterial counts in the sputum. Chest physiotherapy (the mechanical percussion and postural drainage of lung secretions) are the mainstays of treatment in patients with purulent secretions. In addition, several studies have shown that bronchodilators, such as beta-adrenergic agonists and anti-cholinergic agents (eg, albuterol, which was used in our patient), have short term benefits in the treatment of patients with CF and lung disease.[18,19] The infiltration of neutrophils into the lung tissue of patients with CF and the resulting release of DNA contribute to the increased viscosity of the sputum from patients with CF. The administration of DNase to patients with purulent sputum and airway obstruction increases the clearance of sputum and decreases the frequency of symptoms associated with lung dysfunction. The administration of pancreatic enzymes, especially in CF patients with a dysfunctional exocrine pancreas, is essential for good nutrition in these patients. Pancreatic enzymes are given enterally with meals and the number of capsules is adjusted based on body weight gain and loss data and the presence or absence of abdominal cramping and fat in the stool.[2] Because malabsorption of fat can occur in patients with CF, they are at increased risk of fat-soluble vitamin deficiencies. In newly diagnosed patients with CF, nearly 50% have been shown to be deficient in the fat-soluble vitamins A, D, or E.[20,21] Clinical abnormalities associated with vitamin A deficiency are rare, and since vitamin D levels are dependent on the amount of exposure to sunlight, as well as intake, decreased bone mineralization is seen usually in older, less well nourished patients who are taking corticosteroids.[2] Vitamin E deficiency is rarely seen clinically; however, vitamin K deficiency can result in a coagulopathy. Therefore, a multivitamin and additional vitamin E should be given, along with pancreatic enzyme replacement therapy, to patients with CF which should lead to the normalization of serum albumin, retinol, and 25-hydroxyvitamin D levels.[20] In children with CF, constant monitoring of the serum concentrations of the fat-soluble vitamins is recommended as deficiencies of these vitamins, especially vitamin E, can occur even with vitamin replacement therapy.[21] For example, in this patient, vitamin E deficiency (α-tocopherol) was the only fat soluble vitamin seen to be deficient [**T1**]. In addition, children must receive adequate immunizations, including yearly immunization against influenza. In patients with CF and a 1-second forced expiratory volume (FEV_1) of less than 30%, lung transplantation is the most common treatment option; however, the shortage of lung donors limits its use.

Follow-up and Treatment ____

The patient presented in this case study was started on 1 Ultrase capsule with each feeding to be titrated up to 2 capsules as tolerated. Ultrase is an oral pancreatic enzyme supplement prepared from porcine pancreas. Each Ultrase capsule contains lipase (~4,500 U), amylase (~20,000 U), and protease enzymes (~25,000 U). The patient was also started on fat-soluble vitamin replacement therapy (2 cc of a preparation containing vitamins A, D, E, and K given once/day). In addition, albuterol treatment and chest physiotherapy were started with appropriate instructions to his parents. Pulmicort (budesonide, a synthetic steroid) therapy, which had been given by nebulizer (0.25 mg once a day), was continued. Pulmozyme therapy [Dornase alfa, an inhalation solution of recombinant human deoxyribonuclease I (rhDNase)], however, was withheld at this time, with the proviso that if recurrent cough and/or increased sputum production were to occur, Pulmozyme therapy would be considered. Our patient's otitis media was treated with Augmentin (200 mg/5 cc, dosed at three-quarter teaspoon BID for 14 days). His reflux disease was treated with Zantac (1.5 cc p.o. BID). Lastly, dietary changes included changing formulas from Neocate to Pediasure and the addition of baby foods.

Keywords

cystic fibrosis, cystic fibrosis transmembrane conductor regulator gene, failure to thrive, enzyme replacement therapy

References

1. Ravel R. *Clinical Laboratory Medicine: Clinical Application of Laboratory Data*. St. Louis, MO: Mosby, 1995:724.

2. Welsh MJ. Cystic Fibrosis. In: Cecil RL, ed. *Cecil Textbook of Medicine*. Philadelphia: W.B. Saunders, 2000:401-405.

3. Fraser R, Pare J, Pare P, et al. Radiologic signs in the diagnosis of chest disease. In: Fraser R, Pare P, eds. *Diagnosis of Diseases of the Chest*. Philadelphia: W.B. Saunders, 1988:472-537.

4. Baskin LB, Wians FH Jr. Elder F. Preconception and prenatal screening for cystic fibrosis. *MLO Med Lab Obs*. 2002;34:8-12.

5. Heim RA, Sugarman EA, Allitto BA. Improved detection of cystic fibrosis mutations in the heterogeneous U.S. population using an expanded, pan-ethnic mutation panel. *Genet Med*. 2001;3:168-176.

6. Haddad J Jr, Gonzalez C, Kurland G, et al. Ear disease in children with cystic fibrosis. *Arch Otolaryngol Head Neck Surg*. 1994;120:491-493.

7. Ozcelik T, Ozgirgin N, Ozcelik U, et al. Ear, nose and throat findings in cystic fibrosis patients. *Turk J Pediatr*. 1997;39:51-54.

8. Orenstein DM, Winnie GB, Altman H. Cystic fibrosis: A 2002 update. *J Pediatr*. 2002;140:156-164.

9. Kerem E, Reisman J, Corey M, et al. Prediction of mortality in patients with cystic fibrosis. *N Engl J Med*. 1992;326:1187-1191.

10. Nielsen OH, Thomsen BL, Green A, et al. Cystic fibrosis in Denmark 1945 to 1985. An analysis of incidence, mortality and influence of centralized treatment on survival. *Acta Paediatr Scand*. 1988;77:836-841.

11. Phelan P, Hey E. Cystic fibrosis mortality in England and Wales and in Victoria, Australia 1976-80. *Arch Dis Child*. 1984;59:71-73.

12. Cystic fibrosis in the United Kingdom 1977-85: An improving picture. British Paediatric Association Working Party on Cystic Fibrosis. *BMJ*. 1988;297:1599-1602.

13. Curtis JR, Burke W, Kassner AW, et al. Absence of health insurance is associated with decreased life expectancy in patients with cystic fibrosis. *Am J Respir Crit Care Med*. 1997;155:1921-1924.

14. Schechter MS, Margolis PA. Relationship between socioeconomic status and disease severity in cystic fibrosis. *J Pediatr*. 1998;132:260-264.

15. Rubin BK. Exposure of children with cystic fibrosis to environmental tobacco smoke. *N Engl J Med*. 1990;323:782-788.

16. Collinson J, Nicholson KG, Cancio E, et al. Effects of upper respiratory tract infections in patients with cystic fibrosis. *Thorax*. 1996;51:1115-1122.

17. FitzSimmons SC. The changing epidemiology of cystic fibrosis. *J Pediatr*. 1993;122:1-9.

18. Konig P, Poehler J, Barbero GJ. A placebo-controlled, double-blind trial of the long-term effects of albuterol administration in patients with cystic fibrosis. *Pediatr Pulmonol*. 1998;25:32-36.

19. Konig P, Gayer D, Barbero GJ, et al. Short-term and long-term effects of albuterol aerosol therapy in cystic fibrosis: a preliminary report. *Pediatr Pulmonol*. 1995;20:205-214.

20. Sokol RJ, Reardon MC, Accurso FJ, et al. Fat-soluble-vitamin status during the first year of life in infants with cystic fibrosis identified by screening of newborns. *Am J Clin Nutr*. 1989;50:1064-1071.

21. Feranchak AP, Sontag MK, Wagener JS, et al. Prospective, long-term study of fat-soluble vitamin status in children with cystic fibrosis identified by newborn screen. *J Pediatr*. 1999;135:601-610.

Fatal High Fever in a 42-Year-Old Woman

Zhaohai Yang, Meredith A. Lakey, Stephanie D. Reilly

Department of Pathology, University of Alabama at Birmingham, Birmingham, AL

Patient: 42-year-old Caucasian woman with a history of substance abuse, remote trauma, and chronic pain controlled with an indwelling morphine pump.

Chief Complaint: Nausea, vomiting, and diarrhea for 3 days with decreased oral intake and urine output.

History of Present Illness: The patient's initial complaints were attributed to morphine withdrawal. Shortly after the morphine pump was refilled at her doctor's office, the patient developed acute abdominal pain and was taken to the emergency department (ED). On arrival, she was noted to be severely agitated with a blood pressure of 155/110 mm Hg, a pulse of 129 beats/min, a temperature of 97.2°F, and a respiratory rate of 44 breaths/min. Following a grand mal seizure, the patient was given succinylcholine (100 mg IV) and intubated for airway protection. She became rigid 5 minutes after administration of the drug, and her heart rate increased to 185 beats/min. Her rectal temperature was 107.9°F and increased to 108.7°F 40 minutes later. The patient was treated with ice packs, cooling blankets, acetaminophen, lorazepam, ceftriaxone, baclofen, and dantrolene. She was transferred to a tertiary care medical center. Her hospital course was complicated by altered mental status, disseminated intravascular coagulation (DIC), shock liver, and multiple episodes of cardiopulmonary arrest. She expired 3 days after transfer.

Past Medical/Surgical History: Chronic obstructive pulmonary disease, pancreatitis, multiple falls with fractures, paraplegia, and chronic pain treated with an indwelling intrathecal morphine pump.

Social History: The patient was married and had a longstanding history of tobacco, alcohol, and drug abuse with multiple admissions for drug rehabilitation.

Autopsy Findings: Postmortem examination revealed rhabdomyolysis with myoglobin accumulation in the distal renal tubules, submassive centrilobular hepatic necrosis (Image 1), and patchy hyaline membrane deposition in the lungs. Biventricular dilatation of the heart and bilateral pleural effusions were noted. Hemorrhage was present in the lungs, stomach, adrenals, and subarachnoid space of the spinal cord.

T1. Principal Laboratory Findings

Test	Patient's Result		Reference Interval
	Day 1	Day 3	
Hematology			
WBC count	22.9	19.3	4.0-11.0 × 10³/mL
Hematocrit	49	38	39-50%
Platelet count	115	56.7	150-400 × 10³/mL
Coagulation			
Prothrombin time	30.5	27.8	12.6-14.6 sec
INR	2.89	2.57	0.88-1.12
Partial thromboplastin time	47.0	38.0	25.0-35.0 sec
Fibrinogen	ND	214[a]	220-498 mg/dL
D-dimer	ND	>20,000[a]	110-240 ng/dL
Chemistry			
Sodium	144	147	133-145 mmol/L
Potassium	2.1	6.8	3.3-5.1 mmol/L
Chloride	114	108	96-108 mmol/L
CO₂	16	16	23-29 mmol/L
Arterial pH	7.25	7.31	7.35-7.45
BUN	25	40	6-19 mg/dL
Creatinine	1.5	3.2	0.7-1.3 mg/dL
Glucose	75	113	70-100 mg/dL
Calcium	6.2	5.7	8.4-10.2 mg/dL
Phosphate	1.9	9.1	2.7-4.5 mg/dL
Lactate	3	9.4	0.7-2.1 mmol/L
Creatine kinase (CK)	7,432	105,000	35-250 U/L
Albumin	ND	3.1	3.4-5.0 g/dL
Total bilirubin	ND	5.4	0.0-1.0 mg/dL
Aspartate aminotransferase (AST)	ND	3,961	0-37 U/L
Alanine aminotransferase (ALT)	ND	10,662	6-45 U/L

[a]Day 2 result; no data on Day 3. WBC, white blood cell; INR, International Normalized Ratio; BUN, blood urea nitrogen; ND: no data.

Questions

1. What are this patient's most striking clinical, laboratory, and histopathologic findings?

2. How do you explain these findings?

3. What is the patient's most likely diagnosis?

4. What is the pathogenesis of this patient's disease?

5. What is the genetic basis of this patient's condition?

6. What are the diagnostic modalities for susceptible individuals?

7. What is the appropriate treatment for this disease?

8. What are the complications and prognosis for this disease?

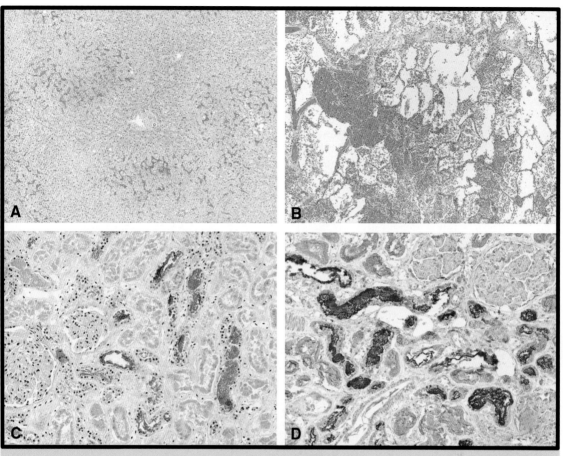

Image 1_Histopathology findings indicating submassive centrilobular hepatic necrosis (**A**), hemorrhages in pulmonary tissue as an example of hemorrhages involving multiple organs (**B**), and myoglobin deposition in renal tubules (**C**; H&E stain) and (**D**; myoglobin immunostain).

Possible Answers _____

1. Key findings include extremely high fever after administration of succinylcholine with rapid progression to DIC; multiple electrolyte disturbances; lactic (metabolic) acidosis; markedly elevated liver enzymes; acute renal failure; markedly increased creatine kinase (CK) level (**T1**); submassive centrilobular hepatic necrosis (**Image 1A**), hemorrhages involving multiple organs (**Image 1B**), and myoglobin deposition in renal tubules (**Images 1C** and **1D**).

2. High fever and rhabdomyolysis cause DIC and multisystem organ failure. All of the patient's abnormal clinical, laboratory, and morphologic findings can be linked to this constellation of conditions, including a markedly elevated total

CK from rhabdomyolysis with myoglobin deposition in the kidneys and liver necrosis. The diffuse hemorrhage may be explained by DIC. Her electrolyte disturbances, in addition to her acidosis, likely resulted in cardiac arrest.

3. ***Most likely diagnosis:*** malignant hyperthermia (MH). Malignant hyperthermia is a hypermetabolic state characterized by muscle rigidity, rhabdomyolysis, hyperthermia, and sympathetic hyperactivity. Although rhabdomyolysis can be caused by many conditions such as drugs (including opiates), alcohol, infection, seizures, and hypokalemia,[1,2] the extremely high fever immediately following succinylcholine administration suggests MH as the most likely cause of this patient's clinical and laboratory findings. The incidence of MH in the general population is estimated to be between 1/20,000 and 1/50,000.

It is typically a fulminant life-threatening disease triggered by potent inhalational anesthetics and/or succinylcholine.

4. Altered regulation and abnormally increased release of calcium from the sarcoplasmic reticulum into the sarcoplasma leads to a rise of intracellular calcium which causes uncontrolled aerobic and anaerobic metabolism and sustained muscle contraction, leading to metabolic acidosis, muscle rigidity, and hyperthermia. If untreated, ATP depletion eventually causes muscle cell death (rhabdomyolysis), leakage of muscle contents (myoglobin, calcium, potassium, and phosphate, etc) into the bloodstream, and dysfunction of multiple organs.[1-3]

5. Malignant hyperthermia is an inherited, pharmacogenetic disorder of the skeletal muscle. Mutations in sarcoplasmic reticulum ryanodine receptor gene (*RYR1*) account for about 50% of cases, and the inheritance pattern is autosomal dominant. Other genes implicated in MH include the voltage-dependent sodium channel and subunits of the dihydropyridine receptor. Malignant hyperthermia is also associated with Duchenne muscular dystrophy, carnitine palmitoyl transferase deficiency, hypokalemic periodic paralysis, and possibly other types of myopathies.[2,3]

6. The current gold standard for the diagnosis of MH is the caffeine halothane contracture test, which is performed on freshly biopsied muscle in 1 of about 30 muscle biopsy centers worldwide (8 in the United States and Canada). It has a sensitivity of near 100% and a specificity of 80% to 93%.[3-5] A less invasive, less expensive molecular test for the *RYR1* mutation has been introduced recently. Though highly specific, its sensitivity is only 30%. Molecular testing is primarily indicated for patients with a positive contracture test, a history of MH, or a positive family history.[3,4]

7. A high index of clinical suspicion is essential. Treatment measures include hyperventilation, immediate physical cooling measures (eg, ice packs, cooling blankets, cold fluid lavage of body cavities), aggressive intravenous fluid to maintain urine output greater than 300 mL/hour, prompt correction of electrolyte disturbances, and early dantrolene infusion, repeated as necessary.[1,2]

Dantrolene binds to the calcium channel, RYR1, and causes its closure, thus reversing the calcium influx. Use of this drug has contributed greatly to a dramatic decline in MH-related mortality and morbidity. The MH Association of the United States recommends that all hospitals, ambulatory centers, and offices where general anesthesia is administered have a full supply of dantrolene (36 vials) immediately available.[4]

8. Early complications of MH include hyperkalemia, hypocalcemia, and hepatic inflammation. Hepatic dysfunction occurs in about 25% of rhabdomyolysis cases. Other complications can occur later in the disease course, including acute renal failure and DIC. Acute renal failure occurs in about 15% of patients and is caused by mechanical obstruction of the renal tubules by myoglobin deposition, the toxic effect of iron, and hypovolemia. Severe hyperkalemia can cause cardiac arrhythmia and possibly cardiac arrest.[1,2] The development of DIC confers a dismal prognosis.

Keywords

malignant hyperthermia, disseminated intravascular coagulation, rhabdomyolysis, succinylcholine, liver necrosis

References

1. Sauret JM, Marinides G, Wang GK. Rhabdomyolysis. *Am Family Physician.* 2002;65:907-912.

2. Warren JD, Blumbergs PC, Thompson PD. Rhabdomyolysis: A review. *Muscle Nerve.* 2002;25:332-347.

3. Litman RS, Rosenberg H. Malignant hyperthermia: Update on susceptibility testing. *JAMA.* 2005;293:2918-2924.

4. Malignant hyperthermia association of the United States. http://www.mhaus.org. Accessed on December 14, 2006.

5. Miller JD. Malignant hyperthermia. http://www.anes.ucla.edu/dept/mh.html. Accessed on December 14, 2006.

Persistently Elevated Prostate-Specific Antigen Level After Successful Laparoscopic Radical Prostatectomy

Sangtae Park,[1] Jeffrey A. Cadeddu,[1] Jody A. Balko,[2] Marie W. Tortelli,[2] Frank H. Wians, Jr.[2]

Departments of [1]Urology and [2]Pathology, University of Texas Southwestern Medical Center, Dallas, TX

Patient: 67-year-old man.

Chief Complaint: Persistently elevated prostate-specific antigen (PSA) level, 4 months after successful laparoscopic radical prostatectomy.

History of Present Illness: During his annual prostate screening examination, the patient was noted to have a rise in PSA from 3.8 ng/mL in 2004 to 4.4 ng/mL in 2005, using the immunochemiluminometric assay (ICMA) Total PSA (TPSA) assay in the ADVIA Centaur instrument (Bayer Diagnostics, Tarrytown, NY). His digital rectal exam (DRE) was unremarkable with an estimated prostate gland size of 35 g and no evidence of nodules or induration.

Past Medical History: Hypertension, well controlled with Nifedipine; no history of heart disease; no recent vaccinations; and no history of organ transplant or blood transfusions.

Family History: Prostate cancer in an older brother, who died of metastatic disease.

Social History: He is a retired professional, without occupational exposure to animals. He was born on a farm but left in 1957; has never had rodent pets, but did have dogs and cats as pets.

Physical Examination Findings: The patient was well-developed and in no acute distress. His laparoscopic incisions were well-healed. There was no palpable lymphadenopathy in the cervical, supraclavicular, or inguinal chains, and no organomegaly.

Additonal Diagnostic Procedures: Due to the magnitude of the rise in his PSA concentration over a 1-year interval, resulting in a total PSA(TPSA) value >4.0 ng/mL, he underwent a 12-core transrectal prostate biopsy, which demonstrated Gleason Score 3+3 adenocarcinoma in 30% of a single core from the left side. After discussion of treatment options for his low-risk clinical grade T1c prostate cancer, he underwent an uncomplicated bilateral nerve-sparing laparoscopic radical prostatectomy. The final pathology report indicated a 42 g gland with organ-confined Gleason Score 3+3 adenocarcinoma, involving 10% of the gland (pT2cNXMX) and a positive focal margin at the left apex but no extracapsular extension. At the 3 month follow-up visit post-prostatectomy, his mean TPSA value from duplicate determinations was 2.25 ng/mL. Because this TPSA value was well above the functional analytical sensitivity (0.05 ng/mL) of the Beckman Coulter TPSA assay and the TPSA value expected (ie, <0.05 ng/mL) for a patient who underwent a successful radical prostatectomy, repeat TPSA testing on a new serum specimen was performed 2 weeks later at which time the patient's mean TPSA value from duplicate determinations was 2.17 ng/mL (**T1**). He subsequently underwent computed tomography (CT) of the abdomen and pelvis and nuclear bone scan and Prostascint imaging studies. The bone scan revealed increased activity in the left ilium, suggestive of Paget's disease. Computed tomography confirmed Paget's disease of the ilium and no other concerning findings. Prostascint imaging revealed focal positivity in the left supraclavicular area. Physical examination of this area was unremarkable, and follow-up contrast enhanced CT of the neck and chest demonstrated no lymphadenopathy or masses. The apparent discrepancy between the negative imaging studies, suggestive of a successful prostatectomy, and his elevated, post-prostatectomy TPSA value, above 0.05 ng/mL, prompted additional laboratory testing (**T1**) of his serum samples to determine the cause of this discrepancy.

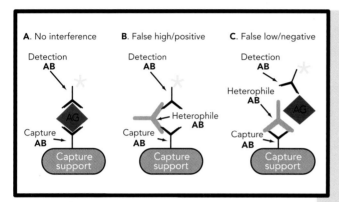

Figure 1_Mechanisms of heterophile antibody (eg, HAMA) interference in 2-site immunometric assays leading to (**A**) no HAMA interference, (**B**) falsely high (or positive) values, or (**C**) falsely low (or negative) values for the antigen (AG), or analyte, being measured. Yellow asterisk indicates the production of a signal based on the nature of the ligand attached to the detection antibody (**AB**). Various ligands used in these assays include substances capable of chemiluminescence, fluorescence, emission of radioactivity, or substrate conversion by enzyme-linked **AB** to a product that can be quantified based on the direct relationship between the quantity of AG captured by the capture **AB** bound to the capture support and the amount of signal produced when the detection **AB** binds to a different epitope (antigenic site) of the AG being quantified than the capture AB. The nature of the ligands attached to the signal AB define the type of immunometric assay as either an immunochemiluminometric assay (ICMA), immunofluorometric assay (IFMA), immunoradiometric assay (IRMA), or immunoenzymetric assay (IEMA), respectively.

Questions

1. What are this patient's most striking clinical and laboratory findings?

2. What is unusual about these findings?

3. How do you explain these findings?

4. What additional laboratory test could be performed to confirm your explanation of these findings?

5. What are some of the ways in which the problem that led to this patient's spuriously increased TPSA concentration can occur?

6. What are some of the ways in which laboratories and manufacturers of diagnostic immunoassays can resolve the problem that led to this patient's spuriously increased TPSA concentration?

7. How effective are the different approaches to identifying and/or resolving the problem that led to this patient's spuriously increased TPSA concentration?

8. What is the incidence of the problem that led to this patient's spuriously increased TPSA concentration?

9. Can adverse consequences occur when the problem that led to this patient's spuriously increased TPSA concentration is unrecognized?

10. Is the problem that led to this patient's spuriously increased TPSA concentration reversible?

Possible Answers

1. The discordance between the patient's detectable TPSA concentration (2.25 ng/mL and 2.17 ng/mL) on 2 separate occasions (**T1**) and

T1. Summary of Patient's PSA Results

Specimen No.	Time PP, mo	Bayer Centaur TPSA Assay TPSA, ng/mL[a]	Beckman Coulter ACCESS TPSA Assay TPSA, ng/mL BC Lab				FPSA, ng/mL[b]	%FPSA	Beckman Coulter ACCESS TPSA Assay TPSA, ng/ml BC Lab with Rgt Lot E + HBR				Bayer Centaur TPSA Assay TPSA, ng/mL[a]
			A	B	C	D			None	X	Y	Z	
-2	-48	3.8											
-1	-24	4.4											
0					Radical Prostatectomy Performed									
1	3		2.25c						1.12	1.03	0.96	0.25	**0.05**
2	3.5			2.17c					1.05	n.d.	n.d.	n.d.	**0.04**
3	4				0.60		2.05	341.7	1.08	n.d.	n.d.	n.d	**0.05**
1R1					0.65		2.37	364.3					
2R1					0.58		2.17	370.5					
3R1					0.57		2.11	370.2					
3D1:2					0.35		2.20	632.8					
3D1:4					0.24		2.12	870.4					
1R2						2.52							
2R2						2.25							
3R2						2.46							

[a] TPSA testing performed at another hospital using the Bayer TPSA assay in the ADVIA Centaur instrument (Bayer Diagnostics, Tarrytown, NY). [b] Using the Beckman Coulter (BC) free PSA (FPSA) assay in the ACCESS instrument (Beckman Coulter, Brea, CA). [c] Mean of duplicate determinations. No., number; PP, post-prostatectomy; R1, repeat test 1; R2, repeat test 2; D, testing performed using a 1:2 or 1:4 dilution (D); HBR, human anti-mouse antiglobulin blocking reagents X, Y, or Z; n.a., not applicable; n.d., not done.

clinical, histopathologic, and imaging results suggestive of a successful radical prostatectomy (RP).

2. Currently, the major therapeutic options for organ-confined prostate cancer include RP, radiation (external beam or brachytherapy), cryoablation, and active surveillance. One of the accepted benefits of RP is that total PSA concentration should be undetectable (ie, less than the functional sensitivity of the assay used to quantify TPSA concentration) post-operatively. Total prostate-specific antigen is an excellent tumor marker for evaluating tumor recurrence status post RP. In clinical practice, detectable TPSA after RP is considered "biochemical recurrence" and mandates consideration of metastatic work-up or adjuvant therapy. After radiation or cryoablation for organ-confined tumors, TPSA should also drop to a nadir level (eg, <0.05 ng/mL). In this case, with pathologically organ-confined, low-grade, low-stage prostate adenocarcinoma, it was extremely unexpected to have detectable TPSA values after RP. Our patient's post-RP TPSA values were approximately 50% of his pre-operative values (T1). This implied that the surgeon had either left half the prostate gland in the patient's body or the laboratory TPSA results were not accurate. Based on the histopathology and post-operative abdominopelvic CT findings, it was considered unlikely that the RP surgical procedure had been unsuccessful. Therefore, the accuracy of the post-prostatectomy TPSA values was investigated further with results as shown in (T1). Additional unusual findings in this case include a free PSA (FPSA) concentration significantly higher (3.4- to 8.7-fold) than the TPSA concentration. Because PSA exists in serum in 2 principal forms, free (FPSA) and protein bound [or "complexed" PSA (CPSA)], and the PSA assay used to quantify the TPSA in our patient's serum samples is an equimolar-response[1] [ie, measures both FPSA and complexed PSA (CPSA) equally, regardless of the ratio of these forms present in the patient's serum specimen] TPSA assay, the [TPSA] = [FPSA] + [CPSA]. Moreover, in patients with prostate cancer, the [CPSA] >> [FPSA].[2,3] Therefore, the FPSA concentration cannot exceed the TPSA concentration in our patient's serum.

3. Based on the information provided in (T1), the most likely cause of this patient's spuriously elevated post-RP TPSA values is the presence in his serum of human anti-mouse antibodies (HAMA). Evidence in support of this conclusion includes: (1) markedly different TPSA values using different lots of TPSA reagents; (2) lack of proportional results with dilution [ie, Specimen No. 3, (T1)]; and (3) the ability of a HAMA blocking reagent (HBR), when added to the patient's serum, to adsorb HAMA and yield TSPA results significantly different from an aliquot of the same serum sample to which the HBR was not added [ie, HBR Reagent Lot "Z", (T1)]. Note that not all HBRs were equally effective in inactivating the HAMA present in our patient's serum.

4. Direct measurement of HAMA in the patient's serum sample. Human anti-mouse antibodies measurement by immunoradiometric assay (IRMA) (Specialty Labs, Santa Monica, CA) of our patient's serum yielded a value of 440 ng/mL, a value ~6-fold higher than the upper limit (74 ng/mL) of the reference range. The fact that this upper limit is relatively high, compared to the likely functional analytical sensitivity of the HAMA IRMA, suggests that most individuals have a certain amount of HAMA in their serum.

5. Circulating anti-animal antibodies, such as HAMA, can arise in humans from 2 sources: iatrogenic and non-iatrogenic.[4] Examples of iatrogenic-induced causes of anti-animal Ab production in humans include: administration of a diagnostic or pharmaceutical agent derived from an animal source, blood transfusion, vaccination, administration of unconventional agents derived from animal sources, and organ transplant patients who receive mouse antibodies (eg, anti-CD3, anti-CD4, or anti-IL-2R)[5-7] for immunoprophylaxis. Examples of non-iatrogenic-induced causes of anti-animal Ab production in humans include: placental transfer to a fetus, occupations involving animal husbandry, pets, and the presence of disease (eg, idiopathic cardiomyopathy) associated with a high incidence of human anti-animal Ab production. We were not able to determine the cause of our patient's high HAMA level.

6. The principal procedures available to **laboratory professionals** in identifying and/or resolving HAMA interference in immunoassay testing are: (1) diluting the patient's serum sample, testing each dilution for the analyte of interest, and observing whether or not the analyte results are linear or non-linear compared to the analyte concentration in an undiluted serum sample (Note: Non-linear results suggest the presence of HAMA; however, 50% of HAMAs are likely to dilute linearly.[8]); (2) re-testing of the patient's serum sample for the analyte of interest using a different immunoassay method. Human anti-mouse antibody interference may affect 1 immunoassay method to a lesser extent than other immunoassay methods (eg, 2-site immunometric assays are especially prone to HAMA interference[4,9]); (3) using a commercially available HBR to remove HAMA interference; or (4) testing for the presence of HAMA in the patient's serum using a HAMA-specific immunoassay method (Note: Unfortunately, there is no universally applicable immunoassay that will measure all different types of HAMA and measure them equally as well in all patient's serum samples). Approaches by **manufacturers** of diagnostic immunoassay methods to limit HAMA interference in their assays include: (1) use of the Fab or $F(ab')_2$ fragment instead of intact immunoglobulin (Ig) as the capture and signal antibodies in 2-site immuometric assays (Note: This approach eliminates interference from anti-animal antibodies with specificity for the Fc portion of an IgG antibody reagent[4]); (2) use of chimeric monoclonal reagent antibodies in lieu of monoclonal antibodies derived from mouse spleen cell-human cancer cell hybridomas; and (3) use of monoclonal reagent antibodies derived from chicken cells such that these antibodies do not have specificity for mouse antibodies. [Note: Such a strategy may simply transfer the problem from HAMA to HACA (human anti-chicken antibodies; however, HACA probably occur less frequently in human serum than HAMA)]. Reagents used in several modern automated immunoassays routinely include nonimmune HBRs. While this strategy has reduced the number of false positive immunoassay results, it is not 100% effective, as demonstrated in this case study. Other physical and chemical techniques used by laboratory professionals and/or manufacturers to remove heterophile Ab interference include ultracentrifugation,[10] precipitation with trichloroacetic acid,[10] and pretreatment of serum with agents such as polyethylene glycol[11] and detergents.[12] However, none of these techniques is universally applicable for all analytes, these techniques are cumbersome, and their reliability is unknown. Moreover, another difficulty is that the problem of solving HAMA interference is a moving target (ie, reagent lots for immunoassays vary over time and HBRs are not equally effective in removing all HAMA interference). In our patient, TPSA testing with reagent lots C, D, and E (all from Beckman Coulter) and reagent lot E with 3 different HBRs gave different results. These findings suggest that the HAMA in our patient's serum had different affinities for the murine antibodies (Ab's) contained in these different reagent lots.

7. Because each of the approaches to identifying and/or resolving HAMA interference have limitations and none are perfect, a multi-pronged approach involving all of the laboratory strategies indicated above is optimal. One explanation for the lack of a "perfect" HBR is the polyspecific nature of heterophile Ab's, such that while many of them can be blocked, others can not. This is because some HAMA are characterized by low-affinity binding, whereas others have higher affinity. Their heterogeneity is explained by the current hypothesis that HAMA are naturally occurring Ab's that arise either by chance or as idiotype-specific antibodies. The HAMA may represent non-specific, weakly-binding antibodies produced by the humoral immune system in the normal Ab production process. In this model, the naïve B cell population generates 10^7-10^8 different Ab's that passively survey the internal milieu for antigens. Once exposed to an antigen, clonal expansion of specific B cells leads to Ab-producing plasma cells and memory B cells. Thus, HAMA simply arise by chance in a given individual's repertoire of 10^7-10^8 naïve Ab's. By contrast, HAMA may represent "idiotypic Ab's." Idiotypic Ab's are those that bind to the idiotope (Id), a site within the variable region of immunoglobulins that binds other Ab's. It is thought that such Id-(anti-Id) interactions regulate humoral immunity. Thus, while idiotypic Ab's are normal regulatory elements of humoral immunity, they can corrupt clinical immunoassays by also acting as interfering HAMA. In the clinical chemistry

literature, the problem of HAMA interference in immunoassay testing has been long recognized.[4,9] Usually, HAMA interference leads to spuriously elevated analyte values, but falsely decreased values can occur, albeit less commonly. The mechanism by which HAMA may produce falsely decreased or increased results in 2-site immunometric assays is shown in **Figure 1**. Finding an easy solution to detect and eliminate HAMA interference in immunoassay testing has been elusive.[13]

8. The incidence of HAMA interference, and spuriously low or high analyte results from this interference, in clinical immunoassays is unknown. Estimates of this interference vary from <1% to as high as 80%.[2] Even if the lowest estimate is correct, the incidence may be rising, however, because of the widespread use of automated 2-site immunometric assays employing monoclonal, mouse spleen cell-derived antibodies and the increasing use of conventional and unconventional agents derived from animal sources (eg, mice) for diagnostic or therapeutic medical purposes. In a recent study published by the Mayo Clinic, 500 serum samples were tested using 8 automated immunoassays for tumor markers. They found that the incidence of heterophile Ab interference ranged from 0.2% (alpha-fetoprotein) to 3.7% (calcitonin).[14] The other tumor markers in this report were gastrin, CA 125, CA 15-3, human chorionic gonadotropin (hCG), TPSA, and FPSA. In an older study that tested free thyroxine and thyrotropin, the incidence of heterophilic interference was 7 out of 21,000 samples (0.033%).[15] The wide range (0.033% to 3.7%) of published values for the incidence of heterophile Ab interference in immunoassay methods for a variety of analytes can be explained by differences in the analytes tested, immunoassay design characteristics (eg, the animal species used to obtain cells for producing reagent monoclonal/polyclonal antibodies), and reagent lots that contain or do not contain HAMA blocking agents.

9. Yes. HAMA can potentially interfere with any clinical immunoassay that uses murine antibodies. In a widely-publicized case, a false elevation in hCG due to HAMA led to unnecessary hysterectomy and lung resection in a 22-year-old woman.[16] In a similar case, a 49-year-old man

with a TPSA concentration of 3.3 ng/mL and Gleason Score 6 prostate cancer underwent unnecessary surgery followed by adjuvant radiation and androgen ablation for 22 months before HAMA was suspected as the cause of his elevated TPSA concentration.[17] Fortunately, our patient was not given unnecessary adjuvant therapy, but his true TPSA will likely never be known due to the high HAMA level in his serum. Based on the 0.2% to 3.7% incidence of HAMA interference in immunoassays for tumor markers reported in the Mayo Clinic study, it is alarming to imagine the extent of the potential psychologic distress and under- or overtreatment of patients with spurious analyte results due to HAMA interference. The present case and those referred to above underscore the importance of teamwork between clinicians and laboratory staff when laboratory results are not consistent with clinical findings or expectations. Clinicians should be aware of heterophilic Ab interference in immunoassay testing and if the laboratory result for a test performed by immunoassay is incongruous with the patient's clinical status, consideration of HAMA is warranted.

10. In our patient, it is unlikely that his serum HAMA interference in our TPSA immunoassay can be completely eliminated. Three HAMA blocking agents were unsuccessful in completely eliminating his HAMA interference using the TPSA immunoassay in the ACCESS instrument. Use of HBRs X, Y, and Z, provided TPSA values that were 8.0%, 14.3%, and 77.7%, respectively, lower than the HBR-untreated serum sample (**T1**); however, none of the TPSA values on the HBR-treated samples were <0.05 ng/mL. However, it is possible that using a TPSA assay from a different manufacturer (eg, Bayer TPSA assay in the ADVIA Centaur instrument) could provide an accurate TPSA value on our patient's serum. When we referred all 3 of our patient's serum samples for testing using the Bayer TPSA assay in the ADVIA Centaur instrument, all values obtained on all 3 of these samples were #0.05 ng/mL (**T1**), confirming that our patient's prostatectomy was successful, and when coupled with our other laboratory data, that HAMA was the most likely cause of his spuriously increased TPSA values using the TPSA reagents and assay in the Beckman Coulter ACCESS instrument. Unlike the Beckman Coulter ACCESS TPSA

assay, which uses both **mouse** monoclonal capture and detection antibodies (see **Figure 1**), the Bayer Centaur TPSA assay uses a mouse monoclonal capture antibody and a **goat** polyclonal detection antibody.[1]

Keywords

prostate cancer, radical prostatectomy, human antimouse antibodies, interference, 2-site immunometric assay, blocking reagent

References

1. Wians FH Jr, Cheli CD, Balko JA, et al. Evaluation of the clinical performance of equimolar- and skewed-response total prostate-specific antigen assays versus complexed and free PSA assays and their ratios in discriminating between benign prostatic hyperplasia and prostate cancer. *Clin Chim Acta.* 2002;326:81-95.

2. Shariat SF, Roehrborn CG, Wians FH Jr. Update on prostate-specific antigen testing for the early diagnosis of prostate cancer. ASCP Check Sample, Clinical Chemistry 2003;43:67-89.

3. Wians FH Jr. The role of prostate-specific antigen testing in the diagnosis, treatment, and follow-up of patients with adenocarcinoma of the prostate. ASCP Check Sample, Clinical Chemistry 1997;37:77-103.

4. Levinson SS, Miller JJ. Towards a better understanding of heterophile (and the like) antibody interference with modern immunoassays. *Clin Chim Acta.* 2002;325:1-15.

5. Abramowicz D, Crusiaux A, Niaudet P, et al. The IgE humoral response in OKT3-treated patients: incidence and fine specificity. *Transplantation.* 1996;61:577-581.

6. Pulito VL, Roberts VA, Adair JR, et al. Humanization and molecular modeling of the anti-CD4 monoclonal antibody, OKT4A. *J Immunol.* 1996;156:2840-2850.

7. Nashan B, Schlitt HG, Schwinzer R, et al. Immunoprophylaxis with a monoclonal anti-IL-2 receptor antibody in liver transplant patients. *Transplantation.* 1996;61:546-554.

8. Ismail AA, Walker PL, Barth JH, et al. Wrong biochemistry results: 2 case reports and observational study in 5310 patients on potentially misleading thyroid-stimulating hormone and gonadotropin immunoassay results. *Clin Chem.* 2002;48:2023-2029.

9. Kricka LJ. Human anti-animal antibody interference in immunological assays. *Clin Chem.* 1999;45:942-956.

10. Liendo C, Ghali JK, Graves SW. A new interference in some digoxin assays: Anti-murine heterophilic antibodies. *Clin Pharmacol Ther.* 1996;60:593-598.

11. Despres N, Grant AM. Antibody interference in thyroid assays: a potential for clinical misinformation. *Clin Chem.* 1998;44:440-454.

12. Muller W, Mierau R, Wohltmann D. Interference of IgM rheumatoid factor with nephelometric C-reactive protein determinations. *J Immunol Methods.* 1985;80:77-90.

13. Ismail AA. A radical approach is needed to eliminate interference from endogenous antibodies in immunoassays. *Clin Chem.* 2005;51:25-26.

14. Preissner CM, Dodge LA, O'Kane DJ, et al. Prevalence of heterophilic antibody interference in 8 automated tumor marker immunoassays. *Clin Chem.* 2005;51:208-210.

15. Ward G, McKinnon L, Badrick T, et al. Heterophilic antibodies remain a problem for the immunoassay laboratory. *Am J Clin Pathol.* 1997;108:417-421.

16. Skolnik S, Sunde S. UW and drug company share blame: *Seattle Post Intelligencer.* Seattle, WA, June 30, 2001, pp 1.

17. Morgan BR, Tarter TH. Serum heterophile antibodies interfere with prostate specific antigen test and result in over treatment in a patient with prostate cancer. *J Urol.* 2001;166: 2311-2312.

Urine Pregnancy Testing in Two Women With Cancer

Tze-Kiong Er,[1,3] Yuh-Jyh Jong,[1] Li-Yu Tsai,[2] Hung-Jung Cheng,[1] Bai-Hsiun Chen[3]

[1]Graduate Institute of Medicine, Faculty of Medicine, College of Medicine, [2]Faculty of Biomedical Laboratory Science, College of Health Sciences, and [3]Department of Laboratory Medicine, Kaohsiung Medical University Hospital, Kaohsiung Medical University, Kaohsiung, Taiwan

	No. 1	No. 2
Patient:	53-year-old woman.	49-year-old woman.
Chief Complaint:	Nausea, vomiting, intermittent abdominal cramping pain for 4 days.	Lower abdominal pain.
Drug History:	Unremarkable.	Unremarkable.
Medical History:	She was previously diagnosed with cancer of the descending colon.	She was previously diagnosed with cervical cancer.
Family History:	Unremarkable.	
Principal Laboratory Findings:	T1	T1

Questions

1. What are the most striking clinical and laboratory findings in these patients?

2. Why is it important to assess pregnancy status?

3. What are some of the causes of false-positive serum and urine pregnancy tests?

4. How would you rule out human or technical error as a possible cause of a false-positive or -negative urine pregnancy test?

5. What can cause discordances between urine and serum hCG test results?

6. What is the most likely diagnosis for these patients?

7. What is the clinical significance of a false-positive urine pregnancy test?

8. Are serum hCG tests unaffected by factors that can cause false-positive test results?

Possible Answers

1. The most striking laboratory findings in both of these patients was a positive urine pregnancy test in patients who, based on their medical history (data not shown), were not expected to have a positive urine hCG pregnancy test.

2. Determination of pregnancy status is important in the work-up of a woman presenting with vaginal bleeding or lower abdominal pain. Women with these symptoms should be screened for pregnancy using a urine pregnancy test, especially prior to undergoing an x-ray procedure. Clinical decisions regarding additional diagnostic

T1. Principal Laboratory Findings

Test	Results on Patient No.		"Normal" Reference Range
	1	2	
Hematology			
WBC count	11.0	11.8	4.0–10.0 × 10³/µL
RBC count	4.6	4.0	4.0–5.5 × 10⁶/µL
Hemoglobin	14.5	12.7	12.0–16.0 g/dL
Hematocrit	43.4	37.6	37.0–47.0%
Platelet count	217	364	130–500 × 10³/µL
Chemistry			
BUN	17.0	n/a	7.0–18.0 mg/dL
Creatinine	1.2	n/a	0.6–1.3 mg/dL
Sodium	138	n/a	136–145 mEq/L
Potassium	3.2	n/a	3.5–5.1 mEq/L
Chloride	96	n/a	98–107 mEq/L
AST	94	n/a	10–42 U/L
ALT	75	n/a	10–40 U/L
CRP	9.8	<5.0	<5.0 µg/mL
Urinalysis			
Color	Yellow	Reddish	Clear
Appearance	Clear	Turbid	Colorless
Specific gravity	1.023	>1.010	1.005–1.025
pH	5.5	5.5	5.0–8.0
Glucose	Neg	Neg	Neg
Bilirubin	Neg	Neg	Neg
Ketones	Neg	4+	Neg
Blood	Neg	2+	Neg
Protein	30	100	Neg (mg/dL)
Urobilinogen	1+	Neg	Neg (EU/dL)
Nitrites	Neg	Neg	Neg
WBCs	Neg	Neg	Neg
Microscopic findings			
RBCs	0–2	25–50	0–2/hpf
WBCs	2–5	25–50	0–2/hpf
Epithelial cells	2–5	5–10	0–2/hpf
Urine pregnancy test	Pos	Pos	Neg (<25 mIU/mL)

WBC, white blood cells; RBC, red blood cell; BUN, blood urea nitrogen; AST, aspartate aminotransferase; ALT, alanine aminotransferase; CRP, C-reactive protein; n/a, not available; EU, Ehrlich Units; hpf, high power field.

testing should be based on the results of the urine pregnancy test and knowledge of those conditions that can cause false-positive screening tests for human chorionic gonadotropin (hCG) in urine and serum, including the presence of serum human anti-mouse antibodies (HAMA) and diseases (eg, colon or cervical cancer) associated with excretion of hCG into the urine.

3. A number of preanalytical conditions, other than pregnancy, including trophoblastic disease and certain non-trophoblastic neoplasms (eg, testicular tumors, prostate cancer, breast cancer, and lung cancer), can cause elevated serum levels of hCG that are then excreted into the urine.[1,2] False-positive urine hCG results have also been reported in patients with nephrotic-range proteinuria and tubo-ovarian abscess.[3,4] Analytical causes of false-positive or false-negative urine hCG tests include human or technical error in the performance of tests and/or the interpretation of test results. We performed pregnancy testing on urine from our patients using the Abbott Testpack Plus (Abbott Laboratories, Chicago) immunochromatographic assay. The principle of this point-of-care qualitative assay is based on the reaction of hCG in the patient's sample with monoclonal anti-hCG capture antibodies contained in the solid support medium to focus any hCG in the patient's specimen as a discrete line in this medium, followed by detection of hCG using a signal antibody conjugated to a substance that imparts a characteristic color to the capture antibody-hCG-detection antibody complex.[10,11] The absence of a colored line in the specific location on the solid support medium when the colored line corresponding to the control is visible indicates a negative result. The capture and signal antibodies recognize 2 of 8 different epitopes on the hCG molecule. The analytical sensitivity of this assay is 25 IU/L.

4. Human or technical error was suspected initially as the cause of the positive urine hCG result on both patients. To rule out such error, testing was repeated on both patients' urine, in duplicate, by each of 2 experienced medical technologists and all results were positive. After discussion with the patients' clinicians, quantitative serum β-hCG testing was performed and the results were 2.6 IU/L (patient No. 1) and 4.5 IU/L (patient No. 2).

5. Because of the discrepancy between the urine and serum hCG results on the patients, we suspected that other hCG molecules (eg, β-core fragments) might be responsible for the false-positive pregnancy tests. Human chorionic gonadotrophin (hCG) is a glycoprotein composed of 2 dissimilar subunits, an α- and β-subunit, held together by charge interactions. Both subunits are needed for biological activity and are common to other hormones (eg, TSH, LH, and FSH); however, the β-subunit determines the specificity of the biological action of the hormones containing these subunits.[5] In the circulation, the bulk of the hCG molecules exist as intact hormone (ie, α/β dimer) with only small amounts of free α- and β-subunits. In urine, however, a large fraction of the immunoreactivity of hCG is due to a metabolic breakdown product of hCG, commonly known as "β-core fragment."[6] This fragment is believed to be a renal degradation product of intact hCG and the free β-subunit.[7] Although this fragment lacks the unique 30-amino acid carboxyl-terminal peptide of the β-subunit of intact hCG, it retains conformational immunological determinants in the urine of pregnant women and some women with various types of cancer sufficient to react with the hCG antibodies used in urine pregnancy tests. Moreoever, the beta-core fragment is virtually undetectable in serum using currently available serum hCG assays.[8] Using Sephadex G100 size exclusion chromatography, Papapetrou and Nicopoulou reported that hCG β-core fragment was present in the urine of patients with uterine cervix, colon, esophageal, or ovarian cancer.[11]

6. ***Most likely diagnosis for both patients:*** *false-positive urine hCG results due to the presence of cross-reacting hCG fragments in the urine of these patients with colon or cervical cancer.*

7. A false-positive urine pregnancy test may place a patient at risk for unnecessary treatment. Our patients point out the need to be aware of colon or cervical cancer as a potential cause of a false-positive urine pregnancy test in women with these conditions who are undergoing pregnancy screening using a urine hCG test. Moreover, it is important to confirm a suspected false-positive urine hCG test using a quantitative serum hCG test.

8. No. Although it is good practice to confirm a suspected false-positive urine hCG result with a quantitative serum hCG test, clinicians need to be cautious of factors that can cause false-positive or false-negative serum hCG results (eg, HAMA). In addition, the cardinal rule of medicine is that if the results do not make sense (eg, given the patient's clinical history and/or the results of other diagnostic procedures or laboratory tests), look for a suitable explanation before treating the patient. Physicians should be very cautious about false-positive results. Indeed, if urine hCG results are not consistent with the patient's clinical history, physicians should contact the laboratory for help in finding an explanation. Such an approach may avoid the misfortune, and considerable malpractice cost, associated with 1 of the most (in)famous cases of failure to consider alternative explanations for positive serum hCG results and to enlist the aid of laboratorians in resolving such results (ie, the Jennifer Rufer case).[12]

Keywords _____

urine pregnancy test, human chorionic gonadotrophin, beta-core fragment

References _____

1. Dawood MY, Saxena BB, Landesman R. Human chorionic gonadotrophin and its subunits in hydatifiform mole and choriocarcinoma. *Obstet Gynecol.* 1977;50:172–181.

2. Braunstein GD, Vaitukaitis JL, Carbone PP, et al. Ectopic production of human chorionic gonadotropin by neoplasms. *Ann Intern Med.* 1973;78:39–45.

3. Levsky ME, Handler JA, Suarez RD, et al. False-positive urine beta-HCG in a women with a tubo-ovarian abscess. *J Emerg Med.* 2001;2:407–409.

4. Kountz DS, Kolander SA, Rozovsky A. False positive pregnancy test in the nephrotic syndrome. *N Engl J Med.* 1989;321:1416.

5. Wu J, Nakamura R. Human circulating tumor markers. Current concepts and clinical applications. Chicago: American Society for Clinical Pathology; 1997:127–176.

6. Davison CM, Kaplan RM, Wenig LN, et al. Qualitative b–hCG urine assays may be misleading in the presence of molar pregnancy: A case report. *Journal of Emerg Med.* 2004;27:43–47.

7. Stricklan TW, Puett D. Contribution of subunits to the function of luteinizing hormone/human chorionic gonadotrophin recombinants. *Endocrinology*. 1981;109:1933–1942.

8. Wehmann RE, Blithe DL, Flack MR, et al. Metabolic clearance rate and urinary clearance of purified beta-core. *J Clin Endocrinol Metab*. 1989;69:510–517.

9. Wehman RE, Nisula BC. Renal clearance of the subunits of human chorionic gonadotrophin in man. *J Clin Endocrinol Metab*. 1980;50:674–679.

10. Chard T. Pregnancy tests: A review. *Hum Reprod*. 1992;5:701–710.

11. Papapetrou PD, Nicopoulou SC. The origin of a human chorionic gonadotrophin–subunit-core fragment excreted in the urine of patients with cancer. *Acta Endocrinologica*. 1986;112:415–422.

12. Bartley N. Woman sues over cancer error. *The Seattle Times*. April 25, 2001.

Nausea, Vomiting, and Decreased Level of Consciousness in a Patient With Chronic Back Pain

Jeffrey W. Oliver,[1] R. Scott Akins,[1] Dale M. Dunn,[1] Brent Farnesworth,[1] Cynthia Jumper,[2] Charles Bradley[1]

Departments of [1]Pathology and [2]Internal Medicine, Texas Tech Health Sciences Center School of Medicine, Lubbock, TX

Patient: 39-year-old male with a history of intractable back pain.

Chief Complaint: The patient was brought to the emergency department via ambulance due to decreased level of consciousness, nausea, and vomiting.

History of Present Illness: The patient had a history of spinal fusion secondary to a spinal injury approximately 2 to 3 years prior to this admission. He subsequently had a history of severe chronic back pain for which he had been prescribed a variety of narcotic analgesics and muscle relaxants. He had been prescribed methadone 1 month prior to admission, but ran out over a weekend and began taking previously prescribed medications. According to family members, he took an estimated 12 hydrocodone/acetaminophen pills (10 mg/500 mg each) and 6 carisoprodol pills (350 mg each) per day for the 3 days immediately prior to this admission.

Social History: The patient's family claimed he had no history of acute or chronic alcohol abuse.

Physical Examination: The patient appeared mildly confused and diaphoretic, and was noted to have mild tremors. His vital signs were: blood pressure, 148/75 mm Hg; pulse rate, 103 beats/min; and normal respiratory rate. Examination of the head demonstrated normal pupillary response and no abnormalities. The cardiovascular system review was negative and the lungs were normal to auscultation. There was no palpable hepatosplenomegaly or abdominal tenderness. The neurological examination was normal, except for the previously noted confusion and slight tremors.

Questions

1. At admission, what are this patient's most striking laboratory results?

2. What is the significance of the patient's elevated serum amylase and lipase on the second hospital day?

3. Based on this patient's history, physical examination, and admission laboratory findings, what conditions should be considered in the differential diagnosis?

4. What is this patient's most likely diagnosis?

5. How should this patient's time-dependent changes in acetaminophen levels be evaluated?

6. How frequent is this patient's condition?

7. What is the pathogenesis of this patient's condition?

T1. Principal Laboratory Findings

Test	Admission	Patient's Result @ Time After Admission, h 24	48	60	72	"Normal" Reference Range
Chemistry						
Sodium	138	141	151	155	157	137-145 mmol/L
Potassium	4.0	5.9	4.3	4.4	4.6	3.6-5.0 mmol/L
Chloride	103	118	122	135	139	99-110 mmol/L
Bicarbonate	17	15	14	13	10	22-30 mmol/L
BUN	6	2	5	7	5	7-17 mmol/L
Creatinine	0.8	0.8	1.0	2.5	3.3	0.7-1.2 mg/dL
Glucose	107	95	154	<20	<20	65-110 mg/dL
Calcium	9.8	9.1	9.9	6.9	7.2	8.4-10.2 mg/dL
Bilirubin, total	2.7	4.1	5.5	4.1		0.2-1.3 mg/dL
ALT	807	1,592	7,227	4,288		21-72 U/L
AST	840	1,668	6,940	3,720		17-59 U/L
ALP	129	160	290	189		38-126 U/L
CK	59					55-170 U/L
CK-MB	1.1					0.7-10.4 ng/mL
Troponin I	<0.3					<2.0 ng/mL
Amylase		500		691		30-110 U/L
Lipase		6,500		4974		23-300 U/L
Acetaminophen	65	35	12			10-30 µg/mL
Ammonia			204	143	288	21-71 µmol/L
dau screen	Pos for opiates					Negative for all drugs screened
Coagulation						
Platelet count		314	238	122	68	140-400 × 10⁹/L
PT		93.2	71.9	92.8	85.4	10.5-13.1 sec
PTT		46.3	42.8	52.4	97.3	23.1-33.8 sec
Fibrinogen					0.27	2.0-4.0 g/L
FDP					>40	<10 µg/L
D-Dimer					0.8-1.6	<0.2 µg/mL

BUN, blood urea nitrogen; ALT, alanine aminotransferase; AST, aspartate aminotransferase; ALP, alkaline phosphatase; CK, creatine kinase; CK-MB, MB isoenzyme of CK; dau, drugs of abuse in urine; PT, prothrombin time; PTT, partial thromboplastin time; FDP, fibrin degradation products.

8. What are the treatment options for this patient's condition?

Possible Answers _____

1. Decreased bicarbonate and BUN; increased total bilirubin and acetaminophen; markedly increased ALT and AST; positive opiate drugs of abuse in urine (dau) screen (**T1**).

2. The patient's elevated serum amylase and lipase levels on the second hospital day suggested acute pancreatitis. In patients with acute pancreatitis, serum lipase concentration increases usually within 3 to 6 hours of onset, peaks at approximately 24 hours, and usually returns to normal

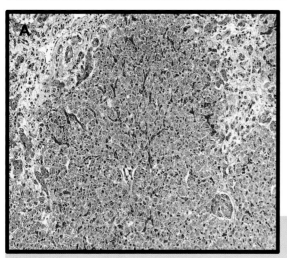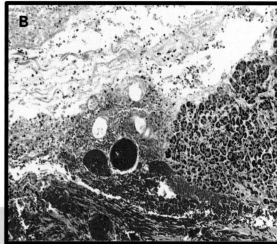

Image 1_Autopsy section of the patient's (**A**) liver, demonstrating widespread hepatocyte submassive necrosis (magnification, 10×) and (**B**) pancreas, demonstrating hemorrhage, fat necrosis, and acute inflammation (hemmorhagic pancreatitis) (magnification, 10×).

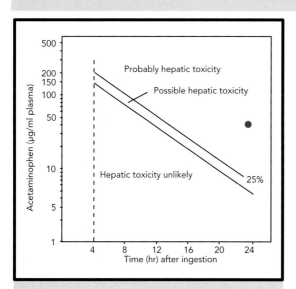

Figure 1_Rumack-Matthew nomogram for evaluating the probability of hepatotoxicity as a function of time and concentration post-ingestion of acetaminophen.[1] Red dot indicates patient's acetaminophen concentration 24 hours after admission.

during a period of 8 to 14 days. Serum amylase concentration also begins to increase within 3 to 6 hours of onset, rises rapidly within 8 hours in 75% of patients, reaches peak concentration in 20 to 30 hours, and increases may persist for 48 to 72 hours. However, in patients with acute pancreatitis, lipase concentration typically increases to a greater extent and remains elevated longer than amylase. Lipase is considered superior to amylase in the assessment of patients with signs and symptoms suggestive of acute pancreatitis.

Therefore, lipase should always be determined whenever amylase is determined when evaluating such patients.[1] In patients with signs and symptoms of acute pancreatitis, pancreatitis is likely when the lipase concentration exceeds 5x the upper limit of normal (ULN) (ie, diagnostic specificity is approximately 85%), but unlikely if the serum lipase concentration is <3× ULN.[1] If lipase values increase significantly over time and/ or lipase and amylase increases are concordant, the likelihood of pancreatitis is also increased.[1]

3. Narcotic overdose or withdrawal, cerebrovascular disease (eg, stroke), other forms of encephalopathy, and drug-induced acute liver failure due to acetaminophen hepatotoxicity.

4. ***Most likely diagnosis:*** *acetaminophen hepatotoxicity.* This patient's markedly increased serum acetaminophen level at admission, with markedly elevated alanine aminotransferase (ALT) and aspartate aminotransferase (AST) values are consistent with hepatocellular injury, while his prolonged PT suggests decreased hepatic synthesis of coagulation factors due to hepatic failure (**T1**). Clinically, the patient's history of recent increased intake of hydrocodone/acetaminophen fits the laboratory data, and the decreased level of consciousness and tremors could be explained by hepatic encephalopathy secondary to hepatic failure. The positive dau screen for opiates is most likely due to the hydrocodone contained in the hydrocodone/acetaminophen tablets taken by the patient.

5. Serum acetaminophen levels at various times post-ingestion of acetaminophen should always be correlated with the probability of hepatotoxicity using the Rumack-Matthew nomogram (**Figure 1**).[2] This nomogram is most applicable in patients who have acutely absorbed a single large dose of acetaminophen, rather than accumulation over several days, which can be equally as toxic.[3] Moreover, this nomogram does not account for potential interactions with other drugs the patient may have taken concurrently with acetaminophen. This patient's history of increased acetaminophen use over several days and concurrent use of carisoprodol made the use of the nomogram less useful, and may or may not have altered his ultimate outcome.

6. Acetaminophen overdose is the most frequent medication inquiry at poison centers in the United States, and is 1 of the most common causes of fulminant hepatic failure.[4] Acetaminophen is readily available over-the-counter as an analgesic and antipyretic in addition to being a common constituent of prescription pain medications combined with opioids.

7. Acetaminophen is metabolized by the liver and is conjugated predominantly with sulfates and/or glucuronides to form nontoxic metabolites which are easily excreted by the kidneys. A toxic intermediate, N-acetyl-p-benzoquinoneimine, is bound normally by hepatocellular glutathione, but high doses of acetaminophen exhaust glutathione reserves and lead to accumulation of this toxic metabolite, which is responsible for hepatocyte necrosis.[5]

8. Basic life support measures are the top priority in the treatment of acute acetaminophen intoxication, and gastric lavage may be helpful immediately post-ingestion. Administration of N-acetylcysteine (NAC) increases the amount of available cysteine, a glutathione precursor. Glutathione then binds N-acetyl-p-benzoquinoneimine to form a nontoxic substance that is cleared by the kidneys.[5] The effectiveness of NAC diminishes with time post-ingestion of acetaminophen. Therefore, NAC should be administered as soon as possible after confirmation of acetaminophen overdose. N-acetylcysteine has been reported by some authors to prevent ongoing liver damage as late

as 24 hours post-ingestion,[6] but others recommend the use of extracorporeal sorbent-based devices for the treatment of acetaminophen overdose in such late-presenting patients.[7] Despite the relative high frequency of acetaminophen intoxication, no consensus exists on the proper dosage, route (oral versus intravenous) of administration, and timing of NAC therapy, or on the effectiveness of charcoal lavage therapy compared to NAC therapy because no large-scale well-controlled study has been conducted to compare the effectiveness of these 2 treatment modalities for acetaminophen intoxication.[8] In our patient, the time elapsed post-ingestion of acetaminophen was unclear at the time of this patient's presentation, so loading (140 mg/kg) and maintenance (70 mg/kg) doses of NAC were administered by nasogastric tube.

Course and Outcome

Despite aggressive therapy, our patient deteriorated, had increased confusion, further increase in serum transaminases levels, hyperkalemia, increased PT and PTT values, and an increased serum ammonia level by the second hospital day (**T1**). He developed tachypnea and hypoxia, and despite ventilatory support, continued to deteriorate. Hypotension, hypoglycemia, disseminated intravascular coagulation, and acute renal failure also developed. On the fourth hospital day, he developed cardiopulmonary arrest and multi-organ failure. The patient's family requested a do not resuscitate (DNR) order, and the patient ultimately became asystolic and died. At autopsy, significant pathologic findings included a moderately sized retroperitoneal hematoma secondary to hemorrhagic pancreatitis, 300 mL of melena in the small bowel and proximal large bowel, and a 1,900 gram liver with capsular and parenchymal mottling. There was no evidence of cholelithiasis. Histologic sections of the liver demonstrated submassive necrosis (**Image 1A**) and acute inflammation, hemorrhage, and necrosis of the pancreas (**Image 1B**). Based on the patient's history, histopathologic findings, and post-mortem toxicology results, no cause of pancreatitis, other than acetaminophen toxicity, was found. Although hemorrhagic pancreatitis is a relatively rare complication of acetaminophen overdose, often overshadowed by the much more common finding of severe hepatic necrosis, this case study adds to the number of patients reported previously who developed acetaminophen-induced hemorrhagic pancreatitis.[9-11]

Keywords

acetaminophen, acute liver failure, hepatotoxicity, hemorrhagic pancreatitis, drug-induced pancreatitis, N-acetylcysteine

References

1. Ranson JH. Etiological and prognostic factors in human acute pancreatitis: A review. *Am J Gasteroenterol.* 1982;77:633-638.

2. Rumack BH, Matthew H. Acetaminophen poisoning and toxicity. *Pediatrics.* 1975;55:871-876.

3. Warraich I, Kumar A, Grewal R, et al. Unresponsive patient admitted to the emergency department. *Lab Med.* 2003;34:724-727.

4. Litovitz TL, Klein-Schwartz W, White S, et al. 1999 annual report of the American Association of Poison Control Centers toxic exposure surveillance system. *Am J Emerg Med.* 2000;18:517-574.

5. Clark J. Acetaminophen poisoning and the use of intravenous N-acetylcysteine. *Air Med J.* 2001;20:16-17.

6. Parker D, White JP, Paton D, et al. Safety of late acetylcysteine treatment in paracetamol poisoning. *Hum Exp Toxicol.* 1990;9:25-27.

7. Ash SR, Caldwell CA, Singer GG, et al. Treatment of acetaminophen-induced hepatitis and fulminant hepatic failure with extracorporeal sorbent-based devices. *Adv Renal Transplant Ther.* 2002;9:42-53.

8. Kozer E, McGuigan M. Treatment strategies for early presenting acetaminophen overdose: A survey of medical directors of poison centers in North America and Europe. *Hum Exp Toxicol.* 2002;21:123-127.

9. Caldarola V, Hassett JM, Hall AH, et al. Hemorrhagic pancreatitis associated with acetaminophen overdose. *Am J Gastroenterol.* 1986;81:579-582.

10. Mofenson HC, Caraccio TR, Nawaz H, et al. Acetaminophen induced pancreatitis. *Clin Toxicol.* 1991;223-230.

11. Farrell J, Schmitz PG. Paracetamol-induced pancreatitis and fulminant hepatitis in a hemodialysis patient. *Clin Nephrol.* 1997;48:132-133.

Unresponsive Patient Admitted to the Emergency Department

Irfan Warraich, Ashwani Kumar, Ratna Grewal, Rodney Tucay, Jeffrey W. Oliver, Dale M. Dunn, Charles A. Bradley[1]

[1]*Departments of Pathology and* [2]*Internal Medicine, Texas Tech University Health Sciences Center, Lubbock, TX*

Patient: 30-year-old woman.

Chief Complaint: She was brought to a hospital emergency department (ED) after being found at home by her children who were unable to arouse her. Empty bottles of Carisoprodol (2-methyl-2-propyl-1,3-propanediol carbamate isopropylcarbamate) and Toradol (Ketorolac Tromethamine) were found near the patient. A bottle containing Paxil (paroxetine hydrochloride) was also found with 2 pills missing from it.

Past Medical History: Significant for recent admission to the same hospital for seizures secondary to cocaine overdose.

Physical Examination: Upon arrival at the ED, she was unresponsive to verbal and deep painful stimuli and was intubated. There was no history of observed seizure activity, fever, or bladder or bowel incontinence. Her vital signs were unremarkable, except for tachycardia with a normal S1, S2, and no murmurs. Pupils were dilated and fixed. She had no papilledema or gag reflex. Her chest was clear to auscultation bilaterally. Neurologic examination revealed a significantly diminished mental status. The patient was unresponsive to pain and exhibited decerebrate posturing with sternal rub. Deep tendon reflexes were exaggerated throughout and had sustained ankle clonus. Mechanical ventilation was initiated, and she was breathing spontaneously above the ventilator rate. She exhibited no withdrawal to pain in all 4 extremities. Electrocardiogram revealed only sinus tachycardia and no widening of QRS complexes. A CT scan of the head was normal. She was admitted to the medical intensive care unit for supportive treatment.

Questions

1. What is(are) this patient's most striking laboratory result(s)?

2. How do you explain this patient's most striking laboratory result(s)?

3. What is (are) this patient's most likely diagnosis(es)?

4. What are the usual causes of and outcomes associated with this patient's condition?

5. How should this patient's condition be treated?

Possible Answers

1. Recent history of seizures secondary to cocaine abuse and ED/hospital admission findings of unresponsiveness to verbal and deep pain stimuli with dilated and fixed pupils and no gag reflex; decreased CO_2; increased BUN, creatinine, and alkaline phosphatase (admission sample only) concentrations; markedly increased AST, ALT, total and direct bilirubin, and CK concentrations; multiple abnormal coagulation tests with results worsening over time; modestly

T1. Principal Laboratory Findings

Test	Hours After Presentation			"Normal" Reference Interval
	0	24	>24	
Chemistry				
Sodium	141	136	140	137-145 mmol/L
Potassium	4.5	4.0	2.3	3.6-5.0 mmol/L
Chloride	107	107	112	99-110 mmol/L
CO_2	16	14	17	22-30 mmol/L
BUN	33	50	46	7-17 mg/dL
Creatinine	1.2	2.3	2.3	0.7-1.2 mg/dL
Alkaline phosphatase	138	120	120	38-126 IU/L
AST	2,101	116	280	14-36 IU/L
ALT	4,766	3,253	1,434	9-52 IU/L
Total bilirubin	7.4	6.1	5.9	0.2-1.3 mg/dL
Direct bilirubin	5.8	5.2	4.6	0.0-0.3 mg/dL
CK	8352			30-135 U/L
Coagulation				
Platelet count	236	114	79	140-400 × 10^3/μL
PT	35.6	41.1	35.1	10.5-13.1 sec
PTT	34.7	67	70.5	23.1-33.8 sec
Fibrinogen	110		115	200-400 mg/dL
Qualitative drug screen - serum				
Ethanol	Neg			Neg
Salicylates	Neg			Neg
Quantitative drug screen - serum				
Acetaminophen	35			10-30 mg/mL
Phenytoin		22.2		10-20 mg/mL
Qualitative drug screen – urine				
TCAs	Pos			Neg

BUN, blood urea nitrogen; AST, aspartate aminotransferase; ALT, alanine aminotransferase; CK, creatine kinase; PT, prothrombin time; PTT, partial thromboplastin time; TCAs, tricyclic antidepressants; Pos, positive; Neg, negative.

increased serum acetaminophen and phenytoin concentrations; and a positive urine drug screen for TCAs [**T1**].

2. These clinical and laboratory findings were suspicious for postictal phase or non-convulsive status epilepticus or drug toxicity due to overdose of either acetaminophen or a TCA (positive urine drug screen for TCAs). However, TCA overdoses are characterized typically by the triad of signs and symptoms associated with coma, convulsions, and cardiac conduction abnormalities

[ie, QRS complex widening, bundle branch block, and atrioventricular (A-V) block]. Our patient had no evidence of convulsions and cardiac conduction abnormalities, suggesting that the positive urine drug screen for TCAs was either a false positive or reflected non-toxic levels of TCAs. On the other hand, acute liver failure (eg, elevated AST, ALT, and bilirubin concentrations), coagulation defects (eg, increased PT and PTT, decreased fibrinogen concentration, and thrombocytopenia), cardiomyopathy (eg, increased total CK), and renal failure (eg,

T2. Clinical Stages of Acetaminophen Toxicity*

Stage	Time Post-Ingestion	Clinical and/or Laboratory Characteristics
I	0.5 to 24 hours	Anorexia, nausea, vomiting, malaise, pallor, diaphoresis
II	24 to 48 hours	Resolution of the above characteristics; right upper quadrant abdominal pain and tenderness; elevated bilirubin, prothrombin time, INR, hepatic transaminases, oliguria
III	72 to 96 hours	Anorexia, nausea, vomiting, malaise may reappear; values for liver function tests peak; FHF with metabolic acidosis, INR >6, and renal dysfunction
IV	4 days to 2 weeks	Resolution of hepatic dysfunction in survivors; oliguric renal failure; death from FHF

*Modified from Linden CH, Rumack BH: Acetaminophen overdose. Emerg Med Clin North Am. 1984;2:103. INR, International Normalized Ratio; FHF, fulminant hepatic failure.

T3. Post-Mortem Blood Drug Findings

Drug	Concentration, mg/mL
Acetaminophen	63
Phenytoin	nd
Valproic acid	5.1
Paroxetine	nd
Meprobamate	nd
Carisoprodol	2.7

nd, none detectable

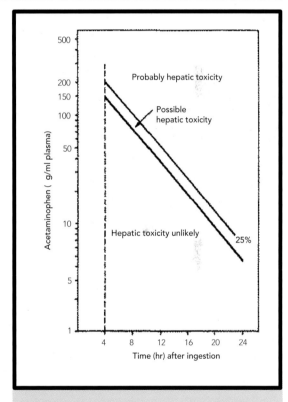

Figure 1_Rumack-Matthew nomogram for evaluating the probability of hepatotoxicity as a function of time and concentration postingestion of acetaminophen (From Rumack BH, Matthew H. Pediatrics. 1975;55;871. In: Rosen P, ed. *Emergency Medicine*, 4th ed. St Louis: Mosby, 1998).

increased BUN and creatinine concentrations) are characteristic findings in phases II (24 to 48 hours post-ingestion) or III (3 to 5 days post-ingestion) of acetaminophen overdose [**T2**].

3. **Most likely diagnosis:** *acute liver failure secondary to acetaminophen overdose.*

Acetaminophen, or N-acetyl-p-aminophenol (APAP), is 1 of the most frequently used medications in the United States. Its use alone or in combination preparations is widespread because of its analgesic and antipyretic properties and presumed safety in recommended doses. However, APAP is responsible for more drug overdose hospitalizations than any other common medication.[1] Acetaminophen is metabolized by hepatocytes. It is usually eliminated as a glucuronide or sulfate conjugate. Following overdose, however, the conjugation pathways become saturated, leading to accumulation of reactive intermediates such as N-acetyl-benzoquinoneimine, mercapturic acid, and probably others.[2] These reactions involve the cytochrome oxidase P-450 system, and the metabolites are normally detoxified by endogenous glutathione. When glutathione stores are depleted, hepatocyte necrosis ensues, typically with a centrilobular distribution. Liver necrosis can result from an acute overdose of a large amount of APAP, or from accumulation over several days.

4. In a study of 94 fatal acetaminophen overdose cases with known reasons for exposure, most were associated with suicidal intentions.[3] However, in 25% of these cases, unintentional therapeutic error and intentional misuse without suicidal intent were the reasons for the overdose. Although the intentions of our patient were not clear, suicidal intent appeared unlikely. Unintentional overdose due to the presumed safety of acetaminophen appeared to be the likely cause. Outcomes in cases of acetaminophen overdose are dependent upon several factors, including the amount of drug ingested and the time period between ingestion and initiation of drug-specific therapy. In cases of delayed treatment, death from irreversible liver failure due to the hepatotoxic effects of reactive acetaminophen intermediates may occur. Thrombocytopenia, as observed in our patient, is a well-reported clinical feature of acetaminophen toxicity and strongly correlates with the degree of hepatotoxicity, although it does not correlate with serum acetaminophen levels.[4] Thus, the finding of thrombocytopenia early in the course of acetaminophen toxicity may help in identifying patients prone to severe hepatotoxicity. Acute renal failure, as observed in our patient, occurs in less than 2% of all acetaminophen poisonings and 10% of severely poisoned patients.[5] Acute tubular necrosis occurring with acetaminophen toxicity has been described previously.[5,6]

5. With N-acetylcysteine (Mucomyst) to stimulate regeneration of glutathione. Early recognition of APAP toxicity is critical since outcomes are improved when antidotal treatment with N-acetylcysteine is started within 8 hours of the overdose. This can be difficult without a clinical history of APAP ingestion. Only nonspecific symptoms of abdominal pain, nausea, and vomiting generally appear within the first 24 hours postingestion. Symptoms often subsequently improve, but liver function tests foretell the acute hepatic failure that typically ensues by about the third day. Serum acetaminophen levels are extremely helpful in the diagnosis, but must be carefully related to the time since ingestion. A seemingly low level may still be a predictor of toxicity if the time since ingestion is long. The Rumack-Matthew nomogram [**Figure 1**] plots this relationship and can be used to assess the need for N-acetylcysteine treatment.[7] However,

treatment with N-acetylcysteine is relatively harmless and should probably be initiated as soon as possible whenever APAP toxicity is suspected. Moreover, the therapeutic window of APAP is narrowed by various associated conditions. These conditions include inherited variations in hepatic enzyme activity, malnutrition,[8,9] ethanol ingestion,[10,11] drug interactions,[12-18] or concomitant medical disorders.[12-18] Of these factors, nutritional factors and drug interactions are more likely to lead to toxicity at conventional doses of acetaminophen. Conditions associated with increased activity of P-450-dependent pathways such as fasting,[10] protein-calorie malnutrition,[8,9] poorly controlled diabetes,[17] and obesity,[18] have been described. Chronic protein-calorie malnutrition, may also lead to low glutathione levels resulting in reduced detoxification.[9] In addition, various drugs that may alter acetaminophen elimination or that stimulate the P-450 microsomal oxidase enzymes include isoniazid, anticonvulsants (eg, phenobarbital, phenytoin), rifampin, and ethanol.[10-16] Severe toxicity has been reported in patients using these drugs concomitantly with APAP, even at low APAP levels.[19] Our patient was treated with phenytoin for her suspected seizure activity; this might have contributed to her morbidity and mortality. In addition, our patient was also taking carisoprodol, which has affected hepatic enzyme activities in rats,[20] and could have interfered with her acetaminophen metabolism. We could not identify other more definite factors contributing to her hepatotoxicity.

Treatment and Course

The patient was treated with phenytoin and N-acetylcysteine. N-acetylcysteine treatment was started approximately 8 hours after the patient presented to the hospital. On the following day, the patient's overall condition deteriorated and she required vasopressor treatment. The neurological examination at that time revealed fixed and dilated pupils, no spontaneous breathing, no spontaneous ocular activity, and a negative cold caloric test. Electroencephalogram revealed a flat tracing suggestive of absent brain activity. These findings suggested brain death. After discussion with the patient's family, ventilatory support was withdrawn and the patient was pronounced dead. Autopsy findings revealed a light yellow-brown homogeneous and congested hepatic parenchyma. The microscopic examination showed extensive microvesicular fatty change with centrilobular congestion and centrilobular necrosis of the hepatocytes. The brain examination revealed moderate global edema of the cerebral hemispheres. No other significant findings were identified. Results of the post-mortem toxicology examination are shown in [**T3**]. In addition, quantitative assay of post-mortem blood samples for alcohols, including ethanol, isopropanol, methanol, and n-propanol, were negative. A qualitative TCA screen and a spot test for salicylates were also negative. The fatal outcome in this case demonstrates that physicians should have high index of suspicion and consider acetaminophen toxicity in any patient who has ingested acetaminophen and has signs of acute hepatic dysfunction, even if acetaminophen levels are not markedly elevated. Moreover, clinicians should avoid focusing too much on a drug(s) associated with a previous history of illicit drug use and remember to correlate the serum acetaminophen level with the time post-ingestion.

Keywords

acetaminophen, acute liver failure, N-acetylcysteine, Rumack-Matthew nomogram

References

1. MJ Smilkstein. Acetaminophen. In: L.R. Goldfrank, ed, *Toxicologic Emergencies*, 6th ed. Stamford, CT: Appleton and Lange. 1998:541–542.

2. Corcoran GB, Mitchell JR, Vaishnar YN, et al. Evidence that acetaminophen and N-hydroxyacetaminophen form a common arylating intermediate, N-acety-p-benzoquinoneimine. *Mol Pharmacol*. 1980;18:1557-1562.

3. Litovitz TL, Klein-Schwartz W, Dyher KS, et al. 1997 annual report of the American Association of Poison Control Centers Toxic Exposure Surveillance System. *Am J Emerg Med*. 1998;16:443-497.

4. Fischereder M. Thrombocytopenia following acute acetaminophen overdose. *Am J Hematol*. 1994;453:258-259.

5. Prescott LF. Paracetamol overdosage: Pharmacological considerations and clinical management. *Drugs*. 1983;25:290-314.

6. Curry RW, Robinson JD, Sughrue MJ. Acute renal failure after acetaminophen ingestion. *JAMA*. 1982;247:1012-1014.

7. Rumack BH, Matthew H. Acetaminophen poisoning and toxicity. *Pediatrics*. 1975;55:871-876.

8. Zhang W, Parentau H, Greenly RL, et al. Effect of protein-calorie malnutrition on cytochromes P450 and glutathione S-transferase. *Eur J Drug Metab Pharmacokinet*. 1999;24:141-147.

9. Sauerwein RW, Mulder JA, Mulder L, et al. Inflammatory mediators in children with protein-energy malnutrition. *Am J Clin Nutr*. 1997;65:1534-1539.

10. Whitcomb DC, Block GD. Association of acetaminophen hepatotoxicity with fasting and ethanol use. *JAMA*. 1994;272:1845-1850.

11. Kaysen GA, Pond SM, Roper MH, et al. Combined hepatic and renal injury in alcoholics during therapeutic use of acetaminophen. *Arch Intern Med*. 1985;145:2019-2023.

12. Bray GP, Harrison PM, O'Grady JG, et al., Long-term anticonvulsant therapy worsens outcome in paracetamol-induced fulminant hepatic failure. *Hum Exp Toxicol*. 1992;11:265–270.

13. Nolan CM, Sandblom RE, Thummel KE, et al. Hepatotoxicity associated with acetaminophen usage in patients receiving multiple drug therapy for tuberculosis. *Chest*. 1994;105:408–411.

14. Minton NA, Henry JA, Frankel RJ. Fatal paracetamol poisoning in an epileptic. *Hum Toxicol*. 1998;7:33–34.

15. Chien JY, Peter RM, Nolan CM, et al. Influence of polymorphic N-acetyltransferase phenotype on the inhibition and induction of acetaminophen bioactivation with long-term isoniazid. *Clin Pharmacol Ther*. 1997;61:24-34.

16. Forrest JA, Roscoe P, Prescott LF, et al. Abnormal drug metabolism after barbiturate and paracetamol overdose. *BMJ*. 1974;4:499-502.

17. Song BJ, Veech RL, Saenger P. Cytochrome P450IIE1 is elevated in lymphocytes from poorly controlled insulin-dependent diabetics. *J Clin Endocrinol Metab*. 1990;71:1036-1040.

18. O'Shea D, Davis SN, Kim RB, et al. Effect of fasting and obesity in humans on the 6-hydroxylation of chlorzoxazone: a putative probe of CYP2E1 activity. *Clin Pharmacol Ther*. 1994;56:359-367.

19. Kearns GL, Leeder JS, Wasserman GS. Acetaminophen overdose with therapeutic intent. *J Pediatr*. 1998;132:5-8.

20. Mansour MM, Fathi MM. Effect of chronic administration of meprobamate on different enzymatic activities in liver and serum in rats. *J Drug Res*. 1989;18:189–200.

Worsening Shortness of Breath in a 62-Year-Old Man

Matthew R. Plymyer

Department of Pathology, Easton Hospital, Easton, PA

Patient: 62-year-old man.

Chief Complaint: Worsening shortness of breath.

History of Present Illness: The patient had experienced worsening shortness of breath (dyspnea) over the past 2 years. Based on clinical and radiographic evidence, it was thought that his shortness of breath was secondary to progressive interstitial lung disease. Therefore, he was referred by his pulmonologist to a thoracic surgeon for video-assisted thoracoscopy with lung biopsy.

Past Medical/Surgical History: The patient had a history of coronary artery disease with myocardial infarction over 10 years ago with no recent history of angina. In addition, he had a history of hypertension, gastroesophageal reflux disease (GERD) with Barrett's esophagus, cholecystectomy, and a lumbar laminectomy. Because of pneumonia, he had been hospitalized 18 months prior to this most recent presentation.

Social History: The patient had been a cigarette smoker, but discontinued smoking after being diagnosed with heart disease. His occupation had subjected him to significant inhalational exposure to graphite dust. There was no history of occupational exposure to any other agents.

Physical Examination: Vital signs: temperature, 98.8ºF; heart rate, 76 beats per minute; respiratory rate, 16 breaths per minute; blood pressure, 142/81 mm Hg. The patient was in no acute distress. He had mild rattles with coughing on pulmonary auscultation. The remainder of the physical examination was unremarkable.

Results of Additional Diagnostic Procedures and Tests: Preoperative chest radiograph showed increased interstitial markings, consistent with interstitial lung disease (**Image 1**). Compared to previous radiographic findings, these radiographic changes had become more prominent over the past 2 years. Electrocardiogram (ECG) showed a normal sinus rhythm with a heart rate of 89 beats per minute, and was unchanged from past ECGs. Video-assisted thoracoscopic biopsy of the right lung showed interstitial fibrosis and emphysema as well as abundant black pigment within macrophages and multinucleated giant cells (**Images 2** and **3**). No polarizable material suggestive of silica was identified in these cells, nor was there evidence of neoplasm, granulomatous disease, vasculitis, viral cytopathic effect, or the presence of microorganisms. Microbiological culture studies performed on lung tissue were negative.

T1. Principal Laboratory Findings

Test	Patient's Result	"Normal" Reference Range
Hematology		
WBC count	5.0	4.8-10.8 × 10³/μL
RBC count	4.72	4.70-6.10 × 10⁶/μL
Hemoglobin	14.5	14.0-18.0 g/dL
Platelet count	168	130-400 × 10³/μL
Coagulation		
PT	12.0	10.9-12.9 sec
INR	1.0	
PTT	27	21-31 sec
Chemistry		
Sodium	139	133-145 mEq/L
Potassium	4.4	3.5-5.0 mEq/L
Chloride	104	96-108 mEq/L
CO₂	24	22-29 mEq/L
BUN	16	6-20 mg/dL
Creatinine	1.1	0.5-1.2 mg/dL
Glucose	118	70-105 mg/dL
Calcium	9.5	8.4-10.2 mg/dL
Total protein	7.7	6.4-8.3 g/dL
Albumin	4.3	3.5-5.0 g/dL
Total bilirubin	0.8	0.0-1.0 mg/dL
ALP	58	40-129 U/L
AST	19	0-37 U/L
ALT	30	0-41 U/L
SaO₂	97%	100%
Microbiology		
Tissue (right lung) culture	No growth	No growth

WBC, white blood cell; RBC, red blood cell; PT, prothrombin time; INR, International Normalized Ratio; PTT, partial thromboplastin time; CO₂, carbon dioxide; BUN, blood urea nitrogen; ALP, alkaline phosphatase; AST, aspartate aminotransferase; ALT, alanine aminotransferase; SaO₂, oxygen saturation.

Questions

1. What are this patient's most striking clinical, laboratory, and radiographic findings?

2. What purpose does video-assisted thorascopic lung biopsy serve in a patient with this constellation of findings?

3. What disease category does this patient's radiographic and biopsy findings suggest?

4. What is this patient's most likely diagnosis?

5. What are the most common signs, symptoms, laboratory, and radiographic features associated with this patient's condition?

6. What are the most appropriate treatment and follow-up for this patient?

Possible Answers

1. Progressive shortness of breath, rattles with coughing, worsening features of interstitial lung disease on chest radiograph, and decreased oxygen saturation (SaO_2). This patient's laboratory findings are striking for what they do not show (ie, except for a modestly decreased SaO_2 value, all other laboratory test results shown in **T1** are within the "normal" reference interval for these tests).

2. The video-assisted thoracic surgery (VATS) technique has become the standard for obtaining lung biopsy material in patients with interstitial lung disease, since it allows the surgeon to visually inspect the lungs to choose a biopsy from the most likely abnormal area and because it has less morbidity (postoperative pain) and results in a shorter hospital stay than more invasive surgical procedures.[1] Interstitial lung disease refers to the presence of inflammation, fibrosis, or both between the tiny air spaces or alveoli of the lungs (the area known as the pulmonary interstitium), causing a distortion of the normal pulmonary microarchitecture.[2] The damage to the pulmonary microarchitecture can be secondary to a wide variety of chronic and acute conditions, including infection, neoplasm, drug reaction, occupational exposure, sarcoidosis, collagen vascular disease (such as rheumatoid arthritis), and numerous others.[2] Because conditions of such differing etiology and treatment implications can cause similar clinical and radiographic findings (**Image 1**), surgical lung biopsy is often necessary to establish or exclude the etiology of these findings.[1]

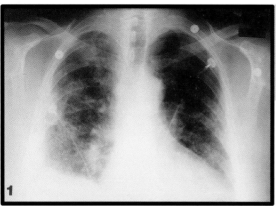

Image 1_Preoperative chest radiograph showing increased white markings in the lungs, especially the right lung, indicative of interstitial lung disease.

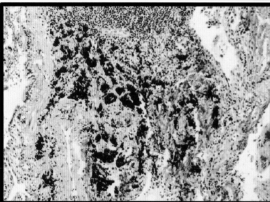

Image 2_Interstitial fibrosis and abundant black pigment [hematoxylin and eosin (H&E) stain, 100× magnification].

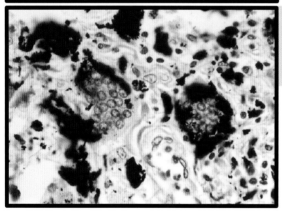

Image 3_Detail of the black pigment, including pigment within the cytoplasm of multinucleated giant cells (H&E stain, 400× magnification).

Pneumoconioses. The lung biopsy in this case did not show evidence of an infectious condition, neoplasm, vasculitis, or granulomas such as those seen in patients with sarcoidosis. The lung biopsy did show interstitial fibrosis and most strikingly, the presence of an extensive amount of dark black pigment within macrophages and multinucleated giant cells (**Images 2** and **3**). These histopathologic features suggest a pneumoconiosis (ie, any nonmalignant chronic lung disease resulting from inhalation and deposition of mineral, metallic, or dust particles in the pulmonary interstitium).[3] The most common environmental agents causing pneumoconiosis are asbestos, silica, and coal,[3] although a variety of other inhaled, dust-borne agents, including forms of carbon other than coal, less commonly cause pneumoconiosis.[4,5] The pneumoconioses are most often seen in the context of occupational lung disorders (ie, any pulmonary disease felt to have been caused by an occupational exposure to any of the aforementioned agents).[4]

3. ***Most likely diagnosis:*** *complicated graphite pneumoconiosis due to occupational exposure to graphite dust.*

As with all of the pneumoconioses, a careful clinical history as to environmental and/or occupational exposure is of paramount importance.[6] In this case, the patient had documented occupational inhalation of graphite dust. Anthracosis, the inhalation and deposition in the lungs of dusts consisting predominantly of carbon, is common in cigarette smokers and those living in urban/industrialized areas. With the exception of the well-known deleterious effects of cigarette smoking, anthracosis due to such environmental exposure generally causes few health problems.[7] Inhaling greater quantities of carbonaceous substances, however, can lead to pulmonary disease, and is often the result of environmental exposure.[7] Although coal miners' pneumoconiosis is the most prevalent occupational exposure-related pulmonary disease due to carbon-based dusts, occupational exposure to other substances such as graphite can less commonly lead to significant health problems.[7] Natural graphite is a crystalline form of carbon which may contain significant quantities of silica.[5,8] Therefore, graphite mining can result in exposure to silica as well as carbonaceous dust.[8] Synthetic graphite is derived from heated coal or coke, and is virtually free of silica.[5,7] Occupational exposure to synthetic graphite (as in the patient presented in this case study) can be seen in the manufacture of steel, lubricants, pencils, electrodes, and other products.[7,8] Millions of workers in the United States may be subject to occupational exposure to natural and synthetic graphite, but the prevalence of pneumoconiosis is probably very low.[8] The pathologic findings are similar in exposure to large amounts of carbon in any form.[7] Simple pneumoconiosis involves deposition of carbon pigment without fibrosis, often as macules scattered throughout the pulmonary parenchyma.[7] Complicated pneumoconiosis (as in the patient presented in this case study) refers to the development of progressive massive fibrosis, defined as a focus of fibrosis and black pigment deposition larger than 1 cm in size.[7]

4. Most patients with graphite pneumoconiosis experience cough, sputum production, and dyspnea, which often worsen as the disease progresses and can lead to right-sided heart failure.[7] On physical examination, the patient may have decreased breath sounds and a few crackles.[7] There are no specific laboratory tests that aid in the diagnosis of graphite pneumoconiosis, although non-specific acute phase reactants such as C-reactive protein (CRP) and fibrinogen may be elevated, hypergammaglobulinemia may be present, and elevated serum rheumatoid factor and antinuclear antibody levels are common.[7] Other laboratory studies may help exclude the many other causes of interstitial lung disease. Radiographic findings vary depending upon the degree of pulmonary damage, and can include small rounded opacities, large nodules, and interstitial fibrosis.[4] Graphite pneumoconiosis is similar clinically and radiographically to coal workers' pneumoconiosis.[5,7,8]

5. There is no specific treatment for pneumoconiosis due to the deposition of carbon dusts.[4] Elimination of the causative agent to avoid further exposure is often helpful, although there can be disease progression even after exposure is eliminated.[3] With progressive massive fibrosis, there is increased risk for chronic respiratory failure, possibly requiring use of supplemental oxygen therapy. In addition, some patients with cough and dyspnea associated with airway limitation may benefit from bronchodilator medications, and patients with hyperresponsive airways may benefit from inhaled corticosteroids.[3] Despite such treatments, patients with progressive massive fibrosis have significantly increased mortality.

Treatment and Course

The patient had already retired from his job at the graphite factory, thereby eliminating the possibility of further graphite exposure. He was discharged home with oxygen therapy and no steroid therapy on the fourth postoperative day following his lung biopsy. He continues to be followed clinically and radiographically, and his disease has remained stable 6 months later.

Keywords

video-assisted thoracoscopy, graphite, pneumoconiosis, interstitial lung disease

References

1. Pearson FG, Cooper JD, Deslauriers J, et al. *Thoracic Surgery*, 2nd ed. Philadelphia: Churchill Livingstone; 2002:103-109.

2. Hess DR, MacIntyre NR, Mishoe SC, et al. *Respiratory Care: Principles & Practice*. Philadelphia: W.B. Saunders; 2002:955-957.

3. Hanley ME, Welsh CH. *Current Diagnosis & Treatment in Pulmonary Medicine*. New York: McGraw-Hill; 2003:325.

4. Fishman AP, Elias JA, Fishman JA, et al. *Fishman's Manual of Pulmonary Diseases and Disorders*, 3rd ed. New York: McGraw-Hill; 2002:205-216.

5. Churg A, Green FH. *Pathology of Occupational Lung Disease*. New York: Igaku-Shoin; 1988:148.

6. Murray JF, Nadel JA, Mason RJ, et al. *Textbook of Respiratory Medicine*, 3rd ed. Philadelphia: W.B. Saunders; 2000:1815-1816.

7. Fraser RS, Colman N, Müller NL, et al. *Fraser and Paré's Diagnosis of Diseases of the Chest*, 4th ed. Philadelphia: W.B. Saunders; 1999:2409-2419.

8. Rom WN. *Environmental Occupational Medicine*, 3rd ed. Philadelphia: Lippincott-Raven; 1998:591.

Hypercalcemia in a 56-Year-Old Female

Kristin A. Pierce, Monte S. Willis, Christopher R. McCudden

Department of Pathology and Laboratory Medicine, University of North Carolina School of Medicine, Chapel Hill, NC

Patient: 56-year-old female.

Chief Complaint: Elevated serum calcium during a recent hospital admission.

History of Present Illness: The patient states that she was recently discharged from the hospital for Bell palsy and was incidentally found to have hypercalcemia. She has been having pain in her legs, constipation, and occasional weakness, but denies any kidney stones, significant weight loss, or abdominal pain. She reports occasional severe headaches. Upon presentation, active medications included: aspirin 81 mg tablet daily, Celexa (20 mg daily), Ezetimibe (10 mg daily), Lisinopril (10 mg daily), metformin (1,000 mg b.i.d.), metoprolol (100 mg b.i.d.), Nexium (40 mg daily), glipizide XL (20 mg daily), nitroglycerine (sublingual p.r.n.), Synthroid (150 mcg daily), Zetia (10 mg daily), Neurontin (600 mg b.i.d.), Flexeril (10 mg p.r.n.), MS Contin (15 mg b.i.d.), Tegretol (200 mg b.i.d.), Valtrex (1,000 mg t.i.d. × 4 days). Known allergies include codeine (hallucination, nausea, vomiting) and ibuprofen (nausea, dizziness). The patient was not known to be taking any herbal supplements or alternative therapy.

Past Medical History: She has a history of diabetes mellitus, hypothyroidism (status post radioactive iodine ablation for hyperthyroidism), chronic obstructive pulmonary disease (COPD), and hypertension. She went through menopause at age 51. The patient also has a history of irritable bowel syndrome (IBS), bilateral footdrop secondary to peroneal nerve injury, and 3 incidences of narcotic overdose (prescription MS Contin). Additional history includes major depressive disorder (on medication) that is in remission. She has had myocardial infarctions and strokes, and in the past month has been hypercalcemic on 3 consecutive occasions.

Social History: She smokes 1–2 packs of cigarettes daily (since age 14). Patient denies alcohol consumption but has visited clinic with odor of alcohol on breath on occasion; she has a history of substance abuse (described above). She is not known to be taking any calcium or vitamin D supplements.

Family History: No known family history of kidney stones, abnormal endocrine disorders, or hypercalcemia.

Physical Examination: Vital signs: blood pressure 143/93 mm Hg; heart rate, 75 bpm; respiratory rate, 18 rpm. Eyes: no lid lag, proptosis, or periorbital swelling. Neck: thyroid is not enlarged. No lymphadenopathy. Lungs: clear to auscultation bilaterally. Heart: regular rate and rhythm without murmurs. Neurological: alert and oriented. Strength was 5/5 of the upper and lower extremities. Reflexes were +2 in the biceps, triceps, brachioradialis, knees, and ankles.

T1. Principal Laboratory Findings

Test	Patient's Result	"Normal" Reference Interval
Hematology		
WBC	11.0	$4.5-11.0 \times 10^9$/L
RBC	4.68	$4.00-5.20 \times 10^{12}$/L
Hemoglobin	15.8	12.0–16.0 g/dL
Hematocrit	45.1	36.0–46.0%
Mean corpuscular volume	96	80–100 fL
Red cell distribution width	13.9	12.0–15.0%
Platelet count	241	$150-440 \times 10^9$/L
Coagulation		
PT	12.1	9.6–12.5 seconds
INR	1.1	
APTT	38.2	27.0–37.1 seconds
Chemistry		
Sodium	137	135–145 mmol/L
Potassium	4.5	3.5–5.0 mmol/L
Chloride	99	98–107 mmol/L
CO_2	26	22–30 mmol/L
BUN	15	7–21 mg/dL
Creatinine	1.0	0.7–1.1 mg/dL
Calcium	11.1	8.5–10.2 mg/dL
Phosphorus	2.9	2.4–4.5 mg/dL
Alkaline phosphatase	214	38–126 U/L
Serum albumin	4,100	3,500–5,000
Hemoglobin A1C	7.9	4.8–6.0%
Endocrine		
Parathyroid hormone	85	12–72 pg/mL
25-OH-vitamin D, total	24	25–80 ng/mL
Serum IgG	1078	600–1,700 mg/dL
Serum IgM	242	35–290 mg/dL
Serum IgA	232	40–400 mg/dL
Serum and urine protein electrophoresis	No monoclonal protein observed	
CSF IgG	2.1	0.5–9.5
CSF albumin	12.7	5.0–50.0
CSF IgG index	0.5	0.3–0.8
Ratio interpretation	Normal permeability; no oligoclonal bands observed	
Toxicology		
Amphetamine	<500	<500 ng/mL
Barbiturate	<200	<200 ng/mL
Benzodiazepine	<200	<200 ng/mL
Cannabinoid	<20	<20 ng/mL
Cocaine metabolite	<150	<150 ng/mL
Methadone	<300	<300 ng/mL
Opiate	≥300	<300 ng/mL
Propoxyphene	<300	<300 ng/mL

aPTT, activated prothrombin time; BUN, blood urea nitrogen; CSF, cerebrospinal fluid; INR, international normalized ratio (specimen sec/normal sec); PTT, prothrombin time; RBCs, red blood cells; WBC, white blood cells.

Questions

1. What are the patient's most striking clinical and laboratory findings?

2. What is the differential diagnosis?

3. What additional laboratory investigations should be performed and why?

4. What is this patient's most likely diagnosis?

5. How would such a patient be managed and why?

6. How is surgical management of this disease assisted by the clinical laboratory?

7. What is the pathophysiology of the disease in the patient presented in this case study?

Possible Answers

1. Significant clinical findings in this patient include bone pain, weakness, and constipation. She is post-menopausal and has a history of hypertension and coronary artery disease; the patient was told that she had a small heart attack approximately 4 years ago, but details are unclear, and she never underwent any diagnostic testing at that time. She also has a history of transient ischemic attacks (TIAs) approximately 2 years ago. Her family history is negative for endocrine disorders and hypercalcemia; however, her

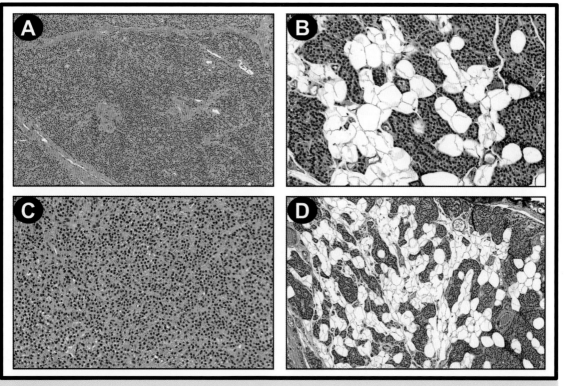

Image 1_A (10× magnification) and **B** (20× magnification): Micrographs of lesion in this patient demonstrating sheets of monotonous eosinophillic cells with poorly-defined cell borders, extensive capillary network, and the absence of stromal fat. **C** (10× magnification) and **D** (20× magnification): Micrographs of normal parathyroid tissue. Note adipose tissue and differentiated secretory cells.

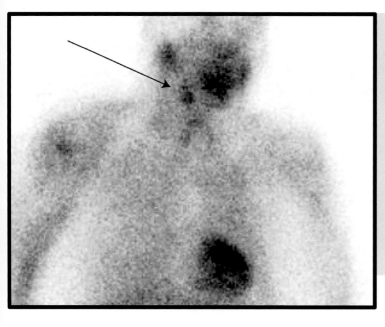

Image 2_ Technetium 99m Sestamibi scan of patient (oblique view). The scan indicates a possible, but not definite, adenoma in the right thyroid bed region (arrow). Also visible are the heart, as well as salivary and parotid glands, which normally display significant uptake of the tracer. Note: there was no uptake by the thyroid due to previous iodine radioablation of the tissue as a treatment for Grave's disease.

laboratory findings reveal elevated total serum calcium, parathyroid hormone, and alkaline phosphatase; her serum phosphorus is low normal. This patient has low total vitamin D, and her chloride is low normal. Despite the hypercalcemia, this patient exhibits no muscular weakness on detailed neurological examination and has no evidence of altered mental status.

2. The differential diagnoses of hypercalcemia at presentation include: primary, secondary, or tertiary hyperparathyroidism, humoral hypercalcemia of malignancy (HHM), hematological malignancies (such as multiple myeloma, leukemia, lymphoma), granulomatous disease (sarcoidosis), altered bone turnover, familial hypocalciuric hypercalcemia, and drug-related causes such as lithium therapy.

In primary hyperparathyroidism (HPT), hypercalcemia is caused by single or multiple parathyroid hormone (PTH)-producing adenomas and is associated with decreased phosphorus and inappropriately-high PTH.[1] Parathyroid hormone is also elevated in secondary and tertiary hyperparathyroidism. In secondary HPT, renal failure inhibits vitamin D synthesis causing hypocalcemia; aggressive treatment of hypocalcemia with supplementary vitamin D and calcium can result in hypercalcemia. Tertiary hyperparathyroidism can result from prolonged renal insufficiency, where parathyroid hypertrophy in response to long-standing excess phosphate and insufficient vitamin D feedback on the parathyroids results in a higher serum calcium set point.[2] To delineate these causes of hypercalcemia, a detailed clinical history can rule out renal failure or drug treatment. In HHM, solid tumors of the breast, lung, or kidney produce parathyroid hormone-related protein (PTH-rp). Parathyroid hormone-related protein is a humoral factor with PTH-like activity (amino acids 1–36 of N-terminus are highly homologous to PTH) that can result in hypercalcemia.[3,4] In HHM, PTH is suppressed in response to elevated PTH-rp, and both hypercalcemia and hypophosphatemia are typically present. Note that PTH-rp may not be detectable in many cases.[4] In cases of multiple myeloma, hypercalcemia is caused by the release of calcium from lytic bone lesions.[5] Multiple myeloma patients typically have normal levels of alkaline phosphatase in serum (when fractures

are not present), which distinguishes this disorder from other causes of bone loss. Other causes of bone loss include Paget's disease[6] and prolonged immobilization.[7] As with myeloma, these diseases result in the release of calcium from bone stores causing hypercalcemia (95% of the calcium in the body is stored in bone). Other causes of hypercalcemia include granulomatous diseases such as sarcoidosis.[8] Patients with sarcoidosis can present with hypercalcemia due to mononuclear cell (macrophage) activation of vitamin D in the lung and lymph nodes. Finally, there are numerous pharmaceutical causes of hypercalcemia. These include vitamin D supplementation, diuretic use, calcium supplementation (milk-alkali syndrome), and lithium therapy. Lithium acts to stimulate parathyroid tissue directly to release PTH-mimicking primary hyperparathyroidism.[9] A detailed drug and supplement history are essential to rule out pharmaceutical causes of hypercalcemia.

3. Additional laboratory tests to assist in differentiating potential causes of hypercalcemia include Sestamibi scan and biopsy. Parathyroid adenomas can be identified with imaging studies such as an MRI or Sestamibi (or Tc99m MIBI) scan. Sestamibi scanning was performed on this patient to attempt to confirm the presence of the disease and to localize the adenoma (**Image 2**). An image of the surgical biopsy is provided in **Image 1**.

4. ***Most likely diagnosis:*** *primary hyperparathyroidism.* Based on the elevated PTH and calcium, the low normal phosphorus, and the pituitary adenoma, the cause of the disorder in this patient is primary hyperparathyroidism. Primary hyperparathyroidism is definitively diagnosed if the hypercalcemia resolves following surgical removal of the adenoma. Up to 90% of primary hyperparathyroidism result from single adenomas; an additional 5% are caused by double adenomas.[10,11] Chief cells are the main constituent of adenomas, which are generally encapsulated and surrounded by normal thyroid tissue half the time. Oxyphil cells compose some adenomas, which are generally larger than those arising from chief cells. Two unusual features of this case are the low total vitamin D and low normal chloride. Usually in patients with primary hyperparathyroidism, vitamin D levels will

be elevated, and patients may also have a mild hyperchloremic metabolic acidosis; however, vitamin D deficiency can occur concomitantly with elevated parathyroid hormone levels and may contribute to a normal or only moderately-increased serum calcium.[1]

5. Parathyroidectomy is the only curative treatment for primary hyperparathyroidism. When patients are asymptomatic, as in the current case, specific indications for surgical removal have been developed and include: a 30% reduction in creatinine clearance; osteoporosis (T score £2.5 at any site); age <50 years; serum calcium >1 mg above reference values; and calciuria >10 mmol/24 hours.[12] Even without surgical indications for treatment, surgery should be offered to patients because disease progression is common (up to 30% of patients), there is an increased risk of bone fractures and cardiovascular morbidity/mortality, and medical follow up is expensive.[13] Conversely, surgery cures >95% of patients, with fewer than 2% experiencing permanent morbidities, and rarely mortalities.[1] Techniques to more accurately localize adenomas, such as parathyroid scintigraphy and ultrasound, have resulted in less-invasive surgeries. Focused parathyroidectomy is currently done in 60% to 75% of patients with primary hyperparathyroidism. Randomized trials have demonstrated that these procedures lower the risk of postoperative hypocalcemia.[14-16] When localization is not possible, as in the present case, bilateral exploration is the procedure of choice. In the present case, Sestamibi imaging allowed the identification of a solitary adenoma, which was subsequently removed (**Image 1**).

6. Intraoperative measurement of serum PTH is currently being widely studied.[17] Because the half-life of PTH is approximately 3 to 5 minutes, decreases in serum PTH should drop soon after surgical removal of the disease gland. The most common criterion for successful removal of an adenoma is a 50% reduction in serum PTH 10 minutes after resection.[1] However, there are reports that intraoperative serum PTH does not commonly identify additional disease glands, and in some cases primary hyper-PTH persists despite an appropriate drop in serum PTH.[18] PTH testing has been adopted in surgical management, making the clinical laboratory essential in this process.

From the perspective of the laboratory, there are several points to consider when instituting an intraoperative measurement of PTH. Approximately 70% of laboratories perform rapid PTH testing in their central laboratory according to a recent College of American Pathologists survey.[19] Only 23% were performing PTH testing in the operating suite, with 6% performing in a satellite laboratory.[19] Performing PTH assays near the operating suite has the advantage of a faster turnaround time and increased visibility for the laboratory. On-site approaches required additional instrumentation, an additional operator, along with >1 hour of set-up time for calibration and instrument checks.[20] Automated systems and technologists in central laboratories generally require less frequent calibrations, and costs have been estimated to be substantially lower.[21] Moreover, 68% of rapid PTH testing sites actually performed testing less than 5 times a month.[19] These factors are important when considering how the laboratory can assist in the surgical management of primary hyperparathyroidism.

7. The underlying pathophysiology for hyperparathyroidism can be identified in only a few patients. Known causes include irradiation exposure and rare genetic abnormalities associated with multiple endocrine neoplasm (MEN) syndromes. A history of radiation to the head and neck an average of 30 to 40 years before the development of hyperparathyroidism has been identified in a number of patients.[22] With doses <300 rads (3 Gy) there is very little risk of developing an adenoma, whereas over 50% develop adenomas when the doses exceeded 12 Gy.[22-24] Given that the present patient has a history of radioiodine ablation of her thyroid (typical doses exceed 12 Gy), it is probable that irradiation is the underlying cause of her primary HPT. In rare cases, there are identifiable monoclonal genetic defects underlying primary hyperparathyroidism. Specific abnormalities include gain-of-function mutations in cyclin D1/PRAD in sporadic tumors, RET for familial tumors, and loss-of-function mutations in MEN1, which occur in sporadic and familial tumors, or HRPT2 for familial ones.[25-27] The PRAD1 genes encode cyclin D1, which is a major regulator of the cell cycle; 20% to 40% of sporadic PTH adenomas overexpress cyclin D1.[28-33] The MEN1 gene

is a tumor suppressor gene, found in nearly two-thirds of patients with MEN type 1 and one-quarter of patients with sporadic primary PTH.[25,34-36] One study has identified mutations in the Wnt-b-catenin signaling pathway in tumors from patients with hyperparathyroidism; these mutations were not observed in patients with secondary hyperplasia.[37]

Patient Follow-up

The primary hypothyroidism was cured with removal of parathyroid adenoma. One week following surgery, the patient's PTH and calcium had normalized: PTH, 34 ng/mL (12–72); total calcium, 8.9 mg/dL (8.5–10.2). To prevent hypocalcemia after parathyroidectomy, the patient was prescribed calcium and vitamin D (600 mg) supplements twice daily. Follow-up studies include a dual energy X-ray absorptiometry (DEXA) bone scan to monitor bone mineral density. Significant loss of bone density can result from prolonged hyperparathyroidism.[38] Her vitamin D and calcium levels 1 month after surgery had normalized to: calcium, 9.1 mg/dL (8.5–10.2); total 25-OH-vitamin D, 18 ng/mL (25–80).

Keywords

Primary hyperparathyroidism, parathyroid, hypercalcemia, adenoma

References

1. Sitges-Serra A, Bergenfelz A. Clinical update: Sporadic primary hyperpara-thyroidism. *Lancet.* 2007;370:468–470.

2. Silver J, Levi R. Cellular and molecular mechanisms of secondary hyperparathyroidism. *Clin Nephrol.* 2005;63:119–126.

3. Casez J, Pfammatter R, Nguyen Q, et al. Diagnostic approach to hypercalcemia: Relevance of parathyroid hormone and parathyroid hormone-related protein measurements. *Eur J Intern Med.* 2001;12:344–349.

4. Rankin W, Grill V, Martin TJ. Parathyroid hormone-related protein and hypercalcemia. *Cancer.* 1997;80:1564–1571.

5. Terpos E, Dimopoulos MA. Myeloma bone disease: Pathophysiology and management. *Ann Oncol.* 2005;16:1223–1231.

6. Siris ES, Lyles KW, Singer FR, et al. Medical management of Paget's disease of bone: Indications for treatment and review of current therapies. *J Bone Miner Res.* 2006;21:94–98.

7. Stewart AF, Adler M, Byers CM, et al. Calcium homeostasis in immobilization: An example of resorptive hypercalciuria. *N Engl J Med.* 1982;306:1136–1140.

8. Adams JS. Vitamin D metabolite-mediated hypercalcemia. *Endocrinol Metab Clin North Am.* 1989;18:765–778.

9. Spiegel AM, Rudorfer MV, Marx SJ, et al. The effect of short term lithium administration on suppressibility of parathyroid hormone secretion by calcium in vivo. *J Clin Endocrinol Metab.* 1984;59:354–357.

10. Bartsch D, Nies C, Hasse C, et al. Clinical and surgical aspects of double adenoma in patients with primary hyperparathyroidism. *Br J Surg.* 1995;82:926–929.

11. Ruda JM, Hollenbeak CS, Stack BC Jr. A systematic review of the diagnosis and treatment of primary hyperparathyroidism from 1995 to 2003. *Otolaryngol Head Neck Surg.* 2005;132:359–372.

12. Bilezikian JP, Potts JT Jr, Fuleihan Gel H, et al. Summary statement from a workshop on asymptomatic primary hyperparathyroidism: A perspective for the 21st century. *J Clin Endocrinol Metab.* 2002;87:5353–5361.

13. Sitges-Serra A, Bergenfelz A. Clinical update: Sporadic primary hyperparathyroidism. *Lancet.* 2007;370(9586):468–470. Clinical update: Sporadic primary hyperparathyroidism 1474–1547X (Electronic).

14. Bergenfelz A, Kanngiesser V, Zielke A, et al. Conventional bilateral cervical exploration versus open minimally invasive parathyroidectomy under local anaesthesia for primary hyperparathyroidism. *Br J Surg.* 2005;92:190–197.

15. Bergenfelz A, Lindblom P, Tibblin S, et al. Unilateral versus bilateral neck exploration for primary hyperparathyroidism: A prospective randomized controlled trial. *Ann Surg.* 2002;236:543–551.

16. Russell CF, Dolan SJ, Laird JD. Randomized clinical trial comparing scan-directed unilateral versus bilateral cervical exploration for primary hyperparathyroidism due to solitary adenoma. *Br J Surg.* 2006;93:418–421.

17. Sokoll LJ. Measurement of parathyroid hormone and application of parathyroid hormone in intraoperative monitoring. *Clin Lab Med.* 2004;24:199–216.

18. Gawande AA, Monchik JM, Abbruzzese TA, et al. Reassessment of parathyroid hormone monitoring during parathyroidectomy for primary hyperparathyroidism after 2 preoperative localization studies. *Arch Surg.* 2006;141:381–384.

19. Hortin GL, Carter AB. Intraoperative parathyroid hormone testing: Survey of testing program characteristics. *Arch Pathol Lab Med.* 2002;126:1045–1049.

20. Sokoll LJ, Wians FH Jr, Remaley AT. Rapid intraoperative immunoassay of parathyroid hormone and other hormones: A new paradigm for point-of-care testing. *Clin Chem.* 2004;50:1126–1135.

21. Johnson LR, Doherty G, Lairmore T, et al. Evaluation of the performance and clinical impact of a rapid intraoperative parathyroid hormone assay in conjunction with preoperative imaging and concise parathyroidectomy. *Clin Chem.* 2001;47:919–925.

22. Tisell LE, Hansson G, Lindberg S, et al. Hyperparathyroidism in persons treated with X-rays for tuberculous cervical adenitis. *Cancer.* 1977;40:846–854.

23. Beard CM, Heath H 3rd, O'Fallon WM, et al. Therapeutic radiation and hyperparathyroidism. A case-control study in Rochester, Minn. *Arch Intern Med.* 1989;149:1887–1890.

24. Schneider AB, Gierlowski TC, Shore-Freedman E, et al. Dose-response relationships for radiation-induced hyperparathyroidism. *J Clin Endocrinol Metab.* 1995;80:254–257.

25. Arnold A, Shattuck TM, Mallya SM, et al. Molecular pathogenesis of primary hyperparathyroidism. *J Bone Miner Res.* 2002;17:30–36.

26. Hendy GN. Molecular mechanisms of primary hyperparathyroidism. *Rev Endocr Metab Disord.* 2000;1:297–305.

27. Shattuck TM, Valimaki S, Obara T, et al. Somatic and germ-line mutations of the HRPT2 gene in sporadic parathyroid carcinoma. *N Engl J Med.* 2003;349:1722–1729.

28. Arnold A, Kim HG. Clonal loss of one chromosome 11 in a parathyroid adenoma. *J Clin Endocrinol Metab.* 1989;69:496–499.

29. Arnold A, Kim HG, Gaz RD, et al. Molecular cloning and chromosomal mapping of DNA rearranged with the parathyroid hormone gene in a parathyroid adenoma. *J Clin Invest.* 1989;83:2034–2040.

30. Hemmer S, Wasenius VM, Haglund C, et al. Deletion of 11q23 and cyclin D1 overexpression are frequent aberrations in parathyroid adenomas. *Am J Pathol.* 2001;158:1355–1362.

31. Hsi ED, Zukerberg LR, Yang WI, et al. Cyclin D1/PRAD1 expression in parathyroid adenomas: An immunohistochemical study. *J Clin Endocrinol Metab.* 1996;81:1736–1739.

32. Rosenberg CL, Kim HG, Shows TB, et al. Rearrangement and overexpression of D11S287E, a candidate oncogene on chromosome 11q13 in benign parathyroid tumors. *Oncogene.* 1991;6:449–453.

33. Vasef MA, Brynes RK, Sturm M, et al. Expression of cyclin D1 in parathyroid carcinomas, adenomas, and hyperplasias: A paraffin immunohistochemical study. *Mod Pathol.* 1999;12:412–416.

34. Agarwal SK, Kester MB, Debelenko LV, et al. Germline mutations of the MEN1 gene in familial multiple endocrine neoplasia type 1 and related states. *Hum Mol Genet.* 1997;6:1169–1175.

35. Friedman E, Sakaguchi K, Bale AE, et al. Clonality of parathyroid tumors in familial multiple endocrine neoplasia type 1. *N Engl J Med.* 1989;321:213–218.

36. Thakker RV, Bouloux P, Wooding C, et al. Association of parathyroid tumors in multiple endocrine neoplasia type 1 with loss of alleles on chromosome 11. *N Engl J Med.* 1989;321:218–224.

37. Björklund P, Akerstrom G, Westin G. Accumulation of nonphosphorylated beta-catenin and c-myc in primary and uremic secondary hyperparathyroid tumors. *J Clin Endocrinol Metab.* 2007;92:338–344.

38. Nakaoka D, Sugimoto T, Kobayashi T, et al. Prediction of bone mass change after parathyroidectomy in patients with primary hyperparathyroidism. *J Clin Endocrinol Metab.* 2000;85:1901–1907.

Growth Delay in an Adolescent Male

Cynthia Z. Liu, Melissa M. Blann, Charles A. Bradley

From the Department of Pathology and Laboratory Medicine, Texas Tech University Health Sciences Center, Lubbock, TX

Patient: 14-and-a-half-year-old male.

Drug History: Unremarkable.

Chief Complaint: He and his parents thought that it was odd that he had been wearing the same size clothes for the past few years. He did not complain of any lack of appetite. The patient presented to the pediatric clinic 5 months later and still complained about being constantly teased by his friends about his height. He had grown only 1 cm during these past 5 months. The differential diagnosis included familial versus constitutional growth delay.

Medical History: He was born after an uneventful pregnancy with a birth weight of 7 lb 11oz.

Surgical History: Orchiopexy/herniorrhaphy at 2 years of age.

Family/Social History: He lived with his mother, adoptive father, and siblings. He performed well in school and sports. His mother was 5 feet 3 inches in height and reached menarche at 12 years of age. His biological father was 5 feet 9 inches in height and had achieved normal pubertal milestones. In addition, his father indicated that several of his relatives had bleeding ulcers, and pancreatic and "neck" tumors.

Physical Examination: His body weight of 93.5 lbs (42.5 kg) was at the 10th percentile and his height of 4 feet 9 inches (145.2 cm) was below the 5th percentile for his age group. He was Tanner stage 1 (no apparent pubertal changes) and the rest of his physical examination was otherwise unremarkable.

Results of Additional Diagnostic Procedures _____

1. A bone age study of his left hand revealed complete agreement between the state of his skeletal maturation and his chronological age.

2. Unenhanced and enhanced T1-weighted magnetic resonance imaging (MRI) scans of his brain and thin scans of the sella region demonstrated an enlarged pituitary gland with a maximum diameter of approximately 1.4 cm. There was heterogeneity of the pituitary gland parenchyma with heterogeneous enhancement consistent with a pituitary gland macroadenoma.

3. A computerized tomography (CT) scan of his abdomen was unremarkable.

Questions _____

1. What is (are) this patient's most striking laboratory result(s)?

T1. Principal Laboratory Findings

Test	Patient's Result	"Normal" Reference Range
TSH	1.22	0.37 - 6.00 µIU/mL
Free T4	0.90	0.92 - 1.57 ng/mL
hGH	0.7	0.7 - 6.0 ng/mL
Prolactin	821	3.6 - 17.9 ng/mL
Calcium	10.4	9.2 - 10.7 mg/dL
PTH	54	10 - 65 pg/mL
FSH	0.4	0.2 - 0.8 mIU/mL
LH	< 0.5	0.5 - 5.3 mIU/mL
Testosterone	18	10 - 572 ng/dL
AFP	< 1.3	< 7.4 ng/mL
HCG, serum	Negative	Negative
IGF-1	112	152 - 540 ng/mL
AM Cortisol	20.1	2.1 - 19.5 µg/dL
Electrolytes	Normal	
Urinalysis	Normal	

TSH, thyroid stimulating hormone; T4, thyroxine; hGH, human growth hormone; PTH, parathyroid hormone; FSH, follicle stimulating hormone; LH, luteinizing hormone; AFP, alpha-fetoprotein; HCG, human chorionic gonadotropin; IGF-1, insulin-like growth factor-1.

2. How do you explain this patient's most striking laboratory test results?

3. Which additional laboratory test(s) should be ordered and why?

4. What is the most likely diagnosis relevant to this patient?

Possible Answer

1. The most striking laboratory finding is a markedly elevated prolactin concentration. Other noteworthy abnormal laboratory findings include slightly or borderline decreased free thyroxine (FT4) and human growth hormone (hGH) concentrations, decreased luteinizing hormone (LH) concentration, and a markedly decreased insulin-like growth factor-1 (IGF-1) concentration.

2. The 4 primary causes of hyperprolactinemia are: 1) physiologic (ie, transient pulses of prolactin); 2) pharmacologic (eg, psychotropic medications); 3) compression of the hypothalamic

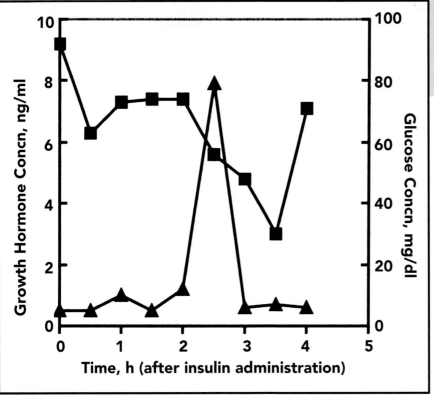

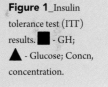

Figure 1_Insulin tolerance test (ITT) results. ■ - GH; ▲ - Glucose; Concn, concentration.

or pituitary stalk; and, 4) prolactinoma. Physiologic, pharmacologic, and hypothalamic/pituitary compression causes of this patient's hyperprolactinemia are ruled out because prolactin concentration is usually <50 ng/mL in physiologic hyperprolactinemia, the patient's drug history was unremarkable and the prolactin concentration is usually <100 ng/mL in pharmacologic hyperprolactinemia, and the prolactin concentration is usually between 20 ng/mL and 100 ng/mL because of compression of the hypothalamus or pituitary stalk. The prolactin concentration is usually >200 ng/mL in patients with hyperprolactinemia due to a pituitary prolactinoma. This patient's prolactin concentration was 821 ng/mL. Moreover, this patient's MRI findings of an enlarged pituitary gland due to a macroadenoma are consistent with the axiom that prolactin levels generally correlate with tumor size. Thus, a pituitary prolactinoma is the most likely cause of this patient's markedly increased prolactin concentration. Prolactinomas are neoplastic growths of lactotroph cells (ie, prolactin-secreting cells of the anterior pituitary gland) and are the most common (approximately 25% to 40%) type of pituitary adenoma. In addition, in men, hyperprolactinemia causes hypogonadism with decreased LH and follicle stimulating hormone (FSH) levels and low testosterone levels. Moreover, although hypothyroidism can cause growth failure, this patient's FT4 level was only slightly decreased and his TSH level was normal, suggesting that hypothyroidism was not the cause of this patient's growth failure. Lastly, although this patient's hGH level was borderline normal, basal GH levels, unlike IGF-1 levels, do not provide a reliable measure of GH reserve capacity. IGF-1 production in the liver and other tissues (eg, bone) is increased by GH and IGF-1 exerts negative feedback inhibition of GH production at the level of both the hypothalamus and the pituitary. Therefore, GH deficiency causes decreased IGF-1 levels and decreased levels of its binding protein, IGFBP-3.

3. Constitutional growth delay was ruled out on the basis of the agreement between his skeletal and chronological age and the absence of hypothyroidism; however, the family history provided by the patient's biological father suggested the possibility of a multiple endocrine neoplasia (MEN) syndrome. The patient's normal serum levels of calcium and parathyroid hormone (PTH), coupled with a normal imaging study of the abdomen, mitigated against an MEN as the cause of this patient's growth delay. GH deficiency is suggested by the borderline normal hGH level, the markedly decreased IGF-1 level in this patient's serum, and the patient's short stature. Short stature is defined as a subnormal height (less than the 3rd percentile) relative to other children of the same sex, age, and ethnicity. Under the age of 2 years, short stature often results from malnutrition. The most common causes in children over 2 years of age are variants of normal growth (ie, familial short stature and constitutional growth delay). The evaluation of children with short stature begins with a good history and physical examination. Nutritional, metabolic, major organ system insufficiency, endocrine, and intrinsic defects must be considered in the differential diagnosis of such children. The selection of follow-up diagnostic tests must be individualized based on the child's overall presentation. Levels of FT4, TSH, and thyroid antibodies must be evaluated in any short child, especially one who is scheduled for provocative tests of GH secretion. Serum IGF-1 and IGF binding protein-3 (IGFBP-3) levels can be helpful, but they are not always diagnostic of GH deficiency. If the levels of IGF-1 and IGFBP-3 are normal, the decision to perform provocative tests of GH secretion is based on growth-related criteria and clinical judgment. If IGF-1 and IGFBP-3 levels are low, the pediatrician should evaluate the child for malnutrition because nutritional status is a regulator of these peptides. A complete blood count, biochemical profile, and a urinalysis should also be performed, as well as a bone age study (left wrist and hand x-ray) to estimate skeletal age and growth potential. An MRI of the hypothalamus and pituitary gland should always be done prior to initiating GH replacement therapy. Consensus guidelines for the diagnosis and treatment of GH deficiency in children and adolescents have been published by the Growth Hormone Research Society.

4. GH deficiency is most frequently assessed using the insulin tolerance test (ITT) to achieve a state of insulin-induced hypoglycemia. Glucose suppresses GH secretion while hypoglycemia stimulates pituitary GH secretion. Both GH and glucose levels are measured at 15 minute or 30

minute intervals after the intravenous administration of an appropriate insulin dose. The patient must be closely monitored during this test for any symptoms of severe hypoglycemia. In children, peak GH values of >10 ng/mL during an ITT are generally considered as normal, values between 7 ng/mL and 10 ng/mL are considered equivocal, and values <7 ng/mL are abnormal. The results of the ITT performed on the patient discussed in this Case Study are shown in **Figure 1**. The patient's peak GH value of 7.9 ng/mL is borderline abnormal.

Most Likely Diagnosis: Secondary GH deficiency due to a prolactin-secreting pituitary macroadenoma.

Treatment and Course

The patient was treated initially with Dostinex (cabergoline; 25 mg biweekly) and his prolactin level decreased. Subsequently, he underwent transsphenoidal exploration with over 99% of the pituitary adenoma cells removed. He was started on growth hormone (Humatrope) therapy (2.1 mg intramuscularly 6 days a week) right after the surgery. Following surgery, his serum prolactin level was decreased but still above the normal reference range. He is currently on Dostinex (0.5 mg twice a week) and Humatrope (2.4 mg 6 days per week) and has reported no adverse side effects. Overall, he has been well since his surgery and is currently undergoing routine follow-up care.

Lower Abdominal Pain, Dyspnea, and Severe Shortness of Breath in a 28-Year-Old Pregnant Woman

[1]Yaseen Samman, [2]Hossam Ghoneim, [3]Ibrahim A. Hashim

[1]*Departments of Medicine,* [2]*Obstetric and Gynecology, and* [3]*Pathology, King Khalid National Guard Hospital, Jeddah, Kingdom of Saudi Arabia*

Patient: 28-year-old pregnant woman.

Chief Complaint: Lower abdominal pain and distention, dyspnea, and severe shortness of breath.

Past Medical History: Induced pregnancies (G5 P2+3) following treatment with clomiphene citrate.

Drug History: No current history of any medications, drugs of abuse, or therapeutic drugs, except clomiphene citrate and other agents used during ovulation induction. The induction protocol involved initial down-regulation of pituitary gonadotropin secretion and inhibition of ovarian steroid secretion with a luteinizing hormone-releasing hormone (LHRH) analogue (Buserelin), followed by stimulation with a follicle stimulating hormone (FSH) preparation, and triggering of ovulation by administration of human chorionic gonadotropin (hCG).

Physical Examination: She was afebrile (temperature: 36°C) with abnormal heart rate (106 beats/min), blood pressure (108/83 mm Hg), and respirations (24/min). Abdominal examination revealed a large distended abdomen that was diffusely tender with positive signs of ascites. She had mild pedal edema. She was admitted to our hospital for further follow-up.

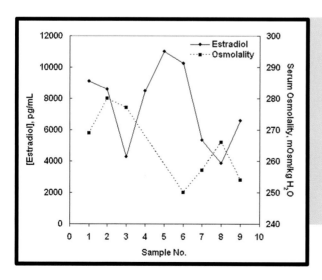

Figure 1_Changes in estradiol and serum osmolality levels in various samples taken on different days (ie, sample numbers do not correspond to hospital day in **T1**) during the patient's 20-day hospital stay.

T1. Principal Laboratory Findings on Admission (Day 0) and During the First 10 Days of the Patient's 20-Day Hospital Stay

Test	Specimen Type	"Normal" Reference Range	Patient's Result on Hospital Day										
			0	1	2	3	4	5	6	7	8	9	10
Sodium (Na+)	serum	135-145 mEq/L	129	128	116	131	123	129	129	131	126	128	130
	urine	<10 mEq/L*			35		91						
Potassium	serum	3.6-5.0 mEq/L	4.2	4.8	6.6	4.5	4.4	4.7	5.0	5.1	4.8	4.6	4.4
CO_2	serum	22-31 mEq/L	22										
Albumin	serum	3.5-5.2 g/dL	3.7	3.7	3.7	2.9	2.9	2.7	2.6	2.6	2.5	3.4	2.6
Glucose	serum	65-110 mg/dL	104						104				
BUN	serum	4-21 mg/dL	23						23				
Creatinine	serum	0.6-1.2 mg/dL	0.9										
β-hCG	serum	<5 mIU/mL†											
Osmolality	serum	270-300 mOsm/kg H_2O	1210						267	276			
	urine	50-1200 mOsm/kg H2O‡	298										
Osmolal Gap§	serum	9-15 mOsm/kg H_2O							0				

*A random or spot urine sodium concentration >10 mEq/L may indicate diuretics, emesis, intrinsic renal diseases, Addison's disease, hypothyroidism, or syndrome of inappropriate anti-diuretic hormone (SIADH) secretion. †Males and non-pregnant females. ‡Depending on fluid intake. §Osmolal Gap = OsmoMeasured – OsmoCalculated; where, OsmoCalculated = 2[Na+] + ([Glucose]/18) + ([BUN]/2.8). BUN, blood urea nitrogen; b-hCG, beta-human chorionic gonadotropin.

In addition to the laboratory data [**T1**], the patient's values for all liver enzyme tests, thyrotropin (TSH), and cortisol were within normal limits; and her hemoglobin (16.7 g/dL), hematocrit (51.5%), and platelet count (599×10^3/mL) values were consistent with hemoconcentration. Serial measurement of serum estradiol concentration was performed during her hospital stay [**Figure 1**].

Results of Other Diagnostic Procedures _____

Cardiovascular examination showed no elevation of jugular vein pressure and normal first and second heart sounds with no murmurs or added sounds. Chest examination showed dullness to percussion in the lower third of the chest posteriorly with decreased air entry and vocal sound vibration. Chest X-ray, with abdominal shield, revealed mild right-sided pleural effusion but no other abnormality.

Questions _____

1. What is(are) this patient's most striking laboratory result(s)?

2. How do you explain this patient's most striking laboratory result(s)?

3. What condition(s) does this patient's laboratory and other findings suggest?

4. What are the principal complications found in this patient's condition?

5. What is(are) the most likely cause(s) of the principal complications found in this patient's condition?

6. Which laboratory and non-laboratory test(s) are appropriate to order on this patient and why?

7. What is the most appropriate treatment for this patient?

Possible Answers

1. Elevated serum β-hCG; hyponatremia with low serum and inappropriately high urine osmolality; and markedly elevated serum estradiol levels (ie, 4,000 to 10,000 pg/mL; normal reference range for premenopausal women: 30 to 400 pg/mL, depending on phase of menstrual cycle). Her serum sodium value decreased from an already low value of 129 mEq/L at admission to 116 mEq/L 48 hours later [**T1**].

2. The elevated serum β-hCG value is consistent with the patient being pregnant. Hyponatremia can be subdivided into 2 types: *dilutional* [due to increased secretion of anti-diuretic hormone (ADH), followed by water retention, and plasma volume expansion] and *depletional* (from renal or extrarenal sodium loss). The most common cause of hyponatremia in hospitalized patients is the syndrome of inappropriate ADH secretion (SIADH); however, other conditions, including congestive heart failure, renal insufficiency, nephrotic syndrome, liver cirrhosis, hypothyroidism, and drugs that stimulate ADH secretion may also cause hyponatremia. The patient's history (eg, the only drugs she was taking were those associated with the ovulation induction protocol), laboratory, and other diagnostic data did not support any of the aforementioned conditions. Her serum was hypo-osmolar (ie, <270 mOsm/kg H_2O). Her urine osmolality (298 mOsm/kg H_2O) was slightly greater than her serum osmolality (267 and 276 mOsm/kg H_2O). There was no significant osmolal gap, and her urine sodium concentration (91 mEq/L on day 4 of her hospital stay) was inappropriately high (ie, 40 to 80 mEq/L). These findings *are typical of patients with SIADH*. Her markedly elevated estradiol values are consistent with *ovarian hyperstimulation syndrome (OHSS)*. Ovarian hyperstimulation syndrome of varying severity is seen following the use of exogenous gonadotropins for induction of ovulation.[1,2] Therefore, the possibility exists that her SIADH was caused by the drugs (eg, clomiphene citrate and gonadotropins) used to induce her to ovulate. This possibility is made less likely by

the fact her serum sodium concentration continued to decrease up to 3 days after admission. Thus, the cause of this patient's hyponatremia is not clear and could be due to defects in the renin-angiotensin system or the involvement of prostaglandins and other endothelial factors. A recent report highlighted a case of severe OHSS with sodium retention, increased plasma renin activity (PRA), and, unlike the patient described in this case study whose urine sodium concentration was inappropriately high, an undetectable urine sodium concentration.[3] Moreover, both renin and aldosterone have been suggested to play a role in the pathogenesis of OHSS.[4] We did not perform renin testing on a plasma sample from our patient. In deciphering the cause of this patient's SIADH, it is interesting to note that her serum estradiol levels were negatively correlated with her serum osmolality [**Figure 1**]. This finding suggests that the steroid, estradiol, and perhaps other steroids may exert an osmoregulatory effect. A recent report of hyponatremia due to SIADH in a patient with an immature ovarian teratoma lends support to this hypothesis.[5] Although the patient's steroid levels were not stated in this report, the serum sodium level returned to normal following resection of the patient's tumor.[5] Thus, it is possible that steroids such as estradiol may be involved in the pathogenesis of hyponatremia.

3. This patient's laboratory and clinical findings are suggestive of *SIADH with OHSS*. This report describes a patient with SIADH in concert with OHSS. Induction of ovulation by administration of exogenous gonadotropins is frequently used in patients being investigated for infertility. Although induction of ovulation is successful in most cases, some degree of hyperstimulation occurs. The most serious is that leading to OHSS, which occurs in approximately 4% of patients undergoing ovulation induction.[1] This syndrome occurs with most methods of ovulation stimulation, and various classifications of its severity have been suggested.[1]

4. Complications of OHSS include fluid depletion, shock, renal failure, thromboembolism, and in some cases, thoracic involvement with acute respiratory distress and pleural effusion.[6] Hyponatremia and sodium retention, evidenced by inappropriately low urine sodium

concentration, have both been reported in patients with OHSS.[5,7] Prior to this report, however, hyponatremia with the low serum osmolality and inappropriately high urine sodium concentration characteristic of SIADH had not been reported in a patient with OHSS.

5. The patient's respiratory distress at presentation was due to the combined effects of a markedly distended abdomen compressing the diaphragm towards the chest and a pleural effusion. A culture of the ascitic fluid was negative for bacterial growth and laboratory analysis of the fluid revealed (parentheses indicate reference range for transudates): white blood cell (WBC) count, 55/mm[3]; red blood cell count (RBC), 101/mm[3]; polymorphonuclear leukocytes, 68%; lymphocytes, 32%; sodium, 130 mEq/L; potassium, 4.8 mEq/L; glucose, 101 mg/dL (>95 mg/dL); lactate dehydrogenase, 126 U/L (<200 U/L); total protein, 39 g/L; and albumin, 25 g/L. These data are suggestive of a hypercellular exudate with transudate glucose and LD concentrations. Because only a few cases have been reported previously, the value of these laboratory findings in identifying patients with SIADH and OHSS is not clear.

6. Plasma renin activity, serum aldosterone, and abdominal ultrasound. The severity of OHSS correlates positively with PRA and measurement of both PRA and aldosterone are useful in ruling out adrenal insufficiency as a cause of hyponatremia. In the patient reported in this case study, adrenal insufficiency was ruled out by the patient's normal cortisol level. Prostaglandins and endothelial factors are thought to have a role in the pathogenesis of OHSS[1]; however, their measurement is not routinely available and is best reserved for research purposes. Abdominal ultrasound examination should be performed to evaluate the ovaries, the extent of ascites, and the viability of any fetuses. Ultrasound testing of our patient's abdomen revealed markedly enlarged ovaries (*left* ovary, 21 × 13 cm; *right* ovary, 21 × 16 cm) occupying most of the abdomen in addition to the ascites and 4 intrauterine gestational sacs.

7. The clinical management of OHSS depends on the severity of the disease.[3] Mild forms of OHSS usually resolve within 2 to 3 weeks, and the

treatment is usually conservative with observation and follow-up. On the other hand severe forms of OHSS require hospital admission and active monitoring of the patient's electrolyte balance, ascites, and respiratory symptoms. The management of hyponatremia depends on the level of the serum sodium concentration and the clinical picture of the patient such as the presence of neurological signs or symptoms. In our patient, although the serum sodium concentration was very low, she did not have any neurological abnormalities which would require prompt administration of hypertonic saline to quickly raise the serum sodium level. Moreover, administration of hypertonic saline is contraindicated in this case because of the patient's hemoconcentration and the possibility of thromboembolic disease. The combination of hyponatremia with low serum osmolality and hemoconcentration is unusual and difficult to explain. Ascites are treated by repeated tapping and removal of the fluid or by inserting a drain. In addition, transfusion of albumin has been used in patients with a severe form of OHSS.[8,9] In patients at risk of developing OHSS, administration of albumin at the time of oocyte collection has been shown to reduce the likelihood of severe OHSS from occurring.[10] We applied this approach to our patient with good success in relieving her symptoms of abdominal discomfort and respiratory distress. Her hypoalbuminemia was corrected by albumin infusion, which increases plasma oncotic pressure and thus limits fluid leakage from the plasma into the intravascular space. Therefore, plasma water retention may explain our patient's hyponatremia.

Treatment and Course

Fluids were restricted and the patient was closely monitored. Although the patient's hyponatremia was asymptomatic, normal saline was infused until her serum sodium concentration exceeded 130 mEq/L. In view of the severity of her ascites, she was continued on fluid restriction. Her hypoalbuminemia was corrected by multiple infusions of 20% human albumin based on her serum albumin level. Four days after admission, she became increasingly short of breath with increased abdominal pain and distension due to the accumulation of ascitic fluid. A therapeutic tap of the ascitic fluid was performed under ultrasound guidance to relieve her severe abdominal discomfort. Due to the rapid accumulation of the ascitic fluid, abdominal tapping to remove ascitic fluid and infusion of albumin was repeated 2 more times based on the patient's symptoms. With the above management, the patient improved progressively and was discharged 20 days after admission. The patient's condition was reviewed during outpatient follow-up visits over the next few weeks. She continued to be stable with minimum ascites and diminishing pleural effusion on ultrasound examination. Moreover, repeat ultrasound examinations during this time period demonstrated diminishing ovarian size (*left* ovary, 16 × 10 cm; *right* ovary, 13 × 5.5 cm). In addition, her pregnancy progressed; however, at 11 weeks gestation, 1 fetus had no heart sounds and was spontaneously aborted. Subsequent ultrasound examinations revealed that the remaining 3 fetuses continued to develop normally. The patient was admitted in labor at 31 weeks gestation and had an emergency Cesarean section. Three healthy male babies were delivered, weighing 3.5, 3.7, and 4.0 pounds. Ten months after delivery, she and her babies were doing well.

Keywords

SIADH, ovarian hyperstimulation, hyponatremia

Reference

1. Golan A, Ron-EL R, Herman A, et al. Ovarian hyperstimulation syndrome: An update review. *Obstet Gynaecol Surv.* 1989;44:430-440.

2. Samman Y, Ghoneim H, Hashim IA. Syndrome of inappropriate ADH as a manifestation of severe ovarian hyperstimulation syndrome. *J Obstet Gynaecol.* 2001;21:201-203.

3. Bangsboll S. Ovarian hyperstimulation syndrome a risk of treatment for infertility. *Nord Med.* 1977;112:236-239.

4. Brindsen PR, Wada I, Tan SL, et al. Diagnosis, prevention, and management of ovarian hyperstimulation syndrome. *Br J Obstet Gynecol.* 1995;102:676-772.

5. Cremisi HD, Mitch, WE. Profound hypotension and sodium retention with the ovarian hyperstimulation syndrome. *Am J Kidney Dis.* 1994;24:854-857.

6. Hanning RV, Strawn EY, Nolten WE. Pathophysiology of the ovarian hyperstimulation syndrome. *Obstet Gynecol.* 1985;66:220-224.

7. Lam SK, Cheung LP. Inappropriate ADH secretion due to immature ovarian teratoma. *Aus N Z J Obstet Gynaecol.* 1996;36:104-105.

8. Al-Mobeireek A, Al-Meshari A, Al-Zamil H, et al. Pleurisy in ovarian hyperstimulation syndrome: A case report. *Saudi Med J.* 1998;19:345- 347.

9. Al-Rahmani M, Leader A, Claman P, et al. Novel approach to the treatment of ascites associated with ovarian hyperstimulation syndrome. *Hum Repro.* 1997;12:2614-2616.

10. Asch RH, Iveryt G, Goldsman MI, et al. The use of intravenous albumin in patients at high risk for severe ovarian hyperstimulation syndrome. *Hum Repro.* 1993;8:1015-1020.

Protein Bands in all Lanes of the Immunofixation Electrophoresis Pattern of Serum From a 50-Year-Old Saudi Woman

Yusra Othman

King Khalid National Guard Hospital, Jeddah, Saudi Arabia

Patient: 50-year-old Saudi woman.

Chief Complaint: Hoarseness, weakness, fatigue, and chronic gum bleeding.

History of Present Illness: She was admitted to the hospital previously and diagnosed with lymphadenopathy, MALT (mucosa-associated lymphoid tissue) subtype non-Hodgkin lymphoma, hypothyroidism, and emphysema.

History of Current Medications: L-thyroxin and Zantac.

Physical Examination Findings: Both eyes were congested and her left eye was swollen. Subsequently, she was seen in an opthalmology clinic and diagnosed with periorbital cellulitis. Review of systems indicated intact central nervous system (CNS) and normal cardiovascular system (CVS) findings. Her abdomen was soft with evidence of splenomegaly and no evidence of any other organomegaly or masses.

Questions

1. What is (are) this patient's most striking clinical and laboratory findings?

2. How do you explain these findings?

3. Why did her initial serum immunofixation electrophoresis (IFE) findings demonstrate a single discrete band in all lanes of the IFE gel?

4. How should her serum be treated to resolve the discrepancy of multiple bands in all lanes of the IFE gel?

5. What is this patient's most likely diagnosis?

6. What is the etiology of this patient's condition?

7. How should this patient's condition be treated?

Possible Answers

1. Fatigue, chronic gum bleeding, splenomegaly, congested and swollen eyes, periorbital cellulitis; anemia (decreased hemoglobin level), increased total protein with decreased albumin, markedly increased globulins, an inverted A/G ratio, and markedly increased serum viscosity; serum protein electrophoresis pattern (SPEP) consistent with a tall, dense band in the gamma region of the SPE gel (**Image 1A**) and abnormal IFE

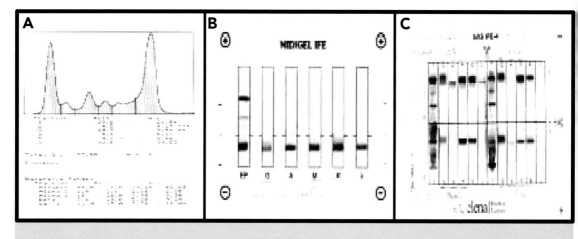

Image 1_Patient's serum protein electrophoresis pattern (SPEP) (**A**), illustrating a tall, dense band in the gamma-region, and immunofixation electrophoresis (IFE) patterns before (**B**) and after (**C**) treatment of the patient's serum with β-mercaptoethanol. In Panel (**C**), the upper left quadrant shows the IFE pattern of the patient's serum pretreated with β-mercaptoethanol for 10 min, while the upper right quadrant shows the IFE pattern of the patient's serum pretreated with β-mercaptoethanol for 30 min. The lower left quadrant shows the IFE pattern of the patient's serum pretreated with β-mercaptoethanol for 60 min. The lower right quadrant shows the IFE pattern of an abnormal control serum of known IgM kappa immunophenotype. Prior to β-mercaptoethanol treatment of the patient's serum, visibly discrete protein bands were observed in all lanes of the IFE gel (**B**), while after treatment of the patient's serum with β-mercaptoethanol, a discrete band of IgM kappa, and some polyclonal IgG, are observed (**C**). Pre-treatment with β-mercaptoethanol for 60 min provided the best resolution of the multiple bands. In all 4 quadrants of panel (**C**), lanes 1-6 represent the lanes to which no antiserum was added (*lane 1*) or to which IgG (*lane 2*), IgA (*lane 3*), IgM (*lane 4*), kappa light chain (*lane 5*), or lambda light chain (*lane 6*) antiserum was added. The horizontal dotted line in panel (**B**) and the solid line in panel (**C**) indicate the point-of-application of serum/antiserum on the IFE gel.

T1. Principal Laboratory Findings

Test	Patient's Result	Reference Interval
Hematology		
WBC count	8.5	4.1-10.9 × 10³/μL
Hemoglobin	9.8	12.0-15.2 g/dL
Platelet count	282	140-450 × 10³/μL
Chemistry[a]		
Total protein	11.2	6.3-8.2 g/dL
Albumin	3.4	3.5-5.2 g/dL
Globulins	7.8	1.3-3.2 g/dL
A/G ratio	0.44	1.5-3.0
IgG	1.72	0.65-1.6 g/dL
IgA	0.11	0.04-0.35 g/dL
IgM	5.84	0.05-0.30 g/dL
Serum viscosity[b]	5.9	1.14-1.34 centipoises

[a]*Liver function tests were normal (data not shown).* [b]*Ordered because her serum appeared highly viscous. WBC, white blood cell; A/G, albumin/globulin.*

findings (ie, protein bands present in all lanes of the IFE gel) (**Image 1B**).

2. Her fatigue is most likely a consequence of her anemia related to chronic gum bleeding, while her congested and swollen eyes with periorbital cellulitis are most likely a consequence of her abnormal protein levels, especially her markedly increased serum globulins and viscosity (hyperviscosity syndrome), and the presence of a large M-protein on SPE. It is not uncommon that opthalmologists order SPE on their patients that present with signs and symptoms of blurred or impaired vision. Moreover, monoclonal proteins are often observed in serum from these patients, which might otherwise go undetected until a later course in their disease. In addition, chronic nasal bleeding and oozing from the gums occur commonly in patients with hyperviscosity syndrome, especially when the serum viscosity is >4 centipoises.[1] Our patient's serum viscosity was 5.9 centipoises (**T1**).

3. Our patient's IFE pattern is classic for the presence of a high concentration of a cryoglobulin that migrates as a single band, precipitates in all lanes of an IFE gel, and is stained with the protein-staining dye used to detect the presence of immunoglobulins in any of the lanes of the SPE gel. This finding, when coupled with her viscous-appearing serum, markedly increased serum viscosity, and presenting symptoms of weakness, fatigue, and bleeding are pathognomonic findings for the large IgM monoclonal protein that is found in the serum of patients with primary (or Waldenström) macroglobulinemia. In serum, IgM immunoglobulin monomers combine to form a pentameric molecule that is large in size. An increased concentration of these molecules causes the serum to become viscous. Moreover, other immunoglobulins (eg, IgG and IgA) can bind to the IgM pentameric complex, thus further explaining the presence of discrete immunoglobulin bands in all lanes of the IFE gel, including the lanes to which anti-IgG and anti-IgA antiserum was added.

4. With the disulfide bond reducing agent, β-mercaptoethanol. The use of β-mercaptoethanol to resolve the serum IFE findings observed in our patient, definitively identify the monoclonal protein in the patient's serum, and produce immunoglobulin information consistent with the results obtained from quantitative measurement of serum immunoglobulins by nephelometry has been described previously.[2-4] After pre-treatment of our patient's serum sample with 10% β-mercaptoethanol for 10, 30, or 60 min, followed by repeat IFE of this mixture, the previously observed multiple bands resolved into fewer bands (**Image 1C**). After pre-treatment of our patient's serum with 10% β-mercaptoethanol for 60 min, a single IgM kappa monoclonal protein band was observed that corresponded with the location of the discrete, dense band found in the electrophoresis lane of the IFE gel [**Image 1C**, lower left quadrant].

5. ***Most likely diagnosis:*** *Waldenström macroglobulinemia (IgM M-protein) in a patient with MALT subtype non-Hodgkin's lymphoma.* To our knowledge, this patient represents the first reported case of Waldenström macroglobulinemia in Saudi Arabia.

6. Macroglobulinemia results from the uncontrolled proliferation of lymphocytes and plasma cells that secrete large amounts of IgM monoclonal protein; however, the cause of this disease is currently unknown. Waldenström macroglobulinemia is an uncommon B-cell lymphoproliferative disorder (lymphoplasmacytic lymphoma) characterized primarily by bone marrow infiltration with a predominantly intertrabecular pattern and an IgM monoclonal gammopathy.[5,6] However, the concentration of the monoclonal IgM M-protein has little or no prognostic relevance in patients with Waldenström macroglobulinemia.[7] Although Waldenström macroglobulinemia is mainly associated with IgM paraproteinemia, it is occasionally associated with IgG and IgA paraproteins.[5,6,8,9] The high molecular weight IgM molecules contribute to the salient symptoms of this disease, including the serious and potentially fatal complications of hyperviscosity syndrome.[10]

7. The treatment for symptomatic hyperviscosity syndrome is daily plasmapheresis [plasma exchange of 3 to 4 L with albumin (in lieu of plasma) replacement] until the patient is asymptomatic. Our patient underwent plasmapheresis and chemotherapy with cyclophosphamide, vincristine, and prednisone with evidence of clinical improvement; however, a computed tomography (CT) scan of her lungs revealed multiple lesions and she was started on MabThera (antibody specific for the CD20 cell surface marker on B cells) therapy.

Keywords

Waldenström macroglobulinemia, hyperviscosity syndrome, monoclonal gammopathy, immunofixation electrophoresis, β-mercaptoethanol

References

1. Widman, F. *Clinical Interpretation of Laboratory Tests.* 9th ed. Philadelphia: FA Davis, 1983, pp 186-187.

2. Keren DF, Gulbranson, R, Cary JL, et al. 2-Mercaptoethanol treatment improves measurement of an IgM protein by capillary electrophoresis. *Clincal Chemistry.* 2001;47:1326-1327.

3. Doinel C, Ropars C, Samon C. Agglutination activities of the subunit of one IgM cold agglutinin treated with various reducing agents. *Eur J Immunol.* 1973;9:563-568.

4. Zemmerman B, Grey HM. Non-covalent interaction between immunoglobulin polypeptide chains: stability to dissociation by denaturant. *Biochemistry.* 1972;1:78-84.

5. Dimopoulos MA, Alexanian R. Waldenström's macroglobulinemia. *Blood.* 1994;83:1452-1459.

6. Dimopoulos MA, Panayoitides P, Moulopoulos LA, et al. Waldenström's macroglobulinemia: clinical features, complications and management. *J Clin Oncol.* 2000;18:214-226.

7. Owen RG, Barrans SL, Richards SJ, et al. Waldenström's macroglobulinemia: development of diagnostic criteria and identification of prognostic factors. *Am J Clin Pathol.* 2001;116:420-428.

8. Jandle JH. Mutiple myeloma and related plasma cell dyscrasias. In: *Blood Pathophysiology.* Boston: Blackwell, 1991:349-370.

9. Rolcke D. Cold agglutination, antibodies, and antigens. *Clin Immunol Immunopathol.* 1974;2:266-280.

10. Waldenström J. Incipient myelomatosis or essential hyperglobulinemia with fibronopenia: a new syndrome? *Acta Med Scan.* 1944;117:216.

Low Serum Albumin and Abnormal Body Shape in a Young Canadian First Nations Woman

Jill Newstead,[1] Sharon E. Card,[1] Andrew W. Lyon[2]

[1]*Department of Internal Medicine, University of Saskatchewan, Saskatoon, Canada* [2]*Department of Pathology and Laboratory Medicine, University of Calgary and Calgary Laboratory Services, Calgary, Canada*

Patient: Obese (271 pounds; height, 65 inches; BMI, 45), 29-year-old woman of Canadian First Nations ancestry.

Chief Complaints: She was referred to a general internal medicine clinic for evaluation of a low serum albumin level (1.5 g/dL) and slight, bilateral lower limb edema.

Prior Medical History: The patient had been admitted to a local hospital with pneumonia 1 year earlier and had a history of arthritic pain in the right knee. There was no other significant medical history, although the patient had an unusual body shape or habitus, including pronounced cellulite deposits on her buttocks and thighs that were disproportionately thick compared to the lipid deposition on her abdomen and trunk [**Image 1**].

Drug History: The patient was taking clindamycin [Cleocin Oral, Cleocin T] 900 mg *tid* for treatment of her right calf cellulitis and celecoxib [Celebrex] (200 mg *od*) for treatment of her right knee arthritis.

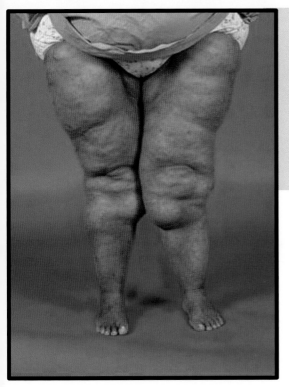

Image 1_The patient's habitus, illustrating the pronounced cellulite deposits on her buttocks and thighs that were disproportionately thick compared to the lipid deposition on her abdomen and trunk.

Questions

1. What (is) are this patient's most striking laboratory result(s)?

2. How do you explain this patient's most striking laboratory result(s)?

3. Which additional laboratory tests should be performed? Why?

Low Serum Albumin and Abnormal Body Shape in a Young Canadian First Nations Woman

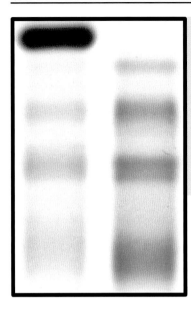

Image 2_Serum electrophoresis pattern illustrating the complete absence of an albumin band in the patient's serum (right lane) compared to normal control serum (left lane).

4. What is this patient's most likely diagnosis?

5. What are the complications associated with this patient's medical condition?

6. What is the most appropriate treatment for this patient?

Possible Answers _____

1. Markedly low serum albumin concentration (1.5 g/dL and <1.0 g/dL on 2 separate occasions) with no evidence of protein loss in the urine and the complete visual absence of an albumin band on protein electrophoresis of the patient's serum [**Image 2**] despite a densitometrically determined albumin concentration of 0.2 g/dL, decreased serum calcium, and increased total and LDL-cholesterol concentrations [**T1**].

2. Acquired disorders associated with markedly low serum albumin levels fall into 2 general categories: a) impaired synthesis of hepatic proteins or b) protein-losing disorders (renal and non-renal). The patient demonstrated no clinical symptoms or laboratory findings consistent with a protein-losing disorder (eg, proteinuria, glomerulopathies, renal diseases, diarrhea, or inflammatory bowel disease). Moreover, there was no evidence of protein malnutrition, malabsorption, or hepatic disease (the patient's hepatic

T1. Principal Laboratory Findings

Test	Patient's Result	"Normal" Reference Range
Hematology		
WBC count	8.2	4.0-11.0 × 10³/mL
Hemoglobin	11.6	13.7-18.0 g/µL
Platelet count	470	150-400 × 10³/µL
Coagulation		
PT (INR)	1.1	0.8-1.2
Chemistry		
Sodium	140	135-146 mEq/L
Potassium	3.5	3.5-5.1 mEq/L
Chloride	106	100-110 mEq/L
Carbon dioxide	27	22-31 mEq/L
Creatinine	0.40	0.51-1.24 mg/dL
Glucose, random	85	65-182 mg/dL
Bilirubin, total	0.2	0.1-1.29 mg/dL
AST	31	10-35 U/L
ALT	27	5-45 U/L
ALK	97	30-100 U/L
Protein, total	6.1	6.0-8.0 g/dL
Albumin	<1.0	3.5-5.2 g/dL
Calcium	7.24	8.40-10.20 mg/dL
Cholesterol, total	227	146-200 mg/dL
Triglycerides	118	54-209 mg/dL
HDL cholesterol	35	35-85 mg/dL
LDL cholesterol	170	77-131 mg/dL
SPE: Albumin	0.2	3.5-5.2 g/dL
Alpha 1	0.7	0.1-0.4 g/dL
Alpha 2	1.4	0.4-0.9 g/dL
Beta	1.6	0.6-1.1 g/dL
Gamma	2.2	1.0-2.2 g/dL
Urinalysis		
Dipstick tests	All negative	Negative

WBC, white blood cell; PT INR, prothrombin time International Normalized Ratio; AST, aspartate aminotransferase; ALT, alanine aminotransferase; ALK, alkaline phosphatase; HDL, high density lipoprotein; LDL, low density lipoprotein; SPE, serum protein electrophoresis.

enzymes and prothrombin time [international normalized ratio] were normal). The patient's markedly low serum albumin concentration with minimal signs of edema and the discrepancy between the initial chemical (1.5 g/dL) and densitometric (0.2 g/dL) albumin values were initially unexplained. However, the patient's low serum albumin concentration did explain her hypocalcemia and hypercholesterolemia. Approximately 45% of total serum calcium is bound to albumin. Consequently, patients with a low serum albumin concentration are expected to have lower serum total calcium concentrations.[1] This predictable relationship between albumin and calcium concentration allows a corrected total calcium concentration to be calculated that is useful for evaluating calcium status in hypoalbuminemic patients[1]:

Corrected calcium, mg/dL = measured calcium, mg/dL + [0.8 × (4 − albumin, g/dL)]

The patient's hypercholesterolmia may be explained, in part, by her low serum albumin concentration. Although the underlying pathophysiologic mechanisms accounting for the association between hypoalbuminemia and dyslipidemia are poorly understood, it was first described in patients with nephrotic syndrome more than 40 years ago.[2,3]

3. Additional diagnostic testing, such as a technetium (Tc)-labeled albumin scan to assess the presence of a protein-losing enteropathy or an albumin catabolic rate study, are not warranted because the serum protein electrophoresis pattern (SPEP) of patients with markedly low serum albumin concentration can provide sufficient information to establish a diagnosis. The SPEP of our patient indicated a complete absence of albumin [**Image 2**] suggestive of congenital analbuminemia. Serum protein electrophoresis methods that use densitometry to quantify serum proteins can detect up to 0.6 g/dL of albumin in analbuminemic sera.[4] Due to the rarity of analbuminemia and the lack of clinical information typically available to clinical chemists/pathologists who interpret a patient's electrophoretic patterns, a SPEP such as that observed on the patient might be interpreted simply as "hypoalbuminemia" rather than the more appropriate interpretation,

"hypoalbuminemia or analbuminemia." Moreover, the discrepancy between chemical and densitometric quantification of albumin concentration can be explained by the differences between these methods of quantification. Chemical methods for the routine measurement of serum albumin concentration use dyes that complex with serum proteins and are prone to generating falsely elevated albumin results in analbuminemic sera, while densitometric methods rely on the absorbance properties of protein-dye complexes in the agarose gel used for protein electrophoresis. The decreased analytical specificity and sensitivity of chemical methods, compared to densitometric methods, for quantifying serum albumin concentration can mislead clinicians when trying to establish a diagnosis of analbuminemia.[4] Quantification of serum albumin concentration by an immunoassay method can be used to confirm the absence of albumin in serum; however, serum protein electrophoresis testing is usually sufficient to establish a diagnosis of analbuminemia.[4] In addition, genetic studies can be used to confirm the cause of hypoalbuminemia in patients who receive intravenous albumin.[5]

4. **Most likely diagnosis:** *congenital analbuminemia.* The patient's markedly low serum total protein concentration, when coupled with the absence of an albumin band by SPE and the clinical findings of no overt edema and abnormal body habitus, suggests a diagnosis of congenital analbuminemia. Lipodystrophy has been proposed as the cause of the abnormal habitus occurring in 30% of post-pubertal females with analbuminemia.[6-9] Congenital analbuminemia is a rare autosomal recessive disorder in which patients have no serum albumin; however, quantification of serum albumin concentration using routine chemical methods may indicate falsely increased concentrations of albumin up to 1.8 g/dL. To date, only 35 other cases of analbuminemia have been reported worldwide. The patient, a member of a First Nations band in the East Central Canadian Province of Saskatchewan, lived in close geographic proximity to 3 other patients with analbuminemia who were not immediately related to her.[4,5] Genetic analysis of 2 of these patients revealed a 2 base pair frameshift mutation in exon 3 of the albumin gene that leads to a premature stop codon and prevents translation

of the albumin gene, resulting in analbumin-emia. This defect has been designated albumin Kayseri.[5] Analysis of the marital patterns in this First Nation band in east central Saskatchewan from 1870 to 1960 revealed a stable population of 190 to 390, largely sustained by within-group marriages.[10] This study suggested that a high degree of consanguinity existed within this community. Analbuminemia is an autosomal recessive disorder and consanguinity is associated with many of the reported cases of analbuminemia.[11,12]

5. Analbuminemia is associated with very few medical complications. Because albumin is important for maintaining plasma colloid oncotic pressure and preventing systemic edema, and for transporting hormones, electrolytes, drugs, metabolites, and free fatty acids, it is surprising that patients with analbuminemia do not demonstrate serious symptoms of this disease such as systemic edema. Analbuminemia is not associated with marked edema because of a compensatory increase in other plasma proteins and the tendency of patients with analbuminemia to have low capillary blood pressure or low-normal blood pressure.[13-17] Clinically, patients with analbuminemia have few symptoms of this disorder other than mild edema, hypotension, fatigue, and occasionally, lipodystrophy. Moreover, patients with analbuminemia are known to have high cholesterol levels; however, there is not enough evidence available in the literature to determine if analbuminemics have an increased risk of atherosclerotic disease. Several reports have suggested that the rarity of analbuminemia may be attributed to the perinatal loss of affected fetuses.[5,8,18,19] In addition, it has been suggested that infants with analbuminemia may be more prone to kernicterus.[8] Because of the obscurity of the diagnosis, patients with analbumemia are prone to misdiagnosis or delayed diagnosis. In addition, patients with analbuminemia who have co-morbid conditions such as diabetes or renal disease will never show albuminuria. It is also possible that some laboratory methods for certain analytes (eg, thyroxine and calcium) may yield clinically misleading results because of the change in the serum matrix when albumin is not present.

6. The most appropriate treatment for patients with analbuminemia is observation. Clinical trials on the efficacy of albumin infusion in patients with analbuminemia have demonstrated a transitory decrease in cholesterol and a variety of plasma proteins; however, no long-term benefit of this therapy has been demonstrated. Moreover, it is not practical to infuse analbuminemic patients with albumin at regular intervals over their lifetime because of the concern about transmission of infectious agents in blood products, the cost of intravenous albumin, and its limited potential to affect outcome.

Treatment and Course

The patient continued to receive Celebrex for her right knee arthritic pain and was doing well despite repeatedly low serum albumin concentration. Due to the lack of evidence indicating a beneficial effect of treatment of hypercholesterolemia in patients with analbumemia, the patient's hypercholesterolemia was not treated

Keywords

analbuminemia, hypoalbuminemia, hypercholesterolemia, edema, protein electrophoresis

References

1. Endres DB, Rude RK. Chapter 39: Mineral and bone metabolism. Burtis CA, Ashwood EA, eds. *Tietz Textbook of Clinical Chemistry.* 3rd ed. Philadelphia: WB Saunders. 1999:1395-1457.

2. Baxter JH, Goodman HC, Havel RJ. Serum lipid and lipoprotein alterations in nephrosis. *J Clin Invest.* 1960;39:455-465.

3. Delvin EE, Merouani A, Levy E. Dyslipidemia in pediatric nephrotic syndrome: Causes revisited. *Clin Biochem.* 2003;36:95-101.

4. Lyon A, Meinert P, Bruce GA, et al. Influence of methodology on the detection and diagnosis of congenital analbuminemia. *Clin Chem.* 1998;44:2365-2367.

5. Galliano M, Campagnoli M, Rossi A, et al. Molecular diagnosis of analbuminemia: A novel mutation identified in 2 Amerindian and 2 Turkish families. *Clin Chem.* 2002;48:844-849.

6. Weinstock JV, Kawanishi H, Sisson J. Morphologic, biochemical and physiological alterations in a case of idiopathic hypoalbuminemia [analbuminemia]. *Am J Med.* 1979;67:132-139.

7. Dammacco F, Miglietta A, D'Addabbo A, et al. Analbuminemia: Report of a case and review of the literature. *Vox Sang.* 1980;39:153-161

8. Boman H, Hermodson M, Hammond CA, et al. Analbuminemia in an American Indian girl. *Clin Genet.* 1979;9:513-526.

9. Berger GMB, Stephan CR, Finestone A, et al. Analbuminemia: Clinical and laboratory features in a South African patient. *South African Med J.* 1985;67:418-422.

10. Meyer D. The development of the marriage isolate among the Pas Mountain Indians. *The Western Canadian Anthropologist.* 1984;1:2-10.

11. The albumin Web site. Register of analbuminemia cases. http://www.albumin.org. Accessed April 13, 2004.

12. Campagnoli M, Rossi A, Palmqvist L, et al. A novel splicing mutation causes an undescribed type of analbuminemia. *Biochim Biophys Acta.* 2002;1586:43-49.

13. Kallee E. Bennhold's analbuminemia: A follow-up study of the first 2 cases (1953-1992). *J Lab Clin Med.* 1996;127:470-480.

14. Russi E, Weigand K. Analbuminemia. *Klin Wochenschr.* 1983;61:541-545.

15. Baldo G, Fellin R, Manzato E, et al. Characterization of hyperlipidemia in 2 patients with analbuminemia. *Clin Chim Acta.* 1983;128:307-319.

16. Dammacco F, Miglietta A, Bonomo L. Analbuminemia. *La Ricerca Clin Lab.* 1979;9:5-12.

17. Baldoo-Enzi G, Baiocchi MR, Vigna G, et al. Analbuminemia: A natural model of metabolic compensatory systems. *J Inh Met Dis.* 1987;10:317-329.

18. Frohlich J, Pudek MR, Cormode EJ, et al. Further studies on plasma proteins, lipids, and dye-and drug binding in a child with analbuminemia. *Clin Chem.* 1981;27:1213-1216.

19. Watkins S, Madison J, Galliano M, et al. A nucleotide insertion and frameshift causes analbuminemia in an Italian family. *Proc Natl Acad Sci.* 1994;91:2275-2279.

Marked Proteinuria in a Young Male

Monte S. Willis, Frank H. Wians, Jr.

Department of Pathology, University of Texas Southwestern Medical Center, Dallas, TX

Patient: 28-year-old male.

Chief Complaint: One week of nausea, vomiting, and dysuria.

Medical History: Five weeks prior to admission, the patient noticed several days of urethral discharge. Subsequently, he noticed bilateral foot swelling, right ankle pain, and erythema which resolved after 3 days, and gross hematuria. One week ago, he had mild throat pain and took an unknown antibiotic. He noted occasional headaches and blurred vision on initial presentation. Upon further questioning after admission to the hospital, the patient reported nighttime polyuria, urinary incontinence, urinary urgency, and a sense of incomplete voiding during the previous several months. A Foley catheter was inserted and a significant post-void residual urine volume was found. The patient had a prior history of gonorrhea and chlamydia urethritis which had been treated several months before. Three months ago he was seen in the ER for a leg injury and was not told that his blood pressure was abnormal at that time. The patient had no history of surgery.

Drug History: The patient was not currently taking any medications.

Family/Social History: The patient had no personal history of kidney disease or cancer; however, he had a family history of hypertension and diabetes. He reported only occasional alcohol consumption, regular marijuana use, no history of IV drug abuse or use of other illicit drugs, and frequent unprotected sexual contact with multiple partners.

Physical Examination: Vital signs included: temperature, 98.6°F; heart rate, 72 beats/min; respirations, 18/min; and blood pressure, 201/132 mm Hg. The patient had 1+ lower extremity edema up to his ankles. The right ankle was currently mildly swollen without erythema or tenderness to palpitation.

Results of Additional Diagnostic Procedures: Continuous ECG (electrocardiogram) monitoring was performed throughout his hospital stay. Left ventricular hypertrophy was found but no other changes were noted (ie, no peaked T-waves indicative of hyperkalemia). A renal ultrasound demonstrated greatly edematous kidneys bilaterally, consistent with hydronephrosis. A serum and random urine electrophoresis were performed. The serum electrophoresis pattern [**Image 1A**] was essentially normal, with an increase in the gamma globulins, which can be seen during infections (due to increased immunoglobulins and other proteins). The urine electrophoresis pattern [**Image 1B**] was consistent with nephrotic syndrome and abnormally resembled the serum protein pattern [**Image 1A**]. Total protein levels in random urine specimens from healthy individuals are typically <20 mg/dL and electrophoresis patterns on these specimens demonstrate the presence of a small amount of albumin, and occasionally, lesser amounts of other proteins. This patient's random urine protein used in the UPEP was 2194.8 mg/dL. This is significantly higher than his presenting urine protein (100 mg/dL). A renal biopsy was initially planned before the ultrasound was performed, and was postponed subsequently until the renal edema resolved. A chest X-ray was performed which was normal.

T1. Principal Laboratory Findings

Test	Patient's Result	"Normal" Reference Range
Arterial blood gases:		
pH	7.39	7.34-7.44
pCO$_2$	36	35-45 mm Hg
pO$_2$	99	75-100 mm Hg
S$_a$O$_2$ (on room air)	96	90-100%
Base excess	-3.2	-2.4-2.3
Total protein	8.6	6.3-8.2 g/dL
Albumin	4.8	3.5-4.8 g/dL
BUN	79	4-21 mg/dL
Creatinine	10.5	0.6-1.2 mg/dL
WBC	7.9	4.1-11.1 × 10^3/mL
Hemoglobin	10.9	13.2-16.9 g/dL
Hematocrit	33.1	39.6-50.2%
Platelets	252	174-404 × 10^3/mL
AST	11	13-40 U/L
ALT	10	10-40 U/L
Alkaline phosphatase	70	38-126 U/L
GGT	31	8-78 U/L
Amylase	20	29-108 U/L
Lipase	48	7-59 U/L
ASO	120	>125 IU/mL
C3 complement	129	88-201 mg/dL
C4 complement	37.8	16-47 mg/dL
Sodium	138	135-145 mEq/L
Potassium	6.3	3.6-4.5 mEq/L
Chloride	104	98-109 mEq/L
Carbon dioxide	18	22-31 mEq/L
Glucose	79	65-110 mg/dL
Magnesium	1.1	1.4-1.8 mEq/L
Phosphorus	5.4	2.4-5.4 mg/dL

S$_a$O$_2$, arterial oxygen saturation; ASO, anti-streptolysin O.

Questions _____

1. What is (are) the patient's most striking findings/laboratory result(s)?

2. How do you explain this patient's most striking findings/laboratory result(s)?

T2. Principal Urine Laboratory Findings

Test	Patient's Result	"Normal" Reference Range
Description	Straw/hazy	Colorless/clear
Specific gravity	1.010	1.002-1.030
pH	7.0	5.0-7.0
Protein	100 mg/dL	Neg
Glucose	Neg	Neg
Ketone	Neg	Neg
Bile	Neg	Neg
Leukocyte esterase	Neg	Neg
Nitrite	Neg	Neg
RBC	11-20	0-3
WBC	3-5	0-5
Squamous epithelial cells	3-5	
Bacteria	Moderate	
Mucus	Rare	
24-h Creatinine	2.5 (0.8-2.8)	0.8-2.8
24-h Protein	17,411	40-150 mg/24 h
Urine culture (Catheter)	No growth after 2 days	

3. Which additional laboratory test(s) are appropriate to order on this patient and why?

4. What condition(s) does this patient's laboratory and other findings suggest?

5. What is the most appropriate treatment for this patient?

Possible Answers _____

1. The most striking findings/laboratory results in this patient are: high blood pressure [201/132 mm Hg; normal systolic/diastolic, (100 to 140)/(60 to 90) mm Hg]; markedly elevated BUN (79 mg/dL) and creatinine (10.5 g/dL) concentrations; decreased hemoglobin/hematocrit values (10.9 g/dL/33.1%); markedly elevated potassium concentration (6.3 mmol/L); decreased carbon dioxide concentration (18 mEq/L), a decreased magnesium concentration (1.1 mg/dL); increased numbers of urine RBCs; and, a

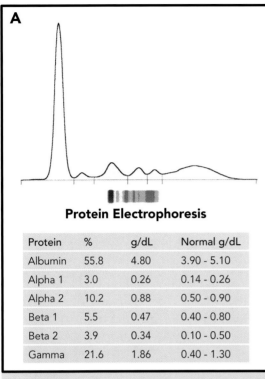

Protein Electrophoresis

Protein	%	g/dL	Normal g/dL
Albumin	55.8	4.80	3.90 - 5.10
Alpha 1	3.0	0.26	0.14 - 0.26
Alpha 2	10.2	0.88	0.50 - 0.90
Beta 1	5.5	0.47	0.40 - 0.80
Beta 2	3.9	0.34	0.10 - 0.50
Gamma	21.6	1.86	0.40 - 1.30

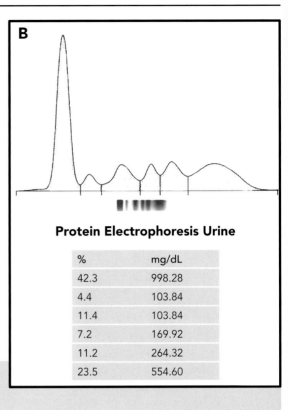

Protein Electrophoresis Urine

%	mg/dL
42.3	998.28
4.4	103.84
11.4	103.84
7.2	169.92
11.2	264.32
23.5	554.60

Image 1_Serum (**A**) and urine (**B**) electrophoresis patterns.

markedly elevated 24-hour urine protein concentration (17.4 **grams**/24 h).

2. This patient was experiencing acute renal failure secondary to urethral obstruction from a gonorrheal and/or chlamydial infection. Urethral obstruction from bacterial infection is much more commonly seen with *E. coli* infections than with organisms associated with sexually transmitted diseases.[1] This is probably due to the uncomfortableness, particularly in males, of the urethritis that accompanies sexually transmitted diseases, causing them to be seen by a physician and treated prior to the development of renal obstruction. Intense pain, due to the distention of the kidney secondary to obstruction (renal colic), can occur if the obstruction develops rapidly. However, when flank pain is absent, the obstruction is likely to have occurred more slowly. This patient's renal ultrasound findings indicated bilateral hydronephrosis (enlarged kidneys), but pain was not a presenting symptom, suggesting that this obstruction occurred slowly. With prolonged obstruction, polyuria and nocturia can occur, as reported by this patient.

During chronic renal obstruction, blood flow decreases. Subsequently, renin, angiotensin, and prostaglandin production increases which leads to systemic vasoconstriction and increased blood pressure. Azotemia (increased BUN concentration) is a result of the dysfunction of the kidney that occurs with hydronephrosis. Structural damage to the kidney tubules and renal parenchymal cell atrophy alter (decrease) sodium and potassium ion transport resulting in urinary sodium loss and hyperkalemia. Our patient's decreased CO_2 concentration and normal plasma pH may be explained by his decreased plasma base excess caused by increased loss of base (bicarbonate) into the urine, which tends to decrease plasma pH. To compensate for the increased bicarbonate loss in the urine and decrease in plasma pH, an increase in CO_2 loss [ie, the removal of excess H^+: $H^+ + HCO_3^- \cdot H_2CO_3 \cdot H_2O + CO_2$ (aqueous solution)° CO_2 (gas phase)] from the plasma via the lungs occurs, which is necessary to maintain plasma pH in the normal range. The increased number of RBCs in the patient's urine (hematuria) and the patient's history of gross hematuria provides the most likely explanation for this patient's decreased hemoglobin and hematocrit values.[2] This patient's markedly elevated 24 h urine total protein concentration (17.4 g/24 h) is consistent with nephrotic syndrome. Nephrotic syndrome is characterized by edema, a 24 h urine total protein concentration of >3.5 g, lipiduria, hypoalbuminemia, hyperlipidemia, and hypercoagulability. Interestingly, this patient's serum total protein and albumin concentrations were high or high normal, despite his marked proteinuria. In addition, his gamma globulin component was increased (**Image 1A**), suggesting that his infection induced the production of proteins (ie, immunoglobulins and other proteins) in adequate concentration to offset protein loss into the urine. Other more common causes of urinary tract obstruction at the level of the urethra include kidney stones, enlargement of the prostate due to benign prostatic hypertrophy (BPH), strictures, and trauma.

3. The laboratory diagnosis of gonococcal infection in men can be validated by the observation of gram-negative intracellular diplococci (GNID) in a urethral exudate. *Neisseria gonorrhoeae*, the principal cause of gonococcal urethritis in men, can be cultured using modified Thayer-Martin or other gonococcal selective media. Polymerase chain reaction (PCR) assays for detecting nucleic acid sequences, using DNA probes that recognize sequences unique to *N. gonorrhoeae* in urethral discharge are also available. Polymerase chain reaction detection is advantageous because it is as sensitive as conventional culture techniques in detecting *N. gonorrhoeae*, and is more cost effective, especially in high-risk males. The disadvantage, however, is that the specimen transport system required for PCR analysis does not allow the specimen to be cultured. In cases of suspected disseminated gonococcal infection, blood culture testing should be performed, even though *N. gonorrhoeae* is rarely recovered.[3] Disseminated gonococcal infection has 2 stages, the first is a bacteremic stage, and the second is the joint-localized stage which manifests as arthritis. Bacteremia generally coincides with hyperthermia and chills along with painful, swollen joints associated with tenosynovitis (inflammation of tendon sheaths). The arthralgias generally involve the knee, elbow, and more distal joints (eg, ankles). Our patient had a swollen ankle that was tender and erythematous

approximately 4 weeks prior to his admission that likely represented the second stage (disseminated) of gonococcal infection.

4. ***Most likely diagnosis:*** *acute renal failure secondary to N. gonorrhoeae urethritis and obstruction.* Acute urethritis is the most common clinical manifestation of gonorrheal infection in males and occurs typically 2 to 7 days after infection. Another common cause of acute urethritis is *Chlamydia trachomatis* infection. Additionally, co-infection with *N. gonorrhoeae* and *C. trachomatis* has been identified in up to 40% of men with acute urethritis.[3]

5. The key to treating urinary tract obstruction is to relieve the obstruction as soon as possible to prevent permanent renal damage and sepsis. In this patient, catheterization relieved the obstruction and doxycycline was successful in treating his gonorrhea infection. Treatment often is required for 3 to 4 weeks. *Neisseria gonorrhoeae* has become resistant to several drugs in different parts of the world, but it is still susceptible to several agents. Adequate treatment is essential to prevent further spread of the disease. The 1998 CDC guidelines for the treatment of gonorrhea recommend several therapeutic regimens, including doxycycline (100 mg twice a day for 7 days) for uncomplicated gonococcal infection.[4] Doxycycline is an ideal drug for this purpose because it is also effective against *C. trachomatis* and co-infection occurs frequently. Alternative drug treatments include single dose (1 g) azithromycin therapy. However, disseminated infections (as in this case) may require longer-term duration of therapy with possibly higher doses.[3] Rapid clearance of the obstruction (ie, catheterization in this case) usually leads to a post-obstructive diuresis, which was seen in this patient. Diuresis is due to the retention of urea in the serum which causes an osmotic diuresis. The increased plasma osmolality triggers the release of anti-diuretic hormone (ADH) and activation of the thirst mechanism. This patient experienced polydipsia during diuresis, which resolved before his discharge, when his fluid input and urine output volumes became approximately equal. The urine that is excreted during diuresis is usually hypotonic and contains large amounts of sodium, chloride, potassium, and magnesium ions. Loss of magnesium in the urine explains

the hypomagnesemia observed in this patient. The potential for volume depletion and electrolyte imbalance, due to excessive Na^+, K^+, PO_4, Mg^{2+}, and water loss in the urine, occurs post-diuresis. When the extracellular fluid volume returns to normal, the diuresis generally abates. Replacement of electrolytes lost during diuresis promotes the return to normovolemia. However, complications from electrolyte imbalances can occur, and the patient should be monitored closely during the diuresis period for evidence of such imbalances. After insertion of the Foley catheter in this patient, his serum creatinine level decreased from 10.5 mg/dL to 3.1 mg/dL over several days. Nausea and vomiting secondary to the uremia in this patient was treated successfully with the anti-emetic agent, Phenergan. Additionally, Kayexalate (a potassium binding resin) was used to treat this patient's hyperkalemia. Following these measures, this patient's electrolyte values returned to normal by the time of discharge, 8 days after admission.

Treatment and Course

The patient was started on long term doxycycline (100 mg, twice a day). The patient's blood pressure remained poorly controlled with trials of Metoprolol and Felodipine, Felodipine alone, or Clonidine and Felodipine. He was discharged and continued on Clonidine and Felodipine therapy, which controlled his blood pressure the best, although poorly. The patient's BUN and creatinine decreased from 79 mg/dL and 10.5 mg/dL on admission to 18 mg/dL and 1.8 mg/dL, respectively, on the day of discharge. The catheter was left in place and the patient

was discharged in fair condition to be followed subsequently as an outpatient.

References

1. Sulowicz W. Can we prevent late complications of urinary tract infections? *Przegl Lek*. 1988;55:58-60.

2. Seifter JL, Brenner BM. Urinary Tract Obstruction. In: Braunwald E, Fauci AS, Kasper DL, eds. *Harrison's Principles of Internal Medicine*, 15th ed. New York, NY: McGraw-Hill, 2001;1627-1629.

3. Ram S, Rice PA. Gonococcal Infections. In: Braunwald E, Fauci AS, Kasper DL, eds. *Harrison's Principles of Internal Medicine*, 15th ed. New York, NY: McGraw-Hill, 2001;931-937.

4. Guidelines for treatment of sexually transmitted diseases. *MMWR*. 1998;47:1.

Acute Alcohol Intoxication

Charles A. Bradley, Ashraf M. Kahn, Ratna Grewal, Dale M. Dunn
Department of Pathology, Texas Tech University Health Sciences Center, Lubbock, TX

Patient 1: A 25-year-old man was brought to the emergency center after being found unresponsive by his family. The family gave a history of the patient having consumed a liter of whiskey earlier that evening on a dare by his friends. He had a previous history of consuming 6 pints of beer per day since the age of 10 years.

Physical Examination: Vital signs: temperature, 98.7°F; respiratory rate, 10 per minute; pulse, 84 beats per minute (bpm); blood pressure, 122/70 mm Hg. He had no gag reflex and no response to pain. He was comatose with pinpoint (meiosis), but reactive pupils. He did not have any needle track marks. He was in respiratory failure and was intubated.

Patient 2: An intoxicated 50-year-old female was brought to the emergency center by emergency medical service (EMS) personnel. She stated that her husband was not allowing her to drink alcohol so she drank "a lot of mouthwash." She stated that she could not get alcohol any other way and she just wanted a drink. She denied drinking alcohol as a suicide attempt. The patient had a 1-year history of alcohol abuse. She denied treatment and/or rehabilitation for alcohol abuse.

Physical Examination: Unremarkable except for slurred and incoherent speech. Vital signs were: temperature, 98.3°F; pulse, 108 bpm; blood pressure, 139/88 mm Hg.

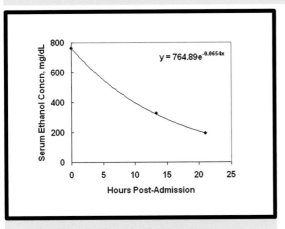

Figure 1_Kinetics of the decline in serum ethanol concentration in Patient 1. The equation for the line-of-best-fit through the data points shown is characteristic of a first-order reaction, where y = serum ethanol concentration and x = hours post-admission.

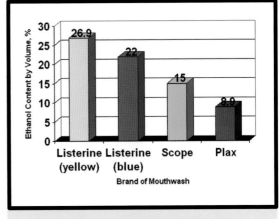

Figure 2_Ethanol content by volume (%) in 4 commercially available brands of mouthwash.

T1. Principal Laboratory Findings			
Test (Serum)	Results For		
	Patient 1	Patient 2	"Normal" Reference Range
Total bilirubin	0.7	n.d.	0.2-1.3 mg/dL
ALT	30	n.d.	21-72 IU/L
AST	46	n.d.	14-50 IU/L
ALP	86	n.d.	25-125 IU/L
LD	554	n.d.	295-535 IU/L
GGT	165	n.d.	8-78 IU/L
Amylase	n.d.	30	30-300 IU/L
Sodium	n.d.	147	137-145 mmol/L
CO_2	n.d.	20	22-32 mmol/L
Ethanol @ hrs post-admission*			
0	761 (0.76)	391 (0.39	
13.3	325 (0.32)	n.d.	
21.0	192 (0.19)	n.d.	

*Quantified using the alcohol dehydrogenase method in the Vitros 950 chemistry analyzer (values in parentheses are % concentration). ALT, alanine aminotransferase; AST, aspartate aminotransferase; LD, lactate dehydrogenase; ALP, alkaline phosphatase; GGT, gamma-glutamyl transferase; n.d., not done.

Questions

1. What are these patients' most striking clinical and laboratory results?

2. How do you explain these patients' most striking clinical and laboratory results and any differences between them in Patient 1 versus Patient 2?

3. What condition(s) do the clinical and laboratory results of these patients suggest?

4. What are the potential complications of these patients' condition(s)?

5. What was the most likely source of the ethanol ingested by Patient 2?

Possible Answers

1. The vital signs and presentation of Patient 1 (ie, depressed respirations and respiratory distress requiring intubation and the comatose state of this patient) were more serious than those of Patient 2. Both Patients 1 and 2 had a markedly elevated serum ethanol concentration; however, the initial serum ethanol concentration for Patient 1 (761 mg/dL) was nearly 2-fold greater than for Patient 2 (391 mg/dL) and remained elevated for more than 24 hours [**Figure 1**]. In addition, the GGT was elevated in Patient 1 and was not performed in Patient 2.

2. Both patients admitted to consuming a large quantity of alcohol or alcohol-containing fluid. Patient 1 consumed nearly a liter of whiskey, while Patient 2 consumed "a lot" of alcohol-containing mouthwash, thus explaining the high ethanol content in the serum of both patients and the higher level in Patient 1, who consumed a purer form of alcohol than Patient 2. Moreover, because Patient 1 had a long history of alcohol abuse, a GGT was ordered, along with other liver function tests. Serum GGT activity is elevated in any form of liver disease (eg, alcoholic cirrhosis) and in the majority of sera from individuals who are heavy drinkers. The serum GGT level reflects the toxic effects of alcohol on microsomal structures within hepatocytes. Because other liver function test values (ie, ALT, ASP, ALP) on serum from Patient 1 were within normal limits, the increase in this patient's GGT activity is most likely related to his acute alcohol ingestion rather than the presence of significant alcoholic cirrhosis in this 25-year-old man, despite a 15-year history of alcohol abuse. In any event, the serum alcohol level in the serum of both patients was significantly higher than the legal limit (ie, 0.08% or 0.10%) established by most states in the United States as consistent with "under the influence of alcohol." On admission, the alcohol concentration in the serum from Patient 1 (0.8%) was approximately 10-fold higher than the legal limit, while in Patient 2 (0.4%) it was approximately 4- to 5-fold higher.

3. ***Most likely diagnosis:*** *acute ethanol intoxication.*

In published case reports, individuals who have survived high levels of serum alcohol intake have been in the age range of 22 to 63 years.[1,2] Lindblad and Olsson reported that patients with blood alcohol levels above 500 mg/dL had a 50% survivability rate.[1] Patient 1 had a serum alcohol level above 500 mg/dL and survived. It has been suggested that survival of individuals with such a high alcohol level is related to the development of tolerance to alcohol.[1] Alcohol tolerance takes a significant number of years to develop and is related to the enhanced activity of liver enzymes involved in alcohol degradation. Thus, individuals who have developed tolerance to alcohol tend to be in an older age group. Moreover, individuals who survive after ingestion of a large amount of alcohol are likely to demonstrate a myriad of clinical disorders. Berild and Hasselbalch reported on an individual with a blood alcohol level of 1,127 mg/dL (1.1%) who survived but had hemorrhagic pancreatitis, disseminated intravascular coagulation (DIC), pneumonia, and a bleeding gastric ulcer.[3] The serum alcohol level in Patient 1 was not as high as 1,127 mg/dL and the principal clinical abnormality experienced by Patient 1 was respiratory depression, which was resolved quickly, with no signs or symptoms of acute pancreatitis or DIC [ie, values for amylase, lipase, and coagulation tests were within normal limits (*data not shown*)]. Finally, alcohol degradation tends to follow *first*-order (non-linear) kinetics in chronic alcoholics and individuals who have ingested a large quantity and survived; and *zero*-order kinetics (ie, alcohol levels decline at a constant rate independent of the dose) in individuals who ingest moderate amounts of alcohol and in alcoholics who abstain from alcohol intake.[2] A possible explanation for this phenomenon is that prolonged ingestion of ethanol induces the microsomal ethanol oxidation system (MEOS) of the liver.

At high blood ethanol concentrations, the MEOS assumes greater importance in the metabolism of ethanol than the alcohol dehydrogenase (ADH) enzyme system. In addition, it has been proposed that the MEOS and ADH systems act synergistically when the serum ethanol level is high (eg, in acute alcoholics and in chronic alcohol abusers who have developed tolerance) as a mechanism for promoting increased ethanol metabolism by first-order kinetics.[2,4-6] Although Patient 1 had a history of alcohol abuse, the decline in his serum ethanol concentration followed zero-order kinetics [**Figure 1**], suggesting that he had not yet developed tolerance to alcohol. In support of this suggestion, Patient 1 exhibited a comatose state and severe respiratory depression, conditions that are less likely to occur in individuals with tolerance and a similar ethanol level. Patient 1 indicates that survivability with high levels of serum alcohol is possible in young individuals with no evidence of tolerance and zero-order alcohol degradation kinetics.

Alcohol intoxication accompanied by respiratory failure can be life-threatening from a number of complications, including respiratory depression or aspiration pneumonia syndrome. Therefore, it is important to institute prompt supportive therapy to avoid aspiration and reverse respiratory depression. With appropriate medical therapy, young individuals can survive high serum alcohol levels despite lack of tolerance.[7]

The mouthwash ingested by Patient 2 is the most likely source of the ethanol she ingested. Therefore, we determined the ethanol content in 4 popular brands of mouthwash [**Figure 2**]. Moreover, we estimated the amount of mouthwash she could have ingested to achieve a serum (blood) alcohol content of 391 mg/dL (0.391%) as follows:

ingestion of 8 fluid ounces (fl oz) of whiskey (100 proof or 50% ethanol by volume) produces a blood alcohol level of 0.2%.[8] If we assume that Patient 2 ingested Listerine (yellow) brand mouthwash with an ethanol content (26.9%) approximately half that of 100 proof whiskey, then the amount (V_f) of mouthwash ingested is given by:

$$V_0/0.391\% = 8 \text{ fl oz }/0.2\%$$

$$V_0 = (8 \times 0.391)/0.2 = 15.64 \text{ fl oz}$$

V_f = final volume of Listerine (yellow) ingested = 15.64 × 2 = 31.28 fl oz or ~32 fl oz or *1 quart* [multiplication by 2 is necessary because Listerine (yellow) contains approximately half the ethanol content of 100 proof whiskey]

The medium-size container of Listerine (yellow) contains 1 quart 1.8 fl oz of mouthwash.

Keywords

alcoholism, tolerance, intoxication

References

1. Lindblad B, Olsson R. Unusually high levels of blood alcohol. *JAMA*. 1976;236:1600-1602.

2. Hammond DB, Rumack BH, Rodgerson DO. A report of unusually high levels in a living patient. *JAMA*. 1973;226:63-64.

3. Berild D, Hasselbalch H. Survival after a blood alcohol of 1127 mg/dL. *Lancet*. 1981;2:363.

4. Winek CL, Murphy KL. The rate and kinetic order of alcohol elimination. *Forensic Sci International*. 1984;25:159-166.

5. Bogusz M, Pach J, Stasko W. Comparative studies on the rate of ethanol elimination in acute poisoning and in controlled conditions. *J. Forensic Sci.* 1977;22:446-451.

6. Baselt RC, Cravey RH. *Disposition of Toxins and Chemicals in Man.* 4th ed. Foster City, CA: Chemical Toxicology Institute. 1995,293-296.

7. Knight B. *Forensic Pathology,* 2nd ed, London, England: Edward Arnold. 1996;548-549.

8. Sidney K. *Handbook of Emergency Toxicology.* 3rd ed. Springfield, IL: Charles C Thomas Pub Ltd. 1970;259.

Conflicting Blood and Urine Ethanol Results

Dennis C. Wooten, Joseph Susa, Leland Baskin

Department of Pathology, University of Texas Southwestern Medical Center, Dallas, TX

Patient: 70-year-old man.

Family History: Non-contributory.

Chief Complaint: The patient presented at the hospital emergency department complaining of shortness of breath and altered mental status.

Medical History: He had a history of diabetes mellitus (treated with oral medication), hypertension (treated with captopril), paraplegia with bilateral lower extremity contractures resulting from a motorcycle accident 5 years ago at which time he had bilateral subdural hematomas. The patient also had a neurogenic bladder which resulted in a history of urinary retention and incontinence. Additionally, the patient had residual altered mental status, secondary to his motorcycle accident.

Drug History: He denied abusing alcohol or drugs. He quit using alcohol 15 years ago after years of heavy use.

Physical Examination: The patient was very somnolent. His vital signs were stable. He had diffuse abdominal tenderness, diffuse bilateral pulmonary rhonchi, and bilateral contractures in the lower extremities.

Principal Laboratory Findings: Whole blood and urine toxicology screens, along with several other laboratory tests [**T1**], were ordered. Except for a positive urine ethanol test, no drugs of abuse were detected in this patient's blood or urine.

Treatment and Results of Additional Diagnostic Procedures: He was admitted to the hospital because of a high index of suspicion for an acute myocardial infarction (AMI), pneumonia, and urosepsis. The patient was treated with ampicillin and sulbactam; however, his myocardial infarction, indicated by electrocardiography, was not treated with heparin or acetylsalicylic acid due to his guaiac positive stool. Hyphae and budding yeast cells, consistent with a fungal urinary tract infection (UTI), were detected upon microscopic examination of his urine. Beta hemolytic Gram-positive cocci in chains grew in urine culture and were identified subsequently as Streptococcus agalactiae. In addition, Candida albicans was identified in a fungal culture of his urine. Due to his proteinuria, urine protein and immunofixation electrophoresis were performed. Non-selective proteinuria without a monoclonal component was reported. A chest radiograph showed persistent blunting of the left costophrenic angle, consistent with pleural disease, and evidence of early congestive heart failure.

T1. Principal Laboratory Findings		
Test	Patient's Result	Reference Range
Serum:		
Sodium	134	135 to 145 mmol/L
Potassium	4.2	3.6 to 5.0 mmol/L
Chloride	109	98 to 109 mmol/L
Bicarbonate	13	22 to 31 mmol/L
BUN	37	7 to 21 mg/dL
Creatinine	1.8	0.6 to 1.2 mg/dL
Glucose	396	65 to 110 mg/dL
Total CK	244	40 to 210 U/L
CK-MB	9	0 to 3 ng/mL
CK-MB Index	37	0 to 3
Troponin I	4.9	<0.1 ng/mL
Whole Blood:		
Hemoglobin	7	13.2 to 16.2 g/dL
Hematocrit	21	40% to 52%
WBC	16.7	4.1 to 10.9 × 10³/mL
Platelet count	301	140 to 450 × 10³/mL
Arterial pH	7.29	7.34 to 7.44
pCO₂	35	35 to 45 mm Hg
HCO₃	16	22 to 26 mmol/L
HbA1c	7.2	3.2% to 5.6%
Ethanol[a]	<10	<10 mg/dL
Urine:		
Glucose	1,000 mg/dL	Negative
Protein	100 mg/dL	Negative
Ketones	Negative	Negative
24-hr Protein	2,206	40 to 150 mg/24 hr
Blood	Moderate	Negative
Leukocyte esterase	Large	Negative
Nitrite	Negative	Negative
Ethanola	20.9	<10 mg/dL
Stool:		
Guaiac	Positive	Negative

[a]*Quantified using an H-P 6890 gas chromatograph (Hewlett-Packard, Wilmington, DE)*
BUN, blood urea nitrogen; CK, creatine kinase; WBC, white blood cell count; Hb, hemoglobin.

Questions

1. What are this patient's most striking laboratory results?

2. How do you explain these results?

3. What is the significance of diabetes mellitus and a positive urine ethanol test?

4. Under what conditions would ethanol be produced in the urine?

5. What types of organisms may produce ethanol in urine prior to and after collection?

Possible Answers

1. The patient's serum bicarbonate, BUN, creatinine, glucose, total CK, CK-MB (and calculated CK-MB Index), and troponin I findings; whole blood hemoglobin (Hb), hematocrit (Hct), white blood cell count (WBC), arterial pH, and HbA1c, and ethanol findings; urine glucose, protein, blood, and leukocyte esterase results; and, positive stool guaiac are the most striking laboratory results. The negative whole blood ethanol result is significant in relationship to the positive urine ethanol finding.

2. These results are explained by the patient's history of diabetes mellitus complicated by diabetic nephropathy (increased serum BUN and creatinine, and urine protein), poor glycemic control (increased HbA1c), metabolic acidosis (decreased serum bicarbonate and whole blood arterial pH), AMI (increased total CK, CK-MB, CK-MB Index, and markedly elevated troponin I), UTI (elevated WBC, large amount of urine leukocyte esterase activity), and a bleeding diathesis (decreased Hb and Hct; moderate amount of blood in the urine; positive stool guaiac).

3. Complications of diabetes mellitus are among the most common reasons for emergency room visits and hospitalizations. Such patients often present with mental status changes accompanied by symptoms of altered respiratory, renal, and cardiac function. Mental status changes often

prompt physicians to order a toxicology screen, even when patients and their family members deny any substance abuse. In this case, the patient denied ethanol ingestion, which was confirmed by a negative whole blood ethanol test; however, his urine tested positive for ethanol. Diabetics with poor glucose control, glycosuria, and a UTI may be mistakenly considered alcohol abusers if ethanol is detected in their urine during routine emergency room visits. This case illustrates that a UTI, especially with a fungal etiology, should be considered when a glycosuric diabetic patient denies ethanol abuse, tests negative for blood ethanol, but tests positive for urine ethanol. The near epidemic proportions of diabetes mellitus in the United States make it important for medical professionals to be aware that some diabetics may test positive for urine ethanol when they are not abusing alcohol.

4. This patient's urinary retention, incontinence, and severe glycosuria, accompanied by a bacterial and fungal UTI, suggest that urine glucose fermentation was occurring in the patient's bladder. Fermentation of glucose in urine may result in the formation of ethanol. This was confirmed when the patient's whole blood ethanol was negative but his urine tested positive. The conditions necessary for ethanol production in the urine include sufficient time, a suitable substrate (eg, glucose), and the presence of microorganisms capable of producing ethanol from the substrate. In patients that meet these criteria, the first morning urine is more likely than a random urine specimen to be positive for ethanol because the urine will have been in the bladder for 6 to 8 hours, an adequate time period for detectable ethanol production to occur.

5. A wide variety of microorganisms are capable of generating ethanol from glucose. This fermentation is characteristic of yeasts and is more uncommon in bacteria.[1-3] Moreover, conflicting ethanol results between various body fluids have been reported previously in both living patients and in forensic cases involving postmortem analyses.[4-7] The Embden-Meyerhof (EM) glycolytic pathway is the major route of ethanol formation in many microorganisms, especially yeasts.[1] In this pathway, pyruvate, the end-product of glucose metabolism, is converted to acetaldehyde and carbon dioxide by pyruvate

decarboxylase, and the acetaldehyde is reduced to ethanol by the enzyme, alcohol dehydrogenase, as summarized below:

EM pathway: Glucose $\rightarrow$ $\rightarrow$ CO_2 + Pyruvic acid

Pyruvate decarboxylase: Pyruvic acid $\rightarrow$ Acetaldehyde

Alcohol dehydrogenase: Acetaldehyde $\rightarrow$ Ethanol

References

1. Corry JEL. Possible sources of ethanol ante- and post-mortem: its relationship to the biochemistry and microbiology of decomposition. *J Appl Bacteriol.* 1978;44:1-56.

2. Ball W, Lichtenwalner M. Ethanol production in infected urine. *New Engl J Med.* 1979;301:614.

3. Saady JJ, Poklis A, Dalton HP. Production of urinary ethanol after sample collection. *J Forensic Sci.* 1993;38:1467-1471.

4. Alexander WD, Wills PD, Eldren N. Urinary ethanol and diabetes mellitus. *Diab Med.* 1988;5:463-464.

5. Alexander WD. Postmortem urinary alcohol is unreliable in diabetes. *Br Med J.* 1998;317:206.

6. Pounder D. Dead sober or dead drunk? *Br Med J.* 1988;316:87.

7. Urry FM, Wong Y-W. Current issues in alcohol testing. *Lab Med.* 1995;26:194-197.

Needle-Shaped Urine Crystals

Monte S. Willis, Frank H. Wians, Jr., Steven Kroft, Leland B. Baskin

Department of Pathology, University of Texas Southwestern Medical Center, Dallas, TX

Patient: 49-year-old male.

Physical Examination: Unremarkable.

Chief Complaint: The patient was admitted to a tertiary care medical center from a community hospital because of ongoing metabolic acidosis and an increased anion gap secondary to ethylene glycol ingestion.

History of Present Illness: Approximately 36 hours prior to admission, the patient had ingested approximately 6 ounces (180 mL) of Prestone brand antifreeze (ethylene glycol) in an attempt to kill himself. After consuming this fluid, he stated that he felt drunk and had difficulty walking.

Past Medical History: The patient had been diagnosed with ankylosing spondylitis in 1982.

Drug History: Vicodin (acetaminophen/hydrocodone bitartrate), prescribed for pain as needed.

Family History: Mother had diabetes mellitus.

Social History: The patient denied ethanol or illicit drug use. He smoked 2 packs of cigarettes per day for the last 30 years. He was a Vietnam-era veteran and was recently certified as eligible to receive health care benefits from the Veterans Administration (VA) medical facilities. He had been diagnosed previously with post-traumatic stress disorder. He and his wife recently moved to Texas from Nevada and had been having marital problems. She had kicked him out of their home 1 week prior to hospital admission, and he had been living in his car. He had been married 4 times, divorced 3 times, and stated that he had 8 children by 2 of the wives and was behind on child support. He admitted feeling depressed but had never been diagnosed with clinical depression.

Questions _____

1. What is (are) this patient's most striking laboratory result(s)?

2. How do you explain this patient's most striking laboratory results?

3. What condition(s) does this patient's laboratory and other findings suggest?

4. How should this patient's condition(s) be treated?

T1. Relevant Laboratory Findings

Test	Patient's Result	"Normal" Reference Range
Serum		
Sodium (Na+)	140	135-145 mEq/L
Potassium (K+)	4.7	3.6-5.0 mEq/L
Chloride (Cl-)	113	98-109 mEq/L
Carbon dioxide (CO$_2$)	12	22-31 mEq/L
Glucose	93	65-110 mg/dL
Anion gap	15	5-20 mEq/L
Osmolality, measured	305	270-300 mOsm/kg H$_2$O
Osmolality, calculated	290	
Osmolal gap	15	-6 to +6 mOsm/kg H$_2$O
Calcium	9.6	8.4-10.2 mg/dL
Blood urea nitrogen (BUN)	16	4-21 mg/dL
Creatinine	1.2	0.6-1.2 mg/dL
Ethylene glycol	Neg	Neg
Methanol	Neg	Neg
Isopropanol	Neg	Neg
Ethanol	Neg	Neg

Arterial Blood		
pH	7.29	7.34-7.44
pCO$_2$	27	35-45 mm Hg
pO$_2$	92	75-100 mm Hg
HCO$_3$-	15	22-26 mmol/L
Base excess	-9.6	-2.4 to 2.3
S$_a$O$_2$ (on room air)	96	90%-100%
O$_2$ content	20	18-22 mL/dL
Hemoglobin	14.8	13.2-16.2 g/dL
Urine		
Drug screen*	Neg	Neg
Color/clarity	Straw/hazy	Colorless/clear
Specific gravity	1.025	1.002-1.030
pH	5.0	5.0-7.0
Protein	30 mg/dL	Neg
Glucose	Neg	Neg
Ketone	Neg	Neg
Bile	Neg	Neg
Blood	Neg	Neg
Urobilinogen	0.2	0.1-1.0 EU
Leukocyte esterase	Neg	Neg
Nitrite	Neg	Neg
RBC/WBC/bacteria	0/0/occasional	0-3/0-5/none
Crystals	Many needle-shaped	

*Amphetamines, barbiturates, benzodiazepines, cannabinoids, cocaine metabolite, opiates. S$_a$O$_2$, arterial oxygen saturation

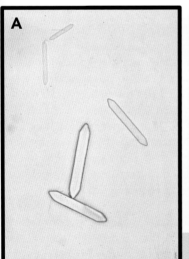
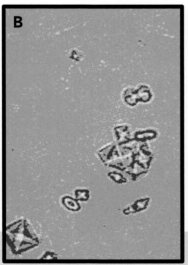
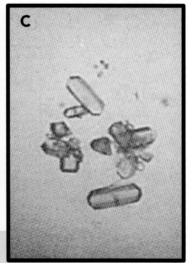

Image 1_Photomicrographs of **A)** the calcium oxalate monohydrate crystals found in our patient's urine, **B)** representative envelope-shaped calcium oxalate dihydrate crystals, and **C)** representative prism-shaped hippuric acid crystals which can be easily confused with calcium oxalate monohydrate crystals.

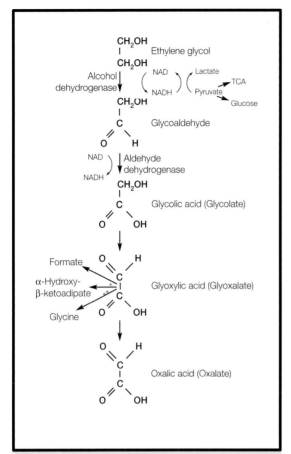

Figure 1_Metabolism of ethylene glycol.[1,13]

*Conversion of glyoxylic acid to α-hydroxy-β-ketoadipate uses thiamine as a cofactor.

**Transmission of glyoxylic acid requiring pyridoxine as cofactor.

Possible Answers

1. The most striking laboratory results include: *serum*, an undetectable level of ethylene glycol, high normal potassium (K^+) concentration, decreased CO_2 concentration, normal anion gap, and an increased osmolality and osmolal gap; *arterial blood*, decreased pH, pCO_2, HCO_3^- concentration, and markedly decreased base excess; *urine*, presence of many needle-shaped crystals [**Image 1**].

2. Undetectable serum ethylene glycol level: Unfortunately, an ethylene glycol level was not obtained on a whole blood sample from this patient during his treatment at the community hospital prior to his transfer to the tertiary care

medical center. The most likely explanation for the absence of ethylene glycol in the patient's serum after his admission to our medical center is a time-dependent decrease in the initial ethylene glycol level. This is due to metabolism and excretion of ethylene glycol and its metabolites in the urine between the time of ingestion and the time that a blood sample was drawn. Ethylene glycol (1,2-ethanediol) is oxidized by alcohol dehydrogenase to glycoaldehyde which is oxidized subsequently to the final product, oxalic acid, via the intermediate metabolites, glycolic acid and glyoxylic acid [**Figure 1**]. Cofactors utilized in this oxidation pathway include pyridoxine, thiamine, and NAD. Because of the tendency of serum oxalic acid to bind calcium, calcium levels should be monitored closely to avoid hypocalcemia and its principal, potentially life-threatening clinical manifestation, tetany. The half-life of the metabolites of ethylene glycol metabolism is 3 to 8 hours and nearly 20% of ingested ethylene glycol is excreted unchanged in the urine.[2] Since this patient had ingested ethylene glycol approximately 36 hours previously, 4 to 12 half-lives had passed, leaving levels undetectable in the blood. The laboratory diagnosis of ethylene glycol intoxication is established by the direct quantification of whole blood ethylene glycol and glycolic acid levels. Both parent compound (ethylene glycol) and the metabolite glycolic acid are measured because the parent compound may not be present at later time points after ingestion whereas the metabolite glycolic acid may still be. Several analytical methods are available to identify and quantify these analytes including chromatographic, enzymatic, and colorimetric methods. Gas chromatography with flame ionization detection is usually the preferred method. Ethylene glycol metabolism produces a metabolic acidosis caused by its organic acid metabolites: glycolic acid, glyoxylic acid, and oxalic acid. Consumption of bicarbonate, caused by the excess contribution of H+ ion from these metabolites, and the formation of hippuric acid, also contribute to the metabolic acidosis.[3] Additionally, the degradation of ethylene glycol inhibits the tricarboxylic acid (TCA) cycle (by exhausting cofactors that are also used in the TCA cycle), which in turn increases lactic acid formation (due to the decrease in pyruvate utilization by the TCA cycle) that further exacerbates the metabolic acidosis (see **Figure 1**).[3]

The profound metabolic acidosis that accompanies ethylene glycol intoxication explains the abnormal serum and arterial blood results.

Decreased pH, pCO_2, HCO_3-, markedly decreased base excess, decreased CO_2, and high normal K+ concentration: The decrease in arterial blood pH, pCO_2, HCO_3^-, and the markedly decreased base excess value are caused by the excess H^+ contributed to the blood by the organic acid metabolites of ethylene glycol. Increased blood H^+ concentration causes the blood pH to decrease and triggers respiratory and renal compensatory mechanisms. Hyperkalemia occurs as intracellular stores of K^+ (and Na^+) are exchanged for the excess H^+ in red blood cells, once the buffering capacity of the major buffering system (ie, hemoglobin) in the body is exceeded. Moreover, HCO_3^- ion concentration, the second most important buffering system in the body (ie, HCO_3^- buffer system), is decreased by the increase in blood H^+ concentration, which, in turn, causes the CO_2 concentration and pCO_2 of the blood to decrease as more CO_2 is expired (increased respiratory rate and tidal volume) to remove excess H^+ concentration and return the pH to normal according to the reaction sequence:

$$H+ + HCO_3\text{-} H_2CO_3 \; H_2O + CO_2 \; (aqueous \; solution) \; CO_2 \; (gas \; phase)$$

Normal anion gap and increased osmolality and osmolal gap: Organic acidemia causes typically an increased anion gap (AG), serum osmolality, and osmolal gap (OG), due to the contribution of organic acid anions to the serum, thus explaining the increased AG observed initially in the patient and his subsequent increased serum osmolality and OG. When the patient was admitted to the tertiary care center, the AG, however, was within normal limits, probably due to the correction in ion concentrations that occurred over the 36-hour period between the initial ingestion of ethylene glycol and obtaining the blood sample on which the values shown in **T1** were obtained. The AG is calculated as: AG = $(Na^+ + K^+) - (Cl^- + CO_2)$. Among the anions that are not included in this formula are anionic proteins, phosphate– and sulfate–containing inorganic acids, and organic anions. When the AG increases above the upper limit of normal

(ie, 20), the increase is most often due to the presence of increased serum anions and less often to decreased cations. When serum albumin concentration is normal, an increase in the AG is usually caused by the presence of phosphate- and sulfate-containing inorganic acids, endogenously produced organic acids (eg, ketoacids, lactic acid, hippuric acid, uremic organic anions), or exogenous acids (eg, salicylate or toxins). Moreover, the organic acidemia that occurred in this patient also explains his increased, measured serum osmolality (305 mOsm/kg H_2O) and OG (15 mOsm/kg H_2O). Osmolality is a measure of the number of solute molecules present in solution (serum) and can be either measured directly using an osmometer or estimated using the equation: Osmolality $(Osmo_{Calculated}) = [2(Na^+) + Glucose/18 + BUN/2.8]$. The OG is calculated as $Osmo_{Measured} - Osmo_{Calculated}$ and is typically 9 to 15 mOsm/kg H_2O. Early in the course of ethylene glycol intoxication, the measured osmolality is abnormally increased because of the extra solutes (parent chemical and metabolites) present in serum from the metabolism of ethylene glycol, which causes the OG to be increased because $Osmo_{Measured} > Osmo_{Calculated}$. In later stages of ethylene glycol intoxication, the OG will return to normal as production of excess solutes decreases and urinary excretion increases.

Presence of many needle-shaped crystals in the urine: The needle-shaped crystals found in the patient's urine are explained by the high concentration of oxalate, the end-product of ethylene glycol metabolism in the body, present in this patient's serum and excreted into the urine, where it forms calcium oxalate monohydrate crystals. The presence of needle-shaped oxalate monohydrate crystals in the urine provides strong presumptive evidence for the diagnosis of ethylene glycol intoxication. Urinary oxalate crystals most commonly take the form of envelope-shaped calcium oxalate *dihydrate* crystals and less commonly as dumbbell-, ovoid-, or needle-shaped calcium oxalate *monohydrate* crystals [**Image 1B**]. Needle-shaped calcium oxalate monohydrate crystals can easily be mistaken for hippurate crystals [**Image 1C**].[5,6] Needle-shaped calcium oxalate monohydrate crystals, however, have rounded ends, and appear longer and narrower than hippuric acid crystals which have more pointed ends, are shorter and wider, and appear as prisms, needles, or rhomboid plates.[7] The crystals found in this patient's urine were needle-like in shape with rounded ends [**Image 1A**]. After approximately 12 to 24 hours post-ethylene glycol intoxication, high levels of oxalate excreted into the urine and calcium oxalate crystals form in vivo and can be deposited in the heart, brain, kidney, lung, and/or pancreas and cause damage to these tissues. In other situations, the small amount of diet-derived oxalate is excreted into the urine and forms the dihydrate oxalate crystals because of an inhibition of monohydrate oxalate crystal formation by macromolecules normally present in the urine.[8] However, when higher levels of oxalate are present (eg, after ethylene glycol intoxication), the monohydrate form appears and may predominate.

3. ***Most likely diagnosis:*** *acute ethylene glycol intoxication with laboratory findings consistent with a late stage of intoxication with this agent.*

There are 3 stages of ethylene glycol intoxication. The first stage lasts 30 minutes to 12 hours and mainly affects the central nervous system. Ethanol intoxication, however, can cause similar effects, including generalized CNS depression, ataxia, speech slurring, and vomiting. Other effects, such as hallucinations, convulsions, and coma, have also been reported. The second stage occurs 12 to 24 hours after ingestion and manifests as a slight increase in blood pressure, tachypnea, and tachycardia which result from the profound metabolic acidosis that can occur. It is in this stage that pulmonary edema,[6,9] related to the increase in the serum concentration of glycolic and glyoxylic acids, as well as the deposition of calcium oxalate crystals in the lungs,[10] may occur. The third stage is seen 24 to 72 hours after ingestion. During this phase, most of the damage from ethylene glycol intoxication occurs to the kidneys. Hematuria and proteinuria are common in this phase as calcium oxalate monohydrate crystals form in the kidneys causing, in some cases, acute tubular necrosis. The degree of acidosis and glycolic acid levels correlate best with the occurrence of renal failure. Calcium oxalate monohydrate crystalluria occurs in 50% of cases of ethylene glycol ingestion.[11,12] Our patient had a mild acidosis (pH = 7.29), modest proteinuria (~30 mg/dL), no hematuria, and calcium oxalate

crystalluria, suggesting the absence of any significant renal failure. Moreover, his BUN and creatinine values were within normal limits (and did not increase over the 2 days subsequent to the day of admission to the tertiary care facility (*data not shown*), further suggesting that severe renal damage had not occurred. Since this patient was seen at the tertiary care facility ~36 hours after the ingestion of ethylene glycol, our patient was most likely in the third stage of ethylene glycol intoxication.

Death has been shown to occur with the ingestion of as little as 100 mL of ethylene glycol[3]; however, there are reports of individuals who have survived ingestion of up to 3,000 mL.[4]

4. In general, treatment modalities for ethylene glycol intoxication are based on the severity of laboratory findings and include: 1) correcting the metabolic acidosis with bicarbonate administration, 2) blocking the metabolism of ethylene glycol to its toxic metabolites using Fomepizole (an inhibitor of alcohol dehydrogenase), and 3) removing ethylene glycol and its metabolites by hemodialysis.[2] If ingestion is acute, aspiration of gastric contents is the first line of treatment followed by administration of activated charcoal. Spontaneous resolution of the metabolic acidosis that accompanies ethylene glycol intoxication does not occur, and large doses of bicarbonate may be required to restore blood pH to within normal limits. Bicarbonate administration also alkalinizes the urine, thereby increasing the excretion of acid metabolites, and decreasing crystal formation. Decreased urine output can be treated with fluids, but it does not enhance the clearance of ethylene glycol. Hypocalcemia can be treated with intravenous (IV) administration of calcium salts. Pyridoxine and thiamine are given to restore the serum levels of these cofactors which are depleted during the metabolism of ethylene glycol (see Figure 1).[2] Generally, treatment with Fomepizole is necessary for any asymptomatic adult with ethylene glycol levels >20 mg/dL. Other indications for treatment include an elevated osmolal gap, an increased anion gap, intoxication in a patient with a history of ethylene glycol ingestion, or any indication of renal toxicity after ethylene glycol ingestion. Hemodialysis can remove ethylene glycol from the blood in as little as 3 hours. Indications for

hemodialysis include an ethylene glycol level of >50 mg/dL, a metabolic acidosis not corrected with bicarbonate therapy, lack of clinical improvement with treatment, or evidence of renal toxicity regardless of ethylene glycol level.[2]

Treatment and Course _____

This patient was given Fomepizole (1 g, IV), thiamine (100 mg), and pyridoxine (500 mg) immediately upon arrival. Both the renal and psychiatric services were consulted, and he was admitted to an inpatient unit of our medical center. Further therapy included aggressive hydration to keep the kidneys functioning and Zoloft (25 mg every day) for treatment of his depression and post-traumatic stress disorder (PTSD). Dialysis was determined to be unnecessary as his renal function (determined by BUN and creatinine levels) was adequate. He was discharged after 24 hours to follow-up care by our psychiatric and medicine services.

References _____

1. Porter WH. Clinical Toxicology. In: *Tietz Textbook of Clinical Chemistry*, 3rd ed., Burtis CA, Ashwood ER, eds., Philadelphia, PA: WB Saunders; 1999:937.

2. Linden CH, Burns MJ. Illnesses due to poisons, drug overdose, and envenomation. In: *Harrison's Principles of Internal Medicine*, 15th ed., Braunwald E, Fauci AS, Kasper DL, et al, eds. New York, NY: McGraw-Hill; 2001:2595-2616.

3. Winchester JF. Methanol, isopropyl alcohol, higher alcohols, ethylene glycol, cellosolves, acetone, and oxalate. In: *Clinical Management of Poisoning and Drug Overdose*, Haddad L, Shannon WB, Winchester JF, eds. Philadelphia, PA: WB Saunders; 1998:491-504.

4. Jacobsen D. New treatment for ethylene glycol poisoning. *N Engl J Med*. 1999;340:879-81.

5. Godolphin W, Meagher EP, Sanders HD, et al. Unusual calcium oxalate crystals in ethylene glycol poisoning. *Clin Toxicol*. 1980;16:479-486.

6. Jacobsen D, McMartin KE. Methanol and ethylene glycol poisonings. Mechanism of toxicity, clinical course, diagnosis and treatment. *Med Toxicol*. 1986;1:309-334.

7. Harber M. Calcium oxalate crystals. In: *Urinary Sediment, A Textbook Atlas*. Chicago, IL: ASCP Press; 1981:40.

8. Wesson JA, Worcester EM, Wiessner JH, et al. Control of calcium oxalate crystal structure and cell adherence by urinary macromolecules. *Kidney Int*. 1998;53:952-957.

9. Parry MF, Wallach R. Ethylene glycol poisoning. *Am J Med*. 1974;57:143-150.

10. Catchings TT, Beamer WC, Lundy L, et al. Adult respiratory distress syndrome secondary to ethylene glycol ingestion. *Ann Emerg Med*. 1985;14:594-596.

11. Jacobsen D, Hewlett TP, Webb R, et al. Ethylene glycol intoxication: evaluation of kinetics and crystalluria. *Am J Med*. 1988;84:145-152.

12. Jacobsen D, Akesson I, Shefter E. Urinary calcium oxalate monohydrate crystals in ethylene glycol poisoning. *Scand J Clin Lab Invest*. 1982;42:231-234.

13. Gabow PA, Clay K, Sullivan JB, et al. Organic acids in ethylene glycol intoxication. *Ann Intern Med*. 1986;105:18.

Neuropathy Following Chronic Use of Denture Adhesive in a 40-Year-Old Patient

Michael F. Neerman,[1] Kathleen Kiefhaber,[1] Richard D. Barrera[2]

[1]*North Texas Poison Center, Parkland Health and Hospital System,* [2]*Department of Surgery, The University of Texas Southwestern Medical Center at Dallas, Dallas, TX*

Patient: 40-year-old male.

Chief Complaint: Pain and numbness in his legs along with persistent nausea.

Past Medical History: The patient has been using denture adhesive for years. The patient stated that he speaks for a living and cannot have loose teeth. Otherwise, he was previously healthy.

Examination Findings: The patient had difficulties flexing his feet. The patient was also suffering from gait problems.

Questions

1. What are this patient's most striking clinical and laboratory findings?

2. How do you explain these findings?

3. What are the principal causes of the most striking laboratory finding in this patient?

4. What is this patient's most likely diagnosis?

5. What laboratory test will be helpful in confirming the diagnosis?

6. What causes this patient's disorder, and how common is it?

7. What is the treatment and management of this disorder?

Possible Answers

1. The laboratory values from the comprehensive metabolic panel, lipid panels, and complete blood count (CBC) are reported in **T1, T2,** and **T3**, respectively. Most of the values are within the normal limits and did not correlate with the patient's history and symptoms. According to the 24-hour urine heavy metal screen (**T4**), however, the patient showed a marked level of zinc with values of 207 µg/dL (ref. 15 to 120 µg/dL) and 2,691 µg/d (ref. 15 to 1,200 µg/d).

2. The patient's laboratory findings insofar as the elevated zinc levels are indicative of hyperzincuria.

3. The average daily intake of zinc for Americans is roughly 5.2 to 16.2 mg, mostly from food.[1] The recommended daily allowance for zinc is 11 mg/d for men and 8 mg/d for women. About 20% to 30% of the zinc ingested is absorbed from the GI tract.[2] Causes of elevated zinc levels include occupational exposure, ingestion of

T1. Comprehensive Metabolic Panel

		Ref
Glucose	95	65–100 mg/dL
BUN	15	8–25 mg/dL
Creatinine	1.1	0.8–1.4 mg/dL
Calculated BUN/creat	14	6–28
Sodium	140	133–146 mEq/L
Potassium	4.4	3.5–5.3 mEq/L
Chloride	104	97–110 mEq/L
Carbon dioxide	22	18–30 mEq/L
Calcium	10	8.5–10.5 mg/dL
Protein, total	7.6	6.0–8.4 g/dL
Albumin	4.7	2.9–5.0 g/dL
Calculated globulin	2.9	2.0–3.8 g/dL
Calculated A/G ratio	1.6	0.9–2.5
Bilirubin, total	0.4	0.1–1.3 mg/dL
Alkaline phosphatase	103	30–132 U/L
AST	10	5–35 U/L
ALT	24	17–56 U/L

BUN, blood urea nitrogen; AST, aspartate aminotransferase; ALT, alanine aminotransferase.

T3. Complete Blood Count

		Ref
WBC	13.8	4.0–11.0 K/Cumm
RBC	5.07	4.10–5.70 M/Cumm
Hemoglobin	16.2	13.0–17.0 g/dL
Hematocrit	46.6	37.0–49.0%
MCV	92	80–100 fL
MCH	31.9	27.0–34.0 UUG
MCHC	34.7	32.0–34.0 g/dL
RDW	14.2	11.0–15.0%
Neutrophils	73	40–74%
Lymphocytes	17	19–48%
Monocytes	7	3–11%
Eosinophils	2	0–7%
Basophils	1	0–2%
Platelets	333	130–400 K/Cumm

WBC, white blood cell; RBC, red blood cell; MCV, mean corpuscular volume; MCH, mean corpuscular hemoglobin; MCHC, mean corpuscular hemoglobin concentration; RDW, red cell distribution width.

T2. Lipid Panel

		Ref
Cholesterol	255	<200 mg/dL
Triglycerides	248	<150 mg/dL
HDL	9	>39 mg/dL
Calculated LDL	176	<100 mg/dL
Risk ratio LDL/ HDL	6.08	<3.55

T4. 24-Hour Urine Heavy Metal Screen

Total volume	1,300 mL	Ref
Cadmium	1.4	0.0–3.3 µg/d
	1.1	0.0–2.6 µg/L
	0.7	0.0–3.0 µg/gCr
Lead	0	0–31 µg/d
	0	0–23 µg/L
	0 µg/gCr	
Copper	25	3–50 µg/d
	1.9	0.2–8.0 µg/dL
	11.8 µg/gCr	
Mercury	0	0–15 µg/d
	0	0–10 µg/L
	0	<35 µg/gCr
Arsenic	21.8	0.0–50.0 µg/d
	16.8	0.0–35.0 µg/L
	10.4 µg/gCr	
Zinc	2,691	150–1,200 µg/d
	207	15–120 µg/dL
	1,285.7 µg/gCr	

poorly treated water flowing through galvanized copper pipes, and overuse of supplements or products containing zinc.

4. **Most likely diagnosis:** *hyperzincuria.* Due to the elevated urinary zinc levels coupled with the patient's history of chronic denture adhesive use containing a zinc compound, oral exposure to the zinc is the likely cause of the patient's elevated zinc level. It can be inferred that the patient also suffers from hyperzincemia due to the high clearance of zinc from the body.

5. Although a 24-hour urine collection is the "gold standard" for detecting metals in the body, a serum analysis should also be performed. Because elevated zinc concentrations cause copper deficiency, a serum copper concentration should always be obtained simultaneously.[1] Whole blood zinc levels exceed serum levels by a ratio of approximately 6:1 to 7:1 because the metal accumulates in the erythrocytes.[3] But because zinc is found everywhere in the environment and laboratory, one must exercise extreme caution to avoid contamination of samples.[1]

6. There are a number of sources leading to elevated zinc levels in the body. Typically, high zinc levels are seen in those who have had environmental exposure to it. Chronic exposure to zinc can engender a reversible sideroplastic anemia and a reversible myelodysplasia-like syndrome.[1] Granulocytopenia and anemia can also be clinical signs with the bone marrow showing vacuolated precursors and ringed sideroblasts[1]; the mechanism is believed to be through a zinc-induced copper deficiency.[4] For example, Willis and colleagues examined 3 cases whereby chronic ingestion of zinc-containing products led to severe neuropathy and neutropenia.[5] The bone marrow findings in all of their cases suggested copper deficiency. Subsequent laboratory testing determined this deficieny to be due to zinc excess. Hepatic or renal toxicity has not been observed in individuals who have consumed excessive amounts of elemental zinc.[6] Furthermore, it has been suggested that exposure to elevated levels of zinc may be important in the pathogenesis of demyelinating diseases,[7-9] possibly causing neurological defects. Overall, however, toxicity from zinc is rare.

7. The treatment for acute oral zinc poisoning is primarily supportive. Hydration and antiemetic therapy should be employed. Insofar as chelation therapy, where the data regarding the efficacy of chelation therapy is lacking, calcium sodium EDTA has been used successfully in a few cases.[10,11] The agent DMPS (sodium 2,3-dimercaptopropane-1-sulfonate) has been shown to be efficacious in increasing the urinary excretion of zinc.[12] Finally, there exists 2 potential zinc-selective chelators, DPESA (4-{[2-{bis-pyridin-2-ylmethylamino)ethylamino]-methyl} phenylmethanesulfonic acid sodium salt and TPESA (4-{[2-{bis-pyridin-2-ylmethylamino) ethyl]-pyridine-2-ymethylamino}-methyl) phenyl]methanesulfonic acid sodium salt,[13] that have shown promise in vitro but further in vivo studies are warranted to assess its clinical utility.[1] Finally, given the plausibility of zinc-induced copper deficiency, serum copper levels should also be determined and replenished if necessary.

Patient Follow-up

The patient was told to discontinue using the product and to seek an alternative dental adhesive that does not contain zinc. Insofar as treatment, chelation therapy was recommended while obtaining zinc levels during the course of chelation.

Keywords

hyperzincuria, zinc, neuropathy, dental adhesive, toxicology

References

1. Ewald MB. Zinc. In: Flomenbaum NE, Goldfrank LR, Hoffman RS, et al, eds. *Goldfrank's Toxicologic Emergencies.* 8th ed. New York, NY: McGraw-Hill; 2006: 1378–1383.

2. Zinc. In: Baselt RC, Cravey RH, eds. *Disposition of Toxic Drugs and Chemicals in Man.* 3rd ed. California: Chemical Toxicology Institute; 1995: 785–787.

3. Minoia C, Sabbioni E, Apostoli P, et al. Trace element reference values in tissues from inhabitants of the European Community I. A study of 46 elements in urine, blood, and serum of Italian subjects. *Sci Total Environ.* 1990;95:89–105.

4. Fiske DN, McCoy HE, Kitchens CS. Zinc-induced sideroblastic anemia: A report of a case, review of the literature, and description of the hematologic syndrome. *Am J Hematol.* 1994;46:147–150.

5. Willis MS, Monaghan SA, Miller ML, et al. Zinc-induced copper deficiency: A report of 3 cases initially recognized on bone marrow examination. *Am J Clin Pathol.* 2005;123:125–131.

6. Goyer RA, Clarkson TW. Toxic Effects of Metals. In: Klaasen CD, ed. *Casarett and Doull's Toxicology—The Basic Science of Poisons.* 6th ed. New York, NY: McGraw-Hill; 2001: 811–867.

7. Kumar N, Ahlskog JE. Myelopolyneuropathy due to copper deficiency or zinc excess? *Arch Neurol.* 2004;61:604–605.

8. Prodan CI, Holland NR. CNS demyelination from zinc toxicity? *Neurology.* 2000;54:1705–1706.

9. Prodan CI, Holland NR, Wisdom PJ, et al. CNS
    demyelination associated with copper deficiency and
    hyperzincemia. *Neurology.* 2002;59:1453–1456.

10. Chobanian SJ. Accidental ingestion of liquid zinc chloride:
    Local and systemic effects. *Ann Emerg Med.* 1981;10:91–93.

11. Potter JL. Acute zinc chloride ingestion in a young child. *Ann
    Emerg Med.* 1981;10:267–269.

12. Torres-Alanis O, Garza-Ocanas L, Bernal MA, et
    al. Urinary excretion of trace elements after sodium
    2,3-dimercaptopropane-1-sulfonate challenge test. *J Toxicol
    Clin Toxicol.* 2000;38:697–700.

13. Kawabata E, Kikuchi K, Urano Y, et al. Design and synthesis
    of zinc-selective chelators for extracellular applications. *J Am
    Chem Soc.* 2005;127:818–819.

Persistent Elevation of CA 19-9 in an Apparently-Healthy 56-Year-Old Woman

Emel Yaman, Ugur Coskun, Suleyman Buyukberber, Banu Ozturk, Ali Osman Kaya, Ramazan Yildiz, Aytug Uner, Deniz Yamac, Mustafa Benekli

Department of Medical Oncology, Gazi University Medical School, Ankara, Turkey

Patient: 56-year-old woman.

Chief Complaint: Anxiety and depression.

History of Present Illness: The patient was referred to the authors' hospital for the evaluation of fatigue, constipation, and a high serum cancer (or carbohydrate) antigen 19-9 (CA 19-9) level (1,400 U/mL) 12 years after her initial CA 19-9 elevation (8,000 U/mL), including a 5-year period during which she was lost to follow-up. Because her thyroid stimulating hormone (TSH, thyrotropin) level was elevated (28 µIU/mL) and her free thyroxine (FT4) level was decreased (0.7 ng/dL), she was considered hypothyroid and treated with levothyroxine. After 6 months of levothyroxine treatment, her TSH level normalized; however, her CA 19-9 level remained increased, with no discernible cause by repeat computerized tomography (CT) scans of her chest and abdomen. She was advised to obtain follow-up CA 19-9 levels and CT scans.

Diagnostic Tests: During her recent admission to the authors' hospital, a CT scan of her abdomen and chest, a mammogram, a whole-body positron emission tomography (PET)-CT scan, an upper gastrointestinal tract endoscopy, and a thyroid ultrasongraphy (US) revealed no abnormalities. The patient declined additional imaging studies by magnetic resonance cholangiopancreatography (MRCP).

Questions

1. What are this patient's most striking clinical and laboratory findings?

2. How do you explain these findings?

3. What is the most likely cause of these findings?

4. What is this patient's most likely diagnosis?

5. What is the clinical significance of this diagnosis?

Possible Answers

1. The absence of any clinical signs and symptoms or CT and PET-CT imaging evidence of a pancreatic (or other tissue site), tumor, despite a long and current history of a markedly-increased CA 19-9 level; a markedly-increased TSH and modestly-decreased FT4 level; increased total- and LDL-cholesterol values; and normal liver function tests, negative serum protein electrophoresis pattern (SPEP), and negative antibodies associated with autoimmune diseases (**T1**).

2. In the absence of clinical or imaging evidence to support the existence of a CA 19-9-secreting tumor to explain this patient's history of a persistently-elevated serum CA 19-9 level, this finding must be categorized as due to: 1) a benign condition; 2) the presence of a tumor not detected by the imaging studies performed; 3) an interferent (eg, human anti-mouse antibodies [HAMA]) in the patient's serum causing a false-positive result; or 4) an incidental finding with no apparent cause. The patient's thyroid function and lipid test results are consistent with hypothyroidism and hypercholesterolemia, respectively. Because lipid clearance may be decreased in hypothyroid patients, serum concentrations of free fatty acids and total cholesterol are increased.[1,2] In the study

T1. Principal Laboratory Findings

Test	Patient's Result	Reference Range
Chemistry		
TSH	2.8	0.4–4.5 µIU/mL
FT4	0.7	0.8–1.8 ng/dL
Total cholesterol	230	100–200 mg/dL
LDL cholesterol	151	<130 mg/dL
Bilirubin, total	1.1	0.2–1.3 mg/dL
Bilirubin, indirect	0.7	0.8–1.3 mg/dL
AST	13	0–40 U/L
ALT	11	0–40 U/L
ALP	69	53–141 U/L
CA 19-9	1,400	<40 U/mL
SPEP	Normal pattern	Normal pattern
Immunology		
ANA	<1:160	<1:160
AMA	<1:160	<1:160
ASMA	<1:80	<1:80
Microbiology		
FOBT	Negative*	Negative

*On 3 stool samples obtained at different times. LDL, low-density lipoprotein; TSH, thyroid-stimulating hormone; FT4, free thyroxine; CA, cancer (or carbohydrate) antigen; ANA, anti-nuclear antibodies; AMA, anti-mitochondrial antibodies; ASMA, anti-smooth muscle antibodies; SPEP, serum protein electrophoresis pattern; FOBT, fecal occult blood test.

by O'Brien and colleagues, hypercholesterolemia was present in 56% of hypothyroid patients, and only 8.5% of these patients had a normal lipid profile.[1]

3. Cancer (or carbohydrate) antigen 19-9 is a glycolipid antigen frequently associated with malignancy. It is commonly elevated in pancreatic cancer; however, increased serum levels of CA 19-9 can be observed in serum from individuals with gastric, colon, biliary, hepatocellular, or non-gastrointestinal cancers.[3] The diagnostic accuracy (ie, sensitivity and specificity) of serum CA 19-9 levels is highest for pancreatic cancer. Usually, CA 19-9 levels above 1,000 U/mL are most often associated with malignant diseases.[4] Although CA 19-9 is not typically elevated in nonmalignant diseases, it can be elevated in some benign liver and renal diseases and in patients with pulmonary or various thyroid diseases, most often thyroiditis.[5-8] In the study

by Maestranzi and colleagues[5] of 150 patients with various types of liver disease, an increased serum CA 19-9 level was found in 84%, 73%, 70%, 61%, and 60% of patients with chronic hepatitis C infection, alcoholic liver disease, chronic hepatitis B infection, primary sclerosing cholangitis, and primary biliary cirrhosis, respectively. Although elevated serum CA 19-9 levels have been reported in patients with hydronephrosis[8] or pulmonary disease (eg, pneumonia and pleural effusions),[9] this patient did not have hydronephrosis or any other urinary or respiratory system abnormality. Moreover, although the patient was hypothyroid, there was no evidence of thyroiditis by thyroid US and PET-CT imaging studies. In addition, in patients with thyroiditis undergoing levothyroxine replacement therapy, serum CA 19-9 levels normalized along with TSH and FT4 levels. This patient's serum CA 19-9 level, however, remained elevated despite normalization of her serum TSH and FT4 levels. Moreover, this patient's long history of an elevated CA 19-9 level, in the presence of current, negative CT and PET-CT imaging studies and despite the patient's refusal to undergo MRCP, suggests the absence of a pancreatic or non-pancreatic tumor to explain this history. Lastly, HAMA are unlikely to cause such marked elevations in CA 19-9 levels, especially when these levels are observed using different CA 19-9 immunoassays. Therefore, the authors were left with an incidental finding with no apparent cause as the most likely explanation for the patient's persistently-increased CA 19-9 levels.

4. ***Most likely diagnosis:*** *unexplained increase in serum CA 19-9 level in an otherwise relatively-healthy individual.*

5. The presence of an increased serum level of CA 19-9 in a relatively-healthy individual, or in individuals with benign diseases, limits the clinical utility of this soluble marker for a specific tumor and its use as a screening test for pancreatic cancer. Although the American Society of Clinical Oncology does not recommend the use of tumor markers in screening for malignancies,[10] they can be misused for this purpose. This case reminds us that soluble tumor markers, such as CA 19-9, can be increased in the absence of malignant conditions, which can lead to expensive and unnecessary follow-up procedures

and can needlessly increase the anxiety levels of patients and their family members. In the study by Osswald and colleagues[11] among patients with elevated CA 19-9 levels, 50% of those patients had malignant diseases, while in 8.8% of the patients there was no explanation for their high CA 19-9 levels. Moreover, the authors found only 1 report of a persistently-elevated CA 19-9 level in an apparently-healthy individual.[12] The patient in that report was a 70-year-old woman with a high CA 19-9 level for a 7-year period. In that study, Kaneko and colleagues[12] found that patients with various diseases had a higher-molecular-weight CA 19-9 in their serum than this apparently-healthy 70-year-old woman. This finding raises the possibility that different isoforms of CA 19-9 may have clinical utility in identifying apparently-healthy individuals with increased CA 19-9 levels.

Keywords _____

CA 19-9, soluble tumor marker, pancreatic cancer, diagnostic accuracy, screening

References _____

1. O'Brien T, Dinneen SF, O'Brien PC, et al. Hyperlipidemia in patients with primary and secondary hypothyroidism. *Mayo Clin Proc*. 1993;68:860–866.

2. Diekman T, Lansberg PJ, Kastelein JJ, et al. Prevalence and correction of hypothyroidism in a large cohort of patients referred for dyslipidemia. *Arch Intern Med*. 1995;155:1490–1495.

3. Atkinson BF, Ernst CS, Herlyn M, et al. Gastrointestinal cancer-associated antigen in immunoperoxidase assay. *Cancer Res*. 1982;42:4280–4283.

4. Ritts RE, Delvillano BC, Go V, et al. Initial clinical evaluation of an immunoradiometric assay for CA 19-9 using NCI serum bank. *Int J Cancer*. 1984;33:339–345.

5. Maestranzi S, Przeimoslo R, Mitchel H, et al. The effect of benign and malignant liver diseases on the tumors markers CA 19-9 and CEA. *Ann Clin Biochem*. 1998;35:99–103.

6. Parra JL, Kaplan S, Barkn JS. Elevated CA 19-9 caused by Hashimoto's Thyroiditis: Review of the benign causes of increased CA 19-9 level. *Dig Dis Sci*. 2005;50:694–695.

7. Schmid KW, Ofner C, Raumsuer T, et al. CA 19-9 expression in subacute (de Quervain's) thyroiditis: An immunohistochemical study. *Mod Pathol*. 1992;5:268–272.

8. Aybek H, Aybek Z, Sýnýk Z, et al. Elevation of serum and urinary carbohydrate antigen CA 19-9 in benign hydronephrosis. *Int J Urology*. 2006;13:1380–1384.

9. Shitrit D, Zingerman B, Shitrit AB. Diagnostic value of CYFRA 21-1, CEA, CA 19-9, CA 15-3 and CA 125 assays in pleural effusions: Analysis of 116 cases and review of the literature. *Oncologist*. 2005;10:501–507.

10. Bast RC Jr, Ravdin P, Hayes DF, et al. Update of recommendations for the use of tumor markers in breast and colorectal cancer: Clinical practice guidelines of the American Society of Clinical Oncology. *J Clin Oncol*. 2001;15: 1865–1878.

11. Osswald BR, Klee FR, Wysocki S. The reliability of highly elevated CA 19-9 levels. *Dis Markers*. 1993;11:275–278.

12. Kaneko Y, Shibata Y, Nakamura H, et al. Extraordinary high elevation of CA 19-9 levels in an apparently healthy subject. *Rinsho Byori*. 1999;47:943–948.

Tumor Markers

Frank H. Wians, Jr.

Professor of Pathology, Clinical and Scientific Consultant, Aston Pathology Lab, University of Texas Southwestern Medical Center, Dallas, Texas

Patient: 55-year-old, African-American male.

Family History: Unremarkable.

Medical History: He characterized his past medical history as "excellent."

Drug History: None.

Chief Complaint: Recently, he had been feeling unusually tired. He complained of anorexia, a poor urinary stream, with some frequency, nocturia, and a post-micturitional dribble.

Physical Examination: Unremarkable.

T1. Principal Laboratory Findings

Test	"Abnormal" Patient's Result	"Normal" Reference Range
CBC with differential	Hct = 29.4	M: 40-52%
	Hb = 9.8	M: 13.2-16.2 g/dL
ESR	8	0-10 mm/h
BUN	32	7-21 mg/dL
Creatinine	3.6	0.5-1.4 mg/dL
BUN/creatine	9:1	>10:1 (prerenal azotemia)
Calcium	8.4	8.9-10.4 mg/dL
Phosphate	5.2	2.4-4.5 mg/dL
Uric acid	8.3	3.9-7.8 mg/dL
Potassium	5.8	3.6-5.0 mEq/L
PSA	8.8	<4.0 ng/mL

T2. Differential Diagnosis of Hypercalcemia

Based on PTH and PTHrP Values

Hypercalcemic	Typical values for condition	PTH	PTHrP
Primary hyperparathyroidism	↑	u.d.	
Hypercalcemia of malignancy	↓		↑

u.d., undetectable.

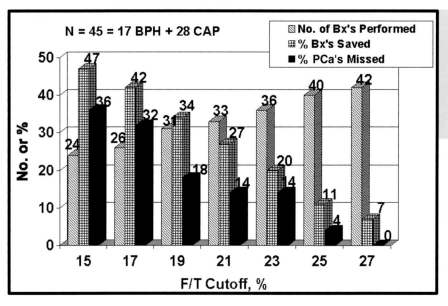

Figure 1_Number of biopsies (Bx's) saved and prostate cancers (PCa's) missed at various F/T cutoffs when 4 ng/mL < total [PSA] < 10 ng/mL.

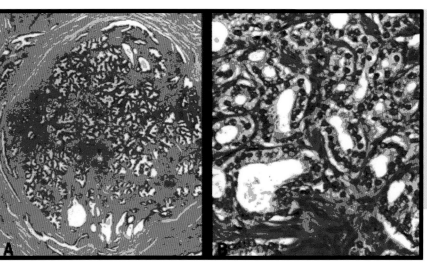

Image 1_(**A**) Nodular proliferation of both stroma and large caliber glands associated with BPH. H&E, low power magnification. (**B**) Small caliber glands with open lumen infiltrating the stroma of a Gleason Score 6 (3 + 3) PCa. H& E, high power magnification.

Questions _____

1. What condition(s) does this patient's chief signs and symptoms suggest?

2. What diagnostic procedures would you include as part of your physical examination of this patient and why?

3. Given the laboratory test findings indicated in **T1**, what do these test results suggest?

4. What additional laboratory test(s) would you order and why?

5. What is the most likely diagnosis in this patient? Results of Additional Diagnostic Procedures: Digital rectal exam (DRE) reveals a rubbery, firm, smooth enlargement of the prostate gland. Intravenous urogram (IVU) reveals both kidneys functioning and bilateral nephrosis (ie, distention of the pelvis and calices of the kidney with urine as a result of obstruction of the ureter) and hydroureter (abnormal distention of the ureter with urine due to obstruction from any cause).

Possible Answers _____

1. Renal failure casued by hydronephrosis resulting from obstruction of the urethra by an enlarged prostate gland.

2. Digital Rectal Exam (DRE) – The American Urological Association (AUA) and the American Cancer Society (ACS) recommend a DRE, in conjuction with a prostate-specific antigen (PSA) test, annually in men beginning at age 50 years, or 40 years in African-American men, or earlier if there is a family history of prostate cancer. Intravenous Urogram (IVU) – to identify possible causes (eg, ureteral obstruction) of post-renal acute renal failure involving X-ray examination of the urinary tract after the IV administration of an opaque medium that is rapidly excreted in the urine.

3. The laboratory test results suggest that the patient is anemic and has acute renal failure (ARF) of the post-renal type. CBC with differential and erythrocyte sedimentation rate (ESR): tiredness and loss of appetite may be due to anemia (decreased hematocrit and hemoglobin) and/or infection (increased WBC and neutrophil count) or inflammation (increased ESR). BUN, creatinine, calcium, phosphorus, uric acid, electrolytes, glucose, total protein, albumin, globulins: these tests evaluate renal function (BUN, creatinine, calcium, phosphorus, uric acid), fluid and electrolyte balance (total protein, albumin, electrolytes), glycemic status (fasting blood glucose), and immune response (globulins). Elevated BUN suggests azotemia which manifests in a number of clinical symptoms, including anorexia. After several days, patients with ARF exhibit: anemia, hypocalcemia, hyperkalemia, hyperphosphatemia, and hyperuricemia. Prostate-Specific Antigen (PSA): Increases in PSA concentration above 4.0 ng/mL are observed frequently in individuals with BPH or PCa; however, the diagnostic sensitivity and specificity of this test alone are inadequate to distinguish between BPH vs PCa. Prostate biopsy is required to make this distinction.

4. Free PSA: PSA exists in serum as either "complexed PSA" (C), a form in which proteinase inhibitors, especially alpha-1-antichymotrypsin (ACT), are non-covalently bound to the PSA molecule, or as, "free PSA" (F), a form in which PSA is not bound to any other protein. The total PSA (T) concentration is the combination of both the complexed and free forms. In addition, the total PSA concentration is increased typically in men with PCa due to a relative increase in the concentration of complexed PSA. In men with BPH, however, the total PSA concentration is increased due to a relative increase in the concentration of free PSA. Therefore, the ratio of free PSA to total PSA (F/T, %) has been used to improve the diagnostic specificity (ie, reduce the number of false positives requiring the additional expense and emotional trauma of a prostate biopsy), with little to no effect on the cancer detection rate, of the total PSA value alone, especially in men with a 4.0 ng/mL < [total PSA] < 10.0 ng/mL [**Figure 1**]. Typically, an F/T ratio >0.25 (or 25%) is more consistent with BPH, while an F/T ratio <0.25 is more consistent with PCa. However, the cutoff value chosen for F/T will vary between laboratories (ie, may differ from 25%) and will, of course, affect the diagnostic specificity (% of Bx's saved) and sensitivity (% PCa's missed) of F/T at that cutoff value [**Figure 1**].

5. Diagnosis: BPH or PCa. Difficulty urinating in a 55 year-old man can often be associated with BPH; however, African-American men have the highest prevalence, the earliest age of onset, and the highest mortality rate from PCa. In addition, the incidence of PCa increases with increasing age, especially in men over the age of 50 years. Moreover, the combination of a DRE and PSA test cannot discriminate between BPH vs PCa – a prostate biopsy is required to make this distinction. Typical histopathological features of BPH and PCa are shown in **Image 1**.

Glossary _____

Anorexia: loss of appetite
Nocturia: excessive urination at night
Post-micturitional: after urination bilateral
Nephrosis: distention of the pelvis and calicies of both kidneys with urine as a result of obstruction of the ureters
Hydroureter: abnormal distention of the ureter with urine due to obstruction from any cause

Transfusion Medicine Overview

Araba Afenyi-Annan and Monte Willis

Over the past 50 years, the discipline of Transfusion Medicine has truly evolved. Initially, the area of blood banking, that is, all aspects related to the collection, storage, and distribution of blood products, had been a predominant focus. Increased concerns about transfusion transmitted disease, led to improved donor screening and the use of nucleic acid testing to identify potentially infectious blood donors very early after infection. The move to component therapy rather than the use of whole blood resulted in increased inventory availability for patient care as well as improved blood product management. Quality systems, including computer laboratory information systems, have played an important role in ensuring the quality of blood products, reducing human error associated with the distribution of incorrect blood products to patients, and improving the turnaround time within which blood products can be provided to patients. With the discovery of the ABO blood group and elucidation of other blood groups, the area of immunohematology was born. Today, blood group serology remains an important and critical area of Transfusion Medicine, allowing for the appropriate labeling of blood products and selection of appropriate blood products to patients. Further, it has been instrumental in the evaluation of adverse effects of transfusion such as acute and delayed hemolytic transfusion reactions. The development of monoclonal antibodies for reagent cells has improved the accuracy and speed of testing patient samples. Testing has moved from the time, labor, and skill intensive tube method to include solid phase technologies which can be coupled with automated data entry systems. The area of transfusion practice has grown to assist clinicians on the appropriate use of blood products, patient evaluation and management with adverse effects of transfusion, as well as improved blood product support to specialized adult and pediatric patient populations. More recently, Transfusion Medicine has broadened to encompass tissue banking, therapeutic apheresis, and the collection, storage, and distribution of hematopoietic progenitor cells (HPCs). Those in the discipline must be well-versed in the pathophysiology of many disease processes, concepts of immunology, histocompatibility, human genetics, chemistry, and molecular techniques.

The cases incorporated into this section represent a spectrum of clinical scenarios involving several different acquired conditions/diseases and areas—immunohematology, blood group serology, and transfusion practice. The cases are arranged by general "Topic Area" followed by a more specific "Topic" to aid the reader in quickly identifying the case studies of interest to their needs.

Representative topic areas/diseases/conditions covered in this section include:

- Causes of discrepant blood typing

- Weak D

- Passively acquired anti-D

- Anti-Hr[b]

- Transfusion support for patients with antibodies to high frequency antigens

- Transfusion support for patients with rare antibodies

- Transfusion support for patients with rare phenotypes

- Delayed hemolytic transfusion reactions

- Positive direct antiglobulin test (DAT)

- Autoimmune hemolytic anemia (AIHA)

- Warm autoantibodies

- Cold agglutinin syndrome (CAS)

- Paroxysmal cold hemoglubinuria (PCH)

- Hemolytic Disease of the Newborn (HDN)

- Neonatal Alloimmune Thrombocytopenia (NAIT)

- IgA Deficiency

As our appreciation of the structure and function of human blood groups has increased, so has our understanding of their role in human disease. For example, the Duffy blood group antigen has long been known to be involved in hemolytic disease of the newborn and hemolytic transfusion reactions. Work in defining the susceptibility to malarial infection with *Plasmodium vivax* showed that the Duffy blood group antigen served as a receptor for malaria infection. A mutation in the promoter region of red blood cell (RBC) Duffy that normally binds the transcription factor GATA-1 leads to the Fy(a-b-) phenotype in people of African descent which is protective against RBC invasion by *Plasmodium vivax* and *P. knowlesi*. Further elucidation of the Duffy antigen structure led to the discovery that the Duffy antigen receptor was expressed on red blood cells (RBCs) as well as non-erythroid cells such as endothelium, brain, spleen, lung, and kidney and serves as a promiscuous chemokine receptor for both C-C and C-X-C type chemokines such as interleukin-8 (IL-8), monocyte chemotactic protein 1 (MCP-1), and regulated upon activation, normal T-cell expressed and secreted (RANTES). Chemokines are a family of small chemotactic cytokines that attract subsets of leukocytes to sites of inflammation. Based on this activity, the 7 transmembrane Duffy protein was renamed the Duffy Antigen Receptor for Chemokines (DARC). *In vitro* and *in vivo* studies suggest that the Duffy antigen expressed on RBCs may play a biologically active role as a chemokine sink and/or reservoir to prevent leukocyte activation in the systemic circulation and impede chemokine dissemination from the blood into other organs where these molecules can induce leukocyte release.[1] RBC Duffy has been implicated as a potential mediator of renal disease in patients with sickle cell disease (SCD)[2] and human immunodeficiency virus (HIV) infection,[3] and worse outcomes in renal transplant patients.[4] In addition, it has been associated with asthma, rheumatoid arthritis, and prostate cancer.[5] Other blood group antigens and disease associations include ABO and malarial infection by *Plasmodium falciparum*, Lewis antigens and gastrointestinal viruses and malignancy,[6,7] and Colton and priapism in SCD patients.[8] Therefore, the accurate determination of blood group antigens on RBCs has important clinical applications and implications beyond guiding transfusion therapy.

Currently, the detection of blood group antigens on RBCs is primarily determined serologically using specific antibodies to detect agglutination as an endpoint. Blood group antigens are made up of a variety of components, including glycolipids, glycoproteins, proteins, and carbohydrates. They can be intrinsic or extrinsic to the RBC membrane. Many advances have been made in understanding the genetic basis of blood groups. The genes and chromosomal locations of blood group systems are largely known, as is that of 17 human platelet antigens. The molecular basis of 29 of 30 blood groups has been clearly delineated (see **Table 1**). Differences in blood group phenotypes are commonly due to single nucleotide polymorphisms (SNPS) in the sequence of the genes encoding blood group structures. A tightly correlated genotype-phenotype relationship exists for most blood groups, allowing for the accurate prediction of blood group antigens by genotype. Blood group genotyping is more commonly being performed in cases where red cells cannot be typed due to auto-antibodies or a recent history of transfusion. Multiple applications of blood group genotyping have been realized in donor centers, reference laboratories, and transfusion services, as outlined in **Table 2**.

Several studies provide experimental proof that genotyping can accurately determine expression of platelet and blood group antigens. A number of common polymerase chain reaction (PCR) based methods are used to genotype the SNPs that determine blood group antigens. Initially genotyping of blood groups was performed by amplification of blood group gene sequences, followed by restriction fragment length polymorphism (RFLP) analysis, where the introduction or loss of restriction sites, were detected based on the SNP present. Next, PCR sequence specific primers (PCR-SSP) were developed, which only allow for production of a PCR product if the sequence of interest is present. However, these analyses are complex, labor intensive, and require post-PCR gel based analyses with inherent risks of errors and contamination. Further advances in PCR technologies have helped bypass these disadvantages and allow for automation by utilizing fluorescent PCR probe based systems. These systems analyze, in real time (as the reaction is occurring), PCR products based on their fluorescent products using DNA binding dyes such as SYBR green and TaqMan technologies. TaqMan assays have the added advantage of using dual-labeled hybridizing probes, including a quencher and flourophore, to ensure PCR primers are more specific. TaqMan has also been applied to the typing of human platelet antigens.[9] Other methods for genotyping blood group antigen SNPs include melting curve analysis as measured by a light cycler and pyrosequencing. Several of these methods allow for multiplexing, running a number of PCR primer pairs in parallel, which can be performed to determine multiple blood group antigens and adapted to analyze multiple samples.[10-13]

While the proof of concept for molecular blood group testing has been established, its application in the real world requires a high-throughput platform that can detect multiple SNPs in multiple blood group systems for multiple patients, donors, and blood products. A number of recent studies have demonstrated how high-throughput platforms, specifically microarrays, can be used to genotype blood group antigens.[14-17] These arrays utilize various forms such as red/infrared colored beads (Luminex XMAP platform), glass arrays (BLOODChip), 384 well plates (GenomeLab SNP), color coded beads (BEADchip), and 3072 bottom-less wells on a stainless steel plate where liquid is held by capillary action and hydrostatic forces (OpenArray, BioTrove Woburn, MA). These systems are summarized in **Table 3**. Large-scale validation studies have shown that high-throughput genotyping is generally very accurate.[14, 16, 17, 18, 19] However, the issue of rare false negative and false positive results, which is a general limitation of molecular technologies, remains. This can be due to the fact genotype may not always reflect phenotype for a variety of reasons. First, an unrecognized polymorphism not targeted by the SNPs of interest may suppress or inactivate expression of a gene. Secondly, the blood group antigen may not be the primary gene product so there may be an indirect relationship between the gene sequence and the blood group antigen. Third, exchange of DNA sequences between homologous genes may lead to variant gene products and the formation of novel blood group antigens. Finally, not all blood group antigens are a consequence of SNPs.[31] An additional, important finding from the large scale-validation studies is to the fact that our understanding of the variability of blood group genetics in larger populations remains incomplete.

Genetic Blood Group Typing: Advancing Transfusion Medicine

Several factors continue to drive the interest in genetic typing of blood group antigens. These include increasing costs of commercial reagents, the labor-intensive procedures associated with hemagglutination testing that require manual data entry, a lack of available antisera for some antigens, and antisera of insufficient volumes or reactivity for testing. Potential barriers to the widespread use of molecular testing include the fact that genotyping may not accurately predict phenotype (limitations described above), as well as lack of standardization of methods, lack of Food and Drug Administration (FDA) approval and regulation in this area, and the concern that current laboratory information systems may not be able to effectively incorporate these data. Today, serology remains the gold standard for blood group antigen identification. However, if blood group genotyping on high-throughput platforms becomes more economically feasible and these other remaining obstacles can be addressed, this could further revolutionize the area of transfusion medicine. If donors and recipients were genotyped for major and minor blood group antigens in less common but relevant systems, as well as high frequency antigens, and/or platelet antigens, individualized transfusion treatment could be provided. Improved antigen matching of blood products may potentially improve patient outcomes as seen in specific disease such as SCD.[20-22] Thus, high-throughput genotyping platforms that meet the high quality standards of blood banking and transfusion medicine may allow the transfusion medicine service to be practically 1 of the first areas in field of medicine to provide personalized therapy.

Table 1. The molecular basis of selected red blood cell group systems.

Blood Group	# of Antigens	Gene Name	Protein Function/Description	Chromosome	Molecular Typing Available?
ABO	4	ABO	Transferase A, alpha 1-3-N-acetylgalactosaminyltransferase; transferase B, alpha 1-3-galactosyltransferase	9q34.2	Yes
MNS	46	GYPA GYPB	Glycophorin A Glycophorin B (Transmembrane protein)	4q31.21	Yes
P	1	Unknown	Unknown	22q11.2 –qter	No
Rh	50	RHD RHCE	Transmembrane proteins	1p36.11	Yes
Lutheran	19	BCAM	Basal cell adhesion molecule	19q13.32	Yes
Kell	31	KEL	Metallo-endopeptidase	7q34	Yes
Lewis	6	FUT3 FUT2	Fucosyltransferases	19p13.32	Yes
Duffy	6	DARC	Chemokine receptor (transmembrane protein)	1q23.2	Yes
Kidd	3	SLC14A1	Urea transporter (transmembrane protein)	18q12.3	Yes

Adapted from: Veldhuisen B, et al., 2009.[23] The genetic basis of the following blood groups are also known: Diego, Yt, Xg, Scianna, Dombrock, Colton, Landsteiner-Weiner, Chido-Rogers, Hh, Kx, Gerbich, Cromer, Knops, Indian, OK, RAPH, JMH, I, Globoside, GIL, and RHAG.

Table 2. Applications of Molecular Testing in Transfusion Medicine

Donor Center	Reference Laboratory	Transfusion Service
• Identify D-negative donors	• Reagent RBCs for antibody detection	• Determine genotype in
• Identify RBC products for special patient populations, ie, patients with sickle cell disease, multiple alloantibodies	» Patient testing	» recently transfused patients
	• Determine dosage of RBC antigens	» patients with autoantibodies
	• Resolution of typing discrepancies	• Genotype fetal DNA to predict risk for HDN
• Expansion of rare donor program	• Predict presence of antigen when no antisera available	• RHD type to predict need for RhIG
• Provide genotypically matched products	» Evaluate risk of HDN	
	» Evaluate need for RhIG or D-negative blood products	• Genotype for human platelet antigen polymorphisms—diagnosis of alloimmune platelet destruction
	• Resolution of unusual serologic findings	
	• Differentiate between allo- and autoantibody	

SCD, sickle cell disease, HDN, hemolytic disease of the newborn, RhIG, Rh immunoglobulin.
Adapted from Hillyer et al., 2008.[24]

Table 3. High-throughput Genotyping Systems for Red Cells and Platelets

Technology	Array Type	Blood Group/Platelet Antigen GENES	Number of Antigens	# SNPs
Open array plates (BioTrove, US) with TaqMan Primers (Applied Biosystems, Inc.)	3072 bottomless wells	RHCH, FY, JK, LU, KEL, DO	6	10 [18]
Luminex xMAP (Luminex, Corp, USA)	Red/infrared beads	MNS, KEL, FY, JK, CO, LU	16	8 [17, 19, 25]
GenomeLab SNPstream (Beckman Coulter, USA)	384 wells	MNS, RHCE, KEL, FY, JK, HPA1, HPA2, HSP5	22	12 [26-29]
GenomeLab SNPstream (Beckman Coulter, USA)	384 wells	MNS, RHD, RHCE, KEL, FY, JK, D1 HPA1	19	12 [15]
BLOODchip (Progenika Biopharma SA, Spain)	Glass	ABO, MNS, RHD, RHCE, KEL, FY, JK, DI, DO, CO	47	116 [29]
Beadchip (Bioarray Solutions, USA)	Colored beads	MNS, RHCE, LU, KEL, FY, JK, DI, DO, CO, SC, LW	24	18 [30]

HPA, human platelet antigen, LU, lutheran; KEL, Kell; Fy, Duffy; Jk, Kidd; DI, Diego, DO, Dombrock; CO, Colton; SC, scianna, LW, Landstein-Wiener. Adapted from: Veldhuisen B, et al., 2009.[23]

To supplement the information provided in the case studies included in this section, readers are referred to the "Suggested Reading" section below for key books and additional articles related to the case study topics selected for inclusion in this section.

Suggested Reading

1. AABB. *Standards for Blood Banks and Transfusion Services*, 25th ed. AABB Press, 2008.

2. AABB. *Technical Manual*, 16th ed. editor John Roback. AABB Press, 2008.

3. Klein H, Anstee DJ. *Mollison's Blood Transfusion in Clinical Medicine*, 11th ed. Blackwell Publishing Ltd, 2006.

4. Hillyer C. *Blood Banking and Transfusion Medicine*. Churchill Livingstone, 2009.

5. Petrides M, Stack G, Cooling L, Maes L. *Practical Guide To Transfusion Medicine*, 2nd ed. AABB Press, 2007.

6. Harmening DM. *Modern Blood Banking And Transfusion Practices*, 5th ed. F A Davis Co., 2005.

7. Issitt PD, Anstee DJ. *Applied Blood Group Serology*, 4th ed. Durham: Montgomery Scientific Publications, 1998.

8. Reid ME, Lomas-Francis C . *The Blood Group Antigen Facts Book*, 2nd ed. Elsevier, 2004.

References

1. Rot A. Contribution of Duffy antigen to chemokine function. *Cytokine Growth Factor Rev.* 2005;16(6):687-694.

2. Afenyi-Annan A, Kail M, Combs MR, Orringer EP, Ashley-Koch A, Telen MJ. Lack of Duffy antigen expression is associated with organ damage in patients with sickle cell disease. *Transfusion.* 2008;48(5):917-924.

3. Liu XH, Hadley TJ, Xu L, Peiper SC, Ray PE. Up-regulation of Duffy antigen receptor expression in children with renal disease. *Kidney Int.* 1999;55(4):1491-1500.

4. Akalin E, Neylan JF. The influence of Duffy blood group on renal allograft outcome in African Americans. *Transplantation.* 2003;75(9):1496-1500.

5. Rot A, Horuk R. Chapter 9 the duffy antigen receptor for chemokines. *Methods Enzymol.* 2009;461:191-206.

6. Rowe JA, Opi DH, Williams TN. Blood groups and malaria: fresh insights into pathogenesis and identification of targets for intervention. *Curr Opin Hematol.* 2009;16(6):480-487.

7. Glinsky GV, Ivanova AB, Welsh J, McClelland M. The role of blood group antigens in malignant progression, apoptosis resistance, and metastatic behavior. *Transfus Med Rev.* 2000;14(4):326-350.

8. Elliott L, Ashley-Koch AE, De Castro L, et al. Genetic polymorphisms associated with priapism in sickle cell disease. *Br J Haematol.* 2007;137(3):262-267.

9. Ficko T, Galvani V, Rupreht R, Dovc T, Rozman P. Real-time PCR genotyping of human platelet alloantigens HPA-1, HPA-2, HPA-3 and HPA-5 is superior to the standard PCR-SSP method. *Transfus Med.* 2004;14(6):425-432.

10. Poulter M, Kemp TJ, Carritt B. DNA-based rhesus typing: simultaneous determination of RHC and RHD status using the polymerase chain reaction. *Vox Sang.* 1996;70(3):164-168.

11. Maaskant-van Wijk PA, Faas BH, de Ruijter JA, Overbeeke MA, von dem Borne AE, van Rhenen DJ, van der Schoot CE. Genotyping of RHD by multiplex polymerase chain reaction analysis of 6 RHD-specific exons. *Transfusion.* 1998;38(11-12):1015-1021.

12. Tax MG, van der Schoot CE, van Doorn R, Douglas-Berger L, van Rhenen DJ, Maaskant-vanWijk PA. RHC and RHc genotyping in different ethnic groups. *Transfusion.* 2002;42(5):634-644.

13. Wagner FF, Bittner R, Petershofen EK, Doescher A, Muller TH. Cost-efficient sequence-specific priming-polymerase chain reaction screening for blood donors with rare phenotypes. *Transfusion.* 2008;48(6):1169-1173.

14. Bugert P, McBride S, Smith G, Dugrillon A, Kluter H, Ouwehand WH, Metcalfe P. Microarray-based genotyping for blood groups: comparison of gene array and 5'-nuclease assay techniques with human platelet antigen as a model. *Transfusion.* 2005;45(5):654-659.

15. Denomme GA, Van Oene M. High-throughput multiplex single-nucleotide polymorphism analysis for red cell and platelet antigen genotypes. *Transfusion.* 2005;45(5):660-666.

16. Beiboer SH, Wieringa-Jelsma T, Maaskant-Van Wijk PA, etal. Rapid genotyping of blood group antigens by multiplex polymerase chain reaction and DNA microarray hybridization. *Transfusion.* 2005;45(5):667-679.

17. Hashmi G, Shariff T, Seul M, et al. A flexible array format for large-scale, rapid blood group DNA typing. *Transfusion.* 2005;45(5):680-688.

18. Hopp K, Weber K, Bellissimo D, Johnson ST, Pietz B. High-throughput red blood cell antigen genotyping using a nanofluidic real-time polymerase chain reaction platform. *Transfusion.* 2010;50(1):40-46.

19. Hashmi G, Shariff T, Zhang Y, et al. Determination of 24 minor red blood cell antigens for more than 2000 blood donors by high-throughput DNA analysis. *Transfusion.* 2007;47(4):736-747.

20. Vichinsky EP, Luban NL, Wright E, Olivieri N, Driscoll C, Pegelow CH, Adams RJ. Prospective RBC phenotype matching in a stroke-prevention trial in sickle cell anemia: a multicenter transfusion trial. *Transfusion.* 2001;41(9):1086-1092.

21. Tahhan HR, Holbrook CT, Braddy LR, Brewer LD, Christie JD. Antigen-matched donor blood in the transfusion management of patients with sickle cell disease. *Transfusion.* 1994;34(7):562-569.

22. Castilho L, Rios M, Bianco C, Pellegrino J Jr, Alberto FL, Saad ST, Costa FF. DNA-based typing of blood groups for the management of multiply-transfused sickle cell disease patients. *Transfusion.* 2002;42(2):232-238.

23. Veldhuisen B, van der Schoot CE, de Haas M. Blood group genotyping: from patient to high-throughput donor screening. *Vox Sang.* 2009;97(3):198-206.

24. Hillyer CD, Shaz BH, Winkler AM, Reid M. Integrating molecular technologies for red blood cell typing and compatibility testing into blood centers and transfusion services. *Transfus Med Rev.* 2008;22(2):117-132.

25. Hashmi G. Red blood cell antigen phenotype by DNA analysis. *Transfusion.* 2007;47(1 Suppl):60S-63S.

26. Denomme GA, Fernandes BJ. Fetal blood group genotyping. *Transfusion.* 2007;47(1 Suppl):64S-68S.

27. Avent ND, Martinez A, Flegel WA, et al. The BloodGen project: toward mass-scale comprehensive genotyping of blood donors in the European Union and beyond. *Transfusion.* 2007;47(1 Suppl):40S-46S.

28. Avent ND. Large-scale blood group genotyping: clinical implications. *Br J Haematol.* 2009;144(1):3-13.

29. Quill E. Medicine. Blood-matching goes genetic. *Science.* 2008;319(5869):1478-1479.

30. Karpasitou K, Drago F, Crespiatico L, Paccapelo C, Truglio F, Frison S, Scalamogna M, Poli F. Blood group genotyping for Jk(a)/Jk(b), Fy(a)/Fy(b), S/s, K/k, Kp(a)/Kp(b), Js(a)/Js(b), Co(a)/Co(b), and Lu(a)/Lu(b) with microarray beads. *Transfusion.* 2008;48(3):505-512.

31. Reid ME, Lomas-Francis C. *The blood group antigen facts book.* 2nd edition. Elsevier, 2004.

Blood Typing and Discrepancies

Laurie J. Sutor

Associate Professor of Pathology, UT Southwestern Medical School, Dallas, TX

Patient: 58-year-old male.

Surgical History: None.

Family History: Not pertinent.

Physical Examination: Unremarkable.

Chief Complaint: The patient donated blood for the first time and was told that he had blood type O, Rh positive. He became upset because when he was hospitalized 5 years previously, he was told he was blood type O, Rh negative. He did not understand why there would be a discrepancy in his blood type and he stated that the blood collection center made a mistake.

Medical History: Bleeding episode from peptic ulcer 5 years ago. Transfused 2 units of O negative red blood cells (RBCs). Otherwise healthy.

Drug History: Ranitidine for peptic ulcer disease.

T1. Principal Laboratory Findings

Test	Hospital (5 years ago)	Blood Collection Center (recently)
Blood type	O	O
	Rh(D) negative	Rh(D) positive
RBC Ab screen	negative	negative
DAT	n.d.	negative

RBC, red blood cells; Ab, antibody; n.d., not done; DAT, direct antiglobulin test.

Questions

1. What RBC antigens are routinely typed during pre-transfusion testing?

2. What conditions, if any, can cause a person's blood type to change?

3. What is another explanation, other than laboratory error, for a blood type discrepancy such as this in a healthy person?

4. What is the importance of identifying the presence of Rh(D) antigen expression in a blood donor?

Possible Answers _____

1. Pre-transfusion testing routinely looks for antigens in the ABO system as well as D in the Rh system. There are 4 common ABO blood types: A, B, O, and AB. Approximately 85% of United States blood donors express D antigen; 15% do not express D and are called "Rh negative."

2. Rare situations exist where a person's blood type may actually change. The most common cause of a blood type change is most likely a hematopoietic stem cell transplantation, where the bone marrow cells of 1 individual are replaced with hematopoietic tissue from another person. Hematopoietic stem cell donors must be matched to their recipient by HLA type, not necessarily by ABO or Rh type. Other rare instances of change in blood type have been recorded. The temporary phenomenon of acquired B antigen with bacterial sepsis changes individuals of blood group A into apparent blood group AB. Also loss of some ABO and Rh blood group antigen expression has been recorded in leukemia. None of these explanations are likely in an apparently healthy person.

3. The Rh(D) type discrepancy in this patient is probably explained by the phenomenon of weak D expression. The Rh(D) typing is performed in 2 steps. The first step, a sort of screening step, mixes anti-D reagent with patient cells and looks for red cell agglutination. Most persons expressing D antigen will test positive by this test. However, a minority of persons with D antigen has a lower number of antigen sites on their RBCs, which are thus not agglutinated by simple incubation with anti-D. These individuals have their D antigen detected only by a second level test using antiglobulin reagent to cross-link RBCs sensitized with the reagent anti-D. This test was called the Du test in past years, but the favored terminology now is to call it a test for weak D expression. Hospitals need only perform the first, screening level of D typing. If no expression of D is detected in this step, the hospital may simply call the patient D negative and transfuse them with Rh negative blood. This procedure saves considerable time and resources that would be needed to perform the second, antiglobulin step. The disadvantage is that more Rh negative blood is transfused than is strictly necessary. Blood collection centers, however, are required to test each donor for weak D expression if they have no reaction in the first level test. Therefore, many individuals who are told they were Rh negative during a hospitalization are actually Rh positive when fully tested in a blood donation situation.

4. D antigen, even in a weakly expressed form, may be able to stimulate anti-D formation when transfused to a D-negative individual. Further, recipients with anti-D may destroy at an accelerated rate transfused RBCs that weakly express D. Therefore, all levels of D antigen expression must be tested in order to properly label RBCs intended for transfusion.

Glossary _____

Blood typing: (Testing "phenotyping") of a person's red blood cells for surface antigen expression. Such antigens may be proteins, glycoproteins, or sugars and vary in expression from 1 individual to the next. The antigens are inherited in Mendelian fashion.

Rh blood group: A group of more than 40 different protein antigens, encoded on chromosome 1 and expressed only on red blood cells. Most persons express some combination of the 5 most common Rh antigens: D, C, c, E, and e. "Rh" comes from Rhesus monkeys which were used in early blood typing experiments.

D antigen: A Rh antigen expressed on the red blood cells of approximately 85% of United States blood donors. Although present in fairly low numbers on the red cell surface (around 20 000 copies per cell), this antigen is 1 of the most immunogenic red cell antigens known when transfused to a person lacking this antigen, stimulating anti-D in nearly 80% of cases.

Pre-transfusion testing: A panel of tests requested prior to transfusion of red blood cells, including ABO and Rh(D) typing and red cell antibody screening. It also may include antibody identification and crossmatching of donor units. The purpose is to ensure transfusion of compatible units; therefore, its synonym is compatibility testing.

Red antibody screen: A blood bank test that looks for "unexpected," clinically significant (usually IgG) antibodies to red cell antigens in patient blood samples. Reagent RBCs from 2 or 3 donors which display all clinically significant RBC antigens are incubated with patient serum or plasma. Antibodies to A or B antigens of the ABO system, which are tested for in the reverse typing for ABO, are excluded from the antibody screen by the use of only group O reagent red blood cells.

Direct antiglobulin test: Also called the direct Coombs' test. A blood bank test that detects immunoglobulin or complement molecules on the surface of RBCs. It is often a marker of immune hemolysis.

Suggested Reading _____

1. Mollison PL, Engelfriet CP, Contreras M. *Blood Transfusion in Clinical Medicine.* 10th ed. Oxford, England: Blackwell Scientific Publications; 1997.

2. Harmening DM. *Clinicial Hematology and Fundamentals of Hemostasis.* 4th ed. Philadelphia, PA: F.A. Davis Company; 2001.

3. McKenzie SB. *Textbook of Hematology.* 2nd ed. Baltimore, MD: Williams & Wilkins; 1996.

Discrepant Blood Typing Results in a 24-Year-Old Woman With a History of an Allograft Bone Marrow Transplant

AJ Goodwin, SL Dudley, SF Bushor, BR MacPherson, MK Fung

Department of Pathology, University of Vermont, Burlington, VT

Patient: 24-year-old woman.

Chief Complaint: New lesion on external genitalia.

History of Present Illness: Patient presented with new papules on vaginovulvar and perianal areas which were increased in size significantly compared to previous lesions. Pap smear at that time was unsatisfactory for analysis. The patient was unable to tolerate a colposcopic exam in office, and thus the procedure was performed in the operating room under general anesthetic. Preoperative blood type and screen performed in the blood bank was abnormal (see below). Biopsies of the lesion demonstrated condyloma acuminatum of the mons pubis, the posterior fourchette, and the labia minora. Cervical biopsy demonstrated high-grade squamous intraepithelial lesion (CIN III).

Past Medical History: The patient was diagnosed with acute myelogenous leukemia (M5 subtype) in 2001. She underwent induction and consolidation chemotherapy and remained in complete remission. Approximately 9 months later, she received an allograft bone marrow transplant. Her allograft bone marrow transplant converted her blood type from O-negative to A-positive, and this was the only information provided at the time of the blood bank type and screen. She now receives dialysis for chronic renal failure. Additional past medical history includes Wolff-Parkinson-White Syndrome with multiple arrhythmias and syncopal episodes. She is status-post 2 ablation procedures. She suffers from migraine headaches, which are well-controlled on Neurontin. She was diagnosed with bipolar disorder. She has a history of gastroesophageal reflux disease, acquired hypothyroid disease [not otherwise specified (NOS)], and deep venous thrombosis.

Past Surgical History: Surgical correction at 8 years of age for a congenital urinary abnormality of the collecting system including 2 ureters in the right kidney. She is status-post adenoidectomy and excision of an atypical mole.

Social History: The patient is married; has a healthy 8-year-old child; and smokes 0.5 pack-per-day, sporadically.

T1. Forward and Reverse Typing Reactions Using RBCs and Serum From the Patient and Known ABO Blood Types

	Forward Typing Antiserum[a]		Rh Type	Reverse Typing RBCs[b]		
ABO Group	Anti-A	Anti-B	Anti D	A_1	B	O
O	–	–		+	+	–
A	+	–		–	+	–
B	–	+		+	–	–
AB	+	+		–	–	–
Patient	4+	0	4+	1+	2+	

			Confirmatory Lectin Test			
	Lectin Test			A_1 Cells		A_2 Cells
Patient's RBCs	–			Lot 1	Lot 2	Lot 1	Lot 2
				4+	4+	–	–

[a]Commercially available anti-serum mixed with patient's RBCs. [b]Commercially available RBCs mixed with patient's serum. RBCs, red blood cells; +, agglutination of RBCs; –, no agglutination of RBCs.

Questions

1. How are the A, B, and O blood groups determined?

2. How should her current ABO blood type be reported?

3. Is there a discrepancy between her forward and reverse typing? If so what is the discrepancy?

4. What are some possibilities for the discrepancy?

5. What is the difference between blood type A subgroups A_1 and A_2?

6. How can this patient's blood typing discrepancy be resolved?

7. What is the most likely explanation for this discrepancy?

8. Does this discrepancy have any significance for her medical care?

Possible Answers

1. The **A blood type** is formed by the addition of N-acetyl-galactosamine (GalNAc) to the H antigen, the **B blood type** from the addition of galalctose to the H antigen, and the **O blood type** when no sugars are added to the H antigen. In the United States, 40% of the Caucasian and 27% of the African-American population are blood type A with the possible genotypes AA or AO. People with blood type A have naturally occurring antibodies against blood type B red blood cells, and these antibodies are predominantly IgM with a small amount of IgG. Unlike most IgM antibodies reactive only at the immediate spin phase of compatibility testing, the ABO IgM antibodies are clinically significant. In the United States, blood type O comprises 45% of the Caucasian and 49% of the African-American population. Only a single genotype (OO) exists for blood type O, and individuals with this blood group are considered "universal blood donors." However, serum from individuals with blood type O contains naturally occurring anti-A, anti-B, and anti-A,B antibodies, with significant amounts in the IgG form.

2. The forward blood typing results (**T1**) demonstrated that she is A-positive, corresponding to the allograft bone marrow transplant she received 2 years ago. Her reverse typing, however, demonstrated that she is blood group O, which was her original blood type prior to her bone marrow transplant. The procedure for forward (or cell) typing uses commercially available

anti-A and anti-B versus the patient cells. In reverse (or serum or back) typing, the patient's serum is tested against commercially available red cells. This form of typing assumes that a person has antibodies against antigens not found on their red blood cells. **T1** illustrates the reaction patterns in routine ABO typing. Her ABO blood group must be reported as indeterminate until further testing is completed. In addition, she must receive only blood group O red blood cells that are cross-match compatible until the discrepancy is resolved between her forward and reverse blood typing results.

3. Yes, she forward types as blood group A, but reverse types as blood group O.

4. The **first possibility**, of particular clinical concern, is that these findings represent repopulation of her bone marrow by her native bone marrow cells. In this situation, her original O-negative red blood cells along with circulating anti-A, anti-B, and anti-A,B antibodies would reoccur. This would be concerning in that she could eventually reject her bone marrow transplant or she might relapse into acute leukemia. A **second possibility** is that the patient may have been passively immunized via plasma-containing products. The half-life of antibodies (such as anti-D) administered to patients is 21 days, and thus a patient who recently received type O or type B plasma or plasma-containing products such as platelets, would have anti-A antibodies which may be detected in the reverse ABO-typing phase of testing. In such a situation, the direct Coombs test is often positive (as is the auto-control). These assays were performed on her sample, and both were negative, and thus it was concluded from the laboratory results that she did not receive blood products resulting in passive immunization. Nonetheless, a full transfusion history is necessary to confirm such a possibility. A **third possibility** for this finding is the presence of an immediate-spin reactive (eg, IgM) alloantibody against the A_1 typing cells. To determine if this is the cause, an antibody screen was performed and was found to be negative. A **fourth possibility** is that the transplanted blood group type is the A_2 subgroup. Type A blood has 2 subgroups, A_1 and A_2, and there is both a qualitative and quantitative difference. The A_1 subgroup contains more A antigen compared to

the A_2 subgroup and, of particular importance, the A_2 subgroups can make antibodies against an A_1 subgroup. In forward typing, the red cells from both an A_1 and A_2 subgroup will react with anti-A, but an ABO discrepancy may present with reverse typing as patients in the A_2 subgroup may show a reactivity against A_1 cells.

5. The difference between blood group A subgroups A_1 and A_2 arises from both biochemical and molecular etiologies. The *ABO* locus is found on chromosome 9 and controls for the 3 common alleles *A*, *B*, and *O*. The *A* and *B* genes encode for glycosyltransferases which determine the final antigen (immunodominant sugar) present on red blood cells. The *O* gene does not produce a functional enzyme, and thus RBCs from individuals with this gene lack A and B antigens. However, group O individuals do have abundant amounts of H antigen, the building block for the A and B antigens. The H antigen is added to RBCs by the product of the *H* gene, a transferase which adds fucose (Fuc) to the number 2 carbon of the terminal galactose of Type 2, 3, and 4 oligosaccharides found on RBCs. The H antigen is also added to Type 1 oligosaccharides which are found in secretions and plasma proteins by a similar fucosyltransferase encoded separately by the *Se* gene, which is located on chromosome 19. Once fucose is added, the *A* and *B* gene-specific transferases can add the immunodominant sugars. The transferase of the A_2 subgroups is less efficient at adding the immunodominant sugars to the GalNAc sites, and this transferase can only add them to Type 1 and 2 oligosaccharides. The transferase present in individuals with the A_1 subgroup is able to add them to Types 1, 2, 3, and 4 oligosaccharides, and it is able to do so much more efficiently than the transferase present in individuals with the A2 subgroup. It is these differences which result in increased A antigen expression on RBCs from individuals with the A_1 subgroup and is the basis for serological distinction between A_1 and A_2 blood types.

6. This patient's blood typing discrepancy can easily be resolved by testing with a lectin produced by the plant *Dolichos biflorus*. This naturally derived lectin is a glycoprotein with a molecular weight of about 120 kDa and consists of 4 subunits of approximately equal size. This

lectin has carbohydrate specificity toward linked N-acetylgalactosamine, and thus it is approximately 5,000 times more active in agglutinating blood group A_1 cells versus A_2 cells. In our patient, the results of this simple serological test will determine if her blood type following bone marrow transplantation was of the A_1 or A_2 subgroup. If she was an A_2 subgroup following her allograft bone marrow transplant then this would explain the discrepancy between her forward and reverse blood typing results. After performing the lectin test, the results indicated that she was transplanted with A_2 cells during her bone marrow transplant, and she has developed anti-A_1 antibodies (**T1**).

7. *Most likely explanation for patient's discrepant forward and reverse blood typing results:* prior allograft bone marrow transplant from a blood group A bone marrow donor of the A_2 subgroup and subsequent development of anti-A_1 by the patient who received this transplant.

8. Yes. In theory, because her serum contains anti-A_1 antibodies, one might believe that possible future red cell transfusions for this patient need to be performed using only A_2 red cells. In practice, however, anti-A_1 is seldom, if ever, a cause of hemolytic transfusion reactions and therefore of minimal clinical significance. However, anti-A_1 antibodies are usually IgM and cold reactive, and may interfere with immediate spin crossmatches with otherwise compatible A_1 red cells. Plasma-containing products are less of a concern as the A_1-type products will not contain any antibodies against A_2 red blood cells. In general, discrepancies between forward and reverse typing results require that the final interpretation of the patient's ABO blood type not be rendered until the discrepancy is resolved. If a patient requires immediate transfusion, O red cells of the patient's Rh type must be administered. Additional pretransfusion samples may be necessary to resolve the discrepancy and should be obtained.

Keywords

ABO discrepancy, lectin, Dolichos biflorus, H antigen, immunodominant sugar, alloantibody, allograft bone marrow transplant

References

1. Brecher ME. *AABB Technical Manual*, 14th ed. Bethesda, MD: American Association of Blood Banks; 2002: 271-285.

2. Mollison PL, Engelfriet CP, Contreras M. *Blood Transfusions in Clinical Medicine,* 10th ed. Boston:Blackwell; 1997: 481.

Aberrant Blood Grouping Results in a Patient With Splenomegaly and Thrombocytopenia

Nancy L. Sapanara, Vanlila Swami, Emmanuel C. Besa

Departments of [1]Pathology and Laboratory Medicine, and [2]Medicine, Medical College of Pennsylvania Hospital and Drexel University College of Medicine, Philadelphia, PA

Patient: 43-year-old male.

Chief Complaint: The patient presented to our outpatient laboratory for pre-operative blood work prior to splenectomy. He had persistent thrombocytopenia that was felt to be secondary to hypersplenism. An appropriately labeled blood sample was sent and received in the blood bank for type and cross.

History of Present Illness: The patient had presented 8 months earlier with anemia, thrombocytopenia, and splenomegaly. He was diagnosed with kappa light chain-restricted chronic lymphocytic leukemia (CLL) with high CD38 expression, Rai stage IV. Complete remission was achieved after treatment with cyclophosphamide, fludarabine, and rituximab.

Past Medical History: No significant history other than as above.

Physical Examination: The pertinent positive finding on physical examination was an enlarged spleen extending to the iliac crest. The patient was afebrile and without palpable lymphadenopathy.

T1. Patient's Forward and Reverse Blood Grouping and Rh Testing Results

Reaction Conditions	Forward Grouping		Rh Grouping			Reverse Grouping	
	Anti-A	Anti-B	Anti-D	Dᵘ	Rh control	A₁ Cells	B Cells
Immediate spin	0	0	0	0	0	0	0
Incubation 5 min, RT						0	0
Incubation 10 min, 3°C						0	0
Incubation 60 min, RT						vw+	vw+

RT, room temperature; 0, no reaction; vw+, very weakly positive

T2. Principal Laboratory Findings

Test	Patient's Result	"Normal" Reference Range
Hematology		
WBC count	12.1	$4.0\text{-}10.8 \times 10^3/\mu L$
Hemoglobin	14.3	14.0-18.0 g/dL
Hematocrit	42.9	42.0-52.0%
MCV	94.8	80-94 fL
Platelet count	33	$150\text{-}450 \times 10^3/\mu L$
Differential		
Neutrophils	69	42-75%
Bands	30	0-5%
Monocytes	1	5-10%
Chemistry		
Sodium	139	133-145 mEq/L
Potassium	4.2	3.3-5.1 mEq/L
Chloride	102	96-108 mEq/L
Bicarbonate	23	22-29 mmol/L
BUN	20	6-19 mg/dL
Creatinine	0.9	0.5-1.2 mg/dL
Glucose	90	70-110 mg/dL
Total protein	6.1	5.9-8.4 g/dL
Albumin	4.7	3.2-5.2 g/dL
Globulins*	1.4	2.5-3.5 g/dL
Blood Bank		
Antibody screen	Neg	Neg
Direct Coombs test	Neg	Neg

Calculated from total protein concentration – albumin concentration.
WBC, white blood cell; MCV, mean cell volume; BUN, blood urea nitrogen.

T3. Results of Additional Blood Group Antigen Testing

Test	Reaction With Blood Group Antigen			
	C	E	c	e
Patient's RBCs	0	0	4+	3+
Positive control	3+	2+	4+	2+
Negative control	0	0	0	0

0, no reaction.

4. What other tests can be done to confirm this patient's blood group and the presence of hypogammaglobulinemia?

5. What are other possible causes of ABO discrepancies?

Possible Answers

1. The discrepancy between forward (group O) and reverse (group AB) ABO blood typing results [**T1**]; decreased globulins; mildly increased WBC count; markedly decreased platelet count; and modestly increased blood urea nitrogen (BUN) concentration [**T2**]. The failure of expected agglutination reactions to occur during forward and reverse typing is called an "ABO discrepancy." Discrepant forward and reverse ABO grouping results should be brought to the attention of the blood bank director and reviewed in tandem with the patient's clinical history, which in this case, indicated the diagnosis, chronic lymphocytic leukemia (CLL). To enhance the reverse group reaction, the tubes were incubated at room temperature for 5 minutes, and at 3°C for 10 minutes. The results in all 4 tubes were still negative [**T1**]. Repeat testing provided the same results. While not standard procedure, the reverse group typing was repeated after a 60 minute incubation at room temperature, and the results were very weakly positive for both A_1 and B reagent RBCs [**T1**].

2. Hypogammaglobulinemia is known to occur in patients with CLL as a result of both leukemia-related immune dysfunction and therapy-related

Questions

1. What is (are) this patient's most striking laboratory result(s)?

2. How do you explain this patient's most striking laboratory result(s)?

3. What is this patient's blood group and Rh type?

T4. Possible Causes of Aberrant Blood Group Typing Reactions

Factors Affecting Typing Reaction

Type of Aberrant Result	Forward	Reverse
Positive	Acquired B antigen in patients with: • gastric or colon cancers • intestinal obstructions • other conditions (eg, inflammatory bowel disease; UTI with *E. coli* 086; pancreatic cancer, primary and metastic)	Unexpected antibody present in blood grouping reagent that may react with an unknown, unexpected patient antigen Genetic chimerism (cis-AB) (rare)
	Rouleaux formation due to: • elevated globulin • elevated fibrinogen • Wharton's jelly • dextran/plasma expanders	Unexpected ABO antibody in patient's serum such as: • anti-A1 in A subgroups (including A2B) • anti-B in cis-AB individuals • anti-H in A1 and A1B individuals
	Polyagglutination: • microbial-associated (ie, T polyagglutination) • nonmicrobial-associated (ie, Tn activation)	Rouleaux formation due to: • elevated globulin • elevated fibrinogen • Wharton's jelly • dextran/plasma expanders
	Autoagglutination due to: • potent cold autoantibodies	Unexpected alloantibody in the patient's serum that may react with an unknown, unexpected reagent RBC antigen
	Antibody-coated RBCs due to: • warm autoantibodies • transfusion reaction	Cold reactive allo- or auto-antibodies that may agglutinate reagent red blood cells
	Acrflavin antibodies	
Negative	Weak A or B subgroups causing weak or mixed field agglutination reactions or no reaction	Weak or missing antibodies in patients with: • hypogammaglobulinemia • newborn or elderly • immunodeficiency • innunosuppresion • congenital deficiency (agammaglobulinemai)
	Excess blood group-specific soluble substances in blood samples from patient's with: • gastric cancer • pancreatic cancer • mucinous ovarian cysts	Genetic chimerism (cis-AB) (rare)
	Antigen depression due to disease	

*Excluding technical and human error. UTI, urinary tract infection.

immunosuppression. The deficiency in humoral immunity is largely responsible for CLL patients' increased risk of infection-related morbidity and mortality, especially by encapsulated microorganisms.[1] The overall decrease in antibody production that occurs during immunosuppression also causes a decrease in ABO antibody levels. Weak, or missing, ABO antibodies due to CLL-related hypogammaglobulinemia are the most logical explanation for the failure of

the patient's serum to react against the A_1 and B cells at immediate spin. Moreover, hypogammaglobulinemia following rituximab therapy has been reported previously.[2-4] In each of these reports, however, the disease being treated was post-transplant lymphoproliferative disorder not CLL. Nevertheless, it is possible that rituximab therapy contributed to the development of hypogammaglobulinemia in the CLL patient. The decreased globulin value may also be a manifestation of the patient's hypogammaglobulinemia. An elevated WBC count may be related to a variety of conditions, including infection, stress (physical or emotional), and hematologic disorders. Thrombocytopenia may result from decreased production or increased consumption of platelets caused by immune- and nonimmune-mediated mechanisms. In this patient with marked splenomegaly, increased platelet sequestration by the spleen is the most likely cause of thrombocytopenia. Changes in intravascular volume due to hypogammaglobulinemia is the most likely cause of this patient's slightly increased blood urea nitrogen (BUN) concentration.

3. Group O, Rh-negative.

4. To confirm the patient's blood type, additional cell typing can be done to rule out the presence of an inhibitory substance in the patient's blood that could cause all reactions to appear negative. When we tested the patient's RBCs using anti-C, anti-E, anti-c, and anti-e antisera, his RBCs were found to have both c and e antigens, thus ruling out the presence of a global inhibitor in his blood [**T3**]. The patient's Rh phenotype is rr, the most common phenotype found in Rh-negative white (Caucasian) blood donors.[5] To confirm and characterize this patient's hypogammaglobulinemia, serum protein electrophoresis and/or quantification of serum levels of the 3 principal serum immunoglobulins, IgA, IgG, and IgM, could be performed. Quantification of these immunoglobulins in our patient's serum indicated a marked decrease in IgA [<14 mg/dL (reference interval: 81-463 mg/dL)], IgG [82 mg/dL (reference interval: 694-1618 mg/dL)], and IgM [<5 mg/dL (reference interval: 48-271 mg/dL)]. The etiology of hypogammaglobulinemia is often related to a hematologic malignancy such as CLL or lymphoma, but it may also be the result of immunosuppressive drug therapy (eg, after transplantation), congenital X-linked agammaglobulinemia, transient hypogammaglobulinemia of the newborn, or an immunodeficiency disorder.

5. The most common cause of an ABO discrepancy is human or technical error; however, other causes include weak or missing antibodies, weakly reacting antigens, unexpected antibodies or acquired antigens, rouleaux or agglutination due to plasma or protein abnormalities, and the presence of cold or warm autoantibodies [**T4**]. In general, reverse typing false negative results are more common than forward typing false negative results. Examples of **human or technical errors** that may result in an ABO discrepancy include mislabeled or misidentified specimens, mixed-up specimens, failure to follow correct procedures including failure to use the reagents properly and failure to add the appropriate reagents, contaminated reagents, and the use of cell suspensions that are either too heavy or too light. **Weak or missing antibodies** in the patient serum due to hypogammaglobulinemia can cause unexpected negative results on reverse typing. Incubation at room temperature, and at 3°C to 4°C if the reaction remains negative, may enhance the reaction between weak antibodies and their respective antigens. Although our sample was only initially incubated at room temperature and at 4°C for 5 and 10 minutes, respectively, other protocols require incubation at room temperature for 30 minutes and at 4°C, if needed, to further enhance the reaction.[6] Neutralization of reagent antibodies may cause weak or false-negative reactions on forward typing. In the presence of excess blood group-specific substance (BGSS), the reagent antibodies are neutralized, leaving minimal or no free antibodies to react with a patient's RBCs. If the sample is suspended in plasma or serum, repeating the test on the same sample suspended in saline may resolve the discrepancy by washing away the excess BGSS.[7] Excess BGSS has been associated with carcinoma of the stomach and pancreas.[7] There is, however, at least 1 case where excess BGSS was identified in the serum, cyst fluid, and ascites of a woman with mucinous cystadenoma of the ovary.[8] After surgical resection of the cyst, the serum BGSS returned to a normal level. Weak antigens are less common than weak or missing antibodies, but when encountered, they too may cause aberrant typing reactions. **Weakly reacting antigens** that may be present include subgroups of A and/or B. Group A is subdivided into A_1 and A_2 phenotypes, which together represent approximately 99% of group A individuals, and several rare A phenotypes, A_3, A_x, A_{end}, A_m, A_y, and A_{el}, which comprise the remaining 1%. The rare A subgroups may yield negative, weak, or mixed-field agglutination reactions upon testing with anti-A, putting the patient at risk of being mistyped as group

O. Similarly, B subgroups B_3, B_x, B_m, and B_{el} demonstrate variable reactivity to anti-B. The presence of **unexpected antibodies** may also produce confusing results. For example, anti-A_1 may be present in up to 8% of blood group A_2 individuals and in 22% to 35% of blood group A_2B individuals,[6] causing a positive reaction to A_1 cells during reverse typing. This discrepancy may be resolved by repeating the forward typing using anti-A_1 lectin reagent instead of the usual anti-A reagent. Group A_1 cells will react with both anti-A_1 lectin and anti-A, but group A_2 cells will only react with anti-A. A negative reaction with anti-A_1 will confirm the suspicion that one is most likely working with group A_2 cells. In addition to blood group A_2, some of the rare A subgroups can also produce anti-A_1. If a positive reaction to A_1 cells is observed on reverse typing and this finding is coupled with an absent or weak reaction to anti-A on forward typing, a patient will erroneously appear to be group O. Finally, an unusual case has been reported in which a transfusion-naïve blood group A_1 individual produced anti-A_1 autoantibodies.[9]

Acquired B antigens are another important, although uncommon, cause of ABO discrepancies. The B antigen is acquired as a result of bacterial enzymatic activity that modifies N-acetylgalactosamine, the immunodominant sugar on A red blood cells, to D-galactosamine. D-galactosamine is similar enough to D-galactose, the immunodominant sugar of B red blood cells, to cause reactivity with most anti-B reagents, but not with autologous anti-B. Acquired B antigens are most commonly seen in conditions where the breakdown of normal bowel mucosa allows bacterial enzymes to enter the systemic circulation. The underlying disease state is often gastric cancer,[10] colon cancer,[11] or intestinal obstruction,[7] but the acquired B phenomenon has been reported in patients with inflammatory bowel disease,[12] urinary tract infection with *E. coli* O86,[13] and pancreatic cancer[14] as well. ABO typing reactions may be misinterpreted as positive in the presence of rouleaux formation or polyagglutination. **Rouleaux** may be attributable to conditions in which there are elevated levels of globulin, such as multiple myeloma, elevated levels of fibrinogen, or in the presence of dextran, other plasma expanders, or Wharton's jelly.[7] In case of the latter, repeating the tests on the same sample after washing the patient's RBCs with saline may resolve the discrepancy by removing the Wharton's jelly. **Polyagglutination** is caused by an alteration in the RBC membrane that enables agglutination to occur in the presence of most ABO-compatible sera. Alteration of the RBC membrane may occur by microbial- or nonmicrobial-associated methods. In either case, normal carbohydrate residues are removed from the RBC membrane causing exposure of what are called hidden, or "cryptantigens." Cryptantigens then react to naturally occurring IgM antibodies in the patients' serum and cause agglutination.[15] **Cold autoantibodies** may be potent enough to cause agglutination of the patient's RBCs used in forward grouping, as well as the reagent cells used in reverse grouping. To resolve the forward grouping problem, the patient's RBCs could be incubated at 37°C, then washed with saline that has also been warmed to 37°C. If warming methods are unsuccessful, dithiothreitol (DTT) can be used to remove IgM-related agglutination.[6] For reverse-grouping discrepancies, the reagent RBCs may need to be warmed to 37°C before mixing with the patient's serum. If IgM-related agglutination still occurs, adsorption may be required to remove IgM antibody from the serum. **Warm autoantibodies** may also cause ABO discrepancies; however, they typically yield weaker reactions than those observed with cold antibodies. When warm autoantibodies are suspected to be the cause of false-positive results in forward grouping, elution may be required to remove bound immunoglobulin from the RBCs. Last, RBCs may become coated with warm antibodies after a transfusion reaction, secondary to the use of certain drugs such as alpha-methyldopa, or in patients with warm autoimmune hemolytic anemia.[7]

Patient Outcome

Given our patient's profound hypogammaglobulinemia, splenectomy was postponed so that he could first receive replacement doses of intravenous immunoglobulin (IvIg). Later, he underwent splenectomy with removal of a 1,550-gram spleen, without complication. It showed no evidence of CLL by histologic examination or flow cytometry. The patient's platelet count recovered; however, he remained hypogammaglobulinemic.

Keywords

ABO discrepancy, hypogammaglobulinemia, chronic lymphocytic leukemia, forward grouping, reverse grouping

References

1. Tsiodras S, Samonis G, Keating MJ, et al. Infection and immunity in chronic lymphocytic leukemia. *Mayo Clinic Proceedings*. 2000;75:1039-1054.

2. Imashuku S, Teramura T, Morimoto A, et al. Prolonged hypogammaglobulinemia following rituximab treatment for post transplant Epstein-Barr virus-associated lymphoproliferative disease. *Bone Marrow Transplantation*. 2004;33:129-130.

3. Castagnola E, Dallorso S, Faraci M, et al. Long-lasting hypogammaglobulinemia following rituximab administration for Epstein-Barr virus-related post-transplant lymphoproliferative disease preemptive therapy. *J Hematotherapy Stem Cell Res*. 2003;12:9-10.

4. Verschuuren EA, Stevens SJ, van Imhoff GW, et al. Treatment of posttransplant lymphoproliferative disease with rituximab: The remission, the relapse, and the complication. *Transplantation*. 2002;73:100-104.

5. Beadling WV, Cooling L, Henry JB. Immunohematology. In: Henry JB. *Clinical Diagnosis and Management by Laboratory Methods*. Philadelphia: W.B. Saunders; 2001:660-717.

6. ABO, H, and Lewis blood groups and structurally related antigens. In: Brecher ME, Ed. *AABB Technical Manual*. 14th ed. 2002;271-293.

7. Harmening DM, Firestone D. The ABO blood group system. In: Harmening DM. *Modern Blood Banking and Transfusion Practices*. Philadelphia: F.A. Davis; 1999:90-125.

8. Kominato Y, Fujikura T, Takizawa H, et al. Investigation of blood group A substance in the circulation of a patient with ovarian cyst. *Exp Clin Immunogenet*. 1991;8:24-28.

9. Rogers VB, Reid ME, Ellisor SS, et al. Auto-anti-A1: Another cause of ABO discrepancy. *Transfusion*. 1981;21:92-95.

10. Beadling WV, Cooling L, Henry JB. Immunohematology. In: Henry JB. *Clinical Diagnosis and Management by Laboratory Methods*. Philadelphia: W.B. Saunders; 2001:660-717.

11. Northoff H, Wolpl A, Bewersdorf H, et al. An ABO-blood group abnormality leading to the detection of a colon-carcinoma. *Blut*. 1983;46:161-164.

12. Roth S, Todd CE, Shaw D. Transient acquired blood group B antigen associated with diverticular bowel disease. *Acta Haematologica*. 1987;77:188-190.

13. Vojvodic S. Acquired B antigen in a pregnant woman belonging to the A1 blood group: Case report. *Medicinski Pregled*. 2001;54:490-492.

14. Itzkowitz SH, Yuan M, Ferrell LD, et al. Cancer-associated alterations of blood group antigen expression in the human pancreas. *J Nat'l Cancer Inst*. 1987;79:425-434.

15. Walker PS. Polyagglutination. In: Harmening DM. *Modern Blood Banking and Transfusion Practices*. Philadelphia: F.A. Davis; 1999:474-488.

Anti-D Antibody in the Serum of an Rh-Positive Vietnamese Woman

Mahnaz Shahidi-Asl, Karen C. Kirkley, Yuan S. Kao

Blood Bank, Department of Pathology, Medical Center of Louisiana, New Orleans, LA

Patient: 38-year-old woman.

Drug History: None.

Family History: Unremarkable.

Chief Complaint: A Vietnamese woman was admitted to the emergency room (ER) of our hospital for a gunshot wound to her abdomen and umbilicus with perforation of the transverse colon and small intestine. She was intubated and packed red blood cells (PRBCs) and fresh frozen plasma (FFP) were ordered by ER physicians. Initially, the blood bank did not know the patient's gender, age, or ethnic background. Because no blood sample was available for typing and crossmatching, blood components were issued under the "Emergency Release of Blood Products" protocol. Under this protocol, in the event of a severe loss of blood that threatens the life of the patient and prompts a request for uncrossmatched blood, O, Rh negative PRBCs are issued if the ABO/Rh type of the patient has not been determined. If there is difficulty in obtaining a blood sample or in determining the patient's ABO/Rh type, additional group O, Rh positive blood units will be emergency issued as needed.

Past Medical History: No information was available at the time of admission. Subsequently, the patient's husband indicated that she had no prior health problems, no history of pregnancy, and, to his knowledge, had never been transfused.

Physical Examination: Upon arrival in the ER, she was in shock with atrial fibrillation.

Principal Laboratory Findings: On the day of admission and over the next 2 days, the patient received the blood products shown in **T1**. After receiving 9 units of PRBCs on the day of admission, a blood sample was obtained for ABO/Rh typing and an antibody screen, with the results shown in **T2**. On day 7 post-admission, another blood specimen was obtained for repeat ABO/Rh typing and antibody screening which again demonstrated a mf-reaction of her RBCs with anti-B and anti-D antisera; however, the reaction was weaker between the patient's serum and known Rh(D) positive panel RBCs.

Questions

1. Based on the information in **T2**, what is the patient's ABO and Rh blood type?

2. Why did the patient's RBCs demonstrate mixed field agglutination with anti-D and anti-B antisera?

3. How is the presence of anti-D in the serum of an Rh positive person explained?

4. How do you explain the strong initial anti-D reaction of our patient's serum with Rh positive panel RBCs?

5. What other information pertaining to our patient would have been useful to know prior to

T1. Patient's Blood Product Transfusion History

Day No.	Patient's ABO/ Rh Status	No. of Units Transfused	ABO/Rh Type of Units		
			PRBCs	FFP	Platelets*
1	Unknown	9	O neg (8); O pos (1)	None	None
2	B/Rh(D)?	29	B neg (4)	B pos (8)	B neg (4); B pos (6); AB pos (7)
3	B/Rh(D)?	13	B neg (3)	B pos (10)	None

*Pooled from random donors. PRBCs, packed red blood cells; FFP, fresh frozen plasma; Rh(D)?, D antigen status unknown; neg, negative for D antigen; pos, positive for D antigen.

T2. Patient's Forward and Reverse Typing Agglutination† and Antibody Screening Results

Patient's RBCs Reacted With			Patient's Serum Reacted With		Antibody Screening
Anti-A	Anti-B	Anti-D	A_1 Cells	B Cells	
0	2+ (mf)†	1+ (mf)	4+	0	Positive*

*Antibody identified subsequently, using a panel of RBCs with known antigens, as anti-D. Ab, antibody, RBCs, red blood cells; mf, mixed field agglutination. †Grading of agglutination results was performed according to the criteria:[1]

Grade	Description
4+	one solid agglutinate, clear background
3+	several large agglutinates, clear background
2+	medium size agglutinate, clear background
1+	small agglutinates, turbid background
W+	tiny agglutinates, turbid background no agglutination or hemolysis
M+	negative macroscopically, a few (6 – 8) agglutinates in each microscop field
(mf)	mixed field; usually agglutinates in a "sea" of unagglutinated cells but can range from 4+ to micscopic
H	complete hemolysis, no cell remain
1+H	some hemolysis, button shakes out as 1+

T3. Relationship Between Serum Antibody (Agglutinin) Titer and Quantitative Antibody Concentration[5]

Agglutinin Titer, Units	Antibody Concn, mg/mL
1	0.0007
8	0.0056
64	0.047
512	0.38
4,096	3.0

Concn, concentration.

T4. Frequency of Rh Haplotypes in Various Ethnic Groups[6]

	Haplotype Frequency (%) in		
	Caucasians	African Americans	Asians
R^1 (CDe)	0.42	0.17	0.70
r (cde)	0.37	0.26	0.03
R^2 (cDE)	0.14	0.11	0.21
R^o (cDe)	0.04	0.44	0.03

Example: Frequency of r (cde) haplotype in Asians = 0.03% = 0.0003 = 3/1000 = 1/333 (1 in 333 Asians possess this haplotype).

the initial ABO/Rh typing performed on this patient's blood?

6. What should be done to clarify this patient's Rh type?

7. What is the frequency of Rh(D) antigen expression in different ethnic groups?

Possible Answers _____

1. Based on the mixed field (mf) agglutination observed with the patient's RBCs against anti-B and anti-D antisera and the strong (4+) reaction of her serum with known Rh(D)-positive panel RBCs, it was concluded that the patient was a group B, Rh(D)status unknown whose serum contained anti-D.

2. Mixed field agglutination is usually characterized by small agglutinates in a "sea" of unagglutinated cells but can range from 4+ to microscopically weak reactions. This patient's initial blood sample showed mixed field agglutination with both anti-B and anti-D antiserum because of the presence of 2 types of RBCs in the patient's blood—the patient's own group B and transfused group O positive RBCs—and the dilution effect on these cells caused by transfusion with 8 units of group O negative PRBCs.

3. The possibilities include: the "partial D" RBC phenotype with the presence of a weakly reactive antibody in the patient's serum that mimics the reaction of anti-D with Rh positive RBCs, passive administration of anti-D through a donor unit, false positive antibody screening reactions resulting from use of the wrong reagents, polyagglutinable red cells which may be agglutinated by any reagent containing human serum, autoagglutinins, and abnormal proteins in the patient's serum which may cause false-positive reactions when unwashed panel RBCs are tested. The concept that the D antigen consists of multiple, individually determined constituents arose from observations that some people with D-positive red cells produced alloanti-D that was nonreactive with their own cells. Red cells from these patient's lack certain antigenic determinants (epitopes) of the D antigen complex and have been referred to in the past as "D mosaic" or "D variant." Currently, this RBC phenotype is referred to as "partial D." In individuals with the "partial D" RBC phenotype, anti-D is produced against missing epitopes when the patient is transfused with RBCs containing these epitopes or acquires them during fetal-maternal hemorrhage. Weakly reactive anti-LWab or anti-LWa may mimic anti-D by reacting with D-positive cells but not with D-negative cells. A D-positive person whose serum contains a weakly reactive anti-LWa may be indistinguishable on initial serologic testing from an individual with a partial-D antigen who has made anti-D. Anti-LW can be easily differentiated from anti-D by testing the patient's RBCs against anti-LW and anti-D antisera after treatment of the RBCs with a sulfhydryl reagent such as dithiothreitol (DTT). The LW antigens are destroyed by DTT, whereas the D antigen is unaffected. In addition, anti-LW usually occurs in the serum of patients whose RBCs lack the LW antigen following transfusion or fetal-maternal transmission of RBCs containing the LW antigen.[2]

4. The possibility that the presence of anti-D in our patient's serum was due to the use of the wrong reagents during antibody screening was eliminated because the screening reactions were repeatedly positive. Moreover, monoclonal anti-D reagents were used in testing the patient's RBCs, thereby eliminating the possibility of polyagglutination as the cause of the D-positive reactions because polyagglutination only occurs with polyclonal reagents. In addition, serum from the patient's initial blood sample demonstrated the presence of a strong anti-D antibody; however, samples of blood from this patient taken later showed the gradual disappearance of anti-D from her serum. Thus, the most likely explanation for the initial presence of a strong anti-D antibody in her serum is that it was acquired passively during transfusion of a unit of O negative RBCs containing anti-D.

5. The patient's transfusion and pregnancy history is very important. Most Rh antibodies result from immunization during transfusion or pregnancy. In the Rh system, the D antigen is the most effective immunogen followed by c and E antigens. The D antigen may be the most potent immunogen of all RBC antigens. Various studies[3] have shown that when Rh negative individuals are transfused with 1 or more units of Rh positive RBCs, more than 80% of them will form anti-D antibodies in their serum within 2 to 5 months. Other studies[4] have indicated that when Rh negative recipients are transfused with 1 mL to 40 mL of Rh positive RBCs, 15% to 30% of these individuals will produce anti-D antibodies. Moreover, despite the high immunogenicity of the D antigen, 20% to 30% of Rh negative

individuals repeatedly exposed to the D antigen never form anti-D antibodies. These individuals are called "non-responders." If we assume that our patient is Rh negative and her husband's comment that she had never been transfused previously or been pregnant was accurate, the presence of anti-D in our patient's serum could not be explained by immunization during transfusion or pregnancy.

6. Retrospectively screen for the presence of anti-D in all 8 group O, Rh negative RBC units transfused to this patient. When this was done, anti-D was detected in 1 of these units—the unit that had been transfused approximately 30 minutes after her admission to the ER and prior to the collection of the initial blood sample for compatibility testing. Packed RBCs are prepared by removing approximately 80% of the plasma from a unit of whole blood. Between 200 and 250 mL of plasma are usually removed from units collected in Citrate-Phosphate-Dextrose-Adenine (CPDA-1) anticoagulant. An extra 50 mL of plasma can be removed from units drawn in CPD plus Adenine-Saline (CPDA-S). The PRBCs prepared from units collected with CPDA-S usually have only about 50 mL of plasma left in them. The donor PRBCs transfused to our patient were prepared in CPDA-S. Thus, despite the marked dilution of the approximately 50 mL of plasma, received by our patient from the single donor unit containing anti-D, by the patient's total plasma volume (approximately 3,000 mL), the patient's serum demonstrated the presence of a strong anti-D antibody. We speculate, therefore, that our patient passively acquired a relatively high concentration of anti-D antibody from transfusion of this anti-D positive donor unit. The serum concentration of an antibody is assessed by its titer. We did not perform an anti-D titer on our patient's serum. Therefore, we were not able to estimate the concentration of anti-D in the donor unit using the information provided in **T3**. However, the reactivity of the patient's serum with Rh positive RBCs after transfusion of 9 units of PRBCs and the administration of resuscitation fluid suggests a high concentration of anti-D in the residual plasma of the single donor unit of PRBCs positive for anti-D that was transfused to our patient. Unlike plasma products from donors whose serum contains alloantibodies, PRBCs from such donors can be used for transfusion.

7. Because the frequency of Rh haplotypes differs between various ethnic groups, the Rh genotype will also vary among these groups. Compared to Caucasians and African Americans, Asians have a very low gene frequency for the "r (cde)" haplotype [**T4**] which increases the odds of their being Rh(D) positive. Four months after being discharged, our patient was readmitted to the hospital for surgical reversal of a right-sided colostomy and revision of a tracheostomy scar. At that time, her preoperative blood sample typed as group B, Rh positive and her serum antibody screen was negative.

Keywords

anti-D antibody, ABO/Rh type

References

1. *Technical Manual*, American Association of Blood Banks (AABB), 11th ed. Bethesda, MD: AABB Press; 1993:612.

2. Lomas CG, Tippett P. Use of enzymes in distinguishing ant-LWa and anti-LWab from anti-D. *Med Lab Sci.* 1985;42:88-89.

3. Petz LW, Swisher SN, et al. *Clinical Practice of Transfusion Medicine*, 3rd ed. New York: Churchill Livingston; 1996:111.

4. Mollison PL, Engelfriet M, Contreras M. *Blood Transfusion in Clinical Medicine*, 10th ed., Oxford, England: Blackwell Science; 1997:169.

5. Wiener AS, Wexler IB, Hurst JG. The uses of exchange transfusion for the treatment of severe erythroblastosis due to A-B sensitization, with observations on the pathogenesis of the disease. *Blood.* 1949;4:537.

6. Mourant AW, Lpec AC, Domaniewska-Sobozak K. *The Distribution of Human Blood Groups and Other Polymorphisms*, 2nd ed. London, England: Oxford University Press; 1976:351-505.

A Rare Red Cell Phenotype in a 36-Year-Old Woman

Lisa Senzel, Christine Lomas-Francis

Laboratory of Immunohematology, New York Blood Center, New York, NY

Patient: 36-year-old woman.

Chief Complaint/History of Present Illness: Patient underwent a routine pre-surgery antibody screen and identification.

Past Medical History: Gravida 5, para 5; no history of transfusion; blood type O negative.

Questions

1. What is this patient's red blood cell (RBC) antigen phenotype?

2. What is unusual about this patient's RBC antigen phenotype?

3. What antibody is present in this patient's serum, and what is its significance?

4. Is this patient an immunologic "non-responder," since she never made an anti-k antibody despite 5 pregnancies and deliveries?

5. Should this patient receive k-negative blood even though she has not thus far made anti-k?

Possible Answers

1. (D-C-E-)c+/K+k-/Jk(a+b-)/Fy(a+b+)/Le(a-b+)/M-N+S-s+/P1-.

2. The patient's RBCs are K+k-. This phenotype has a prevalence of only 1 in 500. This patient's RBCs lack the k antigen, formerly known as Cellano, which is a high-incidence antigen. Only 0.2% of donors are negative for the k antigen. In contrast, 9% of donors are K+k+ and over 90% are K-k+.

The K- phenotype is correctly called "big K negative," but is colloquially (and incorrectly) called "Kell negative." This patient's phenotype is "little k negative." Although most laboratories do not perform phenotyping for little k antigen, antigen and antibody testing on this patient's blood was performed at a referral laboratory where the anti-k reagent was available for antigen typing.

3. The patient's serum contains anti-M reactive only at 4°C. A dosage effect is present, with only double-dose M+ (M+N-) cells showing reactivity. Many individuals have anti-M, and in many of these cases it has occurred naturally. In most cases of anti-M, the presence of this antibody is not clinically significant and can be ignored for transfusion purposes. On very rare occasions, however, potent IgG anti-M, that is active at 37°C, has caused hemolytic disease of the newborn (HDN). In addition, the rare patient with anti-M that causes agglutination of M-positive red cells at 37°C should be transfused with M-negative blood as a precaution. Most anti-M antibodies are IgG, but only react below body temperature in causing direct agglutination of M-positive red cells. About 20% of random donors are M-negative. Technical problems with this antibody in the compatibility test can usually be avoided by performing the test strictly at 37°C. This patient does not require M-negative blood.

T1. Patient's Serum Antibody Panel Results

| | RBC Antigen System | | | | | | | | | | | | | | | | | | | PAP/PEG/LISS | | | Saline | |
| | Rh-hr | | | | | Kell | | Kidd | | Duffy | | Lewis | | MNSs | | | | P | | | | | | |
RBC ID#	D	C	E	c	e	K	k	Jk^a	Jk^b	Fy^a	Fy^b	Le^a	Le^b	M	N	S	s	P1	37°C	IAT	CC	RT	4°C
1	+	+	0	0	+	0	+	0	+	+	0	0	+	+	0	0	+	+	0	0	3+	0	1+
2	+	+	0	0	+	+	0	+	0	0	+	0	+	+	+	0	+	+	0	0	3+	0	0
5	+	0	+	+	0	0	+	0	+	+	+	+	0	0	+	+	0	0	0	0	3+	0	0
6	+	0	+	+	+	0	+	+	0	0	0	+	0	0	+	0	0	+	0	0	3+	0	0
10	0	w	0	+	+	0	+	+	0	0	+	0	0	+	0	0	+	0	0	0	3+	0	1+
12	0	0	0	+	+	+	+	0	+	+	+	+	0	+	0	+	+	0	0	0	3+	0	1+
Auto Ctrl																			0	0	3+	0	0
Cord RBCs																						0	0
Phenotype	0	0	0	4+	4+	4+	0	4+	0	4+	4+	0	4+	0	4+	0	4+	0					

RBC, red blood cells; ID#, identification number; PAP, papain; PEG, polyethylene glycol; LISS, low-ionic strength saline; RT, room temperature; w, weakly (reactive); IAT, indirect antiglobulin test; CC, control cells; Ctrl, control.

4. Fetal-maternal hemorrhage (FMH) of at least 1 cc generally must occur for a woman to become immunized to fetal blood group antigens.[1] This amount of FMH is unusual, occurring in only 4% of all deliveries.[2] Even when this degree of FMH occurs, if the mother is blood group O and the baby is another ABO type, fetal cells may be rapidly cleared from the maternal circulation because of maternal anti-A,B. Finally, this woman received Rh immune globulin after all pregnancies, making it unlikely that she would become immunized to D antigen, and possibly preventing exposure to other fetal red cell antigens as well. Therefore, based on her history, we cannot predict whether she is a "non-responder."

5. In some countries, but not in the United States, girls and women in their childbearing years are given blood matched not only for ABO and D, but for Kell and for Rh antigens as well.[3] However, when extensively phenotyped-matched blood is given to patients who are not immunized to red cell antigens, this can deplete the supply of rare blood, which is needed for those patients who are alloimmunized. Usual practice dictates giving k-antigen-positive blood for this patient and reserving k-negative blood for the future in case she does form anti-k. On the other hand, if the patient plans to have more children, transfusion with k-positive blood could lead to her forming anti-k, which could subsequently cause HDN. The few reports of HDN due to anti-k were in previously transfused women.[4,5] Ideally, the patient should donate autologous units to be stored as frozen blood. Her siblings should be tested, and if k-negative, should be asked to become donors of rare blood. If this patient does form anti-k and requires k-negative blood, the frequency of O-negative, k-negative donors would be ~3 in 10,000 ($0.15 \times 0.002 = 0.0003$) O donors.

Keywords

phenotype, Kell, anti-k, hemolytic disease of the newborn, non-responder

References

1. Ochsenbein-Imhof N, Ochsenbein AF, Seifert B, et al. Quantification of fetomaternal hemorrhage by fluorescence microscopy is equivalent to flow cytometry. *Transfusion.* 2002;42:947-953.

2. Sebring ES, Polesky HF. Fetomaternal hemorrhage: incidence, risk factors, time of occurrence, and clinical effects. *Transfusion.* 1990;30:344-357.

3. International forum of authors. Red cell transfusions and blood groups. *Vox Sang.* 2004;87:210-222.

4. Mollison PL, Engelfriet CP, Contreras M. *Blood Transfusion in Clinical Medicine.* Cambridge, MA: Blackwell Science; 1997:417.

5. Bowman JM, Harman FA, Manning CR, et al. Erythroblastosis fetalis produced by anti-k. *Vox Sang.* 1989;56:187-189.

A 43-Year-Old Postpartum Woman With a Rare Antibody

Eiad Kahwash, Jill Leonard, Lisa Machor, William Lockwood

Department of Pathology and Laboratory Medicine, University of Louisville, Louisville, KY

Patient: 43-year-old, gravida IX/para 8008 African American woman.

Family History: Unremarkable.

Surgical History: Unremarkable.

History of Present Illness: The patient was admitted to the labor and delivery service at 39 4/7 weeks gestational age for induction of an intrauterine pregnancy. She followed a normal labor curve and delivered a live viable male infant with Apgar scores of 9 and 9. Her postpartum course was uncomplicated. On postpartum day 2, her vital signs were stable, her lungs were clear, breasts were non-tender, her legs showed no cyanosis or edema, and the fundus was normal. She was afebrile, ambulating, had good urine output, and her pain was well controlled.

Past Medical History: Chronic hypertension, a history of postpartum hemorrhage requiring red blood cell transfusion, a positive serum antibody screen for anti-C, and no history of allergies.

Drug History: Prenatal vitamins (1 tablet/day), Motrin (600 mg tablets; 1 every 6 hours), Colace (100 mg tablets; 1/day), and iron sulfate (300 mg tablets, twice/day with meals).

Questions

1. What is (are) this patient's most striking laboratory result(s)?

2. How do you explain this patient's most striking laboratory result(s)?

3. What is anti-hr^B?

4. What antigens can be associated with the hr^B- antigen?

5. What type of blood should be transfused to patients with anti-hr^B in their serum? Why?

6. What blood type would be most appropriate for transfusion of the patient presented in this case study? Why?

Possible Answers

1. The patient's most striking laboratory results are decreased hemoglobin and a positive antibody screen for anti-hr^B.

2. Her mild anemia is probably related to her pregnancy. The increase in plasma volume that occurs in pregnant women is relatively greater than the concomitant increase in RBC mass resulting in hemodilution and a decrease in hemoglobin concentration.[1] The increased blood volume serves 2 purposes: it facilitates fetal and maternal exchange of respiratory gases, nutrients,

T1. Principal Laboratory Findings

Test		Patient's Result	"Normal" Reference Range
Hematology			
Hemoglobin		10.9	12-16 g/dL
Hematocrit		32.0	33.5-46.1%
Platelet count		265	150-400 x 10³/mL
White blood cell count		5.9	4.0-11.0 x 10³/mL
Differential:	neutrophils	62.2	40-60%
	lymphocytes	26.5	20-40%
	eosinophils	1.3	0.0-5.0%
	monocytes	10	2.0-8.0%
MCV		81.9	81.2-98.3 fL
Blood Bank			
ABO/Rh type O positive		n.a.	
Indirect antibody screen		Positive	Negative
Antibody identification		Anti-hrB	n.a.
Direct antiglobulin test		Negative	Negative
IgG		Negative	Negative
C₃d		Negative	Negative
Eluate		Not Indicated	Negative

MCV, mean corpuscular volume; n.a., not applicable.

and metabolites; and it reduces the impact of maternal blood loss at delivery. Anti-hr^B, a rare antibody, has been found exclusively in the serum of individuals who have been transfused previously with donor red blood cells, most of whom were pregnant women.

3. Anti-hr^B is an antibody to a partial e-antigen. The e-antigen consists of several epitopes and is a high incidence antigen that is found in more than 98% of the general population. It is called "partial e-antigen" when it lacks 1 or more of its epitopes, a situation seen more often in African Americans than in whites.[2] Shapiro and colleagues first described anti-hr^B in 1972.[3] These investigators found a serum sample that reacted with all red blood cells but with a weaker reaction with R2R2 cells (DcE/DcE) than with e-antigen positive red blood cells. The serum contained antibody activity against a majority of e-antigen

positive RBCs and the antibody isolated from this serum was named anti-hr^B. Subsequently, it was noted that anti-hr^B was found in the serum of many African Americans with sickle cell disease who had received multiple RBC transfusions. However, hr^B-antigen is not the only partial e-antigen that has been found. The hr^S-antigen is another partial e-antigen. Therefore, the designations e-positive/hr^B-negative and e-positive/hr^S-negative have been applied to those individuals whose red blood cells are e-positive but lack hr^B or hr^S antigen, respectively. It had been noted that not all red blood cells with partial e-antigen react with anti-hr^B and anti-hr^S antibodies. Thus, it is believed that the hr^B and hr^S antigens are not the only partial e-antigens, leading to the use of the terms, anti-hr^B- and anti-hr^S-like antibodies. It is also important to note that individuals have been identified whose RBCs are partial e-antigen positive and both hr^B- and hr^S-antigen negative.[2]

4. The majority of individuals whose RBCs are hr^B-antigen negative are VS-antigen positive, suggesting a possible antithetical relationship between the hr^B and VS antigens.[4] However, individuals whose RBCs are both hr^B- and VS-antigen negative have been identified.[2] Therefore, it appears that the hr^B- and VS-antigens are encoded by different alleles, suggesting that a third allele exists. Another possibility is that the genetic arrangement that produces the VS-antigen often, but not always, results in lack of production of the hr^B-antigen.

5. ABO- and Rh-specific, hr^B-antigen negative RBCs because anti-hr^B defines an antigen of high frequency in the Rh system that has been reported to be associated with severe transfusion reactions.[5] Blood units for transfusion of individuals whose serum contains anti-hr^B may be found by crossmatching blood units from hr^B-antigen negative donors with the patient's ABO type and Rh group and selecting only those units that are non-reactive with the patient's serum. Due to the rarity of the hr^B-antigen negative blood type however, patients with anti-hr^B should consider autologous blood donation in anticipation of any future blood needs and should register in the American Rare Donor Program. In addition, family members, especially siblings, should be screened as possible sources of additional hr^B-antigen negative blood.

Serum from the patient presented in this case study contains anti-hr^B; however, there was no current evidence of her serum containing anti-C. The previously identified anti-C reported by our hospital's laboratory was not detectable at the Red Cross laboratory. Since anti-hr^B typically reacts strongly with R_1R_1 RBCs and weakly with R_2R_2 RBCs, our laboratory may have been seeing the anti-hr^B all along. Blood units for transfusion of the patient could be found by crossmatching C- and hr^B-antigen negative donors of the patient's ABO type (O) and Rh group (Rh-positive) and selecting only those units whose RBCs are non-reactive with the patient's serum. Based on the frequency of the C- and hr^B-antigens in the general population (ie, 32% of all Caucasians are C-antigen negative and less than 2% are hr^B-antigen negative), the percentage of C- and hr^B-antigen negative individuals in the overall population of blood donors is less than 1%.[6] Moreover, because blood units from hr^B-antigen negative donors are so rare, the blood supplier should be kept informed of any antici-pated need for RBC components in individuals whose serum contains anti-hr^B.

Acknowledgment

Supported in part by the Norton Healthcare Community Trust Fund #22-07.

Keywords

Partial e-antigen, anti-hr^B

References

1. The Merck Manual of Medical Information. Home edition. Section 22. Women's health issues. Section 22, Chapter 257. http://www.merck.com/mrkshared/mmanual_home/ sec 22/243.jsp. Accessed May 7, 2004.

2. Issitt PD, Anstee DJ. *Applied Blood Group Serology*. 4th ed. 1998;369-376.

3. Shapiro M, LeRoux M, Brink S. *Haematologia*. 1972;6:121.

4. Blancher A, Ried ME, Tossas E, et al. (abstract). *Transfusion*. 1995;35:23S.

5. Ried ME, Øyen R, Marsh WL. *Seminars in Hematology*. 2000;37:203.

6. American Association of Blood Banks. *Technical Manual*, 14th ed. Rh system. 2002;14:297.

A 24-Year-Old Woman With Abdominal Pain

Pete Pelletier

Department of Clinical Laboratory Sciences, Northern Michigan University, Marquette, MI

Patient: 24-year-old woman.

Surgical History: None.

Family History: Unremarkable.

Chief Complaint: Abdominal pain.

Social History: She denied the use of alcohol, tobacco, or illicit drugs.

History of Present Illness: The patient presented to the emergency department (ED) with right upper quadrant pain. Ultrasound examination of the liver, gallbladder, and biliary tract was unremarkable, and a cholelescintigraph [heptoiminodiacetic acid (HIDA) scan] demonstrated a decreased ejection fraction of 7%. She was admitted to surgery and underwent a laparoscopic cholecystectomy the next day. She appeared to do well post-operatively; however, her hemoglobin dropped from 13.4 g/dL (reference interval: 12.9-15.5 g/dL) pre-operatively to 8.6 g/dL post-operatively. She subsequently developed symptoms of lethargy and weakness.

Medical History: The patient was a G1P1 woman who had an unremarkable vaginal delivery 4 years prior to this ED visit. She denied any history of previous blood or blood product transfusions.

Physical Examination: Moderate abdominal tenderness concentrated in the right upper quadrant, with a very positive Murphy's sign (a sign of gallbladder disease associated with interruption of the patient's deep inspiration when the physician's fingers are pressed deeply beneath the right costal arch below the hepatic margin).

T1. Principal Laboratory Findings

Test	Patient's Result	Reference Interval
Blood Bank		
ABO/Rh type	O positive	n.a.
Indirect antibody screen	positive	negative
Antibody identification	anti-Rh17	n.a.

n.a., not applicable.

Questions

1. What is (are) this patient's most significant laboratory finding(s)?

2. How do you explain the patient's most striking laboratory finding(s)?

3. What are some of the clinical and transfusion medicine-related implications associated with the presence of this antibody in the patient's serum?

T2. Patient's Family Members and Patient's Antigen Screening Results

Family Member	RBC Antigen Tested												
	D	C	c	E	e	S	s	K1	k	Fya	Fyb	Jka	Jkb
Mother	+	0	0	0	0	+	0	+	0	+	+	+	0
Father	+	0	+	+	0	+	+	+	+	+	+	+	0
Sister #1	+	0	0	0	0	+	+	+	+	+	+	+	0
Sister #2	+	0	+	+	0	+	0	+	0	+	+	+	0
Sister #3	+	0	+	+	0	+	+	+	0	+	0	+	0
Patient	+	0	0	0	0	+	+	+	+	+	+	+	0

RBC, red blood cell; +, positive; 0, negative.

4. What are the most appropriate actions for the laboratory and clinical staff?

5. Which of this patient's family members are suitable as blood donors for this patient?

6. How does the D—deletion phenotype occur?

7. What is the antigen specificity of an antibody made by a D—individual sensitized by RhCE-positive red blood cells?

Possible Answers

1. The significant post-operative decrease in her hemoglobin concentration and a positive antibody screen for anti-Rh17.

2. Her anemia is the result of post-operative blood loss and hemodilution from intravenous (IV) fluids administered during laparoscopy. Although laparoscopy is a minimally invasive procedure, a small percentage of patients who undergo this procedure can experience marked blood loss. Nearly all patients who undergo laparoscopy are given IV fluids. This results in an increase in blood volume and subsequent hemodilution. The presence of anti-Rh17, a rare alloantibody, is most likely due to sensitization during her prior pregnancy. Since the Rh phenotype of the patient is D—, exposure to fetal cells possessing normal Rh antigens (C, c, E, e) would provide an adequate sensitizing event.[1]

3. Anti-Rh17 (anti-Hr_o) is a monospecific IgG alloantibody, which reacts with a common determinant on the RhCE protein. This antibody is detected best with antiglobulin testing, and will react with both normal and enzyme-treated red blood cells.[2] Moreover, this antibody has been implicated in transfusion reactions, as well as mild to severe hemolytic disease of the newborn. Due to anti-Rh17's specificity, blood products must be of a compatible Rh deletion phenotype and lack RhCE antigens.[3] The American Red Cross (ARC) lists the frequency of compatible donor units for patients with anti-Rh17 in their plasma as <1 compatible unit/10,000 donor units, the lowest frequency category used by the ARC when categorizing the availability of recipient-compatible blood units/products.

4. Given the possible transfusion conundrum related to an antibody against such a high frequency antigen, it is important to act fast in resolving the situation. Communication between the clinical and laboratory staff is essential. Every attempt must be made to limit any additional blood loss. This includes restricting the number and volume of blood draws. Surgery is generally contraindicated. If surgery is the only lifesaving option, use of an intraoperative blood salvaging device is essential. Due to the patient's rare Rh phenotype and the genetics of the Rh blood group antigens, all available family members should be evaluated by antigen typing to find a possible blood donor.

5. The patient's mother and sister #1, because only the red blood cells of these immediate family members were negative for the RhCE antigens (T2).

6. The genetic events which produce the D-- phenotype are not completely defined. The current understanding is that recombination of portions of the RhD gene with the RhCE gene accounts for the overexpression of RhD antigens and the lack of RhCE antigens. Previously, it was thought that the D-- phenotype could only be inherited by consanguineous homozygosity; however, inheritance by compound heterozygosity has also been recently demonstrated.[4] Although molecular gene analysis would be necessary to confirm the pattern of inheritance in our patient, the familial antigen types of our patient's first-degree family members (**T2**) suggest inheritance by compound heterozygosity.

7. Since the RhCE antigens include the Rh17 antigen determinant, anti-Rh17 is capable of reacting with any cells containing the CcEe antigens. Owing to the lack of uniformity in genetic recombinant events, the extent of recombination varies from 1 individual to the next. Consequently, not all D-- individuals produce identical alloantibodies following a sensitizing event with cells containing RhCE antigens. The specific alloantibody produced by any individual is governed in part by the nature of that individual's recombination event and the sensitizing immunogen to which the individual is exposed. As a result, not all anti-Rh17 alloantibodies are created equal, but they are capable of reacting with all forms of the RhCE antigen (ie, C, c, E, and e antigens).[5]

Treatment and Course

The patient recovered without the need for blood transfusion and was advised to enroll in the rare donor program offered by the ARC.

Acknowledgment

The author thanks Portneuf Medical Center, Pocatello, ID, for their cooperation with this case.

Keywords

anti-Rh17, Rh deletion phenotype, alloantibody, consanguineous homozygosity, compound heterozygosity

References

1. Issit PD, Anstee DJ. *Applied Blood Group Serology.* 4th ed. Miami: Montogomery Scientific Publishers. 1998;376-378.

2. American Association of Blood Banks. *Technical Manual,* 14th ed. Rh System. 2002;14:306-307.

3. Avent ND, Reid ME. The Rh blood group system: A review. *Blood.* 2000;95-2:375-384.

4. Huang CH, Peng J, Chen HC, et al. RH locus contraction in a novel Dc-/D-- genotype resulting from separate genetic recombination events. *Transfusion.* 2004;44:853-858.

5. Denomme GA, Ryan G, Seaward PGR, et al. Maternal ABO-mismatched blood for intrauterine transfusion of severe hemolytic disease of the newborn due to anti-Rh17. *Transfusion.* 2004;44:1357-1359.

An Antibody Against a High Frequency Antigen

Peter Bauer, Eiad Kahwash, Dave Krugh, Melanie S. Kennedy

Department of Pathology, The Ohio State University, Columbus, OH

Patient: 42-year-old Caucasian woman.

Allergies: Lisinopril.

History of Present Illness: The patient initially presented to an outside hospital with a 5-week history of persistent cough, hyperglycemia, a worsening right plantar foot ulcer which formed following a local burn, and symptoms attributable to chronic renal insufficiency (CRI). The foot ulcer and symptoms of CRI were considered complications of previously diagnosed type II insulin-dependent diabetes mellitus. Despite intravenous antibiotic therapy and radiographic studies that were negative for osteomyelitis, the patient's clinical status progressively worsened ultimately leading to septic shock, presumably stemming from the infected foot ulcer. An unexplained normochromic, normocytic anemia was also noted. The patient was subsequently transferred to our facility for further treatment.

Chief Complaint: Multiple organ system dysfunction. It was discovered that the patient had been anemic over the last year with a hemoglobin value averaging 7 to 8 g/dL (normal reference interval: 12 to 16 g/dL) and had been taking oral vitamins and iron supplements. The last red blood cell transfusion the patient recalled receiving occurred during coronary artery bypass graft surgery a few years prior to her current admission date.

Past Medical History: Significant for severe coronary artery disease and distant myocardial infarction, both complicated by ischemic cardiomyopathy and congestive heart failure (ejection fraction averaging 31%, normal reference interval: 45% to 70%), type II diabetes requiring insulin, hypertension, and hypothyroidism.

Past Surgical History: Coronary artery bypass graft of 5 vessels, right transmetatarsal amputation of the second through the fifth toe on her right foot due to gangrene and abscess formation.

Medications: Current medications included ciprofloxacin, nafcillin, simvastatin, pioglitazone, losartan, synthroid, carvedilol, ranitidine, dopamine drip, and an insulin regimen.

Social History: She denied the use of alcohol, tobacco, or illicit drugs.

Family History: Father: coronary artery disease; Mother: diabetes, hyperlipidemia, and hypertension.

Review of Systems: Negative for bleeding, bruising, epistaxis, hematemesis, melena, hematuria, or back pain.

T1. Principal Laboratory Findings

Test	Patient's Result	"Normal" Reference Interval
Arterial Blood Gases		
pH	7.48	7.35-7.45
pCO$_2$	30.6	21-48 mm Hg
pO$_2$	52.7	80-100 mm Hg
HCO$_3$	22.6	22-26 mmol/L
Total CO$_2$	23.5	19-24 mmol/L
O$_2$ saturation	90.5	94-98%
Hematology		
WBC count	4.7	4.0-10.0 × 10^3/μL
RBC count	2.52	4.2-5.4 × 10^6/μL
Hemoglobin	7.6	12.0-16.0 g/dL
Hematocrit	23.9	37-47%
MCV	94.7	82-99 fL
MCHC	31.9	32-36 g/dL
RDW	22.5	11.5-14.5%
Platelet count	126	150-400 × 10^3/μL
Reticulocyte count	7.4	0.2-2.0%
Blood smear evaluation	Granulocytosis with left shift (myelocytes and metamyelocytes), toxic granulation, and an occasional Dohle body; normocytic, normochromic RBCs with mild anisopoikilocytosis; unremarkable platelet morphology	
Chemistry		
Sodium	143	132-146 mmol/L
Potassium	4.3	3.3-5.3 mmol/L
Chloride	114	96-106 mmol/L
CO$_2$	23	24-30 mmol/L
Anion gap	11	8-12
BUN	12	12-24 mg/dL
Creatinine	1.89	0.70-1.30 mg/dL
Glucose	108	65-115 mg/dL
Phosphorus	3.8	2.5-4.5 mg/dL
Magnesium	1.8	1.8-2.5 mg/dL
Calcium	9.0	8.6-10.4 mg/dL
Haptoglobin	33	20-320 mg/dL
LD	215	0-199 U/L
Osmolality	300	280-300 mOsm/kg
Coagulation		
PT	16.5	12.0-15.0 sec
INR	1.4	0.8-1.2
PTT	31	23-32 sec
Microbiology		
Blood culture	Coagulase-negative	
Staphylococcus spp.	No growth	

WBC, white blood cell; RBC, red blood cell; MCV, mean corpuscular volume; MCHC, mean corpuscular hemoglobin concentration; RDW, red blood cell distribution width; BUN, blood urea nitrogen; LD, lactate dehydrogenase; PT, prothrombin time; INR, international normalized ratio; PTT, partial thromboplastin time.

T2. Principal Blood Bank Findings

Test	Patient's Result
ABO/Rh(D) typing	A positive
Antibody screen	Positive
Antibody identification	Anti-E, Anti-c, Anti-Kell
	Anti-Jk^a, Anti-C^w, Anti-Co^a
Direct antiglobulin test (type of antiserum):	
polyspecific	Positive
IgG	Negative
C3d	Negative
Eluate antibody screen	Negative

T3. Laboratory Findings After Transfusion of 1 Unit of Co^a Antigen-Positive Packed Red Blood Cells (PRBCs)*

Test	Day 0-BT†	Day After Transfusion of a Single Unit of Co^a Antigen-Positive PRBCs										
		0	1	2	3	4	5	6	7	8	9	10
Hemoglobin	6.1	6.9	6.8	6.8	7.2	6.9	6.6	6.7	7.8	7.3	7.3	7.6
Hematocrit	17.7	20.6	20.0	20.1	21.5	21.0	20.8	21.1	24.6	22.2	22.6	23.9
BUN	18	16	16	16	16	14				14	13	12
Creatinine	2.23	2.29	2.14	2.13	2.13	1.94				1.77	1.92	1.89
Total bilirubin		0.9	1.0	1.0	1.0							
Direct bilirubin		0	0	0	0							
LD		166	168	180	175	194	194	172	192	192		
Urine blood		Neg					Neg				Neg	Neg

*3 Co^a antigen-negative PRBC units were transfused prior (2 units 5 days prior and 1 unit 3 days prior) to the transfusion of a single unit of Co^a antigen-positive PRBCs. †0-BT, day 0 before transfusion of the single unit of Co^a-positive PRBCs. BUN, blood urea nitrogen; LD, lactate dehydrogenase; Neg, negative.

Questions

1. What is the most remarkable antibody present in this patient's serum?

2. What is the approximate frequency in the general population of the antigen related to this antibody?

3. What are some of the features of this antibody?

4. What are some of the features of the antigen associated with this antibody?

5. What are some of the clinical and transfusion medicine-related implications related to the presence of this antibody?

Possible Answers

1. An alloantibody to the Co^a antigen [**T2**].

2. The Co^a antigen is present in approximately 99.8% of Caucasians with a gene frequency of 0.959.[1] Individuals negative for the Co^a antigen but positive for the Co^b antigen comprise approximately 0.2% of the general population.

3. Formation of antibodies to antigens in the Colton blood group system is usually immune mediated, occurring secondary to exposure to antigen-positive blood from transfusion or pregnancy. These antibodies are most commonly of the IgG isotype, although a case of IgM anti-Co^b has been reported.[2] Moreover, they demonstrate variable ability to bind complement.[2] Rare examples of transient anti-Co^a and anti-Co3 production have been documented in antigen-positive patients suffering from autoimmune or lymphoproliferative disorders in whom antigen expression was temporarily depressed.[3] In addition to antibodies specific for Colton antigens Co^a, Co^b, and Co3, found in Co$^{(a-b-)}$ patients, a fourth antibody (Co3-like antibody) has been isolated which only reacts with cells expressing both Co^a and Co^b together, a reaction that is not separable by differential adsorption.[3] Reactions involving antibodies to Co^a are of variable severity and have been implicated in transfusion reactions ranging from mild delayed hemolytic

reaction to life-threatening cases of hemolytic disease of the newborn (HDN) and acute hemolysis.[4] In similar fashion, reactions involving anti-Co^b also demonstrate a range of severities including both delayed and acute hemolytic transfusion reactions. Antibodies against the Co3 antigen may potentially produce a similar spectrum of reactions as listed above.[3,5] In vivo studies that document accelerated destruction of Co-antigen positive cells in the presence of anti-Co^a or anti-Co^b would indicate that selection of Co-antigen negative blood for transfusion is warranted.[3]

4. The codominantly inherited genetic sequences responsible for encoding the Colton antigens exist as polymorphisms of the AQP1 gene located on the short arm of chromosome 7 (7p14).[3] The product of this gene is a transmembrane water channel protein, aquaporin-1 (AQP-CHIP), which is found in the membranes of erythrocytes and renal epithelial cells of the proximal tubule, but is absent in lymphocytes, monocytes, and granulocytes. Further characterization of this protein indicates that Co^a and Co^b antigens correspond to the respective presence of alanine or valine at position 45 within the first extracellular loop of aquaporin-1.[2,3] The expression of the Co3 antigen is dependent on the absence of both the Co^a and Co^b antigens, while the presence of the fourth antigen (to which the Co3-like antibody is directed) results from a neoantigen forming interactions between Colton antigens Co^a and Co^b.[2]

5. Since the presence of anti-Co^a has been implicated in acute in vivo hemolysis, or at the very least decreased survival of transfused Co^(a+) cells, the transfusion of Co^a-antigen negative blood is required in such cases.[2,5] However, due to the relative rarity of Co^a-antigen negative red blood cells, adequate time should be given to secure Co^a-antigen negative red blood cells, in the event that transfusion at some point is deemed necessary. Our patient required multiple red blood cell transfusions that included 3 units of Co^a-antigen negative red blood cells. Unfortunately, the patient required additional transfusion support, and because of the clinical urgency and unavailability of Co^a-antigen negative red blood cells a fourth red blood cell unit was transfused, which was antigen negative for all respective alloantibodies, except anti-Co^a. The patient tolerated the transfusion of the Co^a-antigen positive red blood cells well and there were no signs and/or symptoms of acute or delayed hemolysis [**T3**]. The patient did not require any additional red blood cell transfusions.

Keywords

Co^a antibody, alloantibody, aquaporin-1

References

1. Mollison PL, Engelfrief CP, Contreras M. *Blood Transfusion in Clinical Medicine.* 9th ed. Boston: Blackwell Science, 1993.

2. Daniels G. *Human Blood Groups.* 2nd ed. Boston: Blackwell Science, 2002.

3. Issitt PD, Anstee DJ. *Applied Blood Group Serology.* 4th ed. Durham, NC: Montgomery Scientific Publications.

4. Savona-Ventura C, Grech ES, Zieba A. Anti-Co3 and severe hemolytic disease of the newborn. *Obstet Gynecol.* 1989;73:870-872.

5. Lacey PA, Robinson J, Collins ML, et al. Studies on the blood of a Co (a-b-) proposita and her family. *Transfusion.* 1987;27:268-271.

Evaluation of a Possible Transfusion Reaction With a Positive Direct Antiglobulin Test in a 29-Year-Old Male

Mark R. Steciuk, Michelle R. Brown, J. Barry Freeman, Shu T. Huang
Department of Pathology, University of Alabama at Birmingham, Birmingham, AL

Patient: 29-year-old male.

Past Medical History: Negative.

Chief Complaint/History of Present Illness: The patient underwent orthopedic surgery for a left tibia/fibula fracture sustained in a motor vehicle collision. Postoperatively, he simultaneously received 2 units of red blood cells. Towards the end of the transfusion, the patient developed fever and chills. His temperature increased from 100°F to 102.1°F, pulse increased from 123 to 125, and oxygen saturation decreased from 100% to 92% on room air. His blood pressure was stable and there was no dyspnea.

Past Surgical History: Previous surgery of the left lower extremity.

T1. Transfusion Reaction Workup Results

	Pretransfusion	Posttransfusion
ABO/Rh	O Positive	O Positive
Plasma color	Red[a]	Straw
DAT	Negative	Weak positive (confirmed microscopically)
Urine Hgb	Trace	Negative
Antibody screen (Gel)	Negative	Negative
Antibody screen (PEG)	Negative	Negative
Urine RBCs	0–2/HPF	Not performed
Abbreviated crossmatch (Unit 1)	Compatible	Compatible
Abbreviated crossmatch (Unit 2)	Compatible	Compatible
Full crossmatch Unit 1	Compatible	Compatible
Full crossmatch Unit 2	Incompatible	Incompatible
Elution	Not applicable	Panreactive (1+)[b]

[a]An improperly-collected, hemoglobin-tinged specimen was used for pretransfusion testing due to difficulty of recollection. Normal haptoglobin and indirect bilirubin levels support the absence of in vivo hemolysis.
[b]Positive (1+) with all panel cells tested.
DAT, direct antiglobulin test; Hgb, hemoglobin; PEG, polyethylene glycol; RBCs, red blood cells; HPF, high power field.

Questions _____

1. Why was an elution performed?

2. Which laboratory test should be performed next?

3. Did the transfusion of the second unit cause the patient's symptoms?

4. Did a transfusion reaction occur and, if so, what kind of reaction was it?

5. How should the clinician be advised regarding the cause of the patient's symptoms?

6. What further actions are necessary on the part of the laboratory?

7. Why was this not detected prior to the transfusion of blood products?

8. How common is this occurrence?

Possible Answers _____

1. In order to identify the nature of the antibody bound to the patient's red blood cells, an elution should be performed whenever a positive direct antiglobulin test (DAT) is encountered. A panreactive antibody, as seen in this case, suggests a warm autoantibody[1,2]; however, other possibilities, such as an antibody to a high incidence antigen, should be considered. In this case, an alloantibody to high incidence antigen is not a possibility, since this would have been identified by the antibody screen performed routinely by the blood center.

2. In this case, there are seemingly conflicting results. The posttransfusion DAT is weakly-positive, and the elution is consistent with a warm autoantibody. However, the pre- and post-transfusion antibody screens were negative by 2 different methods. The origin of the antibody bound to the red cells in the posttransfusion sample, which was not in the pretransfusion sample, is unclear. The appropriate next step is to run a DAT on the full crossmatch-incompatible unit. As expected, the DAT on this unit was positive (2+); thus, the antibody was bound to the

red cells in the donor unit and remained bound to the donor cells after the transfusion. This explained both the weak-positive DAT in the posttransfusion sample as well as the full cross-match incompatibility. The donor in this case likely had a warm autoantibody bound to his red cells, thereby explaining the positive posttransfusion DAT and the panreactive elution results. If the DAT on the transfused unit had been negative, a plausible next step would be a full minor crossmatch, although an antibody in the donor's serum should have been discovered at the originating blood center unless that antibody showed specificity to a low-incidence antigen.

3. The transfusion of the "incompatible" unit was no more likely to have caused the patient's symptoms than the first unit. Since the autoantibody remained bound to the donor red cells, if it were to cause hemolysis only the donor red cells would be affected. Furthermore, the autoantibody would only cause hemolysis in the recipient if it caused hemolysis in the donor. The donor did not have a hemolytic anemia, or he would have been ineligible to donate on the basis of his hematocrit. Therefore, it is highly unlikely that there will be hemolysis in the recipient, and it is safe to conclude that the autoantibody is clinically insignificant.

4. It is difficult to answer this question with the given information. The differential diagnosis includes 2 possibilities: febrile transfusion reaction, and coincidental fever. Although the donor units were leukoreduced, a febrile transfusion reaction is a distinct possibility; however, it is also possible that the patient's symptoms were coincident with the transfusion. This is especially likely given that less than 24 hours had elapsed since the patient's surgery. Follow up revealed that the patient continued spiking fevers over the next 24 hours, and atelectasis was seen on his chest radiograph. This information suggests that the patient's symptoms were coincident with the transfusion, stressing the importance of reviewing the vital signs prior to, during, and following transfusion. The patient's fever subsided, and he was discharged to home 4 days later.

5. The clinician should be advised that a hemolytic transfusion reaction did not occur. The autoantibody bound to the red cells of the donor unit

caused the positive posttransfusion DAT. It should also be emphasized that the transfusion of a DAT-positive donor unit is not likely to be clinically significant. The competing possibilities of coincidental fever, versus febrile transfusion reaction, should be discussed with the advice to consider giving the patient acetaminophen prior to future transfusions if fever seems clinically likely. It should be noted that the posttransfusion DAT was very weakly positive. Routine microscopic examination of the DAT is not required. In this case, the technologist was suspicious of a weak reaction on visual examination and confirmed the weak reaction microscopically. It is open to debate whether such reactions should be reported or whether they are so weak as to be clinically insignificant. It is the policy of the authors' institution to investigate and report such findings, especially given the gravity of a possible hemolytic transfusion reaction.

6. No further testing is necessary, although the blood center from which the unit in question was obtained should be informed that the unit had a positive DAT, and a review of the donor's records is warranted. In this case, the donor was a 39-year-old male with a negative antibody screen. The incidence of warm autoantibodies increases with age.[1] Even though the donor in question is relatively young, a warm autoantibody is not an unreasonable proposition.

7. Required pretransfusion compatibility testing includes an ABO and Rh type and antibody screen on the donor unit.[3] A DAT is not routinely performed. The recipient must have a current type and antibody screen. If the antibody screen is negative, and the recipient does not have a history of any clinically-significant antibodies, an abbreviated crossmatch may be performed.[4] Alternatively, if sufficient history is available, the recipient may be eligible for an electronic crossmatch. If the patient's current antibody screen is positive, or if there is a history of a clinically-significant antibody, a full crossmatch is required. As stated above, antibody screening of donor units is required transfusion practice, but, in this case, an antibody was not detected in the donor unit. It is likely that it was negative because the autoantibody was bound to the patient's red cells and not present in the serum. Since a DAT is not routinely performed on donor units, the antibody was not detected.

8. It has been estimated that between 1 out of 1,500 and 1 out of 14,000 donors are DAT positive.[5-7] A relatively large percentage of DAT-positive individuals have negative antibody screens. One study found that 13 out of 20 DAT-positive units from healthy donors had a negative antibody screen[8] because antibodies are bound to red cells and are not free in the serum at detectable levels.[2] Because blood centers do not routinely perform a DAT on donor units, these would not be detected during component preparation. Furthermore, since this is clinically insignificant for the recipient, it would likely only be detected if there was a coincidental transfusion reaction or an unexplained incompatible full crossmatch. Therefore, the rate at which cases like this come to the attention of a transfusion medicine service is low.

Acknowledgments

The authors would like to acknowledge Dr. Marisa B. Marques for her helpful suggestions on the preparation of this manuscript.

Keywords

transfusion reaction, direct antiglobulin test, elution, blood donation

References

1. Wheeler CA, Calhoun L, Blackall DP. Warm reactive autoantibodies. Clinical and serological correlations. *Am J Clin Pathol.* 2004;122:680–685.

2. Reardon JE, Marques MB. Laboratory evaluation and transfusion support of patients with autoimmune hemolytic anemia. *Am J Clin Pathol.* 2006; 125:S1–S7.

3. Code of Federal Regulations (CFR). Title 21 CFR Part 640.5. Washington, DC: US Government Printing Office; 2007.

4. American Association of Blood Banks (AABB). *Standards for Blood Banks and Transfusion Services.* 24th ed. Bethesda, MD: AABB; 2006.

5. Gorst DW, Rawlinson VI, Merry AH, et al. Positive direct antiglobulin test in normal individuals. *Vox Sang.* 1980;38:99–105.

6. Mehta K, Taylor H, Holland B. Positive direct antihuman globulin test in normal blood donors. *N J Med.* 1987;84:265–267.

7. Bellia M, Georgeopoulos J, Tsevrenis V, et al. The investigation of the significance of a positive direct antiglobulin test in blood donors. *Immunohematol.* 2002;18:78–81.

8. Stratton F, Rawlinson VI, Merry AH, et al. Positive direct antiglobulin test in normal individuals. II. *Clin Lab Haematol.* 1983;5:17–21.

Delayed Hemolysis

Laurie J. Sutor

Associate Professor of Pathology, UT Southwestern Medical School, Dallas, TX

Patient: 25-year-old African-American male.

Chief Complaint: Severe back pain 10 days following surgery to remove infected hip prosthesis. Medical and Surgical History: Sickle cell anemia. History of transfusion therapy on 5 occasions in the past (3 for intractable pain crisis, 1 for acute chest crisis). Hospitalized at another facility 4 months prior for bilateral hip replacement surgery following avascular necrosis of both femoral heads. Current admission is for removal of left hip prosthesis because of chronic infection with drainage. Patient was transfused 3 units of RBCs 1 day prior to surgery.

History: Sickle cell anemia in father. Diabetes mellitus in mother.

Drug History: Chronic pain medications, including codeine-containing prescriptions. Currently on IV antibiotics.

Physical Examination: Patient in moderate distress. Pallor. Mild fever at 38.2°C. Drain present in left hip region with pale pink, non-cloudy drainage.

T1. Principal Laboratory Findings

Analyte	Pre-transfusion	Pre-op*	Current
Hematology			
Hematocrit	23%	30%	21%
(NRR: 40-52%)			
Blood bank			
Blood type	B, Rh pos		B, Rh pos
Antibody screen	neg		pos
Antibody ID	n.a.		anti-E; anti-Jkᵃ
DAT	n.d.		3+ pos
Donor blood			
Antigen type	n.d.		2 units E-pos; 1 unit Jkᵃ pos

*After transfusion of 3 units of RBCs. Pre-op, pre-operative; NRR, normal reference range; pos, positive; neg, negative; n.a., not applicable; n.d., not done; ID, identification; DAT, direct antiglobulin test.

Questions

1. What diagnosis can be made based on the prior and current blood bank tests?

2. Are the anti-E and anti-Jk^a new or previously existing antibodies?

3. How can this situation be prevented in the future?

Possible Answers

1. The patient is having immune hemolysis as demonstrated by the fall in hematocrit, new detection of red cell antibodies and positive DAT. Tests for bilirubin and LD would probably be elevated, if done, but are not essential to make the diagnosis. Since the patient is 11 days out from his transfusion, this hemolysis is classified as delayed in nature, making this a classic delayed hemolytic transfusion reaction. The fever and back pain may be symptoms of the delayed hemolysis or might also represent a sickle cell pain crisis. These 2 scenarios are often difficult to differentiate.

2. The anti-E and anti-Jk^a are pre-existing antibodies. Red cell antibodies when stimulated de novo are generally not detected for 1 to 2 months following transfusion. Red cell antibodies detected within 1-2 weeks of a transfusion, especially in a known previously-transfused patient, are most likely pre-existing antibodies that had dropped in titer to below the detectable limits of routine pre-transfusion screening tests. These antibodies are then quickly stimulated in an anamnestic reaction by the administration of antigen-positive units of red blood cells. The blood that was transfused in this patient was compatible by all available tests at the time it was administered. No error was made in the issuing of the blood. Only in retrospect can the units be determined to actually have been incompatible. Kidd antibodies (anti-Jk^a and anti-Jk^b) are especially notorious for dropping below detectable levels and causing subsequent immune hemolysis.

3. This scenario might have been avoided if the blood bank records from the prior hospitalization at another institution (for the hip replacement surgery) had been available. Blood bank records indicating prior red cell antibody formation are used to assure continued transfusion of antigen-negative blood, even if the antibody in question is no longer detectable in routine tests. Red cell antibodies should be considered to have a life-long presence. Another way to avoid delayed hemolytic transfusion reactions is to carefully instruct the patients on the presence of any red cell antibodies, and provide them with a wallet card or med-alert bracelet with this information.

Hemolytic Reactions

Hemolytic reactions occur when the recipient's serum contains antibodies directed against the corresponding antigen found on donor red blood cells. This can be an ABO incompatibility or an incompatibility related to a different blood group antigen.

Disseminated intravascular coagulation (DIC), renal failure, and death are not uncommon following this type of reaction.

The most common cause for a major hemolytic transfusion reaction is a clerical error, such as a mislabelled specimen sent to the blood bank, or not properly identifying the patient to whom you are giving the blood. **DO NOT ASSUME IT IS SOMEONE ELSE'S RESPONSIBILITY TO CHECK!**

Allergic Reactions

Allergic reactions to plasma proteins can range from complaints of hives and itching to anaphylaxis.

From: The University of Utah Medical School's web site:

http://www-medlib.med.utah.edu

Unusual Antibody Reactions in a 55-Year-Old Man

Justin N. Steinert,[1] Julie Kirkegaard,[2] Jigar S. Patel[1,2]

Department of [1]Blood Bank, University of Kansas Hospital, Kansas City, KS and [2]Department of Immunohematology, Community Blood Center of Kansas City, Kansas City, MO

Patient: 55-year-old Caucasian man.

Drug History: History of alcohol abuse.

Medical History: Back surgery in 1974 and 1979; suspected alcohol induced cirrhosis; and complications due to cirrhosis including variceal bleeding, hypersplenism, and thrombocytopenia.

History of Present Illness: Patient was admitted to another local hospital with bleeding gastric varices. Three units of compatible packed red blood cells (RBCs) were transfused. Patient was then transferred to our facility 2 days later for possible placement of a transjugular intrahepatic portosystemic shunt (TIPSS).

Clinical Course: On day of admission, 2 units of RBCs were ordered. The patient's antibody screen was positive, and an antibody workup revealed an allo anti-C (**T1**) antibody. No RBC units were transfused. A type and crossmatch were ordered on day 4 of his hospitalization. An antibody screen and identification revealed an increase in reactivity (**T1**). The patient's serum samples were sent to the Community Blood Center of Kansas City (CBCKC) for further workup with results as shown in **T2a**, **T2b**, and **T2c**. On day 6 of his hospitalization, 1 unit of compatible RBCs was transfused. Subsequently, the clinical staff suspected a febrile nonhemolytic transfusion reaction.

Principal Laboratory Findings: **T1** and **T2**, **Figure 1**, and **Image 1**. In addition, the patient's haptoglobin level was <6 mg/dL (reference range: 16-200 mg/dL) on day 5 of his hospitalization.

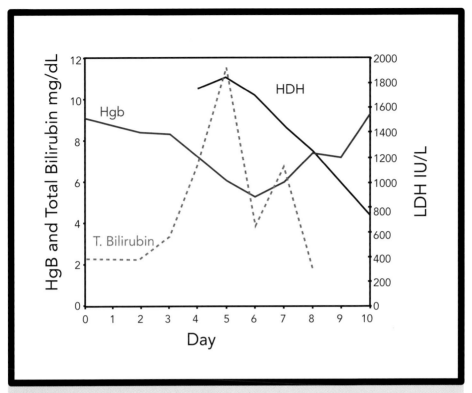

Figure 1_Patient's hemoglobin (Hgb), total bilirubin, and lactate dehyrogenase (LDH) levels over days 0 (admission)-10 of his hospital stay. The patient was transfused with 1 unit of compatible RBCs on days 5, 7, and 8 and with 3 units on day 8.[6]

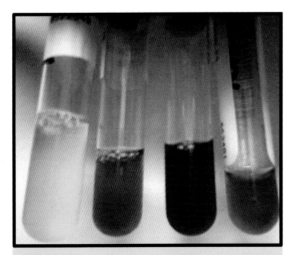

Image 1_Patient's plasma on (left to right) day of admission, day 4, day 6, and day 8, demonstrating increasing hemoglobinemia.

T1. Patient's Serum Antibody Panel Results at UKH on Day of Admission and on Day 4 of Hospitalization

	RBC Antigen System																									
	Rh-hr					Kell						Duffy		Kidd		Lewis		MNS				Lutheran		Gel IAT	
RBC ID #	D	C	E	c	e	K	k	Kp^a	Kp^b	Js^a	Js^b	Fy^a	Fy^b	Jk^a	Jk^b	Le^a	Le^b	S	s	M	N	Lu^a	Lu^b	Day 1	Day 4
1	+	+	0	0	+	0	+	0	+	0	+	+	0	+	0	0	0	0	+	+	+	0	+	4+	4+
2	+	+	0	0	+	0	+	0	+	0	+	+	0	0	+	+	0	+	+	+	0	0	+	4+	4+
3	+	0	+	+	0	0	+	0	+	0	+	0	+	+	+	0	0	+	+	+	0	0	+	0	3+
4	+	0	0	+	+	0	+	0	+	0	+	0	0	+	+	0	0	0	+	+	0	0	+	0	3+
5	0	+	0	+	+	0	+	0	+	0	+	+	+	+	0	0	+	0	+	+	+	0	+	4+	4+
6	0	0	0	+	+	0	+	0	+	0	+	0	+	+	0	0	+	0	+	+	+	0	+	0	3+
7	0	0	0	+	+	+	+	0	+	0	+	0	+	+	+	+	0	0	+	+	+	0	+	0	3+
8	0	0	0	+	+	0	+	0	+	0	+	+	0	+	+	+	0	+	0	0	+	0	+	0	0
9	0	0	0	+	+	0	1+	0	+	0	+	+	+	0	+	0	+	+	0	0	+	0	+	0	1+
10	0	0	0	+	+	0	+	0	+	0	+	+	0	+	0	0	+	+	+	+	0	0	+	0	4+
11	+	+	0	0	+	+	+	0	+	0	+	0	+	+	+	0	+	+	0	+	+	0	+	4+	4+
Auto Ctrl																								+/-	

UKH, University of Kansas Hospital; RBC, red blood cells; ID #, identification number; IAT, indirect antiglobulin test; Ctrl, control.

T2a. Antibody Panel Results at CBCKC on Patient's Hospital Day 4 Serum Sample
(Panel 1: RBC Samples 1-11)

RBC ID #	Rh-hr					Kell						Duffy		Kidd		Lewis		MNS				Lutheran		Other Tests Ficin	
	D	C	E	c	e	K	k	Kp^a	Kp^b	Js^a	Js^b	Fy^a	Fy^b	Jk^a	Jk^b	Le^a	Le^b	S	s	M	N	Lu^a	Lu^b	37°C	IAT
1	+	+	0	0	+	0	+	0	+	0	+	0	+	+	0	0	+	+	+	+	+	0	+	3+	*
2	+	+	0	0	+	+	+	0	+	0	+	+	0	0	+	+	0	+	0	+	0	0	+	3+	*
3	+	0	+	+	0	0	+	0	+	0	+	0	+	+	+	0	+	0	+	+	+	0	+	0	0
4	+	0	0	+	+	0	+	0	+	0	+	0	0	+	0	0	0	+	+	0	+	0	+	0	0
5	0	+	0	+	+	0	+	0	+	0	+	0	0	+	+	0	0	+	+	+	0	0	+	2+	*
6	0	0	0	+	+	0	+	0	+	0	+	+	+	+	0	+	0	0	+	0	+	0	+	0	0
7	0	0	0	+	+	+	+	0	+	0	+	0	+	+	0	+	0	+	+	+	0	0	+	2+	1+
8	0	0	0	+	+	0	+	0	+	0	+	+	0	+	0	0	+	0	+	+	+	0	+	+/-	0
9	0	0	0	+	+	0	+	0	+	0	+	0	0	0	+	0	+	+	0	0	+	0	+	0	0
10	0	0	0	+	+	0	+	0	+	0	+	0	+	+	+	+	0	0	+	0	+	0	+	0	0
11	+	+	0	0	+	0	+	0	+	0	+	0	+	0	+	+	0	0	+	0	+	0	+	2+	*
Auto Ctrl																									
Phenotype^a	4+	0	4+	4+	4+	0						3+	0	3+	3+			0	3+	0					

^{a}Performed on pretransfusion sample. *, indicates agglutination after washing. CBCKC, Community Blood Center of Kansas City; RBC, red blood cells; ID #, identification number; IAT, indirect antiglobulin test; Ctrl, control.

T2b. Antibody Panel Results at CBCKC on Patient's Hospital Day 4 Serum Sample
(Panel 2: RBC Samples 12-22)

RBC ID #	Rh-hr D	C	E	c	e	Kell K	k	Kpᵃ	Kpᵇ	Jsᵃ	Jsᵇ	Duffy Fyᵃ	Fyᵇ	Kidd Jkᵃ	Jkᵇ	Lewis Leᵃ	Leᵇ	MNS S	s	M	N	Lutheran Luᵃ	Luᵇ	LISS 37°C	IAT	Saline RT	4°C	EE/PEG IAT
12	0	0	0	+	+	+	+	0	+	0	+	+	+	+	+	+	0	+	+	+	+	0	+	3+	*	3+	3+	*
13	0	0	0	+	+	+	+	0	+	0	+	+	0	0	+	+	0	0	+	0	+	0	+	0	(+)	0	3+	0
14	0	0	0	+	+	+	+	0	+	0	+	0	+	+	0	0	+	+	0	0	+	0	+	2+	*	r	3+	+
15	+	0	+	+	0	0	+	0	+	0	+	+	0	+	+	+	0	0	+	+	+	0	+	3+	*	4+	4+	*
16	+	0	+	+	0	+	+	0	+	0	+	+	+	+	0	+	0	+	+	+	0	0	+	4+	*	4+	4+	*
17	+	0	+	+	+	0	+	0	+	0	+	+	+	0	+	0	+	0	+	+	0	0	+	4+	*	4+	4+	*
18	+	+	0	0	+	+	+	0	+	0	+	0	+	+	+	+	0	0	+	0	+	0	+	4+	*	4+	4+	*
19	+	+	0	0	+	+	+	0	+	0	+	+	0	0	+	0	+	+	+	+	+	0	+	4+	*	4+	4+	*
20	+	+	+	+	+	+	+	0	+	0	+	+	+	+	+	+	0	+	0	+	+	0	+	4+	*	4+	4+	*
21	0	0	+	+	+	0	+	0	+	0	+	0	+	+	+	0	+	+	+	+	+	0	+	4+	*	4+	4+	*
22	+	+	0	0	+	+	0	0	+	0	+	+	+	+	0	0	+	0	+	0	+	0	+	4+	*	4+	4+	*
Auto Ctrl																								0	0	0	1+	3+

*, indicates agglutination after washing. CBCKC, Community Blood Center of Kansas City; RBC, red blood cells; ID #, identification number; LISS, low-ionic strength saline; RT, room temperature; EE, ether eluate; PEG, polyethylene glycol; IAT, indirect antiglobulin test; r, rough; Ctrl, control.

T2c. Antibody Panel Results at CBCKC on Patient's Hospital Day 4 Serum Sample
(Panel 3: RBC Samples 1-19)

RBC ID #	Rh-hr					Kell						Duffy		Kidd		Lewis		MNS				Lutheran		LISS		Prewarm	EE/PEG
	D	C	E	c	e	K	k	Kp^a	Kp^b	Js^a	Js^b	Fy^a	Fy^b	Jk^a	Jk^b	Le^a	Le^b	S	s	M	N	Lu^a	Lu^b	37°C / IAT		IAT	IAT
1	+	0	+	+	0	0	+	0	+	0	+	+	0	+	0	0	+	0	+	0	+	0	+		0		
2	0	0	+	+	+	0	+	0	+	0	+	+	0	0	+	0	+	0	+	0	+	0	+		0		
3	0	0	0	+	+	0	+	0	+	0	+	+	0	+	+	+	0	+	+	+	+	0	+		*	(+)	
4	+	0	+	0	+	0	+	0	+	0	+	+	0	+	0	+	0	+	+	+	0	0	+		*	1+	
5	0	0	0	+	+	0	+	0	+	0	+	0	0	+	0	0	+	0	+	+	0	0	+		*	1+	
6	+	0	0	+	+	0	+	0	+	0	+	0	+	+	0	0	+	0	0	+	+	0	+	0	(+)	(+)	0
7	0	0	+	+	+	0	+	0	+	0	+	0	+	0	+	+	0	0	+	0	+	0	+		*	1+	
8	+	0	+	+	0	0	+	0	+	0	+	+	0	0	+	0	+	+	+	+	+	0	+		*	1+	
9	0	0	+	+	+	0	+	0	+	0	+	0	+	0	+	0	+	0	+	0	+	0	+		*	1+	
10	0	0	0	+	+	+	+	0	+	0	+	+	0	+	+	0	+	0	0	+	+	0	+		*		
11	+	0	+	0	+	+	+	0	+	0	+	+	0	+	0	0	+	0	+	+	+	0	+		*		
12	+	0	0	+	+	0	+	0	+	0	+	0	+	0	+	0	+	0	0	+	+	0	+	0	0		
13	0	0	0	+	+	0	+	0	+	0	+	0	+	+	0	+	0	0	+	0	+	+	+	0	2+		
14	0	0	0	+	+	0	+	0	+	0	+	0	+	0	+	+	0	0	+	0	+	0	+	+w	2+		2+
15	0	0	0	+	+	0	+	0	+	0	+	+	0	0	+	0	+	0	+	0	+	0	+	0	0		0
16	+	0	+	+	+	0	+	0	+	0	+	+	0	0	+	0	+	+	+	+	+	0	+	0	0		
17	0	0	0	+	+	+	+	0	+	0	+	0	+	0	+	+	0	+	+	+	+	+	+	0	0		
18	0	0	0	+	+	0	+	0	+	0	+	0	0	0	+	+	0	0	+	0	+	0	+	+s	(+)		0
19	+	+	0	0	+	0	+	0	+	0	+	+	0	+	+	0	+	0	+	0	+	0	+				0

*, indicates agglutination after washing. RBC, red blood cells; ID #, identification number; LISS, low-ionic strength saline; EE, ether eluate; PEG, polyethylene glycol; IAT, indirect antiglobulin test.

Questions

1. What is (are) this patient's most striking clinical and laboratory findings?

2. How do you explain these findings?

3. What is the mechanism by which a delayed hemolytic transfusion reaction occurs?

4. What is this patient's red blood cell (RBC) antigen phenotype?

5. What antibodies are present in the patient's serum, and what is their significance?

6. How should this patient be treated?

Possible Answers

1. Presence of alloantibody on day of admission (**T1**), presence of multiple antibodies on day 4 (**T1, T2a, T2b, T2c**), anemia (decreasing hemoglobin levels) (**Figure 1**), increases in total bilirubin and lactate dehydrogenase (LDH) (**Figure 1**), decreasing haptaglobin, increasing visible hemolysis in the patient's plasma (**Image 1**).

2. Our patient's anti-C was formed as an immunological response to a previous allogeneic RBC transfusion, which may have been received during his back surgeries or variceal bleeding episodes. The presence of multiple antibodies in his plasma on day 4 of his hospitalization is most likely an anamnestic response of antibodies that were not detectable prior to the current transfusion episode. The decreasing hemoglobin levels accompanied by a post-transfusion rise in serum total bilirubin and LDH levels are indicative of RBC hemolysis resulting from an immune response, commonly known as a delayed hemolytic transfusion reaction (DHTR). The patient's low haptoglobin level on day 5 could have been caused by the release of free hemoglobin into the plasma, which is then bound by haptoglobin. The haptoglobin-hemoglobin complex is then transported to either the liver or reticuloendothelial system (RES) where it is degraded.[1] Our patient's failing liver must also be taken into

account, and the patient's decreased haptoglobin level may also have been a consequence of decreased hepatic production.

3. A DHTR is most often the result of an anamnestic response in a patient who has been previously sensitized by transfusion, pregnancy, or transplant. In such patients, antibody is not detectable because of very low titers.[2,3] Delayed hemolytic transfusion reactions have an occurrence rate of 1:2,500 units transfused with a mortality rate of 1:600,000.[2] With our patient, 1 of the antibodies present in his serum, anti-C, retained its titer at a level high enough to be easily identified. However, his serum contained multiple additional antibodies that were not detectable until approximately 6 days post transfusion. The presentation of these antibodies was consistent with the normal delayed response time of 3 to 7 days after the transfusion of compatible RBCs. Once the patient developed a sufficient titer of these antibodies, the transfused RBCs became coated with antibody and were removed from the circulation via the extravascular hemolytic pathway. *Extravascular hemolysis* begins typically with an IgG antibody attaching to a RBC surface antigen resulting in sensitization of the RBCs and their subsequent removal by the RES, most commonly in the spleen, but also in the liver.[2] RBC hemolysis usually leads to an increase in unconjugated bilirubin in the plasma accompanied by an increase in serum LDH concentration due to release of LDH from RBCs. When red cell destruction becomes severe enough, the RES may become overwhelmed and intravascular hemolysis can occur. Moreover, certain subtypes of IgG antibodies can activate complement and lead to intravascular RBC lysis. In addition to the findings associated with extravascular hemolysis, *intravascular hemolysis* is marked by hemoglobinemia, hemoglobinuria, and a decreased serum haptoglobin level. Our patient's plasma demonstrated evidence of hemolysis over the course of several days (**Image 1**).

4. D+,C-,E+,c+,e+;K-;Fy(a+,b);Jk(a+,b+);S-,s+,M-

5. The patient's plasma contains multiple antibodies: anti-C, anti-K, anti-Js^a, anti-Fy^b, and anti-M. In addition to these alloantibodies, the patient's serum also contained a cold autoagglutinin. Cold autoagglutinins are not typically clinically

significant; however, they may cause difficulties with the identification of other antibodies that may be present. Anti-C is generally an IgG antibody and most often reacts at the anti-human globulin (AHG) phase of antibody testing but can appear at 37°C. Anti-C has been implicated in hemolytic transfusion reactions. K and Js[a] antigens belong to the Kell blood group system. Antibodies against these antigens react best at the AHG phase and are of the IgG subtype. Moreover, anti-K and anti-Js[a] are capable of causing a transfusion reaction. When an ether elution procedure was performed (**T2b and T2c**), it showed that anti-Fy[b] and anti-M were present on the surface of the patient's RBCs. Anti-Fy[b] antibodies are usually IgG, react best at the AHG phase of antibody testing, and are able to bind complement.[2] Anti-Fy[b] has been implicated in transfusion reactions and albeit rare, has also been known to cause DHTRs.[2,4] Duffy antibodies often show a dosage effect, but this is not always the case due to inheritance patterns of the Duffy antigens. Care must be taken when using a dosage effect to rule out the possibility of either anti-Fy[a] or anti-Fy[b] antibodies.

6. The patient's antibodies, anti-C, anti-K, anti-Js[a], and anti-Fy[b], are unlikely to be naturally occurring and require either a prior transfusion or pregnancy to form; however, anti-M may appear with or without a stimulus. Anti-M is generally thought of as an IgM cold-reacting antibody; however, most anti-M antibodies appear to be IgG or have an IgG component.[2,4,5] Anti-M, whether IgM or IgG, does not bind complement.[5] Anti-M antibodies that react at colder temperatures (ie, room temperature and 4°C) and dissociate when subjected to 37°C or in the AHG phase of antibody testing, generally are not considered clinically significant. Our patient's anti-M continued to show reactivity after pre-warming (**T2c**) and thus must be considered a clinically significant antibody. The presence of anti-M in the eluate confirms its classification as clinically significant. The eluate results provide serologic evidence of anti-Fy[b] and anti-M antibodies as the likely cause of our patient's extra- and intra-vascular hemolysis.

7. No treatment is usually needed for DHTR other than the selection of compatible RBCs that are antigen-negative for the patient's corresponding antibodies.[3] If complications become severe enough, treatment should be extended to include measures taken during an immediate hemolytic transfusion reaction. This may include the use of diuretics to maintain urine output and prevent renal failure, intravenous fluids, vasoactive drugs to maintain intravascular volume and pressure, and blood component therapy if the patient is experiencing disseminated intravascular coagulation (DIC).[2,3] Only ~1% of donor RBCs will be negative for C, K, Js[a], Fy[b], and M antigens, making it difficult to find compatible units for transfusion in our patient. Thus, if transfusion is necessary in patients with antibodies against the aforementioned constellation of antigens, sufficient time should be allowed to obtain compatible donor units.

Keywords

alloantibody, anamnestic response, delayed hemolytic transfusion reaction, phenotype, Kell antigen group

References

1. Radtke J. Proteins. In: Anderson SC, Cockayne S, eds. *Clinical Chemistry Concepts and Applications.* 4th ed. New York, NY: McGraw-Hill. 2003:213.

2. Harmening DM, ed. *Modern Blood Banking and Transfusion Practices.* 4th ed. Philadelphia, PA: FA Davis. 1994:166-167,184,380-385.

3. Jones SL, ed. *Clinical Laboratory Pearls.* Philadelphia, PA: Lippincott Williams & Wilkins. 2001:42-49.

4. Brecher ME, ed. *Technical Manual.* 15th ed. Bethesda, MD: American Association of Blood Banks. 2005:340.

5. Unger PJ, Laird-Fryer B, eds. *Blood Group Systems: MN and Gerbich.* Arlington, VA: American Association of Blood Banks. 1989:19.

6. Immel CC, McPherson M, Hay SN, et al. Severe hemolytic anemia due to auto anti-N. *Immunohematology: Journal of Blood Group Serology and Education.* 2005:21;63.

The Antibody That Came in From the Cold

Jason Nash, David Krugh, Melanie S. Kennedy

Division of Transfusion Medicine, Ohio State University Medical Center, Columbus, OH

Patient: 62-year-old Hispanic male.

Physical Examination: Non-contributory.

Chief Complaint: Chest pain.

Medical History: History of 2 hemolytic transfusion reactions initially occurring after transfusion of 2 units of packed red blood cells and again after transfusion of a single unit of packed red blood cells. Each reaction was similar and consisted of hematuria and jaundice. The history was also significant for pancytopenia, myelodysplastic syndrome, coronary artery atherosclerosis, hypertension, angina, and a 40 pack/year history of smoking.

Family History: Diabetes mellitus and coronary artery atherosclerosis in his grandmother. Coronary artery atherosclerosis in his brother. Cerebrovascular accident in his father.

Drug History: Metoprolol, isosorbide dinitrate, recombinant erythropoietin.

Principal Laboratory Findings: See **T1**. ABO/Rh: O, D+, C+, E-, c+, e+ (most probable genotype: R2r). Antigen Profile: K-, S-s+, Fy(a+b+), Jk(a+b-), P1+.

Questions

1. What does the serologic profile suggest?

2. What additional serologic testing may be helpful in the workup of this patient?

3. What medical condition(s) is/are associated with someone having this serologic profile?

4. How should this patient be medically treated?

5. How should this patient be transfused in the future?

Possible Answers

1. The serologic profile is suggestive of a cold-reactive autoantibody. Cold autoantibodies are nearly always reactive at temperatures below 37°C and have their maximal reactivity below 30°C. Cold autoantibodies can be broadly classified as benign or pathologic. Benign autoantibodies may be demonstrated in the serum of most healthy individuals when testing is performed at 4°C. As their name suggests, benign cold autoantibodies are of no clinical significance because they are not active at physiologic temperatures. Pathologic cold autoantibodies can cause hemolytic anemia ranging from mild to life threatening in clinical severity. Cold hemagglutinin disease

T1. Antibody Screen and Red Cell Panel Reactivity*

Results on Procedure	Testing Phase	7/26/01	8/6/01	9/28/01
LISS	IS	1+ to 3+	0	
	37°C	+/-w to 2+	0	
	AHG	2+ to 3+	1+ to 2+	
	Interpretation	positive	positive	
PEG	IS		0	0
	AHG		2+	1+
	Interpretation		positive	positive
Saline	IS			0
	37°C			0
	AHG			0
Ficin	IS	2+ to 3+		
	37°C	2+ to 3+		
	AHG	2+ to 3+		
Solid Phase	Reactivity			4+
	Interpretation			positive
Allogeneic Adsorbed Serum	Saline	negative		
4°C Incubation	IS		3+	
	Interpretation		positive	
DAT	Polyspecific antisera	negative	microscopic positive	negative
	Anti-IgG	ND	negative	ND
	Anti-C3b, C3d	ND	microscopic positive	ND
Auto-Control		positive	positive	positive
Eluate			negative	

*Antibody reactivity noted in all panel cells tested. LISS, low ionic strength saline; PEG, polyethylene glycol; DAT, direct antiglobulin test; IS, immediate spin; AHG, anti-human globulin; ND, not done.

may be chronic and idiopathic or acute and transient. Serologic workup generally reveals a positive direct antiglobulin (Coombs) test with polyspecific antisera (anti-IgG, anti-C3b, C3d) and monospecific antisera (anti-C3b, C3d), due to the coating of red blood cells with complement. Also the patient's red blood cells will agglutinate upon combination with patient's serum at room temperature.

2. Additional serologic tests that may be helpful in the workup of this patient include an antibody titer and thermal amplitude study. The initial serologic workup had been performed at an outside reference laboratory (approximately 4 months prior) at the time of each hemolytic episode (7/26/01 and 8/6/01), before the patient was referred to our institution. Our blood bank repeated the antibody screen (9/28/01) and performed an antibody titer and thermal amplitude studies. The cold reactive antibody

in this patient's serum showed no reactivity at 37°C or 34°C. At 20°C the antibody titer was 1:1, and at 4°C the titer was 1:32. Therefore, at the time that testing was done in our laboratory, the workup showed a cold reactive antibody with a thermal amplitude of 4°C, and significantly less reactivity than that found at the outside facility. At this time the antibody was felt to be clinically insignificant.

3. The serologic profile of this patient's serum can occur secondary to events such as infection with *Mycoplasma pneumoniae* or Epstein-Barr virus (ie, infectious mononucleosis). Cold autoantibodies may be primary or idiopathic, where no easily identifiable trigger for their production is found. Production of the autoantibody can begin either late in the course of the active infection or in the convalescent stage of the disease. Primary cold autoantibodies tend to be responsible for more severe disease manifestations due to their

higher thermal amplitude, higher titer, and their monoclonal origin. Cold autoantibodies that are produced secondary to a concomitant or preceding infection generally have a lower thermal amplitude, low titers, and are usually polyclonal. Notable also is the transient nature of secondary cold autoantibodies. Production of the antibody eventually stops and the patient no longer shows signs of disease.

4. No specific medical treatment is used in the management of patients with cold autoantibodies. Of greatest concern is the need for future transfusion, which may cause a hemolytic transfusion reaction as seen in our patient. Steroid treatment is largely without merit, but in patients with a low antibody titer and a wide thermal amplitude, steroids may be of some benefit in suppressing antibody formation.

5. Subsequent transfusions for this patient should not present a problem since the cold autoantibody appears to have declined in titer and thermal amplitude with time. Since the patient had previous hemolytic episodes, our recommendation was to give a 15 to 25 mL test dose of red blood cells and then draw a blood sample to visually inspect for hemolysis and perform a direct antiglobulin test. Assuming no hemolysis and a negative direct antiglobulin test, the transfusion could continue. Additionally, we recommended that future infusions be administered with a blood warmer if the cold autoantibody is still reactive, and crossmatching requires using the pre-warming technique.

Muscle Weakness and Fatigue in a Woman With Recurrent Upper Respiratory and Urinary Tract Infections

Eiad Kahwash, Peter Bauer, Dave Krugh

Department of Pathology, The Ohio State University, Columbus, OH

Patient: 57-year-old Caucasian woman.

Chief Complaint: The patient was referred to our facility for further evaluation of her deteriorating clinical status.

History of Present Illness: The patient had been admitted to an outlying facility for complications stemming from an upper respiratory infection (URI) beginning 3 weeks previously, for which a course of oral antibiotics was prescribed. In addition, the patient complained of symptoms attributable to a previously diagnosed urinary tract infection (UTI), which had since recurred. Multiple therapeutic modalities, including administration of steroids, intravenous immunoglobulin (IVIG), cyclophosphamide (Cytoxan), and plasmapheresis were implemented; however, her anemia and respiratory status worsened and progressed to multisystem organ failure.

Past Medical History: Diabetes, hypertension, and multiple prior hospital admissions for upper respiratory and urinary tract infections.

Past Surgical History: Cholecystectomy, dilation and curettage, and arthroscopy of the left elbow and left knee.

Social History: Quit cigarette smoking approximately 10 years ago; occasional alcohol use.

Family History: Mother died at age 68 due to carcinoma of the breast. Father living, age 77, with Parkinson's disease and head/neck carcinoma.

Allergies: Penicillin, sulfa drugs, nitrofurantoin (Macrodantin), and tetanus toxoid.

Review of Systems: Positive for shortness of breath, weakness, fatigue, fevers, chills, urine discoloration, and constipation. She denied chest pain, headaches, blurred vision, nausea, vomiting, and/or weight loss.

Physical Examination: Normal except for mild abdominal distension; tympanic to percussion, jaundice, petechiae on both thighs and lower trunk, bilateral lower extremity edema, and severe weakness of the lower extremities.

Results of Other Diagnostic Procedures: Computed tomography (CT) scans of her chest and abdomen demonstrated bilateral ground-glass infiltrates and ascites, respectively.

T1. Principal Non-Immunohematology Laboratory Findings

Laboratory Test		Patient's Result	"Normal" Reference Range
Hematology/Coagulation			
WBC count		10.3	4.0-11.0 × 10³ μL
Differential:	Neutrophils	94	40-60%
	Lymphocyctes	3	20-40%
	Monocytes	3	2.0-8.0%
Hemoglobin		7.2	12-16 g/dL
Platelet Count		101	150-400 × 10³ μL
PT		27.5	11.2-15.0 seconds
INR		2.5	0.8-1.2
PTT		35	24.4-32 seconds
Chemistry			
Sodium		138	135-145 mmol/L
Potassium		3.4	3.5-5.0 mmol/L
Chloride		91	98-109 mmol/L
BUN		41	7-21 mg/dL
Creatinine		1.3	0.6-1.2 mg/dL
Glucose		76	65-115 mg/dL
Calcium		8	8.4-10.2 mg/dL
Ammonia		101	<60 μmol/L
Total bilirubin		42.2	0-1.5 mg/dL
Direct bilirubin		28.3	0-0.3 mg/dL
Alkaline phosphatase		538	8-78 U/L
GGT		1,314	5-85 U/L
ALT		107	0-60 U/L
AST		148	13-40 U/L
LD		2,337	100-190 U/L
Urinalysis			
Protein		Positive	Negative
Blood		Large	Negative

WBC, white blood cell; PT, prothrombin time; INR, International Normalized Ratio; PTT, partial thromboplastin time; BUN, blood urea nitrogen; GGT, gamma-glutamyltransferase; ALT, alanine aminotransferase; AST, aspartate aminotransferase; LD, lactate dehydrogenase.

T2. Principal Immunohematology Findings

Laboratory Test		Patient's Result	"Normal" Reference Range
Indirect antibody screen		Positive*	Negative
Direct antiglobulin test		Positive†	Negative
Cold autoantibody titer		>1:2000	≤ 1:32
Thermal amplitude cold autoantibody titer @ °C:	20	1:128	
	32	1:8	
	34	1:2	
	37	1:1	

*For the cold autoantibody, anti-I. †C3b only.

Questions

1. What are this patient's most striking clinical findings and laboratory results?

2. How do you explain this patient's striking laboratory clinical findings and laboratory results?

3. Which additional tests should be performed and why?

4. What is the most likely diagnosis?

5. What are the treatment options for this patient?

6. What is the mechanism of action and potential side effects of Rituximab therapy?

Possible Answers

1. Ground glass pulmonary infiltrates; abdominal ascites; neutrophilia; marked anemia (hemoglobin <10 mg/dL); increased PT and INR; modestly increased PTT; slight hypokalemia and decreased chloride; increased BUN; increased ammonia; markedly increased liver function tests, including: total and direct bilirubin, alkaline phosphatase, GGT, ALT, AST, and especially LD; protein and a large amount of blood in the urine [T1]; positive indirect and direct antiglobulin tests; and the presence of a high titer cold autoantibody (anti-I) with a wide thermal amplitude [T2].

2. Ground glass pulmonary infiltrates are consistent with our patient's URTI, complicated by pneumonia. Neutrophilia, electrolyte disturbances (ie, potassium and chloride), protein and blood in the urine, increased BUN and ammonia, and markedly increased values for a variety of liver function tests were most likely due to the combination of the patient's urinary tract and upper respiratory tract infections, worsening renal and liver function, and a hemolytic anemia induced by the patient's high titer of anti-I antibody. Intravascular hemolysis would also contribute to the presence of hemoglobin in the urine and a markedly increased serum LD concentration from release of the LD-1 and LD-2 isoenzymes found in relatively high concentration in red blood cells (RBCs).

3. Peripheral blood microscopic analysis, with or without WBC immunophenotyping by flow cytometry; bone marrow biopsy and hematological examination; hemoglobin electrophoresis; direct antiglobulin test (DAT); cold autoantibody thermal amplitude studies; cryoglobulin testing; Ham's test; the osmotic fragility test; quantitative serum haptoglobin; and *Mycoplasma pneumoniae*, cytomegalovirus (CMV), Epstein-Barr virus, antinuclear (ANA), and antimitochrondrial antibody (ANCA) tests.

Because cold autoantibodies may occur normally in some individuals and in others as a result of a variety of conditions [eg, mycoplasma pneumonia (>80% of cases), listeriosis, infectious mononucleosis, acute CMV infection, subacute bacterial endocarditis, malaria, trypanosomiasis, syphilis, collagen vascular disease, and hematolymphoid malignancies], the presence of these autoantibodies alone may not account for a patient's anemia. Moreover, anti-I and anti-H are the most frequently encountered unexpected antibodies in serologic tests performed at room temperature. Therefore, additional laboratory tests are needed to further define the nature of the patient's anemia. These tests might include: peripheral blood and bone marrow examination for the presence of abnormal cells characteristic of hematolymphoid malignancies; hemoglobin electrophoresis for hemoglobinopathies; DAT for evidence of in vivo RBC sensitization by circulating antibody, suggestive of immune-mediated hemolytic anemia; cold autoantibody thermal amplitude studies; cyroglobulin testing, including clonality by immunofixation electrophoresis (IFE) of any cryoglobulin detected by routine protein electrophoresis; the Ham's test for paroxysmal nocturnal hemoglobinuria (PNH); the osmotic fragility test for hereditary spherocytosis and red cell membrane abnormalities; quantitative serum haptoglobin determination to assess the extent of any intravascular hemolysis; the ANA test for collagen vascular disease; and a variety of other antibody tests indicative of infection by a specific bacterial or viral organism. Cryoglobulin testing and testing for cryoglobulin-like antibodies (eg, P1 blood system antibodies to RBC antigens), including assessment of clonality by IFE of any cryoglobulin detected by routine protein electrophoresis, may also be useful. The majority of cold agglutinins due to infection with *Mycoplasma pneumoniae* are polyclonal (eg, IgM anti-I), while those that occur secondary to hematolymphoid malignancies are typically monoclonal. Test results used to substantiate the intravascular nature of a hemolytic anemia include decreased serum haptoglobin and increased indirect bilirubin and LD concentrations, hemosiderinuria, and hemoglobinuria. Moreover, examination of a stained peripheral blood smear might demonstrate polychromatophilia, anisocytosis/poikilocytosis, macrocytosis, spherocytes, and red cell fragments consistent with ongoing hemolysis due to a specific cause.

Many of the tests indicated above were performed on our patient; however, the results of these tests did not entirely explain the source or cause of the patient's cold autoantibody,

hemolytic anemia, and markedly abnormal liver function tests. In this patient, while *M. pneumoniae* was highly suspected due to recurrent URIs, it was excluded by a negative serum *M. pneumoniae* antibody titer. In addition, negative immunoglobulin M (IgM) antibody titers for CMV and Epstein-Barr virus excluded CMV infection or infectious mononucleosis as the cause of our patient's acute illness. Moreover, collagen vascular disease was excluded by a negative ANA test. On the other hand, this patient's positive DAT due to complement (C3) (with subsequent identification of the cold-reactive autoantibody, anti-I) in our patient's serum was consistent with an autoantibody-induced hemolytic anemia. This finding alone, however, does not explain our patient's markedly elevated liver function tests. Our patient's markedly elevated liver enzymes with high total and direct bilirubin values suggest the presence of liver disease, including that caused by hematolymphoid malignancies.[1] Thus, our patient underwent a transcutaneous liver biopsy in an attempt to explain her ascites and the abnormal laboratory test results. Pertinent biopsy findings included the presence of a marked, diffuse (primarily intracanalicular) bile stasis and portal tract expansion by lymphocytes not associated with piecemeal necrosis. Immunohistochemical analysis demonstrated a mature lymphoid population expressing CD20, bcl-2, and CD43 cell surface markers, while staining negative for CD3 and CD23. These findings, in conjunction with the histopathological findings from the liver biopsy, were highly suggestive of B-cell lymphoma.

4. ***Most likely diagnosis:*** *Cold autoantibody-induced hemolytic anemia secondary to B-cell lymphoma involving the liver.*

5. Being kept in a warm environment, drug therapy, splenectomy, plasma exchange, and monoclonal antibody therapy. It is important that the patient be kept in a warm environment and that all blood and/or blood components and intravenous fluids administered to the patient be warmed to normal body temperature to avoid or limit in vivo RBC sensitization by the patient's cold autoantibody, especially during circulation through distal areas. In addition, high-dose steroid therapy (not helpful in the majority of cases because cold autoantibodies are usually of the IgM class of

immunoglobulins), splenectomy (usually ineffective because sensitized RBCs can also be cleared by the liver), and plasma exchange (helpful only as a temporizing measure in acute situations because antibodies removed during this process are eventually replaced) are other treatment options. Cold autoantibody-induced hemolytic anemia, secondary to B-cell lymphoma, may show improvement following the administration of the monoclonal antibody (anti-CD20) preparation, Rituximab.[2-4]

6. Rituximab is a bioengineered hybrid murine/human monoclonal antibody directed against the CD20 antigen found on both normal and malignant B lymphocytes. The binding of Rituximab promotes the immune-mediated destruction of B lymphocytes. Rituximab is given at a dose of 375 mg/m² by intravenous infusion once per week for a period of 4 weeks. Serious side effects include hypoxia, pulmonary infiltrates, acute respiratory distress syndrome, myocardial infarction, and cardiogenic shock. Other adverse reactions are tumor lysis syndrome, severe mucocutaneous reactions, and prolonged impairment of the humoral immune system leading to an increased risk of viral and bacterial infections.[2-4]

Treatment and Course

Rituximab therapy was initiated in an attempt to decrease or halt the production of the circulating cold autoantibody. Based on serial antibody screens, the treatment was effective as no demonstrable cold autoantibody was detectable following 12 days of therapy. Unfortunately, the patient succumbed to complications stemming from a disseminated *Pseudomonas* infection 4 weeks after the initiation of Rituximab therapy.

Keywords

cold autoantibody, B-cell lymphoma, hemolytic anemia, Rituximab

References

1. Wallach, JB. *Interpretation of Diagnostic Tests*, 7th ed. Boston: Lippincott, Williams and Wilkins; 2001.

2. Zaja F, Iacona I, Masolini P, et al. B-cell depletion with Rituximab as treatment for immune hemolytic anemia and chronic thrombocytopenia. *Haematologica.* 2002;87:189-195.

3. Delgado J, Bustos JG, Jimenez-Yuste V, et al. Anti-CD20 monoclonal therapy in refractory immune thrombocytopenic purpura. *Haematologica.* 2002;87:215-216.

4. Bauduer F. Rituximab. A very efficient therapy in cold agglutinins and refractory autoimmune haemolytic anaemia associated with CD-20 positive, low-grade lymphoma. *Br J Haematol. 2001;112:1083-1090.*

Hemolytic Anemia in a 5-Year-Old Child

Kathleen Nicol,[1] Nawwar Swedan,[1] Phylis Moder,[1] Samir Kahwash,[1] Melissa J. Rose,[2] Bryce Kerlin[2]

Departments of [1]Laboratory Medicine and [2]Hematology/Oncology, Children's Hospital and Ohio State University, Columbus, OH

Patient: 5-year-old male.

Chief Complaint: Dark urine and fever.

Past Medical History: Recent history of upper respiratory infection (URI), following a spell of severe cold weather and a snow storm, requiring treatment with erythromycin. Otherwise, he was previously healthy.

Physical Examination Findings: On hospital admission, the patient was febrile (40°C), lungs were clear to auscultation, and the heart rate was regular. There was no edema or jaundice.

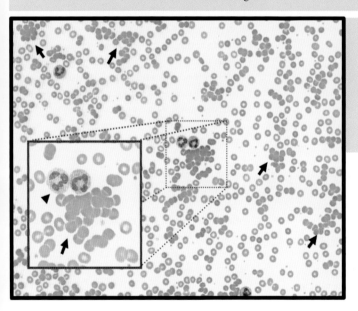

Image 1_Patient's peripheral blood smear showing red cell clumping (arrows) and the absence of schistocytes [inset demonstrates neutrophils with toxic granulation and Döhle bodies (arrowhead)].

Questions _____

1. What are this patient's most striking clinical and/or laboratory findings?

2. How do you explain these findings?

3. What are the principal causes of anemia?

4. What is this patient's most likely diagnosis?

5. What laboratory test will be helpful in confirming the diagnosis?

6. What causes this patient's disorder, and how common is it?

7. What are the treatment and management of this disorder?

Possible Answers _____

1. Dark urine and fever; markedly reduced RBC count, hemoglobin level, and hematocrit; reticulocytosis on hospital day 1 that resolved by hospital day 3 following transfusion of 5 doses of packed RBCs on day 1 (3 doses) and days 2 (1 dose) and 4 (1 dose); markedly elevated ESR, LD, and bilirubin (total, direct, and indirect) levels; a reduced haptoglobin level; a red and hazy urine containing detectable amounts of protein, ketones, urobilinogen, and a large amount of occult blood, along with microscopic findings of a large number of RBCs/hpf; positive antibody findings for Epstein-Barr virus viral capsid antigen IgG antibody (EBV VCA IgG Ab) and EBV nuclear antigen (NA) IgG antibodies; and positive direct antiglobulin test (DAT), using anti-C3 antiserum only, and strongly positive 3-cell antibody screen findings at 4°C (**T1**).

2. All of this patient's clinical and laboratory findings are consistent with an in vivo hemolytic syndrome in a patient with an inflammatory condition (elevated ESR, probably due to recent URI), prior infection with EBV, positive DAT, and strongly positive 3-cell antibody screen findings at 4°C suggestive of RBCs coated with a cold-reactive autoantibody.

3. When classified by pathophysiology, anemia can be divided into 3 major categories: (1) anemia of decreased production, (2) anemia of increased destruction (hemolytic), and (3) combined decreased production and increased destruction, as in some hemoglobinopathies. The first category includes nutritional deficiencies (for which iron deficiency is by far the most common type of anemia in children), anemia of chronic disease, aplastic anemia, and anemia of myelodysplastic or myelopthisic disorders. The second category, the hemolytic anemias, can be further divided, based on etiology, into 2 separate groups—anemia due to an RBC membrane or enzyme defect or to immunologic factors extrinsic to the red cells. Immune hemolytic anemias generally have characteristic clinical findings including rapid onset and progression, dark urine, and jaundice, with or without splenomegaly. Laboratory findings (eg, increased LD and indirect bilirubin, and decreased haptoglobin)

are important in confirming a hemolytic process and in establishing an immunologic etiology (eg, antiglobulin test results). Immune-mediated anemias can be further subdivided into primary autoimmune hemolytic anemia (AIHA) and secondary AIHA. In primary AIHA, there is no identifiable underlying illness, and the hemolytic anemia is the only clinical finding. Moreover, there are 3 forms of primary AIHA: warm-reactive AIHA, cold AIHA (CAIHA), and paroxysmal cold hemoglobinuria (PCH). The possible causes of CAIHA include cold agglutinin syndrome (CAS), PCH, and drug-induced immune hemolytic anemia.[1,2] Complement fixation and thermal reactivity at 4°C can be seen with both CAS and PCH. Cold agglutinin syndrome is usually the result of an auto-reactive IgM antibody that causes intravascular hemolysis via complement-mediated formation of a RBC membrane attack complex (MAC) and extravascular hemolysis via reticuloendothelial destruction of RBC-complement complexes. Although IgG antibodies generally do not bind and activate the complement system, the autoantibody associated with PCH [ie, Donath-Landsteiner (DL) antibody] is a unique IgG antibody that has a low thermal affinity, binds complement with high-affinity, and produces intravascular hemolysis via complete activation of the complement system through the MAC. While CAS may cause either mild, subacute, or severe acute hemolysis, PCH should be suspected clinically anytime there is severe, acute hemolysis.[3]

4. ***Most likely diagnosis:*** *paroxysmal cold hemoglobinuria (PCH).* Due to the brisk, severe intravascular hemolysis associated with the patient's history of recent cold exposure, PCH is the most likely cause of the patient's CAIHA.

5. The serological Donath-Landsteiner (DL) test is designed to confirm the diagnosis of PCH by demonstrating the presence of the DL antibody in the patient's serum. The DL Ab is directed toward the P-antigen complex that is located on the surface of red blood cells.[4,5] Serum from the patient is cooled to 4°C to 5°C, followed by the addition of P1 antigen-positive RBCs. If DL antibody is present in the serum, it reacts with the P-antigen positive RBCs. Upon warming of this mixture to 37°C (ie, body temperature), the DL antibody dissociates from the RBCs, but

T1. Principal Laboratory Findings

Test		Patient's Result on Hospital Day[a]				Reference Interval
		1[b]	2	3	4	
Hematology						
WBC count		7.4, 6.7	10.6	14.4	11.7	$5.5\text{-}15.5 \times 10^3/\mu L$
RBC count		2.73, 2.39	2.11	2.79	1.71	$3.9\text{-}5.3 \times \text{s}10^6/\mu L$
Hemoglobin		8.5, 7.4	6.3	8.2	5.1	11.5-13.5 g/dL
Hematocrit		22.6, 19.6	17.1	22.6	14.0	34-40%
MCV		82.3, 82.3	81.0	80.9	81.9	75-88 fL
RDW		14.1, 14.1	15.4	15.3	15.3	10.0-14.1%
Reticulocytes		1.0, 5.7		1.6		0.4-1.8%
Platelet count		176, 170	232	217	166	$140\text{-}440 \times 10^3/\mu L$
ESR		44				0-15 mm/h
PBS findings		Red cell clumping; no schistocytes; neutrophils with toxic granulation and Dohle bodies (Image 1)				
Chemistry						
LD		8,311				400-1,250 U/L
Aldolase		22.7				3-12 U/L
Bilirubin:	Total	4.7				0.1-1.0 mg/dL
	Direct	1.2				<0.6 mg/dL
	Indirect	3.5				0.1-1.0 mg/dL
Haptoglobin		<9				33-171 mg/L
Urinalysis						
Color and appearance		Red and hazy				Clear and straw colored
Myoglobin		Negative				Negative
Protein		100				0 mg/dL
Ketones		10				0 mg/dL
Urobilinogen		4				<1.1 EU/dL
Occult blood		Large				Negative
Microscopic findings:	RBCs	68				0-2/hpf

Stool occult blood	Negative	Negative
WBCs	1	<6/hpf
Immunology		
EBV VCA Ab: IgG	Positive >1:160	Negative <1:10
IgM	Negative <1:10	Negative <1:10
EBV NA Ab, IgG	Positive >1:160	Negative <1:4
Parvo B19 Ab: IgG	Negative	Negative
IgM	Negative	Negative
Rapid strep & Gen probe tests	Negative	Negative
Mycoplasma Ab, IgG & IgM	Negative	Negative
ANA screen & titer	Negative	Negative
Blood Bank		
IAT	Negative	Negative
DAT antiserum: Polyspecific	1+	Negative
Anti-IgG	Negative	Negative
Anti-C3	2+	Negative
3-Cell Ab screen @ 4°C	4+	Negative

aPatient was transfused with packed red blood cells (RBCs) on days 1 (3 doses), 2 (1 dose), and 4 (1 dose), and on day 1 also received intravenous immune globulin (IVIG). bHematology values on day 1 were obtained at 2 different times. WBC, white blood cell; MCV, mean corpuscular volume; RDW, red cell distribution width; ESR, erythrocyte sedimentation rate; PBS, peripheral blood smear; LD, lactate dehydrogenase; EU, Ehrlich Units; hpf, high power field; EBV, Epstein-Barr virus; VCA, viral capsid antigen; NA, nuclear antigen; ANA, anti-nuclear antigen; Ab, antibody; Ig, immunoglobulin; IAT, indirect antiglobulin test; DAT, direct antiglobulin test; C3, complement component 3.

T2. Donath-Landsteiner Test

Mixture Tested	Presence or Absence of Hemolysis at Incubation Time and Temperature		
	30 min @ 4°C followed by 60 min @ 37°C	60 min @ 37°C	90 min @ 37°C
Patient's serum + P1 positive RBCs	Positive	None	None
Patient's serum + P1 positive RBCs + normal saline	Slight	None	None
NHS + P1 positive RBCS	None	None	None

P1, P1 antigen; RBCs, red blood cells; NHS, normal human serum.

activates the classic complement pathway prior to detaching. Complement is normally present in the patient's sera (or can be provided by adding fresh plasma, a rich source of complement). Because of the complete activation of complement through the C9 complement component, formation of the MAC occurs, and the sensitized red cells are hemolyzed rapidly resulting in in vitro hemolysis similar to the intravascular hemolysis that occurs in vivo. When the DL test was performed on serum from the patient, the test was positive (ie, the characteristic biphasic temperature response of no hemolysis at 4°C, but hemolysis at 37°C was observed), the degree of hemolysis produced was reduced by dilution with normal saline, and normal human serum (NHS) lacking the DL antibody did not react with P1 positive RBCs to produce hemolysis. Moreover, no hemolysis was observed when the patient's serum was incubated for 90 minutes at only 37°C (**T2**).

6. Paroxysmal cold hemoglobinuria is an acquired type of AIHA that is caused by the presence of the DL antibody in the patient's serum. The DL antibody is directed against the P-antigen complex (a glycosphingolipid) on the surface of RBCs. The stimulus for the production of this antibody has been postulated to be an antigen with a structure similar to the P-antigen on human RBCs and some infectious agents, including *Treponema pallidum* (the causative agent of syphilis) and measles and mumps viruses.[6] In the latter half of the 19th century, the most common cause of PCH was congenital or tertiary syphilis. However, with modern antibiotic therapy to effectively treat syphilis, this secondary cause of PCH has been almost totally eliminated. The DL antibody is usually produced within 2 to 3 weeks of an acute viral or febrile illness and may persist for several years after such an illness. Moreover, there are reports of an association between DL antibody and various malignancies; however, except in rare cases, there is no apparent disease-related association.[7-9] Development of DL antibodies has also been reported following measles immunization and in an adult affected with PCH following chicken pox.[6] PCH occurs most commonly in children and constitutes a major proportion (up to 40%) of AIHA cases in children younger than 5 years. Most children usually develop a single, brief, post-viral hemolytic episode. There is no predilection for sex or race. Lack of awareness of the signs, symptoms, and laboratory findings associated with PCH may lead to a failure to recognize and diagnose this syndrome in both children and adults.

7. The mainstays of treatment for PCH are supportive care and avoidance of cold. All exposed portions of the body should be covered, ingestion of cold substances (such as popsicles or ice cream) should be discouraged, and the room in which affected individuals reside should be warmed to ≥70°F. Pre-warmed, packed RBC (PRBC) transfusions for life-threatening hemolysis and symptomatic anemia may be indicated, especially to maintain adequate renal blood flow.[3] However, because nearly all donor blood is P-antigen positive, this blood should be used for transfusion, rather than searching for P antigen-negative components (only 1 in 200,000 donor units are P-antigen negative). Transfusion with P antigen-negative blood, as well as administration of intravenous immune globulin (IVIG) or other temporary support measures, should be considered for patients who fail to respond to pre-warmed, unscreened PRBC units. Administration of steroids is unlikely to benefit the patient and are generally not useful. Overall, it is very important to treat the underlying cause of the infection, malignancy, etc, that caused the development of DL antibodies.[10] In addition, hydration, alkalinization of the urine, and other supportive care measures may become necessary to prevent renal insufficiency due to nephrotoxic hemoglobinemia. With an underlying infectious disease that is controllable or self-limited, the process may resolve spontaneously and quickly without the development of DL antibodies. However, patients with PCH may be in acute distress, with obvious pain, jaundice, fever, and hemodynamic compromise. Pallor, icterus, and urticaria may be seen as well. The latter are postulated to be due to DL antibody binding to P-antigen found on lymphocytes and skin fibroblasts. Moreover, the aforementioned clinical findings may be the only ones present unless they are accompanied by those due to a specific underlying illness.[3]

Patient Follow-up

In addition to RBC transfusions and administration of IVIG, the patient received a 2-week course of corticosteroids. By this time the hemoglobin and reticulocyte counts had stabilized. Eleven weeks after discharge, the DAT was negative, and he was clinically asymptomatic.

Keywords

cold autoimmune hemolytic anemia, paroxysmal cold hemoglobinuria, Donath-Landsteiner antibody

References

1. Petz LD, Garratty G. *Acquired Immune Hemolytic Anemias.* New York, NY: Churchill Livingstone; 1980: 37-50.

2. Sivakumaran M, Murphy PT, Booker DJ, et al. Paroxysmal cold haemoglobinuria caused by non-Hodgkin's lymphoma. *Br J Haematol.* 1999;105:278-279.

3. Ware RE. *Autoimmune Hemolytic Anemia.* In: Nathan DG, Orkin SH, Ginsburg D, Look AT, eds. *Nathan and Oski's Hematology of Infancy and Childhood.* 6th ed. Philadelphia: Saunders; 2003:521-559.

4. Donath J, Landsteiner K. Uber paroxysmale haemoglobinurie. *Munchen Medicine Wochenschr.* 1904;51:1590-1593.

5. Göttsche B, Salama A, Mueller-Eckhardt C. Donath-Landsteiner autoimmune hemolytic anemia in children. A study of 22 cases. *Vox Sang.* 1990;58:281-286.

6. Papalia MA, Schwarer AP. Paroxysmal cold haemoglobinuria in an adult with chicken pox. *Br J Haematol.* 2000;109:328-329.

7. Prasad AS, Berman L, Tranchida L, et al. Red cell hypoplasia, cold hemoglobinuria and M-type gamma G serum paraprotein and Bence Jones proteinuria in a patient with lymphoproliferative disorder. *Blood.* 1968;31:151-165.

8. Sharara AI, Hillsley RE, Wax TD, et al. Paroxysmal cold hemoglobinuria associated with non-Hodgkin's lymphoma. *South Med J.* 1994;87:397-399.

9. Thomas AT. Autoimmune hemolytic anemias. In: Lee GR, Foerster J, Lukens J, Paraskevas F, Greer JP, Rodgers GM, eds. *Wintrobe's Clinical Hematology.* 10th ed. Baltimore, MD: Williams & Wilkins; 1999:1233-1263.

10. Rausen AR, LeVine R, Hsu TC, et al. Compatible transfusion therapy for paroxysmal cold hemoglobinuria. *Pediatrics.* 1975;55:275-278.

Management of Hemolytic Disease of the Newborn

JoAnna D. Williams, David Krugh, Sandra Dietrich, Richard O'Shaughnessy, Melanie S. Kennedy

Departments of Pathology and Obstetric & Gynecology, The Ohio State University, Columbus, OH

Patient: Pregnant (G4P2011) 29-year-old Hispanic woman who presented at 16 weeks gestation.

Medical History: Her first pregnancy ended in a miscarriage during the first trimester. The patient did not receive Rh(D) immune globulin following the miscarriage. The child from her second pregnancy died less than 1 week after birth due to hemolytic disease of the newborn (HDN). Her third pregnancy resulted in a healthy child with no complications. There is no history of any blood transfusions. All of her children had the same father.

Family History: Non-contributory.

Drug History: None.

Physical Examination: Gravid uterus, otherwise unremarkable.

T1. Principal Laboratory Findings

Test	Results
Mother	
ABO/Rh(D) type	Group O Rh(D) Negative
Antibody screen	Positive
Antibody identification	Anti-D
Antibody titer	Saline-Negative; AHG-1:16
ΔOD_{450} @ 19 wks G.A.	0.02 (Liley Graph Zone 1)
Father	
Most probable genotype	CDE/cde (R_zr)
Fetus (G4)	
Most probable genotype*	cde/cde

*Based on Rh(D) genotyping of amniotic fluid fetal cells. ΔOD_{450} delta density at 450 nm; G.A., gestational age.

T2. Typical Follow-up of ΔOD_{450} Results Based on Liley Graph (Zone) Findings

Zone	Repeat Amniocentesis and Amniotic Fluid $\Delta OD450$ Measurement at
I	2 to 3 week intervals
IIa	10 to 14 day intervals, if there is a decreasing trend in $\Delta OD450$ values, with probable delivery at 36 to 38 weeks G.A.
IIb	7 to 10 day intervals, if there is an increasing trend in $\Delta OD450$ values
III	N/A (if G.A. >18 weeks, immediate intrauterine transfusion is indicated and delivery as soon as the L/S ratio is satisfactory)

G.A., gestational age; N/A, not applicable; L/S, lecithin:sphingomyelin [an L/S ratio >2.0 or 2.5 typically indicates fetal lung maturity and a reduced probability of neonatal respiratory distress syndrome (RDS)].

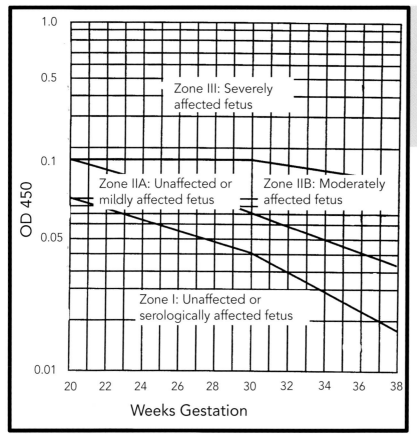

Figure 1_Modified Liley Graph-The Ohio State University Medical Center.

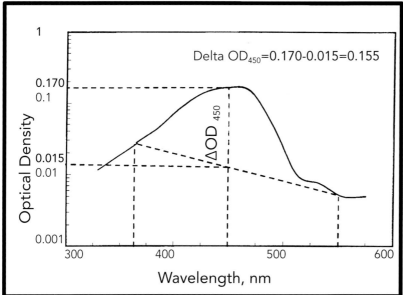

Figure 2_Representative (ie, not from the patient discussed in this case study) amniotic fluid tracing from a recording spectrophotometer illustrating the determination of the ΔOD_{450} value. Note that absorbance is plotted on a logarithmic scale.

In Figure 2: Delta OD_{450}=0.170-0.015=0.155

Questions _____

1. What is the significance of an anti-D antibody in a pregnant woman?

2. Which laboratory test(s) is(are) used in the management of pregnant women with anti-D antibodies and why?

3. What is the principle of the amniotic fluid ΔOD_{450} test and how are the results of this

test used in the management of pregnancies at increased risk for HDN?

4. Based on the results in **T1**, what impact will the mother's Rh(D)-antibody have on her current pregnancy?

5. Why was this mother's Rh(D)-antibody clinically significant (ie, fatal) in her second pregnancy but not in her third?

Possible Answers

1. Anti-D antibodies belong to the immunoglobulin G (IgG) class and are capable of crossing the placenta and entering the fetal circulation. In a pregnant woman whose blood contains these antibodies and who is carrying a fetus that has inherited the Rh(D)-antigen [ie, whose RBCs are Rh(D) positive], these antibodies can attach to the fetal RBCs and destroy them, resulting in HDN.[1] The severity of the anemia that can occur in HDN typically correlates with the amount of antibody (titer) in the mother's serum. Clinical outcomes range from mild anemia, jaundice, hepatosplenomegaly, and mild bleeding diatheses to marked acid-base abnormalities, kernicterus, hydrops fetalis, and miscarriage.

2. Anti-D titer of the mother's serum, Rh phenotype of the father, and ΔOD_{450} value on amniotic fluid. The anti-D titer establishes the severity of maternal isoimmunization, which correlates with the degree of intrauterine fetal anemia that may occur. The Rh phenotype of the father establishes whether or not he possesses the Rh(D)-antigen as well as his zygosity. The spectrophotometric ΔOD_{450} test provides an indication of the extent of intrauterine hemolysis that may be occurring. The ΔOD_{450} test provides an estimate of the concentration of bilirubinoid pigments, principally bilirubin, present in amniotic fluid, resulting from the in vivo destruction of fetal RBCs. The mother's anti-D titer was saline negative but 1:16 with anti-human globulin (AHG). The father's most probable genotype was DCE/dce, $R_z r$. The ΔOD_{450} value was 0.02 (Liley Chart Zone 1 - unaffected or serologically affected) at 19 weeks gestational age [**T1** and **Figure 1**]. Because the mother's anti-D titer was less than 1:32, she should be followed with

repeat serial titers every 2 to 3 weeks. If her titer rises to 1:32 or higher, then an amniocentesis (after 18 weeks gestation) should be performed followed by an amniotic fluid ΔOD_{450} determination. Based on the father's heterozygosity for the Rh(D)-antigen and the patient's history, an amniocentesis would be warranted to determine the inheritance of the D antigen through allele-specific gene amplification studies on fetal cells in the amniotic fluid. Other methods of monitoring for fetal anemia include Doppler assessment of middle cerebral artery peak velocity and fetal hemoglobin via cordocentesis.[2] These 2 methods are used more frequently on patients who have had a previously affected fetus, because Rh(D) titers in subsequent pregnancies become less accurate in assessing the degree of intrauterine fetal anemia.

3. Bilirubin, the end-product of the breakdown of RBC hemoglobin, absorbs maximally at a wavelength of 450 nm. Amniotic fluid can contain pigments related (bilirubinoid) or not related to bilirubin that absorb near the wavelength maximum for bilirubin or provide a higher background level of absorbance than would occur if these pigments were not present. Subtracting the spectrophotometric absorbance at the point perpendicular to the absorbance at 450 nm that intersects a line drawn between the absorbance values at 365 nm and 550 nm corrects for the presence of these non-bilirubin pigments.[3] The difference (or delta) in absorbance [formerly called optical density (OD)] between the absorbance value at 450 nm and the absorbance at the intersection of the perpendicular is the ΔOD_{450} value [**Figure 2**]. To gauge the severity of the fetal anemia, the x,y-pair consisting of the gestational age (G.A.) and ΔOD_{450} value is plotted on the graph developed by Liley[4] for this purpose [**Figure 1**]. There are 3 zones on the "modified" Liley graph[4] associated with increasing degree of severity and different follow-up options [**T2**].

The modification shown in [**T2**] splits Zone II into IIA and IIB. Zone I is consistent with an unaffected or serologically affected fetus. Zone IIa is indicative of an unaffected or mildly affected fetus. Zone IIb is consistent with a moderately affected fetus. Zone III is indicative of a severely affected fetus with a hemoglobin level generally less than 8.0 g/dL. Treatment options based on the Liley graph findings include repeat amniocentesis and ΔOD_{450} measurements at various intervals or fetal intrauterine transfusion [**T2**]. If an intrauterine transfusion is necessary, cytomegalovirus (CMV)-negative, irradiated, antigen negative [for any respective fetal antibody(ies) present] RBCs are used to correct the fetal anemia. Once initiated, intrauterine transfusions must be repeated at 7 to 21 day intervals until delivery. Red cells for transfusion often come from the pregnant mother if she and her fetus are ABO-compatible. The transfusion is done using ultrasound to guide a 20 to 22 gauge needle into the umbilical vein of the cord or, alternatively, into the fetal peritoneal cavity if the fetus is not hydropic. Intrauterine transfusion into the fetal umbilical vein is the preferred technique since pre- and post-transfusion hematologic parameters can be measured and monitored. Fetal transfusions can be given as early as 18 weeks gestational age; however, a program of intrauterine transfusions is not started after 34 weeks gestational age because preterm delivery at that point may carry less risk.

4. None. Because the fetus has not inherited the Rh(D) antigen, it is not at risk for HDN due to the presence of maternal anti-D antibody. However, the mother should be followed with routine prenatal care including a repeat antibody screen at 28 weeks to rule out formation of other red cell antibodies.

5. The mother formed the anti-D antibody after being exposed to the Rh(D) antigen during the miscarriage of her first pregnancy. She did not receive Rh(D) immune globulin at any time during that pregnancy or after her miscarriage. The child from her second pregnancy was Rh(D) positive. Because the mother had been previously sensitized to Rh(D), the Rh(D) antibodies in her blood caused a severe in utero hemolytic disease, ultimately resulting in the death of the neonate within 1 week of birth. The third child was Rh(D) negative and was therefore unaffected by the mother's anti-D antibody. The mother does not need to receive Rh(D) immune globulin during or after her current or future pregnancies because she has already formed the anti-D antibody.

References

1. Narang A, Jain N. Haemolytic disease of newborn. *Indian J Pediatr*. 2001; 68(2):167-172.

2. 2.Divakaran TG, Waugh J, Clark TJ, et al. Noninvasive techniques to detect fetal anemia due to red blood cell alloimmunization: a systematic review. *Obstet Gynecol*. 2001;98(3):509-517.

3. Glasser L, Finley PR. Body Fluids VI: Amniotic fluid and the quality of life. *Diag Med*. 1981;Sep/Oct:31-43.

4. Svendsen EK. Pigment index in amniotic fluid (Liley's method) in Rh-immunization. *Acta Obstet Gynecol Scand*. 1966;45(suppl):99-101.

Is it Really Anti-D and Anti-C or Is it Anti-G?

Nada Rikabi,[1] Lisa Dunn-Albanasse,[2] Dave Krugh,[1] Diane Snider,[1] Kristi Frenken,[2] Karen Rossi,[2] Richard O'Shaughnessy,[2] Melanie S. Kennedy[1]

Departments of [1]Pathology and [2]Obstetrics & Gynecology, Maternal-Fetal Medicine, The Ohio State University, Columbus, OH

Patient: 36-year-old Caucasian woman.

Surgical History: Splenectomy.

History of Present Illness: The patient is a G3P3, group B Rh(D) negative woman, treated appropriately with Rh(D) immune globulin (RhIg) therapy after the birth of her first and second infants. The patient presented in her third pregnancy at 12 2/7 weeks of gestation with a positive antibody screen for anti-D and anti-C. The titer against R1R1 cells initially was 1:8, increasing to 1:16. The anti-D titer against R2R2 cells was 1:4.

Medical History: Thrombotic thrombocytopenia purpura (TTP), treated on multiple occasions with plasma exchange and with plasma infusions [**T1**], deep venous thrombosis, supraventricular tachycardia, and adenomatous polyps of the small bowel.

Family History: Divorced, remarried with 3 children. The patient is adopted and therefore had no knowledge of her family's medical history.

Drug History: Enoxaparin, switched to heparin at 36 weeks of gestation; nitrofurantoin; iron supplementation; and prenatal vitamins.

Results of Additional Diagnostic Procedures: An amniocentesis was performed at 20 weeks gestational age (G.A.) and a delta OD450 analysis performed on amniotic fluid yielded a value of 0.07 (with a hemoglobin peak present in the scan), corresponding to a Liley chart zone of 1 (ie, unaffected or mildly affected fetus for intrauterine hemolysis). Fetal cells in the amniotic fluid were tested by polymerase chain reaction (PCR) for gene sequences corresponding to Rh antigens. PCR testing was positive for D and negative for C antigen gene sequences. At 24 weeks and 2 days G.A. (ie, 24 2/7), anti-G and anti-C were identified in the patient's serum. At 27 6/7 weeks G.A., RhIg was administered to the mother.

Questions

1. Should all prenatal patients presenting with possible anti-D and anti-C in their serum be routinely evaluated to determine the presence of anti-G rather than anti-D?

2. How can anti-G be identified in the laboratory?

3. What is the risk for hemolytic disease of the newborn (HDN) in prenatal patients with anti-G as opposed to anti-D?

4. In this case, if the infant required an intrauterine transfusion or an exchange transfusion, what type of blood would be appropriate for transfusion?

T1. Patient's Transfusion History

Year/Month of Transfusion and Number of Units Transfused

Blood Component Transfused	1992 Aug	1993 Oct	Dec	1994 Jan	1996 Feb	1997 Apr	May	1998 Feb	1999 Feb	2000 Jul	Aug	Sep
Platelet pheresis units	1[a]	0	0	0	0	0	0	0	0	0	0	0
Pooled platelets	1[a]	0	0	0	0	0	0	0	0	0	0	0
FFP	12	43	0	0	14	2	2	0	0	0	0	0
CPP	0	0	6	6	124	62	12	91	2	8	80	0
RBCs	4[a] + 1[b]	0	0	0	2[a]	2[a]	0	1[a]	2[a]	0	2[b]	3[a]

[a]B Rh(D) negative. [b]O Rh(D) negative. FFP, fresh frozen plasma; CPP, cryoprecipitate-poor plasma; RBCs, red blood cells.

T2. Patient's Obstetrical History

Mother					Neonate(s)[a]	
Pregnancy[a]	Ab Screen	G.A. @ Delivery	RhIg Given[b]	Probable Paternal Genotype	HDN Status	Rh(D) Type
G1P1	Neg	40	Yes	n.a.	Unaffected	Positive
G2P3	Neg	40	Yes	n.a.	Unaffected	Negative (twins)
G3P4	Pos	39	Yes	R_2r	Unaffected	Positive

[a]Each pregnancy resulted from 3 different men. [b]Rh(D) immune globulin (RhIg) was administered at ~28 weeks gestational age (G.A.) or at delivery for all 3 pregnancies. Ab, antibody; HDN, hemolytic disease of the newborn; n.a., not available.

T3. Patient's Antibody Screening Results at Various Gestational Ages

	Antibody Titer at Gestational Age, wk						
Ab Testing Phase[a]	12 2/7	16 3/7	22	22	25 2/7	27 6/7	32 1/7
Saline	Neg	Neg	Neg	Neg	Neg	Neg	Neg
AHG	1:8	1:16	1:4	1:16	1:16	1:8	1:8

[a]Antibody (Ab) screening cells were genotype R_1R_1 for all maternal serum Ab screening performed at all gestational ages (G.A.) except at 22 weeks G.A. when both R_1R_1 and R_2R_2 cells were used. AHG, anti-human globulin.

T4. Antibodies Remaining After Sequential Reaction of Serum Containing Anti-D, Anti-C, and/or Anti–G Antibodies With R_0r and r'r Genotype-Specific Red Blood Cells

Serum Containing the Antibodies	Antibodies Remaining After Reaction With R_0r and r'r Cells			
	R_0r (cDe, G positive) 1st Adsorption →	1st Elution →	r'r (Cde, G positive) 2nd Adsorption →	2nd Elution
D, C, and G	D and G	D and G	G	G
D and C	D	D	None	None

Perinatal Transfusion Issues>Hemolytic Disease of the Newborn/Anti-G vs. Anti-D and Anti-C

Is it Really Anti-D and Anti-C or Is it Anti-G?

5. How could the identification of anti-G in a pre-natal patient with an apparent anti-D and anti-C be of help in some legal issues?

6. Is the patient a Rh(D) immune globulin (RhIg) candidate?

Possible Answers

1. Yes. Routine evaluation to differentiate anti-D, anti-C, and anti-G should be done on alloimmunized pregnant women presenting serologically with an apparent anti-D and anti-C in their serum. Anti-G should be suspected when (1) the obstetrical and transfusion history conflicts with formation of anti-D and -C, (2) the pregnant woman has received appropriate Rh(D) immune globulin (RhIg) therapy, (3) the biological father of the infant is Rh(D) negative, and/or (4) the antibody titer of anti-C is significantly higher than the anti-D titer. In 1 case report, the laboratory investigation of a G7P3 woman, who received appropriate RhIg therapy after her last pregnancy, presented with a positive antibody screen with an apparent anti-D and anti-C. Anti-G was suspected because more reactivity was observed with the C(+)D(-) red blood cell sample than with the C(-)D(+) red blood cell sample. Further testing with D(+)G(-) red blood cells showed no reactivity, leading to the exclusion of anti-D.[1] In another study, a G4P1 pregnant woman who had received RhIg therapy when indicated was shown to have anti-D and anti-C with a higher titer of anti-C than anti-D (1:32 versus 1:4, respectively). Adsorption and elution studies proved that the patient had anti-C and anti–G, but no anti-D. Retrospective analysis of sera from 6 other pregnant women with anti-D and anti-C was done; 2 had anti-D, anti-C, and anti-G, 3 had anti-D and anti-G with no anti-C, and 1 had anti-C and anti-G with no anti-D.[2] In another report, 27 pregnant women who were initially identified as having anti-D and anti-C underwent further testing by adsorption/elution techniques in the presence of polyethylene glycol (PEG) using R_0r, r'r, and rGr red blood cells. Anti-C and anti-G with no anti-D were noted in 4 of 27 (14.8%) samples.[3] In our case, anti-G was suspected due to higher titers of anti-D and anti-C compared with anti-D, as well as the lack of history of sensitization [all red blood cells

transfused were Rh(D) negative and RhIg was administered appropriately when indicated]. Since the differentiation of anti-D and anti-G is important in the management and prognosis of a pregnancy complicated by the presence of these antibodies, it should be performed whenever anti-D and anti-C are identified.

2. By testing serum with an appropriate panel of genotypic red blood cells. The G antigen is present on all red blood cells that are C+, since C(+)G(-) red blood cells have not been found. The G antigen is present also on most (not all) D antigen positive red blood cells, since D(+)G(-) red blood cells have been found. The G antigen (weak) is present on Rh(D) positive weak red blood cells. In summary, the G antigen would be absent from C(-)D(-) red blood cells and would be present on most C+ or D+ red blood cells. Because of the way these 3 antigens are expressed, anti-G appears serologically identical to anti-D and anti-C. In a pregnant patient with an apparent anti-D and anti-C, sequential adsorption and elution studies using r'r (Cde) and R_0r (cDe) red blood cells can be done to confirm the presence or absence of anti-G [**T4**]. It is important to mention that rarely, individuals may have red blood cells that are D negative, C negative, but G positive. These cells may have a C-like component known as (C^G) that can react with anti-C. Because of the possibility of this reaction, these rare cells should not be used to detect the presence or absence of anti-G.[2]

3. The risk of HDN is small but finite. The number of case reports of anti-C and/or anti-G without a concomitant anti-D during pregnancy is limited, precluding a complete evaluation of the risk for HDN in these patients. However, it is known that anti-C alloimmunization occurs less frequently than anti-D and even though anti-C may cause serious HDN, it is usually less severe. Anti-G rarely presents with a high titer that may affect the fetus and require medical intervention (ie, amniocentesis or intrauterine transfusion). In 1 study, adsorption and elution testing was performed on serum from 27 pregnant women with apparent anti-D and anti–C and 4 of the 27 samples (14.8%) showed anti-G and anti-C without anti-D. None of the newborn children from these pregnancies were affected with HDN or needed postpartum management.[3] In another case report,

a 35-year-old Rh(D) negative primigravida who had received 4 units of Rh(D) negative allogeneic red blood cells had a history of positive anti-D and anti-C antibody screens as part of her prenatal workup. Additional studies by a different laboratory showed the presence of anti-G and possible anti-C with no anti-D. At 22 weeks gestation, titers were 1:64 against r'r red blood cells and 1:16 against R_2R_2 red blood cells. Amniocentesis indicated that the fetus did not appear to be affected by intrauterine hemolysis. The mother delivered a healthy infant at 36 weeks gestation. The infant had a positive direct antiglobulin test (DAT) with an acid eluate revealing the presence of anti-G. The total bilirubin (highest value) was 11.9 mg/dL at 5 days postpartum and no further management was needed.[4] In contrast to these findings, among 28 sera from alloimmunized women with anti-D and anti-C, 2 contained titers of anti-G consistent with moderate to severe HDN by the chemiluminescence test. It was also noted in this study that fetal hemolysis due to anti-G was more likely to occur in r'r (C-positive, D-negative) fetuses.[5] In another study, an Rh(D) negative woman with a history of multiple transfusions of Rh(D) negative blood in the past was thought to have anti-D and anti-C. Prenatal workup revealed that the patient had an anti-G rather than an anti-D. At 32.5 weeks of gestation, the mother delivered an affected fetus with moderately severe HDN.[6] We conclude that even though hemolytic HDN due to anti-G is very uncommon, it should still be considered when more reactivity is observed with C(+)D(-) than with the C(-)D(+) antibody screening red blood cells.

4. Cytomegalovirus (CMV) seronegative, irradiated group O Rh(D) negative (rr) red blood cells would be indicated. The transfused red blood cells must be D and C antigen negative and consequently G antigen negative. The differentiation of anti-D, anti-C, and anti-G for routine transfusion is not necessary, since most Rh(D) negative, C antigen negative red blood cells would be G antigen negative. If the mother is the donor for intrauterine transfusion, frozen deglycerolized red blood cells allows multiple aliquots to be frozen and then thawed as needed.

5. When the medical and transfusion history are inconsistent with the finding of an apparent anti-D and anti-C in an Rh(D) negative pregnant

woman and the biological father is Rh(D) negative. In such cases, questions about paternity may arise. If anti-D is not present (only anti-C and/or anti-G) RhIg should be given at appropriate times. Therefore, correct antibody identification and appropriate RhIg administration are extremely important in preventing medicolegal situations.[3]

6. Yes. Pregnant women with anti-G and without anti-D in their serum are considered candidates for prophylactic RhIg therapy at 28 weeks gestation, at delivery if the infant is Rh(D) positive, and when clinically indicated (eg, for the risk of sensitization with amniocentesis) to prevent formation of anti-D and potential severe complications in future pregnancies. In our case, the patient continued to receive RhIg therapy, which could have been erroneously excluded if the possibility of an existing anti-G rather than an anti-D antibody was not considered. Our patient delivered a healthy newborn at 39 weeks gestation who typed as A Rh(D) positive and had a negative DAT. No therapeutic interventions were required.

Keywords

anti-D, anti-C, anti-G, Rh immune globulin, hemolytic disease of the newborn

References

1. Judd J. Summary of RAP Session Serologic Controversies (Two G, not CD). *AABB News*. December 2000.

2. Shirey R, Mirabella D, Lumadue J, et al. Differentiation of anti-D, -C, and -G: clinical relevance in alloimmunized pregnancies. *Immunohematology*. 1997;37:493.

3. Palfi M, Gunnarsson C. The frequency of anti-C and anti-G in the absence of anti-D in alloimmunized pregnancies. *Transfusion Med*. 2001;11:207-210.

4. Cash K, Brown T, Strupp A, et al. Anti-G in a pregnant patient. *Transfusion*. 1999;39:531-533.

5. Hadley AG, Poole GD, Poole J, et al. Hemolytic disease of the newborn due to anti-G. *Vox Sang*. 1996;71:108-112.

6. Yesus YW, Akhter JE. Hemolytic disease of the newborn due to anti-C and anti-G masquerading as anti-D. *Am J Clin Pathol*. 1985;84:769-72.

Thrombocytopenia in a Neonate

Maria A. B. Reed, Nada Rikabi, Dave Krugh, Sandra Dietrich, Karen Rossi, Eric Knudtson, Richard O' Shaughnessy, Melanie S. Kennedy

Departments of [1]Transfusion Medicine and [2]Obstetrics & Gynecology, Maternal-Fetal Medicine, The Ohio State University, Columbus, OH

Patient: 33-year-old Caucasian pregnant woman.

Social History: Unremarkable.

History of Present Pregnancy: This patient is a G3P2, group A Rh(D) positive pregnant woman who had previously delivered an infant (G1) with petechiae at birth and a markedly low platelet count ($12 \times 10^3/\mu L$; normal reference range: $150-400 \times 10^3/\mu L$). This infant was treated with intravenous immune globulin and random platelet transfusions. Because of this history, early in her third pregnancy, her serum was screened for the presence of platelet antibodies. The maternal platelet antibody screen was positive for anti-human platelet antigen (HPA)-1a and class I human leukocyte antigen (HLA) antibodies. The maternal platelet antigen type was HPA-1b/1b and the paternal antigen type was homozygous HPA-1a. The patient chose monthly ultrasound testing and periodic cordocentesis to assess fetal platelet count and to decrease the risk of delivery-related complications. Cordocentesis was performed to assess the infant's platelet count at 26 5/7 weeks and 33 weeks gestational age (GA). The fetal platelet count was $176 \times 10^3/\mu L$ and $169 \times 10^3/\mu L$, respectively. The fetal platelet antigen type was HPA-1a/1b. The fetus (G3) was delivered vaginally and had a platelet count of $213 \times 10^3/mL$.

Past Obstetrical History: During her second pregnancy, ultrasound was performed at 6, 10, and 18 weeks GA and no gross abnormalities were noted. Amniocentesis was performed at 21 weeks GA and polymerase chain reaction (PCR) testing confirmed that the fetus was platelet type HP-1a/1b. The fetal platelet count was monitored by 4 serial cordocentesis performed between 21 and 34 weeks GA. Fetal platelet counts ranged from $110-129 \times 10^3/\mu L$. No medical therapy was provided during this pregnancy because the fetal platelet counts remained above $100 \times 10^3/\mu L$. The infant (G2) was delivered vaginally and had a platelet count of $146 \times 10^3/\mu L$.

Past Surgical History: Knee surgery.

Allergies: Codeine.

Family History: Unremarkable, no family history of neonatal thrombocytopenia.

Questions

1. What is the most likely diagnosis in the neonate from her third pregnancy? How did this pregnancy differ from most who have delivered a neonate with this disorder?

2. What is the most common antibody associated with this disorder?

3. How is an infant born with this disorder managed?

4. How should pregnancies with a history of an affected sibling with this disorder be managed?

5. How should the potential transfusion needs of a mother with a history of delivering a neonate(s) with this disorder be managed?

T1. Platelet Alloantigens Implicated in Neonatal Alloimmune Thrombocytopenia[2]

Alloantigens	Synonyms	Phenotype Frequency
		(%)*
HPA-1a	Zw^a , PL^{A1}	97.9
HPA-1b	Zw^b , PL^{A2}	26.5
HPA-2a	Ko^b	99.3
HPA-2b	Ko^a , Sib^a	14.6
HPA-3a	Bak^a , Lek^a	87.7
HPA-3b	Bak^b	64.1
HPA-4a	Pen^a , Yuk^b	99.9
HPA-4b	Pen^b ,Yuk^a	0.2
HPA-5a	Br^b , Zav^b	99.2
HPA-5b	Br^a , Zav^a , Hc^a	20.6
Sr^a (private antigen)		<1
MO (private antigen)		<1
Yu^a (private antigen)		<1

*Caucasian population.
HPA, human platelet antigen.

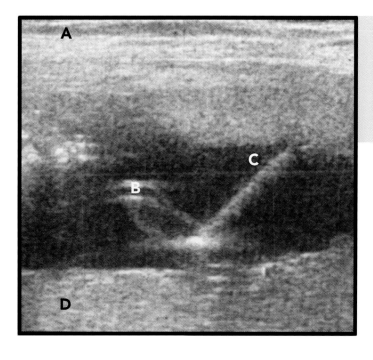

Image 1_Ultrasound view of a cordocentesis illustrating the location of the (**A**) uterine wall, (**B**) umbilical vein, (**C**) 22 gauge spinal needle, and (**D**) the placenta.

Possible Answers

1. **Most likely diagnosis:** *neonatal alloimmune thrombocytopenia (NAIT).*

   An infant presenting with petechiae, purpura, bleeding, and/or unexplained thrombocytopenia at birth is highly suggestive of NAIT. This is a relatively rare disease of the newborn with an estimated incidence of 1 in 1,500–5,000 live births. It is a diagnosis of exclusion, after ruling out autoimmune disease, maternal drug ingestion, maternal immune-mediated thrombocytopenia purpura (autoimmune thrombocytopenia purpura), neonatal sepsis, or other causes of thrombocytopenia in a newborn infant. Typically, there is neonatal thrombocytopenia and the maternal platelet count is normal. The condition may result when platelet antibodies are produced by the maternal immune system after exposure to the fetal platelet antigen inherited from the father, but absent from the mother, or after exposure to a platelet antigen after transfusion.[1] The platelet antibodies (IgG) are produced by the mother's B-cells, cross the placenta, and bind to antigens on the fetal platelets. These platelets are then removed from the fetal circulation by the fetal reticuloendothelial system, causing thrombocytopenia. The placental transfer of maternal platelet antibodies can occur as early as 14 weeks GA, with maximum platelet antibody transfer at 18 to 19 weeks of gestation. Therefore, platelet destruction with thrombocytopenia and intracerebral hemorrhage can occur early in pregnancy. Unlike hemolytic disease of the newborn due to red blood cell alloimmunization, NAIT can severely affect the first-born infant in 60% of cases.[2] The rate of recurrence in infants from subsequent pregnancies is more than 75%, and the degree of thrombocytopenia in subsequent infants is usually as severe as in the preceding affected sibling. The severity has been reported to be directly related to the antibody titer.[2,3] However, the use of a platelet antibody titer has not been accepted as standard of care in the clinical management of pregnant women with a history of delivering infants affected with NAIT. This case is unusual and may support the hypothesis that another mechanism may directly relate to the severity of neonatal thrombocytopenia in NAIT because the patient delivered 2 NAIT-unaffected neonates (G_2 and G_3) from subsequent pregnancies after delivering her first NAIT-affected neonate (G_1). The recurrence rate of NAIT is 50% if the father is heterozygous and 100% if the father is homozygous for a HPA allele.[4] Moreover, the severity of NAIT can vary from no observable symptoms (ie, thrombocytopenia is discovered incidentally) to severe intracerebral hemorrhage.[1] Intracerebral hemorrhage, the major complication of NAIT, occurs in 10% to 20% of affected infants with 25% to 50% of those cases occurring in-utero.[5,6] Infants with intracerebral hemorrhage have been reported to develop spasticity, cerebral palsy, hypotonia, cortical blindness, developmental delays, seizure, and psychomotor retardation.[5]

2. The most common platelet-specific antigen implicated in NAIT is HPA-1a, occurring in 78% of cases [**T1**]. The HPA-1a antigen is not as antigenic as the red blood cell D antigen; thus a lower incidence occurs despite the absence of prophylactic therapy.[7] Studies have shown an association between Class II HLA antigen alloimmunization, particularly DR52a, and alloimmunization against HPA-1a. Similarly, DR6 and alloimmunization against HPA-5b seem to be associated. Other platelet-specific antigens implicated in NAIT include HPA-5b (18% to 19% of cases), HPA-4 (3% to 4% of cases), HPA-2a, and HPA-3a.[2,8] Neonatal alloimmune thrombocytopenia may also be caused by maternal anti-HLA antibodies.[9-11] In 85% of cases, a maternal antibody can be detected to a specific platelet antigen, although the absence of detectable antibodies does not exclude a diagnosis of NAIT. A number of techniques are used to phenotype platelets and detect maternal platelet antibodies. The most commonly used are enzyme-linked immunosorbent assay (ELISA), radioimmunoprecipitation, mixed passive hemagglutination, flow cytometry, monoclonal antibody-specific immobilized platelet assay (MAIPA), and DNA-based assays.

3. Routine prenatal screening for NAIT is not performed; thus, it will be undetected, unless prenatal ultrasound testing detects intracerebral hemorrhage, or the infant has symptoms of thrombocytopenia at birth that lead to platelet testing.[2] The severity of thrombocytopenia ($<20 \times 10^3/\mu L$) and the presence of bleeding will

determine the mode of treatment. If a platelet transfusion is necessary, the infant should receive a platelet transfusion using platelets obtained from the mother who is an excellent source of antigen-negative platelets. The maternal platelets (platelet antigen negative) should be saline washed to remove any circulating platelet antibodies and should be irradiated to prevent graft versus host disease. Moreover, platelets obtained by apheresis and suspended in saline provide more platelets than can be obtained from a whole blood unit. If the mother is unable to donate platelets, the infant may require allogeneic antigen-negative platelets, which should be cytomegalovirus (CMV) negative and irradiated. If maternal or allogeneic antigen negative platelets are not available, high doses of intravenous immunoglobulin can be used as an alternative treatment.[2] The response to intravenous immunoglobulin therapy will be slower than occurs typically following platelet transfusion, providing less immediate response, but better long term increase in the platelet count. If antigen-negative platelets are not available and there is an emergent need for platelet transfusion, random platelet concentrates (CMV negative and irradiated) can be used as there will be an adequate response in 40% of cases. In addition, if NAIT is left untreated, the thrombocytopenia may last for 2-3 weeks and resolve spontaneously.

4. Obstetrical management should begin early in the pregnancy, ideally in the first trimester, to allow time for platelet antigen and antibody testing to be performed. Fetal platelet phenotyping is crucial if the father is heterozygous for the platelet antigen as only 50% of the infants will be affected. Fetal platelet typing by amniocentesis can be done as early as 14 weeks GA, while cordocentesis can be performed as early as 17 to 18 weeks GA [**Image 1**] and at intervals throughout the pregnancy to obtain fetal platelet counts to assess the need and urgency for therapy. The risk (<1%) of hemorrhage or other complications from cordocentesis is less than the overall risk (10% to 30%) of intracerebral hemorrhage from thrombocytopenia.[4] This case emphasizes the value of obtaining a fetal platelet count by cordocentesis. This patient would have received unnecessary treatment through 2 pregnancies if she had been treated on history alone. At each cordocentesis, maternal or allogeneic

antigen-negative platelets should be available in case fetal transfusion for thrombocytopenia is required. If fetal thrombocytopenia is profound ($<100 \times 10^3/\mu L$), high doses (1 g/kg) of intravenous immunoglobulin should be given to the mother weekly or twice weekly. Additional interventions include the use of corticosteroids and intrauterine transfusions of antigen-negative platelets. Scheduled delivery is important to decrease the possibility of intracerebral hemorrhage at birth and immediately postpartum. If the mother desires a vaginal delivery, a cordocentesis must be done prior to delivery to obtain a fetal platelet count. A cesarean section is required when the fetal platelet count is either unknown or below $50 \times 10^3/\mu L$ to decrease the risk of intracerebral hemorrhage from trauma at birth. Vaginal delivery is generally considered safe when the fetal platelet count is above $50 \times 10^3/\mu L$. When the fetal platelet count is below $50 \times 10^3/\mu L$, intrauterine, saline-suspended, antigen-negative platelet transfusion can be performed to allow for vaginal delivery within the next 4 days due to the half-life of the transfused platelets.

5. Most normal deliveries in pregnant women with a history of delivering a neonate(s) affected with NAIT do not require the use of blood and/or blood components. However, it is advisable to have antigen-negative, saline-suspended platelets (maternal and/or allogeneic) available in case of maternal or fetal complications.

Keywords

neonatal alloimmune thrombocytopenia, cordocentesis, human platelet antigen

References

1. Rothenberger S. Neonatal alloimmune thrombocytopenia. *Therapeutic Apheresis.* 2002;6:32-35.

2. Goldman M, Filion M, Proulx C, et al. Neonatal alloimmune thrombocytopenia. *Transfusion Med Rev.* 1994;8;123-131.

3. Jaegtvik S, Husebekk A, Aune B, et al. Neonatal alloimmune thrombocytopenia due to anti-HPA 1a antibodies; the levels of maternal antibodies predicts severity of thrombocytopenia in the newborn. *BJOG.* 2000;107:691-694.

4. Bussel J, Berkowitz R, McFarland J, et al. Antenatal treatment of neonatal alloimmune thrombocytopenia. *N Engl J Med.* 1988;319:1374-1377.

5. Sharif U, Kuban K. Prenatal intracranial hemorrhage and neurologic complications in alloimmune thrombocytopenia. *J Child Neurol.* 2001;16:838-842.

6. Kaplan C, Forestier F, Daffos F, et al. Management of fetal and neonatal alloimmune thrombocytopenia. *Transfusion Med Rev.* 1996;10:233-240.

7. Bussel J, McFarland J, Berkowitz R. Antenatal management of fetal alloimmune and autoimmune thrombocytopenia. *Transfusion Med Rev.* 1990;4:149-162.

8. Glade-Bender J, McFarland JG, Kaplan C, et al. Anti-HPA-3a induces severe neonatal alloimmune thrombocytopenia. *J Pediatr.* 2001;138:862-867.

9. Grainger JD, Morrell G, Yates J, et al. Neonatal alloimmune thrombocytopenia with significant HLA antibodies. *Arch Dis Child Fetal Neonatal Edu.* 2002;86:200-201.

10. Del Rosario ML, Fox ER, Kickler TS, et al. Neonatal alloimmune thrombocytopenia associated with maternal anti-HLA antibody; a case report. *J Pediatr Hematol Oncol.* 1998;20:252-256.

11. Onishi S, Okubo S, Matsuzaki T, et al. Report of 2 cases of neonatal alloimmune thrombocytopenia caused by anti-HLA antibody and their screening using umbilical cord blood. *Rinsho Ketsueki.* 1992;33:42-47.

A Patient With a Low IgA Level Requiring Transfusion During CABG Surgery

Gifford Lum, Paula Szuflad, Michael D'Amarino

Pathology and Laboratory Medicine Service, VA Boston Healthcare System, Boston, MA

Patient: 71-year-old Caucasian man.

Chief Complaint: Bradycardia.

History of Present Illness: Patient was admitted to the medical service with asymptomatic bradycardia (heart rates between 33 and 55 beats/minute). Results of cardiac catheterization showed 2-vessel disease with 90% focal stenosis of the mid- and 40% stenosis of the distal-left main coronary artery and 95% stenosis of the mid-left anterior descending coronary artery. The right coronary artery showed a proximal lesion and 50% stenosis, while the posterior descending coronary artery showed focal stenosis (70%). The patient was referred for coronary artery bypass graft (CABG) surgery.

Prior Medical History: The patient had a history of stroke with left-side hemiparesis; impotence, secondary to vascular insufficiency; deep vein thrombosis and pulmonary embolism with placement of a Greenfield filter; anemia from chronic disease; and benign prostatic hyperplasia.

Additional Diagnostic Procedures: Coronary artery bypass graft surgery was recommended for this patient because of severe 2-vessel coronary artery disease. Because of the possibility of an anaphylactic transfusion reaction, the blood bank was consulted regarding blood product availability. A sample of the patient's blood was submitted to the American Red Cross (ARC) Reference Laboratory for IgA testing, using a more sensitive assay than immunonephelometry, and testing for anti-IgA antibodies. Before results for these tests were available, however, surgeons elected to perform CABG surgery on this patient. The patient was transfused with 2 units of washed RBCs during surgery without incident. In addition, 1 unit of IgA-deficient fresh frozen plasma (FFP) was procured from the ARC and its American Rare Donor Program, and a procedure for washing platelet units was set up in the blood bank. The patient did not require administration of FFP or platelet units. After the CABG surgery had been performed, the IgA (>0.05 mg/dL, but <6.7 mg/dL) and anti-IgA (negative) results were received from the ARC Reference Laboratory.

Questions

1. What is this patient's most striking laboratory result?

2. Why was there a concern about the possibility of an anaphylactic transfusion reaction in this patient?

3. What methods are commonly used for measuring IgA concentration?

4. What is the definition of IgA deficiency?

5. What illnesses are most often associated with IgA deficiency?

6. What is the prevalence of IgA deficiency in the blood donor population?

T1. Principal Laboratory Findings

Test	Patient's Result	"Normal" Reference Range
Hematology		
RBC count	4.04	4.7-6.1 × 10⁶/μL
Hemoglobin	12.5	14-18 g/dL
Hematocrit	36.6	40-52%
Special Chemistry		
Protein, total	7.1	6.0-8.5 g/dL
SPE:		
Albumin	4.20	2.98-5.47 g/dL
Alpha-1-globulin	0.42	0.29-0.86 g/dL
Alpha-2-globulin	0.90	0.51-1.28 g/dL
Beta-globulin	0.37	0.47-1.11 g/dL
Gamma-globulin	1.24	0.63-1.66 g/dL
Quantitative Ig's: IgG	1400	751-1560 mg/dL
IgA	<6.7	82-453 mg/dL
IgM	101	46-304 mg/dL

RBC, red blood cell; SPE, serum protein electrophoresis; Ig's, immunoglobulins.

T2. Characteristics of Selected Methods for Quantifying Serum IgA Concentration

Method	LLD, mg/dL	Assay Time, h
Nephelometry or turbidimetry	6-7	<1
PHAI	0.05	3-5
ELISA	0.005	5-6

LLD, lower limit of detection; PHAI, passive hemagglutination inhibition; ELISA, enzyme-linked immunosorbent assay.

7. What is the significance of the detection of anti-IgA antibodies in patients with IgA deficiency?

8. What stimulates the production of anti-IgA antibodies?

9. What is the frequency of anaphylactic transfusion reactions and associated mortality in IgA-deficient patients?

10. How should patients with IgA deficiency and/or a previous history of anaphylactic transfusion reaction be managed?

Possible Answers

1. An undetectable IgA level (**T1**).

2. Because of the patient's undetectable IgA level, there was a concern that the patient might have anti-IgA antibodies that would react with IgA in any transfused products and cause an anaphylactic transfusion reaction. The first description of anaphylactic transfusion reactions associated with anti-IgA antibodies was reported in 1968 in *Lancet* and included 6 case studies with serious reactions following the administration of blood, plasma, or gamma globulin.[1] These 6 patients were divided into 2 groups: Group I, 3 patients who were IgA deficient with anti-IgA of broad reactivity, who experienced severe anaphylactic transfusion reactions; Group II, 3 multiply transfused patients with an anti-IgA of more limited specificity, who experienced less severe anaphylactoid reactions consisting of urticaria, wheezing, diffuse rashes, and tachycardia.[1]

3. The 3 most commonly used methods for the quantitative determination of serum IgA concentration are nephelometry (or turbidimetry), passive hemagglutination inhibition assay (PHAI), and enzyme-linked immunosorbent assay (ELISA) (**T2**). The basic principle of nephelometric and turbidimetric assays for quantifying IgA concentration is light scatter at various angles by immune complexes formed between IgA (antigen) in the patient's serum and anti-IgA (antibody) antiserum added to the patient's serum. Passive hemagglutination techniques use hemagglutination as the end point of the antigen-antibody reaction, while ELISA methods use a capture antibody bound to the well of a microtiter plate to "capture" antigen (eg, IgA) and a signal antibody, containing an enzyme "signal," that recognizes a different epitope on the antigen than the capture antibody. The addition of substrate specific for the enzyme attached to the signal antibody results in the production of a color whose intensity is directly proportional to the amount of antigen present. Among these methods for the quantitation of IgA concentration, ELISA methods provide the best analytical sensitivity [ie, lower limit of detection (LLD) <0.005 mg/dL] (**T2**). Nephelometric or turbidimetric methods are used routinely in most

T3. Frequency of IgA Deficiency in Various Populations

| Country | Criterion for IgA deficiency, [IgA, mg/dL] | IgA-Deficient Individuals | | | |
		Number	Age, y	Frequency[a]	Reference
Austria	1	3,056		1:382	9
USA	1	6,240		1:416	16
USA	1	73,569	>17	1:651	17
France	1	15,200		1:3,040	18
Japan	1	222,597	16-69	1:31,800	8
USA	2	3,024		1:3,024	19
Sweden	4	6,695	>17	1:670	20
Israel	4	1,803		1:1,803	21
USA	5	6,240		1:328	16
France	5	15,200	20-60	1:2,171	18
China	5	33,171		1:4,146	22
Japan	5	222,597	16-69	1:18,550	8
USA	6	5,764		1:480	23
Spain	6.7	1,956	2-18	1:163	24
Austria	7	7,293	12-66	1:486	25
Israel	8	1,803	>17	1:1,803	21

[a]In blood donor population.

T4. Frequency of Anti-IgA Antibodies in IgA-Deficient Patients

| No. of IgA-Deficient | No. of IgA-Deficient Patients With | | Total | % | Reference Patients Studied |
	Class-Specific IgA Antibodies	Limited Specificity IgA Antibodies			
113	13	0	13	11.5	17
57	6	4	10	17.5	26
156	29	10	39	25.0	27
11	0	3	3	27.3	28
19	6	1	7	36.8	16
139[a]	61	4	65	46.8	4

[a]Includes 80 patients with [IgA] < 0.05 mg/dL and 59 patients with low (0.05-75 mg/dL) IgA levels.

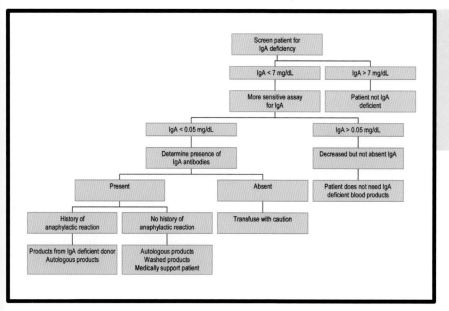

Figure 1_Possible algorithm for managing the transfusion needs of patients with IgA deficiency and/or anti-IgA antibodies in their serum.

clinical laboratories for the quantitation of serum IgA concentration because these methods are rapid, easy to use, and are amenable to automation. According to the data in the College of American Pathologists (CAP) 2004 Diagnostic Immunology Survey Set-B Summary, 93.6% (712 of 760) of participating laboratories used nephelometric or turbidimetric methods for the quantitation of IgA, with the majority (55.2%) of these laboratories reporting the use of nephelometry over turbidimetry.[2]

4. IgA deficiency is defined clinically as a serum IgA level <7 mg/dL in males or females older than 4 years of age, but with normal serum IgG and IgM and in whom other causes of hypogammaglobulinemia (eg, drug-induced, infectious diseases, chromosomal abnormalities, and malignancy) have been ruled out.[3] Severe IgA deficiency has been defined generally as a selectively undetectable IgA concentration of <0.05 mg/dL.[4] The ARC American Rare Donor Program (ARDP) uses this definition to classify blood donors as IgA deficient. IgA deficiency with concomitant lack of secretory IgA is the most common form of primary immunodeficiency in the western world.[5]

5. The most common illnesses associated with IgA deficiency are recurrent sinopulmonary infections, including sinusitis, otitis media, pharyngitis, bronchitis, and bronchopneumonia. Gastrointestinal tract disorders may also be associated with selective IgA deficiency, including a 10-fold increased risk of celiac disease, pernicious anemia, milk intolerance, malabsorption syndrome, and mucosal infections due to acute diarrhea caused by bacteria, viruses, or *Giardia lamblia*.[6]

6. IgA deficiency is more prevalent in patients with autoimmune disease than in healthy individuals, possibly due to impaired immunoglobulin switching or a maturational failure of IgA-producing lymphocytes.[7] Moreover, the incidence of IgA deficiency varies not only with the population examined, but also with the analytical sensitivity of the IgA method used to screen individuals for IgA deficiency and the IgA cutoff value used to classify individuals as IgA deficient (**T3**). At an IgA cutoff value of 1 mg/dL, the incidence of IgA deficiency varies from a high of 1:382 in the Austrian population to a low of 1:31,800 in Japanese blood donors.[8,9] These findings suggest a strong genetic component for inheritance of IgA deficiency.[10]

7. The demonstration of anti-IgA antibodies has been the *sine qua non* for the diagnosis of anaphylactic transfusion reactions in IgA-deficient patients. These preformed antibodies to transfused IgA may be class-specific (anti-IgA), subclass-specific (Anti-IgA$_1$ or –IgA$_2$), or allotype-specific [Anti-IgA$_{2m(1)}$ or anti-IgA$_{2m(2)}$].[11] The most severe anaphylactic transfusion reactions are usually associated with class-specific

antibodies in severely IgA deficient patients. The subclass and allotype-specific antibodies (generally referred to as antibodies of "limited specificity") are associated with less severe transfusion reactions, frequently seen in patients with low or, in some instances, normal levels of IgA.[12] Moreover, anti-IgA antibodies are usually of the IgG class, but may also be IgM or IgE class.[10] Anti-IgA antibodies have also been found in sera from healthy individuals with frequencies ranging from 2% to 59%.[10] The broad range of the frequency of anti-IgA antibodies in serum from healthy individuals has been attributed to methodological differences in the detection of anti-IgA antibodies, which hinders the assessment of the clinical significance of detecting anti IgA antibodies.[10] The frequency of anti-IgA antibodies in sera from IgA-deficient individuals can range from 11.5% to 46.8% (**T4**). Based on data from a recent, large study in the United Kingdom, a frequently quoted estimate for the detection of anti-IgA antibodies in IgA-deficient patients is 33%.[11]

8. It is currently unclear what stimuli lead to the production of anti-IgA antibodies; however, it is known that some cases are associated with a history of exposure to IgA antigen from a variety of sources.[13] In a long-term follow-up study of the development of anti-IgA antibodies in healthy IgA-deficient adults (n=159), there was no correlation between exposure to IgA antigen and the development of anti-IgA antibodies in 42% of these subjects with severe IgA deficiency ([IgA] <0.05 mg/dL) and a history of IgA exposure from pregnancy, blood transfusion, or immunoglobulin injection. Only 24% of these individuals had anti-IgA antibodies in serum from follow-up samples.[13] In this same study, serum from 45 blood donors with decreased serum IgA did not contain anti-IgA antibodies, compared to 30 of 159 (19%) patients with severe IgA deficiency whose serum was positive for anti-IgA antibodies. Moreover, the anti-IgA concentration in the serum from these 30 individuals remained fairly constant over a median follow-up period of 19 years (ie, only 6 of these 30 patients showed increases in IgA antibody concentration, with 4 of them showing significant increases).[13]

In a study of the prevalence of anti-IgA antibodies in 83 individuals with selective IgA deficiency, elevated concentrations of anti-IgA antibodies were detected in 25% to 30% of healthy individuals or those who had non-rheumatoid diseases.[14] However, the prevalence was 50% in those with rheumatoid arthritis, 77% in those with juvenile rheumatoid arthritis, and 100% in those with systemic lupus erythematosus. The authors of this study suggested an association between autoimmune (or immune) dysregulation, selective IgA deficiency, and the production of anti-IgA antibodies.[14] Based on a study of 32,376 random blood donors, the frequency of class-specific IgA antibodies in IgA-deficient patients was 1:1,200 (ie, 27 of 87 IgA-deficient donors had class-specific anti-IgA antibodies in their serum).[4] This same study found that there was a high incidence (76.3%) of class-specific anti-IgA antibodies in severely IgA-deficient patients with a history of anaphylactic transfusion reaction.[4] In addition, these authors reported that 21.7% of 97 asymptomatic IgA blood donors or their IgA-deficient family members had class-specific IgA antibodies in their serum.[4] This finding suggests that the presence of anti-IgA antibodies may overestimate the number of patients at risk for an anaphylactic transfusion reaction.[4]

9. IgA anaphylactic transfusion reactions are rare events, with an estimated occurrence rate of 1:20,000 to 1:100,000 transfusions.[12,15] As discussed previously, the frequency of detecting anti-IgA antibodies (1:1,200) exceeds the observed frequency of anaphylactic transfusion reactions suggesting that the presence of anti-IgA antibodies in a patient's serum is not a good predictor of the risk for an anaphylactic transfusion reaction.[11] In the United States population, 1:1,200 individuals will have severe IgA deficiency and anti-IgA antibodies in their serum. The prevalence of major analphylactic transfusion reactions in the United States population is approximately 2.4%.[11] Since the publication in 1968 of the first report of 3 cases of anaphylactic transfusion reactions associated with anti-IgA antibodies,[1] Sandler and colleagues described 30 additional cases in 1995.[12] In 2002, Vyas reported that at least 42 cases of anaphylactic transfusion reactions caused by anti-IgA were reported to his group at the University of California at San Francisco.[15] To date, there have been no documented cases of mortality due to

anti-IgA-associated anaphylactic transfusion reactions.

10. If there is sufficient time to workup a patient with IgA deficiency, the first step should be to determine whether the patient has detectable levels of IgA and/or anti-IgA antibodies in their serum. If the patient has a low, but detectable, level of IgA (ie, >0.05 mg/dL, but <7 mg/dL), there is no need to transfuse the patient with any special blood product. If the patient has an undetectable concentration of IgA in their serum and is negative for the presence of anti-IgA antibodies, the patient should be transfused with caution. If the patient is severely IgA deficient, has anti-IgA antibodies in their serum, but no history of anaphylactic transfusion reaction, the patient may receive autologous products, washed RBCs/platelets, and should be supported medically. In a patient with severe IgA deficiency, who is positive for the presence of anti-IgA antibodies in their serum and with a history of anaphylactic transfusion reaction, washed RBCs, autologous products, or plasma products from an IgA-deficient donor should be transfused when needed. The aforementioned products are available through the ARC American Rare Donor Program. The release of IgA-deficient plasma is made on a case-by-case basis in consultation with the ARDP medical staff.[11] Washed platelet-pheresis products may be used; however, such products are technically difficult to prepare and have only a 4-hour expiration after preparation. The ARDP maintains a registry of IgA-deficient donors in their apheresis program for situations in which washed plateletpheresis products are unavailable, not feasible, or contraindicated in patients who have previously experienced a reaction to washed platelet products.[11] If there is an emergent need for transfusion in a patient who has been screened for IgA concentration by conventional nephelometric methods and is considered IgA-deficient, and there is no prior history of an anaphylactic transfusion reaction, the likelihood of an adverse reaction is low since the estimated occurrence of anaphylactic reactions is approximately 1:20,000 to 1:100,000 transfusions. If, however, there is a history of an anaphylactic transfusion event, then the patient should receive autologous units, washed RBCs, or IgA-deficient blood products. **Figure 1** provides a decision-making guide for managing the transfusion needs of patients with IgA deficiency and/or anti-IgA antibodies in their serum.

Keywords

IgA deficiency, anti-IgA antibodies, anaphylactic transfusion reaction

References

1. Vyas GN, Perkins HA, Fudenberg HH. Anaphylactoid transfusion reactions associated with Anti-IgA. *Lancet.* 1968;2:312-315.

2. College of American Pathologists, Surveys 2004 S-B Diagnostic Immunology. College of American Pathologists, Northfield, IL, 2004.

3. Conley ME, Notarangelo LD, Etzioni A. Diagnostic Criteria for Primary Immunodeficiencies. Representing PAGID (Pan-American Group for Immunodeficiency and ISID (European Society for Immunodeficiences). *Clin Immunol.* 1999;93:190-197.

4. Sandler SG, Eckrich R, Malamut D, et al. Hemagglutination Assays for the Diagnosis and Prevention of IgA Anaphylactic Transfusion Reactions. *Blood.* 1994;84:2031-2035.

5. Hammarström L, Vorechovsky I, Webster D. Selective IgA deficiency (SigAD) and common variable immunodeficiency (CVID). *Clin Exper Immunol.* 2000;120:225-231.

6. *Samter's Immunologic Diseases,* 5th ed. Frank MM, Austen KF, Claman HN, et al, eds. Boston: Little, Brown and Company, 1995, pp. 410-411;1153-1154.

7. Primary Immunodeficiency Diseases Report of an IUIS Scientific Committee. International Union of Immunological Societies. *Clin Exper Immunol.* 1999;118:S1.

8. Kanoh T, Mizumoto T, Yasuda N, et al. Selective IgA deficiency in Japanese blood donors: frequency and statistical analysis. *Vox Sang.* 1986;50:81-86.

9. Winter PM, Manndorff P. The frequency of IgA-deficiency in the Austrian population. A protocol for large-scale screening by ELISA and a study on 3056 blood donors. *Infusionstherapie.* 1988;15:221-224.

10. Lilic D, Sewell WAC. IgA deficiency: what we should-or should not- be doing. *J Clin Pathol.* 2001;54:337-338.

11. Vassallo RR. IgA anaphylactic transfusion reactions: I. Laboratory diagnosis, incidence, and supply of Ig-A deficient products. *Immunohematol.* 2004;20:226-233.

12. Sandler SG, Mallory D, Malamut D, et al. IgA anaphylactic transfusion reactions. *Transf Med Rev.* 1995;9:1-8.

13. Koistinen S, Tolo H, Hirvonen M, et al. Long-term follow-up of anti-IgA antibodies in healthy IgA-deficient adults. *J Clin Immunol.* 1995;15:194-198.

14. Petty RE, Palmer NR, Cassidy JT. The association of autoimmune diseases and anti-IgA antibodies in patients with selective IgA deficiency. *Clin Exp Immunol.* 1979;37:83-88.

15. Vyas GN. Discussion – Is it possible to administer IVIG (or IMIG) to an IgA-deficient patient with anti-IgA who has had a previous anaphylactic reaction to IVIG? California Blood Bank Society web site, http://www.cbbsweb.org/enf/ivig_igdeficiency .html. Accessed January 21, 2003.

16. Clark JA, Callicoat PA, Brenner NA, et al. Selective IgA deficiency in blood donors. *Amer J Clin Pathol.* 1983;80:210-213.

17. Vyas GN, Perkins HA, Yang YM, et al. Healthy blood donors with selective absence of immunoglobulin A: prevention of anaphylactic transfusion reactions caused by antibodies to IgA. *J Lab Clin Med.* 1975;85:838-842.

18. Frommel D, Moullec J, Lambin P, et al Selective serum IgA deficiency. Frequency among 15,200 French blood donors. *Vox Sang.* 1973;25:513-518.

19. Cassidy JT, Burt A, Petty R, et al. Selective IgA deficiency in connective tissue diseases. *N Eng J Med.* 1969;280:275.

20. Bachmann R. Studies on the serum gamma-A-globulin level. 3. The frequency of A-gamma-A-globulinemia. *Scand J Clin Lab Invest.* 1965;17:316-320.

21. Sharon R, Amar A. IgA deficiency in Israeli blood donors. *J Clin Pathol.* 982;35:582-583.

22. Feng L. Epidemiological study of selective IgA deficiency among 6 nationalities in China. *Zhonghua Yi Xue Za Zhi.* 1992;72:88-90.

23. Huntley CC, Stephenson RL. IgA deficiency:family studies. *NC Med J.* 1968;29:325-331.

24. Pereira LF, Sapina AM, Arroyo J, et al. Prevalence of selective IgA deficiency in Spain: More than we thought. *Blood.* 1997;90:893.

25. Weber-Mzell D, Kotanko P, Hauer AC, et al. Gender, age and seasonal effects on IgA deficiency; a study of 7293 Caucasians. *Euro J Clin Invest.* 2004;34;224-228.

26. Holt PD, Tandy NP, Anstee DJ. Screening of blood donors for IgA deficiency: A study of the donor population of south-west England. *J Clin Path.* 1977;30:1007-1010.

27. Koistinen J, Cardenas RM, Fudenberg HH. Anti-IgA antibodies of limited specificity in healthy IgA deficient subjects. *J Immunogenet.* 1977;4:295-300.

28. Wells VJ, McNally MP, King MA. Selective IgA deficiency in Australian blood donors. *Austr NZ J Med.* 1980;10:410-413.

Microbiology Overview

Dominick Cavuoti

This section contains representative case studies from the major classes of microbial pathogens causing infections in humans:

+ Bacteria

+ Fungi

+ Parasites

+ Viruses

The majority of the cases deal with organisms whose presence in the human host would never be construed as contamination or insignificant. Additionally, some of the cases deal with organisms that are less commonly seen in the typical clinical microbiology laboratory but this certainly depends on the patient population and geographic locale. However, the cases emphasize the integral role the clinical microbiologist and microbiology laboratory play in the diagnosis and management of infectious diseases. To further expand on the relationship between the microbiologist, clinician and patient, some basic tenets of laboratory utilization are presented below, with a primary focus on specimen collection in relation to commonly submitted specimens such as blood, sputum, wounds, and abscesses.

It is useful to think of laboratory testing as a series of events. Traditionally, microbiologists have been concerned with the identification of bacterial, fungal, parasitic, and/or viral agents in human body fluids and tissues (analytic phase) but it is clear that what happens before the identification occurs on the specimen submitted for analysis (pre-analytic phase) and after (post-analytic) are just as important. The diagnosis of a presumed infectious disease begins with a thorough physical examination and history of the illness. A differential diagnosis is generated, and appropriate ancillary studies are performed as necessary to narrow the differential diagnosis. Specimens are collected and submitted to the Microbiology laboratory, and empiric antimicrobial therapy may be started pending the results of the microbiologic studies. In the laboratory, the specimen is examined by a variety of methods in order to identify the offending agent(s). When indicated, antimicrobial susceptibility tests are performed. Once an etiologic agent is identified, directed therapy can be instituted.

In the pre-analytic phase of the process of identifying the organism(s) associated with the patient's disease, the health care provider must decide beforehand if the laboratory results generated from the submitted specimen will be used to alter patient management, if indicated. If not, then there is no reason to submit the specimen for testing. If testing is deemed necessary and likely to contribute to positive patient outcome for the care of the patient then a well collected specimen will yield the most useful information. Clinical Microbiology laboratories typically have a document that describes specimen collection requirements but if there are any questions about how to collect a specimen and they are not addressed in this document, the laboratory should be contacted before collection of the specimen. Consultation with a clinical microbiologist, if available, is also recommended to assist with appropriate test selection. The basic principles of specimen collection are summarized in **Table 1**:

Table I. Principles of Specimen Collection for Microbial Testing

- Collect specimens from the actual site of the infection

- Meticulous attention to aseptic technique is necessary to avoid contamination

- Submit a sufficient quantity of specimen for testing

- Tissue, fluids, and needle aspirates are superior to specimens collected with swabs

- Submit the specimen in the appropriate container for the testing requested

- Ensure that the information on the requisition/order matches that on the specimen container and that the source of the specimen is clearly stated

- Whenever possible, specimens should be collected before the administration of antibiotics

- Transport specimens to the laboratory as soon as possible after collection

- Appropriate smears should be performed as part of the analysis, when indicated

The use of proper aseptic technique when collecting specimens cannot be overstated. Nowhere is this more important than in the collection of blood cultures. Coagulase negative staphylococci can be bloodstream pathogens but the majority of these isolates are contaminants whose presence in blood cultures has led to unnecessary antibiotic therapy. Studies have shown (see **Suggested Reading**) that well trained and dedicated teams of phlebotomists have been able to lower blood culture contamination rates, which, in turn, has led to a decrease in the unnecessary administration of antibiotics and decreased hospital costs. However, any specimen that has the potential to come in contact with mucosal or skin flora should be collected with the utmost care.

Swabs are commonly used collection devices for a variety of specimens; however, they are appropriate for only a few. Their main utility is for sampling mucosal surfaces such as nasal swabs for *Staphylococcus aureus* carriage, peritonsillar fossae for streptococcal pharyngitis, and nasopharyngeal swabs for respiratory viruses or *Bordetella pertussis*. The main drawback of swabs is that they hold only a limited volume of specimen. Additionally, they cannot sample the deep portion of a wound without coming into contact with surface contaminants from the superficial portion of the wound, and some organisms do not survive the transport time from collection to receipt in the laboratory.

Tissues, fluids, and specimens collected by needle aspiration often yield the most useful information. For example, aspirated abscess contents, of sufficient volume, submitted in a capped syringe with the air expressed can be used for routine aerobic, anaerobic, fungal, and mycobacterial testing.

A sterile container with a tight fitting lid is appropriate for most specimens. If anaerobes are suspected, an approved transport device with pre-reduced transport media that ensures an anaerobic environment or the previously mentioned capped syringe with the air expressed are acceptable. In some instances, direct inoculation of media at the bedside is recommended (eg, corneal scrapings or blood cultures).

In addition to all of the pertinent patient information, the requisition should also state, as specifically as possible, the source of the specimen. Terms such as wound, abscess, or lesion are unacceptable as they do not state the anatomic location. The information on the requisition must match the information on the specimen label.

Ideally, specimens should be submitted to the Microbiology laboratory within 2 hours of collection. Sterile fluids such as joint fluid, cerebrospinal fluid (CSF), or pleural fluids should be submitted even sooner. Most specimens (eg, stool, urine, and sputum samples) can be refrigerated if a delay in transport to the Microbiology laboratory is anticipated. However, some organisms (eg, *Neisseria gonorrhoeae*, *Neisseria meningitidis*, *Haemophilus*, and anaerobes) are sensitive to cold so specimens suspected of harboring these agents should **not** be refrigerated. In addition, never refrigerate CSF, genital, or eye specimens.

Once in the Microbiology laboratory, a variety of rapid direct testing methods can be performed while tests requiring long incubation times at various temperatures (eg, cultures) or other tests are in progress. For example, a well prepared and interpreted Gram stain remains an excellent tool for rapidly diagnosing common bacterial infections which can help guide empiric therapy. Moreover, the results of the Gram stain can be used to assess the quality of the specimen. A Gram stain that shows a predominance of inflammatory cells and necrotic debris confirms that the specimen is representative of the infected site while a Gram stain smear that shows a predominance of squamous epithelial cells represents a contaminated specimen whose culture results cannot be considered valid.

When a quality specimen is submitted, the chances of getting an accurate, clinically relevant result are high. However, another tool to ensure appropriate test utilization and submission of a quality specimen to the Microbiology laboratory is the use of specimen rejection criteria. These criteria are usually listed in the laboartory's specimen collection document. Some commonly used rejection criteria are listed in **Table 2**:

Table 2. Commonly Used Specimen Rejection Criteria in the Microbiology Laboratory

- Requisitions and specimen labels do not match or the specimen is unlabeled

- Prolonged transport of the specimen without proper storage

- Improper container (eg, specimen for anaerobes in an aerobic culture device)

- Leaking, cracked, or broken container

- The specimen is unsuitable for the requested testing (eg, stool or vaginal samples submitted for culture of anaerobes)

- Duplicate specimens on the same day for the same request (except sterile fluids or tissues)

- Specimen received plated on outdated or dried out media

- Sputum specimens consisting of oropharyngeal secretions

- Routine bacterial stool cultures on patients in-house over 3 days

No health care provider likes to hear that a specimen on their patient has been rejected but the consequences of accepting inadequate and/or inappropriate specimens can be detrimental to patient care. These criteria are used to ensure that the specimen that arrives in the Microbiology laboratory is correctly identified, properly collected, and appropriate for testing requested.

For additional information regarding specimen collection guidelines and quality assurance procedures used to ensure appropriate utilization of the resources of the Microbiology laboratory, readers are referred to the "Suggested Reading" section below for books and additional articles related to these subjects.

Suggested Reading

1. McKenna R, Keffer J. *The Handbook of Clinical Pathology,* 2nd ed. Chicago: ASCP Press, 2000.

2. Wilson ML. Clinically Relevant, Cost Effective Clinical Microbiology: Strategies to Decrease Unnecessary Testing. *Am Clin Pathol.* 1997; 107(2):154-157.

3. Murray PR. *Manual of Clinical Microbiology,* 9th ed. Washington, DC: ASM Press, 2007, pp. 43-54.

4. Miller JM. *A Guide to Specimen Management in Clinical Microbiology,* 2nd ed. Washington, DC: ASM Press.

5. Schreckenberger P. Lowering *Laboratory Costs: Practical Guidelines for Optimal Processing and Evaluation of Specimens for Clinical Microbiology Testing.* ASCP Teleconference, 2005.

6. Barenfanger J. Quality Assurances: Decreasing Clinically Irrelevant Testing from Clinical Microbiology Laboratories, Part 1. *Clin Microbiol Newsletter.* 2006; 28(3):17-24.

7. Barenfanger J. Quality Assurances: Decreasing Clinically Irrelevant Testing from Clinical Microbiology Laboratories, Part 2. *Clinical Microbiol Newsletter.* 2006; 28(4):25-29.

8. Wilson ML. General Principles of Specimen Collection and Transport. *ClinInfect Dis.* 1996; 22:766-77.

9. Gander RM, Byrd L, DeCrescenzo M, Hirany S, Bowen M, Baughman J. Impact of Blood Cultures Drawn by Phlebotomy on Contamination Rates and Health Care Costs in a Hospital Emergency Department. *J Clin Microbiol.* 2009; 47(4):1021-1024.

10. Peterson LR, Hamilton JD, Baron EJ, et al. Role of Clinical Microbiology Laboratories in the Management and Control of Infectious Diseases and the Delivery of Healthcare. *Clin Infect Dis.* 2001; 32:605-611.

11. Reisner BS, Woods GL. Chapter 50: Specimen Collection and Processing for Microbiology. In: McClatchey KD. *Clinical Laboratory Medicine,* 2nd ed. Philadelphia, PA: Lippincott, Williams and Wilkins, 2002: 1059-1073.

12. Murray PR, Witebsky FG. Chaper 17: The Clinicain and the Microbiology Laboratory. In: Mandell GL, Bennett JE, Dolin R. *Mandell, Douglas, and Bennett's Principles and Practice of Infectious Diseases,* 7th ed. Philadelphia, PA: Churchill Livingstone Elsevier, 2010: 233-265.

A 14-Year-Old Male With Abdominal Pain

Elliot Carter, Andrea G. Kahn, Tara N. Evans

Department of Pathology, University of South Alabama, Mobile, AL

Patient: 14-year-old male.

Past Surgical History: None.

Family History: Unremarkable.

Chief Complaint: Abdominal pain.

Past Medical History: Noncontributory.

History of Present Illness: The patient described a history of subjective recurrent low-grade fevers and epigastric abdominal pain associated with a 10-pound weight loss. A travel history obtained at the time of admission to the hospital revealed that the patient had gone on a camping trip 2 weeks prior to the development of his symptoms. He reported drinking fresh water from a stream while on the trip.

Physical Examination: Moderate abdominal tenderness concentrated in the epigastric region.

Diagnostic Studies: The patient was admitted to the hospital where he underwent upper gastrointestinal endoscopy with biopsies. Histologic examination of the biopsy specimens from the esophagus, stomach, and duodenum showed no significant pathologic changes. A computed tomography (CT) scan of the abdomen revealed a 5.0×4.0 cm mass in the liver which appeared cystic and multilocular (**Image 1A**). A fine-needle aspiration (FNA) of the lesion yielded a light brown viscous material (**Image 1B**). Gram stain and bacterial, fungal, and mycobacterial cultures were performed using this material. Cytologic examination of the aspirated material showed sheets of acute inflammatory cells and necrosis.

Questions

1. What are this patient's most striking clinical and laboratory findings?

2. How do you explain this patient's most striking clinical and laboratory findings?

3. What is this patient's most likely diagnosis?

4. How are different organisms within this group distinguished from one another?

5. What is the treatment for hepatic abscesses caused by this group of organisms?

Possible Answers

1. Recurrent low-grade fever, epigastric abdominal pain, a 10-pound weight loss, moderate abdominal tenderness concentrated in the epigastric region; leukocytosis with a marked left shift, positive Gram stain and bacterial culture for a catalase-negative/Voges-Proskauer-positive organism that hydrolyzed esculin or arginine and that did not produce acid from inulin, sorbitol, or mannitol that was identified as belonging to the *Streptococcus anginosus* group of bacterial organisms (**T1**).

2. Gastritis, inflammatory bowel disease, and acute appendicitis were initially included in the differential diagnosis. Imaging studies, however,

T1. Principal Laboratory Findings

Test		Patient's Result	"Normal" Reference Range
Hematology			
WBC count		18.2	$4.0\text{-}11.0 \times 10^3/\mu L$
RBC count		4.21	$3.8\text{-}5.2 \times 10^6/\mu L$
Hemoglobin		42.1	33.8-45.6 g/dL
Hematocrit		13.0	11.6-15.6 g/dL
MCV		92	81-95 fL
Differential:	Neutrophils	55	40.0-80.0%
	Bands	22	0.0-6.0%
	Lymphocytes	16	15.0-50.0%
	Monocytes	4	2.0-11.0%
	Eosinophils	3	1.0-7.0%
Microbiology			
Gram stain		Gram-positive cocci in chains	
Cultures:	Bacterial	Small white colonies on blood agar	
	Fungal	No growth	
	Mycobacterial	No growth	
Biochemical tests:	Catalase	Negative	
	Voges-Proskauer	Positive	
	Esculin	Positive for hydrolysis	
	Arginine	Positive for hydrolysis	
	Inulin/sorbitol/mannitol	Negative for acid production	
ID of organism:	*Anginosus* group *Streptococcus*		

WBC, white blood cell; RBC, red blood cell; MCV, mean corpuscular volume.

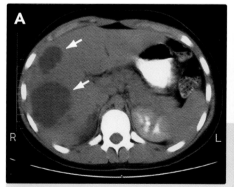 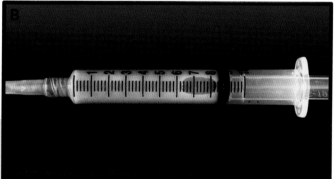

Image 1_The patient's computed tomography (CT) and fine-needle aspiration (FNA) findings illustrating **A**) a multilocular cystic lesion (arrows) of the liver by CT and **B**) the light brown viscous material obtained from FNA of the liver lesion.

revealed a cystic liver lesion which raised suspicion of an abscess, possibly an amoebic abscess due to the history of freshwater consumption on a recent camping trip. No history of diarrhea suggestive of *Entamoeba histolytica* infection was present, although up to 50% of cases of amoebic liver abscess are unassociated with preceding confirmed intestinal amebiasis. Culture of the aspirated material from the patient's cystic lesion showed an organism within the "*Streptococcus anginosus* (formerly *milleri*)" group. Streptococci of the *anginosus* group are facultatively anaerobic, catalase negative, gram-positive cocci which show variable hemolysis on blood agar. Three species of streptococci are found within the *anginosus* group: *S. intermedius, S. anginosus*, and *S. constellatus*.[1] The clinical importance of the identification of these organisms from patient samples depends upon the clinical setting. *S. intermedius, S. anginosus*, and *S. constellatus* may be found as part of the normal flora of the oropharynx. They are isolated commonly from the oral cavity, nasopharynx, and throat of asymptomatic carriers and may also be found in the gastrointestinal and genitourinary tracts. Despite their frequent presence as benign colonizing agents, these organisms have been identified as causative agents of significant infections in humans.

3. **Most likely diagnosis:** *hepatic abscess due to infection with S. intermedius.* The organisms comprising the "*S. anginosus*" group have been documented as the causative agents of bacteremia, head and neck infections, pleural empyema, endocarditis, cellulitis, subcutaneous abscesses, genitourinary tract infections, and abscesses of the brain and liver.[2,3] *S. anginosus* and *S. constellatus* have a widespread spectrum of disease with *S. anginosus* being particularly prevalent as a cause of genitourinary tract infections. *S. intermedius* shows a particular predilection for hepatic and cerebral abscess formation.

4. Biochemically, *S. intermedius* can be distinguished from *S. constellatus* and *S. anginosus* by its production of β-galactosidase, β-D-fucosidase, β-N-acetylglucosaminidase, β-N-acetylgalactosaminidase, α-D-glucosidase, sialidase, and hyaluronidase. Differentiation of *S. constellatus* from *S. anginosus* relies on the

demonstration of α-glucosidase, β-glucosidase, and hyaluronidase production.

5. Drainage of the abscess, whether laparoscopically or percutaneously, and appropriate antimicrobial therapy are the important elements of treatment in cases such as this one. In general, organisms of the "*S. anginosus*" group are susceptible to penicillin, ampicillin, cefotaxime, vancomycin, trimethoprim, and ciprofloxacin. Some strains may show resistance to erythromycin and clindamycin.

Keywords

epigastric, empyema, endocarditis, cellulitis, Streptococcus milleri group, hepatic abscess

Glossary

Epigastric: pertaining to the upper middle region of the abdomen
Empyema: accumulation of pus in the thoracic cavity
Endocarditis: inflammation of the endocardial lining of the cardiac valves or cardiac chambers
Cellulitis: suppurative inflammation of the deep subcutaneous tissues and muscle

References

1. Whiley RA, Beighton D, Winstanley TG, et al. *Streptococcus intermedius, Streptococcus constellatus*, and *Streptococcus anginosus* (the *Streptococcus milleri* group): association with different body sites and clinical infections. *J Clin Microbiol.* 1992;30:243-244.

2. Chua D, Reinhart HH, Sobel JD. Liver abscess caused by *Streptococcus milleri. Rev Infect Dis.* 1989;2:197-202.

3. Yamamoto M, Fukushima T, Ohshiro S, et al. Brain abscess caused by *Streptococcus intermedius*: Two case reports. *Surg Neurol.* 1999;51:219-222.

Misleading Gram Stain Findings on a Smear From a Cerebrospinal Fluid Specimen

Brian J. Harrington,[1] Mary Plenzler[2]

[1]*Department of Public Health, Medical College of Ohio,* [2]*Microbiology Department, Promedica Laboratories, The Toledo Hospital, Toledo, OH*

Patient: 18-year-old female.

Chief Complaint: The patient presented to the emergency department (ED) complaining of severe headache, pain in her legs, nausea, vomiting, and fluid leaking from the site of a previous surgery on the central nervous system (CNS).

Past Medical History: Central nervous system surgery approximately 6 weeks prior. She had been seen in the ED twice in the past 2 weeks with migraine headaches and sinusitis. She underwent a spinal tap on both of these occasions, and cerebrospinal fluid (CSF) cultures showed no growth.

History of Present Illness: The patient was taken to surgery, the previous CNS surgical incision was opened, and a large amount of CSF that had pooled under the incision was collected and submitted to the laboratory. The laboratory requisition that accompanied this pink and hazy fluid indicated a diagnosis of "meningitis" and requests for Gram stain, cell count, glucose, total protein, and culture and susceptibility testing.

Drug History: Prior to obtaining the CSF specimen, the patient was taking rofecoxid (Vioxx), dexamethasone (Decadron), and famotidine (Pepcid). After the CSF specimen was collected, she was placed on vancomycin and cefotaxime therapy.

Questions _____

1. What are this patient's most striking laboratory results?

2. How do you explain this patient's most striking laboratory findings?

3. What organism would you suspect from the initial Gram stain findings [**Image 1A**]?

4. If the gram-negative cocci observed upon re-examination of the initial Gram stain [**Image 1B**] had been seen on the initial examination of this smear, would this finding have raised questions or doubts regarding the presence of gram-positive cocci on the smear?

5. What genera of bacteria have been reported to be prone to under-decolorization in the Gram stain procedure?

6. What precautions, if any, can be taken to reduce the risk of these gram-negative bacteria staining gram-positive?

7. What is the mechanism for gram-negative organisms to appear gram-positive after a Gram staining procedure?

T1. Principal Laboratory Findings – Cerebrospinal Fluid (CSF)

Test	Patient's Result	"Normal" Reference Range
Chemistry and Hematology		
Appearance	Slightly xanthochromic	Clear and colorless
Glucose	3	40-70 mg/dL
Total protein	648	15-45 mg/dL
RBC count	11801	0/µL
WBC count	6514	<5/µL
Neutrophils	89%	
Lymphocytes	2%	
Monocytes	9%	
Microbiology		
Gram stain (spun sediment)	WBCs present with a few gram-positive cocci [**Image1A**]	
Culture, chocolate agar	1 colony of a gram-negative rod	
Thioglycollate broth	gram-negative rods/coccobacilli	
Re-review of initial Gram stain	Rare gram-negative coccobacilli [**Image 1B**]	
Chocolate agar	1 colony that was subcultured to MacConkey agar	
MacConkey agar subculture	Lactose non-fermenter	
Gram stain of growth from colony on TSA with 5% sheep's blood	[**Image 1C**]	
ID of organism*	*Acinetobacter calcoaceticus/baumanii complex*	

Drug susceptibility					
	Amikacin	S	Cefuroxime	R
	Ampicillin	R	Chloramphenicol	R
	Ampicillin/ sulbactam	S	Ciprofloxacin	S
	Cefazolin	R	Gentamicin	S
	Cefepime	S	Imipenem	S
	Cefotaxime	S	Levofloxacin	S
	Ceftazidime	S	Tobramycin	S
	Ceftriaxone	S	Trimethoprim/ sulfamethoxazole	R

| Repeat cultures on days 3 and 5 | No growth | |

*Using Vitek instrument (bioMerieux Inc., Durham, NC).
RBC, red blood cell; WBCs, white blood cells; TSA, trypticase soy agar; ID, identification; S, susceptible; R, resistant

8. What is this patient's most likely diagnosis?

Possible Answers _____

1. Markedly decreased CSF glucose with markedly increased total protein, high WBC count with

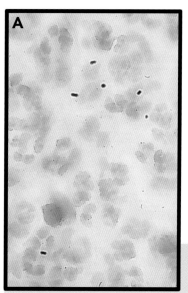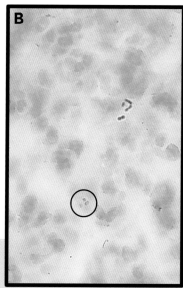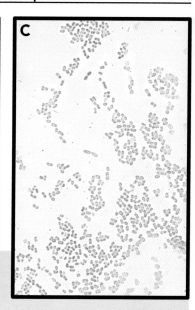

Image 1_Gram-stain findings illustrating the presence of (**A**) white blood cells and a few gram-positive cocci in the cytocentrifuged sediment of the patient's CSF, (**B**) rare gram-negative cocci (circle) in another field of the Gram stain shown in (**A**), and (**C**) many gram-negative cocci and coccobacilli in the Gram-stained smear of a colony from the TSA blood agar culture. (All images are oil immersion with 100× objective.)

89% neutrophils, and the presence of a large number of polymorphonuclear leukocytes and bacteria in the Gram-stained smear [**Image 1A**] of the CSF sediment.

2. The CSF chemistry and hematology results are compatible with those seen typically in patients with bacterial meningitis. In addition, the Gram-stained smear of the cytocentrifuged sediment from the patient's CSF specimen demonstrated the presence of purple, possibly encapsulated, cocci, including diplococci. Moreover, the quality of the Gram stain appeared satisfactory, with adequate decolorization of the cellular material, which was evenly spread on the slide [**Image 1A**].

3. The initial Gram stain findings are consistent with the morphological and Gram stain characteristics of *Streptococcus pneumoniae*.

4. No, because bacterial meningitis caused by multi-organisms is rare and only a few intracellular gram-negative bacteria were observed that could have been gram-positive organisms with damaged cell walls. On the other hand, the patient was leaking fluid from the site of a previous surgery, which could have been the portal of entry for more than 1 type of bacterial organism.

5. The phenomenon of gram-negative organisms appearing gram-positive because of under-decolorization after Gram staining has been reported for several organisms and species including *Escherichia coli, Proteus mirabilis, Klebsiella pneumoniae,*[1] and *Neisseria,*[2] *Moraxella (Branhamella),*[3-5] and *E. coli* and *Acinetobacter* species.[6] With the exception of the report by Ainsworth and colleagues,[3] which involved organisms seen in smears of sputum specimens, all of the aforementioned examples of the underdecolorization phenomenon occurred in organisms isolated from blood culture media. Snyder, however, noted Gram staining problems with *Neisseria* spp. in spinal fluid and urogenital specimens.[7] Other authors have indicated problems with *Moraxella catarrhalis,*[8] the *Neisseria* group,[9,10] and *Acinetobacter* spp.[10-12]; however, these authors did not specify the type of clinical material from which these organisms or species were isolated. Moreover, the underdecolorization problem with *Acinetobacter* spp. isolated from blood culture media is now noted in the latest edition of the American Society for Microbiology's *Manual of Clinical Microbiology.*[13]

6. In 2 reports involving *Moraxella* spp., attention was given to the decolorization step in the Gram stain procedure.[3,5] Ainsworth and colleagues[3] tried different reagents and times, but neither publication mentioned the iodine reagent used. In a follow-up letter, Das and colleagues reported that stabilized (polyvinyl-pyrrolidone) iodine was used routinely with many problems and with under-decolorization of various organisms, including *Acinetobacter* spp.[14] Perry and colleagues noted that the under-decolorization of enteric gram-negative rods was related more to the use of stabilized iodine than to the decolorizers used. Therefore, they recommended the use of Gram's iodine and 95% ethanol as a decolorizer.[1] The problems reported by Harrington with under-decolorization of *E. coli* and *Acinetobacter* spp. were also noted when stabilized iodine was used.[6] However, the iodine reagent used in the case reported here was the traditional iodine solution, not the stabilized iodine reagent. Also, the decolorizer was acetone, which is generally considered to be a fast or rapid decolorizer and faster than a 1:1 mixture of 95% ethanol and acetone (intermediate) or 95% ethanol alone (slow). Ainsworth and colleagues found optimal decolorization of *M. catarrhalis* in sputum smears using a 1:1 mixture of 95% ethanol and acetone for 20 seconds or acetone alone for 10 seconds.[3] Snyder recommended using acetone for 5 to 10 seconds on the basis of its rapid decolorization of gram-negative bacteria and its effectiveness in removing crystal violet from background material while not decolorizing truly gram-positive bacteria, even with prolonged exposure.[7] Two recent postings on the American Society for Microbiology DivC listserver (L. Fairbanks and J. Soxman. November 2003. Re: Gram stain: *Moraxella catarrhalis*.) cite many years of experience using acetone in the Gram stain procedure in which Gram-variable staining of *Acinetobacter* spp. remained a problem, even with this rapid decolorizing reagent. Thus, regardless of the Gram stain reagents used, or the medium in or on which they are grown, or the clinical material they are in, members of the *Neisseria/Moraxella/Acinetobacter* group are prone to under-decolorization during the Gram stain procedure. In the cases of *Neisseria* spp. and *Moraxella* spp., the typical bean-shaped cells and especially the double-bean pairing of cells, if appearing gram-positive, may arouse suspicion of under-decolorization. With *Acinetobacter* spp., the cells typically are not bean-shaped but more oval and coccobacillary in shape, and under-decolorization is less likely to be suspected. The correct staining of control smears, whether performed concurrently or not, is no assurance that all organisms in various smears will stain correctly. Also, as shown by the case presented here, the excellent decolorization of the human cellular material, even in the thicker parts of the smear [**Image 1A**, **Image 1B**], cannot be relied upon to indicate that some gram-negative bacteria are under-decolorized. Thus, they may appear convincingly gram-positive and present an identification problem until culture or subculture results are available. It should also be noted that gram-positive organisms staining gram-negative are a common finding in clinical specimens and in cultures (eg, the pink rods seen in populations of *Bacillus* spp. and *Clostridium* spp., some pink cocci in chains of purple cells of *Streptococcus* spp., some pink cells of *Staphylococcus* spp. when intracellular in pus). This finding can be explained by the age of the cells and/or damage to their cell wall.

7. No mechanism has been proposed that convincingly explains why or how gram-negative bacteria retain the crystal violet/iodine complex and appear gram-positive in an appropriately-processed Gram-stained smear. In a case reported by Meyer and Shope,[4] where *Moraxella catarrhalis* in a blood culture was reported as "gram-positive cocci," a notation was made of a "poorly decolorized Gram-stained smear." Clearly, under-decolorization of bacteria due to inadequate penetration of the decolorizer used during a Gram stain procedure into parts of a smear, either due to the thickness of the smear and/or the exposure time to the decolorizer, may occur and should be avoided.

8. *bacterial meningitis from infection with Acinetobacter calcoaceticus/baumanii complex.* Identification of this organism by Gram stain of a CSF smear was complicated by the under-decolorization phenomenon whereby certain gram-negative bacteria appear gram-positive after the Gram staining procedure.

Keywords

Gram stain, meningitis, under-decolorization, Acinetobacter, Moraxella, Neisseria

References

1. Perry JL, Matthews JS, Sheets TJ. Gram stain procedure for optimal microscopic interpretation of positive blood cultures. Abstr. C 74, 93rd General Meeting of the American Society for Microbiology, 1993.

2. Shooter JR, Howles MJ, Baselski VS. Neisserial infections in dialysis patients. *Clin Microbiol Newsl.* 1990;12:15-16.

3. Ainsworth SM, Nagy SB, Morgan LA, et al. Interpretation of gram-stained sputa containing *Moraxella (Branhamella) catarrhalis. J Clin Microbiol.* 1990;28:2559-2560.

4. Meyer GA, Shope R. *Moraxella (Branhamella) catarrhalis* bacteremia in children. *Clin Pediatr.* 1995;34:146-150.

5. Das K, Shah S, Levi MH. Misleading gram stain from a patient with *Moraxella (Branhamella) catarrhalis* bacteremia. *Clin Microbiol Newsl.* 1997;19:85-88.

6. Harrington BJ. Letter to the Editor. *Clin Microbiol Newsl.* 1997;19:191.

7. Snyder B. A critical review of pitfalls in the Gram stain with a proposed rapid technic. *Lab Med.* 1970;1:41-44.

8. Reyn A. Gram-negative cocci and coccobacilli. In: Buchanan RE, Gibbons NE, eds. *Bergey's Manual of Determinative Bacteriology.* Baltimore: Williams and Wilkins, 1974:427-444.

9. Wilson G, Wilkinson AE. *Neisseria, Branhamella* and *Moraxella.* In: Parker MT, ed. *Topley and Wilson's Principles of Bacteriology, Virology and Immunity.* Baltimore: Williams and Wilkins 1983:156-172 (volume 2).

10. Barenfanger J, Drake CA. Interpretation of gram stains for the nonmicrobiologist. *Lab Med.* 2001;32:368-375.

11. Parker MT. *Chromobacterium, Flavobacterium, Acinetobacer,* and *Alkaligenes.* In: Parker MT, ed: *Topley and Wilson's Principles of Bacteriology, Virology and Immunity.* Baltimore: Williams and Wilkins 1983:263-271 (volume 2).

12. Allan DA, Hartman BJ. *Acinetobacter* species. In: Mandell GL, Bennet JE, Dolin R, eds. *Principles and Practice of Infectious Diseases.* New York: Churchill Livingstone, 1995:2009-2013.

13. Schreckenberger PC, Daneshvar MI, Weyant RS, et al. *Acinetobacter, Achromobacter, Chryseobacterium, Moraxella,* and other nonfermentative gram-negative rods. In: Murray PR, Baron EJ, Jorgensen JH, et al. eds. *Manual of Clinical Microbiology.* Washington: American Society for Microbiology Press, 2003:749-779.

14. Das K, Shah S, Levi MH. Reply to letter. *Clin Microbiol Newsl.* 1997;19:191.

Worsening Symptoms of Fever, Chills, Cough, Fatigue, and Muscle Soreness in Visitors to Washington, DC

Angelica Black

Air Force Institute of Technology Civilian Institution Programs, Department of Medical and Research Technology, University of Maryland School of Medicine, Baltimore, MD

Patients: A 36-year-old mother and her 8-year-old daughter sought medical care in a hospital emergency room while on vacation in Washington, DC.

Chief Complaint: Both mother and daughter complained of sudden onset and worsening symptoms of fever, chills, cough, fatigue, and muscle soreness. The daughter also suffered from nausea, vomiting, stomach cramps, and diarrhea.

History of Present Illness: Both mother and daughter felt well and healthy when they arrived in the nation's capital 2 days prior to their hospital visit. Their symptoms began the day before their hospital visit and severely worsened overnight.

Physical Exam Findings: Temperature, 102.7°F (mother); 103.9°F (daughter). Physical examination of the daughter revealed stridor and lower extremity cyanosis.

Additional Diagnostic Procedures: Chest x-rays were performed on the daughter and showed bilateral infiltrates and consolidation consistent with pneumonia. Additionally, sputum samples were collected from both patients and sent to the laboratory for microscopic examination and culture.

Questions _____

1. What are these patients' most striking clinical and laboratory findings?

2. How do you explain these findings?

3. What is the most likely diagnosis for both patients?

4. Why is it important for health care professionals to be able to recognize the signs and symptoms of the disease affecting these patients?

5. What is the significance of the geographic location of this case in regard to the suspected organism causing their disease?

6. How is the suspected disease contracted?

7. What are the 3 most common forms of this disease?

8. Why is it important this disease be recognized as early as possible?

9. What routine procedures can medical technologists perform to reinforce a suspicion of the organism causing the disease affecting these patients?

10. What are the laboratory test criteria for the diagnosis of this disease?

11. At what point should infection control personnel and public health officials be notified when

T1. Principal Laboratory Findings

Test	Results		Reference Range
	Mother	Daughter	
Hematology			
WBC count	10.2	21.6	3.6-11.1 × 10³/µL
Neutrophils	73	92ᵃ	43-72%
Hemoglobin	12.8	13.2	12.0-16.0 g/dL
Hematocrit	39	39	36-48%
Platelet count	181	79	165-353 × 10³/µL
Coagulation			
PT	14.2	22.8	10.8-13.9 sec
PTT	33.3	36.5	21.0-34.0 sec
Fibrinogen	170	147	168-441 mg/dL
Chemistry			
Sodium	140	139	135-145 mEq/L
Potassium	4.3	4.5	3.4-5.0 mEq/L
Chloride	104	106	98-110 mEq/L
CO₂	23	28	21-29 mEq/L
Glucose	104	93	75-110 mg/dL
BUN	16	12	7-18 mg/dL
Creatinine	0.9	1.1	0.7-1.2 mg/dL
Bilirubin, total	1.3	1.9	0.2-1.3 mg/dL
AST	42	55	8-39 U/L
ALT	54	65	9-52 U/L
Microbiology			
Sputum gram stain	n.d.ᵇ	Bloody with gram-negative bacilliᶜ	Negative

ᵃWith left shift. ᵇNot done. Sputum specimen was unsuitable for analysis due to >10 epithelial cells/low power field. ᶜMany small, plump, ovoid gram-negative rods exhibiting bipolar staining with a characteristic "closed safety pin" appearance.
PT, prothrombin time; PTT, partial thromboplastin time; BUN, blood urea nitrogen; AST, aspartate aminotransferase; ALT, alanine aminotransferase.

individuals present with the signs and symptoms characteristic of the patients presented in this case study?

12. What factors are important in helping health care professionals differentiate naturally occurring disease from disease resulting from a bioterrorism event?

Possible Answers _____

1. The most striking clinical findings were the sudden onset and rapid progression of symptoms consistent with pneumonia in previously healthy individuals. The most striking laboratory findings were leukocytosis with neutrophilia and a left shift and the presence of gram-negative bacilli in a bloody sputum from the daughter consisting of many small, plump, ovoid gram-negative rods exhibiting bipolar staining with a characteristic "closed safety pin" appearance (**T1**).

2. The characteristic staining of the organism found in the daughter's sputum should alert the medical technologist that they may be dealing with *Yersinia pestis*, the cause of plague. *Yersinia pestis* is a small ovoid gram-negative bacillus that characteristically exhibits bipolar staining and resembles a "closed safety pin."[1]

T2. Comparison of Various Characteristics of Naturally Occurring Versus Pneumonic Plague

Characteristic	Type of Plague	
	Naturally Occurring	Primary Pneumonic
Transmission	Typically occurs through the bite of an infected flea or by direct contact with an infected animal	Occurs through the inhalation of aerosolized bacteria
Incubation period 2-8 days	2-4 days	
Geographic distribution	Associated with rural areas inhabited by rodents	Infection (sudden onset of symptoms in previously healthy individuals) may occur in a non-endemic area
Disease hallmark	Buboes typically develop close to site of infection; however, they may be absent in primary septicemic plague	Hemoptysis
Symptoms	Malaise and acute high fever; skin lesions at the site of the flea bite; may advance to systemic infection or cause thromboses (purpuric lesions)	Fever, cough, malaise, dypsnea, bilateral infiltrates or pulmonary consolidation; severe infection that progress rapidly to septicemia and shock

3. **Most likely diagnosis:** infection with *Yersinia pestis*.

4. In light of recent terrorist events in the United States, including the September 11, 2001 attacks on the World Trade Center and the intentional release of anthrax via the postal system, it has become increasingly important for health care professionals to be able to recognize illnesses associated with a bioterrorism event. The Centers for Disease Control and Prevention (CDC) have categorized biological agents based on the risk they pose to the population. Agents of the highest concern are those that can be disseminated or transmitted easily, result in high mortality rates, will most likely cause panic and social disruption, and require public health preparedness.[2] *Yersinia pestis*, the cause of plague, is 1 of these agents. The use of this organism as a bioterrorism agent is considered probable because it is readily available and can easily be produced in large quantities.[3] It is expected that *Yersinia pestis* will be used in aerosol form thereby creating a plague outbreak that is both deadly and contagious. It is also important to note that plague still occurs naturally. Therefore, it is essential that health care professionals be able to differentiate between naturally occurring plague and plague resulting from the intentional release of aerosolized *Yersinia pestis*.

5. Plague does not occur naturally in the eastern United States. Plague is endemic in states west of the Rocky Mountains, most commonly in New Mexico, Colorado, Arizona, and California.[4] However, Washington, DC is an attractive potential target for bioterrorism.

6. Plague is an infectious disease that primarily affects squirrels, rats, prairie dogs, and other rodents. It is generally transmitted to humans and other animals through the bites of plague-infected fleas. It can also be transmitted by direct contact with an infected animal or by inhalation of infected respiratory droplets. Domestic cats that are allowed to roam freely are especially susceptible to plague infection. Such cats pose a significant health risk to their owners by transmitting the disease directly (eg, bites, scratches, coughing) or transporting infected fleas into the home.[5]

7. Plague generally manifests in 3 forms, *bubonic*, *septicemic*, and *pneumonic*. **Bubonic** plague is the most common form of plague, and it typically results from the bite of an infected flea. Once introduced into the body, the organism multiplies in the skin and tissue then migrates through the lymphatic system. Symptoms associated with bubonic plague include sudden onset of fever, chills, headache, malaise, and exhaustion.[6] Frequently, patients develop buboes, which are

enlarged and extremely tender lymph nodes. The lymph nodes involved are usually those that are closest to the site of infection. **Septicemic** plague results from the direct inoculation of the organism into the blood stream. It can also develop secondary to complications of bubonic or pneumonic plague. Patients with primary septicemic plague generally do not develop buboes because severe bacteremia develops before lymph node involvement. Clinical manifestations include rapid onset of severe bacteremia, septic shock, thrombosis, mild disseminated intravascular coagulation, and purpuric skin lesions.[7] **Pneumonic** plague is a pulmonary infection that occurs from the inhalation of infectious respiratory droplets or aerosolized organisms of *Yersinia pestis*. It may also develop secondary to bubonic or septicemic plague. Unlike the bubonic or septicemic forms of plague, pneumonic plague is person-to-person transmissible. It is characterized by the acute and severe onset of fever, chills, malaise, and myalgias. Patients generally present with a productive cough, chest pain, and increasing dyspnea. Hemoptysis (bloody sputum) is a classic symptom. Chest x-rays usually demonstrate bilateral infiltrates and consolidation. Gastrointestinal symptoms such as nausea, vomiting, diarrhea, and abdominal pain may also be present.[5] Additionally, patients may exhibit coagulation abnormalities such as thrombocytopenia, low-grade disseminated intravascular coagulation, and hypofibrinogenemia.[7] Hematologic findings include moderate leukocytosis with greater than 80% neutrophils and an increase in the number of bands.

8. The incubation period for *bubonic* plague ranges from 2 to 8 days.[6] If the disease goes untreated, the infection may spread to the lungs or blood. The mortality rate for untreated bubonic plague ranges from 50% to 60%; however, the rate improves to less than 5% with treatment. Symptoms of *septicemic* plague develop rapidly upon infection, and the disease is 100% fatal if not treated. *Pneumonic* plague has a short incubation period that ranges from 2 to 4 days.[7] Once symptoms begin to develop, the disease progresses rapidly and eventually leads to respiratory collapse, shock, and multiple organ failure. Early detection and immediate treatment are necessary for survival. *Pneumonic* plague is 100% fatal if left untreated and is almost always fatal if the disease is not treated within 24 hours of respiratory symptom onset.[5] Even with treatment, chances for survival are less than 50%.[8]

9. Diagnosis of a suspected plague case requires identification of *Yersinia pestis* from a direct smear or culture of a clinical specimen (eg, blood, lymph node, sputum, cerebrospinal fluid). Specimens submitted for evaluation should be collected prior to antibiotic administration. Additionally, it is recommended that laboratories process these specimens under biological safety level II (BSL-2) precautions. As previously mentioned, *Yersinia pestis* is a small ovoid gram-negative bacillus that characteristically exhibits bipolar staining and resembles a "closed safety pin." Enhanced bipolar staining is seen with Wayson's and Wright's stain. *Yersinia pestis* grows optimally at room temperature and can be cultured on routine media. Cultures incubated at 37°C will grow much slower, and as a result, colonies are usually too small to be seen at 24 hours. Characteristic "hammered copper" and "fried egg" colony morphologies are typically seen at 48 hours and 72 hours, respectively. Commercial and automated biochemical identification systems are not recommended for further identification because these slow growing bacteria will appear inert. Laboratory personnel can also perform oxidase, catalase, and urease tests. *Yersinia pestis* will be catalase positive and oxidase and urease negative.[1]

10. According to the CDC, the following laboratory test criteria are required for the diagnosis of suspected, presumptive, and confirmed plague cases. A case of plague is considered suspect when a patient exhibits symptoms consistent with plague and the organism is seen on a direct smear from a clinical specimen. Presumptive and confirmatory laboratory diagnosis is generally performed by public health laboratories. Presumptive diagnosis requires positive immunofluorescent staining of the *Yersinia pestis* F1 antigen or an anti-F1 titer greater than 1:10. Lastly, confirmatory diagnosis requires bacteriophage lysis of an isolated culture, 2 positive serum samples that show a 4-fold difference in anti-F1 titer, or a single serum sample has an F1 titer greater than 1:128 and the patient has no history of exposure to *Yersinia pestis*.[9]

11. Whenever plague is suspected, hospital infection personnel and public health officials should be notified immediately. Standard infection control precautions should be used in all cases of suspected plague. Additionally, pneumonic plague requires that hospital personnel employ droplet precautions and isolate the patient.[8] Notification of the public health department will trigger a comprehensive epidemiological investigation. The purpose of the investigation is to confirm the case, identify the source and mode of transmission, identify others who may have been in contact with the patient or the source, and develop control and prevention strategies.[5]

12. Manifestations of plague resulting from the use of aerosolized *Yersinia pestis* differ substantially from naturally occurring disease. Naturally occurring plague should be suspected when the disease manifests in the bubonic form. It should also be considered if the patient recently traveled to or lives in a plague endemic area. Outbreaks of naturally occurring bubonic plague will generally be preceded by an increased number of rodent infections and deaths. Conversely, plague resulting from the use of aerosolized *Yersinia pestis* will present in the pneumonic form. A bioterrorism event should be suspected if the infection occurs in an area of the country that is not endemic of plague or if a large number of previously healthy individuals become critically ill with severe pneumonia and hemoptysis. Symptoms of pneumonic plague and bubonic plague are similar with the exception of lymphadenitis (bubo formation) which typically accompanies bubonic plague.[3] **T2** contrasts the characteristics of naturally occurring and primary pneumonic plague following exposure to aerosolized *Yersinia pestis*.

Keywords

plague, closed safety-pin appearance, buboes, hemoptysis

References

1. CDC. Basic protocols for level A laboratories for the presumptive identification of *Yersinia pestis*. http://www.bt.CDC.gov/agent/plague/#laboratory. Accessed December 2, 2005.

2. CDC. Category A biological agents. Available at: http://www.bt.CDC.gov/agent/agentlist-category.asp#a. Accessed December 2, 2005.

3. Inglesby, TV, Dennis, DT, Henderson, DA, et al. Plague as a biological weapon: Medical and public health management. *JAMA*. 2000;283:2281-2290.

4. Imported plague-New York City, 2002. *MMWR*. 2003;52:725-728.

5. Plague training module. http://www.bt.CDC.gov/agent/plague/trainingmodule. Accessed December 2, 2005.

6. Cobbs, CG, Chansolme, DH. Plague. *Dermatologic Clinics*. 2004;22:303-312.

7. Clem, A, Galwankar, S. Plague: A decade since the 1994 outbreaks in India. *J Assoc Physic India*. 2005;53:457-464.

8. Reilly, CM, Deason, D. Plague: A naturally occurring bacterial species can be weaponized. *Am J Nursing*. 2002;102:47-50.

9. Laboratory test criteria for the diagnosis of plague. http://www.CDC.gov/ncidod/dvbid/plague/lab-test-criteria.htm. Accessed December 2, 2005.

Neck Pain and Rash in an 18-Year-Old Student

Monte Willis, Michael Roth, Peter Gilligan

Department of Pathology & Laboratory Medicine, University of North Carolina, Chapel Hill, NC

Patient: 18-year-old Caucasian college student.

Chief Complaint: Headache and skin rash.

History of Present Illness: The patient reported having a sore throat within the past week. One day prior to admission, he experienced nausea and vomiting. On the day of admission, while attending class, he noticed "spots" on his arms, legs, trunk, and abdomen. Shortly before his presentation to the emergency department, he developed fatigue, headache, neck pain, and photophobia.

Past Medical History: The patient had no history of abdominal pain, tick bites, sick contacts, sexually transmitted diseases, or recent travel. The patient received quadravalent Neisseria meningitidis vaccination at the County Health Department 6 months prior to his admission.

Family History: Non-contributory.

Physical Examination: Vital signs: temperature, 36.8°C; heart rate, 114 beats per minute; respiratory rate, 24 per minute; blood pressure, 88/34 mm Hg. Pertinent physical examination findings included tachycardia, hypotension, and purpuric lesions on his arms, legs, trunk, and genitals (**Image 1**). He was acutely ill in appearance, but oriented with nuchal rigidity on neurologic examination (positive Brudzynski and Kernig signs).

Results of Additional Diagnostic Procedures: An echocardiography revealed mild left ventricular enlargement with decreased function [estimated ejection fraction = 30% (Normal >60%)]. A chest x-ray demonstrated pulmonary edema.

Questions

1. What are this patient's most striking clinical and laboratory findings?

2. How do you explain this patient's most striking clinical and laboratory findings?

3. What condition(s) is (are) suggested by this patient's most striking clinical and laboratory findings?

4. What additional test(s) should be ordered on this patient and why?

5. What is this patient's most likely diagnosis?

6. How is this patient's condition typically treated?

Possible Answers

1. Clinically, the most striking findings in this patient are purpuric skin lesions located on his legs, arms, trunk, and genitals; tachycardia;

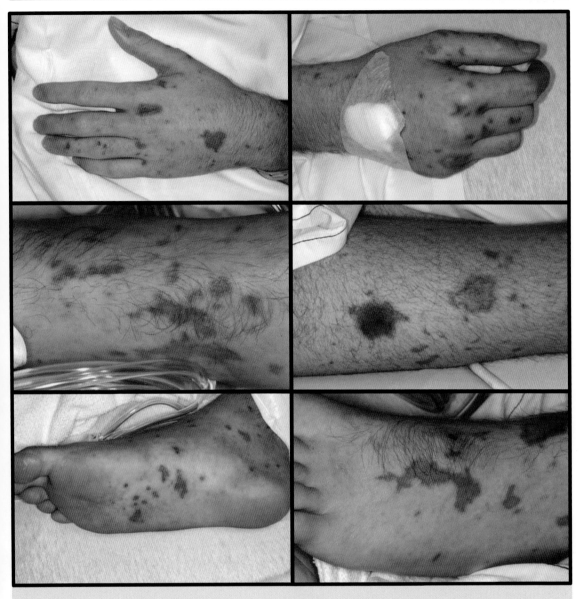

Image 1_The patient's skin lesions during the first 24 hours after admission to the hospital. The distribution of the rash was over his entire body.

hypotension; and nuchal rigidity. Significant laboratory findings include normocytic anemia, thrombocytopenia, prolonged PT and PTT, elevated D-dimer, decreased fibrinogen and ATIII activity, elevated creatinine, decreased calcium, magnesium, phosphorus, and an elevated AST and ALT (**T1**).

2. **Purpura** represents bleeding into the skin and mucosal membranes resulting in a dark (purple) non-blanching rash that may be caused

by a variety of conditions. Generally purpura may be categorized by 3 major etiologies: 1) vascular disorders (eg, viral illnesses, sepsis); 2) abnormalities in platelet number and function (eg, infections, autoimmune diseases); and 3) disorders of coagulation (eg, von Willebrand disease, proteins C, S, antithrombin III deficiencies).[1] **Nuchal rigidity** is the inability of a patient to place their chin to their chest passively without involuntary muscles spasms preventing it. This represents inflammation of the meninges,

T1. Principal Laboratory Findings

Test	Patient's Result	"Normal" Reference Interval
Hematology		
WBC count	5.4	$4.5\text{-}11.0 \times 10^9$/L
	28.4 (24 hours)	
	46.7 (48 hours)	
RBC	3.51	$4.50\text{-}5.90 \times 10^{12}$/L
Hgb	11.6	
Hct	33.0	41.0-53.0%
MCV	94	80-100 fL
Platelets	87	$150\text{-}440 \times 10^9$/L
	67 (24 hours)	
	46 (48 hours)	
Chemistry		
Sodium	136	135-145 mmol/L
Potassium	4.1	3.5-5.0 mmol/L
Chloride	104	98-107 mmol/L
CO_2	22	22-30 mmol/L
BUN	19	7-21 mg/dL
	36 (24 hours)	
Creatinine	2.7	0.8-1.4 mg/dL
Calcium	7.0	8.5-10.2 mg/dL
Magnesium	1.0	1.6-2.2 mg/dL
Phosphorus	1.4	2.4-4.5 mg/dL
AST	51	15-45 U/L
	673 (24 hours)	
ALT	48	
	484 (24 hours)	10-40 U/L
ALP	126	65-260 U/L
GGT	45	13-68 U/L
CK	181	70-185 U/L
CK-MB	1.2	0.0-6.0 ng/ml
Lactate dehydrogenase	874	340-670 U/L
Troponin T	<0.029	0.000-0.029 ng/ml
PTT	84.1	22.6-32.4
PT	20	11-14
INR	1.8	
D-dimer	23.4	0.0-0.5
Fibrinogen	107	150-504
ATII activity	59	70-118

WBC, white blood cell; RBC, red blood cells; HCT, hematocrit; MCV, mean corpuscular volume; BUN, blood urea nitrogen; AST, aspartate aminotransferase; ALT, alanine aminotransferase; ALP, alkaline phosphatase; GGT, gamma-glutamyl transferase; CK, creatine kinase MCV, mean corpuscular volume.

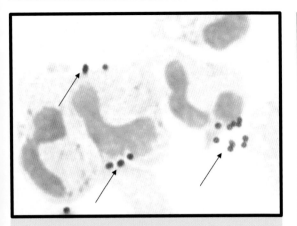

Image 2_Gram stain of a representative CSF with multiple intracellular gram-negative diplococci (arrows) in neutrophils identified as Neisseria meningitidis. 1,000× magnfication.

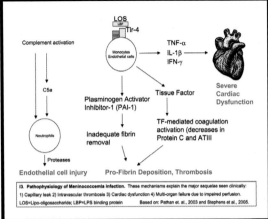

Figure 1_Pathophysiology of meninococcemia infection. These mechanisms explain the major sequelae seen clinically: 1) capillary leak, 2) intravascular thrombosis, 3) cardiac dysfunction, 4) multi-organ failure due to impaired perfusion. LOS=Lipo-oligosaccharide; LBP=LPS binding protein. Based on: Pathan, et al, 2003 and Stephens et al, 2005.

the delicate membranes that cover the brain, and is often the result of an infectious agent. **Normocytic anemia**, or the decrease in normal sized red cells, may be associated with several diseases such as chronic inflammation (infection, connective tissue disease), chronic renal failure, endocrine failure, hepatic disease, or blood loss. Significantly decreased platelets (**thrombocytopenia**) can be caused by: 1) decreased platelet production; 2) splenic sequestration, hypersplenism; and 3) increased platelet destruction. Decreased production may be seen in processes that affect the bone marrow directly such as leukemia, viral infections, and radiation. Increased platelet destruction can be non-immune or immune mediated. Non-immune mediated destruction is seen in disseminated intravascular coagulation (DIC) and thrombotic thrombocytopenia (TTP), while immune mediated destruction is seen in alloimmune thrombocytopenia, post-transfusion purpura, and idiopathic thrombocytopenic purpura (ITP).[1] A **prolonged PT and PTT** suggests that an excessive activation of the coagulation cascade has occurred, resulting in the formation of fibrin. This activation of the coagulation cascade is further evidenced by the decreased fibrinogen, which is used to make a fibrin matrix for clotting. Factors that prevent coagulation (specifically anti-thrombin III) are decreased in this patient. When D-dimer, a degradation product of fibrin, is elevated, fibrinolysis is occurring. A prolonged PT and PTT, decreased fibrinogen and anti-thrombin III, and an elevated D-dimer in the context of this patient's history

is highly consistent with DIC. Moreover, DIC leads to purpura fulminans, thrombocytopenia, and normocytic anemia described above and can result from bacterial sepsis/meningitis.

Creatinine is continuously released from muscle and cleared by renal excretion. Its elevation can be an indicator of decreased renal function. Decreased circulating **calcium** may be associated with decreased PTH secretion or with hyperphosphatemia leading to calcium precipitation. Decreased circulating **magnesium** is generally associated with a decreased intake, an increased loss due to renal magnesium wasting, and acute myocardial infarction.[2] Decreased phosphorous can be due to inadequate intestinal phosphate absortion, excessive kidney excretion, or the shift of phosphorous from extracellular to intracellular compartments.[3] Hypocalcemia is commonly associated with critically ill patients and correlates with the severity of illness.[4,5] Decreased magnesium has also been associated with sepsis.[6] Decreased **phosphorous** levels are associated with malnutrition, refeeding syndrome,[3] sepsis, trauma, diuretics, and steroid therapy.[7,8] The transaminases aspartate aminotransferase (AST) and alanine aminotransferase (ALT) are sensitive indicators of liver injury and are used to detect diseases such as hepatitis. Alanine aminotransferase is found mainly in the liver, while AST can be found in the liver as well as muscle, organs, and erythrocytes. Acute elevations of AST and ALT, such as those seen in this case, are seen in disorders with extensive hepatocellular injury such as viral hepatitis, ischemic liver injury (eg, severe cardiac dysfunction, shock, sepsis), or drug/toxin mediated liver injury.

3. In patients with clinical findings suggestive of meningitis (fever, headache, nuchal rigidity), the differential diagnosis should include bacterial meningitis, viral meningitis, encephalitis, focal infections (brain abscess and subdural empyema), and infectious thrombophlebitis. Fever, headache, and nuchal rigidity occur in >90% of meningitis cases along with mental status changes in >75%. Each of these infections can start with a fever and headache in a previously healthy individual.[9] In community-acquired bacterial meningitis in adults, *Streptococcus pneumoniae* (51%), *Neisseria meningitidis* (37%), *Listeria monocytogenes* (4%) are the most common etiologies.[9] Profound alterations in consciousness are less common in viral meningitis than that seen in bacterial meningitis. Meningitis is unique from other brain infections such as encephalitis, focal infections, and infectious thrombophlebitis, which largely result in focal neurological deficits. The patient in this case had symptoms consistent with meningitis (nuchal rigidity, headache, mental status changes) in addition to evidence of bacteremia that possibly initiated the diffuse intravascular coagulation and skin purpura.

4. The early recognition of acute infections of the nervous system is necessary to initiate antimicrobial therapy quickly, which can be lifesaving. Therefore, the identification of the offending organism is most important. In this patient, blood culture should be performed in order to isolate an infectious cause of this patient's possible meningitis and shock (**Image 2**). Since the patient was in DIC, a lumbar puncture for CSF was not performed because of the high risk of bleeding. Aerobic blood cultures turned positive within 24 hours and gram-negative diplococci were identified on a Gram stain smear of the blood cultures. The blood cultures were plated on chocolate blood agar at 35°C in 5% CO_2. The organisms were found to be oxidase-positive and had the ability to utilize maltose and glucose. The culture was sent to the State of North Carolina Public Health Laboratory, as required by law, where serogrouping was performed.

5. **Most likely diagnosis:** *Neisseria meningitidis* bacteremia and meningitis.

In the United States, sporadic *Neisseria meningitidis* meningococcal disease presents in approximately 1/100,000 people per year.[10] There are 2 peak ages of infection: infants 3 to 9 months of age in whom protective antibodies have not yet formed (10 to 15 cases/100,000 infants/year) and teenagers subjected to crowded conditions such as dormitories and barracks (<1 case/100,000 people/year).[10] The patient in the present case is a college student living in a dormitory. The highest incidence of disease occurs during the winter months when respiratory viral illnesses are at their peak.

Neisseria meningitidis (meningococcus) is subdivided or grouped based on the antigenic structure of the capsular polysaccharides (A, B, C, Y, W-135). Meningococci colonize the upper respiratory tract of about 10% of healthy individuals.[11] Infection occurs by either direct contact or by respiratory droplets. Meningococci are internalized by non-ciliated mucosal cells and/or cross them to enter the submucosa and the blood stream. However, it is not essential that the organisms infect the blood for survival.[10] The virulence traits of meningococcus include an anti-phagocytic capsule and outer membrane proteins such as LOS (lipo-oligosaccharide or endotoxin) and pili to facilitate adhesion.[10] Multiple host factors play a role in keeping *N. meningitidis* at bay in the nasopharynx. To prevent growth, antibodies with bactericidal activity are needed, in addition to opsonic antibodies and phagocytes. These antibodies are serogroup specific, usually of IgG or IgM, and generally bind the capsular surface.[10] Genetic associations with host determinants of meningococcus infection have been made with multiple genes involved in the innate immune system.[12] Meningococcus infection is a complex interaction between bacterial virulence factors and genetically determined host responses.

If *N. meningitidis* is able to enter the blood stream from the upper respiratory tract, replication occurs either slowly or rapidly. Slow growth allows the bacteria to seed in sites such as the meninges, joints, and pericardium. Rapid proliferation is associated with meningococcemia resulting in petechiae, purpura, DIC, and shock. When meningococci enter the blood, 2 main diseases result: 1) meningitis; 2) fulminant meningococcemia (purpura fulminans). In people who develop blood stream invasion, approximately 55% will experience meningitis alone, approximately 30% will have meningitis and meningococemia, and approximately 15% will have only fulminant meningococcemia (without meningitis). Based on this patient's clinical signs and symptoms, he had meningitis (headache, nuchal rigidity) and bacteremia (hypotension, tachycardia, purpuric rash). Based on his clinical presentation and laboratory findings of thrombocytopenia, DIC, elevated AST/ALT, and identification of meningococcus in the blood, the most likely diagnosis is fulminant meningococcemia/meningitis.

Neisseria meningitidis infection results in the most rapid form of septic shock and differs from other organisms by the prominence of hemorrhagic skin lesions and the consistent development of DIC. The dominant pro-inflammatory molecule that mediates meningococcal disease is its endotoxin (specifically its lipid A moiety). The outer membrane of meningococci contains lipo-oligosaccharide (LOS) that is loosely connected to the underlying peptidoglycan.[10] The loosely connected LOS accounts for its shedding as the bacteria grow at a much faster rate than other gram-negative bacteria. The active component in LOS, however, is identical to that of lipopolysaccharide (LPS) found in other gram-negative bacteria. The detectable plasma endotoxin is 10 to 1,000-fold greater in patients with meningococcal bacteremia than other gram-negative bacteria and may account for the more fulminant disease that meningococcus causes compared to sepsis caused by other gram-negative bacteria.[10]

The major pathways of meningococcus pathogenesis are outlined in **Figure 1**. Endotoxin is released from meningococci and activates the immune system by 3 major pathways. First, LOS interacts with toll-like 4 (Tlr-4) receptors on monocytes, neutrophils, and endothelial cells releasing cytokines and other mediators.[13] Meningococci also invade endothelial cells

directly producing pro-inflammatory molecules as well as upregulating adhesion molecules for leukocytes.[13] The main pro-inflammatory mediators that have been identified include TNF-α, IL-1β, IFN-γ, and IL-8.[13] The second major pathway involves the coagulation system. Pro-coagulant and anti-fibrinolytic mechanisms are activated in meningococcemia, resulting in the tendency for fibrin deposition and thrombosis.[13] Upon activation by LOS, monocytes synthesize tissue factor in addition to pro-inflammatory cytokines. This uncontrolled activation of the coagulation cascade results in clotting and deficiencies in regulators of the cascade: protein S, protein C, and anti-thrombin III.[13] Moreover, fibrin deposition is favored by the anti-coagulant tendency from the excessive plasminogen activator inhibitor-1 (PAI-1) released from endothelial cells and platelets.[13] Plasminogen activator inhibitor-1 inhibits the formation of plasmin and the degradation of clotting. Bilateral acute adrenal gland hemorrhage can result in adrenal insufficiency in meningococci infection. This clinical scenario is referred to as the Waterhouse-Friderichsen syndrome and is rare. More commonly, partial adrenal insufficiency results and the patient is unable to mount a normal hyper-cortisolemic response to stress, increasing the risk of mortality and morbidity.[14] The third major pathway in the pathogenesis of meningococcus involves the activation of classical complement pathway by antibodies and/or mannan binding lectin or by the alternative complement pathway, which leads to endothelial cell damage. These mechanisms explain the capillary leak (hypotension), intravascular thrombosis, cardiac dysfunction, and multi-organ failure that may be seen in meningococcal infections.

6. Patients with meningococcemia should be treated with a third-generation cephalosporin (eg, cefotaxime or ceftriaxone). The third-generation cephalosporin should be combined with agents to cover bacteria that can cause similar symptoms (eg, *S. pneumoniae* and *H. influenzae*) until the etiologic agent can be identified. Penicillin G remains an acceptable alternative for confirmed meningococcal disease. However, it should be noted that an increased prevalence of meningococci with reduced penicillin susceptibility has been reported.[15] Upon admission the patient was treated empirically for meningitis

with ceftriaxone, vancomycin, and doxycycline. Upon identification of meningococcemia, the vancomycin and doxycycline were discontinued.

Meningococcal disease is associated with a high morbidity and mortality.[16] Approximately 500,000 cases occur worldwide, of which approximately 10% result in death.[17,18] Of the patients that survive, deafness, seizures, amputation, and mental retardation can result.[19-22]

Vaccination. Eighty to ninety percent of immunocompetent adults vaccinated with quadravalent meningococcal polysaccharide vaccine against serotypes A, C, W-135, and Y develop protective immunity. Children >3 years of age may be vaccinated with multiple doses to prevent serogroup A infection. The duration of the adult immunity is estimated to be less than 5 years.[10] There is currently no vaccine for serogroup B because its polysaccharide is not sufficiently immunogenic.[10] While the patient described in this case study DID receive a meningococcal vaccine within the past 6 months, it was not protective because he was infected with serogroup B meningococcus as determined by the North Carolina State Public Health Laboratory.

Chemoprophylaxis. Since the attack rate for household contacts is >400-fold more than the general population, close contacts should be treated with prophylactic antimicrobials. Ciprofloxacin is the most frequently used agent. Rifampin may be used in children but it should be noted that rifampin-resistant meningococcal isolates have been reported.[23]

Patient follow-up. Over the first 4 days of the patient's hospitalization, normalization of his PT/PTT, LFTs, creatinine, and thrombocytopenia occurred. Clinically his mental status returned to normal as well. Adrenal insufficiency was ruled out as the patient underwent a low- and high-dose co-syntropin stimulation test, to which the cortisol response was appropriately increased. Since the patient was at increased risk for seizures after his meningococcemia, an EEG was performed and his risk for seizures was thought to be low. The patient's purpura fulminans was treated symptomatically and was beginning to resolve by the time the patient was discharged on day 11. The leading cause of

morbidity and mortality in sepsis is the myocardial depression, which generally lasts 7 to 10 days and has been shown to be mediated by the pro-inflammatory cytokines released in response to LPS such as TNF-α, IL-β, and IFN-γ.[24] On day 2, the patient had an estimated cardiac output (ejection fraction) of 30% (normal >60%). By day 11, his cardiac function was still impaired, although improved (45%). While he was well enough to be discharged, he was still experiencing significant cardiac dysfunction that would eventually return to normal. The patient was treated as a heart failure patient until another echo could be performed in 4 to 6 weeks. Lastly, a complement panel looking for deficits for the terminal complement components was performed and found to be normal. People with these deficiencies are more prone to infections with meningococcus.

Keywords

Neisseria meningitidis, meningococcus, lipo-oligosaccharide, endotoxin, cytokines, DIC, toll-like receptor 4, vaccination

References

1. Gurevitch AW, Zipperstein K. Dermatologic problems in the intensive care unit. In: *Bongard FS, ed. Current Critical Care Diagnosis & Treatment*. 2nd ed. New York: The McGraw-Hill Companies, Inc; 2003.

2. Bongard FS, Sue DY. Fluids, electrolytes, & acid-base. In: *Bongard FS, ed. Current Critical Care Diagnosis & Treatment*. 2nd ed. New York: The McGraw-Hill Companies, Inc; 2003.

3. Schade Willis T, Boswell R, Willis MS. Refeeding syndrome in a severely malnourished child. *Lab Med.* 2004;35:548-552.

4. Gauthier B, Trachtman H, Di Carmine F, et al. Hypocalcemia and hypercalcitoninemia in critically ill children. *Crit Care Med.* 1990;18:1215-1219.

5. Zivin JR, Gooley T, Zager RA, et al. Hypocalcemia: A pervasive metabolic abnormality in the critically ill. *Am J Kidney Dis.* 2001;37:689-698.

6. Lote K, Andersen K. Hypocalcemia and hypomagnesemia in meningococcal septicemia. *Tidsskr Nor Laegeforen.* 1977;97:1667-1669.

7. Menezes FS, Leite HP, Fernandez J, et al. Hypophosphatemia in critically ill children. *Rev Hosp Clin Fac Med Sao Paulo.* 2004;59:306-311.

8. Antachopoulos C, Papassotiriou I. Hypophosphatemia in meningococcal sepsis. *Pediatr Nephrol.* 2004;19(2):237-239

9. van de Beek D, de Gans J, Spanjaard L, et al. Clinical features and prognostic factors in adults with bacterial meningitis. *N Engl J Med.* 2004;351:1849-1859.

10. Stephens DS, Munford RS, Wetzler LM. Meningococcal infections. In: Kasper DL, Braunwald E, Fauci AS, et al, eds. *Harrison's Principles of Internal Medicine.* 16th ed. New York: McGraw-Hill Companies, Inc.; 2005.

11. Yazdankhah SP, Caugant DA. *Neisseria meningitidis*: An overview of the carriage state. *J Med Microbiol.* 2004;53:821-832.

12. Emonts M, Hazelzet JA, de Groot R, et al. Host genetic determinants of *Neisseria meningitidis* infections. *Lancet Infect Dis.* 2003;3:565-577.

13. Pathan N, Faust SN, Levin M. Pathophysiology of meningococcal meningitis and septicaemia. *Arch Dis Child.* 2003;88:601-607.

14. Bosworth DC. Reversible adrenocorticol insufficiency in fulminant meningococcemia. *Arch Intern Med.* 1979;139:823-824.

15. Antignac A, Ducos-Galand M, Guiyoule A, et al. *Neisseria meningitidis* strains isolated from invasive infections in France (1999-2002): Phenotypes and antibiotic susceptibility patterns. *Clin Infect Dis.* 2003;37:912-920.

16. Thorburn K, Baines P, Thomson A, et al. Mortality in severe meningococcal disease. *Arch Dis Child.* 2001;85:382-385.

17. Tikhomirov E, Santamaria M, Esteves K. Meningococcal disease: Public health burden and control. *World Health Stat Q.* 1997;50:170-177.

18. Balmer P, Miller E. Meningococcal disease: How to prevent and how to manage. *Curr Opin Infect Dis.* 2002;15:275-281.

19. Offit PA, Peter G. The meningococcal vaccine-public policy and individual choices. *N Engl J Med.* 2003;349:2353-2356.

20. Pollard AJ, Levin M. Vaccines for prevention of meningococcal disease. *Pediatr Infect Dis J.* 2000;19:333-345.

21. Kirsch EA, Barton RP, Kitchen L, et al. Pathophysiology, treatment and outcome of meningococcemia: a review and recent experience. *Pediatr Infect Dis J.* 1996;15:967-979.

22. Tzeng YL, Stephens DS. Epidemiology and pathogenesis of *Neisseria meningitidis.* *Microbes Infect.* 2000;2:687-700.

23. Nolte O, Muller M, Reitz S, et al. Description of new mutations in the rpoB gene in rifampicin-resistant *Neisseria meningitidis* selected in vitro in a stepwise manner. *J Med Microbiol.* 2003;52:1077-1081.

24. Court O, Kumar A, Parrillo JE. Clinical review: Myocardial depression in sepsis and septic shock. *Crit Care.* 2002;6:500-508.

Aortic Valve Insufficiency in a 45-Year-Old Male

Monte Willis, Michael Roth, Peter Gilligan

Department of Pathology & Laboratory Medicine, University of North Carolina, Chapel Hill, NC

Patient: 45-year-old male.

Family History: Unremarkable.

Chief Complaint: Feeling under the weather, unable to go to work.

Past Medical History: Patient was referred from an outside hospital for evaluation of his aortic valve insufficiency. A transthoracic echocardiography study performed at an outside hospital within the previous week was not diagnostic for endocarditis and multiple blood cultures were negative. The patient has a history of ethanol abuse and poor dentition.

Physical Examination: Vital signs: temperature, 36.2°C; heart rate, 110 beats per minute; respiratory rate, 20 per minute; blood pressure 90/60 mm Hg. Skin: No rash. Extremities: No clubbing, cyanosis, edema. Pulmonary: Clear to auscultation bilaterally. Cardiac: Tachycardic with regular rhythm, 5/6 diastolic murmur (aortic area). Extremities: Unremarkable. Neuro: Alert and oriented, cranial nerves intact.

Results of Additional Diagnostic Procedures: Chest x-ray: Bilateral pleural effusions and diffuse interstitial prominence, consistent with interstitial edema. A transthoracic echocardiogram performed at admission identified severe aortic and mitral valve regurgitation. EKG: Normal.

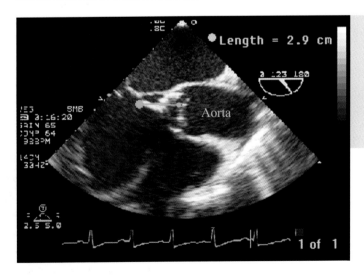

Image 1_Transesophageal echocardiographic study of the patient described in this study. Vegetation (Green Line) on the aortic valve was present and floating freely upon transesophageal echocardiography in this patient upon presentation.

T1. Principal Laboratory Findings

Test	Patient's Result	"Normal" Reference Interval
Hematology		
WBC count	9.5	$4.5-11.0 \times 10^9/L$
RBC	3.51	$4.50-5.90 \times 10^{12}/L$
HCT	34.2	41.0-53.0%
MCV	93	80-100 fL
Platelets	170	$150-440 \times 10^9/L$
Chemistry		
Sodium	137	135-145 mmol/L
Potassium	3.4	3.5-5.0 mmol/L
Chloride	110	98-107 mmol/L
CO_2	21	22-30 mmol/L
BUN	6	7-21 mg/dL
Creatinine	0.7	0.8-1.4 mg/dL
TSH	3.36	0.46-4.68 microIU/ml

WBC, white blood cell; RBC, red blood cells; HCT, hematocrit; MCV, mean corpuscular volume; BUN, blood urea nitrogen; AST, aspartate aminotransferase; ALT, alanine aminotransferase; ALP, alkaline phosphatase; GGT, gamma-glutamyl transferase; CK, creatine kinase.

T2. Diagnostic (Duke) Criteria of Infective Endocarditis

1. Positive valve culture or histology   OR

2. 2 major criteria:

    a. Typical organism

    b. Positive echocardiography for vegetations

    c. Abscess or valve dehiscence   OR

3. 5 of 6 minor criteria:

    a. Valvular heart disease or IV drug abuse

    b. Fever greater than 38°C

    c. Vasculitis

    d. Skin lesions

    e. Suggestive echocardiography (but not definitive)

    f. Positive blood culture   OR

4. 1 major and 3 minor criteria

Adapted from: Durack DT, et al. Am J Med. 1994;96:200-209.

Questions

1. What are this patient's most striking clinical and laboratory findings?

2. How do you explain this patient's most striking clinical and laboratory findings?

3. What additional test(s) should be ordered on this patient and why?

4. What is this patient's most likely diagnosis?

5. How is this patient's condition typically treated?

Possible Answers

1. Significant clinical findings in this patient include tachycardia (HR>100), hypotension, 5/6 diastolic murmur, a history of prior and current dental disease, including tooth extractions on the day of admission, transesophageal echocardiogram with severe aortic and mitral valve regurgitation, pulmonary edema, and a normal EKG. Significant laboratory findings include multiple negative blood cultures (outside hospital), normocytic anemia, and a normal white cell count.

2. **Sinus tachycardia** (>100 beats/minute) in the absence of arrhythmia is a physiologic response to stress. Causes include fever, anxiety, exercise, thyrotoxicosis, hypoxemia, hypotension,

T3. Etiologic Agents Found in Native-Valve Infective Endocarditis

Pathogen	Native Valve	Prosthetic Valve
	Patient age 16-60 years old	<60 days (60 days-12 months) after procedure
Streptococcus spp.	45-65%	1 (7-10)%
Staphylococcus aureus	30-40%	20-24 (10-15)%
Coag-neg staphylococci	4-8%	30-35 (30-35)%
Enterococcus	5-8%	5-10 (10-15)%
Gram-neg bacilli	4-10%	10-15 (2-4)%
Fungi	1-3%	5-10 (10-15)%
Culture neg/HACEK* organisms	3-10%	3-7 (3-7)%
Diptheroids	<1%	5-7 (2-5)%
Polymicrobial	1-2%	2-4 (4-7)%

Adapted from: Mylonakis et al. N Engl J Med. 2001;345(18):1318.
*HACEK: Haemophilus spp., Actinobacillus actinomycetemcomitans, Cardiobacterium hominus, Eikinella la corrodens, Kingella kingae.

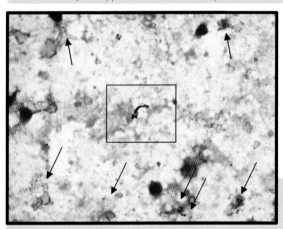 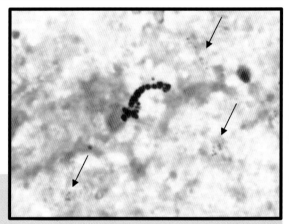

Image 2_Mitral valve biopsy Gram stain seen at 100× (left) and 400× (right) demonstrates gram-positive cocci in chains. Distributed throughout the biopsy preparation, gram-positive cocci that stain poorly are present (arrows) and may represent the results of pre-surgical antibiotic therapy.

congestive heart failure, or volume depletion. **Hypotension** can result from shock, a clinical syndrome characterized by hypoperfusion (and hypo-oxygenation) of organs. Shock has a variety of causes, generally categorized by hypovolemic shock (inadequate circulating volume, plasma volume loss, or excessive water and electrolyte loss), septic shock (infection), or neurogenic shock (drugs, spinal anesthesia). Lastly, cardiogenic shock can cause hypotension due to impaired contractility (mitral insufficiency, aortic insufficiency, dilated cardiomyopathy, acute myocardial infarction), decreased preload (right ventricular infarction, pulmonary embolism, pericardial tamponade), excessive afterload

(malignant hypertension, aortic stenosis, hypertrophic cardiomyopathy). **Aortic regurgitation** (AR) results from aortic valve cusp thickening and shortening, which prevents complete closing during diastole. This results in a diastolic murmur, which represents the backflow of blood through the incompletely closed aortic valve. Nearly two-thirds of patients with AR have a history of rheumatic disease, which is mainly associated with mitral valve defects.[1] Rheumatic disease less commonly causes isolated aortic valve disease. Other causes of aortic regurgitation include congenitial membrane subaortic stenosis (thickened valve leaflets), rheumatoid spondylitis, congenital bicuspid valves, prolapse

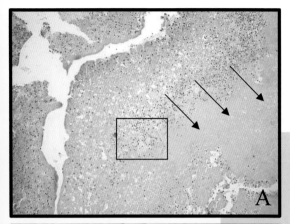

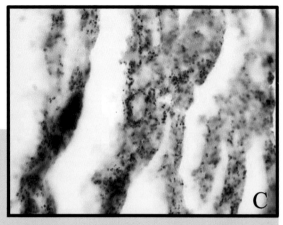

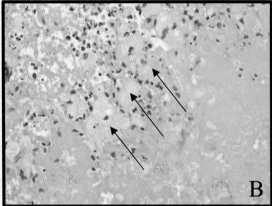

Image 3_Histology of the aortic valve removed for placement of a prosthetic valve. Low power view of the valve (**A**) and the fibrin-platelet-bacterial vegetation (arrows), mag 100×. High power view of the boxed area in **A** is shown in **B**, mag 400×. A pleiomorphic cellular infiltrate at the valve/vegetation border can be seen including histiocytes (arrows). A tissue Gram stain reveals sheets of gram-positive cocci (dark purple) within the vegetation (**C**), mag 100×.

secondary to ventricular septal defects, and congenital fenestrations of the aortic valve.[1] Primary aortic root disease resulting in the separation of the aortic valve leaflets can cause aortic regurgitation. Aortic root disease may manifest in Marfan's syndrome, idiopathic dilation of the aorta, syphilis, ankylosing spondylitis, and severe hypertension, which may develop into progressive AR. Acute aortic regurgitation can also result from infective endocarditis which can occur on valves previously damaged by rheumatic disease, congenitally deformed valves, and on occasion a normal aortic valve.[1] The most common causes of **pulmonary edema** include heart failure and volume overload. The functional consequence of pulmonary edema is the failure of gas exchange due to the excess fluid in the lungs.

3. **Echocardiography** should be performed in patients where the suspicion of endocarditis is high. Transesophageal echocardiogram (TEE) is able to anatomically confirm the presence of a vegetation and determine its size in >90%

of patients with endocarditis. Transesophageal echocardiograms can also be used to assess for abscesses and determine cardiac function. Transesophageal echocardiogram has a higher sensitivity of detection cardiac valve vegetations than transthoracic echocardiography (TTE). The patient in the present case underwent both transthoracic and transesophageal echocardiography, both of which revealed a markedly thickened, bicuspid aortic valve. Moreover, large filamentous and highly mobile vegetations were noted on the 2 aortic cuspids and on the chordae of the medial papillary muscle just adjacent to the mitral valve (**Image 1**). The large aortic valve vegetation measured approximately 29 mm in length. The vegetation adjacent to the mitral valve was multilobular and measured approximately 20 mm in length. Significant aortic and mitral valve insufficiency was identified by Doppler mode. No abnormalities were identified on the right side of the heart. A cardiac MRI was additionally performed to evaluate the patient for abscess formation. There was no evidence of abscess formation by either echo or MRI.

Blood cultures should be performed because identification of an organism is critical for both the diagnosis of endocarditis and selection of appropriate antibiotics.[2] In the absence of prior antibiotic treatment, 3 blood cultures should be collected from different venipuncture sites over 24 hours. If the cultures are negative, additional blood cultures should be performed after 48 to 72 hours and the laboratory notified that they should look for fastidious organisms by extending the incubation time.[1,2] Patients with deteriorating hemodynamics should be treated empirically for endocarditis. Peripheral blood cultures were collected from 2 sites on day 1 and the day after admission in the present case. Aerobic and anaerobic cultures were negative after 1 week. **Serological tests** can help determine the identification of organisms that are difficult to recover by blood culture. In the United States, serology testing for *Coxiella burneti* is used with some frequency, while additional testing for *Brucella* and *Bartonella* is used with more frequency in other parts of the world. **Studies to assist in the management** of endocarditis include CBC, creatinine, chest radiograph, EKG, and cardiac catherization in patients who undergo valve replacement to assess for coronary artery disease. The indications for surgery with endocarditis include heart failure, uncontrolled infection, significant valve dysfunction, artificial valve replacement, abscess formation, or recurrent emboli.[3] The decision to replace this patient's valve was based on his significant aortic and mitral valve dysfunction. The patient underwent cardiac catherization, which identified a 75% blockage in his left anterior descending coronary artery. A head CT with contrast was performed to identify possible septic emboli and was negative. **Direct examination** of pathogens can identify vegetations by microscopic examination, culture, special stains, and PCR identification. On day 5 of the patient's hospital stay, he underwent surgery to replace/repair his aortic and mitral valve in addition to coronary artery bypass surgery on his left anterior descending coronary artery. The aortic and mitral valves were sent to microbiology for direct examination and culture. The valves were minced, placed on slides, and Gram stained. Gram-positive cocci in chains were abundant throughout the specimens (**Image 2**). Both aortic and mitral valves were processed for histology (**Image 3**) and demonstrated fibrosis with

focal areas of granulation tissue, fibrinopurulent exudates, and acute inflammation consistent with endocarditis. Tissue Gram stains showed sheets of gram-positive cocci when stained with a modified Brown and Brenn Gram stain. Aerobic and anaerobic cultures of the aortic and mitral valve were negative after 1 week as were cultures for fungus, *Legionella,* and *Actinomyces.*

Molecular detection. Currently few laboratories have the capability to detect bacteria other than *Chlamydia trachomatis* and *Neisseria gonorrhoeae* by molecular means. However this is a potentially powerful alternative to diagnosing infections from internal body sites such as cardiac vegetations in a patient with culture negative endocarditis.[4-11] In this approach, primers with a broad range are used to amplify specific regions of the 16S rRNA gene. The resulting amplicons are then sequenced and the obtained sequence is matched with known sequences for specific organisms. If the obtained sequence matches a known organism sequence, the patient is considered infected by this organism.

4. ***Most likely diagnosis:*** *infective endocarditis due to viridins streptococci.*

The **Duke Criteria** are used to diagnose infective endocarditis using both clinical and laboratory findings (**T2**).[12] Infective endocarditis can be diagnosed in 4 ways. The diagnosis can be made if there is positive valve culture or histology. In the present case, gram-positive cocci in chains were identified from the valves removed during surgery, which confirms the diagnosis of infective endocarditis. A patient can also be diagnosed if they have 2 major criteria: 1) typical organism present; 2) positive echo for vegetations; 3) abscess/valve dehiscence OR 5 of 6 minor criteria: 1) valvular heart disease; 2) fever; 3) vasculitis; 4) skin lesions; 5) suggestive echo; 6) positive blood culture. Lastly, the diagnosis of infective endocarditis can be made if 1 major and 3 minor criteria are met. The presence of gram-positive cocci in chains in the present case is suggestive of *Streptococcus* and *Enterococcus* spp., both of which have been implicated in infective endocarditis (**T3**). In native valve infective endocarditis, 45% to 65% are caused by *Streptococcus* species, while 5% to 8% are caused by *Enterococcus* species.[2] Of the *Streptococcus* spp.

implicated in endocarditis, 75% are due to viridans group streptococcus, 20% to *Streptococcus bovis*, and the remaining 5% are due to other *Streptococcus* spp. Viridans group streptococcus are found mainly in the oral cavity, where trauma to the tissues can precipitate bacteremia. The severity of periodontal disease and the intensity of the trauma play a role in the magnitude and frequency of bacteremia. *Enterococcus* bacteremia, on the other hand, is associated with examination and instrumentation of the gastrointestinal and genitourinary tract.[13] The patient in the current study had 2 negative aerobic and anaerobic blood cultures in addition to a negative aortic valve biopsy culture plated both aerobically and anaerobically. Therefore, the history of poor dentition in this patient, along with the gram-positive cocci in chains detected in the vegetation itself, leads to the likely conclusion that this patient had viridans streptococcus endocarditis.

The incidence of infective endocarditis continues to rise with a yearly incidence of around 15,000 to 20,000 new cases in the United States.[14] The incidence of community-acquired infective endocarditis (IE) on native-valves in the United States and western Europe is approximately 1.7 to 6.2 cases per 100,000 people per year.[2] Men are affected almost twice as much as women (1.7:1), and the median age is 47 to 69 years.[2] When endocarditis is associated with intravenous drug use, the incidence is approximately 150 to 2000 per 100,000 people per year.[2] Multiple conditions predispose people to IE including diabetes mellitus, hemodialysis (long-term), and poor dental hygiene.[2] The most common cardiovascular disease associated with infectious endocarditis is mitral valve prolapse (100 per 100,000 person with IE per year).[2] Rheumatic heart disease, as a result of group A streptococcus infection in the young, is the most common predisposing factor leading to IE in the world.[2]

Endothelial cells in the vasculature are resistant to bacteria and thrombus formation unless they are injured. Endothelial cell injury may result in turbulent flow that can be conducive to either infection or the development of platelet-fibrin thrombus (non-bacterial thrombotic endocarditis).[1] The formation of a thrombus can also serve as a place where bacteria can attach during episodes of bacteremia. Organisms found in endocarditis (**T3**) enter the blood from skin, mucosal surfaces, or discrete infections. Most bacteria adhere directly to thrombi except more virulent bacteria such as *S. aureus*, which can adhere to the endothelial cells/sub-endothelium directly.[1] The proliferating organisms at the valve site induce tissue factor (TF) which is released from monocytes and/or endothelial cells, initiating the coagulation cascade, leading to fibrin deposition at the site. This leads to the formation of "vegetation," which is composed of inflammatory cells, bacteria, fibrin, and platelets. Adherence of organisms is achieved by receptors that bind fibronectin in many gram-positive bacteria, a fibrinogen/fibrin binding protein on *S. aureus* (clumping factor), and glucan binding protein on streptococci.[1] *Streptococcus mutans* has additionally been shown to be able to bind and activate plasminogen, which could be part of the pathogenesis by which extracellular matrix molecules are degraded.[15] Organisms deep in the vegetation are metabolically active and resistant to antibiotics. The organisms are continuously released into the circulation and cleared by the immune system or re-colonize the vegetation. Endocarditis may arise as a result of vegetation embolization on the heart valve, damage to cardiac structures, and tissue injury due to circulating immune complexes. Embolized vegetation can lead to infection and/or infarction to distant sites such as the extremities and brain.

Patients with infective endocarditis have non-specific cardiac and non-cardiac symptoms. Heart murmurs represent cardiac pathology, specifically valvular damage. Significant regurgitant murmurs can lead to heart failure. The patient in the present study had a significant diastolic murmur as a result of his aortic and mitral valve insufficiency. Thirty to forty percent of patients have a murmur upon presentation and congestive heart failure occurs in as many people as well.[1] If the infection extends into the adjacent myocardial tissues, form abscesses, and extend through the epicardium, pericarditis can occur. Abscesses adjacent to the aortic valve can lead to disruption of the conductive system and heart block. Emboli can break off and end up in the coronary arteries resulting in myocardial infarction, although this is rare.[16] Hematogenous spread of infection can lead to focal infection in the skin, kidneys, meninges, and muscle. Arterial emboli are apparent in nearly 50% of patients clinically, particularly in patients with vegetations that are >10 mm in diameter.[17] Antibiotic treatment decreases embolic event rates that are 13/1,000 patient days in the first week to 1.2/1,000 patient days in the third week.[17] Mimicking the more severe embolic lesions are Janeway lesions (under fingernails) and Osler nodes seen in *S. aureus* endocarditis. Systemic emboli occur in 22% to 50% of endocarditis cases.[18] Of these, 60% to 70% involve the central nervous system, which result in severe and potentially lethal manifestations.[18]

The patient described in this case had his aortic valve replaced, which places him in another risk category of infective endocarditis. While prosthetic valve endocarditis presents the same way as native valve endocarditis does, the symptoms can be overlooked as morbidity associated with the surgery to replace the valve. The types of infections that occur during this time are significantly different from native valve infections and should be treated appropriately. Specifically, the most common infection within the first year is coag-negative staphylococcus.[2] The patient was started on coumadin on post-operative day #2 in order to reduce emboli formation in the new prosthetic aortic valve. He was released several days later with an INR of 2.9 (goal 2 to 3).

5. Left untreated, patients with infective endocarditis are at high risk for death. Therefore, it is important to institute therapy as quickly as possible. Bacterial vegetation is avascular and the bacteria are not proliferating, which makes eradication with antibiotics extremely difficult. Since complete eradication is necessary for therapy, antimicrobial therapy has to be bactericidal and long term.[1] In the present case, the aortic valve was replaced, the mitral valve repaired, and the vegetations removed. However, prolonged antibiotic therapy based on the presumed organisms needed to be given. Most viridans streptococcus species are susceptible to penicillin. However, recent studies have identified an increase in resistance to penicillin.[19,20]

Native valve therapies. If the viridans streptococci are penicillin susceptible (MIC <0.1 mg/mL), penicillin G or ceftriaxone is recommended.[2] Gentamicin can be given concomitantly in some cases, but is not recommended in patients with abscesses, extracardial foci, or prosthetic valve endocarditis.[2] In streptococcus species with a penicillin MIC >0.5 and enterococcus species, penicillin G (or ampicillin) with gentamicin for 4 to 6 weeks should be given.[2] In these patients, 6 weeks of antibiotic therapy is recommended if the symptoms have been longer than 3 months or if other complications such as myocardial abscess are present.[2] In native valve endocarditis where the culture is negative, antibiotics generally given include penicillin, ampicillin, ceftriaxone, or vancomyin in combination with an aminoglycoside.[2] The patient described is the present case was treated with vancomycin and tobramycin to be continued for 6 weeks in accordance with these previous studies. Both peak and trough drug levels were to be followed weekly to ensure that adequate drug levels were being achieved.

Prognosis. Mortality and morbidity are generally related to the patient's other diseases and endocarditis-related organ damage and not antibiotic failure.[1] Survival for patients with native valve endocarditis caused by viridans streptococci, HACEK organisms, or enterococci range from 85% to 90%.[1] A high rate of mortality (40% to 50%) is seen in prosthetic valve replacement if it occurs within the first 60 days.[1] Mortality is lower (10% to 20%) for later onset prosthetic valve infection.[1]

Prevention. Prophylactic antibiotics should be given to patients at risk for endocarditis undergoing procedures that have a high probability of inducing bacteremia (dental procedures likely to cause bleeding, tonsillectomy/adenoidectomy, surgery on infected tissues, surgery of airways/GI/GU tracts). The evidence for the benefit of antibiotic prophylaxis is modest and unproven.[21,22] It has been estimated that patients requiring penicillin are 5 times more likely to die from anaphylaxis than infective endocarditis.[22] Only one-half of patients with native valve endocarditis are diagnosed following a procedure.[1] However, maintaining dental hygiene is important for patients at risk for infective endocarditis.[1] In fact, poor dental health itself is a significant risk factor for the development of endocarditis. Since the patient in this study had an ongoing history of dental disease, and his endocarditis source was likely from his oral flora, it is important that the patient resolves his dental problems. The rate of relapse in native valve penicillin-susceptible viridans streptococci is less than 2%; the relapse rate for enterococci is 8% to 20%.[2] These facts emphasize the need to resolve his dental problems, which also place him at a greater risk for relapse with his prosthetic valve.

Keywords

Infective endocarditis, viridins streptococcus, Enterococcus

References

1. Karchmer AW. Infective Endocarditis. In: *Kasper DL, Braunwald E, Fauci AS, et al., eds. Harrison's Principles of Internal Medicine.* 16th ed. New York: McGraw-Hill Companies, Inc.; 2005.

2. Mylonakis E, Calderwood SB. Infective endocarditis in adults. *N Engl J Med.* 2001;345:1318-1330.

3. Cabell CH, Abrutyn E, Karchmer AW. Cardiology patient page. Bacterial endocarditis: the disease, treatment, and prevention. *Circulation.* 2003;107:e185-187.

4. Rovery C, Greub G, Lepidi H, et al. PCR detection of bacteria on cardiac valves of patients with treated bacterial endocarditis. *J Clin Microbiol.* 2005;43:163-167.

5. Goldenberger D, Kunzli A, Vogt P, et al. Molecular diagnosis of bacterial endocarditis by broad-range PCR amplification and direct sequencing. *J Clin Microbiol.* Nov 1997;35:2733-2739.

6. Grijalva M, Horvath R, Dendis M, et al. Molecular diagnosis of culture negative infective endocarditis: clinical validation in a group of surgically treated patients. *Heart.* Mar 2003;89:263-268.

7. Houpikian P, Raoult D. Diagnostic methods current best practices and guidelines for identification of difficult-to-culture pathogens in infective endocarditis. *Infect Dis Clin North Am.* 2002;16:377-392.

8. Ohara-Nemoto Y, Tajika S, Sasaki M, et al. Identification of Abiotrophia adiacens and Abiotrophia defectiva by 16S rRNA gene PCR and restriction fragment length polymorphism analysis. *J Clin Microbiol.* 1997;35:2458-2463.

9. Qin X, Urdahl KB. PCR and sequencing of independent genetic targets for the diagnosis of culture negative bacterial endocarditis. *Diagn Microbiol Infect Dis.* 2001;40:145-149.

10. Wilck MB, Wu Y, Howe JG, et al. Endocarditis caused by culture-negative organisms visible by Brown and Brenn staining: utility of PCR and DNA sequencing for diagnosis. *J Clin Microbiol.* 2001;39:2025-2027.

11. Fournier PE, Raoult D. Nonculture Laboratory Methods for the Diagnosis of Infectious Endocarditis. *Curr Infect Dis Rep.* 1999;1:136-141.

12. Durack DT, Lukes AS, Bright DK. New criteria for diagnosis of infective endocarditis: utilization of specific echocardiographic findings. Duke Endocarditis Service. *Am J Med.* 1994;96:200-209.

13. Blanco-Carrion A. Bacterial endocarditis prophylaxis. *Med Oral Patol Oral Cir Bucal.* 2004;9 Suppl:44-51; 37-43.

14. Tak T, Dhawan S, Reynolds C, et al. Current diagnosis and treatment of infective endocarditis. *Expert Rev Anti Infect Ther.* 2003;1:639-654.

15. Jones MN, Holt RG. Activation of plasminogen by Streptococcus mutans. *Biochem Biophys Res Commun.* 2004;322:37-41.

16. Beldner S, Bajwa A, Kaplan B, et al. Septic coronary embolism. *J Interv Cardiol.* 2002;15:301-304.

17. Vilacosta I, Graupner C, San Roman JA, et al. Risk of embolization after institution of antibiotic therapy for infective endocarditis. *J Am Coll Cardiol.* 2002;39:1489-1495.

18. Murtagh B, Frazier OH, Letsou GV. Diagnosis and management of bacterial endocarditis in 2003. *Curr Opin Cardiol.* 2003;18:106-110.

19. Prabhu RM, Piper KE, Baddour LM, et al. Antimicrobial susceptibility patterns among viridans group streptococcal isolates from infective endocarditis patients from 1971 to 1986 and 1994 to 2002. *Antimicrob Agents Chemother.* 2004;48:4463-4465.

20. Smith A, Jackson MS, Kennedy H. Antimicrobial susceptibility of viridans group streptococcal blood isolates to eight antimicrobial agents. *Scand J Infect Dis.* 2004;36(4):259-263.

21. Oliver R, Roberts GJ, Hooper L. Penicillins for the prophylaxis of bacterial endocarditis in dentistry. *Cochrane Database Syst Rev.* 2004:CD003813.

22. Seymour R. Is penicillin prophylaxis effective against bacterial endocarditis? *Evid Based Dent.* 2004;5:46.

A Young Woman Presenting With Acute Onset of Chest Pain

Matthew R. Plymyer, Mark R. Rice

Department of Pathology, Easton Hospital, Easton, PA

Patient: 36-year-old Caucasian woman.

Chief Complaint: Acute onset of right-sided chest pain.

History of Present Illness: The patient presented to the emergency department early in the morning after having acute onset of pain in the right side of her chest beginning several hours earlier while rolling in bed. The pain was sharp, non-radiating, and worse when breathing. The patient reported no recent injury, but reported 1 week of insomnia of unknown cause; she denied fever, chills, diaphoresis, dizziness, nausea, or vomiting.

Past Medical/Surgical History: The patient reported no chronic internal illnesses (such as hypertension or diabetes) and was taking no regular medications. She did report having had surgical repair of a left clavicle fracture and bilateral minor foot surgery, both many years previously. Upon further discussion with a pulmonary medicine specialist, the patient also noted a history of chronic dental and gum disease, including a dental abscess within the past month.

Family/Social History: The patient was married, had no recent travel history, denied unusual exposure to livestock, birds, or bats, and had no known exposure to tuberculosis. She reported smoking 1.5 packs of cigarettes per day for 23 years, listed herself as a "social drinker" of alcoholic beverages, and reported drinking 3 cups of caffeinated beverages each morning. Additional family history was unremarkable.

Physical Examination: The patient was alert and cooperative, but looked short of breath and was holding her left shoulder. Vital signs: temperature, 97.2°F; pulse, 90 per minute; respiratory rate, 16 per minute; blood pressure, 115/82 mm Hg. Her room air oxygen saturation was 100%. Poor dentition and inflamed gums were noted. Breath sounds were decreased bilaterally, but the lungs were otherwise clear to auscultation and percussion. Heart rate was regular with no murmurs. No extremity swelling was present.

Results of Other Initial Diagnostic Tests: Electrocardiogram (ECG) showed no significant abnormalities, venous ultrasound study of both legs showed no evidence of thrombosis, and a chest radiograph showed a possible right lung infiltrate. Computerized tomography (CT) scan of the chest showed no evidence of pulmonary embolus, but did show a mass (3.2 cm in greatest dimension) with an apparent liquid center in the right lung and some mildly enlarged lymph nodes in the right lung hilum [**Image 1**].

T1.Principal Laboratory Findings

Test*		Patient's Result	"Normal" Reference Range
Hematology/Coagulation			
WBC count		13.3	4.8-10.8 × 10³/L
Differential: segmented neutrophils		74%	35-80%
	bands	9%	0-10%
	interpretation	left shift	
Platelet count		506	130-400 × 10³/L
Hemoglobin		12.0	12.0-16.0 g/dL
Prothrombin time		12.6	10.9-12.9 s
D-dimer		<0.20	<0.20 g/mL
ESR		38	0-20 mm/h
Chemistry			
CK-MB	S1	0.7	<5.9 ng/mL
	S2	4.2	<5.9 ng/mL
Troponin I	S1	<0.3	<0.5 ng/mL
	S2	<0.3	<0.5 ng/mL

*All tests included in a metabolic panel and a calcium determination were within the reference limits for these tests.
WBC, white blood cell; ESR, erythrocyte sedimentation rate; CK-MB, MB isoenzyme of creatine kinase; S, sample. Samples 1 and 2 were obtained at 8:45 am and 8:40 pm on hospital day #1, respectively.

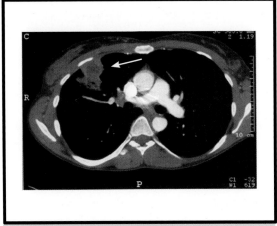

Image 1_Computerized tomography (CT) scan of the patient's chest demonstrating the presence of a mass (arrow) in the right lung measuring 3.2 cm in greatest dimension extending to the pleural surface. The mass has a liquid-density center, suggestive of an abscess and/or a necrotic neoplasm.

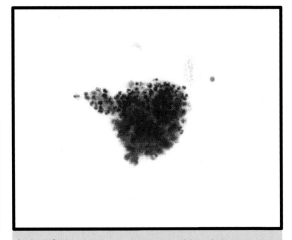

Image 2_Fine needle aspiration biopsy of the right lung mass illustrating the presence of neutrophils, histiocytes, and filamentous bacteria morphologically suggestive of *Actinomyces* (Papanicolaou stain, 400× magnification).

Questions

1. Based upon the patient's clinical presentation, were the laboratory tests and other diagnostic studies ordered on this patient appropriate? Why or why not?

2. What condition(s) does(do) the patient's clinical presentation, medical history, laboratory, and diagnostic test results suggest?

3. What procedure would be appropriate for evaluation of this patient's lung mass?

4. What additional follow-up or work-up might be prudent for this patient?

5. What is this patient's most likely diagnosis?

6. What is the most appropriate treatment for this patient?

Possible Answers

1. Yes. The patient is a young woman with relatively sudden onset of right-sided chest pain with a "pleuritic" character (ie, the pain worsens with breathing). Patients presenting with acute chest pain pose a common and often difficult diagnostic challenge, with numerous possible etiologies including cardiovascular, pulmonary, and gastrointestinal diseases.[1] Those conditions which could pose immediate and serious danger to the well-being of the patient need to be investigated quickly, such as the possibility of myocardial infarction (MI) or pulmonary embolism.[1] Ordering cardiac enzymes and an ECG reflect appropriate concern for myocardial infarction. Likewise, concern for pulmonary embolism prompted the D-dimer assay, the venous ultrasound of the legs (to look for blood clots which could send emboli to the lungs), and a CT scan of the chest (to look for evidence of emboli in the lungs). Finally, the complete blood count, ESR, chest radiograph, and chest CT scan seem appropriate to investigate the possibility of pulmonary disease, including infectious conditions.

2. The clinical presentation suggests a number of possibilities, as discussed above. The negative myocardial enzymes and normal ECG effectively exclude myocardial infarction and related entities. Likewise, the negative D-dimer assay, negative venous ultrasound of the legs, and lack of CT evidence of pulmonary embolus virtually eliminate the possibility of pulmonary embolism.[2] The elevated leukocyte count with "left shift" and elevated ESR suggest an inflammatory or infectious etiology. The chest CT documented a mass with a liquid center in the right lung, possibly representing a lung abscess or a necrotic

neoplasm. Lung abscesses can be caused by a number of bacteria, mycobacteria, fungi, or parasites, and may co-exist with partially necrotic neoplasms or areas of infarction.[3] Symptoms and physical findings of lung abscess often overlap with pneumonia, and most diagnoses are made radiographically.[3] A very important part of this patient's clinical history is that of periodontal disease and recent periodontal abscess. Aspiration of organisms in patients with periodontal disease is a well-established cause of pneumonia and lung abscesses[3] in such patients and is likely to have occurred in our patient.

3. Fine needle aspiration (FNA) biopsy. Fine needle aspiration biopsy is a relatively quick and non-invasive technique to both investigate the composition of a lung mass (inflammatory, neoplastic, or both) and to obtain material for microbiological culture studies. Standard sputum collections for cultures are often contaminated by oral flora[3] and the composition of the normal and diseased oral flora is very complex, with organisms such as *Streptococcus, Peptostreptococcus, Veillonella, Lactobacillus, Corynebacterium*, and *Actinomyces* comprising more than 80% of the normal flora.[4] Many of the same organisms which can contaminate sputum specimens are possible pathogens if aspirated into the lungs. Evaluation of a lung mass by FNA biopsy avoids the possibility of oral contamination and is therefore preferable to sputum cultures in determining whether a specific microbiological organism is the cause of a lung abscess.[3] Computed tomography-guided FNA biopsy of our patient's right lung mass was performed on hospital day #2. Cytologic findings included numerous neutrophils and histiocytes [**Image 2**], consistent with an inflammatory process, such as a lung abscess. No definitive evidence of malignancy was found. Groups of filamentous bacteria morphologically suspicious for *Actinomyces* were noted on the cytology slides [**Image 2**]. Material was obtained during the FNA biopsy for aerobic, anaerobic, fungal, and mycobacterial cultures. Pure (4+) growth of viridans group *Streptococcus* was the only organism recovered.

The viridans group of *Streptococci* includes many of the species found in the oral cavity, such as *S. mutans, S. sanguis, S. mitis*, and *S. salivarus*.[5] Lung abscesses associated with viridans *Streptococci* are rare.[6] There are reports, however, of viridans *Streptococci* as the only isolated pathogen in lower respiratory tract infections, although they often occur together with other organisms such as anaerobes.[4] Interestingly, the cytology slides prepared from our patient's lung mass demonstrated the presence of filamentous bacteria resembling *Actinomyces*; however, *Actinomyces* was not isolated by culture.

4. Serial chest radiographs (conventional and/or CT) and serum measurement of biochemical markers of lung cancer. In 10% to 15% of cases of lung abscess there is underlying carcinoma.[7] In this case, the FNA biopsy showed no diagnostic evidence of malignancy, but the entire mass can never be completely sampled by this technique. Serial chest radiographs during the course of antibiotic treatment are helpful in following the size of the abscess and in documenting healing. Even after completion of an appropriate antibiotic course, however, there may be a residual sterile cavity or fibrosis.[3] If the radiographic appearance of the lung abscess does not improve, additional testing (eg, serum M2-PK measurement) to exclude malignancy may be necessary. Type M2 pyruvate kinase (M2-PK) is a serum marker of lung cancer.[8] Moreover, if the abscess improves but there is a residual radiographic abnormality (eg, scarring), future chest radiographs must be interpreted with the patient's history in mind.

5. ***Most likely diagnosis:*** lung abscess due to viridans group streptococcal infection secondary to chronic periodontal disease.

6. Penicillin and other β-lactam antibiotics are the preferred treatment for viridans streptococcal infections.[4] Resistant strains are common and are usually found in immunocompromised and hospitalized patients. Community-acquired infections are generally susceptible to penicillin.[4] Although our patient may have been co-infected with *Actinomyces*, penicillin is effective against this organism as well.[3] Finally, in patients with possible co-infection with β-lactamase-producing organisms (eg, anaerobes), treatment with a combination of a β-lactam antibiotic plus a β -lactamase inhibitor (eg, amoxicillin/clavulanate) can be used.[3] At least 6 months of oral antibiotic therapy are often necessary to successfully treat patients with viridans streptococcal infection.[3]

Treatment and Course

The patient was begun on oral Augmentin (amoxicillin/clavulanate) therapy and was discharged on hospital day 3 feeling improved with significant decrease of her chest pain.

Keywords

chest pain; fine needle aspiration; viridans group Streptococci; Actinomyces

References

1. Braunwald E, Fauci AS, Kasper DL, et al. *Harrison's Principles of Internal Medicine*, 15th ed. New York: McGraw-Hill; 2001:60-64.

2. Beutler E, Coller BS, Lichtman MA, et al. *Williams Hematology*, 6th ed. New York: McGraw-Hill; 2001:1735-1741.

3. Murray JF, Nadel JA. *Textbook of Respiratory Medicine*, 3rd ed. Philadelphia: W.B. Saunders; 2000:1004-1031.

4. Mandell GL, Bennett JE, Dolin R. *Mandell, Douglas, and Bennett's Principles and Practice of Infectious Diseases*, 5th ed. Philadelphia: Churchill Livingstone; 2000:689-698, 2167-2172.

5. Henry JB. *Clinical Diagnosis and Management by Laboratory Methods*, 20th ed. Philadelphia: W.B. Saunders; 2001:1093-1096.

6. Koneman EW, Allen SD, Janda WM, et al. *Color Atlas and Textbook of Diagnostic Microbiology*, 5th ed. Philadelphia: Lippincott-Raven Publishers; 1997:592-593.

7. Cotran RS, Kumar V, Collins T. *Robbins Pathologic Basis of Disease*, 6th ed. Philadelphia: W.B. Saunders; 1999:722.

8. Schneider J, Velcovsky H-G, Morr H, et al. Comparison of the tumor markers M2-PK, CEA, CYFRA 21-1, NSE, and SCC in the diagnosis of lung cancer. *Anticancer Res. 2000;20:5053-5058.*

The "Perfect Storm"

Jaffar Alfardan,[1] Frank H. Wians, Jr.,[1] Robert F. Dons,[3] Kathleen Wyne[2]

[1]*Departments of Pathology and* [2]*Division of Endocrinology and Metabolism, Department of Internal Medicine, University of Texas Southwestern Medical Center, Dallas, TX, and* [3]*Endocrinology Nuclear Medicine Associates, P.A., San Antonio, TX*

Patient: 60-year-old African-American woman.

Chief Complaint: Exacerbation of tremors, sweating, and palpitations over the past week.

History of Present Illness: This patient presented to the emergency department (ED) with nausea, vomiting, watery diarrhea, sweating, tremor, jitteriness, chills, and palpitations of 1 week duration. The patient reported a 60-pound weight loss during the past 2-year period, chronic thinning of hair, and intermittent palpitations. She reported no shortness of breath, cold or heat intolerance, eye changes, difficulty swallowing, or current use of any medications.

Medical History: The patient reported no history of diabetes, hypertension, or heart disease. A review of her medical record indicated that she had presented 2 years earlier with a diffusely enlarged thyroid gland and was diagnosed with hyperthyroidism. At that time, she was admitted to the hospital and treated with propylthiouracil (PTU), steroids, and beta-blockers, but was subsequently lost to follow up.

Family History: Her father had hyperthyroidism and a daughter has Grave disease. There was no family history of hypertension, diabetes mellitus, or coronary heart disease.

Physical Examination: The patient was diaphoretic, cachectic, and had icteric sclera. Her vital signs were: temperature, 36.2°C (97.2°F); blood pressure, 160/103 mm Hg; pulse (heart rate), 196 beats per minute (bpm); and respiratory rate, 16 breaths per minute. She had a non-tender enlarged thyroid with a right side nodule and bilateral bruit. Cardiac examination revealed a Grade III/IV systolic murmur radiating to the axilla and an elevated jugular venous pressure. A prominent tremor in the extremities was noted.

Additional Diagnostic Testing: Chest x-ray demonstrated a small bilateral pleural effusion with prominent pulmonary vasculature. An electrocardiogram (ECG) demonstrated atrial fibrillation while an echocardiogram showed decreased right and left ventricular function and a left ventricular ejection fraction (LVEF) of only 15% (normal: >50%). A computed tomography (CT) scan, without contrast, of her head was negative for any evidence of bleeding.

Questions

1. What are this patient's most striking clinical and laboratory findings?

2. How do you explain this patient's most striking clinical and laboratory findings?

3. What are the possible etiologies of this patient's disease?

4. What is this patient's most likely diagnosis?

T1. Principal Laboratory Findings

Test	Patient's Value	"Normal" Reference Range
Hematology		
WBC count	15.5	4.1-11.1 × 10³/μL
Hemoglobin	12.0	12.0-15.2 g/dL
Hematocrit	38.0	36.8-48.7%
Differential: Neutrophils	84	36-72%
Bands	11	0-11%
Metamyelocytes	2	None
Lymphocytes	2	20-51%
Monocytes	1	4-11 %
PBS review	Positive for toxic granulation	Negative for toxic granulation
Platelet count	227	174-404 × 10³/μL
Chemistry		
Sodium	135	135-145 mmol/L
Calcium	9.1	8.4-10.2 mg/dL
Glucose	38	65-110 mg/dL
Bilirubin, total	3.1	0.2-1.3 mg/dL
Albumin	3.7	3.5- 5.3 g/dL
Ferritin	564	7-282 ng/mL
ALP	185	38-126 U/L
AST	47	10-40 U/L
ALT	46	8-78 U/L
Lactate	6.7	0.7-2.1 mmol/L
TSH	<0.1	0.4-4.5 μIU/L
T3	548	60-181 ng/dL
FT4	9.30	0.76-1.79 ng/dL
T-Uptake ratio	>2	0.8-1.1
Thyroid peroxidase antibody	Negative	Negative
Troponin I	<0.1	<0.1 ng/mL
BNP	408	<100 pg/mL is generally not consistent with the diagnosis of decompensated heart failure

WBC, white blood cell; PBS, peripheral blood smear; ALP, alkaline phosphatase; AST, aspartate aminotransferase; ALT, alanine aminotransferase; BNP, B-type natriuretic peptide; TSH, thyroid stimulating hormone, T3, triiodothyronine; FT4, free thyroxine

5. What was the precipitating factor that caused this patient's recent ED visit?

6. What is the pathogenesis of this patient's condition?

7. What *clinical* findings are associated typically with this patient's condition?

8. What *laboratory* findings are associated typically with this patient's condition?

9. How is this patient's condition diagnosed?

10. How should this patient's condition be treated?

11. How should the patient's response to therapy be monitored?

T2. Precipitating Factors of Thyroid Storm[a]	
Infection (*most common cause*)	Toxemia of pregnancy
Surgery (*thyroidal and non-thyroidal*)	Parturition
Radioactive iodine therapy	Severe emotional stress
Iodinated contrast dyes	Acute manic crisis
Withdrawal of anti-thyroid treatment	Pulmonary embolism
Amiodarone therapy	Cerebral vascular accident
Thyroid hormone overdose	Bowel infarction
Diabetic ketoacidosis	Acute trauma
Congestive heart failure	Tooth extraction
Hypoglycemia	Vigorous palpation of thyroid gland

[a]Adapted from Ref 2.

12. What is the expected response of total tri-iodothyronine (TT3), free thyroxine (FT4), and thyroid stimulating hormone (TSH) levels in patients who respond appropriately to treatment for thyrotoxicosis?

13. What caused the discrepancy between our patient's TT3 and FT4 levels in response to treatment?

14. What is the prognosis for individuals with this patient's condition?

15. What is the incidence of this patient's condition in the hospitalized population?

Possible Answers

1. Nausea, vomiting, watery diarrhea, sweating, jitteriness, chills, and palpitations of 1 week duration; a 60-pound weight loss during the past 2-year period; chronic thinning of hair; intermittent palpitations; icteric sclera; enlarged thyroid; atrial fibrillation; and a markedly decreased LVEF. Increased WBC count, increased neutrophils, metamyelocytes present, decreased lymphocytes, and neutrophil toxic granulation; hypoglycemia; hyperbilirubinemia; increased ferritin, ALP, lactate, BNP values; increased T3, FT4, T-Uptake values with an undetectable TSH concentration.

2. This patient's clinical signs and symptoms are classical for hyperthyroidism, including sympathetic nervous system overactivity (eg, fever, tachycardia, diaphoresis, tremor, weight loss, atrial fibrillation, and heart failure) and an enlarged thyroid gland. Her striking laboratory findings complement her most striking clinical findings, including hyperbilirubinemia and icteric sclera, hypoglycemia, left-sided heart failure and increased BNP, and thyroid function test values (ie, markedly increased T3 and FT4 values and an undetectable TSH value) which are pathognomonic of hyperthyroidism. In addition, her high WBC count with a left shift and toxic granulation on the peripheral blood smear, and hyperferritinemia suggested an acute bacterial infection (sepsis).

3. Thyrotoxicosis, Graves disease, uncomplicated hyperthyroidism, and thyroid storm. Thyrotoxicosis is an all-inclusive term for all causes of thyroid-induced hypermetabolism, while the term hyperthyroidism is reserved for thyroid-induced hypermetabolic states resulting from increased synthesis and release of thyroxine (**T4**) and triiodothyronine (**T3**) by the thyroid gland.[1] Graves disease is the most common cause of hyperthyroidism and, not surprisingly, of thyroid storm as well. However, other pathologic conditions of the thyroid, such as toxic multinodular goiter, toxic adenomas, and hypersecretory thyroid carcinoma, are also associated with thyroid storm.[2] Graves disease is an autoimmune process whose symptoms wax and wane over time.[3] Thus, many patients stop taking their antithyroid medications when their symptoms wane and never receive definitive therapy (ie, radioactive iodine ablation of the thyroid gland or thyroidectomy). Thyroid crisis can occur in these patients due to a variety of precipitating factors (**T2**). However, the 'surgical crisis' which followed subtotal thyroidectomy in these patients was a common cause of thyroid crisis before the availability of drugs to achieve adequate pre-operative control of thyroid hormone levels.[4] Thyroid storm, also called accelerated hyperthyroidism or thyrotoxic crisis,

T3. Criteria for Scoring Signs and Symptoms Suggestive of Thyroid Storm[a]

Criterion		Point Value
Body temperature (°F):	99.0-99.9	5
	100.0-100.9	10
	101.0-101.9	15
	102.0-102.9	20
	103.0-103.9	25
	>104.0	30
CNS effects:	Absent	0
	Mild (*agitation*)	**10**
	Moderate (*delirium, psychosis, lethargy*)	20
	Severe (*seizure, coma*)	30
GI-hepatic dysfunction:	Absent	0
	Moderate (*diarrhea, nausea, vomiting, abdominal pain*)	10
	Severe (*unexplained jaundice*)	**20**
Tachycardia (heart rate, bpm):	90-109	5
	110-119	10
	120-129	15
	130-139	20
	≥140	**25**
CHF:	Absent	0
	Mild (*pedal edema*)	5
	Moderate (*bibasilar rales*)	10
	Severe (*pulmonary edema*)	**15**
Atrial fibrillation	Absent	0
	Present	**10**
Precipitant factor	Negative	0
(see **T2**)	Positive	**10**

[a]*For each criterion and highest grade of signs and symptoms associated with the patient being evaluated, add the value of points assigned to each criterion to achieve a composite score (range of composite scores: 0-140). Interpret composite score and probability of thyroid storm as follows: <25, thyroid storm unlikely; 25-44, suggestive of impending thyroid storm; ≥45, highly suggestive of thyroid storm (Adapted from Ref 6). CNS, central nervous system; GI, gastrointestinal; CHF, congestive heart failure.* **Bolded values** *indicate the criteria and point values (composite score = 10+20+25+15+10+10 = 90) associated with the patient presented in this case study.*

is defined as a sudden life-threatening exacerbation of thyrotoxicosis associated with systemic decompensation.[1,3] Hyperthyroidism and thyroid storm are caused by excess synthesis and release of thyroid hormones resulting in both high free and total T3 and T4 levels and feedback inhibition of TSH. High thyroid hormones level, especially the active forms (ie, FT3 and FT4), are responsible for the various hypermetabolic and sympathetic nervous system overactivity

manifestations in such patients. Typically, however, the laboratory findings alone can only tell clinicians if slow-onset hyperthyroidism is likely due to non-compliance or under-treatment with antithyroid medications. However, laboratory findings characteristic of hyperthyroidism, when coupled with rapid and severe (life-threatening) onset of the clinical manifestations of hyperthyroidism, as occurred in our patient, favor a diagnosis of thyroid storm over uncomplicated

T4. Effect of Various Substances on FT4 and TT3 Results Using the ICMA Method in the ADVIA Centaur Immunoassay Instrument[a]

Substance (Interferent) Added	Amount Added, mg/dL	% Change in FT4 concn	% Change in TT3 concn
Phenytoin	4	+ 7.9	+ 2.1
Phenylbutazone	30	+ 7.6	+ 2.6
Aspirin	50	+ 1.2	- 1.6
PTU	4	+ 0.9	+ 4.4
Sodium salicylate	50	+ 0.3	- 0.5
MMI	0.4	+ 0.2	- 1.2

[a]Adapted from Ref 16. FT4, free thyroxine; TT3, total triiodothyronine; ICMA, immunochemiluminometric assay; concn, concentration; PTU, propylthiouracil; MMI, methimazole; +, indicates analyte values were higher in samples containing the substance added compared to the same sample in the absence of any added interferent; -, indicates analyte values were lower in samples containing the substance added compared to the same sample in the absence of any added interferent.

hyperthyroidism. A clinical scoring scale has been proposed to categorize cases of severe hypermetabolic syndrome as "suggestive of impending" or "highly suggestive of" thyroid storm based on the severity of the patient's signs and symptoms in the categories: body temperature (thermoregulatory dysfunction), central nervous system (CNS) effects, gastrointestinal (GI)-hepatic dysfunction, tachycardia [cardiovascular system (CVS) dysfunction], congestive heart failure (CHF) and atrial fibrillation, and precipitant history.[6] When our patient's clinical signs and symptoms were evaluated according to the scoring criteria for assessing the probability of thyroid storm, a score of 90 (ie, highly suggestive of thyroid storm) was obtained (**T3**).

4. **Most likely diagnosis:** *thyroid storm.*

5. Thyroid storm in this patient was most likely precipitated by sepsis. Thyroid storm is usually precipitated by an acute illness, including stroke, infection, trauma, diabetic ketoacidosis, toxemia of pregnancy or parturition, recent surgery (especially, surgery involving the thyroid gland), and treatment with radioactive iodine.[3,5] Intravenous administration of exogenous iodine in contrast dye prior to CT scan or angiography may also precipitate thyroid storm.[6,7] Therefore, evaluation of an enlarged thyroid gland should be performed using ultrasonography in lieu of a CT scan. Emotional stress and vigorous palpation of the thyroid gland have also been reported to precipitate thyroid storm.[6,8] A summary of the precipitating factors of thyroid storm is provided in (**T2**).

6. The pathogenesis of thyroid storm is not completely understood; however, several factors seem to play a role in its development. The marked increase in thyroid hormone levels is not the critical factor in the etiology of thyroid storm because most studies revealed no difference in thyroid hormone levels with uncomplicated hyperthyroidism and thyroid storm. The acute discharge of thyroid hormones and rapid change in their concentrations explain many cases of hyperthyroidism.[6,9,10] Examples of such cases include post-surgical patients, or patients receiving 131-iodine (^{131}I) therapy, or in patients in whom treatment with thionamides or lithium is withdrawn suddenly. The interaction of excess levels of catecholamines and thyroid hormones has also been implicated in the pathogenesis of thyroid storm and supported by the signs and symptoms of sympathetic nervous system hyperactivity which occurs in these patients which are relieved by treatment with beta-blockers.[2-5] It has also been suggested that factors such as infection or hypoxemia can enhance cellular responses to thyroid hormones.[2,3,8] Moreover, the mechanism by which some of these factors precipitate the crisis that accompanies thyroid storm may be related to cytokine release and acute immunologic disturbances.[5]

7. Patients with thyroid storm present typically with severe hypermetabolic syndrome, including fever, which can be severe and is almost always present, profuse sweating, tremulousness, and restlessness. Marked tachycardia and/or arrhythmia which may be associated with pulmonary edema or congestive heart failure, even in the absence of prior heart disease, is also often present. However, arrhythmia is unusual in younger patients with thyroid storm because they typically do not have any underlying structural heart

disease, but they can progress to congestive heart failure and pulmonary edema with sustained and prolonged hyperthyroidism.[6,7] Systolic hypertension with widened pulse pressure occurs commonly during the initial stages of thyroid storm, while postural hypotension and shock can also occur due to volume depletion in patients with vomiting and/or diarrhea.[8] Gastrointestinal manifestations of thyroid storm include vomiting, diarrhea, abdominal pain, intestinal obstruction, hepatomegaly, splenomagaly, and jaundice. As the disease progress, CNS manifestations increase, including increased agitation and emotional lability, confusion, delirium, marked psychosis, seizures, stupor, and coma. These symptomatologies are associated classically with a history of thyrotoxicosis, goiter, or exophthalmos and are sufficient to diagnose thyroid storm and to institute immediate treatment prior to laboratory confirmation.[3,5,8] However, in older patients, especially those with multinodular goiter, thyroid storm may present as masked or "apathetic" thyrotoxicosis.[8]

8. Laboratory abnormalities associated with patients with thyroid storm include modest hyperglycemia in the absence of a history of diabetes mellitus, marked leukocytosis with a left shift, even in the absence of infection, although leukopenia can occur in patients with Graves disease, and mild hypercalcemia, due to hemoconcentration and the effect of thyroid hormones on bone resorption. In addition, thyroid storm can lead to hepatic dysfunction and high lactate dehydrogenase (LD), AST, and bilirubin levels.[3,8] Moreover, a high serum cortisol value is an expected finding in thyrotoxic individuals, and the finding of an abnormally low cortisol level in a patient with Graves disease should raise suspicion of coincident adrenal insufficiency especially in a hypotensive patient with an electrolyte imbalance. Importantly, it is inappropriate to wait for a serum cortisol level prior to administering treatment to a patient in thyroid crisis because the adrenal reserve in such patients is often exceeded even in the absence of adrenal insufficiency.[8]

9. The diagnosis of thyroid storm is based mainly on clinical criteria. Most studies have shown that thyroid hormone levels in patients with thyroid storm are not significantly higher than those observed in patients with uncomplicated thyrotoxicosis.[11] Moreover, differentiating between uncomplicated hyperthyroidism and thyroid storm solely on the basis of laboratory findings is extremely difficult.[8] In the study by Brooks and colleagues,[12] significantly higher serum free T4 levels, but not total T4 levels, were found in patients with thyroid storm. Usually, both total and free thyroid hormone levels are elevated, and TSH is undetectable, in patients with hyperthyroidism.[3] Moreover, patients with thyroid storm may have normal T3 levels and thus resemble the findings in patients with non-thyroidal illness and the "sick euthyroid syndrome" (also called the "low T3 syndrome)[11]. Such a circumstance may obscure the diagnosis of coexisting thyrotoxicosis in the first few hours of the initial evaluation of a patient without a previous history of hyperthyroidism. In such patients, finding an increased 2-hour radioiodine uptake (RIU) value, supplemented with a rapid T4 determination, can discriminate between patients with thyroid storm and those with sick euthyroid syndrome. If results of TSH and FT4 testing are rapidly available, RIU testing may be deferred but will still be needed to definitively differentiate between thyrotoxic thyroiditis and primary hyperthyroidism.

10. Treatment of patients in thyroid storm includes, but is not limited to, the administration of drugs such as PTU, potassium iodide, broad-spectrum antibiotics, steroids, propanolol, furosemide, and angiotensin converting enzyme (ACE) inhibitors to control the patient's symptoms of hyperthyroidism, sepsis, hypervolemia, cardiac conduction abnormalities, and heart failure. Treatment of thyroid crisis is likely to be most effective when implemented using a 4-pronged approach: (1) blocking the release and synthesis of new thyroid hormone using iodides, thionamides, and steroids; (2) blocking the effects of existing, excessive circulating levels of T4 and T3 using beta-blockers; (3) treating any precipitating factors; and, (4) treatment of any underlying decompensation, such as fever, heart failure, or shock.[6,8] The **first arm** of the pharmacologic treatment of this disease is aimed at inhibiting synthesis and release of thyroid hormone. Thionamide antithyroid drugs, such as PTU and methimazole (MMI), prevent synthesis of thyroid hormones. These agents are

administered orally, through a nasogastric tube, or rectally, as there are currently no available parenteral forms. Due to its inhibitory effect on T4 to T3 conversion, PTU (200-400 mg q4-6h) is believed to act faster than MMI (20 mg q4h) and, therefore, is the drug of choice in the treatment of thyroid crisis.[2,3,8] The administration of a loading dose (500-1,500 mg) of PTU as soon as thyrotoxicosis is recognized will improve the patient's symptoms and help lower the thyroxine levels faster. The loading dose should be administered before initiating any other therapy (eg, use of a beta-blocker) as it will have more impact on improving the patient's symptoms and lowering heart rate. Moreover, such high doses of MMI may cause a dose-related agranulocytosis for which the only treatment option is surgical removal of the thyroid gland. The doses of PTU and MMI used in the treatment of thyroid storm are much higher than the doses used to treat uncomplicated thyrotoxicosis. Because thionamide drugs have no effects on the release of preformed T3 and T4 from the thyroid gland, agents such as inorganic iodine or lithium carbonate should be used in the treatment of thyroid storm.[8] Treatment with stable iodide in the form of a saturated solution of potassium iodide (SSKI), ipodate, or lugol solution is initiated 1 hour after administration of PTU and continued for a few days. The sequence of administration of these drugs is extremely important, because administration of iodine prior to a thionamide drug results in incorporation of administered iodine into newly formed thyroid hormone, which could exacerbate the condition (Wolff-Chaikoff effect).[5,8] Emergency radioactive iodine ablation therapy, coupled with subsequent high-dose oral iodine, is an option; however, there is a risk of temporarily worsening the patient's thyroid storm. Therefore, this option should be avoided and reserved only for those cases of thyroid storm in which the patient cannot take the antithyroid medication and surgical removal of the thyroid gland is not an option. Dexamethasone in large doses (2 mg PO every 6 hours) is given to inhibit the release of thyroid hormones from the thyroid gland and to prevent the peripheral conversion of FT4 to T3. In successful cases, the combined use of PTU, iodide, and dexamethasone can restore the serum T3 level to normal in 24 to 48 hours.[3] The **second arm** of the pharmacologic intervention strategy

in patients with thyroid storm is aimed at antagonizing the peripheral adrenergic actions of thyroid hormones, especially tachycardia, which can cause high-output heart failure in some patients. Such therapy also provides improvement in the patient's symptoms of agitation, convulsions, psychosis, tremor, diarrhea, fever, and diaphoresis. To achieve this improvement, large doses of beta-blockers (eg, propanolol, 20-80 mg, q4-6h po or IV) may be required due to the severity of the patient's symptoms and the increased metabolic clearance of the drug.[8] Because it has been documented that propranolol is very effective in decreasing the peripheral conversion of T4 to T3, it is the beta-adrenergic blocker drug of choice in the treatment of patients with thyroid storm.[5] If heart failure is present, labetalol or carvedilol is a safer alternative to propanolol. However, regardless of which beta-blocker is used, in the acute setting, the goal of therapy is not to normalize or to reduce the patient's heart rate to less than 100 bpm. While the use of multiple loading doses of labetalol, or rapidly increasing the infusion rate of esmolol, may be necessary to achieve clinical results, this treatment approach should be used cautiously. Beta-adrenergic receptors are upregulated in the setting of hyperthyroidism. Once these receptors are saturated in the presence of rapidly increasing levels of labetolol or esmolol, circulatory collapse may occur. To acutely reduce circulating thyroid hormone levels, peritoneal dialysis, plasmapheresis, and experimental hemoperfusion using charcoal columns have been attempted; however, these options are reserved typically for the most severe cases of thyroid storm.[8] The **third arm** of the treatment strategy for thyroid storm recognizes the importance of identifying and treating the events that precipitated the thyroid storm. In some patients, conditions like ketoacidosis, pulmonary thromboembolism, or stroke may underlie thyrotoxic crisis, especially if the patient is obtunded or psychotic. Such patients should receive the same aggressive treatment as those without these conditions. In some patients, a careful search for a source of infection is necessary and the empirical use of broad-spectrum antibiotics may be warranted while waiting for culture results.[8] The **final arm** of the treatment strategy for thyroid storm includes supportive care. All patients with thyroid storm should be monitored in an intensive care unit especially during the initial stages of this crisis.[2] Specific supportive measures include the administration of intravenous fluid (IVF) containing 10% dextrose to correct dehydration and hypernatremia, and provide glucose. Reversal of hyperpyrexia can be achieved using acetaminophen, wet ice packs, and fans. Salicylates, however, should not be used as they displace T3 and T4 from TBG and transthyretin [also known as thyroxine-binding prealbumin (TBPA)] which can worsen the thyroid storm.

Treatment and Course _____

In the ED, our patient was started on intravenous fluids, an esmolol drip, PTU (1,000 g po loading dose, followed by 200 g q4h), propranolol (40 mg po), and dexamethasone (4 mg IV bid). She was then started on potassium iodine (60 mg po tid). Furosemide and captopril therapy was initiated to control her heart failure and broad-spectrum antibiotics to control sepsis. She was transferred to the cardiac care unit (CCU) for close monitoring. Shortly after admission to the CCU, she was noted to be unresponsive with bradycardia and then asystole. Chest compression, epinephrine, and atropine were instituted with restoration of the patient's pulse rate to 80 beats per minute. She was intubated, beta-blockers were discontinued, and she was started on dopamine. Thyroid function tests were obtained and her total T3 level was noted to have dropped significantly (from 548 ng/dL to 300 ng/dL), while her FT4 level increased inexplicably to >12 ng/dL. However, when the serum sample on which the FT4 result of >12 ng/dL was diluted, the FT4 value obtained, after correcting this value for the dilution factor, was 5.0 ng/dL. Despite the aggressive therapy instituted in this patient, over a 2-day period, she progressed to decompensated heart and respiratory failure and died.

11. Free T4 and total T3 levels are the best indicators of response to treatment in patients with thyrotoxicosis, as TSH suppression may persist for months after the initiation of treatment.[11] Moreover, thyrotoxicosis may persist solely due to FT3 excess, hence the need for monitoring FT3 and TT3 levels in these patients.[14]

12. The expected response in patients treated for thyrotoxicosis using PTU and potassium iodine therapy is a parallel reduction in serum TT3 and FT4 levels and an increase in TSH level from undetectable to a level appropriate for the level of free thyroid hormones (FT3 and FT4) in the patient's blood at the time a blood sample is obtained for TSH testing. As expected, our patient's post-treatment TT3 dropped by 45% (from 548 ng/dL to 300 ng/dL). Unexpectedly, however, her FT4 level not only did not decrease in parallel with the decline in TT3 concentration, it increased to >12 ng/dL. The lack of clinical improvement in her condition, despite aggressive therapy, was a testament to the severity of her thyroid storm and consistent with the relatively slow response expected from such therapy.

13. The effect of drugs used in the treatment of our patient and their effect on the equilibrium between FT4 levels and the amount of T4 bound to the thyroid hormone binding proteins, thyroid binding globulin (TBG), thyroxine-binding prealbumin (TBPA), and albumin. More than 99.9% of T4 in the plasma is reversibly bound to these binding proteins, especially TBG, while the remainder is free in the circulation (FT4) as the metabolically active hormone and the precursor of T3.[13,15] The accuracy of FT4 measurements by immunoassay methods depends on the patient's diluted serum sample, and the standards used to obtain a calibration curve, having similar dissociation characteristics when bound to thyroid hormone binding proteins and the same protein binding characteristics as the tracer used in these assays. Most immunoassay methods for estimating serum FT4 concentration are minimally affected by moderate variations in serum TBG concentration, but not extreme variations, qualitative or quantitative albumin abnormalities, or the effect of circulating competitors for T4 binding to TBG.[16] Drugs such as furosemide, salicylates, phenytoin, phenylbutazone, carbamazepine, non-steroidal anti-inflammatory agents, aspirin, salsalate, meclofenamate, and heparin can displace T4 and T3 from thyroid hormone binding proteins.[17,18] The magnitude and direction (ie, increase or decrease) of various drug interferents in the measurement of FT4 using the immunoassay method in the Bayer ADVIA Centaur instrument is shown in (**T4**).[17] Heparin can increase the concentration of non-esterified

fatty acids in whole blood which displace T4 from TBG and lead to spuriously high estimates of circulating FT4 concentration.[19] Moreover, certain drugs can lead to spuriously low FT4 estimates in immunoassays that require higher dilutions of the patient's serum sample because displacement of endogenous FT4 from its binding proteins depends on the relative concentrations of FT4 and competitive inhibitors, such as drugs, and drugs usually have a lower protein binding ratio (eg, furosemide, 98%) than T4 (99.9%).[11]

14. If the appropriate therapeutic measures are implemented in patients with thyroid storm, and these measures are successful, these patients usually improve in 1 to 2 days and recover within a week.[3,5,8]

15. The incidence of thyroid storm is difficult to estimate mainly because there are no definitive and universally-accepted criteria for its diagnosis and the results of the laboratory tests performed typically in patients with suspected thyrotoxicosis are similar in patients with thyroid storm or uncomplicated thyrotoxicosis.[2,6] Moreover, early diagnosis of hyperthyroidism and the advent and effectiveness of anti-thyroid drugs have reduced the annual incidence of thyroid storm to 1% to 2% of all hospital admissions for thyrotoxicosis. Nevertheless, the mortality rate in patients with thyroid storm remains high and ranges between 20% to 30%, even with prompt and aggressive treatment.[2,5,6] Mortality in these patients is typically due to arrhythmia, heart failure, or hyperthermia.[6,7]

Keywords _____

hyperthyroidism, thyrotoxicosis, thyroid storm, free thyroxine, triiodothyronine, thyroid binding globulins

References _____

1. Roth RN, McAuliffe MJ. Hyperthyroidism and thyroid storm. *Emerg Med Clin North Am.* 1989;4:873-883.

2. Sarlis NJ, Gourgiotis L, Thyroid emergencies. *Rev Endo Metab Disord.* 2003;4:129-136.

3. Stathatos N, Wartosfsky L. Thyrotoxic storm. *Encyclopedia of Endocrine Diseases.* 2004;4:573-576.

4. Laresen PR, Kronenberg HM. *Williams Textbook of Endocrinology*, 10th Edition, 413-414.

5. Kasper DL, Braunwald E. *Harrison's Principles of Internal Medicine*, 16th Edition 2005, 2113-2120.

6. Burch HB, Wartofsky L. Life-threatening thyrotoxicosis. Thyroid storm. *Endocrinol Metab Clin North Am.* 1993;22:263-277.

7. Klein I, Ojamaa K. Thyrotoxicosis and the heart. *Endocrinol Metab Clin North Am.* 1998;27:2751-2762.

8. Martini L. *Encyclopedia of Endocrine Diseases.* 2004;4:573-575.

9. Jacobs HS, Mackie DB, Eastman CJ, et al. Total and free triiodothyronine and thyroxine levels in thyroid storm and recurrent hyperthyroidism. *Lancet.* 1973;2:236-238.

10. Tietgens ST, Leinung MC. Thyroid storm. *Med Clin North Am.* 1995;79;169-184.

11. Hawkins RC. Furosemide interference in newer free thyroxine assays. *Clin Chem.* 1998;44:2550

12. Brooks MH, Waldstein SS. Free thyroxine concentrations in thyroid storm. *Ann Intern Med.* 1980; 93:694-697.

13. Fischer HRA, Hackeng WHL, Schopman W, Silberbusch J. Analysis of factors in hyperthyroidism, which determine the duration of suppressive treatment before recovery of thyroid stimulating hormone secretion. *Clin Endocrinol.* 1982;16:575-585.

14. Braverman LE. Evaluation of thyroid status in patients with thyrotoxicosis. *Clin Chem.* 1996;42:174-178.

15. Fisher D. Physiological variations in thyroid hormones: physiological and pathophysiological considerations. *Clin Chem.* 1996;42:135-139.

16. Stockigt JR. Free thyroid hormone measurement: a critical appraisal. *Endocr Metab Clin N Am.* 2001;30:265-289.

17. FrT4, ADVIA Centaur Assay Manual 2003-07.

18. Dons RF. *Endocrine and Metabolic Testing Manual*, 3rd edition. CRC Press, 1997.

19. Mendel CM, Frost PH, Kunitake ST, et al. Mechanism of the heparin-induced increase in the concentration of free thyroxine in plasma. *J Clin Endocrinol Metab.* 1987;65:1259-1264.

Acute Diarrhea in a Young Traveler

Monte S. Willis, Sumi G. So

Department of Pathology, University of Texas Southwestern Medical Center, Dallas, TX

Patient: 36-year-old male.

Past Surgical History: Tonsillectomy at age 5.

Chief Complaint: The patient reported having fevers, chills, and diarrhea for 1 week.

History of Present Illness: The patient reported that he recently spent 47 days in India and during that time followed a strict vegetarian diet and drank only bottled water; however, he did eat some "well-cooked" indigenous foods. He indicated that he felt good until the last day of his trip when he became acutely ill and fatigued. His symptoms included headaches, fevers with a temperature of up to 39.0°C, chills, and 6 to 8 episodes of diarrhea per day. He reported that his diarrhea was clear without visible blood and did not have an "unusually" foul odor. A few days prior the patient had been diagnosed with Giardia, Endolimax, and Blastocystis hominis at another hospital, and was treated with ciprofloxacin with no resolution of his symptoms. He reported to our emergency room because of continuing diarrhea and fever.

Past Medical History: No prior hospitalizations were reported and the patient was currently taking acetaminophen to control his headaches and fever.

Family/Social History: The patient was unemployed and reported that he was an author of several books. He had traveled to India for religious reasons and had not previously traveled outside of the United States. He denied alcohol, tobacco, or illegal substance abuse. Both of his parents, 2 brothers, and 2 sisters were alive and healthy, while another sister had multiple sclerosis.

Physical Examination: Vital signs: temperature, 39.6°C; blood pressure, 111/89 mm Hg; heart rate, 139 bpm; respiration rate, 16 respirations per minute. The patient appeared ill, cachetic, and was shaking. In addition, he was tachycardic and his rectal exam was guaiac positive. The physical examination was otherwise unremarkable. He was admitted to our hospital for additional diagnostic procedures and laboratory tests.

Results of Additional Diagnostic Procedures and Laboratory Tests: A chest X-ray demonstrated increased vascular markings bilaterally. Fungal blood cultures were negative. Aerobic and anaerobic blood cultures were positive for gram-negative rods identified as *Salmonella typhi*. Urine culture was negative. Stool culture was negative for *Salmonella*, *Shigella*, and *Campylobacter* spp; however, *Candida albicans* growth was heavy. Analysis of the stool for ova and parasites (O&P) was negative; however, many red blood cells were present.

T1. Principal Whole Blood and Serum Findings

Test	Patient's Result	"Normal" Reference Range
Hematology/Coagulation		
WBC count	3.7	4.5-11.1 × 10³/µL
Neutrophils	81	35%-80%
Lymphocytes	9	20%-50%
Monocytes	4	2%-12%
Eosinophils	0	0%-7%
Basophils	1	0%-2%
Hemoglobin	13.6	11.7-16.0 g/dL
Hematocrit	39.7	35%-47%
Platelet count	176	150-450 × 10³/µL
MCV	81.2	82-105 fl
MCHC	34.4	31-35 g/dL
PT	11.9	9.8-11.9 s
PTT	29.5	23.0-32.5 s
Chemistry/Immunology		
Sodium	123	135-145 mmol/L
Potassium	3.9	3.6-5.5 mmol/L
Chloride	88	98-109 mmol/L
CO₂	25	22-31 mmol/L
BUN	8	7-21 mg/dL
Creatinine	0.9	1.6-1.2 mg/dL
Glucose	101	65-110 mg/dL
Calcium	8.4	8.4-10.2 mg/dL
Magnesium	1.3	1.4-1.8 mEq/L
Phosphorus	1.6	2.4-4.5 mg/dL
AST	567	13-40 U/L
ALT	392	10-40 U/L
LD	960	100-190 U/L
Amylase	27	29-108 U/L
Lipase	42	7-59 U/L
Bilirubin, total	2.0	0.2-1.3 mg/dL
Bilirubin, direct	1.0	0.0-0.3 mg/dL
Protein, total	5.0	6.3-8.2 g/dL
Albumin	2.4	3.5-5.2 g/dL
HCV Ab	NR	NR
HBsAb	NR	NR*
HAV Ab, IgM	NR	NR
HIV-1,2 Ab	NR	NR

For individuals not immunized with a hepatitis B vaccine. MCV, mean corpuscular volume; MCHC, mean corpuscular hemoglobin concentration; PT, prothrombin time; PTT, partial thromboplastin time; BUN, blood urea nitrogen; AST, aspartate aminotransferase; ALD, alanine aminotransferase; LD, lactate dehydrogenase; HCV, hepatitis C virus; Ab, antibody; HBsAb, hepatitis B surface antibody; HAV, hepatitis A virus; NR, nonreactive.

Questions

1. What is (are) this patient's most striking laboratory result(s)?

2. How do you explain this patient's most striking laboratory result(s)?

3. Which additional test(s) should be performed? Why?

4. What is (are) the most likely diagnosis(es)?

5. What is the most appropriate treatment for this patient?

Possible Answers

1. The most striking laboratory findings in this case are: **serum**, markedly decreased sodium and chloride concentrations and abnormal liver function tests (LFTs), including markedly increased LD, AST, and ALT, increased total and direct bilirubin, and decreased total protein and albumin. During his hospitalization at our medical facility and treatment for *S. typhi* infection, his LFT values decreased (*data not shown*).

2. Hyponatremia (sodium concentration <135 mEq/L) can be particularly serious when the sodium concentration is below or near 120 mEq/L, a limit close to our patient's sodium value of 123 mEq/L. The symptoms of hyponatremia are primarily related to the effects of low sodium concentration on the central nervous

T2. Principal Urine Findings

Test	Patient's Result	"Normal" Reference Range
Urine Dipstick Tests		
Specific gravity	1.004	1.002-1.030
Color	Yellow	
Clarity	Clear	
pH	7.0	5-7
Protein	30 mg/dL	Neg
Glucose	Neg	Neg
Ketone	Neg	Neg
Bile	Neg	Neg
Blood	Neg	Neg
Urobilinogen	0.2	0.1-1.0 EHR U/dL
Leukocyte esterase	Neg	Neg
Nitrite	Neg	Neg
Microscopic Findings		
RBCs	None	0-3/hpf
WBCs	None	0-5/hpf
Bacteria	Occasional	None

hpf, high power field.

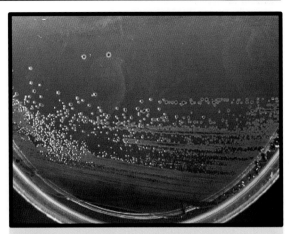

Image 1_Growth of *S. typhi* on Hektoen enteric agar demonstrating characteristic colonies with black centers. Similarly appearing colonies can be seen on xylose-lysiine-deoxycholate (XLD) and bismuth sulfite agars as well. (*Image courtesy of Rita Gander, PhD, University of Texas Southwestern Medical Center, Dallas, TX.*)

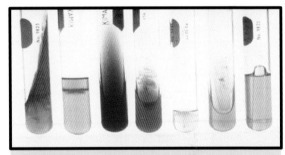

Image 2_Principal biochemical reactions of *Salmonella typhi* include from left to right: triple sugar iron, positive (slant contains H_2S); indole, negative; citrate, negative; lysine, positive; motility, negative; urease, negative; dextrose, negative

system (CNS) and include lethargy, apathy, confusion, disorientation, depression, psychosis, focal neurologic deficits, ataxia, and seizures.[1] This patient's sodium and chloride loss are likely due to the loss of water and sodium from diarrhea, with a greater relative loss of sodium. Such "hypovolemic hyponatremia" is also seen after vomiting, GI suction or drainage, and "third spacing" of fluids after intra-abdominal sepsis, bowel obstruction, pancreatitis, or burns. The patient's increased liver function tests (LD, AST, ALT, total and direct bilirubin) were not due to infection with hepatitis A, B, or C viruses because all hepatitis tests associated with these viruses were negative. A potential cause of his increased transaminases (AST and ALT) was the overdosing of Tylenol (acetaminophen) the patient was taking to relieve his fever. Moreover, increased transaminases are also found in patients with *S. typhi* infection and this patient had positive blood cultures (aerobic and anaerobic) for *S. typhi*. Liver involvement

(hepatomegaly) has been shown to be a consistent finding in patients with typhoid fever, especially during the second and third weeks of infection.[2] Alkaline phosphatase, AST, and ALT levels are increased in >90% of patients with *S. typhi* during the second and third week of infection whereas only 11% to 56% of patients have elevated levels of these enzymes during the first week of infection.[2] These findings suggest that liver involvement is a common feature after the first week of infection with *S. typhi*.[2] The spectrum of hepatic dysfunction in patients with typhoid fever includes increased bilirubin concentration that acute hepatitis, particularly in children, can mimic.[3] Moreover, these LFT values decreased (*data not shown*) during his

T3. Typical Characteristics of Enteric Fever Caused by Various Bacterial Species

Causative Bacteria	Mode of Transmission	Affected Individuals	Clinical Findings	Source[a] of Positive Cultures and Other Laboratory Findings[b]
Salmonella	Travel to tropical areas (eg, India)	Young adults	Bradycardia, splenomegaly, rose spots, conjunctivitis	B, BM, U, F; Leukopenia, Positive serological tests
Yersinia	Pet exposure	Older adults	Chronic liver disease, arthritis, erythema nodosum	B, F, J Positive serological tests
Campylobacter	Pet exposure	Older adults	Stigmata or chronic liver disease, phlebitis	B, F Positive serological tests
Brucella	Animal contact (cattle, sheep); unpasteurized milk	Butchers	Unremarkable	B, BM; Leukopenia, Positive serological tests
Francisella	Animal (rabbits) contact; Vector (ticks) exposure	Variable	Severe prostration, splenomegaly	Positive serological tests

[a]B, blood; BM, bone marrow; U, urine; F, feces; J, joint fluid.
[b]For example, serological tests such as those that identify the presence of serum antibodies (eg, Widal test) to specific bacterial antigens.

hospitalization after this patient's antibiotic treatment for *S. typhi* infection was initiated, further corroborating liver dysfunction as a primary symptom of this disease. Our patient's decreased serum total protein and albumin values were most likely due to his recent poor nutritional status (ie, not eating) and his liver dysfunction.

3. Additional testing might include testing for stool Hemoccult and leukocytes; *Giardia* antigen; *Clostridium difficile* and *Escherichia coli* 0157:H7 toxin tests; cultures using specialized media; O&P analyses; and further radiographic studies to discriminate between gastrointestinal (GI) anatomic abnormalities and tumors, obstructions, fistulas, or inflammatory bowel disease as the cause of disease.[4] Other laboratory tests for diagnosing *S. typhi* infection include the Widal test for *S. typhi* antibodies to the O (surface polysaccharide) and H (flagellar) antigens of *Salmonella* species; an enzyme-linked immunosorbent assay (ELISA) to detect different antigens of *S. typhi*; immunoelectrophoresis and polymerase chain reaction (PCR) methods; WBC count with differential; LFTs; urinalysis; and a chest radiograph.[5]

Hemoccult and fecal leukocyte testing are useful in determining if an inflammatory or infectious process is present. Both of these tests should be performed because the results of a guaiac test alone for hemoglobin can be misleading. Bleeding in the absence of fecal leukocytes is indicative of amebiasis, malignancy, or bowel ischemia. If the stool O&P analysis is negative for *Giardia* organisms and the index of suspicion for giardiasis is high, a *Giardia* antigen test can be useful. A stool test for *Clostridium difficile* toxin in patients with a history of antibiotic use may be useful because this toxin can be detected up to 10 weeks after antibiotic therapy and occurs in 25% to 40% of patients on long-term antibiotic treatment.[4] Cephalosporins, penicillins, and clindamycin are commonly implicated antibiotics associated with a positive stool *C. difficile* toxin test. A positive *C. difficile* toxin test, however, is most often associated with pseudomembranous colitis.[4] If hemolytic uremic syndrome (HUS) is suspected, a stool *E. coli* 0157:H7 toxin test is appropriate. Stool cultures have a low diagnostic sensitivity for enteric pathogens and their use has been questioned. Evaluation of stool for ova and parasites would be appropriate if the travel history included a stay in areas where *Entamoeba histolytica* or *Cryptosporidium* are endemic or visits to day care centers where individuals infected with *Cryptosporidium* or *Giardia* were present.[4]

In our patient, both aerobic and anaerobic blood cultures were positive for *S. typhi* while urine and fecal cultures were negative for bacteria. When attempting to identify enteric pathogens such as *Shigella* and *Salmonella* spp, selective growth medias are used such as Hektoen enteric (HE) agar or xylose-lysine-deoxycholate (XLD) agar, both of which are designed to inhibit the growth of *E. coli* and other coliform organisms.[6] When this patient's blood was cultured on MacConkey agar, clear, colorless colonies formed because *S. typhi*, a lactose non-fermenter, is unable to utilize the available lactose. The growth of colonies with a black center occurred on HE agar [**Image 1**]. Although many *Salmonella* serotypes are not distinguishable by biochemical characteristics, *S. typhi* possesses unique biochemical traits. It produces only trace amounts of hydrogen sulfide (H_2S) on the slant and butt in TSI (triple sugar iron) agar culture.[6] Moreover, *Salmonella typhi* strains are negative in the following reactions: indole, citrate, motility, urease, and gas formation in dextrose, but are able to utilize lysine [**Image 2**].

In patients with *S. typhi* infection, when acute and convalescent serum samples are compared, a 4-fold or greater increase in antibody titer by the Widal test is considered positive for an acute infection.[5] Immunoelectrophoresis and PCR methods have been used primarily in the research setting and have shown only limited success in diagnosing infection with *S. typhi*. Leukopenia has been reported in 16% to 46% of patients with *S. typhi* infection.[7,8] Moreover, in 2 studies of a series of cases, 67% of patients with *S. typhi* infection had no eosinophils on a peripheral blood smear.[9,10] This finding is helpful in distinguishing between helminth (ie, parasitic worms) and *S. typhi* infection in geographic areas where infection with helminths is endemic as eosinophilia is commonly observed in patients with helminth infections. Liver function test (eg, AST, ALT, bilirubin, alkaline phosphatase) values are typically elevated, and may be striking, in patients with *S. typhi* infection, while typical urinalysis findings in such patients include proteinuria, pyuria, and the presence of casts.[5]

4. ***Most likely diagnosis:*** enteric fever caused by *Salmonella typhi* infection.

Infection with enteric pathogens, such as *S. typhi*, is characterized by a clinical syndrome consisting of abdominal pain along with fever, which makes it distinct from that seen in patients with acute gastroenteritis. These pathogens generally inhabit the GI tract and cause 1 of 3 clinical syndromes: 1) enteric fever, 2) mesenteric adenitis, or 3) eosinophilia. Enteric fever is the most serious of these syndromes, caused by several different bacteria, and is characterized by the presence of fever, headache, splenomegaly, abdominal pain, bacteremia, and occasionally a skin rash.[5]

Enteric fever occurs as an acute syndrome in which the initial symptoms include fever, headache, abdominal pain, bradycardia, splenomegaly, and leukopenia.[5] This syndrome is typified by typhoid fever, which is caused by infection with *Salmonella typhi*, although other *Salmonella* spp. [eg, *S. hirschfeldii* (previously called *S. paratyphi* C) and *S. choleraesuis*] can cause a similar clinical syndrome [**T3**]. Typhoid fever is a major problem in areas where sanitation is poor and fecal contamination of food and water occurs. Enteric fever occurs more commonly in children and young adults in the United States and elsewhere. Since humans are the only reservoir for *S. typhi*, a history of travel to a geographic area where sanitation is poor or direct contact with an infected or carrier individual is important information to health care providers. During 1985 to 1994, 72% of all cases (2,445) of enteric fever in the United States were acquired abroad.[11] The majority of these cases (80%) were acquired from travel in Mexico, India, Philippines, Pakistan, El Salvador, and Haiti.[11,12]

When the bacteria that cause enteric fever are ingested, they are able to survive the acidic environment of the stomach and gain access to the small intestine where they penetrate the intestinal epithelium. They multiply in the lymphoid tissue and further disseminate by either the lymphatic system and/or the blood. Species of *Salmonella* can grow inside cells of the lymph nodes, spleen, liver, and bone marrow.

The symptoms of *S. typhi* infection begin with relapsing fevers, which eventually become constant during the first few days of infection. Most patients report headache and fever as common symptoms, and both constipation and diarrhea have also been reported to occur.[7-9,13] Fever occurs in 90% of cases; however, bacteriologic confirmation of typhoid fever has occurred in patients without fever.[7,8] While the classical symptoms of *S. typhi* infection are remitting and subsequently become constant during the first week of infection, deviations from this pattern are found in areas where infection with this organism is endemic.[10,13] Other findings suggestive of enteric fever are a relative bradycardia and the presence of "rose spots" (ie, skin lesions consisting of erythematous macules or papules) which are observed in more than half of all light-skinned patients with enteric fever and less frequently in dark-skinned patients.[5] Rose spots are observed more frequently, however, in patients with *S. typhi* infection than in patients with enteric fever caused by other bacterial organisms.[14,15]

The laboratory diagnosis of enteric fever is made by isolating the infectious organism from a blood, bone marrow, stool, and/or urine culture. Cultures of blood, stool, or urine need to be obtained before antibiotics are administered. Patients with the most severe disease are the most likely to have positive cultures. Moreover, bone marrow cultures have been found to be positive when blood cultures are negative, and stool cultures are positive in less than half of all patients with enteric fever, while urine cultures are even less likely to be positive.[5] Interestingly, culture of the rose spots has been reported to be positive in almost two-thirds of patients with enteric fever even after antimicrobial therapy has been initiated.[16]

Antimicrobial susceptibility testing is important to selecting the most appropriate drug therapy for treatment of patients with enteric fever, especially when the patient has a history of travel to an area where enteric fever is endemic and resistance to the bacterial organisms that cause this fever is more common. Susceptibility testing for *S. typhi*, however, does not necessarily predict drug efficacy as the organism is localized intracellularly.[5] In 1 study, 14% of patients in New Delhi, India with positive blood cultures for *S. typhi* did not respond to ciprofloxacin, even though susceptibility testing demonstrated sensitivity to this drug.[17]

5. Patients with enteric fever should be treated empirically even before the diagnosis is confirmed by culture. Ampicillin, trimethoprim-sulfamethoxazole (TMP-SMX), and chorampheni-col are often used in the treatment of enteric fever; however, isolates of *S. typhi* resistant to these drugs are becoming more common around the world.[5] Chloramphenicol and TMP-SMX are used in patients with organisms that are not sensitive to ampicillin. Other widely used drugs in the treatment of enteric fever include fluoroquinolones (eg, ciprofloxican or ofloxacin); however, there are reports of resistance to these antibiotics as well.[5] Fluoroquinolones are well tolerated, are able to reach high concentrations in phagocytic cells and bile, and result in a faster response than cephalosporins. However, they are contraindicated in children because of the potential damage to cartilage and tendons. Third generation cephalosporins (eg, ceftriaxone) and the monobactam, aztreonam, are also effective in treating patients with enteric fever.

Vaccination against *S. typhi* is recommended for travelers to geographic areas where typhoid fever is endemic or to remote areas where proper food and water storage is difficult. Moreover, vaccination is helpful in preventing disease when exposure to chronic carriers of typhoid fever is likely. The vaccine consists of an oral preparation of an attenuated live strain intended for individuals over the age of 6 and a parenteral inactivated vaccine that can be used in individuals over the age of 2. Oral vaccination requires 4 separate doses every other day and provides protection for 5 years. It is about 70% effective and is well tolerated.[5] The parenteral polysaccharide Vi-antigen vaccine offers 70% protection with 1 dose for those who must travel immediately.[5]

Treatment and Course _____

The patient's symptoms were initially diagnosed as giardiasis, and for this reason the patient was placed on metronidazole q.i.d. During the course of his hospitalization, stool cultures revealed the presence of *Salmonella typhi*. Gastroenteritis from *S. typhi* infection was thought to have contributed to the patient's ill appearance, diarrhea, and abnormal laboratory values. The *Giardia* infection was a non-related infection, which had co-incubated with the bacterial infection with *Salmonella* species. The patient was placed on a second-generation cephalosporin (for which antimicrobial susceptibility testing determined bacteria sensitivity) intravenously and then orally to finish a 14-day course of drug therapy as an outpatient. The patient's diarrhea resolved by hospital day 4, and he was tolerating oral medications by the time he was discharged. The patient's hyponatremia was treated with intravenous physiological saline and his sodium, chloride, phosphorous, potassium, and magnesium levels were normal by the time he was discharged. He was afebrile for 48 hours prior to discharge, appeared well, and was discharged with instructions to remain on antibiotic therapy with the second-generation cephalosporin.

References

1. Gibbs MA, Wolfson AB, Tayal VS. Electrolyte Disturbances. In: *Rosen's Emergency Medicine: Concepts and Clinical Practice.* Rosen P, Marx J, Hockberger R, et al, eds. St. Louis: Mosby, 2002:1724-1744.

2. Morgenstern R, Hayes PC. The liver in typhoid fever: always affected, not just a complication. *Am J Gastroenterol.* 1991;86:1235-1239.

3. Shetty AK, Mital SR, Bahrainwala AH, et al. Typhoid hepatitis in children. *J Trop Pediatr.* 1999;45:287-290.

4. Gough JE, Clement PA. Diarrhea. In: *Rosen's Emergency Medicine: Concepts and Clinical Practice.* Rosen P, Marx J, Hockberger R, Walls R, eds. St. Louis: Mosby, 2002:201-208.

5. Pearson RD, Guerrant RL. Enteric fever and other causes of abdominal symptoms with fever. In: *Mandell, Douglas, and Bennett's Principles and Practice of Infectious Diseases.* Mandell G, Douglas RG, Bennett JE, et al, eds. Philadelphia: Churchill Livingstone, 2000:1136-1150.

6. Koneman EW, Allen SD, Janda WM, et al. *The Enterobacteriaceae. Color Atlas and Textbook of Diagnostic Microbiology.* Philadelphia: Lippincott Williams & Wilkins, 1997:171-252.

7. Wicks AC, Holmes GS, Davidson L. Endemic typhoid fever. A diagnostic pitfall. *Q J Med.* 1971;40:341-354.

8. Hoffman TA, Ruiz CJ, Counts GW, et al. Waterborne typhoid fever in Dade County, Florida. Clinical and therapeutic evaluation of 105 bacteremic patients. *Am J Med.* 1975;59:481-487.

9. Kamat SA, Herzog C. Typhoid: Clinical picture and response to chloramphenicol. Prospective study in Bombay (1972). *Infection.* 1977;5:85-91.

10. Gulati PD, Saxena SN, Gupta PS, et al. Changing pattern of typhoid fever. *Am J Med.* 1968;45:544-548.

11. Mermin JH, Townes JM, Gerber M, et al. Typhoid fever in the United States, 1985-1994: Changing risks of international travel and increasing antimicrobial resistance. *Arch Intern Med.* 1998;158:633-638.

12. Ryan CA, Hargrett-Bean NT, Blake PA. *Salmonella typhi* infections in the United States, 1975-1984: Increasing role of foreign travel. *Rev Infect Dis.* 1989;11:1-8.

13. Samantray SK, Johnson SC, Chakrabarti AK. Enteric fever: an analysis of 500 cases. *Practitioner.* 1977;218:400-408.

14. Wahab MF, Robertson RP, Raasch FO. Paratyphoid A fever. *Ann Intern Med.* 1969;70:913-917.

15. Meals RA. Paratyphoid fever: A report of 62 cases with several unusual findings and a review of the literature. *Arch Intern Med.* 1976;136:1422-1428.

16. Gilman RH, Terminel M, Levine MM, et al. Relative efficacy of blood, urine, rectal swab, bone-marrow, and rose-spot cultures for recovery of *Salmonella typhi* in typhoid fever. *Lancet.* 1975;1:1211-1213.

17. Sinha A, Sazawal S, Kumar R, et al. Typhoid fever in children aged less than 5 years. *Lancet.* 1999;354:734-737.

Recurrent Headache and Febrile Attacks in a Young Woman

Ibrahim A. Hashim,[1] Mohammed Nabil Richi[2]

[1]*Departments of Pathology, and* [2]*Internal Medicine, King Khalid National Guard Hospital, Jeddah, Kingdom of Saudi Arabia*

Patient: 24-year-old woman.

Chief Complaint: Headache, photophobia, painful and stiff neck, nausea and vomiting (5 to 6 episodes).

Past Medical History: Two years ago, the patient presented twice to the emergency department (ED) over a 2-week period with clinical signs and symptoms suggestive of meningitis. Laboratory investigation of her cerebrospinal fluid (CSF) showed decreased glucose and increased total protein, findings suggestive of bacterial meningitis; however, the CSF cell count was low and no bacterial growth was obtained. Antibiotics were administered and the patient was discharged.

Drug History: No current history of any medications, drugs of abuse, or therapeutic drugs. No other drug history was noted apart from Coproxamol and antibiotics (Augmentin, gentamicin, bezylpenicillin, and chloramphenicol) taken at various times following her earlier admission to the ED.

Physical Examination: The patient was febrile (temperature, 38°C), mildly bradycardic (pulse: 80 bpm), borderline hypertensive (blood pressure, 140/80 mm Hg), with neck stiffness, negative Kernig sign (a sign of meningitis in which the patient, in the sitting posture or when lying with the thigh flexed upon the abdomen, cannot completely extend the leg), and no photophobia.

Results of Other Diagnostic Procedures: A computed tomography (CT) scan of the brain was performed and showed a small calcified lesion to the left of the torculax in the posterior fossa which looked like an old lesion (possibly an old granuloma, tuberculous or listerial infection, or a residue of some incident in childhood or infancy) of no current clinical significance. Overall, CT findings on this admission were similar to those obtained during her first presentation to the ED 2 years ago. There was no evidence of hydrocephalus, abscesses, or cysts.

Questions _____

1. What is(are) this patient's most striking laboratory result(s)?

2. How do you explain this patient's most striking laboratory result(s)?

3. What condition(s) does (do) this patient's laboratory and other findings suggest?

4. What are the principal complications found in this patient's condition?

5. What is(are) the most likely cause(s) of the principal complications found in this patient's condition?

6. Which laboratory and non-laboratory test(s) are appropriate to order on this patient and why?

7. What is the most appropriate treatment for this patient?

T1. Principal Laboratory Findings

Test	Patient's Result	"Normal" Reference Range
Serum		
Albumin	4.82	3.5-4.8 g/dL
IgG	1,120	694-1,618 mg/dL
Alb/IgG ratio	4.30	
CSF		
Appearance	Turbid*	Clear
Cell count	>2,000 (89% PMNs)	0-5 nucleated cells/mL
Glucose	14.4	40-70 mg/dL
Total protein	1,740	15-45 mg/dL
Albumin	1,650	13.9-24.6 mg/dL
IgG	370	0.5-6.1 mg/dL
Alb/IgG ratio	4.46	
CSF indices[†]: Alb index	342.3	<9.0
IgG index	9.6	0.34-0.58
IgG Synthesis rate	1767	<3.3 mg/day
IgG_{loc}	340	<0.0 mg/dL
Electrophoresis	3 bands[‡]	
Culture	No growth	No growth
LA tests for bacterial antigens	Negative	Negative
Mantoux test[§] for *Mycobacteria* spp.	Negative	Negative
Analysis for *Listeria* spp.	Negative	Negative

*Sample became clear after centrifugation.
[†]CSF indices were calculated according to the formulas:
Alb index = Q_{Alb} × 1000; where, Q_{Alb} = Alb_S/Alb_{CSF}
IgG index = $(IgG_{CSF} × Alb_S)/(IgG_S × Alb_{CSF})$
IgG synthesis rate = $\{[IgG_{CSF} − (IgG_S/369)] − [Alb_{CSF} − (Alb_S/230) × (IgGS/AlbS) × 0.43]\} × 5$
$IgG_{loc} = \{Q_{IgG} − 0.8[Q_{Alb}^2 + (15 × 10^{-6})]^{1/2} + 1.8 × 10^{-3}\} × IgG_S$; where, $Q_{IgG} = IgG_{CSF}/IgG_S$
[‡]An albumin band and bands in the alpha-2 and beta-globulin regions.
[§]At 1:10000 dilution.
CSF, cerebrospinal fluid; IgG, immunoglobulin G; Alb, albumin; PMNs, polymorphonuclear leukocytes; S, serum; IgGloc, local synthesis of IgG; LA, latex agglutination; spp, species.

Possible Answers

1. Markedly increased CSF cell count, total protein, albumin, and IgG values; markedly decreased glucose concentration; markedly abnormal CSF indices; and negative tests for bacterial organisms.

2. The markedly increased CSF nucleated cell count (89% polymorphonuclear leukocytes), when coupled with the patient's presenting signs (meningeal inflammation) and symptoms (headache, recurrent febrile attacks), are suggestive of Mollaret meningitis. The increased CSF total protein and decreased glucose concentrations are consistent with a bacterial meningitis; however, microbiological analysis failed to isolate or identify a causative organism. Moreover, the CSF total protein concentration was markedly higher than that normally seen in patients with bacterial meningitis, while this patient's values for all CSF indices were considerably higher than those observed typically in patients with multiple sclerosis (MS). In addition, this patient's CSF electrophoresis pattern did not demonstrate the presence of oligoclonal bands (o-bands) in the gamma-region. In active disease, o-bands are present on electrophoresis of CSF from 95% of MS cases.[1]

Diagnosing central nervous system (CNS) infection relies heavily on biochemical and microbiological analyses of CSF. Although microbiological identification of an infectious bacterial organism from the culture of CSF from a patient with signs and symptoms suggestive of meningitis provides a definitive diagnosis of bacterial meningitis, most clinical chemistry laboratories also provide measurements of CSF glucose and total protein concentrations, although results for these tests are not always conclusive. More than 80% of CSF protein originates from plasma by ultrafiltration of low molecular weight proteins through the walls of the capillaries in the meninges and choroid plexus. The remainder originates from intrathecal synthesis. Bacterial infection of the meninges normally results in increased CSF total protein levels due to altered permeability of the blood-brain-barrier (BBB) and/or increased intrathecal synthesis of immunoglobulins by activated lymphocytes and/or bacterial proteins from increased growth of bacteria within the meninges and CSF. Because bacteria metabolize glucose for energy, a decreased CSF glucose concentration is suggestive of bacterial infection; however, other non-inflammatory conditions such as a neoplasm can also cause reduced CSF glucose levels. In cases of viral infection or autoimmune encephalitis, glucose levels will remain within the reference range whereas total protein is typically elevated. The negative microbiology findings in our patient may be explained by the patient's broad-spectrum antibiotic treatment. Moreover, the fact that the patient's condition improved over time, concomitant with a decrease in her CSF total protein and an increase in her CSF glucose levels, during antibiotic treatment provides additional evidence in support of bacterial meningitis as the cause of this patient's signs, symptoms, and laboratory findings. Lastly, the similarity between serum and CSF values for the Alb/IgG ratio and the markedly increased Alb index suggest further that changes in the permeability of the BBB are the most likely cause of her markedly increased CSF IgG concentration rather than intrathecal production of IgG, a characteristic finding in patients with MS. The Alb index is a sensitive indicator of abnormalities in the permeability of the BBB.

3. ***Most likely diagnosis:*** *Mollaret meningitis.* This is a rare cause of recurrent aseptic meningitis characterized by numerous febrile episodes that may occur over many years with symptom-free intervals ranging from weeks to years. The condition was described in 1944 and is associated with the presence of epithelial and/or endothelial cells in the CSF. Although Mollaret suspected that the disease symptoms were of viral origin, no viral agent has ever been found. In our patient, 2 prior recurrent febrile episodes occurred over a 2-week period, and this third episode (2 years later) was associated with similar presenting signs and symptoms and biochemical findings except for a much higher CSF total protein concentration in the recent episode. In all episodes, biochemical analysis of CSF showed decreased CSF glucose and increased total protein—a finding suggestive of bacterial meningitis, despite the negative microbiology findings. The failure to show bacterial growth in her CSF during her prior episodes was due most likely to the antibiotic treatment, prescribed by her general practitioner (GP), 1 week prior to her admission to the ED. A week later, her symptoms recurred and her CSF demonstrated a cell count of 300 nucleated cells/mL, a glucose concentration of less than 18 mg/dL, and a total protein concentration of 650 mg/dL.

Several cases of aseptic meningitis have been reported previously. Brunel and colleagues[2] reported a case of a child with 5 episodes of unexplained aseptic neutrophilic meningitis, later attributed to an intracranial epidermoid cyst. Schwartz and Ballentine[3] described a case of a child who presented 10 times with recurrent aseptic meningitis and an intracranial epidermoid tumor was found at autopsy. Becker and deChadarevian[4] described a female who presented at age 6 years with aseptic neutrophilic meningitis and subsequently had 17 febrile episodes over a 42-month period. Although this patient's cranial CT scans were negative on 2 occasions, a subsequent scan revealed the presence of an epidermoid cyst in the posterior fossa. In 1990, Crossley and Dismukes[5] described the case of a 32-year-old man who presented initially in 1972, and during a 14-year period was hospitalized 30 times for recurrent attacks of aseptic meningitis which occurred more frequently during the most recent 4-year period. The mean interval between episodes in the first 9 years was about 237 ± 68 days, while the mean interval during the last 4 years was 97 ± 40 days. Two cranial CT scans during this patient's episodes of meningitis were negative; however, examination of his CSF revealed the presence, on several occasion, of large mononuclear cells originally described by Mollaret as endothelial cells. However, subsequent ultrastructural and immunocytochemical studies indicated a mono-cyte/macrophage lineage for these cells. Thirteen years later, this patient's cranial CT scan revealed the presence of a 2.2 cm mass in the posterior fossa, which proved to be an avascular, well encapsulated cyst that was surgically resected. In the 2 years following excision of the cyst, the patient had no further episodes of meningitis. Cranial CT scans may be negative in patients with Mollaret's meningitis if the CT scan is obtained during episodes of acute meningitis when epidermoid cysts may be empty or very small following extravasation of the cyst fluid into the CSF. It has been suggested that the use of contrast-enhanced CT or nuclear magnetic resonance imaging (MRI) during asymptomatic intervals is useful in visualizing the presence of a cranial cyst(s).[6]

4. The principal complications of meningitis include neuropathy with possible neurological deficit. There is no specific treatment protocol for these patients; however, patients are treated typically with broad-spectrum antibiotics and observed closely. Data on long-term follow-up of these patients are not available in the literature. Our patient had 3 recurrent episodes of aseptic meningitis over a 2-year period and will need to be closely monitored.

5. The cause(s) of Mollaret meningitis, including the etiology of the neurological deficit associated with this disease, is (are) currently unknown.

6. Cerebrospinal fluid electrophoresis and serum interleukin-6 (IL-6) levels. Protein electrophoresis of CSF from patients with meningitis may be useful because in patients with meningitis there is inflammation of the meningeal membrane that leads to increased permeability of the BBB and the leakage of plasma proteins into the CSF. Thus, in these patients, the CSF protein electrophoretic pattern is similar to that of serum. In addition, an increased globulin band may also be observed, indicative of increased CSF intrathecal immunoglobulin synthesis. This patient's mark-edly increased CSF IgG synthesis rate and IgG$_{loc}$ value are consistent with increased intrathecal IgG synthesis, while the markedly increased Alb index is consistent with significant increased permeability of the BBB [**T1**]. Measurement of CSF IL-6 levels may be useful in evaluating patients with meningitis because IL-6 is a useful marker of inflammation. We have shown that elevated CSF IL-6 levels occur in patients with bacterial meningitis but not in those without meningitis or with viral or aseptic meningitis.[7] Despite our patient's increased CSF total protein, suggestive of bacterial meningitis, her CSF IL-6 level was not elevated, lending further support to the diagnosis of aseptic meningitis.

7. There is no known cure for this condition. Patients with Mollaret meningitis are treated typically with broad spectrum antibiotic therapy and conservative follow-up. Both colchicine and indomethacin have been reported to relieve the symptoms of this disease.[8]

Treatment and Course

The patient was treated with antibiotics, recovered well, and was discharged to follow-up over the next few months.

Keywords

cerebrospinal fluid, Mollaret meningitis, CSF indices

References

1. Peter JB, Bowman RL. Intra-blood-brain barrier synthesis of IgG: Comparison of IgG synthesis formulas in a computer model and in 1,629 consecutive specimens. *Neurology.* 1992;42:510-515.

2. Brunel D, Frerebeau J, Astruc J, et al. Meningite puriformoe aseptique, 5 fois recidivante, revelation d'un kyste epidermoid du 3 evntricule. *Lyon Med.* 1972;228:547-551.

3. Schwartz JF., Ballentine JD. Recurrent meningitis due to an intracranial epidermoid. *Neurology.* 1978;28:124-129.

4. deChadarevian JP, Becker WJ. Mollaret's recurrent aseptic meningitis: Relationship to epidermoid cyst. *J Neuropathol Exp Neurol.* 1980;39:661-669.

5. Crossley GH, Dismukes WE. Central nervous system epidermoid cyst: A probable etiology of Mollaret's meningitis. *A J Med.* 1990;89:805-806.

6. Aristegui FJ, Delgado RA, Oleaga ZL, et al. Mollaret's recurrent aseptic meningitis and cerebral epidermoid cyst. *Paediatric Neurology.* 1998;2:156-159.

7. Hashim IA, Walsh A, Hart CA, et al. Cerebrospinal fluid interleukin-6 and its diagnostic value in the investigation of meningitis. *Ann Clin Biochem.* 1995;32:289-296.

8. Wynants H, Taelman H, Martin JJ, et al. Recurring aseptic meningitis after travel to the tropics: A case of Mollaret's meningitis? Case report with review of the literature. *Clin Neurology Neurosurgery.* 2000;102:113-115.

Nocardia Meningitis

Monte S. Willis, Dominick Cavuoti, Rita Gander

Department of Pathology, The University of Texas Southwestern Medical Center, Dallas, TX

Patient: 69-year-old Caucasian male.

Family History: N/A

Drug History: N/A

Chief Complaint: 7-day history of worsening headache, fever, chills, night sweats, and altered mental status on July 30, 2001.

Medical History: Patient was 14 months status post glioblastoma multiforme tumor removal with positive margins in May 2000. Subsequent treatment included radiation therapy and chemotherapy with Temozolomide. An MRI performed on June 18, 2001 revealed residual and recurrent tumor with enlargement of a ring enhancing lesion.

Physical Examination: Diaphoretic and tachypneic with course breath sounds bilaterally in all fields. Neurologically, only response to painful stimuli was present.

Principal Laboratory Findings: The patient underwent a lumbar puncture. Analysis of the CSF revealed the following: glucose <10 mg/dL (Normal 40-70 mg/dL), protein 750 mg/dL (Normal 15-45 mg/dL), nucleated cells 490/μL (79% neutrophils, 12% lymphocytes, and 9% monocytes), and 70/μL RBCs. Gram stain revealed no organisms. Routine aerobic, fungal, and mycobacterial cultures were submitted. On day 2 of incubation, small tan colonies of a thin, branching gram-positive rod were growing on blood and chocolate agar [**Image 1**]. The rods were partially acid-fast, but negative by conventional Ziehl-Neelsen acid fast staining [**Image 2**]. A reference laboratory found the *Nocardia* species to be *Nocardia farcinica* and susceptible to amikacin, ciprofloxacin, linezolid, and sulfamethoxazole (which the patient was given empirically). Resistance to ampicillin, tobrymycin, clarithromycin, and imipenem was also identified.

Questions

1. What is the differential diagnosis for branching gram-positive rods recovered in aerobic culture?

2. Where are *Nocardia* found? What types of patients are at risk for *Nocardia* infections?

3. What are the clinical manifestations of nocardiosis?

4. How are *Nocardia* infections treated?

5. What are side effects that may be seen with treatment?

6. Should identification to species and susceptibilities be performed on *Nocardia* spp.?

7. What is the prognosis of *Nocardia* infection? What is the overall prognosis in this patient?

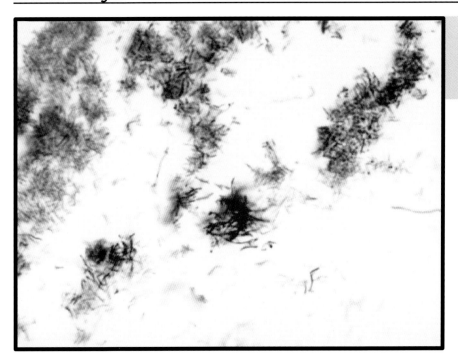

Image 1_Gram stain preparation of growth from colonies on blood agar plate.

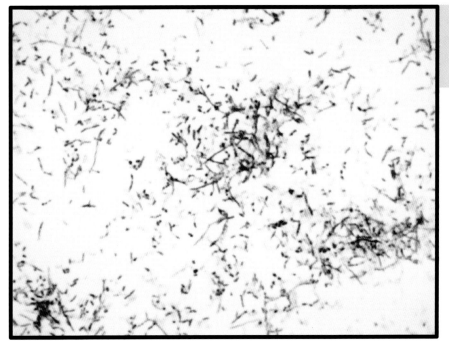

Image 2_Partial acid fast staining of growth from colonies on blood agar plate.

Possible Answers

1. In general, the differential diagnosis for branching gram-positive rods in the United States include *Actinomyces* spp. and *Nocardia* spp. *Nocardia* are partially acid-fast whereas some *Actinomyces* spp. are anaerobic but may be recovered in an aerobic environment after extended incubation.[1]

2. *Nocardia* spp. are found throughout the environment in soil, grasses, straw, grains, and decaying organic materials. Transmission occurs via inhalation of aerosilized dust from these sources. Individuals at increased risk for *Nocardia* infections have a compromised cellular

immunity (due to long-term steroid use, primary immunodeficiency, organ transplantation and immunosuppression therapy, or cytotoxic chemotherapy).[2] In 1976, between 500 and 1000 people were infected with *Nocardia* spp. in the United States, which has undoubtedly increased with increased immunosuppression due to HIV/AIDS, organ transplantation, and chemotherapy.[2] The prevalence is 2-3 times more frequent in men than in women.[2]

3. The 2 main manifestations of *Nocardia* spp. infection are skin lesions and visceral lesions. Primary skin lesions manifest as mycetomas which are uncommon in the United States. Visceral infections are the common form found in the United States. Approximately 75% of these cases involve the lungs and 25% involve the central nervous system (disseminated infection is rare).[2] The lung manifestations include both brochopneumonia and pulmonary abscesses. Of the CNS infections, abscesses are more common than meningitis.

4. The clinical laboratory findings in *Nocardia* meningitis are typical for bacterial meningitis: elevated CSF protein, pleocytosis, and hypoglycorrhachia. The classic presentation is a persistent neutrophilic meningitis with sterile routine aerobic cultures. The frequency with which the CNS is involved has brought about the recommendation that all immunosuppressed patients with pulmonary *nocardiosis* should have a cranial CT, even when asymptomatic.[2]

Empirically, the sulfonamides are the drug of choice, with trimethoprin-sulfamethoxazole (TMP-SMX) being the formulation currently preferred. Clinical improvement is generally seen within 3-5 days after initiation of therapy. In general, immunosuppresive drugs may be continued during antibiotic treatment and the length of treatment depends upon underlying illnesses. A minimum of 3 months of treatment is thought to prevent recurrence that is common with a shorter treatment period. Brain abscesses require surgical debridement in addition to antibiotic therapy.

A susceptibility study of 78 clinical isolates of the *N. asteroides complex* (*N. asteroides*, *N. farcinica*, and *N. nova*) from the United States detected several antibiotic resistance patterns.[4] The first, associated with *N. farcinica*, demonstrated resistance to cefotoxime, ceftriaxone, and cefamandole and accounted for about 20% of isolates. The second, associated with *N. nova*, demonstrated susceptibility to ampicillin and erythromycin and accounted for another 20% of isolates. The last group, associated with *N. asteroides*, demonstrated resistance to broad spectrum cephalosporins, susceptibility to ampicillin and carbenicillin, and intermediate susceptibility to imipenem and accounted for 60% of the isolates.[3]

The patient in this case study improved within 5 days of TMP-SMX treatment and was discharged to home on August 10, 2001 with improved mental status. The decision was made to leave the patient on TMP-SMX indefinitely due to the progressive nature of his tumor. Cultures of *Nocardia* were sent to an outside laboratory for speciation and susceptibility.

Nocardia farcinica is rare but can cause localized and disseminated infections.[5] In a recent review of case reports, only 61% of the patients received adequate antibiotic therapy.[5] *N. farcinica* isolates were found to be susceptible to amikacin, imipenem, ciprofloxacin, and TMP-SMX and resistant to third-generation cephalosporins and aminoglycosides.[5] Although resistance to TMP-SMX has been demonstrated in vitro, it may still be effective in vivo.[5] *N. farcinica* should be kept in mind in patients with indolent *Nocardia* infections not responding to third-generation cephalosporins.[5]

5. Sulfonamide intolerance is seen in up to 55% of AIDS patients.[1] Hypersensitivity reactions may be encountered and require desensitization or the use of alternative drugs. These include amikacin and imipenem or third-generation cephalosporins which have increased CNS penetration and low toxicity compared to sulfonamides.[1]

6. Most clinical laboratories are able to isolate *Nocardia* spp., but final speciation and antimicrobial susceptibility are a challenge because of their slow growth and infrequent isolation. The strains should be referred to specialized laboratories for full identification and susceptibility testing because of the wide variation in susceptibility patterns.

7. The clinical outcome depends on clinical manifestations of *nocardiosis*. With skin involvement, cure rates of nearly 100% are seen, which can be compared with 90% of pulmonary manifestations, 63% of systemic infections, and 50% with brain abscess.[6] This is likely due, in part, to underlying immunosuppression/immunodeficiency or delay in diagnosis.[3] In this particular patient with GBM, the median survival is 1 year, which varies widely depending on histology, response to treatment, and other factors.

References _____

1. Sorrell TC, Iredell JR, Mitchell DH. *Nocardia* species. In: Mandel GL, Douglas R, Bennet JE, eds. *Principals and Practice of Infectious Diseases*. 5th ed. New York, NY: Churchill Livingstone; 2000:2637-2645.

2. Bullock WE. *Norcadiosis*. In: Goldman L, Bennett JC, and Drazen JM, eds. *Cecil Textbook of Medicine*. 21st ed. Philadelphia, PA: W.B. Saunders Company; 2000:1716-1717.

3. Jacobs RF, Schultze GE. Nocardia. In: Berman RE, Kliegman R, and Jenson HG, eds. *Nelson Textbook of Pediatrics*. 16th ed. Philadelphia, PA: W.B. Saunders Company; 2000:824-825.

4. Wallace RJ, Steele LC, Sumter G, Smith JM. Antimicrobial susceptibility patterns of *Nocardia asteroides. Antimicrob Agents Chemother.* 1998;32:1776.

5. Torres OH, Domingo P, Pericas R, Boiron JA, Montiel JA, and Vazquez G. Infection caused by *Nocardia farcinica*: Case Report and Review. *Eur J Clin Microbiol Infect Dis.* 2000;19:205-212.

6. Smego RA Jr, Moeller MB, Gallas HA. Trimethoprin-sulfamethoxazole therapy for *Nocardia* infections. *Arch Intern Med.* 1983;143:711-718.

Glossary _____

Glioblastoma multiforme (GBM): the most common and most aggressive primary brain tumor; a variant of astrocytoma, most common in adults, with a median survival of less than 1 year despite surgery, radiation therapy, and/or chemotherapy; the cause of these tumors is unknown, with familial examples accounting for only 1%, and is more common in older age groups.

Temozolomide: an alkylating chemotherapeutic agent.

Proximal Extremity Weakness and Altered Mental Status

Chad F. Brouse, Monte S. Willis

Department of Pathology, University of Texas Southwestern Medical Center, Dallas, TX

Patient: 65-year-old Liberian woman.

Past Surgical History: None.

Chief Complaint: Four days of progressive weakness and swelling of both arms and upper legs.

History of Present Illness: The patient presented initially to the emergency department (ED) 6 days prior to the current visit with the complaint of progressive weakness and swelling of both arms and upper legs. She stated that she had experienced a similar episode of weakness 1 year earlier that coincided with a "flare" of her polymyositis. Her primary care physician had recently tapered her prednisone to 5 mg/day 1 month earlier (which had previously been 40 mg/day). During this recent ED visit, notable proximal muscle weakness was noted, and she reported periodic difficulty talking because her tongue was numb. The patient was subsequently diagnosed with recurrent polymyositis, her prednisone dose was increased to 60 mg/day, and she was discharged to home. She was brought back to the ED by her family (this visit) with similar symptoms and altered mental status and was hospitalized.

Past Medical History: The patient's past medical history included polymyositis, dermatomyositis, and hypertension all of which had been diagnosed years previously. Her hypertension had been well controlled with medication.

Drug History: Her medications included prednisone, calcium carbonate, metoprolol, and hydrochlorothiazide.

Family/Social History: According to her family and previous records, no family history of diabetes, heart disease, or muscle disease was present. It was noted that she was a refugee from Liberia and had immigrated to the United States "many years ago."

Physical Examination: Her physical examination was normal except for the neurologic findings of upper and lower proximal extremity weakness and unsteady gait. The patient's altered mental status made communication difficult. A left-sided hemiparesis and decreased sensation in her arm were not clearly delineated until 2 days after admission.

Results of Diagnostic Procedures and Additional Tests: Due to her altered mental status, a spinal tap was performed to obtain cerebrospinal fluid (CSF) in order to test for infectious causes of meningitis, including syphilis (VDRL), cryptococcal antigen, cultures (bacterial and fungal), and oligoclonal bands, all of which were negative. The results of screening tests for *Toxoplasma* IgG antibodies by IFA are summarized in [**T1**]. Cerebrospinal fluid indices of antibody, protein, and autoantibody production (ANA, dsDNA, ENA) were also performed. The ANA results are shown in [**T2**]. Autoantibody test results were confirmed by a referral laboratory. Moreover, additional testing for *Toxoplasma* antigens and antibodies was performed by a specialized commercial referral laboratory to delineate further her positive *Toxoplasma* IFA results. In addition, magnetic resonance angiography (MRA), performed after her hospital admission, determined that a right cerebral vascular occlusion involving the anterior and middle cerebral arteries was present.

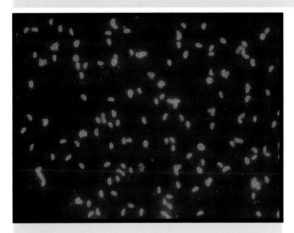

Image 1_Positive *T. gondii* indirect fluorescent antibody (IFA) assay pattern from the patient described in this case study. The patient's serum was added to a glass slide fixed with *T. gondii* tachyzoites followed by incubation and the addition of a fluorescently-labeled [fluorescein isothiocyanate (FITC)] anti-human IgG antibody (400× magnification).

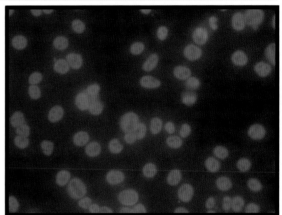

Image 2_Diagnosis of an anti-nuclear antibody (ANA) with a speckled pattern. This assay was performed by adding serum from the patient described in this case study to a glass slide fixed with Hep-2 cells (Hep-2000 ANA, ImmunoConcepts, Sacramento, CA) followed by incubation and the addition of a fluorescently (FITC)-labeled human IgG antibody (400× magnification). The speckled ANA pattern is associated with multiple antigens [ie, Smith (Sm) and ribonuclear protein (RNP)] found in the serum of patients with autoimmune diseases including, systemic lupus erythematosus (SLE), Sjögren syndrome, mixed connective tissue disease (MCTD), and progressive systemic sclerosis.

Questions

1. What is (are) the patient's most striking clinical and laboratory result(s)?

2. How do you explain this patient's most striking laboratory results?

3. What condition(s) does this patient's laboratory and other findings suggest?

4. What are the clinical manifestations of this patient's condition?

5. What is (are) the confounding variable(s) in arriving at this patient's most likely diagnosis?

6. What is the most appropriate treatment of this patient's condition?

Possible Answers

1. Muscle weakness of the proximal arms and legs, left-sided weakness and decreased touch sensation (determined after several days), an unsteady gait, and altered mental status; high titer serum *Toxoplasma* IgG antibody (1:16,384) [**Image 1**], positive CSF *Toxoplasma* IgG antibody titer, positive ANA test (Note: Further investigation

T1. Principal Laboratory Findings

Test		Patient's Result	Reference Interval
Serum			
Toxoplasma antibody:	Total by IFA	> 1:16,384	< 1:256
	IgM by ELISA	0.1	< 2.0
	IgA by ELISA	3.6	< 2.1 (adults)
	IgE by ELISA	Negative	Negative
	Total by S-F dye test	1:8,000	Negative
	IgG AC titer	<1:50	n.a.
	IgG HS titer	1:3,200	n.a.
	AC vs HS titer plot	NAP[a]	
HIV IFA		Negative	Negative
Albumin		3,670	3,484-4,956 mg/dL
IgG		1,660	694-1618 mg/dL
Rheumatoid factor		Negative	Negative (0-20 U/L)
ANA:	Titer	> 1:2,560	< 1:160
	Pattern	Speckled	
Anti-dsDNA		Negative	Negative
Anti-Jo-1		Negative	<1:26
ENA antibody panel[b]		Negative	Negative
CSF			
Toxoplasma antibody:	Total by IFA	1:256	Negative
	Index	5.5[c]	
CSF Albumin		22.5	13.9-24.6 mg/dL
CSF IgG		4.7	0.5-5.9 mg/dL
Albumin index[d]		6.1	0-9
IgG index[e]		0.46	0.34-0.70
IgG synthesis rate[f]		-5.2	< 3.3 mg/dL
IgG$_{loc}$ synthesis rate[g]		-1.91	< 0 mg/dL

[a]*Non-acute pattern based on the x-y plot of the AC (x-axis) versus HS (y-axis) titers.* [b]*Includes antibodies to Smith (Sm), ribonuclear protein (RNP), Sjögren's syndrome A (SSA [Ro]), Sjögren's syndrome B (SSB [La]), scleroderma (Scl)-70, and Jo antigens.* [c]*Toxoplasma antibody index = [CSF Toxoplasma titer/serum Toxoplasma titer] × ([IgG]serum/[IgG]csf) (titers determined by IFA). Interpretation of Toxoplasma antibody index as an indicator of intrathecal IgG synthesis: <1, not indicative; > 1 but < 8, suspicious; > 8, indicative and suggestive of CNS toxoplasmosis.* [d][Alb]csf/[Alb]serum. [e][IgG]csf/[IgG]serum. [f]{([IgG]csf − ([IgG]serum/369)) − ([Alb]csf − ([Alb]serum/230)([IgG]serum/[Alb]serum)(0.43))} × 5. [g]IgGloc = {([IgG]csf/[IgG]serum) − 0.8(([Alb]csf/[Alb]serum)2 + (15 × 10⁻⁶))}1/2 × [IgG] serum. *IFA, indirect fluorescence immunoassay; ELISA, enzyme-linked immunosorbent assay; S-F, Sabin-Feldman; AC, titer determined using acetone-fixed T. gondii tachyzoites; HS, titer determined using formalin-fixed T. gondii tachyzoites; ANA, antinuclear antibodies; dsDNA, double-stranded deoxyribonucleic acid; ENA, extractable nuclear antigens; loc, local.*

into the patient's previous laboratory results uncovered a previously determined high-titer speckled ANA pattern) [**Image 2**], negative RF, anti-dsDNA, anti-Jo-1, ENA antibody panel, and HIV tests, a high titer (1:8,000) *Toxoplasma* antibody by the Sabin-Feldman Dye Test, a low IgM antibody to *Toxoplasma* by an

ELISA method, an elevated *Toxoplasma* IgA by an ELISA method, a negative *Toxoplasma* IgE antibody, a low-titer *Toxoplasma* antibody to acetone-fixed *Toxoplasma* tachyzoites, a high titer toxoplasma antibody to formalin-fixed *Toxoplasma* tachyzoites, and negative or normal CSF tests for: VDRL; cryptococcal antigen;

T2. Characteristics of Various Antibody Isotypes Associated With *T. gondii* Infection*

Antibody Isotype	Characteristics
IgG	Present in serum 1-2 weeks post-infection
	Titer peaks at approximately 6-8 weeks, declines over 1-2 years, but may persist for life
IgM	Present early in infection
	A negative result in immunocompetent patients generally excludes infection
	May persist for 1+ years following infection
IgA	More sensitive for detection of infection of fetus and newborn than IgM antibody
	Perform testing during the first few days of life and retest after 10 days if positive test obtained
	Can persist for months or years following acute infection
	Avidity assay useful in infections during the first trimester of pregnancy
IgE	Presence represents the acute phase of infection in adults, although this antibody isotype may persist in the serum for months
	Positive in cases of congenital infection
	Absence of this antibody isotype does not exclude infection

*Modified from information presented in references 4 and 5.

bacterial, AFB, and fungal cultures; oligoclonal bands; and indices of intrathecal IgG synthesis [**T1**].

2. The patient in this case study had a recent history of polymyositis and a distant history of dermatomyositis. Both poly- and dermatomyositis are characterized by the onset of muscle weakness in a symmetrical manner over weeks to months involving mainly proximal muscles including the pelvic girdle, shoulder girdle, and the neck flexors. Dermatomyositis differs from polymyositis only in that it has a characteristic rash that accompanies or precedes the onset of the muscle weakness. This patient's recent diagnosis of polymyositis was made because she did not have a rash at this presentation, although objective weakness in her upper and lower extremities was present.

This patient's altered mental status had many potential causes with the very limited history available: physical injury (eg, head trauma), systemic infection (eg, pneumonia), intracranial infection (eg, viral or bacterial encephalitis or meningitis), neurosyphilis, fungal infection, parasitic infection (eg, *Toxoplasma* or malarial parasites), intoxication by drugs or poisons, metabolic disorders (eg, hypoglycemia), vascular disorders due to migraine, cerebrovascular disorders

[eg, transient ischemic attack (TIA)], or stroke [cerebrovascular accident (CVA)], cardiovascular disorders (eg, myocardial infarction, congestive heart failure), vasculitis, hematological disorders [eg, anemia, TTP (thrombotic thrombocytopenic purpura)], cerebral degenerative disorders (eg, multiple sclerosis), extracranial neoplasms/space occupying lesions (eg, tumor), or hypersensitivity and autoimmune disorders.[1] Differentiating the cause(s) of this patient's altered mental status was also difficult because of the patient's inability to communicate effectively and her "apparent" symptoms of polymyositis. Cultures and serological tests for bacterial, viral, and parasitic organisms (including *T. gondii*) were performed because of her African country of origin (Liberia) and the potential likelihood of these agents as the cause of her symptoms.

Toxoplasma gondii infection is diagnosed by serological testing for antibodies to this organism; however, many people without apparent disease have antibodies (IgG) against *T. gondii*. This finding is fairly common in immunocompetent individuals who generally have had a mild or subacute infection with *T. gondii*. The prevalence of *T. gondii* in the United States varies regionally; however, 1 American study estimated the overall serological prevalence to be 22.5% and among women of child-bearing age (ie, 15-44 years of age), the prevalence was 15%.[2] This is in sharp contrast to the prevalence in people from Africa, and specifically from Liberia, where greater than 50% of the population have been shown to be seropositive for *T. gondii*.[3]

There are several clinical scenarios in which it is important to differentiate between an acute versus a chronic *T. gondii* infection. For example, if a female becomes infected while she is pregnant, congenital infection of her newborn can be damaging. However, if she had already been exposed to *T. gondii* before the pregnancy, there is no threat to her newborn. Therefore, to differentiate acute from non-acute infection, identification of the antibody isotypes of *T. gondii* is useful.[4]

Acute toxoplasmosis can also be harmful in immunosuppressed patients, where reactivation of *T. gondii* occurs. This includes patients with malignancies, organ transplants, or acquired immunodeficiency syndrome (AIDS). The initial assessment of such patients should include serum testing for *T. gondii*-specific IgG antibodies. If the serum *T. gondii* IgG antibody test is positive, the individual is at risk of reactivation of the disease.[5] When *T. gondii* IgG antibodies are detected in HIV-infected patients with a CD4+ count less than 200/mL, it is prognostic of *Toxoplasma* encephalitis, especially when the titer is >150 IU/mL.[6,7]

In the evaluation of an immunocompetent patient (eg, during pregnancy) for *T. gondii* infection, screening for IgG antibodies to *T. gondii* is a good practice. Since IgM antibodies can be detected for up to 12 months after an acute infection, its usefulness as an indication of acute infection has been questioned. If IgG titers are equivocal, serum from serially collected blood samples should be tested. If IgG titers to *Toxoplasma* are negative (<1:16), then previous *Toxoplasma* infection can be ruled out. A 2-fold rise in antibody titer indicates an acute infection, as does seroconversion from a negative to a positive titer. However, a single high antibody titer is not sufficient for diagnosing toxoplasmosis because of the persistence of a high IgG antibody titer for many years in some individuals.[5]

After an initial infection with *Toxoplasma*, IgG antibodies appear in the serum 1 to 2 weeks later,

peak after 6 to 8 weeks, and decline over the next 1 to 2 years, although in some individuals these antibodies persist for life.[5] The IFA assay used initially to detect IgG *Toxoplasma* antibodies in this patient's serum uses killed organisms as a substrate to detect antibodies against antigens expressed by these organisms [**Image 1**]. False positive IFA results can occur in individuals whose serum contains ANAs, while false negatives can occur in patients with very low *Toxoplasma* antibody titers.[8] The Sabin-Feldman dye test is considered the "gold-standard" test for assessing *Toxoplasma* antibody titer. In this test, live *Toxoplasma* organisms, patient's serum, and complement are mixed together and if the patient's serum contains IgG-specific *Toxoplasma* antibodies, lysis of the organisms occurs. If a positive test occurs, the antibody titer is determined in a manner similar to determining antibody titer by IFA. *Toxoplasma*-specific IgG antibodies can also be determined by ELISA. To differentiate an acute infection from a chronic infection in adults, a differential agglutination test can be performed using formalin- (abbreviated, "HS") or acetone- fixed ("AC") *Toxoplasma* organisms. These agglutination tests require treatment of the patient's serum with 2-mercaptoethanol, which breaks the disulfide bonds in both IgM and IgA antibodies, leaving mainly intact IgG antibodies to assay. An acute pattern demonstrates high titer antibodies to both acetone- and formalin-fixed *Toxoplasma*, while a non-acute pattern demonstrates only high titer antibodies to the formalin-fixed *Toxoplasma* and low titer antibodies to acetone-fixed *Toxoplasma*.

Serum from the patient described in this case study demonstrated high titer IgG *T. gondii* antibodies (1:16,384) by IFA. Since it was discovered that this patient had previously had a positive speckled ANA pattern and ANAs can give false positive IFA results, the Sabin-Feldman dye confirmatory test was performed. This test was positive for high titer (1:8,000) IgG antibodies against *T. gondii*, indicating that her IFA results were a true positive. Moreover, when her serum was assayed, a differential agglutination pattern with high titer (1:3,200) antibodies against formalin-fixed *Toxoplasma* organisms (1:3,200) and low titer (<1:50) antibodies against acetone-fixed organisms were detected, indicating a non-acute infection.

Lastly, this patient's values for the CSF indices (Albumin index, IgG index, IgG synthesis rate, and IgG local synthesis rate) [**T1**] indicate that this patient's IgG antibody production was not occurring intrathecally. Although her CSF:serum *Toxoplasma* IgG antibody index (5.5) was "suspicious for local antibody synthesis," it was not diagnostic of local antibody synthesis and the index value; in this case, it is not reliable because it was determined using CSF and serum IgG antibody values determined by IFA in a patient whose serum was ANA positive, which can give false positive IFA results.

3. **Most likely diagnosis:** *Stroke with the incidental finding of non-acute toxoplasmosis.*

   This patient presented with proximal weakness (consistent with polymyositis) and altered mental status that progressed to left upper extremity weakness, decreased touch sensation, and unsteady gait. These clinical symptoms, when coupled with the MRA findings of right cerebral vascular occlusion in the distribution of the anterior and middle cerebral arteries in the brain, are consistent with a diagnosis of stroke. Serological testing for antibodies to *T. gondii* determined that the patient had non-acute toxoplasmosis; however, this was not realized until several days after the patient was hospitalized and the results of confirmatory testing, performed by a referral laboratory, were made available.

4. Stroke is defined as a neurologic deficit lasting more than 24 hours caused by a deficiency in arterial blood flow to the brain. In contrast, a TIA is defined as a neurologic deficit lasting less than 24 hours, and generally, less than 1 hour.[9] The reason why a clinical distinction is made between a TIA and a stroke is to determine whether brain damage is likely to have occurred so that the extent of any damage (infarction or ischemic necrosis) can be determined quickly.[9] The most common site for atherothrombosis of cerebral blood vessels is the carotid artery bifurcation at the origin of the internal carotid artery. Thrombosis at this site results in symptoms similar to those caused by occlusion of the middle cerebral artery.[9] Occlusion of the anterior cerebral artery (ACA) produces contralateral symptoms of motor and cortical sensory deficiency, including disturbances in gait, speech (eg,

decreased spontaneous speech), and a generalized depression in motor activity.[9] Most strokes involve the middle cerebral artery (MCA) resulting in contralateral hemiparesis and sensory loss in the face and arms. Posterior cerebral artery occlusion can result in contralateral hemiparesis, sensory loss in the legs, as well as vision and memory impairment.[9] The occlusions in this patient's anterior and middle cerebral arteries correlate with the patient's contralateral hemiparesis and sensory loss noted clinically.

5. *Toxoplasma gondii* infection was suspected in this patient as part of the differential diagnosis of muscle weakness and altered mental status. Since the initial *Toxoplasma* antibody screening test by IFA was positive at high titer for IgG antibodies, additional testing by a referral laboratory was performed to determine the nature of the infection (ie, acute versus chronic) to rule out the possibility of *Toxoplasma* encephalitis. These tests were performed or ordered before it was clear that the patient's hemiparesis and sensory deficits were localized to the left side of her body. Nevertheless, the initial and follow-up *T. gondii* antibody testing was necessary to determine the most appropriate treatment for this patient, despite the fact that this patient's toxoplasmosis infection turned out to be unimportant in the selection of that treatment.

Toxoplasma gondii is a parasite found worldwide that commonly causes non-pathologic infection in humans. An understanding of the life cycle of this organism is important in the diagnosis of toxoplasmosis. Three forms of the parasite exist: tachyzoite, cyst, and oocyst. The tachyzoite is the infectious invasive form, the cyst (containing bradyzoites) is found in tissues, and the oocyst (containing sporozoites) is found in the soil and in the feces of mammals of the cat family. The released oocysts from the feces of cats are ingested by a host of mammals, creating a large reservoir of domestic and wild animals. Amplification of the infection, however, occurs in cats where the sexual cycle of the parasite takes place.[4] Humans become infected with *T. gondii* through the ingestion of cysts in raw or uncooked meat (mainly pork and beef), ingestion of mature oocysts in food or water contaminated with cat feces, or through transplacental passage of the parasite from the mother to the fetus, with acute infection of the latter. Transmission through blood transfusion, laboratory accidents, and organ transplantation is less common, and epidemiological evidence exists implicating hematophagous insects as biological vectors of *T. gondii*.[10]

In the United States, the major risk factor associated with *T. gondii* infection is exposure to feces-contaminated water and/or soil by activities such as gardening or the ingestion of undercooked foods which have been contaminated with oocysts or contain cysts. In general, house cats can be vectors for this disease; however, they do not play a major role in the transmission of this disease. Moreover, individuals with predominantly indoor cats fed cooked food (eg, most dry and canned cat foods) are not at risk of acquiring *T. gondii* infection from their cats. It is important, however, that individuals at risk (eg, immunosuppressed individuals and pregnant females) avoid exposure to *T. gondii* by washing their hands frequently, wearing gloves while gardening, cooking meats thoroughly, and avoiding cat feces (litter boxes) used by "outdoor" cats.

The gastrointestinal tract is the major route by which *T. gondii* initially infects its hosts. The tachyzoite form of *T. gondii* is found during primary infection within host cell vacuoles, where the tachyzoites are able to multiply. Here they can multiply every 4 to 6 hours, leading to cell disruption and invasion of nearby cells, or they can be phagocytosed and transported to other areas of the body by the blood and lymphatic systems.[11] Tissue cysts form when tachyzoites enter the cytoplasm of cells and replicate. The most common sites of cyst formation are the central nervous system (CNS) and skeletal, smooth, and cardiac muscles.[12] Bradyzoites released from tissue cysts penetrate epithelial cells in the intestine, spreading first to mesenteric lymph nodes and then to distant organs via the lymphatics and then the blood.

IgG, IgM, IgA, and IgE antibodies are produced in humans in response to *T gondii* infection, and the mainstay of diagnosis of *T. gondii* infection is serologic testing. Since the serum from a relatively high proportion of healthy individuals contains *T. gondii* IgG antibodies, interpretation of serological test results can be challenging. To overcome this challenge, assays for different antibody isotypes have been developed to confirm and differentiate between acute and chronic *T. gondii* infection [**T2**].

In the immunocompetent individual, *T. gondii* infection is symptomatic in approximately 10% of cases, presenting mainly as lymphadenopathy.[13] Some patients experience symptoms such as fever, myalgias, arthralgias, fatigue, headache, sore throat, and rash.[13] The transmission of *Toxoplasma* to the unborn (congenital transmission) has been shown to vary considerably, depending on the gestational age when infected. Nearly 85% of congenital infections are asymptomatic at first but later exhibit signs and symptoms of overt disease such as chorioretinitis or developmental delays. The earlier the infection occurs during development, the more severe the outcome. *Toxoplasma* encephalitis (TE) occurs in patients with AIDS, Hodgkin disease, or after bone marrow transplantation, which is thought to be due to reactivation of a chronic infection. *Toxoplasma* encephalitis patients present with headache, disorientation, drowsiness, hemiparesis, reflex changes and convulsions, and many become comatose.[14] Toxoplasmosis ranks high on the list of diseases which lead to death in patients with AIDS. Approximately 10% of AIDS patients in the United States and up to 30% in Europe are estimated to die from toxoplasmosis.[15] Although in AIDS patients any organ may be involved (including the testes, dermis, and the spinal cord), infection of the brain is most frequently reported. Most AIDS patients suffering from toxoplasmosis have bilateral, severe, and persistent headaches, which respond poorly to analgesics. As the disease progresses, the headache may lead to a condition characterized by confusion, lethargy, ataxia, and coma.[16]

6. The most appropriate treatment for patients with stroke is to maintain them on bed rest for a minimum of 24 hours to avoid postural hypotension. Moreover, hypertension should be treated in a limited step-wise fashion. Passive range of motion exercises should be started early to help maintain mobility and prevent contractures.[9] More intensive physical rehabilitation to improve walking, speaking, dexterity, and to manage daily living activities becomes important thereafter. Additionally, movement of the ankles and legs

should occur to prevent deep venous thrombosis and deep breathing to prevent atelectasis should be encouraged.[9] Anti-thrombolytic therapy may be appropriate for patients who present early with ischemic stroke.[9] Tissue plasminogen activator (TPA) at a dose of 0.9 mg/kg (maximum 90 mg) can be given intravenously, 10% as a bolus, and the rest infused over 1 hour.[9] Anticoagulants and aspirin should not be given for the first 24 hours after TPA therapy is initiated, and blood pressure should be monitored closely. In patients given TPA, there is a significant increase in the occurrence of hemorrhage, although mortality is unchanged; however, at 3 months, the neurologic outcome is significantly improved. Aspirin should be given during the first 24 hours of symptoms in patients who do not get TPA.

The most appropriate treatment for this patient's *T. gondii* infection is no treatment because it is an incidental finding in a patient who formerly lived in Liberia, Africa. However, in patients with *Toxoplasma* encephalitis (as was initially suspected here), sulphadiazine and pyrimethamine (Daraprim) are 2 drugs widely used for treatment of toxoplasmosis.[17] These drugs act against the proliferative forms, or tachyzoites, present during the acute phase of infection or during reactivation of latent foci in immunocompromised hosts, but do not eradicate the encysted form of the parasite. The combination of sulfadiazine and pyrimethamine is considered to be the most effective therapy when administered in 2 phases: acute and maintenance (eg, in AIDS patients). The regimen of choice is sulfadiazine at a dose of 4 to 6 g/day combined with pyrimethamine at a dose of 50 to 75 mg/day for 4 to 6 weeks during the acute phase, and a 50% reduction in the initial dose of both drugs (2 g/day sulfadiazine plus 25 mg/day pyrimethamine) in the maintenance phase. A response is observed in 70% to 95% of cases, and 91% of patients show objective signs of improvement within the first 10 to 14 days of therapy. In refractory cases, diaminodiphenylsulphone, atovaquone, spiramycin, and clindamycin have been used.[10]

Treatment and Course

The patient was placed on bed rest; aspirin therapy was initiated; her blood pressure was monitored closely; and physical and occupational therapy were initiated.

Keywords

stroke, toxoplasmosis, Toxoplasma gondii, serology, parasitology

References

1. Schiff HB, Sabin TD. Alterations in mental state: Coma and acute confusional states. In: Greene HL, ed. *Noble: Textbook of Primary Care Medicine.* St. Louis: Mosby, 2001:1462-1473.

2. Jones JL, Kruszon-Moran D, Wilson M, et al. *Toxoplasma gondii* infection in the United States: Seroprevalence and risk factors. *Am J Epidemiol.* 2001;154:357-365.

3. Omland T, Tonjum A, Frentzel-Beyme RR. Prevalence of *Toxoplasma gondii* antibodies in different populations of native Liberians. *Tropenmed Parasitol.* 1977;28:372-376.

4. Willis MS, Southern P, Latimer MJ. Toxoplasma infection: Making the best use of laboratory tests. *Infect Med.* 2002;19:522-532.

5. Montoya JG, Remington JS. *Toxoplasma gondii.* In: Mandel GL, Douglas R, Bennet JE, eds. *Principles and Practice of Infectious Diseases.* New York: Churchill Livingstone, 2000:2858-2881.

6. Derouin F, Leport C, Pueyo S, et al. Predictive value of *Toxoplasma gondii* antibody titers on the occurrence of *Toxoplasma* encephalitis in HIV-infected patients. ANRS 005/ACTG 154 Trial Group. *AIDS.* 1996;10:1521-1527.

7. Hellerbrand C, Goebel FD, Disko R. High predictive value of *Toxoplasma gondii* IgG antibody levels in HIV-infected patients for diagnosis of cerebral toxoplasmosis. *Eur J Clin Microbiol Infect Dis.* 1996;15:869-872.

8. Araujo FG, Barnett EV, Gentry LO, et al. False-positive anti-*Toxoplasma* fluorescent-antibody tests in patients with antinuclear antibodies. *Appl Microbiol.* 1971; 22:270-275.

9. Pulsinelli WA. Ischemic cerebrovascular disease. In: Goldman L, Bennett JC, Drazen JM, et al, eds. *Cecil Textbook of Medicine.* Philadelphia: W.B. Saunders; 2000:2100-2109.

10. Ferreira MS, Borges AS. Some aspects of protozoan infections in immuno-compromised patients- a review. *Mem Inst Oswaldo Cruz.* 2002;97:443-457.

11. Dubey JP. *Toxoplasma, Neospora, Sarcocystis,* and other tissue cyst-forming coccidia of humans and animals. In: Kreier J, ed. *Parasitic Protozoa.* San Diego: Academic Press; 1993:1-57.

12. Smith JE. A ubiquitous intracellular parasite: the cellular biology of *Toxoplasma gondii*. *Int J Parasitol*. 1995;25:1301-1309.

13. Liesenfeld O, Remington JS. Toxoplasmosis. In: Goldman L, Bennett JC, Drazen JM, eds. *Cecil Textbook of Medicine*. Philadelphia: W.B. Saunders, 2000:1963-1967.

14. Remington JS, Cavanaugh EN. Isolation of the encysted form of *Toxoplasma gondii* from human skeletal muscle and brain. *N Engl J Med*. 1965;273:1308-1310.

15. Luft BJ, Remington JS. *Toxoplasma* encephalitis in AIDS. *Clin Infect Dis*. 1992;15:211-222.

16. Renold C, Sugar A, Chave JP, et al. *Toxoplasma* encephalitis in patients with the acquired immunodeficiency syndrome. *Medicine (Baltimore)*. 1992;71:224-239.

17. Hill D, Dubey JP. *Toxoplasma gondii*: Transmission, diagnosis and prevention. *Clin Microbiol Infect*. 2002;8:634-640.

A 49-Year-Old Man With AIDS, Fever, and Weight Loss

Jill Zyrek-Betts,[1] Haig Donabedian,[2] Robert Booth,[1]

Departments of [1]Pathology and [2]Internal Medicine, Medical University of Ohio, Toledo, OH

Patient: A 49-year-old Caucasian man from Northwest Ohio.

Chief Complaint: Diarrhea and vomiting for the previous 2 weeks, progressing to include fever and chills within the last 2 days. Additionally, he had an unintentional weight loss of 30 pounds during the previous 2 to 4 weeks and was admitted to the hospital.

Past Medical History: Bipolar disease, cocaine abuse, and alcohol abuse.

Radiologic Findings: Computed tomography (CT) scan of the abdomen revealed prominent periaortic lymphadenopathy (**Image 1A**).

Clinical Course: The patient rapidly became hypoxic and required intubation. With an overall poor prognosis, he died within 2.5 weeks of admission.

Autopsy Findings: Autopsy revealed bilateral, diffuse pulmonary granulomas with necrosis, edema, and hemorrhage. Caseating granulomas were also present in the spleen, abdominal periaortic and thoracic perihilar lymph nodes, liver, and bone marrow. Methenamine silver staining showed 3- to 5-μm thin-walled yeast forms within the foamy macrophages in the areas of granuloma formation (**Image 1B**).

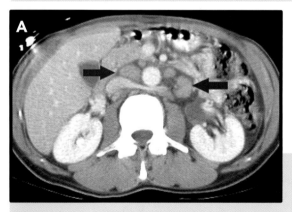
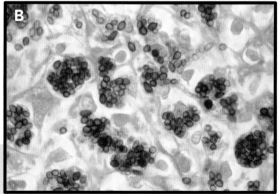

Image 1_CT scan of the abdomen illustrating prominent periaortic lymphadenopathy (arrows) (**A**) and methenamine silver stain of thoracic perihilar lymph nodes illustrating the presence of 3- to 5-μm thin-walled yeast forms within the foamy macrophages in the areas of granuloma formation (magnification, 1,000×) (**B**).

T1. Principal Laboratory Findings

Test	Patient's Result	Reference Interval
Hematology		
WBC count	2.3	4.0-10.0 × 10³/μL
RBC count	3.96	4.3-5.9 × 10³/μL
Hemoglobin	12.2	13.9-16.3 g/dL
Hematocrit	35.7	39-55%
MCV	90.1	80-100 fL
Platelet count	163	100-400 × 10³/μL
Differential count: Neutrophils	85	50-70%
Lymphocytes	2	20-40%
Monocytes	5	2-8%
Eosinophils	3	0-5%
Peripheral blood smear findings	Intracellular yeast	Negative for yeast cells
Coagulation		
Prothrombin time	13.9	12.3-14.8 sec
INR	1.03	0.88-1.12
Partial thomboplastin time	30.1	25.0-35.0 sec
Flow Cytometry/Molecular Diagnostics		
Absolute CD4 T-cell count	1	430-1,185 cells/mm³
Relative CD4 T-cell count	3	40-70%
HIV-1 Western Blot	Positive	Negative
Chemistry		
Sodium	129	136-146 mmol/L
Potassium	3.2	3.4-5.2 mmol/L
Chloride	94	98-108 mmol/L
CO₂	23	22-32 mmol/L
BUN	8	6-21 mg/dL
Creatinine	0.9	0.4-1.6 mg/dL
Glucose	91	70-100 mg/dL
Bilirubin, total	0.3	0.2-1.2 mg/dL
Bilirubin, direct	0.2	0.0-0.3 mg/dL
Aspartate aminotransferase	102	10-39 U/L
Alanine aminotransferase	54	4-42 U/L
Alkaline phosphatase	45	40-125 U/L
Microbiology		
Histoplasma antigen, urine	58.4	<1.0 EIA units
Cultures: BALF	Negative	Negative
Bone marrow	*H. capsulatum*	Negative
Blood	Negative	Negative
Stool	Negative	Negative
Urine	Negative	Negative
Serology		
Cryptococcal antigen	Negative	Negative
EBV Ab to VCA		
IgG	4.44	<0.90
IgM	0.05	<0.90

WBC, white blood cell; RBC, red blood cell; MCV, mean corpuscular volume; INR, International Normalized Ratio; CD, cluster of differentiation; HIV, human immunodeficiency virus; BUN, blood urea nitrogen; EIA, enzymeimmunoassay; BALF, bronchoalveolar lavage fluid; Ab, antibody.

Questions

1. What are this patient's most striking clinical and laboratory findings?

2. What is the patient's most likely diagnosis?

3. How did this patient acquire the disseminated infection associated with the most likely diagnosis?

4. What are the forms of clinical presentation of this patient's disease?

5. What laboratory methods are available for diagnosing this patient's disease?

6. Why is this patient's disease more common in immunosuppressed patients?

7. What is the most appropriate treatment of this patient's disease?

Possible Answers

1. His laboratory results were significant for an alarmingly low T cell subset count, including a

relative CD4 count of 3% and an absolute count of 1 cell/mm³. Confirmatory tests were consistent with a diagnosis of HIV.

A bone marrow biopsy demonstrated a mildly hypercellular marrow. A bone marrow culture demonstrated *H. capsulatum* on day 12, 2 days after his death.

Intracellular yeast was found in the peripheral blood smear. After a histoplasma urine antigen test was found to be positive, the biopsy was reevaluated and a few foamy macrophages and tiny yeast forms were observed.

2. **Most likely diagnosis:** *disseminated histoplasmosis.* Our patient's clinical, radiographic, and laboratory findings are consistent with this diagnosis.

3. *H. capsulatum*, a dimorphic fungus endemic to the Ohio and Mississippi river valleys, infects over 500,000 people in the United States each year with an overall prevalence of approximately 40 million cases.[1] Infection with this organism develops by inhalation of dust particles from soil contaminated with bird or bat droppings that contain the microconidia of the fungus, which subsequently germinate into yeast forms within the lungs.[2] Transmission via person to person contact has not been reported.

4. The clinical presentation of individuals with disseminated histoplasmosis varies based upon the intensity of exposure, as well as the immune status of the individual and pre-existing pulmonary deficiency. Asymptomatic primary infection is the most common form of this disease found in those with a normal immune system.[1] With a high dose inoculum, healthy individuals may develop acute pulmonary histoplasmosis, which may include fever, headache, nonproductive cough, chills, weight loss, malaise, and myalgias. Moreover, mediastinal granulomas, pericarditis, and rheumatologic syndromes are common sequelae. Chronic pulmonary histoplasmosis is most commonly seen in those with preexisting pulmonary abnormalities, such as emphysema. Symptoms resemble those of reactivation tuberculosis and include chronic cough, dyspnea, chest pain, fatigue, fevers, and sweats.[3] In 80% of cases, disseminated histoplasmosis is seen in immunocompromised patients,[1] and has been

an AIDS defining illness since 1987.[4] While HIV infection and a CD4 count of less than 200 cells/mm³ are found typically in patients with this disease, they may instead have lymphoreticular neoplasms or be receiving corticosteroids, cytotoxic therapy, and immunosuppressive agents.

5. While culture is the gold standard for the diagnosis of histoplasmosis infection, some isolates may require 10 to 14 days for recovery from blood culture.[5] Fungal staining of tissue and blood specimens recovers organisms in up to 70% of cases.[5] Bone marrow produces the highest yield of organisms, staining positive in up to 75% of cases of disseminated histoplasmosis.[1] Serologic detection of antigen to *H. capsulatum* occurs in the urine of 90% of patients and in the serum of 70% of patients with histoplasmosis.[4]

6. Neutrophils, macrophages, lymphocytes, and natural killer cells are activated in response to a *Histoplasma* infection. Following infection with this organism, the intracellular parasite can survive within macrophages for an extended period of time.[5] Widely disseminated histoplasmosis is particularly common in immunosuppressed patients since *Histoplasma* infections are controlled by helper T cells that recognize the cell wall antigens of *H. capsulatum* organisms. Moreover, macrophages assist in spreading the organism to the adjacent lymph nodes and throughout the reticuloendothelial system (liver, spleen, lymph nodes, adrenal glands, and bone marrow).

7. Treatment of disseminated histoplasmosis depends on HIV status and severity of disease.[4] Therapy usually requires amphotericin; however, there is evidence suggesting that itraconazole may also be effective in the treatment of this disease.[6,7] In our patient, itraconazole therapy was chosen to minimize toxicity in this desperately ill patient. Unfortunately, the patient died 5 days after therapy was initiated, making the choice of antifungal agent moot. The survival of AIDS patients with disseminated histoplasmosis in the current era of highly effective therapy is unknown. A recent study comparing 2 amphotericin preparations reported that as many as 88% of the patients with disseminated histoplasmosis enrolled in this study had a good response to intravenous, followed by oral, itraconazole

therapy.[8] However, long-term survival rates in this cohort of patients were not addressed.

Keywords

H. capsulatum, disseminated histoplasmosis, microconidia, HIV, amphotericin, itraconazole

References

1. Kurowski R, Ostapchuk M. Overview of Histoplasmosis. *American Academy of Family Physicians*, 2002; Vol. 66, 2247-52.

2. Kumar V, Abbas A, Fausto N. *Robbins and Cotran Pathologic Basis of Disease*, 7th ed. Philadelphia: W.B. Saunders Company. 2005.

3. Wheat LJ, Conces D, Allen SD, et al. Pulmonary histoplasmosis syndromes: Recognition, diagnosis, and management. *Semin Respir Crit Care Med*. 2004;25:129-143.

4. Vathesatogkit P, Goldenberg R, Parsey M. A 27-year-old HIV-infected woman with severe sepsis and pulmonary infiltrates. *Chest*. 2003;123:272-276.

5. Forbes BA, Sahm DF, Weissfeld AS. *Diagnostic Microbiology*, 11th Ed. St. Louis: Mosby. 2002.

6. Brooks JT, Wheat LJ. Histoplasmosis: Update 1998. *AIDS Clin Care*. 1998;10:4-5.

7. Wheat LJ, Kauffman CA. Histoplasmosis. *Infect Dis Clin North Am*. 2003;17:1-19.

8. Johnson PC, Wheat LJ, Cloud GA, et al. Safety and efficacy of liposomal amphotericin B compared with conventional amphotericin B for induction therapy of histoplasmosis in patients with AIDS. *Ann Intern Med*. 2002;137:105-109.

A 36-Pound Weight Loss and Debilitating Painful Rash in a 42-Year-Old Male

Jason A. Bennett, Ted Krafczyk, John G. Thomas, Patricia M. Canfield

Department of Pathology and Laboratory Medicine, West Virginia University Hospitals, Morgantown, WV

Patient: 42-year-old male.

Family History: Unremarkable.

Chief Complaints: Fever, cough that had steadily worsened, intermittent episodes of diarrhea and vomiting that increased in frequency during the past month, a 36-pound weight loss over the previous 5 months, and a debilitating, painful rash that was unresponsive to topical therapies.

Prior Medical History: Smoker with bipolar affective disorder and no history of a positive purified protein derivative (PPD) test. He had a stroke 3 years ago that included left-sided weakness and a normal magnetic resonance imaging (MRI) scan.

Drug History: None presently. Previously, he had been treated with lithium; however, he stopped taking this drug due to a rash that he thought was caused by the lithium.

Physical Examination Findings: Very thin body habitus; excoriated, erythematous raised rash on the distal extremities; oral thrush; mild cervical lymphadenopathy; and bilateral ronchi and wheezes.

Questions

1. What are this patient's most striking clinical and laboratory findings?

2. How do you explain this patient's most striking clinical and laboratory findings?

3. What is this patient's most likely diagnosis?

4. What are the common laboratory methods for establishing HIV infection?

5. What laboratory and clinical findings define this patient's disease?

6. What factors can cause a false negative HIV antibody test?

7. What is the "window period" for HIV antibody detection?

8. What is a useful diagnostic algorithm for laboratory screening for HIV infection?

9. What laboratory test(s) should be used to follow known HIV positive patients?

10. At what CD4 level are patients tested and/or treated prophylactically for *Pneumocystis carinii* pneumonia (PCP)?

Possible Answers

1. All of his clinical findings described under "Chief Complaints" are striking, especially a 36-pound weight loss over the previous 5 months, and a debilitating, painful rash that was unresponsive to topical therapies. Striking laboratory findings

T1. Principal Laboratory Findings*

Test	Patient's Result	"Normal" Reference Range
Hematology		
White blood cell count	3.6	3.4-9.2 × 10³/mL
Absolute neutrophil count	1.7	1.5-6.9 × 10³/mL
Eosinophils	55	1-6%
Immunology		
CD4 count	23	600-2,100 cells/mL
HIV-1,2 antibodies by EIA	Negative	Negative
Western blot	Negative	Negative
HIV-1 p24 antigen	Repeatedly reactive	Negative
HIV-1 provirus, qualitative	Repeatedly reactive	Negative
HIV-1 RNA viral load	>750,000	0 copies/mL
Microbiology		
GMS staining of BAL fluid	Positive for *Pneumocystis carinii*	

*Compiled over a 2-3 month period. CD, cluster designation; HIV, human immunodeficiency virus; Ab, antibody; GMS, Gomori metheneamine silver; BAL, bronchoalveolar lavage; EIA, enzymeimmunoassay; WB, Western blot.

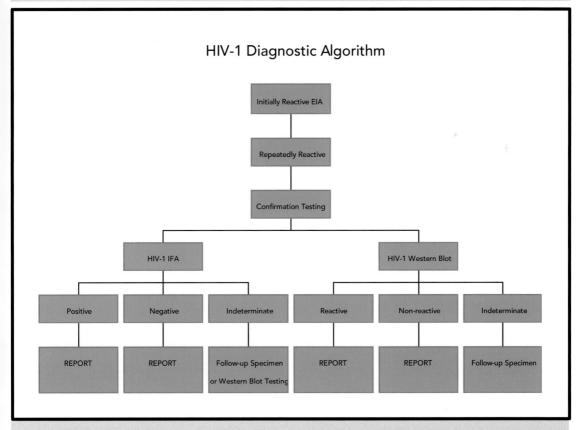

Figure 1_Testing Algorithm for HIV-1 Antibody Detection.

T2. Categories of HIV Infection[2]

Category	Type of HIV Infection	Characteristics
A	Asymptomatic	No ARC- or AIDS-related diseases of the types indicated below and a CD4+ count never <500 cells
B	ARC	Any 1 of the Category B diseases indicated below or a CD4+ count <500 cells, but never <200 cells
C	AIDS	Any 1 of the Category C diseases indicated below or a CD4+ count <200 cells at any time

Category B (ARC-related diseases)	Category C (AIDS-related diseases)
Bacillary angiomatosis Candidiasis, oropharyngeal (thrush) Candidiasis, vulvovaginal; persistent, frequent, or poorly responsive to therapy Cervical dysplasia (moderate or severe)/cervical carcinoma in situ Constitutional symptoms, such as fever (38.5°C) or diarrhea lasting greater than 1 month *Hairy* leukoplakia, oral *Herpes zoster* (shingles), involving at least 2 distinct episodes or more than 1 dermatome Listeriosis Pelvic inflammatory disease, particularly if complicated by tubo-ovarian abscess Peripheral neuropathy	Candidiasis of bronchi, trachea, or lungs Candidiasis, esophageal Cervical cancer, invasive Coccidioidomycosis, disseminated or extrapulmonary Cryptococcosis, extrapulmonary Cryptosporidiosis, chronic intestinal (greater than 1 month duration) Cytomegalovirus disease (other than liver, spleen, or lymph nodes) Cytomegalovirus retinitis (with loss of vision) Encephalopathy, HIV-related *Herpes simplex:* chronic ulcer(s) (greater than 1 month duration); Idiopathic thrombocytopenic purpura or bronchitis, pneumonitis, or esophagitis Histoplasmosis, disseminated or extrapulmonary Isosporiasis, chronic intestinal (greater than 1 month duration) Kaposi sarcoma Lymphoma, Burkitt (or equivalent term) Lymphoma, immunoblastic (or equivalent term) Lymphoma, primary, of brain *Mycobacterium avium* complex or *M. kansasii*, disseminated or extrapulmonary *Mycobacterium tuberculosis,* any site (pulmonary or extrapulmonary) *Mycobacterium,* other species or unidentified species, disseminated or extrapulmonary *Pneumocystis jirovecii* pneumonia Pneumonia, recurrent Progressive multifocal leukoencephalopathy *Salmonella* septicemia, recurrent Toxoplasmosis of the brain Wasting syndrome due to HIV

HIV, human immunodeficiency virus; AIDS, acquired immunodeficiency syndrome; CD, cluster designation; ARC, AIDS-related complex.

Common Causes of False Negative HIV Antibody Tests[1,3-5,7]

Antibody testing performed in the "window period" prior to seroconversion
Antibody testing in very advanced stages of AIDS
Agammaglobulinemia
Immunosuppression due to malignancy or chemotherapy
Replacement transfusion
Infection with HIV subtype O or any strain showing little genetic homology with HIV-1 subtype M

HIV, human immunodeficiency virus; AIDS, acquired immunodeficiency syndrome.

include marked eosinophilia, a markedly decreased CD4+ cell count with a markedly increased HIV-1 RNA viral load, a repeatedly reactive HIV-1 p24 antigen test, but negative HIV-1,2 antibody tests, and a positive GMS stain of BAL fluid for *Pneumocystis jirovecii* [**T1**].

2. This patient's clinical and laboratory findings are most likely due to *Pneumocystis jirovecii* pneumonia in a patient with acquired immunodeficiency syndrome (AIDS). However, there is a disparity between this patient's HIV-1,2 antibody results and the results of additional confirmatory HIV tests, including a markedly increased HIV-1 RNA viral load [**T1**].

3. ***Most likely diagnosis:*** *Pneumocystis pneumonia due to seronegative human immunodeficiency virus (HIV) infection and AIDS.*

4. HIV infection is established by 1 of the following serum-based methods: detection of antibody to the virus by immunoassay [eg, enzymeimmuno-assay (EIA), immunoenzymetric assay (IEMA), or enzyme-linked immunosorbent assay (ELISA)], detection of viral p24 antigen, culturing HIV, or detecting and quantifying HIV RNA. The most commonly performed screening test for HIV infection is the ELISA antibody screening test, which is often the first test performed following a known exposure to HIV. Positive screening tests are then confirmed by other laboratory methods, including immunofluorescent antibody (IFA) detection, Western blot, radioimmunoprecipitation assay (RIPA), virus culture, or polymerase chain reaction (PCR)-based molecular probe assays.[8,10] Some authorities recommend obtaining 2 positive ELISA tests before proceeding to a confirmatory test. Alternatively, ELISA testing for HIV p24 antigen, which is the earliest detectable antigen in HIV infection, can be performed. Disadvantages of antigen detection assays include poor diagnostic sensitivity (only 69% in AIDS patients and as low as 20% in infants <1 month old) and failure to detect p24 antigen in patients with a high level of p24 antibody (which complexes with the p24 antigen).[8]

5. HIV infection is divided into 3 categories (Category A, B, and C) based on degree of severity, assessed by the CD4+ cell count, and progression of the HIV viral infection to include

a variety of concomitant illnesses/diseases [**T2**]. Patients in all categories have documented and confirmed HIV positivity by 1 or more of the HIV antibody detection/confirmatory methods indicated above; however, patients with Category A disease are asymptomatic and have never had a CD4 count below 500. Patients with Category B disease [also referred to as AIDS-related complex (ARC)] have any of the diseases listed in **T2** or CD4 counts less than 500, but never less than 200, while patients with Category C disease have AIDS, as defined by the presence of any of the illnesses/diseases listed in **T2** or a CD4 count less than 200 at any time. Thus, an infection with the HIV virus does not progress to AIDS in all cases.

6. The most common cause of a false negative HIV antibody test occurs when the testing is performed in the "window period" prior to sero-conversion. Other causes include those shown in **T3**. In 1994, 7 cases of HIV infection were identified in France which had atypical Western blot patterns and weak or no seroreactivity by an HIV-1 EIA. Such isolates had been previously loosely grouped as phylogenetic outliers, termed "group O" strain, representing a highly divergent strain from the group M strain that gave rise to the HIV pandemic. The first documented case of HIV group O infection in the United States was identified in April of 1996.[6] Screening tests for HIV-1,2 antibodies, especially those based on the detection of virus envelope (*env*) peptides or the immunoassay "sandwich" method (ie, analyte sandwiched between a capture and a signal antibody), can lack sensitivity for HIV-1 subtype O antibodies. Further epidemiological surveys are required to determine the prevalence and geographic distribution of HIV-1 subtype O infection.[8] In addition, a patient may occasionally fail to produce HIV antibodies indefinitely following the window period of infection.[5,10] The factors which may predispose an otherwise immunocompetent patient to demonstrate this unusual lack of immune response have not been identified.

7. The "window period" refers to the variable period of time following HIV infection when the infected individual is mounting an antibody response to HIV; however, HIV antibodies are not yet detectable in the patient's serum by

the commonly used HIV antibody screening tests. It generally takes up to 3 months, and rarely as long as 6 months, for antibodies to the HIV virus to develop following HIV infection. Approximately 95% of HIV-infected individuals will have detectable antibodies 3 months after infection with HIV. While p24 is the first clinically detectable antigen to appear in the serum of an HIV-infected individual, in many cases it becomes undetectable in the bloodstream following the appearance of HIV antibodies.[8] Moreover, patients in the late stages of AIDS may show continued immunologic deterioration by becoming seronegative for some HIV-1 antibodies. However, antibody to HIV-1 rarely decreases if the disease has not progressed.

8. The most widely accepted diagnostic algorithm for HIV antibody testing involves HIV antibody screening using an ELISA or EIA, followed by Western blot confirmation of any screen-positive serum sample [**F1**]. Generally, a negative HIV antibody screening test at 3 months following exposure to the HIV effectively rules out HIV infection in an asymptomatic patient. If any clinical doubt remains, another blood specimen can be collected from the patient at 6 months and tested again for the presence of HIV antibodies. A positive HIV antibody screening test must be confirmed by IFA, Western blot, or some other confirmatory test.[10] A patient with antibody-confirmed HIV infection should be assigned a disease category [**T2**] and followed with periodic CD4 counts and HIV viral RNA quantitative studies to determine the course of future therapy. The rare patient with diminished CD4 counts and/or any AIDS/ARC-defining illnesses [**T2**] and a negative HIV antibody test after the window period should have viral RNA quantitative testing and/or p24 antigen testing to help confirm the diagnosis and follow the course of the disease. Moreover, an effort should be made to identify a reason for the patient's failure to seroconvert.

9. HIV-positive patients on antiretroviral therapy are followed by repeat CD4+ cell counts and HIV RNA (viral load) testing. Viral load testing is not intended as a primary diagnostic test for HIV infection, and misdiagnoses have resulted from its misuse in this regard.[9] HIV RNA quantitative testing is best applied to follow the efficacy

of antiretroviral therapy and monitor the course of infection. The determination of CD4 cell counts over time is a crucial factor in prognosis, management, and therapeutic decision-making in HIV-infected patients. For example, the risk of developing AIDS or death over a 10-year follow-up period are 5%, 17%, 33%, 55%, and 80% for HIV RNA viral loads of 500 copies/mL or less, 501 to 3,000 copies/mL, 3,001 to 10,000 copies/mL, 10,001 to 30,000 copies/mL, and more than 30,000 copies/mL, respectively.[8]

10. In patients with HIV infection or on immunosuppression therapy, a CD4 count less than 200 cells/mL predisposes these patients to *P. jirovecii* infection and subsequent pneumonia. Trimethoprim-sulfamethoxazole is the therapy of choice for prophylaxis and treatment.

Keywords _____

human immunodeficiency virus, acquired immunodeficiency syndrome, AIDS-related complex, Pneumocystis pneumonia, CD4 count, viral load, window period

References _____

1. Farzadegan H, Polis MA, Wolinsky SM. Loss of human immunodeficiency virus type 1 (HIV-1) antibodies with evidence of viral infection in asymptomatic homosexual men: A report from the Multicenter AIDS cohort study. *Ann Intern Med.* 1988;108:785.

2. The Official US Government Definition of AIDS (1993). http://www.aegis.com/topics/definition.html. Accessed on June 15, 2004.

3. Berrios DC, Hearst N, Coates TJ, et al. HIV antibody testing among those at risk for infection. *JAMA.* 1993;270:1576.

4. Loussert-Ajaka I, Ly TD, Chaix ML, et al. HIV-1/HIV-2 seronegativity in HIV-1 subtype O infected patients. *Lancet.* 1994;343:1393.

5. Persistent lack of detectable HIV-1 antibody in a person with HIV infection: Utah, 1995. *MMWR Morb Mortal Wkly Rep.* 1996;45:181.

6. Rayfield MA, Sullivan P, Bandera CI, et al. HIV-1 group O virus identified for the first time in the United States. *Emerg Infect Dis.* 1996;2:209.

7. Gurtler L. Difficulties and strategies of HIV diagnosis. *Lancet.* 1996;348:176.

8. Peter JB. *Use and Interpretation of Laboratory Tests in Infectious Disease.* 5th ed., 1998.

9. Rich JD, Merriman NA, Mylonakis E, et al. Misdiagnosis of HIV infection by HIV-1 plasma viral load testing: A case series. *Ann Intern Med.* 1999;130:37.

10. Bartlett JG. Serologic tests for the diagnosis of HIV infection. http://www.uptodate.com. Accessed June 15, 2004.

Unusual Organisms in the Bone Marrow of a Patient With Systemic Sarcoidosis

Sandrine Kagialis-Girard,[1] Luc-Marie Gerland,[2] Charles Dumontet,[2] Danielle Treille-Ritouet[2]

[1]*Hematology Laboratory, Hôpital Edouard Herriot and Hôpital Debrousse and* [2]*Hematology Laboratory, Hôpital Edouard Herriot, Lyon, France*

Patient: 34-year-old man.

Chief Complaint: Intermittent fever and abdominal pain of 1 week duration.

Past Medical History: Ten years earlier, the patient had been diagnosed with systemic sarcoidosis (ie, neurosarcoidosis), diabetes insipidus, and neurological bladder disease.

Physical Examination: On admission, the patient was febrile (39.7°C), coughed, and complained of sudden iliac pit pain and dyspnea. Clinical examination revealed jaundice, a petechial purpura, and massive splenomegaly.

Principal Laboratory Findings: (T1). In addition, the results of testing for the activity of various coagulation factors were consistent with results for these factors seen typically in patients with disseminated intra-vascular coagulation (DIC) (data not shown).

Additional Diagnostic Procedures: Abdominal ultrasound revealed hepatic microabscesses, while the results of a bone marrow aspiration revealed necrosis with very few hematopoietic cells and massive infiltration by spherical, encapsulated yeast cells (**Images 1A** and **1B**).

Questions

1. What is (are) this patient's most striking clinical and laboratory finding?

2. How do you explain this patient's most striking clinical and laboratory finding(s)?

3. Why was a spinal tap not performed on this patient?

4. What is this patient's most likely diagnosis?

5. What are the clinical characteristics of this patient's disease?

6. How should this patient's disease be treated?

Possible Answers

1. Hyperthermia, dyspnea, jaundice, petechial purpura, and massive splenomegaly; decreased hemoglobin, MCV, and platelet count; markedly increased total bilirubin and CRP concentrations; a positive cryptococcal antigen test at high titer; positive blood cultures for *Cryptococcus neoformans* (*C. neoformans*); and a necrotic, hypocellular bone marrow with massive infiltrates of *C. neoformans* in a patient with a previous history of sarcoidosis.

T1. Principal Laboratory Findings

Test	Patient's Result	Reference Interval
Hematology		
WBC count	7.7	4.1-10.9 × 10^3/µL
Hemoglobin	8.2	13.2-16.2 g/dL
MCV	62	82-105 fL
MCH	28	28-34 pg
Platelet count	50	140-450 × 10^3/µL
Chemistry		
Bilirubin, total	13.0	0.2-1.3 mg/dL
CRP	19.1	<0.5 mg/dL
Immunology		
Cryptococcal antigen, serum	Pos @ 1:1,000	Negative
Microbiology		
Blood cultures	Pos for *C. neoformans*	Negative

WBC, white blood cell; MCV, mean corpuscular volume; MCH, mean corpuscular hemoglobin; CRP, C-reactive protein; Pos, positive; C. neoformans, Cryptococcus neoformans.

2. The constellation of this patient's clinical and laboratory findings are consistent with cryptococcal infection. Cryptococcal infection, although rare, should be considered in sarcoid patients and hematopathologists should be aware of the morphological characteristics of cryptococcal organisms when reviewing bone marrow smears obtained from these patients.

3. A spinal tap is contraindicated in a patient with DIC. Although cerebrospinal fluid (CSF) was not tested for cryptococcal antigen, the patient's serum was positive for cryptococcal antigen at high titer (**T1**).

4. ***Most likely diagnosis:*** *disseminated cryptococcosis with bone marrow involvement due to long-term immunosuppressive therapy in a patient with sarcoidosis.*

5. *Cryptococcus neoformans* is an opportunistic fungal pathogen frequently present in patients with identifiable underlying predisposing factors or disorders such as sarcoidosis, advanced human immunodeficiency virus (HIV) disease, prolonged immunosuppressive treatment, or other disorders associated with cell-mediated immune dysfunction.[1-8] In rare cases, it has also been described in healthy individuals.[9] Sarcoidosis is an idiopathic granulomatous disease of unknown etiology in which patients

have an increased risk of opportunistic infection related both to sarcoidosis itself and to the use of steroid therapy in the treatment of this disease.[3-6] Systemic cryptococcosis is a life-threatening disease occurring in immunocompromised patients.[8] Cryptococcal meningitis is the most common manifestation of infection with *C. neoformans*; however, other sites can be affected, including the lungs where these organisms can cause fungal pneumonia.[3,7] Bone marrow cryptococcosis is a classical, albeit relatively infrequent, presentation in patients with acquired immunodeficiency syndrome (AIDS) and is only rarely seen in patients with sarcoidosis.[1,2,10] Systemic sarcoidosis is associated with chronic T-cell deficiency which is exacerbated by prolonged steroid therapy in patients with this disease.[3] Moreover, cases of meningeal, skin, and joint cryptococcal infection have been reported in patients with systemic sarcoidosis.[6,11] In our patient, immunosuppression was likely because of prolonged steroid therapy in the treatment of his systemic sarcoidosis. Peripheral blood cytopenias are frequently observed in patients with bone marrow involvement by cryptococcus organisms.[7] Cytopenias have also been reported in patients with cryptococcal meningitis because of hemophagocytic syndrome.[12] In our patient, there was no evidence of hemophagocytosis or granulomatous disease; however, necrosis and infiltration of bone marrow by encapsulated

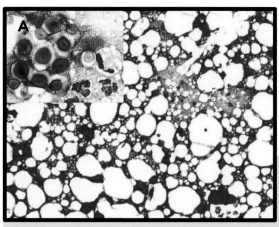
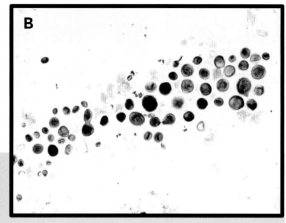

Image 1_Patient's bone marrow illustrating the presence of spherical, encapsulated yeast cells of *C. neoformans* using (**A**) May-Grunwald-Giemsa stain (Inset shows a cluster of these cells) and (**B**) Gomori-Grocott stain (50× magnification).

yeast cells were observed. Our patient presented with anemia and thrombocytopenia, yet the leukocyte count remained normal (**T1**). The presence of numerous cryptococcal organisms in the bone marrow provided a definitive diagnosis for this patient's clinical and laboratory findings. Hematopathologists should be familiar with the morphological characteristics of cryptococcal organisms in bone marrow specimens so that cryptococcosis can be considered as among the possible causes of fever and cytopenia in patients with systemic sarcoidosis.

6. Intravenous administration of flucytosine and amphotercin B is the usual treatment for disseminated cryptococcal infection.

Keywords _____

sarcoidosis, Cryptococcus neoformans, immunodeficiency, opportunistic infection, bone marrow cryptococcosis

References _____

1. Pantanowitz L, Omar T, Sonnendecker H, et al. Bone marrow cryptococcal infection in the acquired immunodeficiency syndrome. *J Infect.* 2000;41:92-94.

2. Wong KF, Ma SK, Lam KW. Acquired immunodeficiency syndrome presenting as marrow cryptococcosis. *Am J Hematol.* 1993;42:392-394.

3. Botha RJP, Wessels E. Crytococcal meningitis in an HIV negative patient with systemic sarcoidosis. *J Clin Pathol.* 1999;52:928-930.

4. Harris TR, Blumenfeld HB, Cruthirds TP, et al. Coexisting sarcoidosis and cryptococcosis. *Arch Intern Med.* 1965;115:637-643.

5. Nottebart HC, McGehee RF, Utz JP. Cryptococcosis complicating sarcoidosis. *Am Rev Respir Dis.* 1973;107:1060-1063.

6. Ross JJ, Katz JD. Cryptococcal menigitis and sarcoidosis. *Scand J Infect Dis.* 2002;34:937-939.

7. Pappas PG, Perfect JR, Cloud GA, et al. Cryptococcosis in human immunodeficiency virus-negative patients in the era of effective azole therapy. *Clin Infect Dis.* 2001;33:690-699.

8. Sepkowitz KA. Opportunistic infections in patients with and patients without acquired immunodeficiency syndrome. *Clin Infect Dis.* 2002;34:1098-1107.

9. Basu S, Marwaha N, Aggarwal V. Images in haematology. Bone marrow cryptococcosis in a human immunodeficiency virus-negative patient. *Br J Haematol.* 2003;120:122.

10. Robert F, Durant JR, Gams RA. Demonstration of cryptococcus neoformans in a stained bone marrow specimen. *Arch Intern Med.* 1977;137:688-690.

11. Mehrany K, Kist JM, Gibson LE. Cryptococcal infection in sarcoidosis. *Int J Dermatol.* 2002;41:773-774.

12. Numata K, Tsutsumi H, Wakai S, et al. A child case of haemophagocytic syndrome associated with cryptococcal meningoencephalitis. *J Infect.* 1998;36:118-119.

Chronic Fever, Chills, Night Sweats, and Dark Urine in a 66-Year-Old Woman

Louis Novoa-Takara, Ranveer Nand

Department of Pathology and Division of Neoplastic Diseases, Medical College of Wisconsin, Milwaukee, WI

Patient: 66-year-old woman from northwestern Wisconsin.

Family History: Noncontributory.

Chief Complaint: Fevers for 4 weeks, chills, night sweats, and dark orange-colored urine.

History of Present Illness: The patient was transferred to our hospital in mid-September for fever of unknown origin of 4 weeks duration and recent acquired hemolytic anemia. She was treated for left thigh thrombophlebitis with cephalexin and indomethacin at another hospital. Lower extremity Doppler ultrasounds were negative for deep venous thrombosis on 3 occasions. Blood cultures were negative. Fevers at home and at the first hospital were as high as 104°F prior to her admission at our hospital where she received 2 doses of ceftriaxone. She was found to have a hemolytic anemia and was given a red cell transfusion. Medicines upon transfer to our hospital included acetaminophen, subcutaneous heparin, iron sulfate, prednisone taper, and multivitamins. She reported hiking in the woods 5 to 6 weeks prior to admission, and had a small rash on her left arm, but did not specifically report any insect bite or tick exposure.

Past Medical History: Splenectomy and partial pancreatectomy for benign pancreatic cystadenoma located in the tail of the pancreas 6 years prior.

Social History: One-half pack per day tobacco use for 40 years; no alcohol. The patient has a pet cat. The patient has no HIV risk factors.

Physical Examination Findings: Vital signs: temperature, 99.2°F; pulse, 74 beats per minute; respiratory rate, 20 breaths per minute; blood pressure, 108/50 mm Hg. Pale conjunctiva, no visible jaundice, but muddy sclerae. No hepatomegaly. No rash currently. Neurologic examination was nonfocal.

Questions

1. What are this patient's most striking clinical and laboratory findings?

2. Based on this patient's history, physical examination, and admission laboratory findings, what conditions should be considered in the differential diagnosis?

3. How does this patient's peripheral blood smear findings contribute to the establishment of this patient's diagnosis?

4. What is this patient's most likely diagnosis?

T1. Principal Laboratory Findings

Test	Patient's Result	"Normal" Reference Range
Hematology		
WBC count	6.3	4.0–10.0 × 10³/µL
RBC count	2.1	4.0–5.2 × 10⁶/µL
Hemoglobin	7.0	12.0–15.0 g/dL
Hematocrit	22.0	37.0–47.0%
MCV	103	80–100 fL
Platelet count	323	150–350 × 10³/µL
Reticulocyte count	0.318	0.024–0.084 × 10⁶/µL
Reticulocyte %	14.9	0.8–2.0%
ESR	113	0–15 mm/h
PBS findings	**Image 1**	
Chemistry		
LD	1070	135–225 U/L
Haptoglobin	30	36–195 mg/dL
CRP	6.7	<0.5 mg/dL
Immunology		
Cold agglutinin screen	Negative	Negative
ANA titer	1:320	1:160
Anti-Sm antibody	Negative	Negative
Anti-dsDNA	Negative	Negative
Lyme antibody screen	Negative	Negative
Urinalysis		
Color/appearance	Dark orange/clear	Straw/clear
pH	6.0	5.0–8.0
Blood	2+	Negative
Bilirubin	Negative	Negative
Blood Bank		
Direct Coombs	2R	Negative
DAT-IgG	2+	Negative
DAT-C3	1+	Negative

WBC, white blood cell; RBC, red blood cell; MCV, mean corpuscular volume; ESR, erythrocyte sedimentation rate; PBS, peripheral blood smear; LD, lactate dehydrogenase; CRP, C-reactive protein; ANA, anti-nuclear antibody; Sm, Smith; dsDNA, double-stranded deoxyribonucleic acid; 2R, 2+ positive with Rouleaux formation; DAT, direct antiglobulin test.

5. What is the epidemiology, clinical presentation, and pathology of this patient's disease?

6. What are the treatment options for this patient?

Possible Answers

1. Fevers, chills, night sweats, dark-colored urine, and acquired hemolytic anemia without thrombocytopenia in a patient with prior splenectomy, recent antibiotic therapy, and recent transfusion (**T1**).

2. The differential diagnosis for fever and autoimmune hemolytic anemia includes neoplasia, drug reaction, rheumatologic disease, glucose-6-phosphate dehydrogenase (G6PD) deficiency, hemolytic transfusion reaction, and infection. The patient had no evidence of a neoplastic condition. This patient was on several drug medications, including cephalexin and ceftriaxone. There are case reports of an association between ceftriaxone and immune hemolysis.[1] Among the rheumatologic disorders, systemic lupus erythematosus (SLE) is most commonly associated with hemolysis;[2] however, the patient's ANA titer was only modestly elevated at 1:320, and her anti-Smith and dsDNA antibody tests were negative (**T1**). She had no history of G6PD deficiency. She had received a recent red cell transfusion; however, her anemia predated the recent red cell transfusion. Workup of her hemolytic anemia indicated a positive direct antiglobulin test (DAT) with anti-IgG (2+) and anti-C3 (1+). Infections include illness due to bacterial, viral, or protozoal organisms.[3] Bacteria associated with hemolysis include *Escheri coli*, *Mycobacterium tuberculosis*, *Clostridium perfringens*, and *Mycoplasma pneumoniae*. *Escheri coli* is associated with hemolytic uremic syndrome (HUS) and thrombocytopenia; however, this patient did not have thrombocytopenia or renal impairment. Moreover, the patient had a normal WBC count and negative blood cultures suggesting that bacterial infection was an unlikely cause of her signs and symptoms. Viruses associated with hemolytic anemia include hepatitis A and B, human immunodeficiency virus (HIV), cytomegalic virus (CMV), and Epstein-Barr virus (EBV). Protozoa include malaria and *Babesia*. Malaria is the most common protozoal illness worldwide, but this patient had no recent history of travel outside the United States.

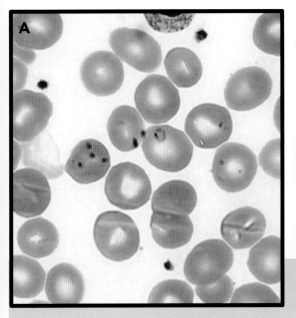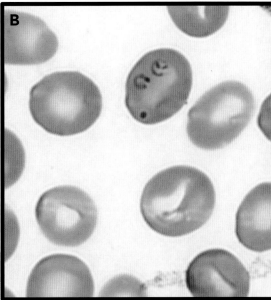

Image 1_Patient's peripheral blood smear (Wright-Giemsa stain; 100× magnification) findings showing (**A**) tetrad of *Babesia* organisms in a red blood cell (RBC) and (**B**) an RBC containing 2 *Babesia* organisms.

3. Examination of the patient's peripheral blood smear provided a way for us to narrow the possibilities constituting the differential diagnosis. The white blood cells were normal in number, differential, and morphology. In addition, abundant platelets were observed, and no schistocytes were seen. However, there were several erythrocyte inclusions on the peripheral blood smear, including fine basophilic stippling, Howell-Jolly bodies, Pappenheimer bodies, and intracellular organisms. Fine basophilic stippling represents precipitated ribosomes and is seen in a variety of anemias. Howell-Jolly bodies are usually single, inkdot-like inclusions that represent nuclear remnants or DNA and are associated with splenectomy. Pappenheimer bodies are small, dense granules that represent iron siderosomes or mitochondrial remnants.[4] Among the organism inclusions in RBCs, the most common are malaria and *Babesia*. Malaria is distinguished by hemozoin pigment and a variety of forms, including trophozoites and gametocytes. The pear-shaped trophozoite-like organisms, without hemozoin pigment, observed in the peripheral blood smear of our patient (**Image 1**) are characteristic of *Babesia* infection but can be confused with malarial organisms. However, the patient's history, including the absence of travel

outside the United States, ruled against malaria as the cause of the patient's sign and symptoms. Moreover, less than 1% of the patient's red cells were infected with a protozoal organism.

4. ***Most likely diagnosis:*** *Babesiosis.*

5. Babesiosis is a protozoal parasitic infection caused by organisms of the genus *Babesia* (eg, *B. microti* and *B. divergens*) and transmitted by ticks from animals to humans. The primary vertebrate host for *B. microti* is the white-tailed mouse. When an *Ixodes dammini* tick feeds on the mouse it acquires the organisms. The organisms multiply inside the tick and are transmit-ted to either deer or humans by a tick bite. Alternatively, transmission can occur by blood transfusion. *Babesia* is the most common transfusion-transmitted protozoal agent in the United States. A long-term study in Connecticut, which reviewed 18 cases of transfusion-associated babesiosis, indicated the risk in that state as 1 per 100,000 units of red blood cells transfused.[5] In Europe, babesiosis is primarily caused by *B. divergens*, whereas in the United States, most cases of babesiosis, particularly those reported from the Great Lakes and Northeast regions of the United States, are due to *B. microti* infection.[6]

Typically, infected individuals become ill 1 to 6 weeks after the tick bite. The spectrum of disease in humans varies from latent infection to fulminant hemolysis.[7] Fatalities have been reported in immunocompromised or splenectomized individuals. The parasites infect red cells and cause intravascular hemolysis. The pear-shaped trophozoites are identified on peripheral blood smears stained with Wright-Giemsa stain.

6. Most patients with babesiosis are treated with clindamycin and quinine. This regimen has been shown to be effective, but has side effects of diarrhea (33%), tinnitus (39%), vertigo (17%), and decreased hearing (28%). The study documenting these side effects recommends atovaquone (750 mg q 12 hours) and azithromycin (500 mg on day 1 and 250 mg every day thereafter) as an alternative drug therapy with fewer side effects.[8] Cases of severe hemolysis are sometimes treated by exchange transfusion.

Patient Follow-up

Digital pictures of the intraerythrocytic organisms found on this patient's peripheral blood smear were sent to the Centers for Disease Control and Prevention (CDC) along with the patient's clinical history. Our presumptive diagnosis, babesiosis, was confirmed by CDC with the identification by polymerase chain reaction (PCR) of *B. microti* in a sample of the patient's blood. The patient was started on clindamycin (600 mg po q 8 hours) and quinine (600 mg po q 8 hours); however, clindamycin was discontinued after 5 days due to diarrhea. She completed her course of quinine therapy. Because of her diarrhea, her antibiotics were changed to levofloxacin and metronidazole for presumed *C. difficile* infection. At a 2-week follow-up visit, the patient reported some problems with hearing; however, her diarrhea had improved.

Keywords

Babesia, intraerythracytic inclusions, autoimmune hemolysis

References

1. Anonymous. Hemolysis from Ceftriaxone. Medical Letter on Drugs and Therapeutics. 2002;44:100–101.

2. Lichtman MA. *Williams Hematology.* 7th ed. New York: McGraw-Hill; 2006.

3. Rosenthal DS. Hematologic Manifestations of Infectious Disease. In: Hoffman R, ed. *Hematology: Basic Principles and Practice.* Vol. 1. Philadelphia: Churchill Livingstone; 2000:2420–2429.

4. Kjeldsberg CR. *Practical Diagnosis of Hematologic Disorders.* Vol. 1. 4th ed. Chicago: ASCP Press; 2006:4.

5. Cable RG, Leiby DA. Risk and prevention of transfusion-transmitted babesiosis and other tick-borne diseases. *Curr Opin Hematol.* 2003;10:405–411.

6. Homer MJ, Aguilar-Delfin I, Telford SR, et al. Babesiosis. *Clin Microbiol Rev.* 2000;13:451–469.

7. Setty S, Khalil Z, Schori P, et al. Babesiosis. Two atypical cases from Minnesota and a review. *Am J Clin Pathol.* 2003;120:554–559.

8. Krause PJ, Lepore T, Sikand VK, et al. Atovaquone and azithromycin for the treatment of babesiosis. *N Engl J Med.* 2000;343:1454–1458.

Eosinophilia in an Indian Farmer

Menka Doomra, Seema Garg, Naveen Kakkar

Department of Pathology, Christian Medical College and Hospital, Ludhiana, Punjab, India

Patient: 38-year-old Indian farmer.

Medical/Drug/Family History: Unremarkable.

Chief Complaint: None. The patient was asymptomatic; however, a routine complete blood count (CBC) was done as an immigration requirement.

Physical Examination Findings: The patient was well built with normal general physical and systemic examinations.

T1. Principal Laboratory Findings

Test	Patient's Result	Reference Range
Hematology		
WBC count	9.8	4.0-11.0 × 10³/L
Hemoglobin	12.4	12.0-16.0 g/dL
Platelet count	150	150-400 × 10³/L
Differential: Neutrophils	48	40-80%
Lymphocytes	14	20-40%
Eosinophils	35	2-6%
Monocytes	3	1-6%
Absolute eosinophil count	3.43	0.02-0.5 × 10⁹/L
PBS findings	Microfilaria present with numerous nuclei throughout the body of the organism that stop well short of the tip of the tail (**Image 1**)	

WBC, white blood cell; PBS, peripheral blood smear.

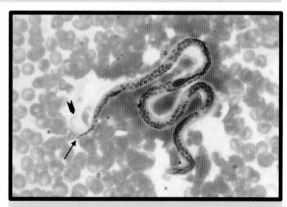

Image 1_Patient's peripheral blood smear, illustrating the presence of the microfilarial organism, Wuchereria bancrofti (Leishman stain; 1,000× magnification). Note the large, empty (ie, no nuclei present) space between where the nuclei in the body end (arrow) and the tip of the tail (arrowhead) of the organism.

Questions

1. What is (are) this patient's most striking clinical and laboratory finding(s)?

2. Given this patient's history and laboratory findings, what is the differential diagnosis?

3. Among the possibilities in the differential diagnosis, what features of the organism found in this patient's blood enable you to suggest the most likely diagnosis?

4. What is this patient's most likely diagnosis?

5. What is the geographical distribution of the organism found in this patient's blood?

6. What are the clinical features and the treatment of the disease caused by the organism present in this patient's blood?

7. What is the life cycle of the organism found in this patient's blood?

8. What is the pathogenesis of the clinical manifestations caused by the organism found in this patient's blood?

9. How is the diagnosis of the organism found in this patient's blood made in the laboratory?

Possible Answers _____

1. Marked eosinophilia and the presence of a parasite (microfilaria) in the peripheral blood smear (**T1 and Image 1**).

2. Parasitic infection with microfilarial larva of *Wuchereria bancrofti, Brugia malayi, Loa loa, Oncocerca volvulus,* or *Dipetalonema perstans.*

3. The microfilariae are the **larval stage** of the parasite and appear as colorless, transparent bodies with blunt heads and pointed tails on unstained peripheral blood preparations. When dead and stained with Romanowsky stain, the microfilariae show certain morphological characteristics, including a hyaline sheath, which is a structureless sac and is longer than the larval body; somatic cells (nuclei) which appear as granules in the central axis of the body of the organism and extend from the head to an area just short of the tip of the tail, and a cephalic space at the anterior end of the organism which is devoid of granules. The continuity of the granules is broken at definite places along the sheath that form anatomical landmarks for locating the nerve ring, oblique space, genital cells, anterior V spot, posterior V spot, and the anal pore of the organism. Sheathed microfilariae of *Brugia malayi* and *Loa loa* can be distinguished from those of *Wuchereria bancrofti* on the basis of the morphology of the tail tip. In the case of *Brugia malayi*, the tail shows 2 discrete nuclei: 1 at the extreme tip of the tail which is slightly bulbous and the other midway between the tip and posterior column of nuclei with a constriction of the tail in between. The microfilariae of

Loa loa contain a column of nuclei extending to the tail tip. The **adult worms** are long filiform shapes found in lymphatic vessels and lymph nodes of man. The head of the worm terminates in a slightly rounded swelling and female worms are longer than male worms. The tail end of male worms is curved, while that of females is narrow and abruptly pointed.

4. ***Most likely diagnosis:*** asymptomatic microfilarial infection by the larval form of *Wuchereria bancrofti*. The morphology of the tail in the organism shown in **Image 1** is consistent with the characteristics of the tail found in *Wuchereria bancrofti*. This parasite belongs to the superfamily, *Filariodea* and subfamily, *Acanthocheilonematinae*.

5. Filariasis is largely confined to the tropics and subtropics, occurring in India (especially along the coast line), West Indies, Southern China, Japan, West and Central Africa, and Central America.

6. The most common clinical presentation of bancroftian filariasis is asymptomatic microfilaremia (especially with mild infection). In symptomatic patients, the clinical manifestation has 2 phases—an acute inflammatory phase of adenolymphangitis and the phase of chronic lymphatic obstruction. The **acute inflammatory phase** is characterized by high fever, chills, and malaise. Intense pain, redness, and edema occur along the lymphatic channels and the draining lymph nodes become enlarged and painful. Any lymph node or any body part can be affected but the common sites include upper and lower extremities, groin, and the axilla. Genital lymphatics are commonly involved in males leading to funiculitis, orchitis, epididymitis, and scrotal pain and tenderness. In the **chronic obstructive phase**, elephantiasis (solid edema) of the affected part occurs in which brawny edema, hyperkeratosis, and fissuring of the skin develops. Genital involvement in males results in the development of hydrocele, scrotal lymphedema, and elephantiasis. In patients with occult filariasis, chyluria, chylothorax, chylous ascites, and chylous diarrhea may also develop. Occult filariasis is a condition characterized by massive eosinophilia, generalized lymphadenopathy,

hepatosplenomegaly, pulmonary symptoms, and the absence of microfilaremia.[1]

7. Man is the definitive host and mosquitoes (Anopheles, Culex, and Aedes species) are the intermediate host of *W. bancrofti*. Sheathed microfilariae ingested by the mosquito during its blood meal collect in the anterior end of the stomach where they cast off their sheath and penetrate the gut wall. Then, they migrate to the thoracic muscles where they rest. Further maturation proceeds through 3 stages. In the third stage, larvae enter the proboscis sheath of the mosquito and infect man during the mosquito's blood meal. The larvae enter the skin of man, migrate into the bloodstream, and eventually reach lymphatic channels where they finally settle down in the inguinal, scrotal, and abdominal lymphatics and begin to grow into adult, sexually mature forms. Fertilization occurs and the gravid female gives birth to larvae. A new generation of microfilariae is created which pass either through the thoracic duct or the right lymphatic duct into the venous system and pulmonary capillaries and then into the peripheral circulation where they can be detected on blood smear examination.

8. The principal lesions that occur during the *acute* inflammatory phase of *W. bancrofti* infection are lymphangitis and lymphadenitis. Both of these occur due to the mechanical irritation caused by motile adult worms residing in afferent lymphatics and the sinuses of lymph nodes and to the toxic metabolites released by growing microfilariae and disintegrating dead worms. In the *chronic* phase of infection, lymphatic obstruction occurs due to mechanical blocking of the lumina by dead worms, endothelial proliferation, inflammatory thickening of the wall of lymphatic vessels, and excessive fibrosis of the lymphatic vessels due to repeated attacks of lymphangitis.

9. The laboratory diagnosis of filariasis can be made using direct or indirect methods. The **direct methods** include visualization of the larval stage (microfilariae) or the adult worm. Microfilariae can be seen in the peripheral blood or other body fluids (eg, urine and ascitic, hydrocele, or lymph fluid). In the peripheral blood, microfilariae can be detected by 3 principal methods: 1) wet smear examination under the microscope where motility can also be seen; 2) examination of a

stained peripheral blood smear which is also useful in species identification based on the morphologic features of the organism, especially the tail end; and, 3) thick or concentrated blood smears, if the diagnosis cannot be made using the other methods. Concentration smears are especially useful in patients who have low parasitemia. In such cases, membrane filtration techniques can also be used to concentrate organisms and promote their detection and identification. Moreover, microfilariae do not remain in the blood stream all the time. In oriental (Indian and Chinese) individuals with filariasis, the microfilariae appear in the circulation between 10:00 PM and 2:00 AM, the optimal time period for obtaining a blood sample for testing. This phenomenon is thought to be related to the nocturnal feeding habits of the mosquito host. However, a single dose of diethylcarbamazine can provoke the microfilariae to appear in the circulation during daytime if blood sampling at night is inconvenient.[2] Adult worms can also be demonstrated in a lymph node biopsy, while calcified adult worms can be visualized on an X-ray. Doppler ultrasonography can also be used to detect the presence of motile adult worms in dilated lymphatics.

The **indirect methods** include: peripheral blood eosinophilia, elevated serum IgE concentration, and the presence of an antifilarial serum antibody. Intradermal and complement fixation tests have been used in the past; however, these tests are unreliable. Among the better methods available for diagnosing infection with *W. bancrofti*, an enzyme linked immunosorbent assay (ELISA) and a rapid format immunochromatographic card test for circulating antigens of *W. bancrofti* permit the diagnosis of microfilaremic and amicrofilaremic (cryptic) infection.[3] A polymerase chain reaction (PCR)-based assay for deoxyribonucleic acid (DNA) gene sequences of *W. bancrofti* is also available.[4] Lastly, radionuclide lymphoscintigraphic imaging of the limbs can demonstrate widespread lymphatic abnormalities both in patients with symptomatic microfilaremia and in those with clinical manifestations of lymphatic obstruction.[5]

Treatment and Outcome

The drug of choice for filariasis presently is ivermectin, given as a 150 to 200 mg/kg single oral dose. The dosage can be repeated after 2 to 3 months. Diethylcarbazine (DEC or Hetrazan) is, however, more widely used especially in developing countries in a strength of 6 mg/kg/day 3 times a day for at least 12 days and preferably for 3 weeks. A lower dose of 2 to 3 mg/kg/day is recommended for the first 3 days to decrease the risk of adverse effects especially hypersensitivity reactions. In the present case, the patient was prescribed DEC but did not return for follow-up.

Keywords

microfilariae, filariasis, Wuchereria bancrofti, lymphangitis, lymphadenitis

References

1. Meyers WM, Neafie RC, Connor DH. Bancroftian and Malayan Filariasis. In: *Pathology of Tropical and Extraordinary Diseases*. Binford CH, Connor DH. eds. Washington DC: Armed Forces Institute of Pathology, 1976:340-355.

2. Chatterjee KD. *Parasitology*. 12th ed. Calcutta: Chatterjee Medical Publishers; 1980.

3. Nuchprayoon S, Porksakorn C, Junpee A, et al. Comparative assessment of an Og4C3 ELISA and an ICT filariasis test: a study of Myanmar migrants in Thailand. *Asian Pac J Allergy Immunol*. 2003;21:253-257.

4. Kanjanavas P, Tan-ariya P, Khawsak P, et al. Detection of lymphatic Wuchereria bancrofti in carriers and long-term storage samples using semi-nested PCR. *Mol Cell Probes*. 2005;19:169-172.

5. Freedman DO, de Almeido Filho PJ, Besh S, et al. Lymphoscintigraphic analysis of lymphatic abnormalities in symptomatic and asymptomatic human filariasis. *J Infect Dis*. 1994;170:927-33.

Fever of Unknown Origin (FUO) and Massive Splenomegaly in an Indian Girl

Naveen Kakkar

Department of Pathology, CMC Hospital, Ludhiana, Panjab, India

Patient: 13-year-old Indian girl from the state of Bihar, India.

Family History: Unremarkable.

Chief Complaint: Fever, weight loss, anorexia, and abdominal discomfort for the past 4 months.

Medical History: Unremarkable.

Drug History: Received 30 intramuscular injections earlier; however, further details were unavailable.

Physical Examination: Thin, febrile (101°F) adolescent with marked pallor, massive splenomegaly to the level of the umbilicus, and mild hepatomegaly.

Questions

1. What are this patient's most significant clinical and laboratory findings?

2. What is this patient's most likely diagnosis?

3. What are the principal clinical features of this patient's condition?

4. What are the geographic and life-cycle characteristics of the organism responsible for this patient's condition?

5. What are the possible causes of this patient's anemia?

6. What laboratory investigations can be carried out to diagnose this patient's condition?

7. In addition to the organism responsible for this patient's condition, what other parasitic organisms can be seen in the peripheral blood and/or bone marrow?

Possible Answers

1. Fever, massive splenomegaly, bicytopenia (anemia and leukopenia), hypoalbuminemia with mild elevation of hepatic enzymes [**T1**], and Leishman Donovan (LD) bodies in the bone marrow aspirate [**Image 1**].

2. **Most likely diagnosis:** *visceral leishmaniasis.*

Leishmaniasis is a systemic illness caused by parasitization of the reticuloendothelial system (bone marrow, liver, spleen, and lymph nodes) by the protozoan—*Leishmania donovani.* *Leishmania donovani* is an obligate intracellular protozoan with 2 developmental stages: promastigote (flagellated) and amastigote (non-flagellated). The promastigote occurs in the vector for this organism, sandflies of the genus *Phlebotomus*, and in culture media, while the amastigote form is seen in man and other hosts (eg, rodents and dogs). Promastigotes are 15 to 26 μm in length and 2 to 3 μm in width and exhibit a prominent flagellum.[1] The amastigote

T1. Principal Laboratory Findings

Test	Patient's Result	"Normal" Reference Range
Hematology		
WBC count	3.0	4.0-11.0 × 10³/µL
Hemoglobin	4.0	12.0-16.0 g/dL
MCV	64	76-96 fL
MCH	20.4	27.0-32.0 pg
MCHC	31.9	29.0-31.0 g/dL
Platelet count	300	150-400 × 1,000/µL
Differential:		
Neutrophils	26	40-80%
Myelocytes	4	
Metamyelocytes	24	
Lymphocytes	46	20-40%
Reticulocyte count	1.5	0.2-2.0%
Chemistry		
Bilirubin, total	1.8	0.5-1.4 mg/dL
Bilirubin, direct	1.4	0.0-0.4 mg/dL
AST	175	5-50 U/L
ALT	308	5-50 U/L
ALP	114	70-230 U/L
Total protein	7.3	6.0-8.4 g/dL
Albumin	1.9	3.5-5.0 g/dL
BUN	79	15-45 mg/dL
Creatinine	1.4	0.7-1.5 mg/dL

WBC, white blood cell; MCV, mean corpuscular volume; MCHC, mean corpuscular hemoglobin concentration; AST, aspartate aminotransferase; ALT, alanine aminotransferase; ALP, alkaline phosphatase; BUN, blood urea nitrogen.

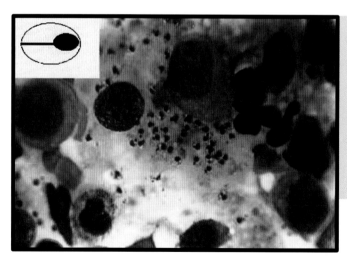

Image 1_Bone marrow aspirate of the patient demonstrating numerous amastigote forms (Leishman Donovan bodies) of *Leishmania donovani* within the cytoplasm of a histiocyte along with a few extracellular forms (magnification, 1,000x). Note the small stub-like projection (arrows) or kinetoplast arising from the nucleus. Inset: Diagrammatic illustration of the amastigote form of *Leishmania donovani*.

form is round (2 to 4 μm in diameter) to oval in shape with a large eccentrically placed nucleus, an internalized flagellum, and a kinetoplast—a rod-shaped, specialized mitochondrial structure [**Image 1**].

3. Patients with visceral leishmaniasis present with intermittent fever of long duration, months to years. Organomegaly is conspicuous, especially splenomegaly, which can be massive if the condition is untreated. Mild to moderate hepatomegaly and lymphadenopathy frequently accompany the enlarged spleen. Cytopenias are common and patients may present with malaise, frequent infections, and bleeding from various sites due to anemia, leukopenia, and thrombocytopenia, respectively. Patients in India may experience hyperpigmentation of the skin which led to the other name for visceral leishmaniasis, Kala-azar, the Hindi word for black fever. Visceral leishmaniasis has a mortality of 10% even if adequately treated. It may also be associated with HIV infection.[2]

4. More than 90% of all cases of visceral leishmaniasis in the world occur in the following countries: Bangladesh, northeastern India (especially the states of Bihar, West Bengal, Uttar Pradesh, and Assam), Nepal, Sudan, North Brazil, China, and Northern Europe. Moreover, other *Leishmania* species (eg, *L. infantum, L. chagasi, L. amazonensis,* and *L. tropica*) can also cause visceral leishmaniasis. In addition, a variety of other *Leishmania* species cause cutaneous and muco-cutaneous lesions.[2,3] Specific species of sandfly transmit disease caused by different species of *Leishmania*. The vector for Indian Kala-azar is the sandfly belonging to the genus *Phlebotomus* and species *argentipes*. The disease can be transmitted by the bite of an infected sandfly, parenterally (blood transfusion or shared needles), and congenitally from an infected mother to her newborn baby. The parasite has an incubation period that varies from a few weeks to 2 years or more. As the infected flies attempt to feed, they regurgitate the parasite's flagellated promastigotes onto the skin of its mammalian host. Promastigotes that enter the blood stream attach to receptors on macrophages, are phagocytosed, and then transform within the acidic environment of the phagolysosomes into the aflagellate amastigote stage which multiplies by binary fission. Sandflies

ingest the amastigote-containing macrophages when they take a blood meal. These then convert to the flagellate promastigote form in the gut of the sandfly and later migrate to the pharynx to further propagate the cycle during a subsequent blood meal by the sandfly.[2]

5. Possible causes of this patient's anemia include: hypersplenism (sequestration of red blood cells, white blood cells, and platelets in the enlarged spleen), extensive bone marrow infiltration by the parasite, bleeding (due to thrombocytopenia), and occasionally autoimmune red cell hemolysis.

6. The laboratory diagnosis of visceral leishmaniasis can be made on the basis of indirect and or direct evidence. Indirect evidence would include: leukopenia, with relative lymphocytosis, monocytosis and eosinopenia, or pancytopenia in the peripheral blood, and positive aldehyde, antimony, or complement fixation tests. The aldehyde and antimony tests, however, are nonspecific and only indicate hypergammaglobulinemia which is seen consistently in all patients with leishmaniasis. Direct evidence would include: the presence of the amastigote (aflagellate) form of *Leishmania donovani* (ie, Leishman Donovan bodies in the cytoplasm of neutrophils or monocytes) in thin or thick film preparations of the peripheral blood, or in aspirates from bone marrow obtained from the sternum or iliac crest, or in aspirates of the spleen or enlarged lymph nodes. Diagnosis by splenic puncture touch preparations can be as high as 98% compared with less than 90% by other procedures. However, because of the risk of bleeding while performing splenic puncture, bone marrow aspiration is routinely done to clinch the diagnosis. Moreover, promastigote (flagellated) forms can be seen in the culture of blood or aspirates from bone marrow, spleen, or lymph nodes using Novy-MacNeal-Nicolle (NNN) media. In addition, polymerase chain reaction (PCR)-based assays have also been developed and are emerging as the method of choice for the diagnosis of leishmaniasis when isolation of amastigote forms by other methods fails. Other direct tests include isoenzyme analysis of cultured promastigote forms, the use of monoclonal antibodies, and detection by molecular methods of leishmaniaspecific DNA sequences using DNA probes.[1]

7. Other than leishmaniasis, malaria, filariasis, trypanosomiasis, babesiosis, and onchocerciasis are diseases in which the parasites that cause these diseases can be visualized in peripheral blood smears.

Keywords

Leishmania donovani, parasite, amastigote, promastigote, leishmaniasis, sandfly

References

1. Manson-Bahr PH. Leishmaniasis. In: *Manson's Tropical Diseases*. 16th ed. London, England: Balliere, Tindall and Cassell. 1966:107-143.

2. Berman JD. Human leishmaniasis: Clinical, diagnostic and chemotherapeutic developments in the last 10 years. *Clin Infect Dis*. 1997;24:684-703.

3. Pearson RD, Sousa AQ. Clinical spectrum of leishmaniasis. *Clin Infect Dis*. 1996;22:1-13.

Fever and Coma in a Young Indian Boy

Reeta Thapa,[1] Naveen Kakkar,[1] Mary John[2]

Departments of [1]Pathology and [2]Medicine, Christian Medical College and Hospital, Ludhiana, Punjab, India

Patient: 15-year-old Indian boy.

Medical/Family History: Unremarkable.

Chief Complaint: High grade fever for 5 days and altered sensorium 16 hours prior to admission.

Drug History: History of abuse of dextropropoxyphene, an opioid derivative.

Physical Examination Findings: The patient was comatose and febrile (102°F) with pallor, mild icterus, moderate hepatosplenomegaly, and brisk deep tendon reflexes.

Questions

1. What is (are) this patient's most striking clinical and laboratory finding(s)?

2. How do you explain these findings?

3. What is this patient's most likely diagnosis?

4. What are the other species of the organism found in this patient's blood?

5. What is the geographical distribution of the organism found in this patient's blood?

6. What are the clinical features of the disease caused by the organism present in this patient's blood?

7. What causes the clinical effects of the organism found in this patient's blood to be more severe compared to other species of this organism?

8. What is the life cycle of the organism found in this patient's blood?

9. How is the diagnosis of the organism found in this patient's blood made in the laboratory?

Possible Answers

1. High-grade fever for several days with altered mental status, icterus, hepatosplenomegaly; severe anemia, mild leukocytosis with left shift, markedly increased LD level, azotemia, mild hyperbilirubinemia; and the presence of malarial trophozoites and crescent-shaped gametocytes in several red blood cells on the peripheral blood smear (PBS) (**T1** and **Image 1**).

2. The constellation of this patient's clinical and laboratory findings, especially the presence of crescent-shaped gametocytes in the PBS, are characteristic of a malarial infection with the protozoan parasite, *Plasmodium falciparum*.

3. ***Most likely diagnosis:*** cerebral malaria due to *Plasmodium falciparum*.

4. *Plasmodium vivax, Plasmodium ovale,* and *Plasmodium malariae.* Plasmodia are protozoa

T1. Principal Laboratory Findings

Test	Patient's Result	"Normal" Reference Range
Hematology		
WBC count	15.9	4.0-11.0 × 10³/L
Hemoglobin	4.1	12.0-16.0 g/dL
Hematocrit	11.4	38-47%
Platelet count	75	150-400 × 10³/L
Reticulocyte count	3.4	0.2-2%
Differential: Myelocytes	22	0%
Metamyelocytes	14	0%
Neutrophils	20	40-80%
Lymphocytes	42	20-40%
Eosinophils	2	0-6%
PBS findings	Many RBCs with malarial trophozoites and crescent-shaped gametocytes (Parasitic Index = 80%) **(Image 1)**	
Chemistry		
Blood urea nitrogen	198	15-45 mg/dL
Serum creatinine	3.1	0.7-1.5 mg/dL
Total bilirubin	3.7	0.5-1.4 mg/dL
Direct bilirubin	2.5	0-0.4 mg/dL
ALT	80	5-50 U/L
AST	310	5-50 U/L
ALP	351	70-230 U/L
LD	4480	230-460 U/L

WBC, white blood cell; PBS, peripheral blood smear; ALT, alanine aminotransferase; AST, aspartate aminotransferase; ALP, alkaline phosphatase; LD, lactate dehydrogenase.

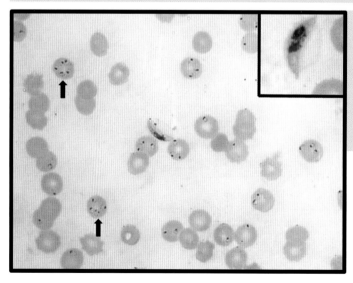

Image 1_Patient's peripheral blood smear, illustrating the presence of trophozoites (arrows) and a crescent-shaped gametocyte (inset) of *P. falciparum* (1,000× magnification).

belonging to the suborder Hemosporina and the class, Sporozoa, that cause malaria in man.

5. Malaria is more prevalent in the tropics and subtropics where optimal conditions exist for the development and growth of the parasite within the mosquito vector. The Anopheles mosquito survives at temperatures between 15°C to 38°C; however, optimal growth of the parasite occurs at 20°C to 30°C and at a minimum of 60% humidity. *Plasmodium falciparum* is most common in Africa, New Guinea, and Haiti and is also seen in South America and East Asia. *Plasmodium vivax* occurs in temperate zones and in large areas of the tropics as well as in Central America and the Indian subcontinent. *Plasmodium malariae* and *Plasmodium ovale* are common in Africa. In North America, Europe, and other regions of the world where malaria has been eradicated, the disease is imported by visitors/travelers from endemic areas.

6. In the early phase of malarial infection, clinical symptoms of disease are typically mild and non-specific, similar to those occurring during an acute viral infection. The classical paroxysms of chills and fever occurring at regular periodic intervals for *P. vivax* (48 h), *P. ovale* (48 h), and *P. malariae* (72 h) are absent in infections with *P. falciparum* in which the pattern of fever is irregular and occurs at 24 to 48 hours. Associated clinical findings with malarial infection include: anemia, mild jaundice, and hepatosplenomegaly. The clinical complications of malarial infection are seen more frequently and are more significant, including life-threatening, in falciparum malaria than other malarial species and include: cerebral malaria, hypotension, hypothermia, acute renal failure, lactic acidosis, acute respiratory distress syndrome (ARDS), and intravascular hemolysis leading to hemoglobinuria.[1]

7. The increased severity of disease symptoms associated with malarial infection by *P. falciparum* is due to the larger parasitic load (ie, more red blood cells are parasitized) caused by this malarial parasite compared to other malarial species. In addition, parasitized red blood cells (RBCs) are rendered sticky by a protein, *P. falciparum* erythrocyte membrane protein (PfEMP), that causes knob-like structures on RBC membranes and increases their adherance to the endothelium

of capillaries and venules. This leads to vascular occlusion and tissue anoxia which causes increased capillary permeability and edema, the primary cause of the cerebral symptoms associated with *P. falciparum* infection.[2]

8. The definitive host for plasmodium species is the mosquito vector, the female anopheles mosquito. Man is the intermediate host. In the human host, sporozoites inoculated during the mosquito bite enter the liver where **pre-erythrocytic schizogony** occurs within the hepatocytes to liberate daughter merozoites into the peripheral circulation. Released merozoites which may be 10,000 to 30,000 in number attach to RBC membranes and enter these cells for the next phase of the life-cycle, **erythrocytic schizogony**. In this phase of the life-cycle, the trophozoites grow by feeding on the hemoglobin of the host RBCs until schizogony occurs with discharge of merozoites into the blood stream. The duration of this phase correlates with the interval between clinical paroxysms of fever. The merozoites infect other RBCs to repeat the cycle while some develop into the sexual forms, the male and female gametocytes which, in the case of *P. falciparum*, are large and crescent-shaped. Once a mosquito ingests a blood meal from an individual whose RBCs contain gametocytes, they fuse to form a zygote, followed by development of an ookinete and an oocyst. The mature oocyst releases 50 to 100 sporozoites into the salivary apparatus of the mosquito and this permits the cycle to continue in the human host during its next human blood meal. Unlike other malarial species, **exo-erythrocytic schizogony** does not occur in *P. falciparum* infection and therefore, relapses do not occur in individuals infected with this malarial species.

9. The diagnosis of malaria in the laboratory can be made by **direct methods** which involve visualization of the parasite or by **indirect methods** that identify the presence of malarial enzymes or antigen.

Direct methods:

a. Thin-smear examination: the malarial parasite is directly visualized by microscopic examination of a thin film of peripheral blood stained with Romanowsky, Giemsa, Leishman, Wright or

Field stain. Malarial ring forms (trophozoites), crescent-shaped gametocytes, or both may be seen in the peripheral blood smear.

b. Thick-smear examination: dehemoglobinized thick smears are used for screening blood for the presence of malarial parasites. However, artifacts and distortion of morphology do not always permit correct identification of the malarial species present. For this reason, examination of a thin and thick smear should always be performed simultaneously when screening a PBS for the presence of malarial parasites. Both smears are examined using the oil immersion lens and the number of parasitized RBCs and parasites are counted in the thin and thick smears, respectively. A minimum of 100 oil immersion fields of the thick smear should be examined before a negative report is released. Thick smears are extremely helpful in cases of low parasite load in which thin-smear examination may be negative.

c. Concentration smears: useful in identifying the presence of a malarial parasite when the degree of parasitemia is low. Thin smears should be visualized simultaneously for identification of the species of malarial parasite present because speciation is difficult using concentration smears.

Indirect methods:

d. Staining the blood smear with fluorescent dyes, especially acridine orange, has been shown to be a sensitive test in the diagnosis of malaria. Compared to Giemsa-stained PBSs, acridine orange-stained PBSs provide higher sensitivity in detecting malarial organisms when the level of parasitemia is low (<1,000 organisms/μL). Rapid results is the major advantage of this method.[3]

e. The plasmodial lactate dehydrogenase (pLD) assay provides better sensitivity in detecting *P. falciparum* than blood-smear examination.[4] Moreover, because this assay can be performed rapidly and is positive only during active infection, it is being used increasingly to identify individuals infected with *P. falciparum*.

f. The detection of histidine rich receptor-2 (HRP-2) antigen using monoclonal antibodies can be used to identify plasmodium infection;

however, this test can be positive even after the active infection has subsided.

g. Polymerase chain reaction (PCR) assays have been used recently to diagnose malarial infection and also during vaccine trials.[5] Although such assays are more sensitive than the gold standard (ie, microscopic examination by thin and/or thick smear) in the detection and identification of malarial parasites, the high cost of these assays can be prohibitive to the economies of developing countries where malaria is rampant.

h. Other serological methods for the detection of malarial organisms include enzyme-linked immunosorbent assays (ELISA), indirect hemagglutination assays, and immunoprecipitation assays; however, these assays are generally cumbersome and not used routinely by most clinical laboratories.

Keywords

plasmodia, parasitemia, cerebral malaria, trophozoite, crescent-shaped gametocyte, schizogony

References

1. Mackintosh CL, Beeson JG, Marsh K. Clinical features and pathogenesis of severe malaria. *Trends Parasitol.* 2004; 20:597-603.

2. Russell C, Mercereau-Puijalon O, Le Scanf C, et al. Further definition of PfEMP-1 DBL-1alpha domains mediating resetting adhesion of *Plasmodium falciparum*. *Mol Biochem Parasitol.* 2005;144:109-113.

3. Keiser J, Utzinger J, Premji Z, et al. Acridine Orange for malaria diagnosis: its diagnostic performance, its promotion and implementation in Tanzania, and the implications for malaria control. *Ann Trop Med Parasitol.* 2002;96:643-654.

4. Odhiambo RA, Odulaja A. New enzymatic assay, parasite lactate dehydrogenase, in diagnosis of malaria in Kenya. *East Afr Med J.* 2005;82:111-117.

5. Ndao M, Bandyayera E, Kokoskin E, et al. Comparison of blood smear, antigen detection, and nested-PCR methods for screening refugees from regions where malaria is endemic after a malaria outbreak in Quebec, Canada. *J Clin Microbiol.* 2004;42:2694-2700.

Fever and Confusion in a 47-Year-Old Man

Pamala F. Jones, Jane Hudson, Sabrina Bryant, Randy Coulter

Department of Medical Technology, University of Southern Mississippi, Hattiesburg, MS

Patient: 47-year-old Caucasian man.

Chief Complaint: Fever, nausea, and worsening confusion after returning from a trip to Nigeria.

History of Current Medications: He was taking a homeopathic medicine for prevention of malaria during his trip to Nigeria.

Past Medical History: Nonsmoker with no history of alcohol abuse and no chronic medical conditions. He had asthma and allergic rhinitis when he was younger and was treated for this condition with immunotherapy for a short period of time.

Questions

1. What are this patient's most striking clinical and laboratory findings?

2. How do you explain this patient's most striking clinical and laboratory findings?

3. What is this patient's most likely diagnosis?

4. What is the most common parasite for this infection?

5. What are some complications of this patient's disease?

6. Would this patient be denied as a blood donor?

7. What drugs could be used for prevention and treatment of this patient's disease?

Possible Answers

1. Fever, nausea, and the developing of worsening confusion; decreased hemoglobin and hematocrit, marked thrombocytopenia, increased BUN, decreased glucose, a markedly increased LD (**T1**); and peripheral blood smear findings of many ring forms and a few schizonts of a malarial parasite in the red blood cells which were of normal size (**Image 1A**).

2. Fever, nausea, and confusion are typical symptoms of a malarial infection, while the high degree of parasitemia and associated destruction of parasite-containing RBCs by cells of organs (bone marrow, liver, and spleen) of the reticuloendothelial system (RES) explains the decreased hemoglobin and hematocrit values, thrombocytopenia, and increased LD concentration. The increased BUN is attributed to renal dysfunction that may result in acute renal failure.[1] Other manifestations of severe malaria are lactic acidosis and hypoglycemia due to the infected red blood cells undergoing

T1. Principal Laboratory Findings		
Test	Patient's Result	"Normal" Reference Interval
Hematology		
WBC count	4.2	$4.8–10.8 × 10^3$/mL
Hemoglobin	12.4	14.0–16.5 g/dL
Hematocrit	35.7	42–52%
Platelet count	16	$150–400 × 10^3$/mL
PBS findings on hospital day:	**1.** Many malarial ring forms; few schizonts (**Image 1A**)	
	2. 80% malarial parasitemia (**Image 1B**)	
	3. 20% malarial parasitemia (**Image 1C**)	
	5. No malarial organisms observed (**Image 1D**)	
Chemistry		
Glucose	55	70–110 mg/dL
BUN	51	6–20 mg/dL
Total protein	4.6	6.7–8.2 g/dL
Albumin	2.1	3.2–5.5 g/dL
AST	66	10–42 U/L
ALT	24	10–60 U/L
LD	671	91–180 U/L

WBC, white blood cell; PBS, peripheral blood smear; BUN, blood urea nitrogen; AST, aspartate aminotransferase; ALT, alanine aminotransferase; LD, lactate dehydrogrenase.

increased anaerobic glycolysis.[2] The patient's travel history is consistent with the possibility of a malarial infection because Nigeria is located in a region of Africa where malarial disease is highly endemic, and both morbidity and mortality from malaria have been estimated by the World Health Organization (WHO) to be ~85% in 2001.[3]

3. **Most likely diagnosis:** *malaria due to infection with P. falciparum.* Among the different species of malarial parasites, *P. falciparum* exhibits the heaviest parasitemia with associated destruction of RBCs.[4,5] The combination of this patient's travel history, and clinical and laboratory findings (especially the number and morphological characteristics of the ring forms observed in the RBCs on the peripheral blood smear and the presence of schizonts with a large number

of merozoites) is consistent with infection with *P. falciparum* species of malaria. Infection with *P. falciparum* occurs in humans when the sporozoites from the salivary secretions of a mosquito infected with the parasite are introduced into the blood of a human during a blood meal.[6] Moreover, the national falciparum prevalence (N*f*P) for Nigeria is ~50%.[3] The N*f*P is calculated as described in Reference 3 and is used to compare and contrast risk among various areas of the world using a metric other than land area to visualize, using a cartogram, variations in infection rates between these areas.[3]

4. The most prevalent infection in the world is malaria, and it accounts for approximately 300 million to 500 million cases per year worldwide.[3] Malaria is a mosquito-transmitted infectious parasitic disease caused by *Plasmodium* protozoa. Of the *Plasmodium* species identified, only 4 species are considered pathogenic for humans (*vivax, ovale, falciparum, and malariae*). The most common malarial parasite is *P. vivax*; however, the multiple ring stages and the schizonts with up to 24 merozoites found in this patient are indicative of the species *P. falciparum*, which is responsible for infecting about 5% of the world's population and causing the deaths of more than 2 million children each year.[2]

5. After an incubation period of about 7 to 10 days, patients infected with *Plasmodium falciparum* may have flu-like symptoms with occurrences of severe diarrhea, chills along with fever, and vomiting. The chills and fever peaks occur on a cycle of 36 to 48 hours. Although *P. vivax* is the most common malarial parasite, *P. falciparum* is the most deadly in untreated patients. This is due to the heavy parasitemia, production of toxic products, and obstruction of blood vessels caused by the crescent shaped gametocytes of this species of malaria. Because hemoglobinuria is often associated with *P. falciparum* infection, the disease caused by this organism is sometimes called "black water fever." Patients may also experience acute renal failure, tubular necrosis, or even death from this infection.[1,4]

6. This patient would be deferred as a blood donor. The American Association of Blood Banks (AABB) requires that potential donors who have been diagnosed with malaria, have traveled to a

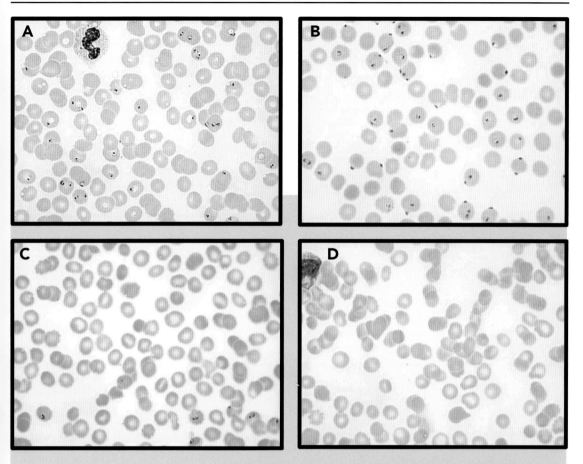

Image 1_Patient's peripheral blood smear findings illustrating (**A**) many ring forms and few schizonts (Wright-Giemsa stain; 1,000× magnification) on day 1 of hospital admission; (**B**) 80% malarial parasitemia on day 2 of hospital admission; (**C**) 20% malarial parasitemia on day 3 of hospital admission; and (**D**) no organisms seen in RBCs on day 5 of hospital admission.

malaria endemic area, or have lived in a malaria endemic area and have symptoms suggestive of malaria be deferred for 3 years after symptoms are no longer apparent.[7] Also, if an individual has lived for 5 consecutive years in areas the Centers for Disease Control and Prevention (CDC) Malarial Branch considers endemic, the individual is deferred as a donor for 3 years after the individual leaves the area.[8]

7. According to the CDC, preventative methods for travelers to areas such as Africa, South America, the Indian Subcontinent, Tajikistan, Asia, and the South Pacific include the use of 1 of the following antimalarial drugs: atovaquone/proguanil, doxycycline, mefloquine, or primaquine.[8] According to the CDC, the most common drugs used in the treatment of malarial parasites include: chloroquine, sulfadoxine-pyrimethamine, mefloquine, atovaquone-proguanil, quinine, and doxycycline.[9] The need for safe, effective, and inexpensive drugs and/or combination drugs against *P. falciparum* in poor endemic countries is urgent.[9] Due to the increasing resistance of malarial parasites to antimalarial drugs, the control of malaria is becoming less and less successful.[10] This patient was treated with chloroquinine and during a 5-day course of therapy, the patient's parasitemia decreased to no organisms observed on his peripheral blood smear on day 5 (**Image 1B, C,** and **D**).

Keywords

malaria, Plasmodium falciparum, black water fever, chloroquine, blood donations

References

1. Zeibig EA. *Clinical Parasitology: A Practical Approach*. 1st ed. Philadelphia: W.B. Saunders; 1997:91–94.

2. Mehta M, Sonawat HM, Sharma S. Malaria parasite-infected erythrocytes inhibit glucose utilization in uninfected red cells. *FEBS Letters*. 2005;579:6151–6158.

3. Hay SI, Guerra CA, Tatem AJ, et al. The global distribution and population at risk of malaria: Past, present, and future. *Lancet Infect Dis*. 2004;4:327–336.

4. Markell EK, John DT, Krotoski WA. *Medical Parasitology*. 8th ed. Philadelphia: W.B. Saunders; 1992:102.

5. Burtis CA, Ashwood ER. *Tietz Fundamentals of Clinical Chemistry*. 4th ed. Philadelphia: W.B. Saunders;1996:308.

6. Baron EJ, Peterson LR, Finegold SM. *Bailey & Scott's Diagnostic Microbiology*. 9th ed. St. Louis: Mosby-Year Book Inc; 1994:823.

7. Brecher ME. *Technical Manual*. 15th ed. Bethesda: AABB;2005:697.

8. Centers for Disease Control and Prevention (2006). Information for the public: Prescription Drugs for Malaria Treatment and Prevention. http://www.cdc.gov/malaria/diagnosis_treatment/treatment.htm. Accessed on July 4, 2006.

9. Meissner PE, Mandi G, Witte S, et al. Safety of the methylene blue plus chloroquine combination in the treatment of uncomplicated falciparum malaria in young children of Burkina Faso. *Malaria Journal*. 2005;4:45.

10. Miao J, Fan Q, Cui L, et al. The malaria parasite *Plasmodium falciparum* histones: Organization, expression and acetylation. *Gene*. 2006;369:53–65.

Recurrent Fever, Chills, and Malaise in a 53-Year-Old Man

Elliot Carter

Department of Pathology, University of South Alabama Medical Center, Mobile, AL

Patient: 53-year-old man who recently returned from a trip to India.

Chief Complaint: Episodic fever, chills, and muscle pain.

Medical History: The patient described a 1-week history of recurrent fever, chills, and malaise. He had also experienced episodic headaches as well as intermittent epigastric pain.

Family History: Unremarkable.

Drug History: None.

Physical Examination: The patient appeared to be in no acute distress but was sweating profusely. His temperature was 102.5°F. He appeared slightly jaundiced. No hepatosplenomegaly was identified.

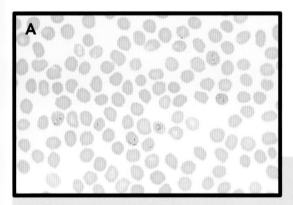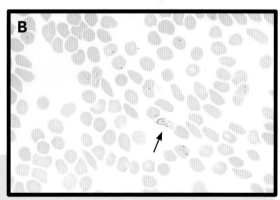

Image 1_Patient's peripheral blood smear demonstrating **A**) multiple erythrocytes containing intraerythrocytic malarial ring forms and **B**) intraerythrocytic malarial ring forms and a banana-shaped gametocyte (arrow).

T1. Principal Laboratory Findings

Test	Patient's Results	"Normal" Reference Range
Hematology		
WBC count	1.9	$4.0\text{-}11.0 \times 10^3/\mu L$
RBC count	3.2	$4.2\text{-}5.9 \times 10^6/\mu L$
Hematocrit	31.7	38.2-50.3%
Hemoglobin	10.0	13.2-16.7 g/dL
MCV	85	82-96 fL
Platelet count	65	$146\text{-}394 \times 10^3/\mu L$
Differential cell count:		
Segmented neutrophils	61	40.0-80.0%
Band neutrophils	10	0.0-6.0%
Lymphocytes	24	15.0-50.0%
Monocytes	3	2.0-11.0%
Eosinophils	2	1.0-7.0%
Chemistry		
ALT	192	30-65 U/L
AST	178	15-37 U/L
Bilirubin, total	12.4	0.2-1.2 mg/dL
Urinalysis		
Hemoglobin	2+	Negative

WBC, white blood cell; RBC, red blood cell; mean corpuscular volume; ALT, alanine aminotransferase; AST, aspartate aminotransferase.

Questions

1. What is (are) this patient's most striking clinical and laboratory finding(s)?

2. Based on this patient's travel history and clinical signs and symptoms, which laboratory test(s) should be performed to diagnose the cause of this patient's illness?

3. What is this patient's most likely diagnosis?

4. What are the characteristic clinical and laboratory features associated with this patient's disease?

5. What is the treatment and outcome of individuals with this patient's condition?

Possible Answers

1. Recurrent fever, chills, malaise, jaundice, and diaphoresis in any individual returning from an area where a variety of endemic diseases is prevalent is striking. In addition, this patient's WBC count was decreased; he was anemic, with a reduced platelet count and a modest shift to the left; his total bilirubin and liver enzymes, ALT and AST, were significantly increased; and he had hemoglobinuria.

2. Malaria is endemic in many parts of the world, and a complete travel history is usually very helpful in establishing the possibility of malarial infection. Geographically, *Plasmodium* spp. are found predominantly in the Indian subcontinent, Southeast Asia, Africa, and Central and South America. Cases seen in the United States, Canada, Australia, and Eastern Europe are usually related to recent travel by the patient to 1 of

these malaria-endemic regions. Therefore, preparation and analysis of thin and thick peripheral blood smears for malarial parasites is strongly indicated in this patient. The blood smears prepared from this patient's blood are shown in **Image 1**.

3. ***Most likely diagnosis:*** *malarial infection with P. falciparum.*

   Based upon the identification of the protozoan forms seen on this patient's peripheral blood smear, the diagnosis of *P. falciparum* malaria was made. Moreover, the patient's symptoms of intermittent relapsing fever and chills are consistent with this diagnosis. Four different species of *Plasmodium* may cause disease in humans, and the identification of a specific species frequently relies upon correlation of the patient's symptomatology as well as morphologic characterization of the *Plasmodium* spp. in the clinical laboratory. Two of the *Plasmodium* spp., *P. ovale* and *P. vivax*, cause enlargement of erythrocytes and are associated with Schuffner's dots (coarse red granules) in the erythrocyte cytoplasm. *P. malariae* and *P. falciparum* do not cause enlargement of erythrocytes and are not associated with Schuffner's dots. These 2 species can usually be distinguished by the presence of banana-shaped gametocytes (seen only in *P. falciparum*) in peripheral blood smears, as well as the relative percentages of erythrocytes involved (>10% for *P. falciparum*; <0.5% for *P. malariae*). **Image 1A** and **Image 1B** show erythrocytes with readily apparent ring forms. The relatively uniform size of the erythrocytes, the absence of Schuffner's dots, and the percentage of involved erythrocytes suggest *P. falciparum* infection. It is the banana-shaped gametocyte seen in **Image 1B** which is diagnostic of *P. falciparum*.

4. Intermittent epigastric pain and relapsing fever, chills, diaphoresis, and muscle aches can occur in patients with malarial infection. Infrequently, patients with malaria may also develop arthralgias, nausea, vomiting, abdominal pain, and hepatosplenomegaly. Although not commonly present, liver abnormalities secondary to *Plasmodium* spp. infection may occur. In addition, hepatosplenomegaly, jaundice, and hyperbilirubinemia occur in some cases of malaria, while liver function tests (ALT and AST) may

be variably elevated. Although not commonly present, liver abnormalities secondary to *Plasmodium* spp. infection may occur. Lastly, like many blood-borne infectious diseases, malaria can cause significant hematologic/coagulopathic sequela. One of these is disseminated intravascular coagulation (DIC). Disseminated intravascular coagulation is 1 of the microangiopathic hemolytic anemias and causes erythrocyte destruction in the microvasculature. In patients with DIC, abnormal coagulation studies as well as anemia and thrombocytopenia are seen. Hemoglobinuria may be seen as a result of hematuria and erythrocyte lysis.

5. Chloroquine is the standard therapy for prophylaxis against, as well as treatment of, malarial infections. Chloroquine-resistant strains of *P. falciparum*, however, exist in many areas of the world, and in these areas, patients may need to be treated with any of a variety of second-line drugs, including quinine and quinidine. The outcome of a malarial infection depends on many factors including the type of *Plasmodium* spp. involved and the underlying health of the patient. Most cases of malaria respond very well to treatment, but chloroquine-resistant malarial strains may require the use of drugs which are not without toxic side-effects. Untreated cases of malaria may be fatal but may also subside completely over time. Relapses of malaria may occur years after infection with *P. vivax* and *P. ovale* due to a dormant hepatic form of the parasite (hypnozoite).

Epigastric Pain, Vomiting, and Diarrhea in a 47-Year-Old Woman

Elliot Carter

Department of Pathology, University of South Alabama Medical Center, Mobile, AL

Patient: 47-year-old Caucasian woman.

Chief Complaint: Epigastric pain and vomiting.

Medical History: The patient described a history of epigastric and abdominal pain of 3 weeks duration. Over the week prior to presentation, she began experiencing intermittent nausea and vomiting as well as diarrhea. She had a previous medical history significant only for asthma.

Family History: Unremarkable.

Drug History: Albuterol (metered-dose inhaler) and prednisone.

Physical Examination: The patient exhibited significant epigastric tenderness. Auscultation of the chest revealed bilateral wheezing.

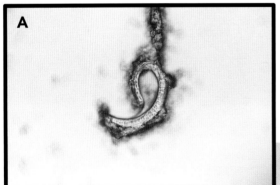 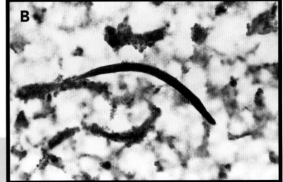

Image 1_*Strongyloides stercoralis* from stool specimen: **A**) Rhabditiform larva (Iodine stain, 40× magnification) **B**) Rhabditiform larva (Trichrome stain, 40× magnification).

T1. Principal Laboratory Findings

Test	Patient's Result	"Normal" Reference Range
Hematology		
WBC count	4.9	4.0-11.0 × 10³/μL
RBC count	3.6	3.8-5.2 × 10⁶/μL
Hematocrit	33.1	33.8-45.6%
Hemoglobin	11.0	11.6-15.6 g/dL
MCV	92	81-95 fL
Differential Count (peripheral blood)		
Segmented neutrophils	35	40-80%
Band neutrophils	22	0-6%
Lymphocytes	19	15-50%
Monocytes	11	2-11%
Eosinophils	13	1-7%
Differential Count (bone marrow)		
Blasts	1.0	0.3-5.0%
Promyelocytes	7	1-8%
Myelocytes	19	5-19%
Metamyelocytes	5.0	13.0-32.5%
Band neutrophils	4	12-30%
Segmented neutrophils	2	7-30%
Eosinophils	31.0	0.5-6.0%
Basophils	1	0-1%
Monocytes	3	0-4%
Normoblasts	19.0	8.5-51.0%
Lymphocytes	8	3-20%
Parasitology		
O & P stool examination	Positive (see **Image 1**)	Negative

WBC, white blood cell; RBC, red blood cell; MCV, mean corpuscular volume; O & P, ova and parasites.

Questions

1. What is (are) this patient's most striking laboratory finding(s)?

2. How do you explain this patient's most striking laboratory findings?

3. What is the significance of the eosinophilia noted on her peripheral blood and bone marrow smears?

4. What is the significance of her medication history to her current illness?

5. What is this patient's most likely diagnosis?

6. What other nematodes would be included in the differential diagnosis of an individual with this patient's clinical presentation?

7. What is the treatment and outcome of individuals with this patient's diagnosis?

Possible Answers

1. Decreased hematocrit and hemoglobin; normal WBC count with peripheral blood shift to the left, and marked eosinophilia in both the peripheral blood and bone marrow smears; and a positive stool O & P test.

2. All of this patient's striking laboratory results are related to her current use of immunosuppressive steroid medications and parasitic infection with *S. stercoralis*. The organism identified in the patient's stool was the rhabditiform larvae of *Strongyloides stercoralis*, a nematode with a widespread geographic distribution but particularly seen in warm, humid climates. The developmental cycle of *Strongyloides* involves 2 larval forms: filariform and rhabditiform. Filariform larvae dwell in the soil and enter the bloodstream through unprotected skin. They migrate via the pulmonary vasculature into the bronchial tree before entering the trachea where they are coughed up and swallowed. In the duodenum, the filariform larvae mature to adult worms which inhabit the mucosa of the small bowel. Adult female worms produce eggs which mature to rhabditiform larvae [**Image 1**] in the small intestine before being passed in the feces. In the soil, the rhabditiform larvae may mature to free-living adult worms or convert to the infective filariform larval stage, thus continuing the infective cycle. In immunocompetent patients, infections with *S. stercoralis* may be mild or asymptomatic. In symptomatic cases, common complaints are itching at the skin site of larval

entry, coughing due to larval migration through the respiratory tract, and abdominal cramping with diarrhea. Anemia, weight loss, and chronic colitis are rare manifestations of *Strongyloides* infection.

3. As with most invasive parasitic infections, *Strongyloides stercoralis* infections cause increased production of eosinophils in the bone marrow and related eosinophilia in the peripheral blood. While patients with parasitic infections usually have elevated eosinophil counts, the counts may be artifactually low due to the use of steroidal medications. Interestingly, hyperinfections with *Strongyloides* may show a lack of eosinophilia, although this may be related to the higher rates of hyperinfection in patients who are chronically immunosuppressed.

4. The patient had been diagnosed with asthma several months previously because of the development of episodic wheezing and shortness of breath. A steroid-based medication was prescribed at that time. Subsequently, the patient developed worsening of her gastrointestinal symptoms. Undoubtedly, the immunosuppressive effects of the steroid therapy exacerbated the patient's *Strongyloides* infection, causing hyperinfection which is characteristic in immunosuppressed individuals. In a hyperinfection state, rhabditiform larvae mature to filariform larvae in the intestinal tract and an autoinfection cycle is initiated.

5. *Most likely diagnosis: parasitic infection with S. stercoralis exacerbated by the concomitant use of immunosuppressive steroids.*

6. The major differential diagnosis in *S.* infection is hookworm infection. *Ancylostoma duodenale* and *Necator americanus* are the hookworm species responsible for the majority of human hookworm infections. Both have a broad geographic distribution, although *Necatur* species appear to be the cause of most hookworm infections acquired in the United States. While the life cycles and symptoms of hookworm and *Strongyloides* infections are similar, hookworms are voracious blood suckers and may cause significant anemias in infected patients. Morphologically, there is little difficulty in differentiating the adult hookworm from that of

Strongyloides due to the marked difference in size (adult hookworms = 7 to 13 mm in length; *Strongyloides stercoralis* = 2 to 3 mm in length). The most difficult morphologic distinction is between the first-stage larval form of hookworm and the rhabditiform larvae of *Strongyloides*; the differences include a shorter buccal cavity and a prominent genital primordium in the *Strongyloides* larvae. The eggs of hookworms and *Strongyloides* are virtually indistinguishable.

7. Antihelminthic agents are the treatment of choice. Thiabendezole, albendazole, and ivermectin have all been used successfully. Prophylactic antibiotic therapy may be used in patients with hyperinfection to prevent gram-negative sepsis. Infections in immunocompetent patients are generally mild and may be asymptomatic. In malnourished, debilitated, or immunosupressed patients, however, the infection may be fatal secondary to multi-organ involvement and sepsis.

Treatment and Outcome

The patient was treated with antihelminthic agents, and her gastrointestinal and pulmonary symptoms ceased, suggesting that her asthma-like breathing difficulty was actually a manifestation of her parasitic infection.

Keywords

eosinophilia, ova & parasites, roundworm, Strongyloides, hookworm, antihelminthic

Periumbilical Rash in an Immunosuppressed Patient

Michael D. White, Monte S. Willis, Franklin S. Fuda, Rita M. Gander, Paul M. Southern, MD

Department of Pathology, The University of Texas Southwestern Medical Center, Dallas, TX

Patient: 70-year-old man, born in Brazil.

Chief Complaint: Shortness of breath.

History of Present Illness: The patient presented with a history of gradual (over several weeks) onset shortness of breath. Six weeks prior to presentation, the patient had undergone a resection of a malignant brain tumor (glioblastoma multiforme).

Past Medical/Family/Social History: Non-contributory.

Drug History: The patient was currently taking steroids (dexamethasone) which were started after his tumor resection.

Physical Examination: The patient presented with fever (38.2°C) and hypotension (blood pressure, 100/50 mm Hg). Other significant findings included atrial fibrillation, blood in his stool, and a periumbilical petechial rash.

Additional Diagnostic Procedures: A chest X-ray identified bilateral diffuse opacities. A bronchoalveolar lavage (BAL) was performed and the fluid obtained was examined microscopically [**Image 1**].

T1. Principal Laboratory Findings

Test	Patient's Result	"Normal" Reference Range
White blood cell count	15.7	4.1-11.1 × 10³/mL
Differential: Neutrophils:		
Segmented	70	50-70%
Bands	20	0-5%
Lymphocytes	10	20-40%
Monocytes	0	0-7%
Basophils	0	0-1%
Eosinophils	0	0-5%

Questions

1. What is (are) the patient's most striking clinical and laboratory finding(s)?

2. How do you explain this patient's most striking laboratory findings?

3. What is this patient's most likely diagnosis?

4. What is the life cycle, epidemiology, and pathogenesis of the organism associated with this patient's condition?

5. What are the clinical manifestations of this patient's condition?

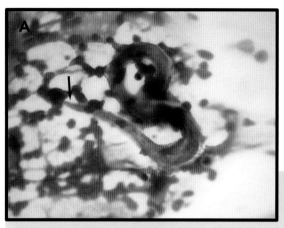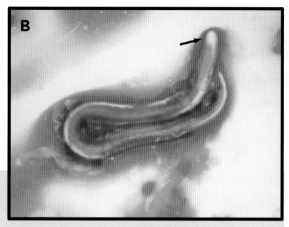

Image 1_Organisms identified in the patient's Pap-stained bronchoalveolar lavage (BAL) fluid from a cytospin preparation (magnification, 1,000×): (**A**) *Strongyloides stercoralis* larval form (generally 300-380 mm) illustrating its characteristic pointed tail (arrow) and (**B**) short buccal cavity (arrow).

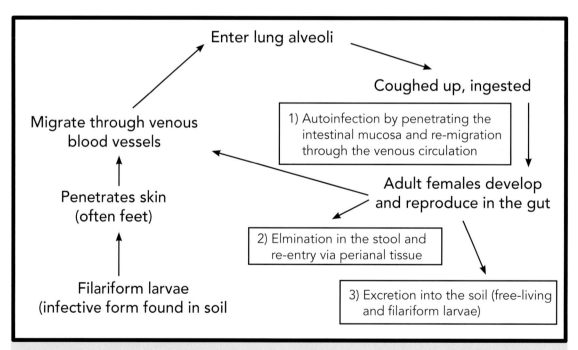

Figure 1_Life cycle of *Strongyloides stercoralis*. Infection with *S. stercoralis* occurs when the free-living filariform larvae found in the soil penetrates the skin and migrates to the lungs via the venous circulation. After entering the alveolar spaces, they are coughed up, swallowed, and mature in the small intestine. Female rhabditiform larvae continue their life cycle by 3 different pathways: 1) development into infective filariform larvae and release from the GI tract (internal autoinfection), 2) release from the bowel and re-entry into the host via penetration of peri-anal skin (external autoinfection), or 3) release eggs and development into infective filariform larvae in the soil.

6. What is the most appropriate treatment of this patient's condition?

Possible Answers

7. The most striking *clinical* findings include fever, hypotension, atrial fibrillation, a bloody stool, and a periumbilical petechial rash. Additionally, his birthplace, Brazil, and a glioblastoma multiforme brain tumor resection 6 weeks prior to presentation, current corticosteroid therapy (dexamethasone), and bilateral diffuse opacities on chest X-ray are also significant. The most striking *laboratory* findings include an increased WBC count with a left shift and no eosinophilia, and the identification of organisms in the Pap-stained bronchoalveolar lavage (BAL) fluid from a cytospin preparation [**Image 1**].

8. A neutrophilic leukocytosis with a left shift, like that found in this patient [total WBC count = $15.7 \times 10^3/\mu L$ with 70% polymorphonuclear leukocytes (PMNs) and 20% bands] generally represents an infectious etiology, possibly of bacterial origin. Patients with viral infections tend to have normal or decreased WBC counts. However, these distinctions are not absolute as some viral infections can be associated with a neutrophilic leukocytosis. Since microscopic examination of the BAL fluid demonstrated the presence of parasites [**Image 1**], it was surprising that eosinophilia was not present. Many helminthic parasites and parasitic infections are associated with a systemic eosinophilia, including *Ascaris lumbricoides*, hookworms, *Strongyloides stercoralis*, trichinosis, and filariasis.

9. *Most likely diagnosis: Strongyloides stercoralis hyperinfection secondary to steroid immunosuppression after glioblastoma multiforme (GBM) tumor resection.*

   Patients with brain tumors are placed on dexamethasone therapy to reduce the intracranial pressure and edema which commonly occurs with brain tumors. However, the side effects of taking corticosteroids include immunosuppression and the possibility that latent parasites can become reactivated. The diagnosis of *S. stercoralis* is based on the identification of larvae in either host tissue, GI, or pulmonary secretions. It

should be noted, however, that diagnosis by serology[1] and molecular probe techniques[2] have been described and may prove helpful because of their increased sensitivity as compared to methods detecting ova and parasites in stool and other body fluids. The principal method for the diagnosis of parasitic infections is the direct examination of stool samples for the presence of parasites. The identification of filariform or rhabditiform larvae in body fluid secretions (gastrointestinal), washings (bronchoalveolar lavage), or sputum can diagnose parasitic hyperinfection syndrome and disseminated parasitic infection. Additionally, peritoneum, kidney, urine, skin, and brain specimens of immunocompromised patients have been used to diagnose parasitic infections.[3] In this case, a Pap-stained cytospin preparation from BAL fluid identified *S. stercoralis* and further suggested a disseminated infection. In patients with a disseminated parasitic infection, laboratory abnormalities can include eosinophilia, although this does not universally occur in immunosuppressed hosts. Since this patient's dexamethasone therapy caused an immunosuppressed state, this may explain his lack of eosinophilia [**T1**]. Complications of *S. stercoralis* infection include secondary fungal or bacterial sepsis (eg, gram-negative rods, enterococcal, or polymicrobial septicemia) thought to be due to the migrating larvae translocating out of the gut. The patient's symptoms of hypotension and fever may be the result of such a syndrome, although his blood cultures did not confirm this. There is an increased risk of *S. stercoralis* hyperinfection in patients taking steroids as a result of reactivation of a dormant infection possibly from decades earlier. Since *S. stercoralis* is not common in the United States and is endemic in this person's country of origin (Brazil), it may be hypothesized that he had a latent infection from childhood that became active with immunosuppression, secondary to his brain tumor and steroid therapy.

10. *Strongyloides stercoralis life cycle* [**Figure 1**]: Infection with *S. stercoralis* occurs when the free-living filariform larval form found in the soil comes in contact with skin. The larvae penetrate the skin and migrate to the small vessels of the lungs by way of the venous circulation.[3] The larvae then travel to the alveolar spaces, are coughed up and swallowed, and further mature into adult

worms in the duodenum and jejunum. Adult females bury deep into the crypts of the duodenum and jejunum and penetrate the mucosa and submucosa to lay their eggs (ova) approximately 28 days after infection.[3,4] Rhabditiform larvae are released from the eggs and passed into the stool, and the infective form (filariform) develops in the soil by either direct transformation from the rhabditiform or indirectly from intermediate, free-living forms: the major route by which these parasites develop. Rhabditiform larvae can be identified by their well-defined muscular esophagus and prominent esophageal bulbs. Unlike other helminthic parasites found in humans, adult worms of *S. stercoralis* reproduce in the GI tract "parthogenetically"[3] (ie, development of a gamete without fertilization) resulting in an increase in worm burden without environmental re-exposure. It is this ability to multiply in the definitive host (ie, humans) that is the basis for the persistence of this organism over many years.[5] Rhabditiform larvae can also develop into the infective filariform larvae in the GI tract or after passage into the feces. When the rhabditiform larvae emerge before being passed through the bowel, internal (in the bowel) or external autoinfection (perianal skin penetration) occurs, which initiates migration to and development in the lungs. If autoinfections become frequent, hyperinfection is said to occur allowing the parasite to migrate and cause pathological changes in areas of the body that they do not normally invade, including the central nervous system (CNS).[3] *Epidemiology:* S. stercoralis infection is endemic in Africa, Asia, Latin America, and areas of Southern and Eastern Europe. Prevalence rates of rhabditiform larvae in stool samples have been shown to vary between >40% in Africa to 1% to 7% in Europe. Endemic infection can be seen in areas of the United States as well, specifically in rural Appalachia and other southern areas, ranging from a prevalence of 0.4% to 3%.[3] The frequency of *S. stercoralis* infection in homosexual men is approximately 3.9%; however, this estimate of prevalence is likely to be low because of the poor sensitivity of a single stool exam.[3] *Pathogenesis:* When the adult worms and larvae penetrate the upper intestine, or when the filariform larvae infect the lungs, an inflammatory response ensues consisting of eosinophil and mononuclear cell infiltrates.[3] Autoinfection leading to high worm burdens and disseminated

strongyloidiasis may occur in patients with decreased cell-mediated immunity.[6] Individuals at risk for autoinfection include those chronically taking steroids, renal transplant recipients, and patients with leukemia or lymphomas.[7,8] Although *S. stercoralis* can persist as a latent infection for decades, it is important to recognize that changes in immune competency can initiate a conversion from asymptomatic disease to hyperinfection. Initially, this patient's diffuse bilateral pulmonary infiltrates caused suspicion for pneumonia (*Pneumocystis carinii*), and he was started on Levaquin. A BAL procedure was performed to identify the specific causative agent. Identification of the causative agent is important because retrospective studies have determined that the diagnosis of *S. stercoralis* infection can be delayed, on average, by as much as 10 weeks.[9] Diagnosis can be made by the detection of larvae in the feces (diagnostic sensitivity: 27% to 73%), duodenal fluid (39% to 76%), sputum, BAL fluid, or lung tissue.[10] Eosinophilia and elevated IgE in the serum can be present and helpful in the diagnosis, but they are commonly absent in hyperinfection syndromes, as in this case (ie, no eosinophilia; quantitative serum IgE testing was not performed).[11] *Strongyloides stercoralis* in the intestine can mimic celiac sprue, peptic ulcer, regional enteritis, or ulcerative colitis, and patients can additionally present with meningitis due to enteric organisms. Moreover, hyperinfection and disseminated strongyloidiasis can look like bacterial or fungal sepsis.

11. The clinical manifestations of *S. stercoralis* infection can be divided into 3 stages: skin invasion, larval migration, and invasion of the intestinal mucosa.[4] However, in both acute and chronic infections, approximately one-third of patients are completely asymptomatic.[4,10] Skin manifestations of *S. stercoralis* infection include a hypersentivity reaction at the site of invasion. Clinically, intestinal bloating, diarrhea without nausea, and epigastric pain may be present. In immunocompromised patients with hyperinfection, pulmonary findings can resemble adult respiratory distress syndrome, including acute shortness of breath and a productive cough, which can be bloody. Fever, fast breathing, and decreased oxygen levels, in addition to respiratory alkalosis, may also be present. Moreover, invasion of the larvae into the CNS, pancreas,

and eye can lead to symptoms due to tissue destruction in these areas. It should be noted that petechial rashes have been reported in patients with hyperinfection due to immunosuppression.[12-14] In fact, periumbilical purpura has been reported in a case of *S. stercoralis* infection,[15] similar to that reported in the patient presented in this case study. In immunocompetent hosts, *S. stercoralis* infection is usually asymptomatic. However, an immediate local skin eruption at the site of entry of the infective larval form may be seen, along with coughing secondary to tracheal irritation at 6 to 9 days as the larvae pass through the lungs. Gastrointestinal symptoms are seen at approximately 18 days post-infection and consist of diarrhea, constipation, GI bleeding (seen in current patient), and epigastric pain. The disease state differs in immunosuppressed patients as they are unable to eliminate the worms from the GI tract and unable to prevent autoinfection. It should be noted that the atrial fibrillation seen in this patient was unrelated to his parasitic infection. Atrial fibrillation is the most common sustained arrhythmia found in adults and has a prevalence of 6% in people older than 75.[16] Thus, the presence of atrial fibrillation in this patient is most likely due to his advanced age (70 years) and not his parasitic infection.

12. The most appropriate treatment for this patient's condition would be thiabendazole (Mintezol). All patients infected with *S. stercoralis* should be treated with thiabendazole at a dose of 25 mg/kg twice a day for 2 days to a maximum of 3 g/day.[4] In patients with the hyperinfection syndrome, it is imperative to identify the parasite early, and treat for 2 to 3 weeks.[4] In endemic areas, immunosuppressed individuals should avoid walking barefoot, have their stools examined, and start treatment if larvae of *S. stercoralis* are detected in fecal samples. If the development of immunosuppression is anticipated, thiabendazole (25 mg/kg/day for 2 days) may be given prophylactically for a month preceding the initiation of immunosuppressive therapy.[3] Thiabendazole is used in the treatment of several helminthic diseases (eg, infection with *Ascaris lumbricoides* or *Necator americanus*), but its mechanism of action has not been fully elucidated. It may act on the helminth enzyme, fumarate reductase.[17]

Treatment and Follow-up

The patient was started on thiabendazole; however, the patient died a few days later due to a cardiopulmonary event.

Keywords

strongyloidiasis, parasitic hyperinfection, parasitic autoinfection, eosinophilia, immunosuppression therapy, thiabendazole

References

1. Sato Y, Kobayashi J, Shiroma Y. Serodiagnosis of strongyloidiasis. The application and significance. *Rev Inst Med Trop Sao Paulo*. 1995;37:35-41.

2. Ramachandran S, Thompson RW, Gam AA, et al. Recombinant cDNA clones for immunodiagnosis of strongyloidiasis. *J Infect Dis*. 1998;177:196-203.

3. Kazura JW. Nematode infections. In: Cecil RL, Goldman L, Bennett JC, Drazen JM, eds. *Cecil Textbook of Medicine*. Philadelphia: W.B. Saunders, 2000:1984-1990.

4. Mahmoud AF. Intestinal nematodes (Roundworms). In: Mandell GL, Douglas RG, Bennett JE, Dolin R, eds. *Principles and Practice of Infectious Diseases*. Philadelphia: Churchill Livingstone, 2000:2938-2943.

5. Grove DI. Strongyloidiasis in allied ex-prisoners of war in southeast Asia. *Br Med J*. 1980;280:598-601.

6. Mahmoud AA. Strongyloidiasis. *Clin Infect Dis*. 1996;23:949-953.

7. Heyworth MF. Parasitic diseases in immunocompromised hosts. Cryptosporidiosis, isosporiasis, and strongyloidiasis. *Gastroenterol Clin North Am*. 1996;25:691-707.

8. Gompels MM, Todd J, Peters BS, et al. Disseminated strongyloidiasis in AIDS: Uncommon but important. *AIDS*. 1991;5:329-332.

9. Woodring JH, Halfhill H, Berger R, et al. Clinical and imaging features of pulmonary strongyloidiasis. *South Med J*. 1996;89:10-19.

10. Gopinath R, Nutman TB. Parasitic diseases. In: Murray JF, ed. *Textbook of Respiratory Medicine*. Philadelphia: Saunders, 2000:1143-1171.

11. Chu E, Whitlock WL, Dietrich RA. Pulmonary hyperinfection syndrome with *Strongyloides stercoralis*. *Chest*. 1990;97:1475-1477.

12. Gelber M, Rodrig J. *Strongyloides stercoralis* hyperinfection. *Harefuah*. 1996; 130:90-92.

13. Simpson WG, Gerhardstein DC, Thompson JR. Disseminated *Strongyloides stercoralis* infection. *South Med J.* 1993;86:821-825.

14. Soroczan W. Strongyloidosis. Specific and nonspecific skin lesions. *Wiad Parazytol.* 1994;40:45-51.

15. Kalb RE, Grossman ME. Periumbilical purpura in disseminated strongyloidiasis. *JAMA.* 1986;256:1170-1171.

16. Akhtar M. Cardic arrhythmias with supraventricular origin. In: Cecil RL, Goldman L, Bennett JC, Drazen JM, eds. *Cecil Textbook of Medicine.* Philadelphia: W.B. Saunders, 2000:234-241.

17. *Mosby's Drug Consult.* Nissen D, ed. St. Louis: Mosby, 2003.

Sore Throat/Fever and Delayed Renal Impairment in a 10-Year-Old Girl

Arthur G. Weinberg

Professor of Pathology and Pediatrics, UT Southwestern Medical School, Dallas, TX.

Patient: 10-year-old white girl.

Chief Complaint: Dark urine and fever.

Medical History: Sore throat and fever 10 days ago that resolved with outpatient treatment. Recent onset of puffy face, malaise, and low grade fever. Noticed cola-colored urine and reduced urine output. No history of skin rash or joint pain. Throat culture negative. Anti-streptolysin O (ASO) titer 664 (reference range, <166 Todd U).

Family History: Unremarkable.

Drug History: Acetaminophen for headache and fever.

Physical Examination: Normally grown child with periorbital edema. Blood pressure 150/98. Temperature 38°C. Skin clear. Heart slightly enlarged with no murmurs. Liver slightly enlarged. The rest of the examination was unremarkable.

T2. Principal Laboratory Findings

Test	Patient's Result	Reference Range
Urinalysis		
Protein	2+	neg
Glucose	neg	neg
Blood	large	neg
Ketones	neg	neg
Nitrite	neg	neg
LE	neg	neg
Sediment	many RBCs	neg
	red cell casts	
	10 WBCs/hpf	
BUN	25	5-18 mg/dL
Creatinine	1.1	0.3-0.7 mg/dL
Albumin	2.3	3.1-4.6 g/dL
Cholesterol	150	125-170 mg/dL
Triglycerides	50	30-86 mg/dL
C3	40	70-206 mg/dL
C4	35	11-61 mg/dL

Questions _____

1. What is the diagnosis?

2. Are the complement studies helpful in this patient?

3. What is the significance of the red cell casts?

4. How are the results of the throat culture and streptococcal serology studies reconciled?

5. What is the cause of the edema and hypertension?

6. What light microscopic changes would most likely be present in the kidney?

Possible Answers _____

1. This patient has a nephritic-appearing urine with pronounced hematuria and proteinuria as well as red cell casts. This followed an apparent bout of pharyngitis. Despite a negative throat culture, there was serologic evidence of a recent streptococcal infection. A diagnosis of acute poststreptococcal (postinfectious) glomerulone-phritis is appropriate in this context. No biopsy is indicated unless the child progresses to renal failure or shows other atypical features.

2. The low C3 and normal C4 indicate that there is complement consumption by the alternative activation pathway, a pattern typical of though not specific for immune-mediated postinfectious glomerulonephritis. A similar pattern occurs in other immune complex–mediated forms of glomerulonephritis such as lupus nephritis, but the clinical presentation of this patient is not consistent with systemic lupus erythematosus.

3. Red cell casts are important in localizing the source of hematuria to the nephron as distinct from bleeding from the lower urinary tract, as would occur with cystitis or a tumor. Red cell casts degenerate rapidly and must be sought promptly in a fresh urine sample.

4. The organisms may have been cleared from the throat by the time that the cultures were obtained. Serologic studies provide a useful means of documenting recent streptococcal infection in the absence of a positive culture. ASO titers are elevated in >90% of patients with streptococcal pharyngitis and begin to rise 1 week after infection. They are a less reliable marker for recent streptococcal skin infection (which may also cause glomerulonephritis), in which instance other anti-streptococcal antibodies may be more sensitive (anti-DNAseB, Wampole's M Streptozyme). The Streptozyme titer may rise more slowly than the ASO titer.

5. Edema and hypertension are often present in patients with acute poststreptococcal glom-erulonephritis. They result from salt and water retention by the kidney with consequent hyperv-olemia and respond promptly to diuresis.

6. Acute poststreptococcal glomerulonephritis is characterized by hypercellular enlarged glomeruli that are infiltrated by neutrophils and monocytes (acute exudative and proliferative glomerulonephritis). Red cell casts are often present in the tubules.

Fever, Weight Loss, Cough, and Chest Pain in a HIV-Positive Man

Asim Diab, Rita Gander, Debra Grant, Dominick Cavuoti, Paul Southern

Department of Pathology, University of Texas Southwestern Medical Center and Clinical Microbiology Laboratory, Parkland Health and Hospital System, Dallas, TX

Patient: 36-year-old African-American homosexual man.

Drug Allergies: Cephalosporins.

Chief Complaint: Shortness of breath, left-sided chest pain that was worse when lying flat, fever, productive cough, generalized muscle weakness, and a 12-pound weight loss.

History of Present Illness: The patient had been admitted previously for ongoing productive cough and fevers and 1 month prior to this most recent admission to our hospital, the patient had been admitted to another hospital where he underwent a bronchoscopy and tuberculosis and Pneumocystis carinii (PCP) pneumonia were ruled out. However, 1 day after discharge from the hospital, the patient presented at our hospital because his symptoms had worsened. He was treated with primaquine and clindamycin for presumed PCP infection. Although his sputum smears were negative for PCP by direct fluorescence assay (DFA), he remained symptomatic. Subsequently, the patient presented on this admission with fever and left-sided chest pain that was worse when lying flat.

Past Medical History: Seven years ago, he had been diagnosed with human immunodeficiency virus (HIV) infection and had taken anti-retroviral drugs only intermittently after receiving this diagnosis. In addition, he had a previous history of histoplasmosis with duodenitis, anal condyloma, and a parvovirus B19 viral infection which led to anemia that required frequent blood transfusions.

Social History: Half-pack a day smoker; occasional ethanol and marijuana use.

Physical Examination: The patient's vital signs were: temperature, 38.1°C; blood pressure, 128/74 mm Hg; and heart rate, 110 beats per minute. He was cachectic and in mild distress. A head-ear-eyes-nose-throat (HEENT) examination showed slight bitemporal wasting, some shotty lymphadenopathy, and no evidence of thrush. The cardiovascular examination demonstrated tachycardia, but was otherwise unremarkable. The lungs were clear to auscultation bilaterally. The abdomen was soft, non-tender, and non-distended with good bowel sounds. The extremities demonstrated no clubbing, cyanosis, or edema.

Additional Tests and Procedures: Given the patient's pulmonary symptomatology, he underwent fiberoptic bronchoscopy to obtain bronchoalveolar lavage (BAL) fluid. The BAL fluid was stained and analyzed with the results shown in **Images 1A-D**. A sonogram of the spleen was normal, while a computed tomography (CT) scan of the abdomen demonstrated patchy basilar lung disease, mild hepatomegaly, and normal kidneys. Chest x-ray showed a left posterobasal infiltrate as well as a retrocardiac infiltrate. A CT scan of the chest, without intravenous contrast, demonstrated no mediastinal or hilar adenopathy and the presence of a small pericardial effusion. In addition, both lower lobes of the lungs demonstrated a patchy consolidation with a ground-glass appearance. No destructive bone lesions were observed.

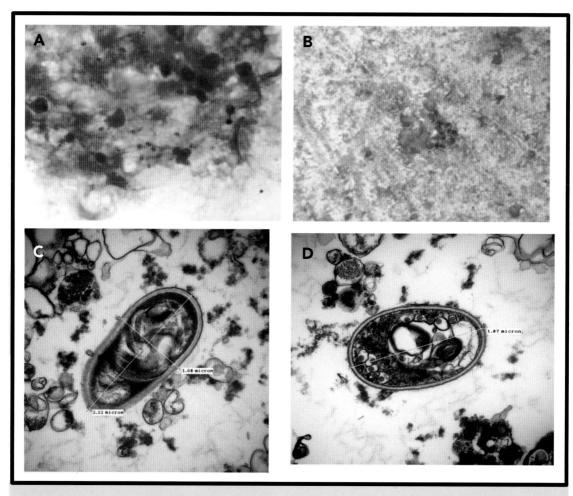

Image 1_Patient's BAL fluid, illustrating stained spores of microsporidia (**A**, Gram stain; 1,000× magnification; **B**, Trichrome modified stain, 1,000× magnification) and (**C, D**) transmission electron micrographs, illustrating the transverse dimensions of a typical microsporidian spore recovered from the patient's BAL fluid.

Questions

1. What are this patient's most striking clinical and laboratory findings?

2. How do you explain this patient's most striking clinical and laboratory findings?

3. What is this patient's most likely diagnosis?

4. What are the forms of presentation of this patient's disease?

5. What laboratory methods are available for diagnosing this patient's disease?

6. Why was fiberoptic bronchoscopy with collection of BAL fluid performed on our patient?

7. What are other pulmonary infectious conditions that can occur in immunocompromised and HIV-infected individuals?

8. What are the measures to prevent infection with the pathogens that can cause infection in immunocompromised and HIV-infected individuals?

9. What is the most appropriate treatment of our patient's disease?

Possible Answers

1. Shortness of breath, left-sided chest pain that was worse when lying flat, fever, generalized muscle weakness, a 12-pound weight loss, and abnormal chest x-ray and CT findings. Markedly decreased RBC count, hemoglobin, hematocrit, absolute and relative CD4 counts, and a markedly elevated HIV-1 RNA viral load (**T1**). Bronchoalveolar lavage fluid positive by light and electron microscopy for the presence of microsporidia spores.

2. Our patient's clinical, radiographic, and laboratory findings are consistent with pulmonary infection. Our patient's marked anemia is most likely a chronic anemia secondary to his parvovirus infection, while the BAL fluid findings (**Images 1A-D**) are consistent with a microsporidia infection. Viral, bacterial, and

fungal cultures from BAL fluid, bone marrow, and blood were repeatedly negative (**T1**). Moreover, his anorectal condyloma is most likely due to human papilloma virus (HPV) infection because HPV infection and anal condylomas are known to occur with increased frequency in HIV-infected homosexual patients.

3. ***Most likely diagnosis:*** *pulmonary microsporidiosis in an immunocompromised, HIV-infected individual.* Microsporidia are obligate eukaryotic intracellular protozoal parasites of the phylum Microspora. Microsporidiosis has been demonstrated in a large number of vertebrate and invertebrate species. In humans, 8 (*Brachiola, Enterocytozoon, Encephalitozoon, Nosema, Pleistophora, Septata, Trachipleistophora,* and *Vittaforma*) of the 150 genera of Microspora have been shown to cause disease.[1,2] Microsporidia are characterized by the production of environmentally resistant spores that vary in size, depending on the species. They possess a unique organelle, the polar tubule or filament, which is coiled inside the spore and can be viewed by ultrastructural analysis using transmission electron microscopy. These resistant spores are the infective form of the disease. The spore infects a host cell by extruding its polar tubule into the cell and injecting the cell with its infective sporoplasm through the polar tubule. Inside the host cell, the sporoplasm undergoes extensive multiplication either by merogony (binary fission) or schizogony (multiple fission). Multiplication can occur either in direct contact with the host cell cytoplasm or inside a vacuole termed a parasitophorous vacuole. In either case, microsporidia develop by sporogony to mature spores. During sporogony, a thick wall is formed around the spore, which provides resistance to adverse environmental conditions. When the spores increase in number and completely fill the host cell cytoplasm, the host cell membrane is disrupted and releases the spores to the surroundings. These free, mature spores can infect new cells, thus continuing the cycle. The microsporidial spores of species associated with human infection measure from 1 to 4 μm and this is a useful diagnostic feature of these organisms. The mode of transmission of microsporidia to humans is not known. Microsporidia are released into the environment in stool, urine, and respiratory secretions by infected animals.

T1. Principal Laboratory Findings

Test	Patient's Result	Reference Interval
Hematology		
WBC count	7.4	$4.1-11.1 \times 10^3/\mu L$
RBC count	2.03	$4.27-5.99 \times 10^6/\mu L$
Hemoglobin	6.4	13.2-16.9 g/dL
Hematocrit	19.1	39.6-50.2%
MCV	94	76.2-98.61 fL
Platelet count	522	$174-404 \times 10^3/\mu L$
Differential count:		
Neutrophils	68	36-72%
Lymphocytes	16	20-51%
Monocytes	15	4-11%
Basophils	1	0-1%
Eosinophils	1	1-7%
Coagulation		
PT	10.3	9.2-12.5 sec
INR	1.0	0.9-1.2
PTT	35.6	24.5-34.5 sec
Flow Cytometry/Molecular Diagnostics		
Absolute CD4 T-cell count	4	$416-1,751/\mu L$
Relative CD4 T-cell count	0.9	31.0-64.0%
HIV-1 RNA viral load	163,000	0 copies/mL
Chemistry		
Sodium	133	135-145 mEq/L
Potassium	4.3	3.6-5.0 mEq/L
Chloride	99	98-109 mEq/L
CO_2	25	22-31 mEq/L
BUN	10	7-21 mg/dL
Creatinine	0.8	0.6-1.2 mg/dL

Test	Result	Reference
Glucose	112	65-110 mg/dL
Bilirubin, total	0.4	0.2-1.3 g/dL
Bilirubin, direct	0.1	0.0-0.3 g/dL
AST	19	13-40 U/L
ALT	24	10-40 U/L
ALP	34	38-126 U/L
Microbiology		
Histoplasma antigen, urine	0.51	<1.0 EIA units
BAL fluid culture	Negative	Negative
Bone marrow culture	Negative	Negative
Peripheral blood culture	Negative	Negative
Serology		
Blastomycin	Ab negative	Negative
Coccidioidin	Ab negative	Negative
Aspergillin	Ab negative	Negative

WBC, white blood cell; RBC, red blood cell; MCV, mean corpuscular volume; PT, prothrombin time; INR, International Normalized Ratio; PTT, partial thromboplastin time; CD, cluster of differentiation; BUN, blood urea nitrogen; AST, aspartate aminotransferase; ALT, alanine aminotransferase; ALP, alkaline phosphatase; HIV, human immunodeficieincy virus; RNA, ribonucleic acid; EIA, enzyme immunoassay.

However, it is not known whether humans are infected from person-to-person contact, the environment, other mammals, or insects.[1]

4. Microsporidia may cause a broad spectrum of disease.[1] In HIV patients, gastrointestinal disease is the most common presentation, and isolated pulmonary disease is rare.[1,2] Patients who are immunocompromised from other diseases are at high risk for microsporidial infection. It is unclear, however, whether infection in immunocompromised individuals is a newly acquired infection or a reactivation of latent infection acquired prior to immunosuppression.[3] Immunocompromised patients may also develop chronic, severe, non-bloody, non-mucoid diarrhea with weight loss and fat malabsorption, or hepatitis and peritonitis. Gastrointestinal microsporidial infection has been documented in several immunocompetent individuals who had only self-resolving traveler's diarrhea.[5] Other less common manifestations of microsporidial infection include keratoconjunctivitis, sinusitis, urinary tract infection, myositis, and lower respiratory tract infections. Rarely, patients can develop cerebral infections, urethritis, cutaneous infections, osteomyelitis, and abscesses. Pulmonary infections have been found primarily with microsporidia from the genus *Encephalitozoon*. Most patients with respiratory tract infections also have systemic or intestinal microsporidiosis, but isolated cases of pulmonary involvement do exist.[1,4] Our patient did not have evidence of extrapulmonary disease. An association between the presence of microsporidia in the lungs and pulmonary symptoms has yet to be determined. It is not known whether pulmonary microsporidiosis is acquired through the aerosol route, by aspiration, or by hematogenous dissemination from the intestine. Unfortunately, prevalence data on microsporidial colonization of the lungs are not known.

5. Laboratory detection of microsporidia can be accomplished using several methods: (1) light microscopy; (2) transmission electron microscopy (TEM); (3) immunofluorescence assay (IFA); and (4) polymerase chain reaction (PCR) molecular techniques. **Light microscopic examination** of stained smears, especially from fecal samples, is an inexpensive method of diagnosing microsporidial infection even though it

does not allow identification of microsporidia to the species level. The most widely used staining technique is the chromotrope-based staining method or a modification of this method. This technique stains the spore and the spore wall a bright pinkish-red color. Often, a belt-like stripe, which also stains pinkish-red, is seen in the middle of the spore.[5] A recently developed "Quick-Hot Gram Chromotrope technique" however, cuts down the staining time to less than 10 minutes and makes any spores more easily visible against the lightly stained background. Using this technique, the spores stain dark violet and the appearance of a belt-like stripe is enhanced. In some cases, dark staining gram-positive granules are also clearly seen.[6] Chemofluorescent agents such as Calcofluor white are also useful in the quick identification of spores in fecal smears. **Transmission electron microscopy (TEM)** is the gold standard for speciating microsporidial organisms.[7] However, TEM is expensive, time consuming, and not feasible for routine diagnosis. **Immunofluorescence assay** methods that use monoclonal and/or polyclonal antibodies are being developed for the identification of microsporidia in clinical samples.[8] **Molecular methods**, mainly PCR techniques, are alternative methods for the laboratory diagnosis of microsporidiosis. However, PCR-based methods are available only in research laboratories and have been successfully used for the identification of *Brachiola algerae*, *Enterocytozoon bieneusi*, *Encephalitozoon intestinalis*, *Encephalitozoon hellem*, and *Encephalitozoon cuniculi*.[8] The principal drawback to these methods is that they do not work well on formalin-fixed samples in long-term storage.

6. Fiberoptic bronchoscopy with collection of BAL fluid was performed on our patient because of his persistent respiratory symptoms of undetermined cause. We detected microsporidial spores in the BAL fluid. The patient was not known to have intestinal microsporidiosis. However, this diagnosis was suspected on examination of the material processed from the BAL fluid, evaluated by Gram stain, and confirmed by chromotrope-2R-modified trichrome stain and by TEM. Microsporidial spores are difficult to identify using conventional hematoxylin and eosin and Papanicolaou stains. Gram stain of sediment from the BAL fluid showed low numbers of

intra- and extra-cellular microsporidian spores, with 0 to 10 spores per field at 1,000x magnification. Some of these spores were gram-positive (**Image 1A**), some were gram-variable with a uniform oval shape, and contained an equatorial belt across the midline of the spore or polar granule (**Image 1A**). Direct microscopy of Gram stained smears of clinical specimens is important in diagnostic microbiology.[9,10] In Gram stained smears of specimens from the respiratory tract, unexpected findings may occur such as the presence of parasitic larvae (eg, *Strongyloides stercoralis*), pseudohyphae, hyphae of filamentous fungi, trophozoites, oocytes of various organisms (eg, *Cryptosporidum parvum*), cysts of *P. carinii*, or spores of microsporidial species. However, a definitive diagnosis based on Gram stain findings will not be possible in every case and the sensitivity of the Gram stain for the detection of these organisms may not be equal to or greater than that of more conventional stains commonly used to identify these organisms in clinical specimens. This case study demonstrates that with experience and an awareness of some unusual findings, some infections, possibly unsuspected clinically, may be detected. This may be especially important in immunosuppressed and immunocompromised patients. The development of reliable differential staining techniques such as Weber's chromotrope-2R-modified trichrome stain, has facilitated the widespread diagnosis of microsporidia by light-microscopy. Moreover, use of chromotrope-2R-modified trichrome stain is preferable to Gram stain in specimens (eg, stool) that contain large numbers of bacteria. In this case study, detection of microsporidia was optimized using a chromotrope-based stain and when clinical specimens, stained using the chromotrope-based stain, were examined by light microscopy, 6 to10 spores per high power field containing clusters of pink microsporidial spores were detected (**Image 1B**). In addition, the ultrastructural characteristics of microsporidia were confirmed by electron microscopy examination of samples prepared from BAL fluid. The presence of spores measuring from 1.87 to 2.22 μm and polar tubules with 5 isofibrillar coils (**Images 1C-D**), suggest that our patient's isolate belonged to the genus, *Encephalitozoon.* However, further immunological, biochemical, and molecular studies are needed to definitively identify the genus and species of the organisms found in our patient's BAL fluid.

7. The spectrum of pulmonary manifestations in an immunocompromised patient in general, and those that can occur in HIV-infected patients in particular, is broad and includes inflammatory, infectious, and neoplastic conditions. Infectious conditions can have viral, bacterial, fungal, or parasitic causes. Cytomegalovirus is the most common cause of viral infections affecting the respiratory tract followed by adenovirus, respiratory syncytial virus, influenza virus, and parainfluenza virus. Bacterial infections that affect both immunocompetent and immunocompromised patients include those caused by *Streptococcus pneumoniae, Haemophilus influenzae*, and *Mycobacterium tuberculosis*. In addition to these common pathogens, many other organisms can cause lower respiratory tract infections, including *Nocardia* spp., *Rhodococcus equi, Legionella* spp., and infection with opportunistic pathogens (eg, *Mycobacterium avium* complex), which are seen almost exclusively in immunocompromised individuals. Fungal causes of pulmonary infections can be localized or disseminated and can be due to *Candida* species, *Histoplasma capsulatum, Cryptococcus neoformans, Blastomyces dermatitidis,* or, most commonly, *P. carinii*. Extrapulmonary spread of *P. carinii* can occur through hematogenous or lymphatic dissemination.

8. Data supporting effective strategies for the treatment of immunocompromised and HIV-positive individuals infected with various pathogens are limited because the mode of transmission and source of infection by these pathogens are uncertain. The presence of infective spores in body fluids and feces suggests that adherance to universal precautions procedures in health care and other institutional settings, with attention to hand washing and other personal hygiene measures, may be helpful in preventing primary infections. Hand washing may be of particular importance in preventing ocular infections, which may occur as a result of inoculation of conjunctival surfaces by fingers contaminated with respiratory fluids or urine.[3] Moreover, there are no standardized methods available to test infectivity of microsporidial spores and to evaluate the efficacy of preventive measures. Microsporidial spores may survive in the environment for months to years

depending on temperature and humidity. Even in a typical hospital room temperature (22°C) environment, microsporidial spores can survive for at least a month.[11] Exposure of microsporidial spores to recommended working concentrations of most disinfectants for 30 minutes, boiling for 5 minutes, and autoclaving at 120°C have been reported to kill these spores.[11] However, freezing may not be an effective means of disinfection because it has been possible to grow *E. hellem* after storing it at -70°C for months.[3]

9. Immune reconstitution using highly active anti-retroviral therapy (HAART) frequently results in the clearance of microsporidia.[12] Supportive care with hydration, correction of electrolyte abnormalities, and nutritional supplementation should also be provided. Current treatment recommendations for microsporidiosis are a 4-week course of oral albendazole (7.5 mg/kg; maximum of 400 mg twice daily). This treatment will lead to clinical improvement of the patient's symptoms and apparent parasitic eradication from stool, urine, respiratory specimens, or conjunctival scrapings from HIV-infected patients with *E. intestinalis*, *E. hellem*, and *E. cuniculi* microsporidiosis.[13] Case reports of patient response to albendazole therapy indicate that treatment failures were rare events in cohorts that included patients with chronic sinusitis or lower respiratory tract infection, urethritis, renal failure, cerebral encephalitozoonosis, or disseminated infection.[14]

Acknowledgments

We thank Lynne Garcia and Ann Cali, PhD for reviewing the electron micrographs, and Elma Cortinas for preparing the electron micrographs.

Keywords

human immunodeficiency virus, immunocompetent, immunocompromised, microsporidial infections

References

1. Weber R, Bryan R, Schwartz D, et al. Human microsporidial infections. *Clin Microbiol Rev.* 1994;7:426-461.

2. Franzen C, Muller A. Microsporidiosis: Human disease and diagnosis. *Microbes Infect.* 2001; 3:389-400.

3. Weber R, Bryan R. Microsporidial infections in immunodeficient and immunocompetent patients. *Clin Infect Dis.* 1994;19:517-521.

4. Schwartz D, Visvesvara M, Leitch L, et al. Pathology of symptomatic microsporidial (*Encephalitozoon hellem*) bronchiolitis in AIDS; a new respiratory pathogen diagnosed from lung biopsy, bronchoalveolar lavage, sputum, and tissue culture. *Hum Pathol.* 1993;4:937-943.

5. Weber R, Bryan RT, Owen RL, et al. Improved light microscopical detection of microsporida spores in stool and duodenal aspirates. *N Eng J Med.* 1992;326:161-166.

6. Moura H, Schwartz DA, Bornay-Linnares F, et al. A new and improved "quick-hot Gram-chromotrope" technique that differentially stains microsporidian spores in clinical samples, including paraffin-embedded tissue sections. *Arch Pathol Lab Med.* 1997;121:888-893.

7. Orestein JM. Microsporidiosis in acquired immunodeficiency syndrome. *J Parasitol.* 991;77:843-864.

8. Visvesvara GS, Leitch GJ, Da Silva AJ, et al. Polycolonal and monoclonal antibody and PCR-amplified small-subunit rRNA identification of a micrsporidian, *Ecephalitozoon hellem*, isolate from an AIDS patient with disseminated infection. *J Clin Microbiol.* 1994;32:2760-2768.

9. Barenfanger J, Drake CA. Interpretation of Gram stains for the nonmicrobiologist. *Lab Med.* 2001;32:368-375.

10. Barenfanger J, Gaydos JM. Gram stain-beyond the basics. *Lab Med.* 2002;33:609-614.

11. Waller T. Sensitivity of *Encephalitozoon cuniculi* to various temperature, disinfectants and drugs. *Lab Anim.* 1979;13:227-230.

12. Carr A, Marriott D, Field A et al. Treatment of HIV-associated microsporidiosis and cryptosporidiosis with combination antiretroviral therapy. *Lancet.* 1998;351:256-261.

13. Molina JM, Oksenhendler E, Beauvais B, et al. Disseminated microsporidiosis due to *Septata intestinalis* in patient with AIDS: Clinical features and response to albendazole therapy. *J Infect Dis.* 1995;171:245-249.

14. Dore GJ, Marriott DJ, Hing MC, et al. Disseminated microsporidiosis due to *Septata intestinalis* in nine patients infected with human immunodeficiency virus: Response to therapy with albendazole. *Clin Infec Dis.* 1995;21:70-76.

Abdominal Pain and Leukocytosis in an Immunosuppressed Patient

Adam C. Seegmiller, Rita M. Gander

Department of Pathology, University of Texas Southwestern Medical Center, Dallas, TX

Patient: 25-year-old Hispanic woman.

Chief Complaint: Abdominal pain.

History of Present Illness: The patient presented to her regular renal clinic appointment complaining of decreased appetite and midepigastric abdominal pain for 2 weeks. She described the pain as episodic in nature, occurring approximately twice daily, and resolving spontaneously. The pain was associated with bloating, but there was no accompanying nausea, vomiting, or diarrhea. The patient had a history of gastroesophageal reflux disease (GERD), but stated that her current pain was different from the pain she experienced during an episode of GERD. Additionally, her pain was not positional and was unchanged by eating.

Past Medical History: Systemic lupus erythematosis (SLE) diagnosed 7 months prior to presentation, stage IV lupusnephritis, steroid-induced diabetes mellitus, hypertension, and a history of GERD.

Past Surgical History: Removal of a benign axillary mass.

Drug History: Prednisone, 60 mg, once daily; hydroxychloroquine, 200 mg, twice daily; lisinopril 20 mg, once daily; glimepiride, 1 mg, once daily; esomeprazole, 40 mg, once daily.

Family/Social History: The patient had no significant family medical history. She has 1 child and denied any history of alcohol, tobacco, or drug abuse. She had a single blood transfusion 7 months prior to presentation.

Physical Examination: Vital signs: temperature, 36.9°C; heart rate, 80 beats per minute; respiratory rate, 20 breaths per minute; blood pressure, 94/63 mm Hg. The patient was in no acute distress. She had a cushingoid appearance with moon facies. The remainder of the physical examination was normal. Of note, the patient's abdomen was soft, non-tender, and non-distended with normoactive bowel sounds.

Results of Additional Diagnostic Procedures and Tests: A bone marrow biopsy revealed a hypocellular bone marrow with increased megakaryocytes, mild anemia, and leukemoid reaction with moderate eosinophilia. Blood and urine cultures were negative for microorganisms. Stool cultures grew normal gastrointestinal (GI) tract flora, but the bacteria were spread between the colonies in a lacy, web-like pattern on the solid growth medium, giving the appearance of "tracks" (**Image 1A**). A selenite broth culture that had been inoculated with the stool sample was centrifuged and a sample of the sediment was analyzed for ova and parasites (O&P) (**Image 1B-1D**).

T1. Principal Laboratory Findings

Test	Patient's Result	"Normal" Reference Range
Hematology		
WBC count	23.0	4.1-11.1 × 10^3/μL
RBC count	3.44	4.01-5.31 × 10^3/μL
Hemoglobin	10.8	12.1-16.1 g/dL
Hematocrit	31.5	36.8-48.7%
Platelet count	122	174-404 × 10^3/μL
Differential: Neutrophils	50	36-72%
Bands	17	0-11%
Lymphocytes	9	20-51%
Monocytes	3	4-11%
Eosinophils	4	1-7%
Basophils	1	0-1%
Myelocytes	16	0%
MCV	91.4	76.2-98.6 fL
ESR	25.0	0-15 mm/h
Coagulation		
PT	10.3	9.2-12.5 sec
INR	1.0	
PTT	28.6	24.5-34.5 sec
Chemistry		
Sodium	136	135-145 mEq/L
Potassium	4.8	3.6-5.0 mEq/L
Chloride	104	98-109 mEq/L
CO_2	24	22-31 mEq/L
BUN	28	7-21 mg/dL
Creatinine	1.5	0.6-1.2 mg/dL
Glucose	110	65-110 mg/dL
AST	9	13-40 U/L
ALT	35	10-40 U/L
Amylase	41	29-108 U/L
Lipase	34	7-59 U/L
CRP	1.0	0.0-0.8 mg/dL

WBC, white blood cell; RBC, red blood cell; MCV, mean corpuscular volume; ESR, erythrocyte sedimentation rate; PT, prothrombin time; INR, International Normalized Ratio; PTT, partial thromboplastin time; BUN, blood urea nitrogen; AST, aspartate aminotransferase; ALT, alanine aminotransferase; CRP, C-reactive protein.

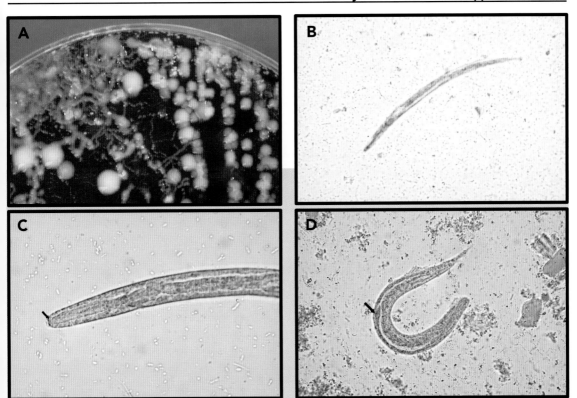

Image 1_A, Bacterial growth from routine culture of our patient's stool on blood agar illustrating the appearance of "tracks" on the agar; **B**, appearance of iodine-stained *Strongyloides stercoralis* larvae from a selenite broth culture; **C**, appearance of iodine-stained *S. stercoralis* larvae from a selenite broth culture illustrating the organism's buccal cavity (arrow); **D**, *S. stercoralis* larva from an iodine-stained stool O&P preparation indicating the organism's prominent genital primordium (arrow).

Questions

1. What are the most striking clinical and laboratory findings?

2. How do you explain the most striking findings?

3. What is the organism recovered from the patient's stool?

4. What other organisms must be ruled out to make a definitive diagnosis?

5. What is this patient's most likely diagnosis?

6. What is the major clinical concern with this diagnosis?

7. What is the most appropriate treatment for this patient?

Possible Answers

1. Decreased appetite and episodic epigastric abdominal pain with bloating; marked peripheral leukocytosis with a significant increase in immature granulocytes; mild anemia; hypocellular bone marrow with moderate eosinophilia; the appearance of "tracks" on the blood agar plate culture of the patient's stool sample; and a positive O&P examination.

2. **Abdominal pain.** The differential diagnosis of epigastric abdominal pain includes several conditions (eg, appendicitis, pancreatitis, biliary obstruction, hepatitis, bacterial, fungal, or parasitic infection). The setting and location of her pain and her benign physical examination, however, rules out a significant number of these conditions. Moreover, the results of the stool culture make parasitic infection the most likely cause of our patient's epigastric abdominal pain. **Leukocytosis.** Our patient's leukocytosis was

characterized by neutrophilia and a marked shift to the left. This kind of neutrophilia can be classified as either primary, where there is no other obvious associated disease, or secondary, where the increase in neutrophils and precursors has a discernible cause.[1] It is unlikely that our patient has a primary neutrophilia because: (1) there are potential secondary causes, and (2) the bone marrow examination showed no evidence of neoplastic or myelodysplastic disease. There are several potential secondary causes of neutrophilia with a left shift, including infection (eg, bacterial), drug-induced neutrophilia, and chronic inflammation. Neutrophilia with a left shift is a common finding in bacterial infections; however, it is an uncommon finding in patients with parasitic infections.[2] Eosinophilia, seen only upon bone marrow examination, is more common in parasitic infections; however, eosinophilia may be suppressed in patients on glucocorticoid therapy.[3] Parasitic infection, glucocorticoid treatment, and a chronic inflammatory condition (eg, SLE) are the most likely causes of our patient's neutrophilia with a left shift. **Anemia.** Our patient's anemia was mild and normocytic with a hypocellular bone marrow. There was no evidence of a hemolytic, myelophthisic (ie, reduction of the cell-forming functions of the bone marrow), or neoplastic process. In the setting of a chronic inflammation, anemia of chronic disease becomes the most likely diagnosis. **"Tracks" in the blood agar stool culture.** The medical technologist reviewing the blood agar culture of our patient's stool astutely recognized the unusual appearance of this culture as suggestive of the presence of a motile organism that was confirmed subsequently by a positive O&P examination.

3. *Strongyloides stercoralis* is the smallest of the intestinal nematodes.[4] Infection with this parasite is extremely common, with a prevalence estimated at approximately 100 million cases worldwide.[5] It is endemic to tropical and sub-tropical regions, but is also seen in some temperate regions, including the southeastern United States.[3,5,6] Humans are infected by filariform larvae, which are found in the soil.[4,5] The larvae invade through the skin into the circulatory system. It is thought that they then migrate to the lungs and up the respiratory tract to the pharynx, where they are swallowed.

They take up residence in the small intestine where they mature into adults. The adult females lay eggs in the intestine, which hatch as rhabditiform larvae that are shed in the stool. In this environment, they develop into the infective filariform larvae and wait to invade a new host. Two additional aspects of the parasite life cycle are important in understanding its interactions with humans. The first is the ability of *S. stercoralis* to reproduce outside of its host. The larvae shed in the stool can develop into adults in the soil and reproduce sexually in the so-called indirect life cycle. The second important aspect is the parasite's ability to auto-infect its host. At some rate, infective filariform larvae develop in the small intestine and infect their host by direct invasion of the GI mucosa or perianal skin. This autoinfection cycle allows the parasite to persist in its host for long periods of time. There are reports of chronic strongyloidiasis in patients decades after their presumed exposure.[7,8] Diagnosis of strongyloidasis is made by the observation of these small (approximately 2 mm long) rhabditiform larvae in the stool (**Image 1B**). *Strongyloides stercoralis* is the only intestinal parasite that sheds larvae in the stool. The other nematodes, including hookworms, *Ascaris, Trichuris,* and *Enterobius,* typically shed ova. Strongyloidiasis, especially the chronic variety, is often asymptomatic,[3] although there may be skin, pulmonary, and GI symptoms in some patients following the pattern of parasite migration in the body.[5] Pulmonary symptoms may include cough and tracheal irritation, resembling bronchitis. Gastrointestinal symptoms include indigestion, abdominal pain, diarrhea, and anorexia.

4. Although *S. stercoralis* is the only intestinal parasite that sheds larvae in the stool, diagnosis in this case is complicated by the fact that the parasite was recovered in a routine stool culture after at least 24 hours of incubation. If a stool sample is allowed to incubate before being processed with preservative, there is concern that the observed larvae may be from the hatched ova of hookworms, which are very similar in appearance to *Strongyloides* larvae.[4] The main differentiating features of *S. stercoralis* are illustrated in **Images 1C-1D**. *Strongyloides* larvae have short buccal cavities (**Image 1C**) in contrast with hookworm larvae, which have appreciably longer

buccal cavities. In addition, they have much more prominent genital primordia (**Image 1D**) than hookworm larvae. This complicating issue can be avoided by requesting an additional stool sample, which is then immediately processed in preservative to prevent development of larvae from the ova of other parasites. In this case, an additional stool sample was received, and the diagnosis of strongyloidiasis was confirmed by the observation of rhabditiform larvae.

5. **Most likely diagnosis:** *gastrointestinal infection by Strongyloides stercoralis.*

6. Although strongyloidiasis causes a relatively minor infection in most people, it can be much more serious, even fatal, in the setting of immune compromise. In immunosuppressed patients, there can be an acceleration of the autoinfection cycle, leading to overwhelming parasite loads, termed hyperinfection,[3,5] which can lead to a number of serious complications. Increased parasite loads in the GI tract cause more frequent and severe manifestations of acute strongyloidiasis symptoms. Additionally, there have been reports of more serious complications, including malabsorption syndrome, GI bleeding, ileus, and small bowel obstruction. Pulmonary manifestations result from transit of parasites through the lungs and may include cough, wheezing, pleuritic chest pain, hemoptysis, and other respiratory complaints. In rare, severe cases, pulmonary infection may progress to pulmonary hemorrhage, which is potentially fatal.[6] A third complication is disseminated infection. *Strongyloides stercoralis* larvae have been detected in multiple organs, including skin, lymph nodes, gallbladder, liver, diaphragm, heart, pancreas, skeletal muscle, kidneys, ovaries, and brain.[3] Finally, *Stronglyoides* hyperinfection is commonly complicated by concomitant bacterial infection. These infections usually involve GI flora that have reached the circulation via the entry site of filariform larvae in the intestinal wall, or perhaps even carried on the surface of the larvae.[3] Such infections have resulted in a gram-negative bacteremia, sepsis, and meningitis. The most common cause of *Strongyloides* hyperinfection in immunosuppressed patients is glucocorticoid therapy. In experimental model systems, glucocorticoid treatment has been shown to increase *Strongyloides* parasite size and fecundity.[9] The

parasites are also found more anteriorly in the GI tract and are cleared at a slower rate. However, the exact mechanism leading to these changes and how they increase the incidence of hyperinfection are unknown. Hyperinfection has also been observed in patients treated with other immunosuppressant medications, although many of these cases are complicated by concomitant glucocorticoid treatment. One exception is cyclosporine. Patients treated with this drug rarely experience hyperinfection, leading some to believe that it has antihelminthic properties.[3] Other settings in which hyperinfection has been reported include human T-cell lymphotropic virus (HTLV-1) infection, solid organ transplant, especially renal transplant patients taking glucocorticoids, hypogammaglobulinemia, and human immunodeficiency virus (HIV) infection. However, many of the patients described in these reports were also taking glucocorticoids, making it impossible to define the exact causative agent of their hyperinfection syndrome.

7. Ivermectin has emerged as the treatment of choice for *Stronglyoides* infection. It has been shown to be as effective, and with fewer side effects, as thiabendazole, the previous most common treatment for *Strongyloides* infection.[10] However, refractoriness to these treatments has been observed, and treatment should be continued until symptoms resolve and stool samples have been cleared of parasite for at least 2 weeks, the approximate length of the autoinfective cycle.[3]

Treatment and Course

Our patient received a 2-day course of ivermectin therapy and experienced complete resolution of both her GI symptoms and leukocytosis. On discharge, her WBC count had dropped to 6800/μL and remained normal during the ensuing follow-up period. Repeat stool O&P examination approximately 1 month after treatment showed no parasites, indicating successful treatment.

Keywords

Strongyloides stercoralis, strongyloidiasis, hyperinfection, leukocytosis, glucocorticoids, immunosuppression

References

1. Curnutte JT, Coates TD. Disorders of phagocyte function and number. In: Hoffman R, Benz EJ, Shattil SJ, et al, eds, *Hematology: Basic Principles and Practice*. 3rd ed. Philadelphia:Churchill Livingstone. 720-762.

2. Hanson CA. Peripheral blood and bone marrow: Morphology, counts and differentials, and reactive disorders. In: *Clinical Laboratory Medicine*, 2nd ed, McClatchey KD, ed. Philadelphia: Lippincott Williams & Wilkins. 797-829.

3. Keiser PB, Nutman TB. *Strongyloides stercoralis* in the immunocompromised population. *Clin Microbiol Rev.* 2004; 17:208-217.

4. Pfaller MA. Parasitology. In: *Clinical Laboratory Medicine*, 2nd ed, McClatchey KD, ed. Philadelphia: Lippincott Williams & Wilkins. 1291-1344.

5. Mahmoud AAF. Strongyloidiasis. *Clin Infect Dis.* 1996;23:949-53.

6. Safdar A, Malathum K, Rodriguez SJ, et al. Strongyloidiasis in patients at a comprehensive cancer center in the United States: a retrospective study covering the years 1971-2001. *Cancer.* 2004;100:1531-1536.

7. Pelletier LL Jr. Chronic strongyloidiasis in World War II Far East ex-prisoners of war. *Am J Trop Med Hyg.* 1984;33:55-61.

8. Gill GV, Beeching NJ, Khoo S, *et al.* A British Second World War veteran with disseminated strongyloidiasis. *Trans R Soc Trop Med Hyg.* 2004;98:382-386.

9. Wilkes CP, Thompson FJ, Gardner MP, et al. The effect of the host immune response on the parasitic nematode *Strongyloides ratti. Parasitology.* 2004;128:661-669.

10. Gann PH, Neva FA, Gam AA. A randomized trial of single- and two-dose ivermectin versus thiabendazole for treatment of strongyloidiasis. *J Infect Dis.* 1994; 169:1076-1079.

Fever and Petechiae in a Middle Aged Male

Seema Garg, Rachna Arora, Naveen Kakkar

Department of Pathology, Christian Medical College & Hospital, Ludhiana, Punjab, India

Patient: 38-year-old man.

Medical History: Unremarkable.

Chief Complaint: Fever for 3 days with body ache.

Family History: Unremarkable.

Physical Examination Findings: Average built male with petechiae over his arms and legs and no organomegaly.

Drug History: He had received antipyretics from a local doctor.

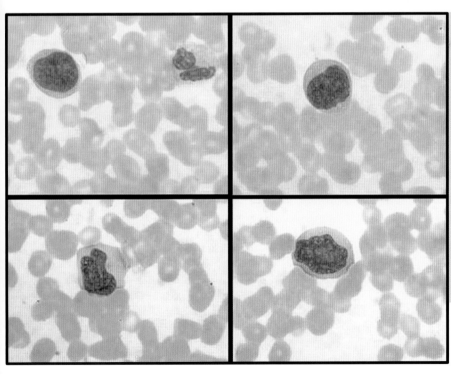

Image 1_Example of 4 fields in the patient's peripheral blood smear (Leishman stain; 1000× magnification) illustrating leukopenia with the presence of atypical, large lymphocytes (virocytes) with coarse nuclear chromatin and abundant basophilic cytoplasm and severe thrombocytopenia. The morphology of the red blood cells is unremarkable.

T1. Principal Laboratory Findings

Test	Patient's Result	"Normal" Reference Range
Hematology		
Hemoglobin	12.3	12.0-16.0 g/dL
Hematocrit	37.9	38-47%
WBC count	3.2	4.0-11.0 × 10³/µL
Platelet count	16	150-400 × 10³/µL
Differential: Metamyelocytes	2	0%
Neutrophils	34	40-80%
Lymphocytes	43	20-40%
Atypical lymphocytes	19	0%
Eosinophils	1	0-6%
Basophils	1	0-1%
PBS findings:	Normocytic, normochromic RBCs; leukopenia with neutropenia; many atypical lymphocytes (virocytes) seen with size 14-20 microns, oval to rounded nucleus with coarse chromatin, and abundant agranular basophilic cytoplasm, and severe thrombocytopenia	
Immunology		
Serological test for dengue virus	Positive	Negative

WBC, white blood cell; PBS, peripheral blood smear; RBCs, red blood cells.

Questions

1. What are this patient's most striking clinical and laboratory findings?

2. How do you explain these findings?

3. What is this patient's most likely diagnosis?

4. What is the causative organism of this patient's disease?

5. What is the geographical distribution of the organism causing this patient's disease?

6. What is the life cycle of the organism causing this patient's disease?

7. What are the clinical features of the disease caused by this organism?

8. How is the laboratory diagnosis made of the disease caused by this organism?

9. What are other conditions in which atypical lymphocytes can be seen on a peripheral blood smear?

Possible Answers

1. Fever with bicytopenia (leukopenia and thrombocytopenia) (**T1**) with atypical lymphocytes in the peripheral blood smear (**Image 1**) and a positive serology test for dengue virus.

2. The constellation of the clinical and laboratory findings in this patient is characteristic of dengue fever.

3. ***Most likely diagnosis:*** *dengue fever.*

4. The dengue virus that causes dengue fever is an arbovirus, with 4 serotypes (1, 2, 3, and 4), belonging to the flaviviridae family. Infection with a particular serotype confers complete immunity against that particular serotype and partially against other serotypes.

5. Dengue fever is a disease of the tropical and subtropical regions of the world affecting urban and semi-urban areas. Currently, dengue fever/dengue hemorrhagic fever (DHF) is endemic in 112 countries of the world, prominent among which are Bangladesh, India, Indonesia, Maldives, Myanmar, Sri Lanka, Thailand, and Vietnam.[1] Other countries in Southeast Asia are also affected. Dengue infection is also seen in the Caribbean islands. In the past few years, dengue infection has occurred in the United States especially among the inhabitants along the Mexican border. Large parts of South America also experience frequent outbreaks of dengue infection.[1,2] Annually, 100 million cases of dengue fever and half a million cases of dengue hemorrhagic fever occur worldwide. Being a re-emergent disease, its geographical distribution has greatly expanded

beyond endemic areas with increasing urbanization, poverty, intercontinental air travel, and the demise of Aedes mosquito eradication programs.

6. Dengue fever is a mosquito-borne infection. Outbreaks often start during the rainy season when the mosquito vector, *Aedes aegypti*, is abundant. The mosquito breeds in water-holding receptacles (desert coolers, vases, discarded containers, coconut husks, or old tires) or in plants close to human dwellings. The reservoir of infection is both man and mosquito. The female mosquito acquires the virus by feeding on an infected human with viremia. After a period of 1 to 2 weeks, the mosquitoes are infective and remain so for their entire life span of 1 to 3 months. In this period, they infect other humans during a blood meal.

7. Typically patients present with sudden onset fever, headache, retro-orbital and back pain, along with severe myalgia, giving rise to the popular term "breakbone fever." Individuals of all ages and both sexes are susceptible to dengue fever. Patients also have a macular rash, lymphadenopathy, and palatal vesicles. The illness usually lasts for 1 week. Additional symptoms usually include anorexia, nausea, and vomiting. Epistaxis and scattered petechiae are commonly seen in uncomplicated dengue. Pre-existing gastrointestinal lesions may bleed during the acute illness. **Dengue hemorrhagic fever** is a severe form of dengue fever caused by infection with more than 1 serotype of dengue virus. The initial infection sensitizes the patient and the subsequent infection by the second serotype invokes a severe hypersensitivity reaction leading to increased plasma capillary leakage and hemostatic derangement. Patients manifest clinically with severe bleeding and shock. Dengue hemorrhagic fever has a high mortality rate.

8. The laboratory diagnosis of dengue fever can be made by either indirect or direct methods. **Indirect methods** include: (1) complete blood count (CBC) and peripheral blood smear (PBS) - CBC shows leukopenia and thrombocytopenia while the PBS shows the presence of atypical lymphocytes (virocytes) with abundant basophilic cytoplasm and enlarged nuclei which are larger with a more immature chromatin than normal lymphocyte; (2) biochemical tests - serum transaminases are frequently elevated; and (3) serological tests for the presence of antibodies to dengue fever virus proteins. Moreover, in DHF, coagulation tests are commonly abnormal. The diagnosis of dengue fever is usually made based on a positive IgM enzyme-linked immunosorbent assay (ELISA) during the recovery phase of the patient's disease or by antigen detection by ELISA or reverse transcriptase-polymerase chain reaction (RT-PCR) identification of viral ribonucleic acid (RNA) during the acute phase of the infection.[3] Among the **direct methods**, viral isolation from human sera is cumbersome and very difficult. Hence, alternative techniques like mosquito cell culture, mosquito inoculation, and RT-PCR assays have been attempted for diagnosing dengue infection, especially in endemic areas.[4]

9. Infection with Epstein-Barr virus, hepatitis A, cytomegalovirus, measles, mumps, Herpes zoster, Herpes simplex, and human immunodeficiency virus (HIV) can also show atypical lymphocytes in a peripheral blood smear. Noninfectious causes of atypical lymphocytes in the peripheral blood smear include graft-versus-host disease (GVHD), systemic lupus erythematosus (SLE), and Hodgkin lymphoma.[5]

Keywords

Aedes Egypti, atypical lymphocytes, dengue, leukopenia, thrombocytopenia

References

1. Malavigue GN, Fernando S, Fernando DJ, et al. Dengue viral infections. *Postgrad Med J.* 2004;80:588-601.

2. Peter CJ. Infections caused by arthropods- and rodent-borne viruses. In: Kasper DL, Braunwald E, Fauci AS, Hauser SL, Longo DL, Jameson JL, eds. *Harrison's Principles of Internal Medicine.* 16th edition. New York, McGraw-Hill; 2005:1161-1174.

3. Grobusch MP, Niedrig M, Gobels K, et al. Evaluation of the use of RT-PCR for the early diagnosis of dengue fever. *Clin Microbiol Infect.* 2006; 12:395-397.

4. Philip Samuel P, Tyagi BK. Diagnostic methods for detection & isolation of dengue viruses from vector mosquitoes. *Ind J Med Res.* 2006;123:615-628.

5. Bains BJ. *Blood Cells: A Practical Guide.* 3rd ed. London, Blackwell Science; 2002.

Recurrent Hoarseness and Shortness of Breath in an Adult Smoker

Michael Constantinescu,[1] Elba A. Turbat-Herrera,[1] Jianhua Wu,[1] Dorothy Rivette,[1] Kellous A. Price,[2] Robert F. Aarstad,[2] Janice M. Matthews-Greer[1,2]

Departments of [1]Pathology, [2]Otorhinolaryngology, and [3]Pediatrics, Louisiana State University Health Sciences Center, Shreveport, LA

Patient: 67-year-old male.

Chief Complaints: Hoarseness and shortness of breath.

Past Medical History: History of recurrent laryngeal papillomatosis for 8 years, treated with multiple ablative surgical procedures. History of systemic lupus erythematosus, osteoporosis, and smoking for more than 50 years.

Physical/Laryngoscopic Examination: Multiple papillomas were found, located mostly in the subglottic area with minimal involvement of the true vocal cord [**Image 1**]. Ablation of the lesions was performed, and tissue samples were sent for histopathologic analysis.

Principal Histopathology Findings: Tissue samples submitted for histopathology consisted of multiple fragments of pink-tan soft tissue that measured $1.5 \times 0.6 \times 0.5$ cm in aggregate. Microscopically, the tissue had multiple finger-like projections of squamous epithelium with a fibrovascular stromal core. The epithelium revealed scattered cells with slightly enlarged irregular wrinkled nuclei and a surrounding clear cytoplasmic halo [**Image 2A, Image 2B**]. A mild degree of acanthosis was noted and a few scattered inflammatory cells were present. In addition, tissue cut from 1 of the papillomas was tested using the Digene (Gaithersburg, MD) Hybrid Capture-2 assay according to the protocol of the manufacturer for biopsy specimens. The results of this testing demonstrated coinfection of the tissue with both low- and high-risk human papilloma virus (HPV).

Questions

1. Based on this patient's clinical and histopathology findings, what is this patient's most likely diagnosis?

2. What are the clinical features and etiology of this patient's condition?

3. What are the genotypic characteristics of the agent responsible for this patient's condition?

4. What is the most appropriate treatment for this patient's condition?

5. How can this patient's condition be prevented?

Possible Answers

1. ***Most likely diagnosis:*** *Laryngeal papillomatosis due to HPV infection.*

The microscopic diagnosis of this patient's tissue lesion was squamous papilloma of the posterior commissure of the larynx. The cells observed in the tissue with irregular (wrinkled) nuclei surrounded by a clear cytoplasmic halo are known as koilocytes and represent the hallmark of HPV infection. This finding was confirmed by the detection of HPV-specific DNA sequences using the Digene Hybrid Capture-2 assay.

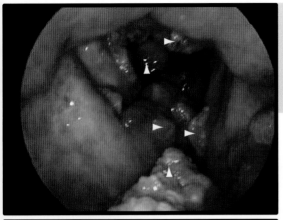

Image 1_Endoscopic (direct laryngoscopic) findings in our patient illustrating multiple polypoid, irregular, or finger-like projections on the laryngeal mucosa (arrowheads).

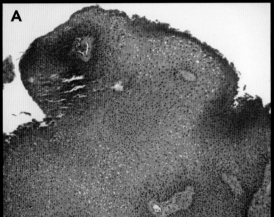

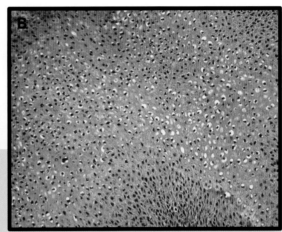

Image 2_Microscopic appearance of 1 of the fragments excised illustrating **A**) the irregular, finger-like configuration of the lesion (hematoxylin-eosin staining, 200× magnification); **B**) squamous epithelium with scattered koilocytes - slightly enlarged cells with wrinkled irregular nuclei (hematoxylin-eosin staining, 400× magnification).

2. Laryngeal papillomatosis (LP) is a rare benign laryngeal neoplasm. Clinically, the principal symptom of LP is hoarseness with or without airway obstruction. The condition has 2 forms: adult- and juvenile-onset. In both forms, the typical location of HPV infection is within the vocal folds of the larynx. Juvenile-onset HPV infection occurs when an infant comes into contact with HPV-infected maternal genital mucosa during delivery.[1] Although not clearly proven, adult-onset HPV infection may be transmitted via orogenital contact. Adult-onset LP occurs usually in individuals 20 years of age or older,[2] and there is a clear male predominance, with the male to female ratio for this disease varying from 2:1 to 4:1. The HPV etiology of LP has been accepted, and HPV genotypes 6 and 11 (associated with low-risk HPV) are the most common types identified in laryngeal papilloma lesions. Other, less commonly associated HPV genotypes include genotypes 16 and 18 (associated with high-risk HPV), both of which are also associated more frequently with progression to malignancy. The HPV genotype 16 appears to be more common in adult- than in juvenile-onset LP. In patients with LP and in patients in remission from LP after treatment, HPV DNA can be identified in both normal and abnormal histologically appearing sites. It is estimated that 3% to 7% of LP cases may result in malignant transformation. Moreover, exposure to radiation and to cigarette smoke increases the risk of malignant transformation. Because genital condylomas (genital warts) are caused more often by HPV genotypes 6 and 11, vertical transmission of juvenile-onset LP has been postulated. However, the rare association of juvenile LP with other common cervical HPV genotypes (eg, 16, 18, 31, 33, and 35) that are commonly found in the cervix challenge this theory.[3] Similarly, orogenital transmission of

HPV in adult-onset LP is not clearly supported by clinical evidence. Whereas coinfection with both high- and low-risk HPV genotypes in the cervix is common,[4] coinfection of the low- and high-risk HPV genotypes is unusual in the laryngeal respiratory mucosa.[5]

3. Human papilloma virus is a DNA virus with oncogenic potential that infects epithelial cells and belongs to the Papillomaviridae family of viruses. More than 100 HPV genotypes have been described and associated with a variety of conditions: genotypes 6, 11, 16, 18, and 70 (anogenital condyloma); genotypes 2, 4, and 49 (verruca vulgaris or wart); genotypes 16, 18, 26, 27, 30, 31, 33-35, 40, 42-45, 51-59, 61-62, 64, 66-69, 71-74 (cervical dysplasia and/or carcinoma); genotypes 6, 7, 11, 60, 63, 65, 78 (respiratory papillomatosis).[6] Mucosal HPV infections are classified as high- or low-risk based on tissue tropism and their malignant transformation potential. The tissue target of HPV is the squamous epithelium. Infection can be latent, subclinical, or clinical. Clinical manifestations of infection develop in most cases within 1 to 8 months after exposure. Oncogenic transformation is associated with the integration of the viral genome into the host DNA. The genetic material of these nonenveloped icosahedral viruses is distributed into early (E1 to E7) and late regions (L1 and L2) of the host DNA. In high-risk HPV infection, the E6 and E7 early regions promote the degradation of the tumor suppressor proteins, p53 and Rb, respectively, in association with other mechanisms of oncogenic transformation.[6]

4. Surgical excision remains the most widely used treatment for LP. The recurrence rates are high and complications include scar formation, bleeding, and infection. The CO_2 laser is both surgically precise and favored over cold instruments.[7] Pharmaceutical agents are also effective in the treatment of HPV, although their effect on respiratory HPV lesions is less well known. The antimetabolic agent, 5-fluorouracil, which inhibits DNA synthesis, has been used topically in the treatment of warts and genital HPV infection. The antiviral agent, Cidofovir, has also been shown to have promise in the treatment of warts and high-grade cervical dysplasia associated with HPV infection. In addition, alpha-interferon,

an immunomodulator that inhibits viral protein synthesis, has also been used successfully in the treatment of HPV infection. The most common side effects of this treatment modality include flu-like symptoms, increased liver transaminase levels, leukocytopenia or thrombocytopenia, and spastic diplegia. Lastly, Imiquimod, another immunomodulator that locally increases cytokine production, also appears to be effective and well tolerated in the treatment of anogenital warts and cervical dysplasia.[6,7]

5. Primary prevention consists of measures to reduce the incidence of HPV infection, including education about safe-sex practices; however, complete protection from HPV infection using barrier protective devices (eg, condoms) is not possible because these barriers do not prevent contact with the entire anogenital region. Screening for HPV infection by Pap smear and more recently by HPV DNA testing has proven successful in preventing both morbidity and mortality due to genital cancer. Smoking cessation also appears to reduce the incidence of the types of tumors associated with genital cancer. Lastly, the therapeutic use of vaccines to prevent high-risk HPV infection is currently undergoing clinical trials.[6]

Keywords _____

papillomatosis, human papilloma virus, koilocytes, coinfection, malignant transformation

References _____

1. Kashima HK, Shah F, Lyles A, et al. A comparison of risk factors in juvenile-onset and adult-onset recurrent respiratory papillomatosis. *Laryngoscope.* 1992;102:9-13.

2. Corbitt G, Zarod AP, Arrand JR, et al. Human papillomavirus (HPV) genotypes associated with laryngeal papilloma. *J Clin Pathol.* 1988;41:284-288.

3. Rimell F, Maisel R, Dayton V. In situ hybridization and laryngeal papillomas. *Ann Otol Rhinol Laryngol.* 1992;101:119-126.

4. Rousseau MC, Pereira JS, Prado JC, et al. Cervical coinfection with human papillomavirus (HPV) types as a predictor of acquisition and persistence of HPV infection. *J Infect Dis.* 2001;184:1508-1517.

5. Lin KY, Westra WH, Kashima HK, et al. Coinfection of HPV-11 and HPV-16 in a case of laryngeal squamous papillomas with severe dysplasia. *Laryngoscope.* 1997;107:942-947.

6. Brentjens MH, Yeung-Yue KA, Lee PC, et al. Human papillomavirus: A review. *Dermatol Clin.* 2002;20:315-331.

7. Derkay CS, Darrow DH. Recurrent respiratory papillomatosis of the larynx; current diagnosis and treatment. *Otolaryngol Clin North Am.* 2000;33:1127-1142.

Mixed Aphasia in an Adult Male With AIDS

Monte S. Willis, Matthew L. Bell, Regina Y. Najera, Frank H. Wians, Jr.

Department of Pathology, University of Texas Southwestern Medical Center, Dallas, TX

Patient: 41-year-old African-American male.

Chief Complaint: A 3-week history of progressive right-sided weakness, confusion, and difficulty speaking (dysarthria).

Past Medical History: The patient had been diagnosed with AIDS a year ago and had been in a slow-speed motor vehicle accident 5 weeks prior to admission. A computed tomography (CT) scan following this accident revealed an area of abnormality in the left frontoparietal lobe that was attributed to trauma sustained during the accident.

Physical and Neurological Examination: The patient was afebrile and alert but disoriented, with mixed aphasia and an inability to follow most commands. Right facial droop was present with rightward tongue deviation and a left gaze preference. There was a right-sided hemiparesis with increased deep reflexes and sustained right-sided clonus. Sensation was intact bilaterally.

Laboratory Findings: A cerebral spinal fluid (CSF) analysis, including viral tests, was ordered; however, the results of the viral tests were not immediately available [**T1**].

Results of Additional Diagnostic Procedures: The CT scan demonstrated diffuse, low attenuation within the left frontal and parietal white matter, mild edema, and no midline shift. Magnetic resonance imaging (MRI) of the head revealed a left frontoparietal mass involving the white matter tract and extending to the corpus callosum [**Image 1**]. The mass was hypointense on **T1**-weighted MRI and hyperintense on **T2**-weighted MRI. There was a mild mass effect and minimal diffuse enhancement. No uptake was seen on a gadodiamide contrast-enhanced MRI scan.

Questions

1. What is (are) this patient's most striking laboratory result(s)?

2. What condition(s) does (do) this patient's laboratory results and history suggest?

3. Which additional test(s) should be performed? Why?

4. What is (are) the most likely diagnosis(es)?

5. Is there any further workup that should be done on this patient?

6. What is the most appropriate treatment for this patient?

T1. Principal Laboratory Findings

Test	Patient's Result	"Normal" Reference Range
CSF total protein	48	15-45 mg/dL
VDRL	Negative	Negative
CMV PCR	Negative	Negative
JCV PCR	Positive	Negative

CSF, cerebrospinal fluid; VDRL, venereal disease research laboratory; CMV, cytomegalovirus; PCR, polymerase chain reaction; JCV, JC virus.

T2. Opportunistic Infectious Causes of CNS Lesions in HIV+ Patients*

Infectious Cause	Frequency, %†
CMV encephalomyelitis‡	20
PML	3
Possible Varicella-zoster	<1
Mycobacterial infections (TB and MAI)	2
Other bacterial infections	4
Mycotic infections	11
Parasitic infections	3.5

Adapted from Burns DK, et al. (Ref. 1).
†Of cases (n = 112) with morphologic CNS abnormalities and infectious causes shown from a cohort of 141 HIV+ patients.
‡Includes both definitive (16%) and presumptive (4%) cases of cytomegalovirus (CMV).
CNS, central nervous system; CMV, cytomegalovirus; PML, progressive multifocal leukoencephalopathy; TB, tuberculosis; MAI, mycobacterium avium intracellulare.

Possible Answers

1. Slightly increased CSF total protein and a positive test for the presence of JC virus (JCV) DNA by polymerase chain reaction (PCR).

2. Prior to receiving the results of the CSF PCR test for JCV, the differential diagnosis might include: primary central nervous system (CNS) lymphoma, toxoplasmosis, progressive multifocal leukoencephalopathy (PML), HIV encephalitis, tuberculosis (TB), cryptococcosis, or herpes simplex virus (HSV) infection. The treatment based on the presumption of any 1 of these disease entities might include dexamethasone, antitoxoplasma drugs, and highly active antiretroviral

T3. Frequency of Various Neurologic Manifestations in Patients With PML

Neurologic Manifestation	Frequency, %*
Hemiparesis	42
Cognitive disturbance	36
Visual field deficits	32
Ataxia	21
Aphasia	17
Cranial nerve defects	13
Sensory deficits	9

*Of patients with PML that demonstrate each neurologic manifestation listed.

therapy (HAART). Additional diagnostic testing might include MRI or brain biopsy. The decision might be made to await the results of the JCV PCR test before initiating drug therapy. When the results of this test came back positive, PML was the most likely choice among those considered in the differential diagnosis.

In a study of postmortem neuropathologic changes from our institution, morphologic abnormalities were found in 112 of 141 consecutive patients with HIV at autopsy.[1] The most common opportunistic infection identified was cytomegalovirus (CMV) found definitively in 23 patients and presumptively in 6 patients (20%). Progressive multifocal leukoencephalopathy was present in only 4 patients (3%). Other opportunistic infectious causes of the morphologic changes in the CNS of patients with HIV are shown in **T2**. Other multi-center prospective studies have found PML to be an uncommon cause of CNS infection in HIV patients (current estimates up to 5%) which has not increased in the era of HAART.[2,3]

Progressive multifocal leukoencephalopathy is a progressive demyelinating disease, first described by Astrom in 1958,[4] that occurs in immunocompromised patients due to infection, in virtually all cases, with JCV. The JC virus belongs to the *Polyoma* genus of the Papovaridae family of small, non-enveloped viruses with icosahedral symmetry and covalently closed, circular, double-stranded DNA.[5] Polyomaviruses differ from papillomaviruses, another member

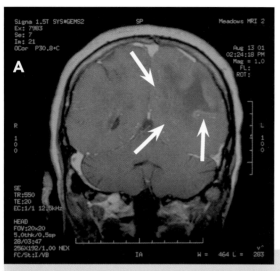
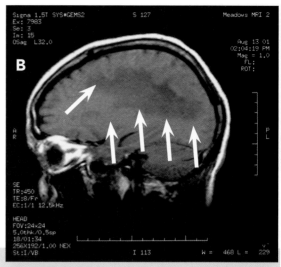
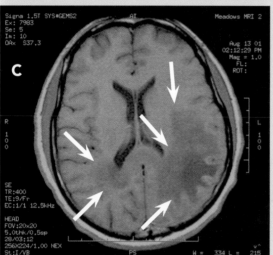
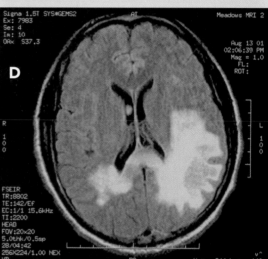

Image 1_Several magnetic resonance imaging (MRI) views of this patient's extensive lesion found in the left frontoparietal lobe. Views **A** thru **C** illustrate the large low signal intensity mass (shown by **T1**-weighted MRI) within the left parietal lobe that extends anterior to the corpus callosum and involves the white matter (outlined by arrows). The extent of the mass shown in View **C** is emphasized by a **T2**-weighted MRI of the same area (View **D**). No contrast enhancement after gadodiamide injection was noted (not shown).

of the Papovaridae family, in both virion and genome size and in the organization of the genome. Polyomaviruses are generally smaller than papillomaviruses. The JC virus shares significant (approximately 70% to 75% of the genome) nucleotide sequence homology with 2 other polyomaviruses, human BK virus (BKV) and simian virus 40 (SV40) found in monkeys. In addition, the genome of JCV consists of approximately 5,000 nucleotide base pairs organized into early, late, and noncoding regions. The early region codes for small and large T-antigens and is important in viral transformation, replication, and regulation of gene expression. The late region codes for 3 viral capsid proteins (V1, V2, and V3), while the noncoding region contains the replication origin, T-antigen binding sites, and transcription regulatory elements. The serum of 80% to 90% of all adults contain antibodies to JCV which are typically acquired between the ages of 10 and 14 years. There is no evidence for an animal reservoir for JCV. Asymptomatic viruria may occur in 10% to 45% of immunosuppressed patients and in 3%

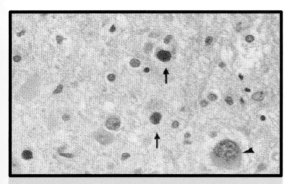

Image 2_Brain tissue biopsy specimen illustrating abnormal oligodendrocytes (arrows) and a bizarre-looking astrocyte (arrowhead) (H&E stain, high power magnification). Courtesy of Neuropathology (ref. 8).

of pregnant women. The diagnostic sensitivity of the JCV PCR test on a CSF sample can be as low as 60%, while diagnostic specificity is nearly 100%. Therefore, a negative JCV PCR test does not rule out the diagnosis of PML while a positive JCV PCR test, when combined with typical clinical and radiographic findings of PML, strongly supports the diagnosis of PML. Typical clinical findings in patients with PML include rapidly progressing focal neurologic deficits (eg, cortical blindness, quadriparesis, profound dementia, and coma) without signs of increased intracranial pressure. In contrast to other demyelinating diseases [eg, multiple sclerosis (MS) and acute disseminated encephalomyopathies], however, the optic nerves and spinal cord of individuals with PML are very rarely affected. Typical radiographic findings on CT include hypodense, rarely enhancing, asymmetric lesions of the cerebral white matter, usually with no mass effect [**Image 1A-C**]. There is increased signal intensity on **T2**-weighted and decreased signal intensity on **T1**-weighted MRI [**Image 1D**]. The MRI is typically more sensitive than CT in detecting a lesion, which is most commonly in the parietal lobe in PML.

3. Plasma CD4 count, repeat CSF analysis and JCV PCR testing, and viral culture. Typically, patients with PML have a CD4 count of <200 cells/mm^3 and those with a count >300 cells/mm^3 have a greater likelihood of prolonged survival. Because a negative JCV PCR test on an initial CSF specimen does not rule out JCV infection, it is useful to repeat the CSF analysis and JCV PCR test at a later time point, especially in patients

for which the index of suspicion for PML remains high. In patients with PML, the CSF cell count is typically <20 cells/mm^3 and the total protein concentration may be slightly elevated. Viral culture of JCV is possible; however, it is hampered by the slow growth of this virus and the lack of susceptible cells, such as primary human fetal glial cells.

4. **Most likely diagnosis:** *progressive multifocal leukoencephalopathy.*

The clinical, laboratory, and radiographic findings related to the patient described in this case study are consistent with a diagnosis of PML. Patients with PML typically present with various neurologic manifestations, some of which are more common than others [**T3**]. Hemiparesis, cognitive disturbance, and visual field deficits occur in approximately one-third or more of patients with PML and all 3 were present in the patient presented in this case study. Moreover, PML can be the presenting manifestation of AIDS and greater than 50% of the deaths due to PML occur in HIV-positive individuals. The patient presented in this case study had been previously diagnosed with AIDS. Prior to the HIV era, PML occurred primarily in older patients with a hematologic malignancy, most commonly chronic lymphocytic leukemia (CLL) or Hodgkin's disease, or in patients with conditions associated with depressed T cell-mediated immunity [eg, organ transplantation or systemic lupus erythematosus (SLE)]. In the HIV era, up to 5% of all HIV-positive individuals will develop PML. The pathogenesis of PML initially requires sustained close contact with a JCV-infected individual. Primary infection, usually occurring at a young age, is often characterized by the absence of any symptoms or only mild symptoms of an upper respiratory infection (URI), affecting mainly the tonsillar tissue. Following primary infection, the virus enters a latent period during which the virus is harbored by cells of the kidney and mononuclear cells in the bone marrow and, possibly, the CNS. Viral reactivation occurs during a period of immunosuppression. A hematogenous route, involving mononuclear B cells, has been proposed as the mechanism for transport of JCV to the CNS. Subsequently, direct JCV infection of oligodendrocytes in the CNS causes these cells to lyse, leading to decreased myelin production and demyelination.

5. Additional, non-laboratory tests on patients with PML would include contrast enhancement imaging studies and tests of neurological function because radiographic evidence of improvement (ie, decrease in size of lesion) and recovery of neurological function are positive predictive factors for prolonged survival. In addition, cytology, histology of a brain biopsy specimen, electron microscopy (EM), fluorescence in situ hybridization (FISH), and immunostaining are other procedures that have been used in the diagnosis of PML. Urine cytology might demonstrate the presence of oligodendrocytes with an enlarged nucleus and a single, large, basophilic intranuclear inclusion. However, urine cytology cannot distinguish between patients with asymptomatic viruria and those with PML or between those with JCV and those with BKV infection. Gross and microscopic histological analysis of a brain biopsy specimen would provide a definitive diagnosis of PML. Gross examination of brain tissue from individuals with PML would typically demonstrate multifocal lesions in the subcortical white matter, located most commonly near the gray-white matter junction. Microscopic examination of stained tissue typically demonstrates multiple, asymmetric foci at various stages of demyelination within the cerebral white matter with axonal sparing. Multiple lipid-laden macrophages, abnormal oligodendrocytes characterized by nuclear enlargement, loss of normal chromatin pattern, and intranuclear accumulation of a deeply basophilic homogenous material (ie, an inclusion body) may also be seen. In addition, there may be bizarre looking astrocytes characterized by marked enlargement, intensely hyperchromatic and irregularly shaped nuclei, and minimal evidence of cerebral inflammation (ie, mature lymphocytes) [**Image 2**]. Electron microscopy might demonstrate the presence of polyomavirus particles in the nuclei of oligodendrocytes and, sometimes, in reactive astrocytes. Immunostaining and FISH might demonstrate the presence of JCV-specific gene sequences or proteins in tissue specimens.

6. There is no accepted treatment for PML. The majority of JCV infections are asymptomatic and therefore do not require treatment. Treatment of

individuals with PML with cytosine arabinoside (Ara-C), potent combinations of antiretroviral drugs (ie, HAART), Interferon-alpha (IFN-a), cidofovir, or topotecan have resulted in either no clinical benefit or mixed success.[6,7] A few patients (<10%) with PML will have spontaneous fluctuations in their clinical course and live for 2 to 3 years after diagnosis; however, most deteriorate rapidly and usually die within 6 months of diagnosis.

Patient's Course

The patient discussed in this case study had 3 generalized tonic clonic seizures followed by rapid deterioration. An emergency CT scan revealed increased cerebral edema, a 1 cm midline shift, and an enlarged ventricle consistent with hydrocephalus. The patient died shortly thereafter, and autopsy findings confirmed the diagnosis of PML.

References

1. Burns DK, Risser RC, White CL. The neuropathology of human immunodeficiency virus infection. The Dallas, TX, experience. *Arch Pathol Lab Med.* 1991;115:1112-1124.

2. Berger JR, Major EO. Progressive multifocal leukoencephalopathy. *Semin Neurol.* 1999;19:193-200.

3. Antinori A, Ammassari A, Giancola ML, et al. Epidemiology and prognosis of AIDS-associated progressive multifocal leukoencephalopathy in the HAART era. *J Neurovirol.* 2001;7:323-328.

4. Astrom KE. Progressive multifocal leukoencephalopathy. Demyelinating viral disease - common complication of AIDS. *Lakartidningen.* 2001;98:4206-4211.

5. Khalili K. Human neurotropic JC virus and its association with brain tumors. *Dis Markers.* 2001;17:143-147.

6. Geschwind MD, Skolasky RI, Royal WS, et al. The relative contributions of HAART and alpha-interferon for therapy of progressive multifocal leukoencephalopathy in AIDS. *J Neurovirol.* 2001;7:353-357.

7. De Luca A, Giancola ML, Ammassari A, et al. Potent anti-retroviral therapy with or without cidofovir for AIDS-associated progressive multifocal leukoencephalopathy: extended follow-up of an observational study. *J Neurovirol.* 2001;7:364-368.

8. Ellison D, Love S, Chimelli L, et al. *Neuropathology.* Barcelona, Spain: Mosby International; 1998;13-15.

An 18-Year-Old Male With Shortness of Breath and Cough

Alexandra Harrington, Richard Komorowski, Steven H. Kroft

Department of Pathology, Medical College of Wisconsin, Milwaukee, WI

Patient: 18-year-old male.

Chief Complaint: Shortness of breath (SoB), cough, fever, and vomiting.

History of Present Illness: The patient presented to the emergency room with complaints of progressive SoB, fever, cough, and vomiting. One day prior to admission, the patient was seen at a clinic for similar complaints. A chest X-ray revealed bilateral infiltrates and the patient was started on oral antibiotics. The patient's symptoms progressively worsened overnight.

Past Medical and Surgical History: None.

Family History: The patient's cousin was recently diagnosed with pneumonia.

Social History: The patient had moved within the last 2 weeks to the Midwest from Arizona to begin military basic training.

Physical Examination: Vital signs: temperature, 100.4°F; pulse, 109 beats per minute; respiratory rate, 26 breaths per minute; blood pressure 111/74 mm Hg; O2 saturation, 99% on non-rebreather mask. The patient was mildly ill-appearing, alert and oriented, flushed, and diaphoretic. Lung exam revealed bilateral coarse breath sounds and scattered rales.

Results of Additional Diagnostic Procedures and Tests: An admission chest X-ray revealed diffuse bilateral fluffy infiltrates, consistent with adult respiratory distress syndrome (ARDS). A pulmonary bronchoscopy was performed shortly after admission, which revealed erythematous bronchi with purulent secretions. Repeat chest X-rays were consistent with progressively worsening ARDS. The patient expired within 12 hours of admission. Post-mortem examination revealed bilateral acute interstitial pneumonitis with focal diffuse alveolar damage, significant pulmonary edema, large bilateral pleural effusions, and reactive hyperplasia of the spleen, and mediastinal lymph nodes.

T1. Principal Laboratory Findings

Test		Patient's Reference	Result Interval
Hematology			
WBC count		14.9	4.5-13.0 × 10³/μL
RBC count		6.2	4.4-5.8 × 10⁶/μL
Hemoglobin		19.1	13.0-17.0 g/dL
Hematocrit		52	40-50%
Platelet count		46	150-350 × 10³/μL
Differential:	Neutrophils	40	
	Bands	35	
	Metamyelocytes	8	
	Lymphocytes	9	
PBS findings	**(Image 1)**		
Coagulation			
PT		17.5	9.3-12.5 sec
PTT		49.0	24.6-37.4 sec
D-dimer		5.7	0.5-2.1 mg/L
Fibrinogen		232	180-350 mg/dL
Arterial Blood Gases			
pH		7.32	7.35-7.45
pO₂		57	80-104 mmHg
pCO₂		33	35-45 mmHg
O₂ saturation		90.3	95.0-98.0%
Microbiology			
BAL fluid:	*Mycoplasma* culture	Negative	Negative
	Fungus culture	Negative	Negative
	Virus culture	Negative	Negative
	Legionella culture	Negative	Negative
	RSV by RT-PCR	Negative	Negative
	Pneumocystis by DFA	Negative	Negative
Blood culture		Negative	Negative
Sputum culture		Negative	Negative
Urine Legionella antigen	Negative	Negative	
Fungal antibody panel	Negative	Negative	
Hantavirus serology	Negative	Negative	

WBC, white blood cell; RBC, red blood cell; PBS, peripheral blood smear; PT, prothrombin time; PTT, partial thromboplastin time; BAL, bronchoalveolar lavage; RSV, respiratory syncytial virus; RT-PCR, reverse transcriptase polymerase chain reaction; DFA, direct fluorescent antigen.

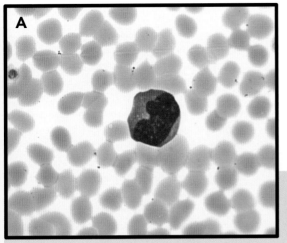

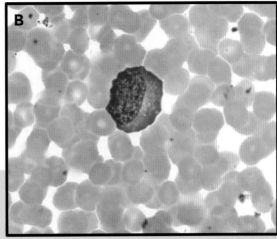

Image 1_Patient's peripheral blood smear findings, illustrating a circulating **A**) immunoblast and **B**) a reactive lymphocyte with more prominent plasmacytic differentiation.

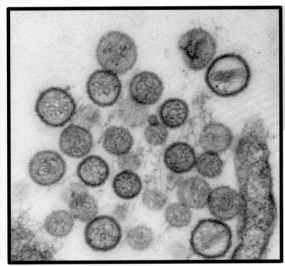

Image 2_An electron micrograph of the sin nombre virus. Courtesy of the Centers for Disease Control and Prevention.

Questions

1. What are the patient's most striking clinical and laboratory findings?

2. How do you explain this patient's most striking clinical and laboratory findings?

3. What is this patient's most likely diagnosis?

4. What additional tests are available to confirm this diagnosis?

5. What is the significance of the "tetrad of hematologic findings"?

6. What is the prognosis and treatment for individuals with this patient's disease?

Possible Answers

1. Fever, tachycardia, tachypnea, diaphoresis, bilateral coarse breath sounds, progressively worsening SoB and cough symptoms, abnormal chest X-rays consistent with a rapidly developing ARDS; leukocytosis with neutrophilia and a left shift, circulating immunoblasts, hemoconcentration, severe thrombocytopenia, prolonged clotting times with a normal fibrinogen, metabolic acidosis with low oxygen saturation, and negative microbiology studies, including cultures and molecular studies (**T1**).

2. The patient's clinical and laboratory findings suggest infection as a cause for his rapidly declining respiratory status. Initially, the differential diagnosis for the causative agent was broad, including bacteria, viruses, fungi, and atypical organisms, such as Pneumocystis and Mycoplasma. Given the patient's recent move from Arizona, a Hantavirus infection was strongly considered. An adenovirus pneumonia was also considered, as adenovirus has been implicated in outbreaks among military recruits. Examination of the patient's hematology results, including a peripheral blood smear review, provided valuable information for narrowing the initially broad differential diagnosis. Our patient's severe thrombocytopenia is one of the most strikingly abnormal hematologic findings. Thrombocytopenia has been associated with many infectious agents, including rickettsiae, parvovirus, Epstein-Barr virus, Cytomegalovirus, human immunodeficiency virus (HIV), Hantavirus, Mycoplasma, Yersinia, and Francisella tularensis.[1,2] In addition to the severe thrombocytopenia, our patient had an elevated hemoglobin and hematocrit, a leukocytosis with neutrophilia, and circulating immunoblasts. These collective findings have been termed "a hematologic tetrad," which in the appropriate clinical setting, is suggestive of Hantavirus cardiopulmonary syndrome (HCPS).[2] Elevated clotting times and metabolic acidosis have also been reported in patients with HCPS.[3] Additional patient history was obtained in this case and revealed that the patient's cousin was diagnosed with Hantavirus infection.

3. **Most likely diagnosis:** Hantavirus cardiopulmonary syndrome.

4. The causative agents of HCPS are members of the genus, Hantavirus and family, Bunyaviridae. The first recognized outbreak of hantavirus infection in the United States occurred in May 1993. The Centers for Disease Control and the health departments of New Mexico, Arizona, Colorado, and Utah began investigating case reports of acute respiratory illness associated with mortality. A previously unrecognized Hantavirus, later named sin nombre virus (SNV), was identified as the causative agent by serology and autopsy studies (**Image 2**).[4] Although SNV is the most common cause of HCPS in the United States, other Hantaviruses have also been implicated. As of July 2005, 396 cases of HCPS in the United States have been confirmed.[5] Hantavirus cardiopulmonary syndrome is clinically characterized by fever, myalgias, non-productive cough, shortness of breath, gastrointestinal symptoms, headache, tachycardia, tachypnea, hypotension, and respiratory compromise secondary to noncardiogenic pulmonary edema.[3]

5. Several laboratory tests are available for the diagnosis of HCPS, including serology, immunohistochemistry (IHC), and molecular techniques. Serologic assays either target a nucleocapsid protein common to all Hantaviruses or target a specific nucleocapsid protein of the SNV. Demonstration of IgM antibodies or a 4-fold or greater rise in IgG antibody titers confirms the

diagnosis.[6] It has been demonstrated that IgM antibodies are present in nearly all patients in the prodromal phase of a Hantavirus infection.[7] The cause of the negative Hantavirus serology in our patient is unclear. Immunohistochemistry can be performed on tissue sections, with lung, kidney, and spleen being the preferred specimens. Positive IHC staining of the Hantavirus antigens within tissue endothelial cells is diagnostic of Hantavirus infection. In the present case, Hantavirus IHC performed on autopsy tissue was positive. Finally, polymerase chain reaction (PCR) assays are available to detect hantavirus gene sequences, and these assays can be performed on blood or tissue specimens. However, such molecular techniques are not widely available. Because Hantavirus does not cause viral cytopathic effect, viral cultures are not routinely performed for diagnosis.

6. The "tetrad of hematologic findings" seen often in patients with HCPS includes (1) thrombo-cytopenia, (2) leukocytosis with neutrophilia and a left shift, (3) hemoconcentration, and (4) circulating immunoblasts and plasma cells.[8] Thrombocytopenia. Early in Hantavirus infection, during the prodrome phase, thrombocytopenia is usually the sole hematologic abnormality.[2] As with most cases of infection-associated thrombocytopenia, the low platelet count is likely secondary to decreased platelet production.[1] Leukocytosis with neutrophilia. The feature of leukocytosis with neutrophilia is interesting in this infection, as most viral infections elicit a reactive lymphocytosis. In contrast to the neutrophilia seen in bacterial infections, neutrophils in HCPS do not show severe toxic granulation.[2] Hemoconcentration. Hemoconcentration, defined as an elevated hematocrit, is a feature seen in patients with severe HCPS and may not be seen in patients with milder presentations.[2] This hematologic feature illustrates the mechanism of the pathogenesis of Hantavirus infections—capillary leak. It is believed that as a result of the viral tropism for endothelial cells and the response of the immune system to the infection, a significant amount of plasma leaks out of the vascular spaces. This concentrates the red blood cells within the vessels. Hemoconcentration, as an indicator of capillary leak, correlates well with the common clinical manifestations of capillary leak, including large pleural effusions and pulmonary edema.[9] Immunoblastosis. The presence of small numbers of immunoblasts, described as medium to large lymphocytes with moderate amounts of deeply basophilic cytoplasm and nuclei with uniform chromatin and variably prominent nucleoli, can be seen in many transient reactive processes.[2] In HCPS, the immunoblasts and plasma cells account for >10% of lymphoid cells. The significant number of circulating immunoblasts seen in HCPS correlates well with the increased number of immunoblasts seen within lung, lymph nodes, liver, and the spleen.[9] These immunoblasts are thought to play a role in the capillary leak syndrome.

7. Hantavirus cardiopulmonary syndrome has a high mortality, ranging from 50% to 75%.[10] Death results from cardiogenic shock and heart failure. Treatment is largely supportive and often includes intensive care unit (ICU) monitoring, mechanical ventilation, and intravenous fluid therapy. Patients who survive the infection are usually without sequela.

Keywords

adult respiratory distress syndrome, Hantavirus cardiopulmonary syndrome, tetrad of hematologic findings

References

1. Beutler E, Coller BS, Lichtman MA, et al (eds). *William's Hematology*. New York: McGraw-Hill; 2005.

2. Koster F, Foucar K, Hjelle B, et al. Rapid presumptive diagnosis of hantavirus cardiopulmonary syndrome by peripheral blood review. *Amer J Clin Path*. 2001;116:665-672.

3. Duchin JS, Koster FT, Peters CJ, et al. Hantavirus pulmonary syndrome: A clinical description of 17 patients with a newly recognized disease. *New Engl J Med*. 1994;330:949-955.

4. CDC. Outbreak of acute illness – Southwestern United States, 1993. *Morbidity and Mortality Weekly Report*. 1993;42:421-424.

5. CDC Web site. http://www.cdc.gov/ncidod/diseases/hanta/hps/index.htm. Accessed on April 10, 2006.

6. CDC: Progress in the development of Hantavirus diagnostic assays – United States. *Morbidity and Mortality Weekly Report*. 1993;42:770-771.

7. Bharadwaj M, Nofchissey R, Goade D, et al. Humoral immune responses in the hantavirus cardiopulmonary syndrome. *J Infect Dis.* 2000;182:43-48.

8. Nolte KB, Feddersen RM, Foucar K, et al. Hantavirus pulmonary syndrome in the United States: A pathological description of a disease caused by a new agent. *Hum Path.* 1995;26:110-120.

9. Colby TV, Zaki SR, Feddersen RM, et al. Hantavirus pulmonary syndrome is distinguishable from acute interstitial pneumonia. *Arch Path Lab Med.* 2000;124:1463-1466.

10. Khan AS, Ksiazek TG, Peters CJ. Hantavirus pulmonary syndrome. *Lancet.* 1996;347:739-741.

Travel-Related Fever Due to an Emerging Infection

Lisa M Sutton,[1] Rita Gander,[1] Paula Revell,[2] and Paul Southern[1]

Department of Pathology, [1]University of Texas Southwestern Medical Center and [2]Children's Medical Center, Dallas, TX

Patient: 8-year-old male.

Past Medical History: None.

Immunizations: Up to date.

Chief Complaint: Fever for 2 weeks and migrating arthralgias.

History of Present Illness: The patient presented with daily cyclic fevers that started after returning from a 2.5-month trip to Dhaka, Bangladesh, to visit family. While in Bangladesh, he developed shoulder pain which migrated to multiple other joints. He complained currently of bilateral thigh pain. He also mentioned that he had had mild nausea, vomiting, decreased appetite, and cough for several weeks.

Family/Social History: Noncontributory.

Medications: Ibuprofen for arthralgias and fever.

Physical Examination: The patient appeared febrile, but was in no acute distress. His temperature was 40.5°C, and he was mildly tachycardic, with a heart rate of 109 bpm. The remainder of his vital signs were within normal limits. Head, ears, eyes, nose, and throat were all unremarkable, with no scleral icterus or lymphadenopathy noted. The cardiovascular system was normal, and his lungs were clear to auscultation. His abdomen was tender to palpation with no organomegaly noted. No skin rash was present. His extremities were tender to palpation, with no obvious joint deformities. His neurologic examination was unremarkable.

Questions

1. What are this patient's most striking clinical and laboratory findings?

2. What should be considered when evaluating a patient with travel-related fever?

3. How do you explain this patient's most striking clinical and laboratory findings?

4. What additional laboratory tests should be ordered and why?

5. What is the patient's most likely diagnosis?

6. Omitting dengue fever, what is the epidemiology, clinical presentation, and pathogenesis of the other condition that may have caused this patient's travel-related illness?

7. What is an appropriate treatment and outcome for this patient?

8. Why should the United States be concerned about this relatively new pathogen?

Possible Answers

1. Fever, migrating arthralgias, normal white blood cell count with mild thrombocytopenia, mildly-elevated liver function tests, and elevated

T1. Principal Laboratory Findings

Test	Patient's Result	"Normal" Reference Range
Chemistry		
Sodium	135	134–146 mEq/L
Potassium	3.6	3.5–5.0 mEq/L
Chloride	100	98–106 mEq/L
Bicarbonate	23	18–31 mEq/L
Total bilirubin	0.4	0.1–1.3 mg/dL
Conjugated bilirubin	0.1	0.0–0.3 mg/dL
BUN	7	5–18 mg/dL
Creatinine	0.5	0.3–0.7 mg/dL
CK	41	21–232 U/L
GGT	78	3–30 U/L
ALT	123	10–50 U/L
AST	103	10–55 U/L
Alkaline phosphatase	265	175–420 U/L
ESR	70	0–15 mm/h
C-Reactive protein	9.2	0.0–1.0 mg/dL
Hematology		
WBC	5.6	$4.5–13.5 \times 10^3/mm^3$
RBC	4.41	$4.50–5.30 \times 10^6/mm^3$
Hemoglobin	11.3	11.5–14.9 g/dL
Hematocrit	32.4	35.0–45.0 %
MCV	73.5	75.0–90.0 fL
MCH	25.6	26.0–34.0 picogram
MCHC	34.9	32.0–36.0 g/dL
RDW	12.6	11.5–15.0%
Platelet	109	$150–475 \times 10^3/mm^3$
Reticulocyte count	2.0	0.5–1.5%
Differential:		
Neutrophils	41	31–61%
Bands	11	0–11%
Basophils	1	0–2%
Monocytes	6	0–10%
Lymphocytes	41	28–48%
Coagulation		
PT	14.9	12.0–15.3 sec
PTT	28.8	26.4–35.2 sec
INR	1.1	

BUN, blood urea nitrogen; CK, creatinine kinase; GGT, gammaglutamyl transferase; ALT, alanine aminotransferase; AST, aspartate aminotransferase; ESR, erythrocyte sedimentation rate; WBC, white blood cell; RBC, red blood cell; MCV, mean corpuscular volume; MCH, mean corpuscular hemoglobin; MCHC, mean corpuscular hemoglobin concentration; RDW, red blood cell distribution width; PT, prothrombin time; PTT, partial thromboplastin time; INR, international normalized ratio.

T2. Microbiology and Virology Findings

Test	Patient's Result	"Normal" Reference Range
Blood cultures	No growth × 5	No growth
Malaria preparations	Negative × 4	Negative
Brucella		
IgM	0.30 IV	<0.89 IV
IgG	0.02 IV	<0.89 IV
Viral DFA (nasal swab):		
Influenza	Negative	Negative
Parainfluenza	Negative	Negative
RSV	Negative	Negative
Adenovirus	Negative	Negative
Viral culture (nasal swab)	*No virus isolated*	*No virus isolated*
Dengue:		
IgM	0.41 IV	<0.89 IV
IgG	6.93 IV	<0.89 IV
Salmonella:		
O Paratyphoid A	1:40	<1:20
O Paratyphoid B	>1:160	<1:20
O Typhoid Group D	>1:160	<1:20
H Paratyphoid a	1:40	<1:20
H Paratyphoid b	<1:20	<1:20
H Typhoid Group D	>1:160	<1:20

IgM, immunoglobulin M; IgG, immunoglobulin G; IV, index value; DFA, direct fluorescent antibody; RSV, respiratory syncytial virus.

erythrocyte sedimentation rate (ESR) and C-reactive protein level (**T1**).

2. The travel history of the patient. Febrile illness is 1 of the most commonly encountered travel-related illnesses. It affects as many as 10% of travelers to developing countries, either during their travel or after returning home.[1] In addition, the majority of post-travel hospital admissions are due to a febrile illness. It is a frequent diagnostic dilemma faced by physicians, and the diagnosis can be difficult since many causes of travel-related febrile illness are seldom seen in the United States.

A recent study by Freedman and colleagues evaluated data from over 17,000 returning travelers who presented at infectious disease clinics worldwide.[2] The authors analyzed the 6 regions of travel most commonly resulting in post-travel illness of any type. Sub-Saharan Africa had the highest number of ill travelers, followed by Southeast Asia and South-Central Asia. Lower numbers of cases were identified in South America, Central America, and the Caribbean. Moreover, the type of disease presentation differed based on where the patient traveled. Systemic febrile illnesses were most often seen after travel to sub-Saharan Africa or Southeast Asia. Acute diarrhea was most common from South-Central Asia, and dermatologic problems were commonly seen after travel to the Caribbean, Central America, or South America. When a patient presents after traveling to any of these regions, it is important to consider diseases found in that region as part of the differential diagnosis.

Whether or not a patient has received immunizations or prophylactic medications before traveling to developing countries should also be considered when evaluating a patient for travel-related fever. When patients travel to visit family, they are less likely to receive prophylactic treatment for a variety of reasons.[3] The patient in this case was visiting family, and he had received all routine vaccines. However, he had not received the typhoid vaccine or malaria prophylaxis recommended for travel to South Asia and was at risk for these infections.[4]

3. The patient presented with a travel-related febrile illness and migrating arthralgias. At presentation, the patient had no obvious cause for his fever, and his initial abnormal laboratory findings were all nonspecific. There are many different etiologies of travel-related fever. Malaria is the most common specific diagnosis observed. Other causes include dengue fever, enteric fever due to *Salmonella* serotype Typhi or *Salmonella* serotype Paratyphi, rickettsial infections, acute schistosomiasis, invasive amebiasis, and mononucleosis.[1] It is also important not to forget cosmopolitan infections. These include common infections seen worldwide, such as respiratory tract infections, bacterial enteritis, skin or soft

tissue infections, genitourinary infections, and tuberculosis.

Freedman's study identified 5 different infections as the most common specific etiologies of travel-related febrile illness: malaria, dengue fever, typhoid fever, Epstein-Barr viral infection, and rickettsial infection.[2] Malaria was the most frequently-identified cause of travel-related illness, and it was predominantly seen in travelers from sub-Saharan Africa; however, positive cases were seen in all of the regions investigated. Dengue fever was seen primarily in Southeast Asia and the Caribbean, but it was also seen in all of the regions investigated. Typhoid fever was primarily seen in South-Central Asia, with a low number of cases observed in the other regions investigated. Epstein-Barr viral infections were seen in low numbers in all regions investigated, while rickettsial infections were identified in low numbers in sub-Saharan Africa and Asia only.

The patient in this case visited Bangladesh, part of South-Central Asia, so one should focus on travel-related diseases (eg, typhoid fever) that are common in this region. Ruling out cosmopolitan infections is the first priority. A malarial infection is also particularly concerning because the patient did not receive malaria prophylaxis. Typhoid fever and dengue fever should be high on the differential list of diagnoses since both are highly prevalent in the region visited by the patient. There have also been recent outbreaks of chikungunya throughout South Asia, but no confirmed cases have been documented in Dhaka, Bangladesh[5]; however, the rapidly increasing number of chikungunya cases in countries neighboring Bangladesh, particularly India, should raise one's suspicion for this disease.

4. Blood cultures should be ordered to help rule out many of the cosmopolitan causes of travel-related fever. This is also an excellent means for diagnosing typhoid fever. Peripheral thick and thin blood smears should be prepared to look for *Plasmodium* species. The patient had a normal urinalysis with no urinary symptoms, so urine cultures were not obtained. Serologic tests can be ordered for dengue fever and chikungunya; however, this may not be the first step in an investigation, as one searches for more-common causes of a patient's travel-related fever. Our

patient's additional laboratory test results are shown in **T2**.

5. **Most likely diagnosis:** *dengue or chikungunya viral infection.* The patient's laboratory workup did not provide any clear-cut answers. All blood cultures were negative. Malaria smears were prepared when the patient spiked a fever and were negative as well. The *Salmonella* antibody study, or Widal test, can be somewhat confusing to interpret as it was positive for both paratyphoid and typhoid antigens. This study is highly nonspecific and is not the most useful method for diagnosing *Salmonella* infections.[6,7] High titers can be due to other *Salmonella* species, and a high prevalence of antibodies have been found among healthy individuals in areas of endemicity.[7] Typically, typhoid fever is diagnosed based on isolation of organisms from blood, urine, or stool. Bone marrow culture is the gold standard but is rarely performed. In our patient, the absence of a positive culture for *Salmonella* means that the serology results can only be interpreted as inconclusive.

Dengue serology was only positive for IgG antibodies. Primary infections typically have an increase in IgM antibodies within 4 to 5 days of fever onset and remain detectable for 3 to 6 months, while IgG antibodies can remain detectable for life.[8] Lack of positive IgM antibodies most likely indicates that the patient has been previously infected and does not have a current infection. However, it could also be due to the patient's delayed presentation or a secondary infection. A secondary infection by a different dengue virus serotype can occur with low-to-absent IgM antibody levels.[8] To confirm a secondary infection, one must document a rapid rise in IgG antibodies. Because a second serology test was not performed on our patient, the presence of a secondary infection could not be determined.

The patient continued to spike fevers for several days, but the diagnostic workup performed was not successful in identifying a source of infection. The patient's symptoms of fever and arthralgias, however, are consistent with dengue fever. Considering that dengue virus is endemic to Bangladesh, this is the most likely diagnosis;

however, without confirming serology, it is reasonable to consider other causes as well.

Chikungunya fever was on the differential of infections that may have caused the patient's illness, especially since infected patients have similar symptoms to those with dengue fever. In recent years, an increasing number of chikungunya fever cases have been seen in South Asia. With the number of these cases reaching over 1 million in the past year, it is logical to explore this possible diagnosis further.

6. Chikungunya viral disease has become a significant problem recently in South Asia and Africa. Numerous travel-related cases have been seen throughout Europe as well. While it is rarely fatal, it can produce long-term crippling effects. The chikungunya virus is a positive-stranded, enveloped RNA virus of the family *Togaviridae* and the genus *Alphavirus*.[9] The primary transmission vector for this virus is the mosquito, including both *Aedes aegypti* and *Aedes albopicus* species. Outbreaks tend to occur during the rainy season when the number of mosquitoes is the highest. The typical transmission cycle is from man to mosquito and back to man. Monkeys and other wild animals have been shown to serve as a reservoir as well. On average, chikungunya fever has an incubation period of 2 to 12 days.[10] Acute symptoms are nonspecific, including fever, headache, fatigue, lymphadenopathy, nausea, vomiting, muscle pain, rash, and migratory joint pain.[9,10] Initial laboratory abnormalities can include leukopenia, thrombocytopenia, and elevated liver and muscle enzymes.[9,11] The acute illness usually lasts 1 to 7 days. A typical rash includes papules and macules on the trunk and limbs with diffuse redness, often accompanied by pruritis.[11] Joint involvement is usually symmetrical and involves multiple joints. Joints typically affected are the small joints of the hands, wrists, ankles, and feet with symptoms including periarticular swelling, pain, redness, and limitation of movement.[9] Large joints are involved less frequently. The hallmark of the disease is the chronic arthralgias that can last for months to years after the initial infection. As many as 5% to 10% of patients experience chronic joint pain, stiffness, and swelling.[9] Younger patients tend to experience a less-severe course.

Chikungunya fever was first observed in Tanzania in 1952, which is where the name was originally coined.[11] The name is derived from the Makonde language, meaning "that which bends up" in reference to the chronic arthralgias. Throughout the 1950s, chikungunya fever epidemics were noted throughout East Africa and Asia. In the 1970s, cases were noted in South Africa; however, from the 1980s to 1999 there was very limited activity observed. In 1999, one of the first reemergences was noted in the Democratic Republic of the Congo, with approximately 50,000 people infected. Throughout the early 21st century, cases were noted in Indonesia and Kenya. In 2005 and 2006, one of the largest outbreaks occurred in the Indian Ocean islands and India. In particular, Reunion Island had more than a 35% incidence with more than 200,000 people infected.[11] The current estimate for the past year is more than 1 million suspected cases.

Diagnosing chikungunya in the United States can be somewhat difficult. Throughout Europe, there are many places that are offering serologic and reverse-transcriptase polymerase chain reaction (RT-PCR) tests. However, in the United States, the Centers for Disease Control and Prevention (CDC) is the only location currently performing diagnostic tests for chikungunya virus infection, and the testing can only be approved through one's state department of health. The CDC is currently offering serologic testing on paired acute and convalescent serum specimens, ideally separated by 2 weeks.[12] If the serology is positive, the results are confirmed using a plaque-reduction neutralization assay. Finally, viral load can be determined by performing RT-PCR testing of patients' serum specimens.

7. Treatment for chikungunya fever is nonspecific. Rest and adequate fluid intake is recommended. Analgesics and anti-inflammatory drugs can be used to help with the fever and arthralgias that accompany this infection.[10] Our patient's fever resolved after 5 days, his arthralgias improved, and he was discharged home. He never received any antibiotics during his hospital stay. Because the patient improved without treatment, the decision was made not to send specimens for chikungunya serology. Therefore, we are not certain that our patient had chikungunya fever.

Nevertheless, if our patient did have acute-phase symptoms of chikungunya fever, the complete resolution of his symptoms combined with his young age gave him an excellent prognosis.[9]

8. Chikungunya viral infections continue to spread to new countries. Recent expansion of this infection to Europe has been documented with local mosquito transmission confirmed in Italy.[13] In 2006, the CDC reported 35 cases of chikungunya in the United States based on positive serology tests.[14] All cases were from patients who had traveled to endemic areas. RT-PCR assays were performed, and 8 serum specimens showed positive results with titers ranging from $10^{3.9}$ plaque-forming units (PFU)/mL to $10^{6.8}$ PFU/mL. All 8 patients had been ill for less than 1 week. The high viremia level seen in the acute phase is particularly concerning because studies have shown that titers of approximately 10^4 PFU/mL in monkeys have resulted in productive mosquito infections.[14] *Aedes albopictus* mosquitoes have been present in the United States since the 1980s, and both *A. aegypti* and *A. albopictus* mosquitoes are well established in several southeastern coastal states.[13,15] It is a real possibility that the infection could be passed on to local mosquitoes.[16] There needs to be greater awareness of this travel-related infection in the United States, as there are likely to be more cases in the future.

Keywords

Chikungunya, migrating arthralgias, viremia, reverse-transcriptase polymerase chain reaction, plaque-forming units

References

1. Bottieau E, Clerinx J, Schrooten W, et al. Etiology and outcome of fever after a stay in the Tropics. *Arch Intern Med.* 2006;166:1642–1648.

2. Freedman DO, Weld LH, Kozarsky PE, et al. Spectrum of disease and relation to place of exposure among ill returned travelers. *N Engl J Med.* 2006;354: 119–130.

3. Wilson ME, Freedman DO. Etiology of travel-related fever. *Curr Opin Infect Dis.* 2007;20:449–453.

4. Arguin PM, Kozarsky PE, Reed C, eds. *CDC Health Information for International Travel 2008.* New York, NY; Elseiver: 2007.

5. No evidence of chikungunya virus in Dhaka, Bangladesh. Health Science Bulletin, ICDDR,B. 2007;5:1–4.

6. Olopoenia LA, King AL. Widal agglutination test 100 years later: Still plagued by controversy. *Postgrad Med J.* 2000;76:80–84.

7. Detrick B, Hamilton RG, Folds JD, eds. *Manual of Molecular and Clinical Laboratory Immunology.* Washington, DC: ASM Press: 2006.

8. Wilder-Smith A, Schwartz E. Dengue in travelers. *N Engl J Med.* 2005;353:924–932.

9. Senevirante SL. CDC Health Information for International Travel. *J Travel Med.* 2007;14:320–325.

10. Centers for Disease Control and Prevention. (2006, Jan 16) Chikungunya Fever Fact Sheet. http://www.cdc.gov/ncidod/dvbid/Chikungunya/ chikvfact.htm.

11. Simon F, Parola P, Grandadam M. Chikungunya infection: An emerging rheumatism among travelers returned from Indian Ocean Islands. Report of 47 cases. *Medicine.* 2007;86:123–137.

12. Centers for Disease Control and Prevention. Update: Chikungunya fever diagnosed among international travelers—United States, 2006. *MMWR.* 2007;56:276–277.

13. Centers for Disease Control and Prevention. *In the News: Chikungunya fever in Italy.* Travel Notice. Sept 11, 2007.

14. Lanciotti RS, et al. Chikungunya virus in U.S. travelers returning from India, 2006. *Emerg Infect Dis.* 2007;13:764–766.

15. Charrel RN, de Lamballerie X, Raoult D. Chikungunya outbreaks—The globalization of vectorborne diseases. *N Engl J Med.* 2007;356:769–771.

16. Turell MJ, Beaman JR, Tammariello RF. Susceptibility of selected strains of *Aedes aegypti* and *Aedes albopictus* (*Diptera: Culicidae*) to chikungunya virus. *J Med Entomol.* 1992;29:49–53.

Undetectable Plasma Creatinine in a Paralyzed Patient Infected With Human Immunodeficiency Virus

Omer Chaudhry,[1] Mary M. Mayo[2] Arshag D. Mooradian[1]

[1]*Department of Internal Medicine and* [2]*Department of Pathology and Clinical Laboratories, Saint Louis University Hospital, Saint Louis, MO*

Patient: 42-year-old African-American man.

History of Present Illness: The police found him lying naked in a ditch, the victim of an apparent assault. He had multiple signs of trauma, including numerous bruises and abrasions on his face and extremities. He was conscious but was confused and combative.

Physical Examination: The patient's vital signs were: temperature, 96.8°F; pulse, 72 beats/min; respirations, 20 breaths/min; blood pressure, 131/88 mm Hg. His oxygen saturation on room air was 96%. He could follow verbal commands but could not communicate. He showed bilateral injected sclera, left periorbital swelling, and bilateral round and reactive pupils. He had a swollen upper lip and limitation in his ability to open his mouth. There was no evidence of any other abnormalities. He was admitted to the hospital for further evaluation.

Past Medical History: Seven years ago, he was diagnosed with human immunodeficiency virus/acquired immunodeficiency syndrome (HIV/AIDS). In addition, he had been treated for Pneumocystis carinii (PCP) pneumonia 4 months prior to this current hospitalization during which time his HIV viral load was 330,000 copies.

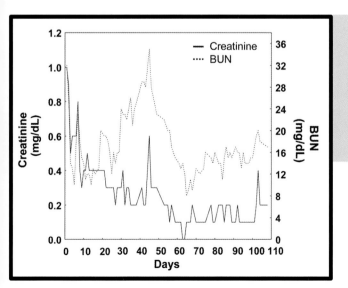

Figure 1_Time course of changes in the patient's plasma creatinine and blood urea nitrogen (BUN) levels during his hospitalization. Creatinine levels were low (<0.2 mg/dL) during hospital days 54 to 100 and undetectable on days 62 and 63.

T1. Principal Laboratory Findings

Analyte	Patient's Result	"Normal" Reference Range
Hematology		
WBC count	9.3	$3.5\text{-}10.5 \times 10^3/\mu L$
RBC count	5.06	$4.30\text{-}5.70 \times 10^6/\mu L$
Hemoglobin	15.4	13.5-17.5 g/dL
Hematocrit	45.3	39.0-50.0%
MCV	89.5	82.0-97.0 fL
MCH	30.4	28.0-34.0 pg
MCHC	34.0	32.0-36.0 g/dL
RDW	14.3	11.2-14.8%
RDW SD	46.4	37-50 fL
Platelet count	272	$150\text{-}400 \times 10^3/\mu L$
MPV	9.0	9.3-12.8 fL
Chemistry		
Sodium	142	135-145 mmol/L
Potassium	3.6	3.5-5.5 mmol/L
Chloride	107	101-111 mmol/L
CO_2	29	20-28 mmol/L
Calcium	9.8	8.7-10.5 mg/dL
Magnesium	2.6	1.58-2.55 mg/dL
Phosphorus	2.7	2.3-5.1 mg/dL
Glucose	161	70-110 mg/dL
BUN	32	5-25 mg/dL
Creatinine	1.0	0.5-1.5 mg/dL
BUN/creatinine	32	7-23
Anion gap	10	11-23
Immunology		
CD3, %	35	64-88%
CD4, %	3	41-57%
CD4 count	20	976-1357/mm³
CD8, %	30	17-45%
CD4/CD8 ratio	0.10	0.70-2.70

WBC, white blood cell; RBC, red blood cell; MCV, mean corpuscular volume; MCH, mean corpuscular hemoglobin; MCHC, mean corpuscular hemoglobin concentration; RDW, red cell distribution width; SD, standard deviation; MPV, mean platelet volume; BUN, blood urea nitrogen; CD, cluster of differentiation.

Questions _____

1. What are this patient's most striking laboratory findings?

2. How do you explain these findings?

3. What is the most common method of measurement of serum/plasma creatinine concentration?

4. What are common interferents in this method?

5. How would you determine whether or not a patient's serum/plasma contains an interfering substance(s) in the method used most commonly to quantify creatinine concentration?

6. What is the most likely explanation for this patient's extremely low and undetectable creatinine levels?

7. What difficulties are presented to the clinician in assessing this patient's renal function?

8. What other test(s) might have proved helpful in this assessment?

Possible Answers _____

1. Markedly decreased CD4 count, very low CD4/CD8 ratio (**T1**); and, persistently low creatinine values during hospital days 54 to 100, including an undetectable creatinine on days 62 and 63 (**Figure 1**).

2. The markedly decreased CD4 count is consistent with the patient's HIV status, high viral load, and very low CD4/CD8 ratio. The finding of undetectable plasma creatinine levels on days 62 and 63 of hospitalization (**Figure 1**) prompted additional laboratory studies to ascertain whether or not the patient's plasma contained any substance(s) that may have interfered in the assay used to measure the patient's creatinine concentration.

3. The Jaffe reaction (or modification of) is the most commonly used method of measuring serum/plasma and urine creatinine concentration. The Jaffe reaction for creatinine determination is based on the formation of a yellow-orange chromogen when picric acid in alkaline solution is added to serum, plasma, or urine:

   Creatinine + picric acid alkaline creatinine-picric acid complex solution

4. The Jaffe method is affected by numerous interferents that can cause creatinine results by this method to be falsely increased or decreased. Examples of interferents include glucose, protein, bilirubin, hemolysis, and lipemia.[1] Modifications to the original Jaffe method and the advent of kinetic enzymatic methods, with and without rate blanking, have reduced the error in creatinine measurement caused by the presence of various interferents.

5. By testing the patient's serum/plasma suspected of containing a substance(s) that interfered in the creatinine assay based on the Jaffe reaction using a creatinine assay based on a different methodology and by performing mixing studies of the patient's serum/plasma with serum/plasma, containing a high creatinine concentration, obtained from another patient. We mixed the patient's plasma with an equal volume of plasma from a patient with chronic renal failure whose plasma creatinine concentration was 3.3 mg/dL. Subsequently, the mixture was tested by 2 different creatinine methods: 1 based on the Jaffe reaction and another based on a coupled-enzyme methodology. Reagents for both methods were obtained from Roche Diagnostics, Indianapolis, IN, and used according to the manufacturer's instructions. According to the manufacturer's product inserts, the enzymatic method is more specific for creatinine and less subject to analytical interferences, particularly bilirubin, than the method based on the Jaffe reaction. The enzymatic method uses a coupled-enzyme reaction with formation of a quinoneimine chromogen that is measured spectrophotometrically. The creatinine values obtained by both creatinine methods in the sample mixture, after correcting for the dilution and the creatinine contributed by each sample used to prepare this mixture, were in excellent agreement with the expected creatinine value, suggesting that the patient's plasma did not contain an interfering substance(s).

6. The extremely low levels of creatinine in this patient were attributed to severe loss of muscle mass secondary to the additive effects of muscle paralysis and cachexia associated with HIV infection. It is generally accepted that bed rest and paralysis are associated with rapid deterioration in muscle mass.[2,3] It is also well known that patients infected with HIV suffer from sarcopenia.[4,5] Thus, the effect of HIV infection in a patient who is paralyzed is likely to augment, or at least be additive to, the effect of paralysis on muscle wasting.

7. For more than 40 years, serum or plasma creatinine concentration has been the most commonly used serum/plasma marker of renal function. However, serum/plasma creatinine measurements are affected by a number of factors not related to renal function, particularly age, gender,

and muscle mass.[6,7] In the patient presented in this case study, the rapid decline in his muscle mass renders his serum/plasma creatinine level essentially useless for monitoring renal function.

8. Alternatives for the assessment of renal function or glomerular filtration rate (GFR) in the patient include measurement of the clearance of exogenously administered substances (eg, inulin, iohexol, or ^{51}Cr-EDTA), which do not require the measurement of plasma creatinine, or the measurement of serum/plasma cystatin C. Cystatin C, a small 122-amino acid-containing protein, is a cysteine protease inhibitor expressed in all nucleated cells.[8] Cystatin C is produced at a constant rate and is freely filtered by the glomerulus. It is reabsorbed by the tubular epithelial cells and subsequently catabolized. Additionally, it is not affected by muscle mass, gender, or age as is creatinine. Because of these features, the plasma concentration of cystatin C can be used as a reliable measure of the GFR.[9] It has been suggested that serum/plasma cystatin C is an ideal endogenous marker for assessing renal function.[9]

Course and Outcome

The patient had multiple neurological problems during his hospital stay, despite an initial electroencephalogram (EEG) which did not show any epileptiform activity. Moreover, multiple testing of cerebrospinal fluid at various stages of his hospitalization did not reveal the etiology of his neurological problems. He received multiple courses of antibiotics, but ultimately it was felt that he had traumatic meningitis and not infectious meningitis. During his hospital stay, he developed status epilepticus and required intubation, mechanical ventilation, and treatment with phenytoin and valproic acid. His seizures were ultimately controlled and he was weaned off the phenytoin and kept on a maintenance regimen of valproic acid. Multiple radiologic scans of his brain and spine revealed subarachnoid hemorrhage and some dilated ventricles consistent with hydrocephalus. On hospital day 8, he developed flaccid paralysis of the lower extremities. Extensive work-up failed to reveal the exact etiology of the paralysis, and it was felt that it was a myelitis related to his HIV infection or another,

unidentified virus. In addition to the medications mentioned above, he was treated with azithromycin and trimethoprim/sulfamethoxazole to prevent opportunistic infections and with famotidine to prevent gastrointestinal ulcers. He was not treated with antiretroviral agents while he was an inpatient. The patient ultimately lapsed into a vegetative state attributed to his traumatic brain injury. He was not able to follow commands or communicate, and he never regained any strength in his lower extremities.

Keywords

creatinine, human immunodeficiency virus, Jaffe reaction, cystatin C, renal function

References

1. Soldin SJ, Henderson L, Hill JG. The effect of bilirubin and ketones on reaction rate methods for the measurement of creatinine. *Clin Biochem.* 1978;11:82.

2. LeBlanc A, Shackelford L, Schneider V. Muscle atrophy during long duration bed rest. *Int J Sports Med.* 1997;18:S283-S285.

3. Kawakami Y, Muraoka Y, Kubo K, et al. Changes in muscle size and architecture following 20 days of bed rest. *J Gravit Physiol.* 2000;7:53-59.

4. Panegyres PK, Papadimitriou JM, Hollingsworth PN, et al. Vesicular changes in the myopathies of AIDS. Ultrastructural observations and their relationship to zidovudine treatment. *J Neurol Neurosurg Psych.* 1990;53:649-655.

5. Kotler DP, Rosenbaum K, Wang J, et al. Studies of body composition and fat distribution in HIV-infected and control subjects. *J Acquir Immune Defic Syndr Human Retroviro.* 1999;20:228-237.

6. Heymsfield SB, Arteaga C, Maccanus C, et al. Measurement of muscle mass in humans: Validity of the 24-hour urinary creatinine method. *Am J Clin Nutr.* 1983;37:478-494.

7. James GD, Sealey JE, Alderman M, et al. A longitudinal study of urinary creatinine and creatinine clearance in normal subjects. Race, sex, and age differences. *Am J Hypertens.* 1988;1:124-131.

8. Abrahamson M, Olafsson I, Palsdottir A, et al. Structure and expression of the human cystatin C gene. *Biochem J.* 1990;268:287-294.

9. Grubb A. Diagnostic value of analysis of cystatin C and protein HC in biological fluids. *Clin Nephrol.* 1992;38:S20-S27.

A 20-Year-Old Male With Sinusitis and Bilateral Lung Opacities

Holly N. Burford, Stephanie D. Reilly

Department of Pathology, University of Alabama at Birmingham, Birmingham, AL

Patient: 20-year-old male.

Past Medical History: None.

Chief Complaint: Headache and neck pain.

History of Present Illness: The patient presented to an outside emergency room with a 5-day history of flu-like symptoms, headache, and stiff neck. He also had a 1-day history of left-sided extremity weakness. A urine drug screen was positive for amphetamine/methamphetamine. Antibiotics were started empirically, and the patient was transferred to our institution.

Social History: Significant for tobacco and methamphetamine abuse.

Physical Examination Findings: At time of transfer: temperature, 37.8°C; pulse, 130 beats per minute; respiratory rate, 24 breaths per minute; blood pressure 93/56 mm Hg. The patient appeared mildly confused but in no acute distress. Cardiac examination revealed tachycardia. Pulmonary auscultation was clear bilaterally. A neurological examination detected decreased strength (2/5) in the upper- and lower-left extremities. Sensation was decreased on the left side. There was also a positive Babinski reflex on the left side. Pupils were equally round and reactive to light; extraocular movements were intact. There was no cervical tenderness to palpation.

Diagnostic Studies: A chest x-ray revealed bilateral lower-lobe infiltrates and diffuse patchy nodules consistent with pneumonia (**Image 1A**). Magnetic resonance imaging (MRI) of the head showed left-sided pansinusitis as well as a right-sided parafalcine subdural empyema (**Image 1B**).

Hospital Course: Two days after admission, the patient underwent evacuation and debridement of the subdural empyema and debridement of the left ethmoid, maxillary, and frontal sinuses. Cultures from a left frontal sinus swab were positive for Peptostreptococcus species. Postoperatively, the patient remained intubated for respiratory failure secondary to worsening bilateral cavitating lung disease (**Image 1C**). The patient was febrile (temperature up to 40.5°C) throughout most of his hospitalization. An ultrasound of the neck 7 days after admission revealed a right internal jugular vein thrombosis with extension into the brachiocephalic vein. The patient's respiratory status improved and he was extubated on hospital day #10. On hospital day #13, the patient experienced severe hemoptysis, collapsed, and was pronounced dead after unsuccessful resuscitation efforts.

Autopsy Findings: Bilateral cavitating lung disease with multiple abscesses and hemorrhage was found (**Image 1D**). Clotted blood was found in both mainstem bronchi and in smaller airways, indicating asphyxiation as the cause of death. The craniotomy skin, bone, and dural flaps were intact. Purulent fluid was present midline in the epidural and subdural spaces. A small thrombus was identified in the right internal jugular vein. Microscopic examination of the lungs revealed diffuse hemorrhage in the airways with necrosis and acute infection in portions of all lobes. Examination of the brain identified focal resolving leptomeningitis.

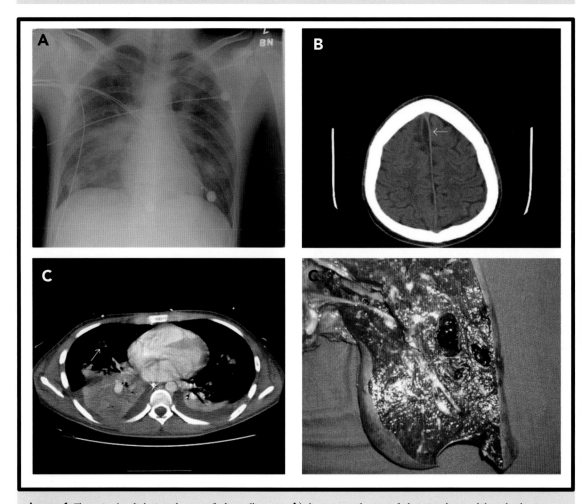

Image 1_The patient's radiologic and autopsy findings, illustrating **A**) chest x-ray at the time of admission showing bilateral pulmonary opacities suggestive of pneumonia; **B**) computed tomography (CT) scan image the day after admission showing a right parafalcine fluid collection consistent with empyema; **C**) CT image on hospital day #6 showing multifocal necrotizing pneumonia; and, **D**) multiple abscesses and hemorrhage of the right lung, confirming at autopsy the clinical impression of cavitating lung disease.

Questions _____

1. What are this patient's most striking clinical and laboratory findings?

2. How do you explain this patient's clinical and laboratory findings?

3. What processes should be considered when a cavitating lung disease is identified?

T1. Principal Laboratory Findings

Test	Patient's Result	Reference Range
Hematology		
WBC count	14.63	4.00–11.00 × 10³/μL
Hemoglobin	12.2	13.5–17.0 g/dL
Hematocrit	35	39–50%
Platelet count	9.9	150.0–450.0 × 10³/μL
MCHC	35	32–36 g/dL
MCV	87	80–96 fL
RDW	14.2	11.0–16.0%
Coagulation		
PT	16.6	12.6–14.6 sec
PTT	42	25–35 sec
INR	1.40	—
D-Dimer	2,796	110–240 ng/mL
Chemistry		
Sodium	140	133–145 mEq/L
Potassium	4.7	3.3–5.1 mEq/L
Chloride	107	96–108 mEq/L
Bicarbonate	20	23–29 mEq/L
BUN	48	6–19 mg/dL
Creatinine	1.6	0.7–1.3 mg/dL
Glucose	58	70–105 mg/dL
AST	35	0–37 U/L
ALT	67	6–45 U/L
Alk phos	153	39–117 U/L
Bilirubin		
total	5.5	0.0–1.0 mg/dL
indirect	1.8	0.0–0.9 mg/dL
direct	3.7	0.1–0.3 mg/dL
Albumin	1.8	3.4–5.0 g/dL
Fibrinogen	533	220–498 mg/dL
LD	257	120–240 U/L

WBC, white blood cell; MCHC, mean corpuscular hemoglobin concentration; MCV, mean corpuscular volume; RDW, red blood cell distribution width; PT, prothrombin time; PTT, partial thromboplastin time; INR, international normalized ratio; BUN, blood urea nitrogen; AST, aspartate aminotransferase; ALT, alanine aminotransferase; LD, lactate dehydrogenase.

4. What condition is suggested by this patient's most striking clinical and laboratory findings?

5. What organisms have been associated with this patient's condition?

6. What are the signs and symptoms of this patient's condition?

7. What is the expected clinical outcome in individuals with this patient's condition?

Possible Answers

1. Mild confusion and altered mental status; decreased strength in the upper- and lower-left extremities; Babinski reflex present on the left side; imaging showing bilateral pneumonia, a left-sided pansinusitis, and a right parafalcine fluid collection consistent with subdural empyema. Abnormal laboratory findings included a positive urine drug screen, decreased hematocrit and hemoglobin, increased white blood cell count, and markedly-decreased platelet count (**T1**).

2. The differential diagnosis for altered mental status includes drug toxicity/overdose, metabolic derangement, structural abnormality/head injury, systemic infection, meningitis, seizures, and psychiatric illness.[1] In this case, the urine drug screen was positive for methamphetamines, which could have contributed to this patient's altered mental status. Infection was the most likely etiology, however, with imaging studies revealing a subdural empyema as well as pansinusitis and pulmonary opacities suggestive of pneumonia. The presence of sinusitis and subdural empyema suggests the possibility of the contiguous spread of a bacterial or fungal sinus infection. The right sided parafalcine subdural empyema would have affected the motor strip and produced the left-sided weakness. The presence of bilateral pneumonia along with the sinusitis suggests several possible etiologies. Upper respiratory viral infections can predispose one to develop both sinusitis, where mucosal edema obstructs the sinus ostia, and a secondary bacterial pneumonia. Another possible etiology of the pneumonia is hematogenous dissemination of infection from a distal site, in this case the

pansinusitis. Aspiration of oropharyngeal bacteria should also be considered in patients with a history of drug abuse. The laboratory abnormalities included increased white blood cell count, decreased hematocrit, markedly-decreased platelet count, and an increased D-dimer level (**T1**). Sepsis/disseminated intravascular coagulation (DIC) can cause thrombocytopenia. With the patient presenting with meningitis-like symptoms, hypotension, and bilateral pneumonia, there is a high probability that sepsis was the cause of the low platelet count. Disseminated intravascular coagulation was probably not fully developed, as the D-dimer level was only 2,796 ng/mL. D-dimer levels in DIC are expected to be more markedly elevated than the level seen in this patient. An early DIC-type picture could also account for the mild anemia.

3. Cavitary lung lesions can be caused by a diverse array of pathologic processes. The differential diagnosis includes infection (bacterial, fungal, and parasitic), septic embolism, pulmonary infarct, neoplasm, vasculitides, congenital anomalies, rheumatoid nodule, and progressive massive fibrosis which occurs with pneumoconiosis.[2] Cavitation which occurs in consolidated lungs is called necrotizing pneumonia. *Staphylococcus aureus*, gram-negative bacteria, anaerobic bacteria, and tuberculosis are common causes of this condition. Cavitation seen with bacterial infection, especially anaerobic bacteria, can evolve into a discrete abscess.[2]

4. ***Most likely diagnosis:*** *Lemierre's syndrome.* In this particular case, the patient's course began with pansinusitis, which spread locally into the central nervous system, resulting in an empyema. The cavitating lung lesions were attributed to septic emboli secondary to the sinusitis; thus, the patient's clinical presentation and laboratory findings are consistent with a diagnosis of Lemierre's syndrome. Lemierre's syndrome is defined as an oral or nasopharyngeal infection associated with jugular vein thrombophlebitis and metastatic infection to the lungs and other sites. It is a rare syndrome, with a reported incidence of 1 in 1 million persons per year;[2] however, a rise in yearly incidence beginning in the 1990s has been reported.[2,3] Lemierre's syndrome most often occurs between the ages of 16 and 19 in previously-healthy individuals.[2] The

most common underlying illness is tonsillitis or peritonsillar abscess, but it has been described in patients with sinusitis, mastoiditis, otitis media, and tooth infections.[3]

5. Classically, Lemierre's syndrome results from an infection by *Fusobacterium necrophorum*, an anaerobic, gram-negative bacterium; however, other organisms have been implicated including *Streptococcus* species, *staphylococci, Eikenella corrodens, Peptostreptococcus* species (as in this case), *Bacteroides* species, and other *Fusobacterium* species.[4]

6. Characteristic signs and symptoms of Lemierre's syndrome include sepsis and high fever within 1 week of the primary local infection.[3] Patients often complain of neck pain and stiffness. Swelling near the angle of the mandible or anterior to the sternocleidomastoid muscle indicates the development of internal jugular venous thrombophlebitis. This has been detected in 26% to 45% of cases.[2] In our case, an ultrasound performed 1 week into the hospital course revealed a thrombus within the right internal jugular vein with extension into the brachiocephalic vein. A central line was in place, so it is unclear whether the thrombus was catheter associated or should be attributed to the infection, or perhaps was due to a combination of the 2. Pulmonary involvement by septic embolization is common in Lemierre's syndrome and reportedly occurs in 79% to 100% of cases.[2] The lung lesions occur early in the course of the illness and cause a pleuritic-type pain with shortness of breath and hemoptysis. Abnormal liver function is detected in 49% of patients.[5] Other manifestations seen in this syndrome include septic arthritis, osteomyelitis, skin and soft tissue abscesses, renal failure, and DIC.[3]

7. When Lemierre first described this syndrome in 1936, the mortality rate was extremely high with 18 of his 20 reported cases succumbing to the disease. With the advent of antimicrobial therapy, the mortality rate has dropped significantly. Current reported mortality rates range from 0% to 18%.[3]

Keywords

Lemierre's syndrome, cavitating lung lesions, Fusobacterium necrophorum

References

1. Ropper AH. Acute Confusional States and Coma. Braunwald E, ed. In: *Harrison's Principles of Internal Medicine.* New York: McGraw-Hill; 132,135.

2. Ryu JH, Swensen SJ. Cystic and cavitary lung disease: Focal and diffuse. *Mayo Clin Proc.* 2003;78:744–752.

3. Riordan T, Wilson M. Lemierre's syndrome: More than a historical curiosa. *Postgrad Med J.* 2004;80:328–334.

4. Kristensen LH, Prag J. Human necrobacillosis, with emphasis on Lemierre's syndrome. *Clin Infect Dis.* 2000;31:524–532.

5. Williams MD, Kerber CA, Tergin HF. Unusual presentation of Lemierre's syndrome due to *Fusobacterium nucleatum. J Clin Micro.* 2003;41;3445–3448.

Abdominal Tenderness in a Male

Monte S. Willis, Frank H. Wians, Jr., Leland B. Baskin

Department of Pathology, University of Texas Southwestern Medical Center, Dallas, TX

Patient: 49-year-old African-American male.

Chief Complaint: Mid-epigastric pain of 1 week duration which radiated to his back.

History of Present Illness: The patient stated that his pain increased when he was recumbent and after he ate meals high in fat content. He denied nausea, vomiting, melena, hematochezia, diarrhea, fever, chills, or night sweats.

Past Medical History: The patient's past medical history included previous positive tests for both the human immunodeficiency virus (HIV) and hepatitis C viruses (HCV) in the mid-1990s. The patient revealed a history of intravenous (IV) drug use. He was taking the anti-retroviral drug dideoxyinosine [Didanosine (ddI)] for his HIV infection.

Physical Examination: Right upper quadrant tenderness and a palpable liver 8 to 9 cm below the costal margin. The physical examination was otherwise within normal limits.

Results of Additional Diagnostic Procedures: A serum protein electrophoresis (SPE) was performed and the densitometric pattern (SPEP) demonstrated hypoalbuminemia, polyclonal gammopathy, and beta-gamma bridging [**Image 1**].

Questions

1. What is (are) this patient's most striking laboratory result(s)?

2. How do you explain this patient's most striking laboratory results?

3. What condition(s) does this patient's clinical and laboratory findings suggest?

4. What are the principal complications found in this patient's condition?

5. Which additional laboratory test(s) are appropriate to order on this patient and why?

6. What is the most appropriate treatment for this patient?

Possible Answers

1. Increased serum amylase and lipase levels; increased liver function tests (AST, ALT, GGT); positive HCV antibodies; prolonged PT and PTT; macrocytosis (MCV >100 fL) without anemia; and an SPEP that demonstrated

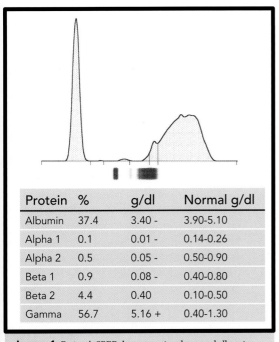

Protein	%	g/dl	Normal g/dl
Albumin	37.4	3.40 -	3.90-5.10
Alpha 1	0.1	0.01 -	0.14-0.26
Alpha 2	0.5	0.05 -	0.50-0.90
Beta 1	0.9	0.08 -	0.40-0.80
Beta 2	4.4	0.40	0.10-0.50
Gamma	56.7	5.16 +	0.40-1.30

Image 1_Patient's SPEP demonstrating decreased albumin and increased gamma-globulin bands and beta-gamma bridging. Subsequent immunofixation electrophoresis (IFE) of this patient's serum demonstrated no M-protein (data not shown).

hypoalbuminemia, polyclonal gammopathy, and beta-gamma bridging.

2. Serum amylase activity is most commonly used in the diagnosis of acute pancreatitis. The level increases 2 to 12 hours after symptoms (ie, RUQ or mid-epigastric pain) begin and plateaus in 3 to 5 days in most cases.[1] When the amylase level is 5-fold higher than the upper limit of the normal range, it is highly specific for pancreatitis.[1] Lipase is also used to aid in the diagnosis of pancreatitis and has similar diagnostic sensitivity (approximately 90%) and specificity (approximately 70%) as amylase. Increased lipase levels, however, remain elevated for a longer period of time than amylase. Using both amylase and lipase increases the specificity to 90%.[1] Increased AST, ALT, and GGT are suggestive of liver dysfunction (eg, hepatitis). This patient's prior history of HCV infection, intravenous drug use, when coupled with his current positive HCV antibody test, suggests chronic HCV infection. The clinical finding of an enlarged liver, palpable beyond the costal border, indicates that this patient has active chronic HCV infection. The prolonged PT

and PTT are consistent with a coagulopathy that is most likely due to his chronic liver disease and subsequent liver dysfunction. The major site of synthesis of the coagulation factors, V, VII, IX, X, XI, XII, XIII, prothrombin, and fibrinogen, is the liver. When liver damage due to hepatitis progresses, the more severe the deficiency in these factors, resulting in prolonged coagulation (ie, increased PT and PTT). Because this patient had a history of chronic hepatitis, an SPE was performed to determine if a monoclonal immunoglobulin might be present. One of the extrahepatic manifestations of HCV infection is an essential mixed cryoglobulinemia. An SPE in a patient with chronic HCV infection is essential to the diagnosis of this condition. Type II (mixed monoclonal) and type III (mixed polyclonal) cryoglobulins are associated with HCV infection and cause disease by multiple autoimmune mechanisms. This patient's SPEP demonstrated a decreased albumin fraction, a polyclonal gammopathy, and beta-gamma bridging, a pattern seen frequently in patients with HCV infection and chronic liver disease [**Image 1**]. Albumin is synthesized in the liver and is therefore decreased in the serum of patients with chronic liver disease, while the increase in the major immunoglobulins (IgG, IgA, and IgM) that accompanies infection causes a polyclonal gammopathy of sufficient magnitude to blur the distinct separation between b- and g-globulin bands [**Image 1**]. Moreover, in patients with liver disease, a significant increase in RBC volume occurs from defective DNA synthesis or accelerated erythropoiesis resulting in thin macrocytes (with increased surface area) with normal volume, which has no effect on other RBC indices.

3. *Most likely diagnosis:* Chronic HCV infection and acute pancreatitis secondary to anti-retroviral drug therapy.

In a patient with HIV infection, pancreatitis can arise from numerous drug and infectious sources.[2] Patients will have elevated amylase and lipase; however, elevated amylase without pancreatic disease may be due to macroamylasemia, which is found in patients with acquired immunodeficiency disease (AIDS).[3] Pancreatitis occurs most commonly in AIDS patients following therapy with pentamidine (used for *Pneumocystis carinii* prophylaxis) or the anti-retroviral drug, ddI. Pentamidine-induced pancreatitis develops after oral or inhalation administration of this drug.[4,5] The severity of disease varies from mild to fatal and is accompanied by dysregulation of glucose metabolism.[5] Therefore, serum glucose levels should be monitored in patients taking this drug. Early trials of ddI demonstrated a 10% incidence of symptomatic pancreatitis in patients receiving this drug.[6] Trimethoprim-sulfamethoxazole is also an occasional cause of drug-induced pancreatitis. Moreover, pancreatitis in AIDS patients can be caused by many infectious agents [eg, cytomegalovirus (CMV), mycobacteria, cryptococcus, and herpes simplex virus (HSV)][2]; however, definitive diagnosis of pancreatitis requires a biopsy of the pancreas which is a difficult procedure and therefore, only infrequently performed. Other potential causes of pancreatitis in patients with HIV infection include lymphoma infiltration of the pancreas and Kaposi's sarcoma[7] which causes pancreatitis by a mass effect or by obstruction of the pancreatic duct.

Co-infection with HCV in patients with HIV infection is variable. In some groups of HIV-infected patients, such as IV drug users and hemophiliacs, the prevalence of co-infection can be as high as 100%, whereas in other groups, such as male homosexuals, the prevalence is just slightly greater than in the general population. Two studies have suggested that HIV/HCV co-infection results in more severe liver damage and a worse prognosis than in patients with only HCV infection.[8,9] In a cohort study of 91 hemophiliacs with HCV/HIV co-infection, 8 developed liver failure over an 18-year follow-up period compared to 0 out of 58 patients with HCV infection alone (P=0.03).[9] Another study compared 66 HCV/HIV co-infected predominantly homosexual men to 132 HIV-infected control patients who were HCV antibody negative and found that HCV co-infection did not adversely affect survival.[8] These conflicting results may be due to several factors such as the duration of the HCV infection before the onset of HIV infection, the route of infection, and other factors. However, there is no evidence that co-infection is beneficial to long-term survival.

Serological testing for HCV infection in immunocompromised patients underestimates the prevalence of disease, and the use of the polymerase chain reaction (PCR) technique to detect HCV RNA becomes necessary for diagnosis.[8] In a study comparing the second-generation antibody tests [Enzyme-Linked Immunosorbent Assay (ELISA)-2 and Radioimmunoblot assay (RIBA-2)] for detecting HCV antibodies versus PCR RNA and branched DNA (bDNA) assays to diagnose HCV infection after liver transplantation, the ELISA-2 assay failed to detect HCV antibodies in 12% of patients that were positive by PCR RNA and bDNA assays. This study demonstrated that second-generation HCV antibody tests had lower diagnostic sensitivity in detecting HCV infection in immunocompromised patients than the nucleic acid tests (NATs). Decreased or undetectable HCV antibody titer to specific HCV antigens (eg, c100-3 and c33c) has been demonstrated in recipients of HCV-positive kidney and bone marrow transplants.[10]

The seroprevalence of HCV antibodies worldwide is approximately 1%, although marked variation exists between various geographic locations such that 0.4% to 11.1% in North America are seropositive while 9.6% to 13.6% of the population in North Africa are seropositive.[11] In 1991, HCV antibody screening of blood donors began and transfusion-related HCV infection declined to the point that non-transfusion-related transmission of HCV is more important today than prior to 1991.[12] In 40% of patients with acute or chronic HCV infection, the most common risk factor is IV drug abuse, while in another 40% of these patients, no risk factor can be identified.[13]

Two major modes of transmission have been identified for HCV – percutaneous (ie, blood transfusion or needlestick inoculation) and non-percutaneous (ie, perinatal and sexual contact). The risk of transfusion-related HCV infection, using first-generation HCV antibody tests to detect the presence of HCV antibodies, is approximately 0.6% (ie, out of a 1,000 HCV antibody-negative patients receiving a blood/blood product transfusion, 6 will have a positive, post-transfusion HCV antibody test).[12] Blood donor and recipient screening with second- and third-generation HCV antibody assays is predicted to reduce the incidence of HCV infection to indistinguishable levels from hospitalized patients who have not received blood transfusions.[14] The prevalence of HCV infection among IV drug abusers is 48% to 90% and the risk of acquiring HCV infection from IV drug abusers is as high as 90%. Unlike the decrease in the prevalence of HCV infection resulting from blood/blood product transfusions, the prevalence of HCV infection among IV drug abusers has not decreased and they remain an important reservoir of this disease.[14] Hemodialysis can be related to endemic cases of HCV infection and the prevalence of HCV seropositivity in hemodialysis patients has been reported to be between 10% and 20%.[11] Serologic assays for HCV antibodies, however, may underestimate the prevalence of HCV infection in dialysis patients and NAT may be necessary for accurate diagnosis in these patients.[11] Health care workers with documented needlestick exposure from an HCV-infected individual have a seroconversion rate of 0% to 4%; however, when HCV testing is performed by PCR, the risk of infection has been reported to be as high as 10%.[11,15,16] Transmission of HCV from an infected health care worker to patients has also been reported.[14]

Non-percutaneous HCV transmission between sexual partners, as well as congenital infections have been reported. The evidence indicates that in sharp contrast to the percutaneous modes of transmission the non-cutaneous modes are very inefficient. This is particularly true for sexual transmission, which clearly occurs, but is rare. Ten percent of patients with a sporadic acute HCV infection report a history of sexual exposure although seroepidemiologic studies have demonstrated the presence of HCV antibodies in the serum of only very low numbers of sexual contacts. For example, HCV antibodies are detected in less than 3% of female sexual partners of male hemophiliacs (most of whom are infected with HCV).[11] Overall, the sexual partners of HCV antibody-positive individuals have a prevalence of HCV antibody positivity of 0% to 27%, while partners without liver disease or high-risk behaviors such as IV drug abuse or many sexual contacts, the prevalence is much lower (0% to 7%).[11] Sporadic HCV infections account for 40% of patients without identifiable risk factors. These infections may result from a common, yet unidentified, route of transmission.

4. There are 3 primary complications of chronic pancreatitis: 1) pseudocysts; 2) pancreatic ascites, and 3) obstruction of nearby organs. A pancreatic pseudocyst is an encapsulated pocket of high concentrations of pancreatic enzymes with chronic inflammation and cirrhosis around it.[1] Pseudocysts are collections of fluid developed during acute pancreatitis that have not resolved. Frequently, they result from pancreatic duct obstruction and can occur in up to 60% of patients with chronic pancreatitis.[1] They can be life threatening because of complications of infection, hemorrhage, and rupture.[1] Large pseudocysts (>5 cm in diameter) should be treated by drainage into the intestinal tract. Effusions in the abdomen or pleura can result from a disrupted pancreatic duct. The serum lipase and amylase levels can be markedly elevated and surgical correction may be needed to return them to normal levels. Lastly, structures near the pancreas can be obstructed. For example, obstruction of the common bile duct can lead to jaundice; the gastric outlet can be obstructed; and the splenic veins can be compressed or thrombosed leading to bleeding.[1]

5. The diagnosis of pancreatitis should include plain X-rays or CT of the abdomen to visualize intraductal calcifications of the pancreas. Abdominal CT may be more sensitive and detect small calcifications missed on plain X-ray in addition to pancreatic duct dilation and pseudocysts. Endoscopic ultrasonography (US) may detect early stages of disease. The most sensitive method for diagnosing chronic pancreatitis is the secretin stimulation test which involves determining the bicarbonate and enzymes released by the pancreas into the duodenum in response to the administration of secretin + (cholecystokinin or cerulean). In a simpler test, trypsin activity is determined in the proximal jejunum after a liquid meal is given; however, neither of these tests is used widely. The diagnosis is generally based on the combination of symptoms, pancreatic function tests, radiologic studies, and endoscopic retrograde cholangiopancreatography (ERCP). If the results of any 2 of these variables are consistent with manifestations of pancreatitis, then the diagnosis is made.[1] For example, if pancreatic calcifications are observed on abdominal film of the abdomen in a patient with chronic upper abdominal pain, the diagnosis is pancreatitis. To

rule out a mild chronic pancreatitis, the duodenal secretin test and ERCP, in addition to endoscopic US, should be performed. Endoscopic retrograde cholangiopancreatography is used to differentiate chronic pancreatitis from adenocarcinoma or cystic tumor of the pancreas. In addition, cytologic testing of percutaneous aspirates, diagnostic laparotomy, surgical resection, and abdominal exploration may all be necessary to provide a definitive diagnosis.

6. The most important task in treating chronic pancreatitis is controlling the abdominal pain. To do this, narcotics are frequently required and should not be withheld even if the patient has an addiction to narcotics, alcohol, or both. Attacks of pancreatitis require hospitalization, withholding all oral intake, IV administration of analgesics, and renewed efforts at alcohol abstinence if appropriate. When chronic intractable pain or intermittent pain is present, a surgical procedure, such as ERCP, or a CT evaluation of the pancreatic ducts should be performed. If duct dilation >8 mm is present, decompression can be attempted by endoscopic stent placement; however, most patients with this finding require permanent duct decompression by surgery. If a dilated duct is absent, a surgical procedure such as a pancreaticoduodenectomy (ie, a Whipple procedure) can be helpful if the ductal changes are found in the head of the pancreas. Gastrointestinal (GI) malabsorption occurs when the secretion of digestive enzymes is decreased by >90%.[1] At this point, fat is not absorbed from the GI tract because lipase is not present resulting in steatorrhea. Malabsorption syndrome can be documented by a stool fat level of >7 g/day. Treatment for steatorrhea (increased level of fat in the stool) is indicated when weight loss not corrected by increased caloric intake occurs. The low potency of porcine pancreatic extracts because of irreversible destruction at gastric pH levels makes steatorrhea difficult to overcome. However, enteric-coated enzymes (Pancrease or Creon) are released in an alkaline environment (duodenum) and are useful in the treatment of steatorrhea when 2 to 3 capsules are taken with every meal.[1]

Hospital Course: The patient was admitted to the hospital, placed on an NPO (nothing by mouth) diet and given morphine for pain. In addition, an NG tube was inserted, and ddI therapy was discontinued. The patient's abdominal pain progressively improved over the next several days and he was released to follow up by an outpatient physician specialist in the treatment of HIV patients for alternative anti-retroviral drug therapy.

References

1. Soergel KH. Pancreatitis. In: Cecil RL, Goldman L, Bennett JC, et al, eds. *Cecil Textbook of Medicine*. Philadelphia: W.B. Saunders, 2000:752-758.

2. Bonacini M. Pancreatic involvement in human immunodeficiency virus infection. *J Clin Gastroenterol*. 1991;13:58-64.

3. Greenberg RE, Bank S, Singer C. Macroamylasaemia in association with the acquired immunodeficiency syndrome. *Postgrad Med J*. 1987;63:677-679.

4. Pauwels A, Eliaszewicz M, Larrey D, et al. Pentamidine-induced acute pancreatitis in a patient with AIDS. *J Clin Gastroenterol*. 1990;12:457-459.

5. Schwartz MS, Cappell MS. Pentamidine-associated pancreatitis. *Dig Dis Sci*. 1989;34:1617-1620.

6. Lambert JS, Seidlin M, Reichman RC, et al. 2′,3′-dideoxyinosine (ddI) in patients with the acquired immunodeficiency syndrome or AIDS-related complex. A phase I trial. *N Engl J Med*. 1990;322:1333-40.

7. Friedman SL, Wright TL, Altman DF. Gastrointestinal Kaposi's sarcoma in patients with acquired immunodeficiency syndrome. Endoscopic and autopsy findings. *Gastroenterology*. 1985;89:102-8.

8. Garcia G, Terrault N, Wright TL. Hepatitis C virus infection in the immunocompromised patient. *Semin Gastrointest Dis*. 1995;6:35-45.

9. Eyster ME, Diamondstone LS, Lien JM, et al. Natural history of hepatitis C virus infection in multitransfused hemophiliacs: effect of coinfection with human immunodeficiency virus. The Multicenter Hemophilia Cohort Study. *J Acquir Immune Defic Syndr*. 1993;6:602-610.

10. Lok AS, Chien D, Choo QL, et al. Antibody response to core, envelope and nonstructural hepatitis C virus antigens: comparison of immunocompetent and immunosuppressed patients. *Hepatology*. 1993;18:497-502.

11. Rall CJ, Dienstag JL. Epidemiology of hepatitis C virus infection. *Semin Gastrointest Dis*. 1995;6:3-12.

12. Donahue JG, Munoz A, Ness PM, et al. The declining risk of post-transfusion hepatitis C virus infection. *N Engl J Med*. 1992;327:369-373.

13. Alter MJ, Hadler SC, Judson FN, et al. Risk factors for acute non-A, non-B hepatitis in the United States and association with hepatitis C virus infection. *JAMA*. 1990;264:2231-2235.

14. Terrault NA, Wright TL. Viral Hepatitis A Through G. In: Sleisenger MH, Fordtran JS, Feldman M, et al, eds. *Sleisenger & Fordtran's gastrointestinal and Liver Disease: Pathophysiology, Diagnosis, Management.* Philadelphia: Saunders, 1998:1123-1170.

15. Kiyosawa K, Sodeyama T, Tanaka E, et al. Hepatitis C in hospital employees with needlestick injuries. *Ann Intern Med.* 1991;115:367-369.

16. Mitsui T, Iwano K, Masuko K, et al. Hepatitis C virus infection in medical personnel after needlestick accident. *Hepatology.* 1992;16:1109-1114.

Weakness of the Extremities in a 40-Year-Old Woman

Ronald Thomason

Esoterix Oncology, Brentwood, TN

Patient: 40-year-old Caucasian woman.

Chief Complaint: Weakness of the extremities.

Medical History: Hepatitis C virus (HCV) infection.

Electromyogram and Nerve Conduction Velocity Findings: Abnormalities indicative of a peripheral neuropathy.

Principal Radiographic Findings: No lymphadenopathy, organomegaly, or extranodal mass lesions identified by CT scan of the abdomen.

T1. Principal Laboratory Findings

Test		Patient's Result	"Normal" Reference Range
EDTA-whole blood			
WBC count		15.5	4.5-11.0 × 10³/mL
Lymphocyte count		28	20-51%
Hemoglobin		14.9	12.0-15.0 g/dL
MCV		100	79-98 fL
Serum			
AST		102	5-40 U/L
ALT		120	7-56 U/L
Total protein		9.1	6.2-8.2 g/dL
Globulins		4.0	2.3-3.5 g/dL
Quantitative Ig's:	IgG	1,880	569-1,919 mg/dL
	IgA	298	61-330 mg/dL
	IgM	782	47-147 mg/dL
Qualitative cryoglobulins		Positive	Negative
RF		Positive (titer = 1:1024)	Negative

EDTA, ethylenediaminetetraacetate; WBC, white blood cell; MCV, mean corpuscular volume; AST, aspartate aminotransferase; ALT, alanine aminotransferase; Ig's, immunoglobulins; RF, rheumatoid factor.

T2. Principal Bone Marrow Findings

Morphology	
Normocellular	
No lymphocytic aggregates	
18% small lymphocytes on differential count	
Few lymphoplasmacytoid cells with rare Dutcher bodies*	
1% plasma cells	
Flow Cytometry	
Monoclonal B-cell population comprising approximately 5% of studied events	
Immunophenotype of B-cell clone:	
Positive markers	*Negative markers*
CD19	CD5
CD20	CD10
HLA-DR	CD23
Kappa	CD45
	Lambda

*Dutcher bodies are periodic acid-Schiff-positive intranuclear pseudoinclusions found in plasma cells in mucosa-associated lymphoid tissue lymphoma, Waldenström macroglobulinemia, and myeloma.[6] CD, cluster of differentiation; HLA, human lymphocyte antigen.

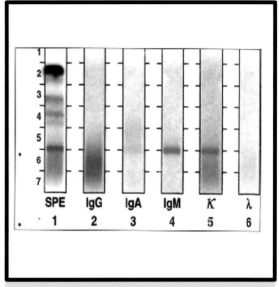

Image 1_IFE pattern of patient's serum.

Questions

1. What are this patient's most striking clinical and laboratory findings?

2. How do you explain this patient's most striking clinical and laboratory findings?

3. What condition(s) is(are) suggested by this patient's most striking clinical and laboratory findings?

4. How is(are) this patient's condition(s) typically treated?

5. Which laboratory test(s) is(are) used to assess the therapeutic response in individuals with this patient's condition(s)?

Possible Answers

1. Peripheral neuropathy with no lymphadenopathy; modest leukocytosis; elevated liver enzymes (ie, AST and ALT); increased serum total protein and globulin concentrations; markedly increased serum IgM concentration; positive cryoglobulin screen; positive RF test; serum M-protein identified by immunofixation electrophoresis (IFE) as IgM kappa [**Image 1**]; and the identification of B cells by flow cytometry with kappa light chain restriction [**Image 2**].

2. All of this patient's most striking clinical and laboratory findings are a consequence of her HCV-associated cryoglobulinemia. Cryoglobulins are immune complexes that precipitate when exposed to cold temperatures. In cryoglobulinemia, tissue deposits of these complexes initiate an inflammatory response, which leads to a wide spectrum of clinical manifestations including purpura, arthralgia, weakness, renal failure, and peripheral neuropathy. Cryoglobulins are classified as types I, II, or III depending on the composition and character of the immune complexes. In type II cryoglobulinemia, the immune complexes are usually comprised of monoclonal IgM bound to polyclonal IgG. The monoclonal IgM has an affinity for the polyclonal IgG and is therefore a monoclonal rheumatoid factor

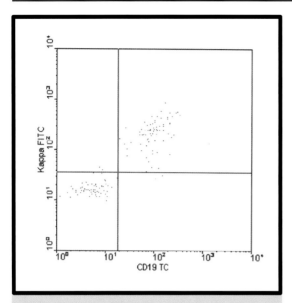

Image 2_Flow cytometric dot plot of the reaction between the patient's bone marrow lymphocytes and CD19 and kappa light chain markers. FITC, fluorescein isothiocyanate; TC, tri-color.

(mRF). Type II cryoglobulinemia is strongly associated with HCV infection, and HCV virions have been shown to be specifically concentrated within the cryoglobulins of patients with these associated conditions.[1] Similar to the patient presented in this study, a substantial proportion of patients with type II cryoglobulinemia are found to have a clonal expansion of B-lymphocytes within the bone marrow.[2-5] Hepatitis C virus does not appear to be directly oncogenic, as it does not possess reverse transcriptase or oncogenes.[3] Instead, the monoclonal B-cell expansions associated with HCV infection are likely an indirect consequence of the infection arising from the persistent polyclonal immune response to the virus. Therefore, the presence of mRF may represent an exaggeration of the natural immune response to HCV.[1] The mRF in type II cryoglobulinemia may be detected as an M-protein by serum protein electrophoresis.[5] Since it is a rheumatoid factor, it may also be detected by rheumatoid factor assays.

3. **Most likely diagnosis:** HCV-associated type II cryoglobulinemia.

   Because increased serum concentrations of monoclonal IgM are characteristic of type II cryoglobulinemia, this condition represents a form of monoclonal gammopathy. As such, the laboratory features of type II cryoglobulinemia overlap with those of lymphoplasmacytic lymphoma (LPL), also known as Waldenström macroglobulinemia. In LPL, a proliferation of monoclonal lymphoplasmacytic cells secretes monoclonal IgM. Similar to LPL, pathologic examination of bone marrow from patients with type II cryoglobulinemia often reveals features of an indolent B-cell lymphoma with multiple nodular aggregates of small to medium-sized lymphocytes present in a random or paratrabecular distribution.[2-5] By immunohistochemical, flow cytometric or gene rearrangement studies, these B-cell expansions are often found to be clonal and exhibit an immunophenotypic profile compatible with LPL.[2,5] Despite these findings, in the usual case, the initial clinical manifestations of type II cryoglobulinemia are more reflective of an inflammatory than a neoplastic condition. This inflammatory response includes the presence of an apparently stable low-grade monoclonal B-cell expansion. This seemingly benign B-cell proliferation appears to be susceptible to malignant transforming mutational events which may over time give rise to overt lymphoma.[3] Such events offer an explanation for the increased risk of overt lymphoma observed in patients with type II cryoglobulinemia. Due to their overlapping features, the distinction between type II cryoglobulinemia and overt lymphoma is not always clear. The distinction is based primarily on the clinical manifestations of the disease and the degree of lymphoproliferation. The clinical picture in type II cryoglobulinemia is dominated by systemic signs and symptoms related to the inflammatory response elicited by cryoglobulin deposition in tissue. In overt lymphoma, on the other hand, the clinical picture is dominated by the effects of the pronounced expansion of the lymphocytic clone and related consequences (ie, lymphadenopathy, organomegaly, extranodal mass lesions, lymphocytosis, bone marrow replacement and failure, and/or serum hyperviscosity due to high monoclonal IgM levels). Due to their overlapping characteristics, however, not all cases of LPL and type II cryoglobulinemia can be easily classified on the basis of clinical features. The patient in this case study showed no clinical features of overt lymphoma. No peripheral lymphadenopathy was observed on physical examination and no central lymphadenopathy, organomegaly, or extranodal mass lesions were detected by CT scan of the abdomen. Therefore, this patient's clinical and laboratory findings were more reflective of type II cryoglobulinemia than LPL.

4. HCV-associated type II cryoglobulinemia is commonly treated with interferon-α (IFN-α). A majority of patients show at least some response to this therapy as measured by decreased cryoglobulin concentration or cryoglobulin-related symptoms.[5] It is speculated that the therapeutic benefit of IFN-α is related to its combined antilymphoproliferative and antiviral actions.[5] Given the availability of a specific therapy, it is important that HCV-associated type II cryoglobulinemia be recognized and diagnosed as early as possible. It should be part of the differential diagnosis in patients with an unexplained IgM M-protein, signs/symptoms of cryoglobulinemia, a positive cryoglobulin assay, and/or an unexplained positive rheumatoid factor assay.

5. Effective therapy for HCV-associated type II cryoglobulinemia should result in a decreased mRF concentration as measured by RF titer, serum protein electrophoresis, or cryoglobulin concentration. Moreover, response to therapy can be assessed by evaluating the patient for remission of the signs and symptoms related to this disorder.

Keywords

hepatitis C virus, cryoglobulinemia

References

1. Agnello V, Chung RT, Lee MK. A role for hepatitis C infection in type II cryoglobulinemia. *N Engl J Med.* 1992;327:1490-1495.

2. Monteverde A, Sabattini E, Poggi S, et al. Bone marrow findings further support the hypothesis that essential mixed cryoglobulinemia type II is characterized by a monoclonal B-cell proliferation. *Leuk Lymphoma.* 1995;20:119-124.

3. Pozzato G, Mazzaro C, Crovatto M, et al. Low-grade malignant lymphoma, hepatitis C virus infection, and mixed cryoglobulinemia. *Blood.* 1994;84:3047-3053.

4. Mussini, Mascia MT, Zanni G, et al. A cytomorphological and immunohistochemical study of bone marrow in the diagnosis of essential mixed type II cryoglobulinemia. *Haematologica.* 1991;76:389-391.

5. Mazzaro C, Franzin F, Tulissi P, et al. Regression of monoclonal B-cell expansion in patients affected by mixed cryoglobulinemia responsive to interferon-a therapy. *Cancer.* 1996;77:2604-2613.

6. Gray Y, Schwartz S. Dutcher bodies in chronic synovitis. *Arch Pathol Lab Med.* 2002;126:199-201.

Viral Meningitis

Karen K. Krisher

Associate Professor of Pathology, Department of Pathology, Children's Hospital Medical Center, Dallas, Texas

Patient: 2-month-old female.

Family History: N/A.

Drug History: N/A.

Chief Complaint: Fever, irritability, diarrhea.

Medical History: Previously healthy infant admitted to the hospital with diagnosis of FUO. Discharged after 72 hr when fever defervesced. Readmitted 24 hr later with elevated temperature of 100.2°F and diarrhea. Empiric therapy with Cefotaxime was initiated in response to symptoms. Cerebrospinal fluid and blood were collected for cultures. Therapy discontinued after 48 hours.

Physical Examination: Unremarkable with the exception of fever.

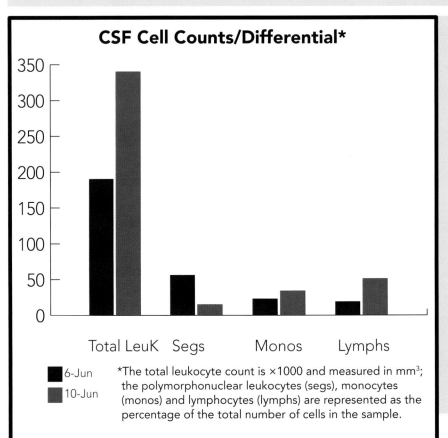

CSF Cell Counts/Differential*

6-Jun
10-Jun

*The total leukocyte count is ×1000 and measured in mm³; the polymorphonuclear leukocytes (segs), monocytes (monos) and lymphocytes (lymphs) are represented as the percentage of the total number of cells in the sample.

Figure 1_ Leukocyte cell count and differentiation for cerebrospinal fluid (CSF) and blood. Red bars represent sample taken June 6 and blue bars represent samples taken June 10. Results show an increase in total leukocyte count in the cerebrospinal fluid. The leukocyte increase corresponds with an increase in lymphocyte count and a decrease in polymorphonuclear (PMN) cell count. Blood results show a similar pattern.

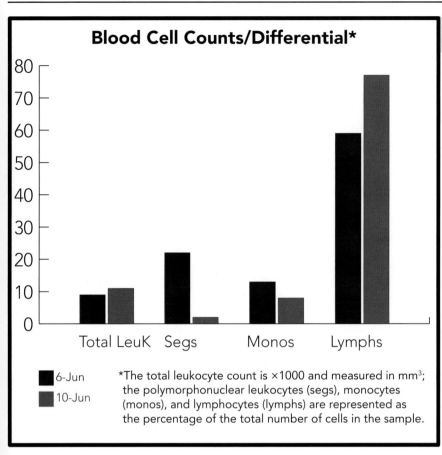

Figure 1_ Continued

Questions _____

1. What information contained in the clinical information is pertinent to the diagnosis?

2. What laboratory procedure(s) is (are) the most helpful in establishing the diagnosis?

3. What was the clinical diagnosis and likely cause of infection?

4. Why did the patient fail to respond to therapy?

Possible Answers _____

1. Information such as the season of the year and the patient's age and symptoms may assist in determining the etiologic agent of infection. Clinical diagnosis of an infection in an infant is often difficult due to the lack of specific symptoms other than fever. In infants, the diagnosis of FUO (fever of unknown origin) can represent a number of conditions. The terminology is often used to represent the presence of fever in association with failure to isolate a bacterial pathogen from the clinical specimen submitted for culture. The more rigorous definition of FUO applies to the presence of fever greater than 38°C for more than 2 weeks with no known cause as determined by clinical history, physical examination, and routine laboratory test. In infants less than 3 months of age, the presence of fever is often indicative of a generalized response to a bacterial infection that is localized in 1 of many locations such as the lung (pneumonia), bone (osteomyelitis), bladder (urinary tract infection), or central nervous system (meningitis). Viral infections are also very common in infants of this age. Since diagnosis is difficult based strictly on clinical symptoms, medical intervention is often dependent upon the results of laboratory testing.

2. When attempting to diagnose an infectious disease, especially in an infant, helpful laboratory tests are the quantitation and differentiation of leukocytes in both the blood and cerebrospinal

fluid (CSF). Elevated leukocyte count and CSF protein level in conjunction with a low CSF glucose level is suggestive of meningitis. A CSF finding of pleocytosis and a normal glucose concentration with no evidence of bacterial organisms may indicate a viral infection. Causative agents of aseptic meningitis include enteroviruses, lymphochoriomeningitis virus, cytomegaloviruses, adenoviruses.

3. Viral meningitis. The CSF findings of this infant are typical of viral meningitis. Although polymorphonuclear leukocytes predominated initially in the CSF, within a week, the lymphocyte count increased beyond that of the earlier PMN count. This sequence was also reflected in the quantitation of the leukocytes in the peripheral blood. The CSF of viral meningitis usually contains from 50-500 leukocytes/mm^3, predominantly lymphocytes. CSF protein is elevated but rarely above 200 mg/dL.

CNS viral infections are classified according to clinical findings as asymptomatic, meningitis, and/or encephalitis. Meningitis denotes an infection localized to the membranes enveloping the brain, the dura mater, pia mater, and arachnoid. Encephalitis is confined to the brain tissue itself. Isolation of viruses from the CSF depends on the strain of virus. One of the more common causes of viral meningitis in children, enteroviruses, are cultivable from CSF within 2-4 days. Other viruses, especially those causing meningoencephalitis are difficult to isolate in culture and diagnosis depends on the demonstration of an antibody response to the particular virus. Specimens for viral culture include CSF, throat swabs, and stool. A serum specimen should be obtained early in the illness and again in 2-3 weeks for serologic identification of the virus.

Enteroviruses cause approximately 85% of all cases of aseptic meningitis. Man is the only known natural host for human enteroviruses which are spread by person-to-person contact through fecal contamination (most common) or aerosol spread from the orophaynx. Infections are more common in the summer months and occur most frequently in pediatric populations.

4. In the interim between the clinical diagnosis and reporting of laboratory tests, empiric therapy with a broad spectrum antibiotic is usually administered to the patient. Failure to respond to therapy is due to several reasons including resistance to the antibiotic agent, inability to achieve adequate levels of the antibiotic in the location of the infection, or infection due to a non-bacterial pathogen that does not respond to antibiotic therapy (such as a virus).

Hematology/Coagulation Overview

Yuri D. Fedoriw

The series of studies that follow represent a brief sampling of both common and more esoteric cases encountered in the practice of diagnostic hematology. Many seemingly unrelated benign and malignant conditions trigger changes of the hematolymphoid system that often represent the first observable indication of disease. While often non-specific, qualitative and quantitative changes in the cellular fractions of peripheral blood may warrant further investigation for autoimmune disease, infection, or drug/toxin exposure. In the context of clinical history, these findings may narrow an otherwise broad differential and guide appropriate diagnostic testing and/or therapeutic intervention. Conversely, many primary benign and malignant hematopoietic disorders are associated with manifestations and effects on classically "non-hematologic" laboratory parameters. Defects in renal function, aberrations in serum protein distribution and electrolyte imbalances can all be associated with hematologic malignancy, and can importantly serve as effective prognostic and predictive markers. As such, some cases of primary hematological disorders and related sequelae are covered in other chapters within this compilation.

Cases within this chapter are divided into the main 'Topic Areas' of coagulation, benign hematology and malignant hematology to provide a possible framework for classification. Paralleling the difficulty in classification of hematologic disease, some of the cases have overlapping features between 'Topic Areas' and are listed subjectively within these groups. Although these examples do not offer a comprehensive review, the cases illustrate the breadth of analytical hematology and hematopathology. The 'Topics' covered represent both congenital and acquired disorders including:

Inherited:

- Hemophilia
- von Willebrand disease
- Transient myeloproliferative disorders
- Hemoglobinopathies
- Red cell membrane defects
- Enzyme deficiency

Acquired:

- Drug effect
- Iron deficiency anemia
- Leukemia/lymphoma
- Myelodyplastic syndromes/myeloproliferative neoplasms

Our evolving understanding of physiologic and pathologic processes demands a near constant re-evaluation of our current classification systems. This assertion holds true in the realms of both benign and malignant hematology, as new discoveries translated into clinical practice are re-shaping our approach to the diagnosis and treatment of disease.

The prognostic and predictive impact of newly identified cytogenetic and molecular features is notably reflected in the most recent 2008 World Health Organization (WHO) classification of acute myeloid leukemia (AML) (**Table 1**). The WHO classification builds on the original French-American-British (FAB) system of the 1970s and 1980s that classified AML into 8 subgroups (M0 through M7) based primarily on morphologic and cytochemical features of the leukemic cells. While successful differentiation and prognostic stratification was partly successful on these grounds, profound clinical heterogeneity was evident within many of the prescribed categories.

With the routine application of cytogenetic techniques, including karyotype analysis and fluorescence in-situ hybridization (FISH), recurring chromosomal aberrations were identified and reported in a subset of AML. While some recurrent translocations, such as the t(15;17)(q22;q12)(PML-RARA), showed excellent concordance with the FAB classification, other abnormalities differentiated morphologically indistinguishable groupings. These findings importantly correlated with disparate disease outcomes, risks of relapse, and therapeutic responses (figure 1). The block in cellular differentiation induced by the protein product of the aforementioned t(15;17), resulting in a fusion of the Promyelocytic Leukemia (PML) and Retinoic Acid Receptor Alpha (RARA) genes, can be directly overcome with the addition of all-trans retinoic acid to a conventional anthracyclin-based chemotherapeutic regimen (for further discussion of Acute Promyelocytic Leukemia, please refer to H-CS25, page 586). Progressive application of technologies has equated to significant clinical consequences, as cases harboring the t(15;17) carry the best prognosis of all AML.

In addition to gross chromosomal changes identified by karyotype or FISH, specific gene mutations have most recently demonstrated prognostic and predictive value. For example, AML with normal cytogenetics harboring internal tandem duplications within the juxtamembrane domain of the fms-related tyrosine kinase 3 (FLT3) shows significantly worse clinical outcome than cases with unmutated FLT3. Conversely, AML with normal cytogenetics and a mutated nucleophosmin (NPM1) gene shows more favorable clinical characteristics. Mutations of numerous other genes including, KIT, RAS, CEBPA, and WT1 are under investigation and may prove to dramatically affect future classification and treatment of disease. Molecular techniques, primarily based on the principles of polymerase chain reaction (PCR), targeting the myriad of genetic defects, serve not only to classify AML upfront, but to sensitively detect specific aberrations that may herald disease relapse after therapy. These assays serve to identify the earliest signs of disease, at stages too early to appreciate by morphologic analysis alone.

As we gather data from the cytogenetic and molecular techniques described above along with other clinically relevant technologies including flow cytometry, immunohistochemistry, gene expression array, comparative genomic hybridization, etc., we are faced with an exponential growth of new information. Processing of those data represents another daunting task, and the outcomes and results of those analyses will likely represent a significant impact on future systems of disease classification.

Suggested Reading

1. Mais DD. *Quick Compendium of Clinical Pathology,* 2nd ed. Chicago: ASCP Press, 2009.

2. Swedlow SH, Campo E, Jaffe ES, et al. *WHO Classification of Tumours of Haematopoietic and Lymphoid Tissues.* Edited by Swerdlow SH; Lyon, France IARC Press, 2008.

3. Gulati G, Caro J. *Blood Cells an Atlas of Morphology.* Singapore: ASCP Press, 2007.

4. Dunphy CH. *Integrated Hematopathology.* Hong Kong: ASCP Press, 2010.

5. *Practical Diagnosis of Hematologic Disorders,* 5th ed. Edited by Kjeldsberg CR. Singapore: ASCP Press 2010.

6. *Laboratory Hemostasis, A Practical Handbook for Pathologists.* Edited by Bennett ST, Lehman CM, Rogers GM. New York: Springer Science 2007.

7. *Clinics in Laboratory Medicine.* Edited by Rinder HM. Philadelphia: Elseiver (Saunders)Press 2009.

8. *Hemostasis and Thrombosis: Basic Principles and Clinical Practice,* 5th ed. Edited by Colman RW, Marder VJ, Clowes AW, George JN, Goldhaber SZ. Philadelphia: Lippincott Willams & Wilkins 2006.

9. *Quality in Laboratory Hemostasis and Thrombosis.* Edited by Kitchen S, Olson JD, Preston FE. Hoboken: Wiley-Blackwell 2009.

10. *Practical Hemostasis and Thrombosis.* Edited by O'Shaughnessy D, Makris M, Lillicrap D. Malden: Blackwell Publishing Ltd 2005.

11. Leonard DG. *Diagnostic Molecular Pathology.* Philadelphia: Elseiver (Saunders) Press 2003.

12. *Haemophilia and Haemostasis: A Case-Based Approach to Management.* Edited by Roberts HR, Carrizosa D, Ma A.Malden: Blackwell Publishing Ltd 2007.

13. Picard C, Silvy M, Gabert J. Overview of real-time PT-PCR strategies for quantification of gene rearrangements in the myeloid malignancies. *Methods Mol Med.* 2006; 125:27-68.

14. Grimwade D. The clinical significance of cytogenetic abnormalities in acute myeloid leukemia. *Best Prac Res Clin Haematol* 2001, 14:497-529.

15. Mrozek K, Marcucci G, Paschka P, et al. Clinical relevance of mutations and gene-expression changes in adult acute myeloid leukemia with normal cytogenetics: are we ready for a prognostically prioritized molecular classification. *Blood.* 2007; 109:431-448.

16. Mrozek K, Bloomfield CD. Chromosome aberrations, gene mutations and expression changes, and prognosis in adult acute myeloid leukemia. *Hematology Am Soc Hematol Educ Program.* 2006:169-77.

17. Gulley ML, Shea TC, Fedoriw Y. Genetic tests to evaluate prognosis and predict therapeutic response in acute myeloid leukemia. *J Mol Diag.* 2010; 12:3-16.

Table 1: Acute Myeloid Leukemias recognized by recurrent cytogenetic and molecular features: 2008 WHO Classification:

AML With Recurrent Genetic Abnormalities
• AML with t(8;21)(q22;q22) *RUNX1-RUNX1T1 (CBFA-ETO)*
• AML with inv(16)(p13q22) or t(16;16)(p13;q22) *CBFB-MYH11*
• APL with t(15;17)(q22;q11–12) *PML-RARA*
• AML with t(9;11)(p22;q23) *MLLT3-MLL* and other balanced translocations of 11q23 (*MLL*)
• AML with t(6;9)(p23;q34) *DEK-NUP214*
• AML with inv(3)(q21q26.2) or t(3;3)(q21;q26.2) *RPN1-EVI1*
• AML (megakaryoblastic) with t(1;22)(p13;q13)*RBM15-MKL1*
• AML with mutated *NPM1**
• AML with mutated *CEBPA**
Provisional entities.

Figure 1: Comparison of 2 morphologically similar cases. Figure 1. Aspirate smears of 2 cases with similar clinical presentations are morphologically indistinguishable. Karyotype analysis demonstrates specific cytogenetic abnormalities, which are now considered critical to classification and impart disparate prognoses.

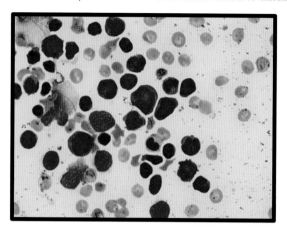 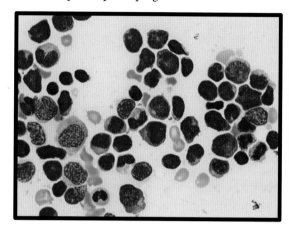

FAB Classification	
M2: AML with granulocytic maturation	M2: AML with granulocytic maturation
Abnormal Cytogenetic Finding	
t(8;21);*RUNX1-RUNX1T1*	t(6;9)(p23;q24);*DEK-NUP214*
WHO Classification	
AML with t(8;21)(q22;q22)	AML with t(6;9)(p23;q24)
Prognosis	
Favorable: excellent long-term survival	Unfavorable

A Neonate With Bleeding and Multiple Factor Deficiencies

Suthida Kankirawatana,[1] Roger L. Berkow,[2] Marisa B. Marques[1]

[1]Departments of Pathology and [2]Pediatrics, University of Alabama, Birmingham, AL

Patient: 1-month-old male infant.

Medications: None.

Chief Complaint: Prolonged bleeding after heel stick blood draws soon after birth.

History of Present Illness: Previous laboratory evaluation revealed prolonged partial thromboplastin time (PTT) of 111 seconds and variable levels of factor VIII, ranging from 4% to 23%. Factor IX level was not determined. According to the mother, the infant was not transfused with any blood products nor had any other bleeding or bruising.

Past Medical History: Infant is a fraternal twin, born by Caesarean section at 36 weeks of gestation (birth weight, 5 lbs 13 oz). Uncomplicated prenatal course, except for hyperbilirubinemia during the first 10 days of life, which resolved with phototherapy.

Family History: Negative for any bleeding problems. Twin sister was asymptomatic, growing, and developing well.

Physical Examination Findings: Temperature 98.6°C; pulse 90/min; blood pressure 77/40 mm Hg; weight 6 lbs 13 oz; length 47 cm. Infant was a normal-appearing, uncircumcised male, who was well-developed, well-nourished, in no acute distress, and without any evidence of bruises or hematoma. The remainder of the examination was normal for age.

T1. Principal Laboratory Findings

Test	Patient's Result	"Normal" Reference Range
Hematology		
WBC count	9.5	5.0-19.5 × 10³/μL
RBC count	2.3	3.0-5.4 × 10⁶/μL
Hemoglobin	7.6	10.0-18.0 g/dL
Hematocrit	22.3	31.0-55.0%
MCV	97.0	85.0-123.0 fL
MCH	33.0	28.0-40.0 pg
MCHC	34.0	29.0-37.0 g/dL
RDW	16.9	<17.0%
Platelet count	358	140-440 × 10³/μL
Coagulation		
PT	13.7	12.6-15.2 sec
INR	1.0	0.9-1.1
PTT	96.1	22.7-36.0 sec
Factor levels: VII	70	50-150%
VIII	<1	50-186%
IX	28	50-150%

WBC, white blood cell; MCV, mean corpuscular volume; MCH, mean corpuscular hemoglobin; MCHC, mean corpuscular hemoglobin concentration; RBC, red blood cell; RDW, red cell distribution width; PT, prothrombin time; PTT partial thromboplastin time; INR, international normalized ratio.

T2. Reference Intervals for Various Coagulation Tests in Healthy Premature (30-36 Weeks Gestation) Infants and Healthy Adults[a]

| Test | Day after birth | | | Adults |
	1	30	180	
Screening Tests				
PT, sec	10.6-16.2	10.0-13.6	10.0-15.0	10.8-13.9
INR	0.61-1.70	0.53-1.11	0.05-1.48	0.64-1.17
PTT, sec	27.5-79.4	26.9-62.5	27.2-53.3	26.6-40.3
TT, sec	19.2-30.4	18.8-29.9	18.9-31.5	19.7-30.3
Clotting Factors With Lower Levels in Young Children Than Adults				
Factor		**%**		
II	20-77	36-95	51-123	70-146
V	41-144	48-156	58-146	62-150
VII	21-113	21-145	47-151	67-143
IX	19-65	13-80	50-120	55-163
X	11-71	20-92	35-119	70-152
XI	8-52	15-71	46-110	67-127
XII	10-66	11-75	22-142	52-164
PK	9-57	31-87	40-116	62-162
HMWK	9-89	16-112	41-125	50-136
Clotting Factors With Similar or Higher Levels in Young Children Than Adults				
Fibrinogen, mg/dL	150-373	150-414	150-360	156-400
VIII, %	50-213	50-199	50-187	50-149
vWF, %	78-210	66-216	54-158	50-158

[a]Modified from Ref. 10. PT, prothrombin time; INR, international normalized ratio; PTT partial thromboplastin time;TT, thrombin time; PK, prekallikrein; HMWK, high molecular weight kininogen.

Questions

1. Given this infant's history and physical examination findings, how should his bleeding disorder be evaluated?

2. Based on clinical and laboratory testing, how are primary hemostasis defects differentiated from secondary hemostasis defects?

3. In terms of laboratory test reference intervals, how should this infant's laboratory results be evaluated?

4. What is (are) this infant's most striking laboratory findings?

5. What is the best interpretation of this patient's laboratory results?

6. How do coagulation factor levels differ in neonates compared with adults?

7. What is this patient's most likely diagnosis?

8. How should this patient's disorder be treated?

Possible Answers

1. For patients who present with bleeding disorders, a complete history (including family history) and physical examination yield the most valuable data to lead to a diagnosis. If the patient is male, X-linked recessive conditions such as hemophilia A or B should be considered,

although other autosomal disorders cannot be ruled out. The age of onset is also helpful. Early-onset vitamin K deficiency can manifest in the first week after birth, while delayed-type deficiency may only appear later at 3 to 4 weeks of life.[1] Other associated symptoms provide important clues to the etiology of bleeding diatheses: a healthy-looking child may harbor congenital factor deficiencies; physical abnormalities of the upper extremities may be observed in congenital platelet disorders such as TAR syndrome or Fanconi's anemia[2]; jaundice, hepatomegaly, poor weight gain, foul-smelling stool may indicate liver disease or a malabsorption syndrome resulting in secondary vitamin K deficiency[3]; and an ill-appearing child may have sepsis syndrome and disseminated intravascular coagulation (DIC). A comprehensive history of medications used by either the neonate or the mother is also important. Prenatal exposure to phenytoin or phenobarbital may predispose an infant to vitamin K deficiency.[4] While a history of bleeding problems in relatives may guide the evaluation of the patient, a negative family history does not exclude a congenital condition. Indeed, 30% of hemophilia cases are due to new mutations.[5]

2. When evaluating specific bleeding symptoms, one should attempt to differentiate between primary and secondary hemostatic problems. **Primary hemostasis defects**, also known as blood vessel or platelet-type bleeding, usually present with petechiae, purpura, and/or mucosal or prolonged bleeding from a small wound.[6] Initial laboratory testing in these circumstances should include a complete blood count (CBC) and examination of platelet morphology. Other tests include platelet aggregation and measurement of von Willebrand factor (vWF) levels. In **secondary hemostasis defects** (or coagulation type-bleeding), patients commonly present with hemorrhages into soft tissue or muscular structures, with hemarthroses or hemorrhage in internal organs.[6] For these types of presentation, initial studies should include a prothrombin time (PT), partial thromboplastin time (PTT), and thrombin time (TT). Prolongation of any of these tests may be the result of a coagulation factor deficiency or, more rarely, a circulating inhibitor. Follow-up testing should include repeating any of these tests that are abnormal using a mixture of patient's plasma and normal human

plasma (ie, a "mixing study"). A correction of the test result to within 10% of the normal human plasma result suggests a factor deficiency, while lack of correction (ie, a persistently prolonged result) suggests the presence of a factor inhibitor.[7] Factor assays or other specialized coagulation tests can then be performed to further characterize the abnormality.

3. The neonatal hemostatic system is physiologically immature as reflected by prolonged coagulation screening tests such as PT and PTT.[8-10] Thus, interpretation of laboratory test results should be based on age-specific reference intervals (**T2**).

4. Decreased RBC count, hemoglobin, and hematocrit; markedly prolonged PTT with a normal PT; markedly decreased factor VIII and low factor IX levels.

5. The patient's anemia may be accounted for by the history of blood losses from heel sticks, and possibly by his history of twin gestation and premature birth which usually lead to lower iron stores compared with full term babies. In addition, at 1 month, he is at the nadir of the physiologic anemia of infancy. A prolonged PTT and normal PT indicate a defect in the intrinsic pathway of the coagulation cascade. The potentially implicated factor deficiencies include factors VIII, IX, and XI.[7] Deficiencies of factor XII, high molecular kininogen, and prekallikrein are not associated with bleeding. Although contamination of the specimen by heparin is also a possibility, a normal TT excludes this possibility. Among bleeding disorders in the general population, hemophilia A (factor VIII deficiency) is 6 times more common than hemophilia B (factor IX deficiency) with an incidence of 1 in 5,000 male births, and comprises 80% to 85% of all cases of hemophilia.[11] Since one-third of cases of hemophilia A or B are due to *de novo* mutations, failure to recognize this possibility can lead to delay in diagnosis and management. However, this infant's test results show low levels of both factors VIII and IX, raising the concern that he could have both hemophilia A and B, which would be an exceedingly rare occurrence.

6. In term newborns, factor VIII activity may be higher on the first day of life than it is in adults,

falling to adult levels by about the tenth postnatal day. In addition, factor VIII-associated antigen levels have been found to be even higher than factor VIII activity, and to not decrease in the first 10 days of life.[12] Thus, it is possible to make a diagnosis of hemophilia A in a neonate if factor VIII levels are low. In our neonate, the variability we observed in postnatal factor VIII levels (*see History of Present Illness*) might have been secondary to a rise in factor VIII associated with postnatal stress, a phenomenon well-documented in non-hemophilic newborns.[13] Since factor VIII is an acute-phase reactant, it might have been released from endothelial cells and caused a higher plasma level than expected. In contrast, a diagnosis of hemophilia B may be masked in the neonatal period because factor IX, like the other vitamin K-dependent factors (II, VII, and X) are normally reduced at birth, especially in preterm infants.[8,9] (**T2**). Thus, although the diagnosis of severe and moderate hemophilia B is possible at birth, confirmation of mildly affected cases is problematic due to overlap of test results in such cases with the normal range. Repeat testing at around 6 months of age may be necessary to confirm or exclude a diagnosis of hemophilia B, unless molecular analysis is used when there is a known familial genetic defect.[14] A normal PT helps exclude vitamin K deficiency as an alternative explanation for low factor IX. In a dubious case of vitamin K deficiency, a factor VII level would be a good indicator, since factor VII is produced solely by the liver and has the shortest half-life of all coagulation factors. Thus, it is the first coagulation factor to decrease in vitamin K deficiency or liver disease.

7. **Most likely diagnosis:** this infant has factor VII and IX levels within the age-specific reference interval for these factors and an undetectable factor VIII level, consistent with the diagnosis of **severe hemophilia A**.

8. Specific treatment for hemophilia A is factor VIII replacement to prevent or treat bleeding symptoms. Current practice in the developed world is to use recombinant factor VIII, since these products are not capable of transmitting viral infections.[15,16] Although desmopressin (DDAVP) is a useful agent for the management of mild hemophilia A in older children, its use is contraindicated during the neonatal period due to

the risk of hyponatremia.[15] Fresh frozen plasma is also not recommended in the treatment of neonatal hemophilia, but may be given in the limited context of acute hemorrhage in a patient with a suspected congenital factor deficiency for whom confirmatory testing is not yet available.[5,14] Further work-up is warranted to confirm the need for genetic counseling. If an individual is the first of his family members with hemophilia A, it is likely that this individual carries a new mutation in the factor VIII gene. However, the likelihood remains that his mother is a carrier of hemophilia A, either by inheritance or through a *de novo* mutation. Thus, in the case of our infant, the mother's factor VIII level should be measured and if it is found to be in the range (40% to 50%) of a carrier, the twin sister's factor VIII level should also be evaluated. If the mother is a carrier, there is a 50% risk of her having another son with hemophilia A and a daughter with the carrier state in each subsequent pregnancy.

Keywords

neonatal bleeding, pediatric coagulation factor ranges, hemophilia

References

1. Sutor AH. New aspects of vitamin k prophylaxis. *Semin Thromb Hemost.* 2003;29:373-362.

2. Alter BP. Bone marrow failure syndromes in children. *Pediatr Clin North Am.* 2002;49:973-988.

3. Demirören K. Intracranial hemorrhage due to vitamin K deficiency after the newborn period. *Pediatr Hematol Oncol.* 2004;21:585-592.

4. Thorp JA, Gaston L, Caspers DR, et al. Current concepts and controversies in the use of vitamin K. *Drugs.* 1995;49:376-387.

5. Conway JH, Hilgartner MW. Initial presentation of pediatric hemophiliacs. *Arch Pediatr Adolesc Med.* 1994;148:589-594.

6. Allen GA, Bertil G. Approach to the bleeding child. *Pediatr Clin North Am.* 2002;49:1239-1256.

7. Bethel M, Adcock DM. Laboratory evaluation of a prolonged APTT and PT. *Lab Med.* 2004;35:285-292.

8. Andrew M, Paes B, Milner R, et al. Development of the human coagulation system in the full term infant. *Blood.* 1987;70:165-172.

9. Andrew M, Peas B, Milner R, et al. Development of the human coagulation system in the healthy premature infant. *Blood.* 1988;72:1651-1657.

10. Male C, Johnston M, Sparling C, et al. The influence of developmental haemostasis on the laboratory diagnosis and management of haemostatic disorders during infancy and childhood. *Clin Lab Med.* 1999;19:39-69.

11. Kulkarni R, Lusher J. Perinatal management of neonates with haemophilia. *Br J Haematol.* 2001;112:264-274.

12. Muntean W, Belohradsky BH, Klose HJ, et al. Factor VIII activity and factor VIII associated antigen in newborns. *Klin Padiatr.* 1977;189:412-413.

13. Maak B, Frenzel J. Factor VIII activity and factor VIII-associated antigen in healthy newborns and in newborns with stressing perinatal factors. *Folia Haematol Int Mag Klin Morphol Blutforsch.* 1982;109:334-345.

14. Chalmers EA. Hemophilia and the newborn. *Blood Rev.* 2004;18:85-92.

15. Williams MD, Chalmers EA, Gibson BES. Guideline: the investigation and management of neonatal haemostasis and thrombosis. *Br J Haematol.* 2002;119:295-309.

16. Dunn AL, Abshire TC. Recent advances in the management of the child who has hemophilia. *Hematol Oncol Clin North Am.*

A 5-Month-Old Male With an Isolated Prolonged Partial Thromboplastin Time

Alde Carlo P. Gavino

Department of Pathology, UT Southwestern Medical Center, Dallas, TX

Patient: 5-month-old Caucasian male.

Physical Examination Findings: No signs of any bleeding.

History of Present Illness: The patient presented for evaluation of a markedly elevated partial thromboplastin time (PTT) that was first detected immediately following birth (**T1**). The level of Factor IX was reported to be unquantifiable "possibly secondary to the presence of inhibitors." On repeat testing (**T1**), the patient's Factor IX level was found to be markedly decreased. An inhibitor screen was performed at this time and was negative.

Medical History: The patient was born without complications by spontaneous vaginal delivery. The pregnancy was unremarkable. The patient had not bled since birth.

Family History: The patient's mother was a symptomatic hemophilia B carrier with a Factor IX level of 16%, and his maternal uncle had moderate hemophilia B with a Factor IX level of 2%.

T1. Principal Laboratory Findings

Test	Patient's Result Initial @ t_0	Repeat @ t_1	Normal Reference Range
PT	13.0	11.1	9.2–12.5 seconds
PTT	104.2	84.7	23.5–33.5 seconds
Inhibitor screen	Not Done	Negative	Negative
Factor IX activity	Uaq[1]	<1%	82–155%

[1]*Unable to quantify possibly secondary to the presence of inhibitors.*

Questions

1. What are this patient's most striking clinical and laboratory findings?

2. What factors should be considered in arriving at differential diagnoses for this patient?

3. What are this patient's differential diagnoses?

4. What is this patient's most likely diagnosis?

5. How is this patient's disease differentiated from the other diseases constituting his differential diagnoses?

6. What is the inheritance pattern and epidemiology of this patient's disease?

7. What are the bleeding manifestations of this patient's disease?

8. How is the confirmatory laboratory test for this patient's disease performed?

9. How is this patient's disease treated?

T2. Classification of the Severity of Hemophilia[1]

Characteristics	Degree of Hemophilia		
	Mild	Moderate	Severe
Distribution of patients, %	30–40	10	50–70
Factor VIII/IX activity, %	6–30	1–5	<1
Pattern of bleeding episodes	Uncommon	4–6/year	2–4/month
Etiology of bleeding episodes	Major trauma Surgery	Minor trauma	Spontaneous

[1]Adapted from Ref 2.

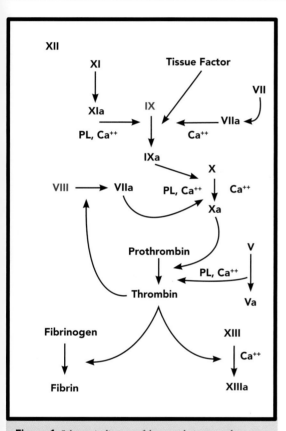

Figure 1_Schematic diagram of the coagulation cascade illustrating the factors whose deficiencies are associated with hemophilia A (Factor VIII) and B (Factor IX). HK, high molecular weight kininogen; PK, prekallikrein; PL, phospholipid.

10. What prophylactic measures are appropriate for this patient's disease?

11. How is dosing of coagulation factor concentrates determined?

12. What complications can arise in the treatment of individuals with this patient's disease?

13. How is coagulation factor inhibitor activity measured?

14. How is information on coagulation factor inhibitor activity used to treat patients whose blood contains these inhibitors?

Possible Answers _____

1. No history of bleeding in a patient with a family history of hemophilia, a markedly elevated partial thromboplastin time (PTT), a normal prothrombin time (PT), a negative inhibitor screen, and a markedly decreased Factor IX level (**T1**).

2. When faced with a patient who presents with an isolated prolonged PTT, the first thing that needs to be determined is whether or not the patient is bleeding. This piece of information is crucial in zeroing in on the cause of the patient's abnormal PTT. Additional pertinent information includes a family history of bleeding disorders, medical illnesses requiring anticoagulation, history of bleeding or clotting, and the pattern of bleeding. Appropriate laboratory testing will usually identify with high accuracy the exact cause of the patient's prolonged PTT and/or bleeding disorder.

3. In a patient who is bleeding: heparin therapy, von Willebrand disease (vWD), hemophilia (Factor VIII or IX deficiency), and Factor XI deficiency. In a patient who is not bleeding: lupus anticoagulant or a deficiency in 1 of the

contact factors (ie, Factor XII, prekallikrein, or high molecular weight kininogen).

4. ***Most likely diagnosis:*** *severe hemophilia B.* Although our patient at presentation had not yet manifested signs and symptoms of bleeding, hemophilia B was the most likely diagnosis given that he was not on heparin therapy, his family history was positive for hemophilia B, and laboratory testing revealed a marked deficiency in Factor IX level. Hemophilia B is usually diagnosed after patients, typically male neonates or infants, with a positive family history or a history of bleeding in their extremities soon after they started to crawl or walk, are tested and found to have a deficiency in Factor IX.

5. Von Willebrand disease (vWD) is a congenital or acquired, qualitative or quantitative, deficiency of von Willebrand factor (vWF), a multimeric protein that plays a pivotal role in hemostasis. Von Willebrand factor is a carrier protein for Factor VIII, and its absence promotes rapid clearance of Factor VIII from plasma.[1] In addition, vWF is an adhesive platelet ligand that anchors platelets to subendothelial collagen exposed by vascular injury.[1] Von Willebrand factor is diagnosed by performing assays for vWF antigen and/or the vWF ristocetin cofactor activity. Factor XI deficiency is most common in Ashkenazi Jews, and patients rarely have spontaneous hemorrhages. Instead, abnormal bleeding usually follows injury or surgery, particularly those involving areas of the body with high fibrinolytic activity such as the oral and nasal cavities and the genitourinary tract.[2] Factor XI activity level is decreased in these patients. Patients with lupus anticoagulant test positively in the laboratory and typically have, instead of bleeding, a history of venous and arterial thromboses. Among the contact factor deficiencies, Factor XII deficiency is most common.[2] Deficiencies in Factor XII and high molecular weight kininogen (a rare disorder) both cause a marked elevation of the PTT.[2] By contrast, prekallikrein deficiency causes the PTT to be only mildly prolonged.[2] When suspecting contact factor deficiency, a Factor XII assay should be performed first (given the fact Factor XII deficiency is most common). Since patients do not bleed and no factor replacement therapy is necessary, contact factor deficiency needs to be accurately diagnosed when present, in order to avoid unnecessary factor infusions.

6. Hemophilia is a hereditary bleeding disorder of specific blood clotting factors (**Figure 1**). Hemophilia A is caused by Factor VIII deficiency and is the most common severe congenital bleeding disorder affecting 1 in 5,000 to 10,000 males.[2] Hemophilia B, on the other hand, is due to Factor IX deficiency and affects 1 in 25,000 to 30,000 males.[2] The genes that encode for Factors VIII and IX are located on the X chromosome. Hemophilia A and B are X-linked recessive disorders that mainly affect males. Females can harbor a defective gene on 1 of their X chromosomes and are then called "carriers." Female carriers may become symptomatic when they have an imbalanced Lyonization of the normal X chromosome, Turner syndrome (46; XO), or if they are daughters of an affected male and a carrier female.[2] The most common genetic defect in hemophiliacs is inversion of intron 22, which is present in 40% to 45% of patients.[2] Other genetic defects have been found to cause a defective Factor VIII or IX protein, and these include severe defects such as large deletions and nonsense mutations, and less severe defects such as small deletions, missense mutations, and splice-site mutations.[3] Of note, one-third of hemophilia cases arise from spontaneous mutations.[2] The majority of hemophiliacs are diagnosed at birth after screening and confirmatory tests, prompted by a positive family history, are performed. Those with spontaneous mutations, by contrast, are diagnosed later (ie, after they present with bleeding symptoms as soon as they begin crawling or walking).

7. Like other clotting factor disorders, hemophilia shares a constellation of bleeding manifestations that may include easy bruising; hemarthrosis; soft tissue hematomas (including bleeding into muscles); excessive bleeding with surgery, trauma, dental extraction, and circumcision; bleeding into the gastrointestinal and genitourinary tracts; epistaxis; poor wound healing; and, uncommonly, umbilical stump bleeding.[2] Based on the plasma factor level, hemophilia is classified into 3 categories: mild, moderate, and severe (**T2**).[2] Mild hemophiliacs usually do not manifest symptoms until they undergo trauma or major surgery, during which time they will

present with prolonged bleeding. They rarely require intravenous factor replacement. Severe hemophiliacs, by contrast, typically present with frequent spontaneous bleeds requiring treatment and/or prophylactic therapy with replacement factor products.

8. When hemophilia is suspected in a patient with a prolonged PTT, Factor VIII or IX assays are completed to confirm the diagnosis. Factor assays involve mixing a patient's plasma with a substrate that is deficient in the specific factor being tested. The degree of correction achieved by this mixture is measured using a PTT-based test. The result is then calculated by comparing it with the degree of correction obtained when various dilutions of assayed normal plasma are mixed with the same factor-deficient substrate.[2] The test is reported as a percentage of normal factor activity. Plasma with 100% factor activity contains 1 U/mL of that factor and 1 unit of a factor is the amount of the factor present in 1 mL of normal pooled human plasma.[2] Typical reference ranges for Factors VIII and IX are 50% to 150% and 82% to 155%, respectively.

9. Prompt and appropriate treatment of hemorrhages and prophylactic therapy are key to the successful management of patients with hemophilia. Both treatment of bleeding episodes and prophylactic therapy to prevent these episodes involve the use of factor concentrates. In the past, coagulation factors were derived from human and animal plasma, putting hemophiliacs at risk for contracting blood-borne infectious diseases. Recombinant factor products have since been developed. Because no human or animal sources are used to manufacture them, recombinant products are free of any blood-borne infectious organisms, virtually eliminating this potential complication of factor replacement therapy. Recombinant Factor VIII products currently available include Recombinate (first generation), Helixate/Kogenate FS and ReFacto (second generation), and Advate (third generation).[4] There is only 1 recombinant Factor IX product commercially available and this is marketed as BeneFIX.[4] For patients with mild to moderate hemorrhages such as those involving the oral and nasal cavities, the goal is to raise Factor VIII levels to at least 30% to 40% and Factor IX levels to at least 30%.[5] When bleeding episodes involve the cranium, bowels, or airways, aggressive factor replacement is imperative. The goal in these life-threatening situations is to promptly normalize Factor VIII or IX levels to 100% to 150% and then to maintain a level between 80% to 100% in the next 5 to 7 days, followed by a vigorous maintenance program.[5]

10. Dosing of factor concentrates is based on the patient's weight and the desired plasma factor level. Factor VIII levels increase by 2% for each unit of recombinant factor/kg used.[2] Thus, to determine the appropriate dose of Factor VIII needed to treat epistaxis in a 20-kg child with severe hemophilia A (Factor VIII level <1%), the following calculation is used: dose of Factor VIII (units) = desired rise in plasma Factor VIII (percent) × body weight (kg) × 0.5. Therefore, to achieve a factor level of 40% in this patient, 400 U (40% × 20 kg × 0.5) of Factor VIII needs to be infused. By contrast, each unit of recombinant Factor IX/kg raises factor activity by 0.8% in adults and 0.7% in children. Thus, the following formula is used when calculating the dose of Factor IX needed to treat epistaxis in a 20-kg child with severe hemophilia B: dose of Factor IX (units) = desired rise in plasma Factor IX (percent) × body weight (kg) × 1.4 (1.25 in adults). To achieve a plasma level of 40%, 1,120 U (40% × 20 × 1.4) of Factor IX needs to be administered to this patient. The half-life of Factor VIII is 12 hours while that of Factor IX is 24 hours.[2] Thus, Factor VIII is given in more frequent doses than Factor IX.

11. Prophylactic therapy of patients with hemophilia constitutes regularly scheduled infusions of clotting factors. This concept was developed in Sweden in 1958.[4] Since then, the prophylactic use of Factor VIII and IX concentrates has become an integral part of the management of hemophiliacs, particularly in developed countries. Studies have shown that many patients benefit from prophylaxis (versus replacing deficient factors only when patients are bleeding) in that it allows patients to have a more normal lifestyle by preventing the majority of bleeding episodes and preventing joint disease secondary to hemarthroses. The optimal time to initiate prophylaxis is controversial. One school of thought advocates that prophylaxis be instituted during the second year of life when the patient is not bleeding or

after the first joint bleed, whichever comes first.[4] It has been shown that early prophylaxis may reduce the frequency of bleeding into joints.[6] However, early prophylaxis may increase the overall cost of therapy and may promote the development of inhibitors.[4] Moreover, since 10% to 14% of patients with severe hemophilia rarely have bleeding episodes, these patients may be over-treated by this early approach.[4] The second school of thought believes that hemophiliacs should be started on prophylaxis only after they have developed a pattern of bleeding.[4] This approach may decrease the overall cost of therapy and also lessen the likelihood of needing a central venous access device.[7] A major concern however is that even just 1 or 2 episodes of hemarthrosis might be enough to cause a slowly progressive arthropathy that might take years before it is recognized clinically.[4] An example of a prophylactic regimen for hemophilia A involves giving 25 U/kg of Factor VIII on Monday and Wednesday and then giving 35 U/kg on Friday (to tide the patient over the weekend). For hemophilia B, because of the longer half-life of Factor IX, the typical dose given is 80 to 100 U/kg twice every week.

12. The development of factor inhibitors in hemophiliacs is a serious complication that results in limited or no response to standard factor replacement therapy. The risk of bleeding in patients with inhibitors is significantly higher than in those without inhibitors.[8] Thus, inhibitors put patients at risk for repetitive joint bleeds that might lead to arthropathy and permanent disability. Inhibitors develop secondary to exposure to exogenously administered coagulation factors. The incidence has been estimated to be as high as 20% to 30% in patients with hemophilia A and to be significantly less (<5%) in patients with hemophilia B.[8] Moreover, the incidence of inhibitor development is higher in severe cases of hemophilia.[8] It is important to note that the prevalence of inhibitors in hemophilia A patients is much lower than the estimated incidence.[3] This is due to the fact that there are patients who develop inhibitors only transiently and also those who are cured by immune tolerance induction. Why some patients develop inhibitors and some do not has been attributed to several factors including genetics, environmental influences, and the type of replacement factor and

therapeutic regimen used.[3,9] A genetic etiology is supported by the fact that inhibitors have a higher incidence among siblings compared with extended relatives and in blacks compared with whites.[9] Furthermore, various human leukocyte antigen (HLA) molecules have been found to be linked to inhibitor development.[3] Inhibitors generally develop within the first 50 days following factor exposure, the median being 9 to 12 days.[3] The risk is greatest after the first (versus subsequent) exposure to replacement factors.[3] As mentioned above, early factor exposure may increase the risk of inhibitor development. Finally, switching from 1 type of factor product to another could induce development of inhibitors.[10] The presence of inhibitors is usually suspected when a patient, who previously showed good response to treatment, fails to respond to an appropriate dose of factor concentrate. To test for this, a factor inhibitor screen is first performed, which, if positive, is followed by a factor inhibitor assay.

13. Factor inhibitor activity is measured in Bethesda Units (BU). One BU is the amount of antibody that neutralizes 50% of Factor VIII or IX in normal plasma.[3] Based on the amount of inhibitor activity present, patients are classified into those with high-titer or low-titer inhibitors. High-titer inhibitors have a peak historical titer of greater than 5 BU and exhibit an anamnestic response to factor re-exposure.[11] By contrast, low-titer inhibitors have a peak historical titer of less than 5 BU and do not increase with factor re-exposure.[11]

14. Low-titer inhibitors are treated by overwhelming them with large doses of factor concentrates.[11] On the other hand, high-titer inhibitors are dealt with using bypassing agents. These agents are referred to as such because they provide factors that "bypass" the steps in the coagulation cascade that require the action of Factor VIII and IX (**Figure 1**). There are 2 bypassing agents currently available: FEIBA (Factor Eight Inhibitor Bypassing Activity) and NovoSeven (Activated Recombinant Factor VII or rFVIIa). FEIBA contains Factors II, IX, and X, activated Factor VII, and small amounts of Factor VIII, and has been shown to be effective in 81% to 96% of bleeding cases.[11,12] It is typically given every 6 to 12 hours, and it can be administered at home. Some of the disadvantages of using FEIBA include the

fact that Factor VIII present in the product may cause an anamnestic response, and that it may cause thromboembolic events, particularly in patients who have obesity, hyperlipidemia, or liver disease.[11] NovoSeven is effective in 92% of bleeding cases.[11] Anamnesis is not associated with the use of NovoSeven because it is devoid of Factor VIII and IX;[11] however, it is very expensive and because of its short half-life, it has to be given frequently. Thrombotic events have also been reported with NovoSeven use, although they are less common than those associated with FEIBA.[11] Unfortunately, no studies have been completed as of yet to compare FEIBA head-to-head against NovoSeven. Until then, the decision to use either product will depend on the clinical situation and the preferences of both patients and clinicians. Patients with high-titer inhibitors may also be treated with immune tolerance induction (ITI). Immune tolerance induction has been shown to be the most effective long-term strategy for the treatment of patients with high-titer inhibitors.[8] Moreover, it remains the only known strategy capable of eliminating inhibitors.[8] Patients treated with ITI receive factor concentrates over an extended period of time, with most dosing intervals ranging from twice per day to every other day. Ideal factor dosages have not been established. The success rate of ITI is estimated to be 60% to 80% in hemophilia A and 36% in hemophilia B.[11] Tolerance can usually be achieved in 1 to 3 years. ITI fails in 29% of patients.[11] Of those successfully treated, 15% will relapse.[11]

Acknowledgments

The assistance provided by Dr. Ravindra Sarode and Kim Miller, RN, in providing helpful suggestions and information related to the content of this case study is gratefully acknowledged.

Keywords

hemophilia B, coagulation factor inhibitor, von Willebrand disease, bypassing agents

References

1. Miller JL, Rao AK. Blood Platelets and von Willebrand Disease. 747-69. In: McPherson RA and Pincus MR, eds. *Henry's Clinical Diagnosis and Management by Laboratory Methods*, 21st ed. Philadelphia, PA: Saunders Elsevier; 2007.

2. Schmaier AH, Thornburg CD, Pipe SW. Coagulation and Fibrinolysis. 729-46. In: McPherson RA and Pincus MR, eds. *Henry's Clinical Diagnosis and Management by Laboratory Methods*, 21st ed. Philadelphia, PA: Saunders Elsevier; 2007.

3. Astermark J. Overview of inhibitors. *Semin Hematol.* 2006;43:S3–S7.

4. Dunn AL, Abshire TC. Current issues in prophylactic therapy for persons with hemophilia. *Acta Haematol.* 2006;115:162–171.

5. Montgomery RR, Gill JC, Scott JP. Hemophilia and von Willebrand Disease, 1547-1576. In Nathan DG, Orkin SH, Ginsburg D, Look AT, eds. *Nathan and Oski's Hematology of Infancy and Childhood*, 6th ed. Philadelphia: WB Saunders. 2003.

6. Astermark J, Petrini P, Tengborn L, et al. Primary prophylaxis in severe hemophilia should be started at an early age but can be individualized. *Br J Haematol.* 1999;105:1109–1113.

7. Van Dijk K, Van Der Bom JG, Bax KN, et al. Use of implantable venous access devices in children with severe hemophilia: benefits and burden. *Haematologica.* 2004;89:189–194.

8. Leissinger CA. Inhibitor development in patients with hemophilia: An overview. *Semin Hematol.* 2006;43:S1–S2.

9. Astermark J. Why do inhibitors develop? Principles of and factors influencing the risk for inhibitor development in haemophilia. *Haemophilia.* 2006;12:52–60.

10. Peerlinck K, Arnout J, Gilles JG, et al. A higher than expected incidence of factor VIII inhibitors in multitransfused haemophilia A patients treated with an intermediate purity pasteurized factor VIII concentrate. *Thromb Haemost.* 1997;77:80–86.

11. Mathew P. Current opinion on inhibitor treatment options. *Semin Hematol.* 2006;43:S8–S13.

12. Young G. New Approaches in the management of inhibitor patients. *Acta Haematol.* 2006:115:172–179.

Prolonged aPTT and Normal PT

Kara Partridge, Ravi Sarode

Department of Pathology, University of Texas Southwestern Medical Center, Dallas, TX

Patient: 63-year-old African American male.

Family History: Unremarkable.

Chief Complaint: Right arm and right eye swelling and bruising.

Medical History: Chronic obstructive pulmonary disease (COPD) and hypertension; no history of bleeding in the past.

Drug History: Albuterol and Atrovent for COPD; Verapamil for hypertension.

Physical Examination: Hematoma of the right arm and right eye soft tissues. Bruising of the neck and chest. No hepatosplenomegaly or lymphadenopathy. Pulses adequate bilaterally. Diffuse wheezes on chest auscultation.

T1. Principal Laboratory Findings

Test	Patient's Result	"Normal" Reference Range
WBC count	16.9	4.1-10.9 × 10³/µL
Hemoglobin	9.7	13.2-16.2 g/dL
Hematocrit	28.6	40%-52%
Platelet count	180	140-450 × 10³/µL
PT	10.8	9.8-11.9 s
aPTT	70.0	24.4-34.5 s

WBC, white blood cell; PT, prothrombin time; aPTT, activated partial thromboplastin time.

Questions

1. What is the differential diagnosis in a patient with a prolonged aPTT, but normal PT?

2. What initial screening test is performed to differentiate between coagulation factor deficiencies and factor inhibitors?

3. What test is used to quantify the amount of factor VIII (FVIII) inhibitor in a patient's plasma?

4. What is the most likely diagnosis in this patient?

5. Which individuals develop FVIII inhibitors?

6. What is the mechanism of the bleeding that occurs in individuals with FVIII antibodies?

7. How are individuals with FVIII inhibitor treated?

Possible Answers

1. A congenital or acquired clotting factor deficiency in the intrinsic pathway of the coagulation cascade or the presence of an inhibitor such

T2. Mixing Study Results

APTT (s)		
Mixture	Patient A	Patient B
PP only	70	70
PP + NPP (1:1), immediate mix	33	45
PP + NPP (1:1), incubated 1h at 37°C	55	45
Interpretation	FVIII inhibitor	LA

Patient A was the patient in this case study, while patient B illustrates for comparison the results of mixing studies in a patient with a LA. aPTT, activated partial thromboplastin time; PP, patient's plasma; NPP, normal pooled plasma; LA, lupus anticoagulant.

T3. Results of Additional Laboratory Tests

Test	Patient's Result	"Normal" Reference Range
Factor VIII coagulant Activity	<1%	50%-150%
Human Factor VIII inhibitor assay	10.0	0.0 BU/mL

BU=Bethesda Units.

as a FVIII inhibitor or a lupus anticoagulant (LA). The aPTT provides information about the adequacy of the function of the intrinsic pathway of the coagulation cascade, while the PT provides information about the tissue factor (or extrinsic) pathway. Therefore, an isolated prolonged aPTT indicates that there is a low level of an intrinsic pathway factor. For example, there may be decreased levels of Factors VIII, IX, XI, or XII. Hemophilia A, which is characterized by a congenital deficiency of FVIII, is a typical example of a bleeding disorder associated with a factor deficiency. Other causes of a prolonged aPTT, but normal PT include the presence of a LA in patients with the antiphospholipid antibody (APA) syndrome, the most common acquired hypercoagulable disorder. Lupus anticoagulant is an antibody to the phospholipid (PL) and protein complex in vivo. This antibody interferes with the coagulation cascade in vitro and prolongs the clotting time. Since the PT reagent contains a large amount of PL, the PT test is generally not affected by LA; however, occasionally, when a very strong LA is present, there is prolongation of the PT as well. In contrast to patients with congenital or acquired Factor VIII deficiencies, patients with LA do not have a history of bleeding tendencies.

2. A mixing study. To differentiate between LA and acquired FVIII inhibitor, the mixing study must be done in 2 steps - immediate mix, and a time- and temperature-dependent mix. A mixing study is performed by mixing the patient's plasma with an equal amount of normal pooled plasma

(NPP). To avoid adding PL from platelet membranes, which can neutralize LA and provide complete correction of the aPTT (ie, a false negative result), it is important that both the patient's plasma and NPP be free of platelets (ie, $<5 \times 10^3/\mu L$). An aPTT is then performed immediately on this mixture. If the aPTT value obtained on the 1:1 mixture of patient's plasma and NPP is normal, it suggests that the patient's plasma contains a factor deficiency (eg, FVIII, FIX, FXI, or FXII). If the aPTT value on this mixture is indicative of incomplete correction, however, it suggests the presence of an immediate-acting inhibitor such as LA when the patient has no history of bleeding tendencies or, rarely, a FIX or FXI inhibitor when the patient has a history of bleeding tendencies. FVIII inhibitor is a time- and temperature-dependent neutralizing antibody, hence the immediate mix aPTT will correct, while the aPTT value obtained on the mixture of patient's plasma and NPP incubated for 1 hour at 37°C will be prolonged. In our patient, the mixing study [T2] demonstrated the presence of a time- and temperature-dependent inhibitor, suggestive of an acquired FVIII inhibitor. Moreover, the FVIII level was <1% [T3], thus confirming the diagnosis of acquired hemophilia.

3. The Bethesda assay. This assay quantifies the amount of inhibitor in a patient's plasma by measuring the functional inhibition of FVIII activity in NPP by the patient's plasma. Results are reported in Bethesda Units (BU) per milliliter of plasma (BU/mL). A Bethesda Unit is the amount of inhibitor that inactivates 50% of the FVIII activity in a mixture of equal amounts of patient's plasma and NPP incubated at 37°C for 2 hours.

4. ***Most likely diagnosis:*** *acquired hemophilia due to an acquired FVIII inhibitor.*

5. Congenital hemophiliacs with alloantibody to FVIII and acquired hemophiliacs with an autoantibody to FVIII. To control bleeding, FVIII concentrate is administered to hemophiliacs. *Alloantibodies* to FVIII develop in 15% to 25% of patients with severe hemophilia A because the FVIII protein is recognized as "foreign" by hemophiliacs with no intrinsic FVIII production. In non-hemophiliacs, acquired *autoantibodies* may develop spontaneously, usually in older adults with no apparent underlying disease, pregnant or postpartum women, or persons with drug reactions, malignancy, or immunologic disorders such as systemic lupus erythematosus (SLE).

6. The failure of FVIII-mediated activation of Factor X, a critical step in the cascade of reactions required for normal clotting to occur. FVIII increases the activation of Factor X by 10,000-fold. Antibodies to FVIII neutralize the activity of FVIII resulting in a bleeding tendency. In hemophiliacs, bleeding occurs primarily in joints and soft tissues, and the presence of inhibitors does not increase the frequency of bleeding. In contrast, patients with spontaneously acquired FVIII autoantibodies often have severe, life-threatening bleeding manifested by large hematomas, gross hematuria, or internal hemorrhage in the organs, including the brain.

7. With high doses of human FVIII concentrates or porcine FVIII (Hyate:C) to achieve hemostasis in patients with low-titer inhibitor levels, with prothrombin complex concentrates (PCC) or recombinant FVIIa (rFVIIa, NovoSeven) to eliminate the requirement of FVIII in the coagulation cascade in patients with high-titer inhibitor levels, with immunosuppressants (eg, corticosteroids, cytoxan) to suppress inhibitor production, and/or with other therapies including extracorporeal immunoadsorption, immune tolerance, and intravenous administration of immune globulin (IVIg). The drug of choice is rFVIIa for patients with high-titer FVIII inhibitor levels because this drug acts through the tissue factor pathway and does not utilize the intrinsic pathway. Prothrombin complex concentrates, which contain activated FXa, are effective as well in achieving hemostasis because the presence of FXa bypasses the need for FVIII. Lastly, it is important, of course, for hemophiliacs to avoid situations that may result in bleeding, including venipuncture, intramuscular injections, minor trauma, and the use of aspirin.

References

1. DellaCroce FJ, Kountakis S, Aguilar EF. Manifestations of factor VIII inhibitor in the head and neck. *Arch Otolaryngol Head Neck Surg.* 1999;125:1258-1261.

Prolonged Bleeding From the Tongue in an Infant

Reade Quinton, Frank Nizzi, Ravindra Sarode

Department of Pathology, University of Texas Southwestern Medical Center, Dallas, TX

Patient: 17-month-old male.

Surgical History: None.

Chief Complaint: The patient presented initially following a profuse 4-day episode of bleeding from his tongue sustained during minor trauma from a fall. His mother related that he tended to bleed for prolonged periods from his immunization sites, but there was no other history of bruising or hematomas. At presentation, his hemoglobin was 7 g/dL, and PT and PTT results were within normal limits. The patient was sent home on iron supplementation and was scheduled for a return visit to be more extensively evaluated for a bleeding disorder. On his second visit 6 weeks later, his hemoglobin value had increased; however, his mother reported that he continued to have exaggerated bleeding from minor scratches and cuts.

Medical History: He was born full term via Cesarean section secondary to breech presentation and was not circumcised.

Drug History: The patient had received antibiotics within the past month for an ear infection.

Family History: The patient lived with his mother, father, and 3-year-old brother. There was no family history of a bleeding disorder.

Physical Examination: There was no evidence of hepatosplenomegaly, lymphadenopathy, pallor, jaundice, hematomas, bruising, or actively bleeding scratches or cuts. The mouth and mucosal membranes were unremarkable, with no evidence of lesions or injury.

Questions _____

1. What is (are) this patient's most striking laboratory result(s)?

2. What condition(s) does (do) this patient's laboratory results and history suggest?

3. Which additional test(s) should be performed? Why?

4. What is (are) the most likely diagnosis(es)?

5. Is there any further workup that should be done on this patient?

Possible Answers _____

1. The most striking laboratory results are a markedly prolonged PTT (74.5 sec) and a PFA-100 (platelet function analyzer) closure time of >300 seconds [**T1**]. Also of note (in view of these

T1. Relevant Laboratory Findings

Test	Patient's Result	"Normal" Reference Range
Hemoglobin	11.7	13.2-16.9 g/dL
MCV	77.0	76.2-98.6 fL
WBC count	7.6	4.1-11.1 × 10³/μL
Platelet count	265	174-404 × 10³/μL
PT	11.6	9.8-11.9 s
PTT	74.5	24.4-34.5 s
PTT, mixing study	53.5	24.4-34.5 s
PTT, mixing study	56.3	24.4-34.5 s (1h incubation at 37°C)
PFA-100 closure +Epi	>300	75-187 s
time +ADP	>300	63-114 s

MCV, mean corpuscular volume; WBC, white blood cell; PT, prothrombin time; PTT, partial thromboplastin time; PFA, platelet function analyzer; Epi, epinephrine; ADP, adenosine diphosphate.

T2. Results of Lupus Anticoagulant Panel

Test	Patient's Result	"Normal" Reference Range
PTT-LA	>200	<50 s
DRVVT screen	59.3	<42 s
DRVVT confirmatory	30.9	<42 s
DRVVT ratio	1.92	<1.30

PTT-LA, partial thromboplastin time-lupus anticoagulant; DRVVT, dilute Russell viper venom time.

T3. Results of vWF Studies

Test	Patient's Result	"Normal" Reference Range
FVIII Level	Decreased[a]	
vWF antigen	37	50%-150%
vWF ristocetin cofactor	<20	50%-150%

[a]An accurate value could not be obtained due to the interference of LA in the PTT-based FVIII assay. vWF, von Willebrand factor.

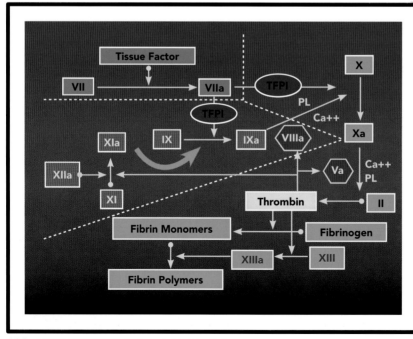

Image 1_ The coagulation cascade.

results) are normal values for the PT and the platelet count.

2. Prolongation of the PTT (or aPTT, activated PTT) reflects a defect in the intrinsic pathway of the coagulation cascade [**Image 1**]. Therefore, possible explanations for this finding include: 1) a clotting factor deficiency (ie, factor VIII, IX, XI, and/or XII); 2) von Willebrand disease (vWD); 3) the presence of an antiphospholipid antibody [eg, a lupus anticoagulant (LA)]; or 4) heparin therapy, which can be excluded in this case because the patient was not on heparin therapy. Moreover, the patient's markedly increased PFA-100 closure times, when coupled with his history of mucocutaneous bleeding, suggests the presence of a primary hemostasis disorder, such as vWD or platelet dysfunction.

3. To distinguish between a hemostasis disorder due to the presence of a factor deficiency versus an inhibitor, a mixing study is typically performed. The patient's plasma is mixed 1:1 with normal pooled plasma (containing normal levels of all clotting factors), and a PTT is performed immediately and after a 1-hour incubation at 37°C. Correction of the PTT to a value similar to the normal control value suggests a factor deficiency, whereas a partial correction (ie, the PTT value decreases but is still higher than the PTT value obtained on the normal control plasma) suggests the presence of an inhibitor. Because some inhibitors (eg, factor VIII inhibitors) are time- and temperature-dependent, they will show immediate correction and then a prolonged PTT using the mixture incubated for 1 hour at 37°C. In this patient's case, the immediate and 1-hour mixing studies showed a partial correction of his initial PTT value (74.5 seconds) to 53.5 and 56.3 seconds, respectively (normal control PTT value = 34.5 seconds) [**T1**]. These results are consistent with the presence of an immediately-acting inhibitor, such as a LA. Therefore, a LA panel was performed, the results of which are shown in **T2**. Lupus anticoagulant was first described in patients with systemic lupus erythematosus (SLE). Lupus anticoagulant is a double misnomer, because in vivo, it causes thrombosis, rather than a bleeding diathesis (ie, it is not an anticoagulant like heparin), and it is found more commonly in patients without rather than with SLE. Thus, in this patient,

it is the most likely cause of his prolonged PTT, but not his symptoms. Lupus anticoagulant is a rather common finding in children with a prolonged PTT, and it tends to be transient in nature, often not causing any symptoms. This acquired nature fits with the patient's history of a normal PTT during his initial evaluation 6 weeks earlier. Diagnosis of a LA requires a positive screening test, followed by a positive confirmatory test. **T2** includes the results of 2 screening tests for the presence of a LA, the PTT-LA, and the dilute Russell viper venom test (DRVVT) and a confirmatory DRVVT. The PTT-LA is performed in a similar manner as a regular PTT; however, a lower amount of phospholipid in the reagent used in the PTT-LA test makes it more sensitive to the presence of an antiphospholipid antibody which causes a marked prolongation of the PTT clotting time. The DRVVT screening test is performed by adding a low concentration of phospholipid and diluted Russell viper venom (an activator of factor X) to the patient's plasma and then performing a clotting time on this mixture. In the presence of a LA, the clotting time is prolonged. To confirm LA, the DRVVT is repeated with excess phospholipids which neutralizes LA and corrects the prolonged clotting time. The DRVVT is considered positive if the ratio of the screening result to the confirmatory result (ie, DRVVT ratio = $DRVVT_{screen}$, seconds:$DRVVT_{confirmatory}$, seconds) is greater than 1.3. In our patient's case, both screening tests and a confirmatory test for a LA were positive (ie, the PTT-LA and DRVVT screening tests were positive, and the DRVVT ratio = 1.92 was greater than 1.30) [**T2**], thus confirming the presence of a LA in this patient's plasma. However, our patient's prolonged epinephrine and ADP PFA-100 closure times must be further evaluated. In this test whole blood passes through a collagen-coated membrane with an aperture coated with either epinephrine or ADP. As the blood passes through the aperture, the instrument measures "closure time" (ie, how fast the aperture closes due to the formation of a platelet clot). When used in conjunction, epinephrine and ADP can rule out the most likely primary hemostasis dysfunction, an aspirin effect. In patients taking aspirin, the PFA-100 clotting time with epinephrine is prolonged, while with ADP it is within normal limits. If the PFA-100 closure time is prolonged in the presence of both epinephrine and ADP, then a primary platelet defect or vWD is likely. Among the principal causes of primary hemostasis defects, vWD is far more common than primary platelet disorders and, therefore, should be ruled out first. Initial evaluation should include vWF antigen and FVIII quantitation and assessment of vWF function using ristocetin cofactor assay. If there is a strong suspicion that a platelet disorder is present, platelet aggregation studies may also be appropriate. In our patient, vWF antigen concentration and ristocetin cofactor activity were abnormally low [**T3**], consistent with both quantitative and qualitative vWF defects.

4. ***Most likely diagnosis:*** *von Willebrand disease with a lupus anticoagulant.* Von Willebrand disease is divided into subtypes based on the presence of quantitative or qualitative vWF defects. Type 1 is a mild form of vWD in which vWF is present, but at a decreased level. Type 2 is defined by a number of qualitative vWF defects, including alterations in platelet binding site domains and/or multimer size. In Type 1 vWD, a decrease in vWF antigen and activity parallel each other. In vWD Types 2-A and 2-B, however, the ristocetin cofactor activity is decreased out of proportion to the decrease in antigen concentration (as seen in our patient). In Type 2-A vWD, only small, abnormal vWF multimers are present, while Type 2-B is associated with increased binding of large vWF multimers to platelet glycoprotein Ib. Type 3 vWD is defined by a total absence of vWF, leading to severe bleeding tendencies such as hemophilia A.

5. Further studies are needed to determine the vWD subtype of this patient. The results of the studies presented in this case suggest that our patient has Type 2 vWD; however, vWF multimer analysis and low-dose ristocetin-induced platelet aggregation (RIPA) studies would provide information on the subtype. The low-dose RIPA assay is used to exclude Type 2-B vWD, in which there is a gain of platelet function with spontaneous binding of platelets to vWF and rapid clearing of platelets and multimers. The presence of small vWF multimers would favor subtype 2-A, while an increased response to low ristocetin concentration would be diagnostic of subtype 2-B. The patient's vWF multimer analysis demonstrated the presence of small molecular weight multimers, while the RIPA studies showed decreased platelet aggregation in the presence of both low and high concentrations of ristocetin. Overall, these studies support a diagnosis of *vWD Type 2-A*.

Profound Normocytic Anemia in a 36-Year-Old Woman With Syncopal Episodes

Jonathan Baker, Yin Xu

Department of Pathology, University of Texas Southwestern Medical Center, Dallas, TX

Patient: 36-year-old Hispanic female.

Family History: Unremarkable.

Chief Complaint: The patient presented to our emergency department complaining of syncopal episodes over the previous 2 days, resulting in a fall and bruising of her left hip. The episodes were preceded by dizziness and palpitations and were accompanied by urinary incontinence. She also complained of nausea, headache, neck pain, and minor vaginal bleeding.

Past Medical History: The patient had no significant past medical history. She was taking no medications and had no known drug allergies.

Physical Examination: She was notably pale, alert, and oriented. Her vital signs were: temperature, 37.9°C; blood pressure, 93/68 mm Hg; pulse rate, 90 beats per minute; and respiratory rate, 16 breaths per minute. The remainder of the physical examination was unremarkable.

Additional Diagnostic Procedures and Tests: The patient's blood smear revealed a normocytic and normochromic anemia with frequent RBC fragments, increased polychromasia, and marked thrombocytopenia (**Image 1**). An electrocardiogram showed normal sinus rhythm. A chest X-ray revealed a prominent right hilum, but was otherwise normal. Her stool was guaiac negative and a urine pregnancy test was negative.

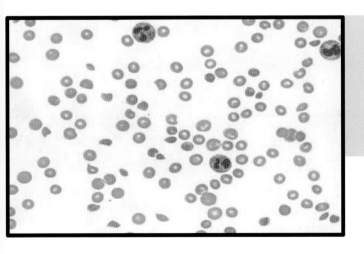

Image 1_Patient's peripheral blood smear demonstrating a profound normocytic and normochromic anemia with reticulocytosis and frequent schistocytes (Wright-Giemsa stain; 500× magnification).

T1. Principal Laboratory Findings

Test	Patient's Result	"Normal" Reference Range
Hematology		
WBC count	12.5	$4.1-11.1 \times 10^3/\mu L$
RBC count	1.98	$4.01-5.31 \times 10^6/\mu L$
Hemoglobin	5.8	12.1-16.1 g/dL
Hematocrit	16.8	36.8-48.7%
MCV	85.2	76.2-98.6 fL
MCH	29.4	24.6-33.4pg
MCHC	34.5	31.6-35.4 g/dL
RDW	18.1	10.8-13.8%
Platelet count	7	$174-404 \times 10^3/\mu L$
Coagulation		
PT	10.7	9.2-12.5 sec
INR	1.0	0.9-1.2
PTT	24.1	24.5-34.5 sec
Chemistry		
Sodium	136	135-145 mmol/L
Potassium	4.0	3.6-5.0 mmol/L
Chloride	101	98-109 mmol/L
CO_2	27	22-31 mmol/L
BUN	21	7-21 mg/dL
Creatinine	0.8	0.6-1.2 mg/dL
Calcium	8.4	8.4-10.2 mg/dL
Phosphorus	3.2	2.4-4.5 mg/dL
Magnesium	1.6	1.4-1.8 mEq/L
Total protein	7.1	6.3-8.2 g/dL
Albumin	4.3	3.5-5.2 g/dL
Bilirubin, total	2.9	0.2-1.3 mg/dL
Bilirubin, direct	0.4	0.0-0.3 mg/dL
AST	34	13-40 U/L
ALT	32	10-40 U/L
GGT	23	8-78 U/L
ALP	105	38-126 U/L
LD	1082	100-190 U/L

WBC, white blood cell; RBC, red blood cell; MCV, mean corpuscular volume; MCH, mean corpuscular hemoglobin; MCHC, mean corpuscular hemoglobin concentration; RDW, red cell distribution width; PT, prothrombin time; INR, International Normalized Ratio; PTT, partial thromboplastin time; BUN, blood urea nitrogen; AST, aspartate aminotransferase; ALT, alanine aminotransferase; GGT, gamma-glutamyl transferase; ALP, alkaline phosphatase; LD, lactate dehydrogenase.

Questions

1. What are this patient's most striking clinical and laboratory findings?

2. How do you explain the patient's most striking clinical and laboratory findings?

3. What condition does this patient's clinical and laboratory findings suggest?

4. What is this patient's most likely diagnosis?

5. What is the pathophysiology of this patient's disease?

6. What is the most appropriate treatment for this patient?

Possible Answers

1. Syncope; a profound normocytic, normochromic anemia with frequent schistocytes; marked thrombocytopenia; elevated indirect bilirubin; markedly elevated LD.

2. **Syncope:** Syncope is a transient loss of consciousness due to reduced cerebral blood flow and is usually caused by 1 of 3 general mechanisms: *disorders of vascular tone or blood volume* (eg, vasovagal, orthostatic hypotension, peripheral neuropathy, antihypertensive or vasodilator drugs, anemia, or blood loss), *cardiovascular disorders,* including cardiac arrhythmias, or *cerebrovascular disease.* Our patient had a profound anemia with low blood pressure, which are the most likely causes of her syncopal episodes. **Anemia:** A normocytic and normochromic anemia can be seen in anemia of chronic disease, blood loss, reduced bone marrow production of RBCs (such as marrow suppression caused by viral infection, toxin, drugs, immunologic diseases, marrow replacement by neoplastic infiltration, or myelodysplasia), or hemolysis (such as immune-mediated hemolytic anemia, microangiopathic hemolytic anemia, or mechanical damage by hypertension in patients with a prosthetic heart valve). In the absence of signs for bleeding, a normocytic anemia with increased polychromasia (reticulocytosis), as occurred

in our patient, suggests a hemolytic anemia. **Thrombocytopenia:** Thrombocytopenia is caused by 1 of 3 mechanisms: decreased bone marrow production of platelets, increased splenic sequestration of platelets, or accelerated destruction or consumption of platelets.[1] The most common causes of decreased platelet production are marrow aplasia, fibrosis, or infiltration by malignant cells, all of which can be diagnosed by bone marrow examination. Approximately one-third of the total platelet mass is normally sequestered in the spleen. When the spleen enlarges, the fraction of sequestered platelets increases and thrombocytopenia results. The most common causes of splenomegaly are portal hypertension due to liver disease and splenic infiltration by tumor cells in myeloproliferative or lymphoproliferative disorders. The most common causes of platelet destruction are immunologic due to viral or bacterial infections, drugs (heparin), and idiopathic thrombocytopenic purpura (ITP). Platelets can be coated with antibodies or complement, and such platelets are then rapidly cleared by macrophages in the spleen or other tissues. Platelet destruction or consumption can also be accelerated by nonimmunologic causes such as abnormal vessels, intravascular prostheses, and fibrin thrombi.[1] Marked thrombocytopenia in conjunction with profound normocytic anemia with frequent schistocytes strongly suggests a consumption of platelets in a microangiopathic hemolytic process. **Elevated indirect bilirubin:** Bilirubin exists in the blood predominantly in 2 fractions: conjugated (or direct) and unconjugated (or indirect). Elevation of the conjugated fraction of bilirubin in the blood is commonly due to liver diseases or biliary obstruction. An isolated elevation of unconjugated bilirubin is infrequently seen in genetic disorders such as Crigler-Najjar and Gilbert's syndrome, and primarily seen in hemolytic anemia, which occurred in our patient. **Elevated LD:** The various isoenzymes of LD are present in various types of cells in liver, lung, myocardium, skeletal muscle, and erythrocytes. Cellular injury causes release of LD into the blood and an elevated serum LD concentration. The combination of our patient's increased indirect bilirubin and normal liver function test results (**T1**) suggests that our patient's hemolytic anemia is the most likely cause of her markedly elevated LD concentration.

3. The patient had an unremarkable past medical history and a normal physical examination except for paleness. Her clinical, laboratory, and morphologic peripheral blood smear findings indicate a microangiopathic hemolytic anemia, possibly due to thrombotic thrombocytopenic purpura (TTP), hemolytic uremic syndrome (HUS), or disseminated intravascular coagulation (DIC).[2] Thrombotic thrombocytopenic purpura is a rare disorder that has been classically characterized by the pentad of findings: fever, thrombocytopenia, microangiopathic hemolytic anemia, transient neurologic deficits, and renal failure.[1] However, only microangiopathic hemolytic anemia and thrombocytopenia are required for the diagnosis of TTP. Hemolytic uremic syndrome and TTP are often difficult to distinguish from each other clinically. Thrombotic thrombocytopenic purpura typically occurs in adults and spares the kidneys, while HUS typically occurs in children and is characterized by the absence of neurologic symptoms and the dominance of acute renal failure. The clinical manifestations of TTP and HUS in adults and children seem to be due to differences in the distribution of microvascular thrombi.[3] Disseminated intravascular coagulation is characterized by widespread intravascular coagulation and the formation of microthrombi that cause bleeding from the consumption of platelets and coagulation factors and the anticoagulant effects of fibrolytic products. In addition to thrombocytopenia, the peripheral blood smear of patients with DIC demonstrates the presence of both schistocytes and spherocytes and coagulation tests (ie, PT and PTT) are commonly abnormally increased. Notably, our patient's PT and PTT values were not increased (**T1**).

4. ***Most likely diagnosis:*** *thrombotic thrombocytopenic purpura (TTP).* Our patient had a microangiopathic hemolytic anemia, thrombocytopenia, and a low fever. Although renal impairment and neurologic changes were not apparent at the time of her admission, they appeared later when her TTP rapidly worsened.

5. Thrombotic thrombocytopenic purpura is caused by a decrease or deficiency of the vonWillebrand factor (VWF) cleaving protease, ADAMTS-13 [13th member of the ADAMTS family of metalloproteases (ie,

metalloproteases containing **A D**isintegrin-like **A**nd **M**etalloprotease with **T**hrombo**S**pondin type I motif)].[4] VonWillebrand factor, a large glycoprotein that is synthesized in endothelial cells and megakaryocytes, promotes platelet adhesion and aggregation. It is produced as a large multimer and assumes a globular form under relatively static conditions, but normally exists in the blood as a series of smaller multimers due to the action of ADAMTS-13. When vascular injury occurs, VWF binds to damaged endothelium and unfolds, enhancing its interaction with platelets to form thrombi. VonWillebrand factor also unfolds in normal circulation when it is exposed to increasing shear stress in arterioles and capillaries. Such unfolding exposes VWF cleavage sites to the action of ADAMTS-13, which cleaves the VWF into smaller multimers. When there is a deficiency of ADAMTS-13, the large VWF multimers unfold in the arterioles and capillaries and induce aggregation of platelets and the formation of microvascular thrombi, which subsequently fragment red cells passing through these areas and result in microangiopathic hemolytic anemia. The deficiency of ADAMTS-13 can be congenital, resulting in chronic relapsing TTP. More commonly, however, the deficiency of ADAMTS-13 is acquired, triggered by infection, drugs (Ticlopidine),[5] and immune system abnormalities [eg, systemic lupus erythematosus (SLE), human immunodeficiency virus (HIV) infection], which lead to an autoimmune reaction to ADAMTS-13 mediated by IgG antibodies. This reaction is usually transient and confined to a single episode.

6. **Management:** The goals of treatment for TTP are to replace the ADAMTS-13 protease and remove the antibodies against it. Plasma exchange accomplishes both of these goals, and should be initiated as early as possible in the treatment of patients with TTP. The introduction of plasma exchange as a treatment for TTP has decreased mortality rates to less than 10%. Previously, TTP was fatal in the majority of cases. Fresh frozen plasma (FFP) infusion can also be used to replace the protease, but it is not as effective as plasma exchange in the treatment of patients with acquired TTP because the antibodies to ADAMTS-13 remain in the patient's plasma. However, FFP infusion has the advantage of speed, and should be utilized until

plasma exchange can begin. Moreover, regular FFP or cryo-poor plasma infusions are sufficient for the treatment of TTP caused by a congenital deficiency of ADAMTS-13. Immunosuppression therapy has also been used with some success in the treatment of TTP, including the use of steroids, Rituxan, and Vincristine. Platelet transfusion is strongly contraindicated in patients with TTP, as it will increase platelet thrombi formation and exacerbate the condition. Moreover, TTP patients generally do not bleed, and therefore, platelet transfusion should only be considered in cases of life-threatening hemorrhage.

Keywords

thrombotic thrombocytopenic purpura, hemolytic uremic syndrome, disseminated intravascular coagulation, von Willebrand factor, schistocyte

References

1. Handin, RI. Harrison's Principles of Internal Medicine, 16th ed. Chapter 101: Disorders of the Platelet and Vessel Wall. The McGraw-Hill Companies, Inc. 2005.

2. Kjeldsberg C, Kojo E-J, Foucar K. Practical Diagnosis of Hematologic Disorders, 3rd ed. Chicago: ASCP Press. 2000;796-798.

3. Hosler GA. Thrombotic thrombocytopenic purpura and hemolytic uremic syndrome are distinct pathologic entities. *Arch Pathol Lab Med.* 2003;127:834-839.

4. Tsai, H-M. Advances in the pathogenesis, diagnosis, and treatment of thrombotic thrombocytopenic purpura. *J Am Soc Nephrol.* 2003;14:1072-1081.

5. Tsai H-M, Rice L, Sarode R. Antibody inhibitors to von willebrand factor metalloproteinase and increased binding of von willebrand factor to platelets in ticlopidine-associated thrombotic thrombocytopenic purpura. *Annals of Int Med.* 2000;132:794-799.

Laboratory Evaluation of Coagulation Inhibitors

Amy L. Adams, Yara M. Audeh, Regina de Luna, Monette S. Baker, Marisa B. Marques

Department of Pathology, Division of Laboratory Medicine, University of Alabama School of Medicine, Birmingham, AL

Patient #	1	2	3	4
Age/Sex: Chief Complaint:	11-year-old female Epistaxis, fever, malaise, and anorexia	43-year-old male Ischemic stroke	11-year-old male Epistaxis that occurred 1 week prior to current evaluation; treated with fresh frozen plasma at another institution where a diagnosis of prothrombin deficiency was made	69-year-old female Easy bruising within the past few weeks
Physical Exam Findings:	Afebrile, well-nourished child with cervical lymphadenopathy		Apparently healthy child in no acute distress with no active bleeding	Large hematoma at the site of an IM injection; multiple ecchymoses in left arm with diffuse swelling
Past Medical History:	Unremarkable	Hypertension	Fever and lymphadenopathy approximately 6 months prior to presentation	Hypertension, diabetes mellitus, rheumatoid arthritis, and asthma
Surgical History:	Tonsillectomy at age 9 years without increased bleeding	None	Circumcision and tonsillectomy without excessive bleeding	Cholecystectomy and hysterectomy without increased bleeding
Family History:	No relatives with a bleeding disorder	Noncontributory	Negative for bleeding disorder	No relatives with a bleeding disorder
Drug History:	Aspirin for fever	Multivitamins	None	Acetaminophen, atenolol, azithromycin, estradiol, glyburide, pravastatin sodium, prednisone, ramipril, and theophylline

Questions _____

1. What are the most striking laboratory results for each of these patients?

2. What are the common causes of an abnormal PTT with a normal PT?

3. What clinical factors should be considered when evaluating patients with abnormal PTT and normal PT results?

4. What is your assessment of the most striking laboratory results for each of the 4 patients presented in these case studies? Include in your assessment the most likely diagnosis for each of the 4 patients presented, how each condition should be treated, and the role of the laboratory in managing these patients.

T1. Principal Laboratory Findings

Test					Reference Range
	1	**2**	**3**	**4**	
Platelet count			287	324	130-400 × 10³/mL
PT, sec	13.8	12.5	25.0	11.2	
PT reference interval, sec	11.3-14.6	11.3-14.6	10.7-13.0	10.7-13.0	
INR			2.3		1.00
Prothrombin activity	82		6		50-150%
PTT	55.0	78.0	62.0	99.5	25.0-34.0 sec
PTT mixing study	43.0		42.0	60.4	Correction to 25.0-34.0 sec
PTT-LA	108.0	90.0	113.0	131.4	36.1-50.1 sec
Staclot® LA delta	20.4		61.5	19.9	<8.0 sec
Thrombin time		16.0	17.0	15.3	<18.0 sec
dRVVT: Check	43.1	78.6	99.2	42.2	29.6-42.9 sec
Mix		56.0			Correction to 29.6-42.9 sec
Sure		37.5	70.2		N/A
ratioª		2.1	1.4		<1.3
Factor VIII activity	135	200		<1%	50-186%
Factor VIII inhibitor	N/A	N/A	N/A	64 BU	Undetectable

ªdRVVT ratio = (dRVVT check)/(dRVVT sure). PT, prothrombin time; INR, International Normalized Ratio; PTT, partial thromboplastin time; LA, lupus anticoagulant; dRVVT, dilute Russell viper venom time; BU, Bethesda units; N/A, not applicable.

T2. Evaluation of Coagulation Test Results for Patients 1 Through 4 Against the ISTH Criteria for the Diagnosis of a Lupus Anticoagulant

Criterion	Patient #			
	1	2	3	4
Prolonged coagulation screening tests (PTT, PTT-LA, or dRVVT)	+	+	+	+
Uncorrectable screening test by mixing study	+	+	+	+
Shortening of abnormal clotting time with addition of excess PL	+	+	+	+
Exclusion of a specific coagulation factor inhibitor	+	+	-	-

+, criterion met; -, criterion not met; ISTH, International Society on Thrombosis and Haemostasis; PTT, partial thromboplastin time; PTT-LA, partial thromboplastin time-lupus anticoagulant; dRVVT, dilute Russell viper venom time; PL, phospholipids.

Possible Answers

1. One or more abnormal screening tests: PT (*Patient #3*), PTT (*Patients #1-4*), PTT-LA (*Patients #1-4*); abnormal PTT mixing study results (*Patients #1-4*); abnormal confirmatory test for the presence of an inhibitor, Staclot® LA delta (*Patients #1, 3, and 4*) and/or dRVVT ratio (*Patients #2 and 3*); low factor VIII activity with an increased factor VIII inhibitor level (*Patient #4*).

2. The most common reasons for prolongation of the PTT with a normal PT are heparin therapy, intrinsic factor deficiencies, presence of a lupus anticoagulant (LA), and/or an intrinsic factor inhibitor (eg, an antibody against factor VIII).

T3. Summary of Most Likely Diagnosis and Rationale for the Diagnosis in Patients #1 through #4

Patient #	Most Likely Diagnosis	Rationale
1	LA with thrombocytopenia*	Fever, malaise, and cervical lymphadenopathy suggest infectious mononucleosis. Viral infections are commonly associated with decreased platelet count, while aspirin is an inhibitor of platelet function and, therefore, a promoter of bleeding such as epistaxis High Staclot® LA delta value Normal PT and prothrombin activity values
2	Antiphospholipid (APL) syndrome	Phospholipid antibodies (eg, LA) are found in 18% of ischemic stroke patients
		dRVVT screening and confirmatory test results consistent with the presence of a less than 44 years old phospholipid inhibitor
3	Acquired prothrombin deficiency due to presence of an LA	Markedly increased Staclot® LA delta value INR > 1.4 Markedly low prothrombin activity level
4	Acquired hemophilia	Occurs typically in individuals over the age of 50
		50% of patients with acquired hemophilia have an associated disorder (eg, RA, SLE, a malignancy, or a drug reaction) Associated with spontaneous bleeding and/or delayed hemostasis Markedly low factor VIII activity Markedly increased factor VIII inhibitor level

Due to the unavailability of the data from the patient's complete blood count (CBC), thrombocytopenia could not be confirmed by a platelet count. RA, rheumatoid arthritis; SLE, systemic lupus erythematosis.

3. When assessing a patient with abnormal coagulation screening tests such as PT and/or PTT, several clinical factors are important to consider in guiding further evaluation in a cost-effective manner: gender, age, drug history, signs/symptoms, and concurrent medical conditions.

4. **Patient #1:** Since this patient is female, the probability of a factor deficiency is low, because the most common factor deficiencies, hemophilia A (deficiency of factor VIII) and hemophilia B (deficiency of factor IX), are X-linked disorders, and therefore only males are affected. Hemophilia carriers have decreased levels of factors VIII or IX, but these patients still have enough factor activity to provide a normal PTT result. Heparin is also an unlikely explanation for this patient's prolonged PTT result because she was not hospitalized and did not have an indwelling catheter. Finally, an antibody to factor VIII is very unlikely because the patient is a child, and specific factor inhibitors occur mainly in older individuals or in association with pregnancy. Thus, the most likely explanation for the prolonged PTT result in this patient is the presence of an LA. The term **lupus anticoagulant** refers to a heterogeneous group of autoantibodies that react with protein-binding phospholipids and thereby affect clotting tests that use a limited supply of phospholipid to form the clot (eg, PTT, PTT-LA, and dRVVT tests).[1] Thus, LAs and anticardiolipin antibodies are called antiphospholipid antibodies. Anticardiolipin antibodies, however, do not prolong clot-based tests and are assayed by ELISA. The International Society on Thrombosis and Haemostasis (ISTH) has defined the following 4 criteria for the diagnosis of LA: (1) at least 1 abnormal screening test (PTT, PTT-LA, or dRVVT) result; (2) lack of correction of the prolonged screening test result after a mixing study has been performed; (3) shortening of an abnormal clotting time with the addition of excess phospholipid (eg, Staclot® LA); and (4) exclusion of a specific factor inhibitor.[2] Evaluation of the coagulation results for *Patient #1* against these criteria indicated that she was likely to have an LA in her plasma [**T2**]. Screening tests such as PTT, PTT-LA, and dRVVT are very sensitive to interference by a phospholipid inhibitor and are typically prolonged in the presence of an LA. Because an abnormal screening test by itself is not specific for LA, additional testing must be done to confirm the diagnosis. A mixing study is helpful

in this scenario and is performed by repeating the initial screening test with the patient's plasma diluted 1:1 with "normal" plasma containing adequate levels of all clotting factors. This mixture would be expected to correct an abnormal screening test result that was due to a specific coagulation factor deficiency. In the case of an abnormal screening test due to the presence of an inhibitor such as an LA, the test result obtained on the mixture will still be abnormal because the inhibitor will interfere with the clotting factors from both plasma sources. The Staclot® LA (Diagnostica Stago M, Parsippany, NJ) test is a commonly used confirmatory test in the workup of a possible LA. Using the Staclot® LA procedure, 2 PTT-based clotting times are performed, 1 with a limited amount of phospholipid (tube 1) and the other with an excess of hexagonal phospholipids (tube 2). If the difference (or delta) between the clotting time values from tubes 1 (low phospholipid) and 2 (excess phospholipid) is greater than 8 seconds, a phospholipid-binding antibody such as an LA may be present. However, a decrease in the clotting time after the addition of excess phospholipid is not specific for an LA because this can happen in other conditions with a prolonged PTT, such as the presence of factor VIII antibodies. Although an LA is more common than any specific coagulation factor inhibitor, factor VIII antibodies are the second most common inhibitors, and their presence must be ruled out in order to establish the presence of an LA. Factor VIII inhibitors are measured with the Bethesda assay, which quantifies the amount of inhibitor based on the ability of the patient's plasma to inhibit the activity of factor VIII present in normal plasma. One Bethesda unit is the amount of antibody capable of decreasing the activity of normal factor VIII by 50%. A positive Bethesda assay in conjunction with a low factor VIII activity confirms the presence of a factor VIII inhibitor. The factor VIII activity for this patient was normal, however, thus ruling out the presence of a factor VIII inhibitor. In this case the patient's prolonged PTT, PTT-LA, and diluted Russell viper venom time (dRVVT) [**T1**], along with a mixing study that did not correct the PTT and a high Staclot® LA delta, confirm the presence of an LA.

Lupus anticoagulants are only rarely associated with bleeding. More often they are asymptomatic or are associated with thrombosis. This patient's PT and prothrombin activity were normal. Therefore, this patient's epistaxis was a "red herring" and may have been due to thrombocytopenia from a viral illness or from the effect of aspirin therapy on her platelets. Most LAs in children are associated with viral infections, are transient, and are not expected to cause thrombosis under these clinical conditions.[3]

Patient #2: Similar to *Patient #1*, the coagulation results for *Patient #2* are consistent with the presence of an LA. The PTT, PTT-LA, and dRVVT results were abnormal, and the dRVVT mixing study did not correct the dRVVT check results [**T1**]. In the case of *Patient #1*, the presence of a LA was confirmed using the Staclot® LA test. For *Patient #2*, the confirmatory test was the dRVVT ratio. The dRVVT is a clotting test that utilizes the ability of Russell viper venom to activate factor X. As a screening test for the presence of an LA, the test is performed with a low amount of phospholipid ("dRVVT check"). If abnormal, the dRVVT may be repeated using a 1:1 mixture of the patient's plasma with normal plasma (ie, plasma known to contain all clotting factors in adequate amounts with no substances that will interfere with any of the components of the coagulation cascade). If an inhibitor is identified by lack of correction in the mixing study, another dRVVT with concentrated phospholipid is performed ("dRVVT sure"). If an LA is present, it will essentially be neutralized by the excess phospholipid, allowing the dRVVT to correct. A "dRVVT check" to "dRVVT sure" ratio greater than 1.3 is consistent with the presence of a phospholipid inhibitor such as an LA. Moreover, the presence of a factor VIII inhibitor in this patient's plasma was ruled out by his high factor VIII activity level, probably due to an acute phase reaction. Because this patient exhibited a thrombotic manifestation (stroke) in conjunction with an LA, this patient can be diagnosed as having the antiphospholipid syndrome (APS). Phospholipid antibodies are found in 18% of ischemic stroke patients younger than 44 years of age. In addition, neurological symptoms are more likely to occur in such patients in the presence of other risk factors, such as hypertension and smoking.[4] Lastly, since this patient's baseline PTT was prolonged due to the presence of an LA, the PTT could not be used to monitor heparin therapy. The anti-Xa (activated factor X) assay is helpful in this situation because it is not affected by the presence of an LA and it provides a very reliable measurement of anticoagulation in a patient receiving heparin. The laboratory should alert the patient's physician to request the anti-Xa assay in this clinical setting.

Patient #3: This patient's prolongation of both the PTT and PT results suggests either the presence of an inhibitor or the deficiency of a specific coagulation factor within the common pathway of the coagulation cascade. However, the abnormal screening tests, the lack of correction with a mixing study, and the abnormal confirmatory test (dRVVT ratio and Staclot® LA delta) results indicate an inhibitor, most likely LA, as the probable culprit [**T1**]. In patients with an LA and bleeding, it is important to check for hypoprothrombinemia. Occasionally, an LA is directed against prothrombin (factor II), leading to immune clearance of this factor from the plasma. In such cases, the prothrombin level is low, and the PT is prolonged. This scenario should be suspected if the INR is greater than 1.4. Because the INR for *Patient #3* was 2.3, while the prothrombin activity was low [**T1**], and all of the ISTH criteria for the presence of an LA were met [**T2**], these findings are highly suggestive of an LA with specificity for prothrombin.

A history of a preceding viral illness is common in patients with an LA, but an episode of bleeding, as seen in *Patient #3*, is not. Lupus anticoagulants are more often associated with thrombosis. If the LA is directed at prothrombin, however, a hypoprothrombinemia can develop resulting in epistaxis, easy bruising, hematoma formation, menorrhagia, and prolonged bleeding after trauma or surgery. As noted in **T1**, the prothrombin activity level was low (6%). This type of acquired prothrombin deficiency is more likely than a congenital form of prothrombin deficiency, as this patient had previously undergone both a tonsillectomy and circumcision without excessive bleeding.

Fortunately, even with acquired prothrombin deficiency, the prognosis of LAs in children is good, as most are transient and resolve without specific treatment.[3] Supportive therapy with management of bleeding episodes as they occur

is the appropriate treatment for this patient. When bleeding episodes occur, fresh frozen plasma (FFP) is used to control bleeding. Fresh frozen plasma contains all of the clotting factors at an activity level of 100%. In vivo, a prothrombin activity level of 20% to 40% is generally adequate for achieving hemostasis. This level is often reached with the amount of prothrombin in FFP, in which case no other treatment is needed. While there is not a specific prothrombin concentrate available, a prothrombin complex concentrate exists which contains, in addition to prothrombin, factors VII, IX, and X. The only currently available formulation on the market is Bebulin, which contains a high level of prothrombin activity. This prothrombin complex concentrate has 2 main advantages over FFP for the treatment of prothrombin deficiency. First, it is safer because it undergoes a viral inactivation process to prevent the transmission of HIV, hepatitis B, and hepatitis C viruses. Second, the concentrate contains a higher level of prothrombin activity in a smaller volume, so less volume needs to be given to the patient to achieve hemostasis. This is particularly important in children or other patients who cannot tolerate excessive fluid. Also, for patients with more severe bleeding or for those being prepared for a surgical procedure, a hemostatic level of prothrombin can be achieved more quickly and with less overall volume. The loading dose of concentrate may be calculated by first determining the patient's blood volume (BV), which is based upon the patient's weight in kilograms. For children and slender adults, BV is presumed to be 70 mL per kilogram of body weight. For obese adults, the BV is estimated using 60 mL per kilogram. Next, the plasma volume (PV) is determined by the following formula:

$$PV = BV \times (1 - Hematocrit)$$

Finally, the dose of concentrate to be given is calculated as follows:

Dose, IU = (Desired % Activity – Current % Activity) $\times$ PV, where 100% activity equals 1 IU/mL.

The amount of each clotting factor present in 1 vial of prothrombin complex concentrate is based upon the amount of factor IX present, measured in international units (IU). For example, a vial of Bebulin should have 120 IU for every 100 IU of factor IX. The package insert for each formulation of prothrombin complex concentrate should specify the total number of units of factor IX in each vial. To assess the appropriateness of the dose, the plasma prothrombin level should be measured approximately 30 minutes after the infusion. Since the presence of an LA is expected to shorten the half-life of prothrombin, it is advisable to check factor levels prior to deciding on subsequent doses.

Patient #4: As with the other 3 patients, the results of the coagulation screening tests (PTT and PTT-LA), the PTT mixing study, and/or the Staclot® LA delta confirmatory test were abnormal [**T1**]. However, this patient's dRVVT test was normal, and the patient had a significant bleeding history, a classic picture of acquired hemophilia. This combination of findings is consistent with the presence of a specific inhibitor to factor VIII, a condition known as acquired hemophilia.[5] This suspicion was confirmed by this patient's extremely low (<1%) factor VIII activity [**T1**]. Acquired hemophilia is a rare condition caused by the development of a neutralizing autoantibody against factor VIII, which leads to factor VIII deficiency. Most patients with acquired hemophilia are over age 50 and about half have an associated disorder such as rheumatoid arthritis, systemic lupus erythematosus, malignancy, or a drug reaction. Peripartum women may also develop IgG anti-factor VIII. Patients with this disease often have a dramatic clinical presentation with spontaneous bleeding and/or delayed hemostasis. Other common sites of bleeding include the gastrointestinal and the urinary tracts. Such patients are usually managed with immunosuppressive agents such as corticosteroids. Serious hemorrhage requires additional treatment. If the level of inhibitor is low, the factor VIII level may be raised with factor concentrates purified from plasma or derived by recombinant technology. In patients with high inhibitor levels (>5 BU), hemostasis may be attained with alternative compounds which bypass the need for factor VIII, such as activated prothrombin complex concentrates or recombinant factor VIIa. If the antibody to factor VIII does not cross-react with porcine factor VIII, this product may also be of benefit to control bleeding. The role of the laboratory in this disease is

to monitor factor VIII and factor VIII inhibitor levels over time.

A summary of the most likely diagnosis and its rationale for each of the 4 patients presented in this case study is included in **T3**.

Keywords

lupus anticoagulant, coagulopathies, acquired hemophilia, antiphospholipid syndrome, acquired prothrombin deficiency

References

1. Greaves M. Antiphospholipid antibodies and thrombosis. *Lancet.* 1999;353:1348-1353.

2. Brandt JT, Triplett DA, Alving B, et al. Criteria for the diagnosis of lupus anticoagulant: An update. *Thromb Haemostas.* 1995;74:1185-1190.

3. Male C, Lechner K, Eichinger S, et al. Clinical significance of lupus anticoagulants in children. *J Pediatr.* 1999;134:199-205.

4. Levine SR, Deegan MJ, Futrell N, et al. Cerebrovascular and neurologic disease associated with antiphospholipid antibodies: 48 cases. *Neurology.* 1990;40:1181-1189.

5. Boggio LN, Green D. Acquired hemophilia. *Rev Clin Exp Hematol.* 2001;5:389-404.

Easy Bruising and Epistaxis in a 30-Year-Old Pregnant Woman

Diana L. Cochran-Black[1] Marta L. Klein[2]

[1]*Department of Medical Technology*, [2]*Physician Assistant, Wichita State University, Wichita, KS*

Patient: 30-year-old Hispanic woman in her 11th week of pregnancy.

History of Present Illness: She presented to her primary care physician for her first prenatal checkup. She had 2 other children and both of those pregnancies had been uneventful. Over the last 5 weeks she noticed that she bruised quite easily and had an occasional problem with epistaxis. She also admitted to some mild vaginal bleeding. She denied any hematuria, constipation, diarrhea, hematochezia, or melena. She also denied any gingival bleeding, chest pain, or shortness of breath.

Physical Examination: She had a variety of bruises at different stages distributed over her lower and upper extremities. No rashes or swelling in her feet were noted. The physician ordered a complete blood count, and it was discovered that the patient's platelet count was 4,000/μL. She was immediately admitted to the hospital for evaluation.

Questions

1. What is (are) this patient's most striking clinical and laboratory finding(s)?

2. How do you explain this patient's most striking clinical and laboratory findings?

3. What is this patient's most likely diagnosis?

4. Why are laboratory tests important in discriminating between the various types of pregnancy-associated thrombocytopenias?

5. What is the appropriate treatment for this patient's medical condition?

Possible Answers

1. Easy bruising, epistaxis, vaginal bleeding, markedly decreased platelet count with normal prothrombin and activated partial thromboplastin times, D-dimer and fibrinogen concentrations, and the absence of any platelet antibody.

2. The possibilities include various types of pregnancy-associated thrombocytopenias: idiopathic thrombocytopenic purpura (ITP), gestational thrombocytopenia (GTP), thrombotic thrombocytopenic purpura (TTP), hemolytic uremic syndrome (HUS), disseminated intravascular coagulation (DIC), and the syndrome of hemolysis, elevated liver enzymes, and low platelet count (HELLP). These possibilities can be differentiated on the basis of characteristic laboratory test findings [**T2**].

3. ***Most likely diagnosis:*** *pregnancy-associated idiopathic thrombocytopenic purpura (ITP).*

   Idiopathic thrombocytopenic purpura, also known as autoimmune thrombocytopenic purpura (AIT), can occur in children and adults. In adults, it is principally a disease of young women. Most women (70%) with this disorder are less than 40 years of age.[1] Idiopathic thrombocytopenic purpura is the

T1. Principal Laboratory Findings

Test	Patient's Result	"Normal" Reference Range
Hematology		
White blood cell count	9.5	4.0–11.0 × 10³/μL
Red blood cell count	4.37	4.0–6.0 × 10⁹/μL
Hemoglobin	13.1	12.0–18.0 g/dL
Hematocrit	36.8	36.0–54.0%
MCV	84.2	80.0–100.0 fL
MCH	30.0	27.0–34.0 pg
MCHC	35.6	33.0–37.0%
Platelet count	4.0	130–400 × 10³/μL
RDW	11.9	11.0–15.0%
MPV	9.4	7.4–11.0 fL
Differential		
Segmented neutrophils	75	40–70%
Lymphocytes	19	15–45%
Monocytes	5	2–10%
Eosinophils	1	0–6%
Red blood cell morphology	Normal	Normal
Coagulation		
Prothrombin time	13.5	11.7-14.2 sec
APTT	30.1	21.2-35.3 sec
Platelet antibody	Negative	Negative
D-dimer	0.22	<0.50 μg/mL
Fibrinogen	375	201-479 mg/dL
Chemistry		
BUN	10	6-20 mg/dL
Creatinine	0.5	0.5-1.2 mg/dL
AST	19	10-42 U/L
ALT	22	10-60 U/L
LD	123	98-192 U/L
Rheumatoid factor	23	0-43 IU/mL

MCV, mean corpuscular volume; MCH, mean corpuscular hemoglobin; MCHC, mean corpuscular hemoglobin concentration; RDW, red blood cell distribution width; MPV, mean platelet volume; APTT, activated partial thromboplastin time; BUN, blood urea nitrogen; LD, lactate dehydrogenase; AST, aspartate aminotransferase; ALT, alanine aminotransferase.

most common autoimmune disorder seen during pregnancy.[2] It occurs in approximately 1 to 2 per 1,000 to 10,000 pregnancies and accounts for 3% of all pregnancy-associated thrombocytopenias.[3-5] Moreover, there is generally no history of exposure to drugs or an infectious agent that can be related to the onset of the thrombocytopenia. Platelet counts are usually less than 30,000/μL in patients presenting with bleeding abnormalities.[6] Clinical symptoms for the disorder include an abrupt onset of easy bruising, petechiae, and bleeding from mucous membranes. Life-threatening bleeding is rare but can occur resulting in hematuria, gastrointestinal bleeding, and intracranial hemorrhage.[7] The normal range for a platelet count in adults is 150,000 to 400,000/μL.[7] Recent studies have demonstrated that the platelet count falls about

T2. Differentiation of Various Types of Pregnancy-Associated Thrombocytopenia Based on Laboratory Test Results

Laboratory Test	Type of Pregnancy-Associated Thrombocytopenia						
	ITP	GTP	TTP	HUS	DIC	HELLP	Patient
Platelet count (x 10³/μL)	<100	70-150	<50	LN to ↓	↓	<100	<50
Platelet antibody	+/–	+/–	–	–	–	–	–
PT and APTT	N	N	N	N	↑	N	N
D-dimer, μg/mL	<0.5	<0.5	<0.5	>0.5	>0.5	>0.5	<0.5
AST and ALT	N	N	N	N	N	↑	N
LD	N	N	↑↑↑	↑↑↑	↑	↑	N
BUN and creatinine	N	N	N or ↑	↑↑↑	N or ↑	↑	N
RBC morphology	N	N	schistocytes	schistocytes, spherocytes, helmet cells	schistocytes	schistocytes	N

ITP, idiopathic thrombocytopenic purpura; GTP, gestational thrombocytopenia; TTP, thrombotic thrombocytopenic purpura; HUS, hemolytic uremic syndrome; DIC, disseminated intravascular coagulation; HELLP (syndrome), syndrome of hemolysis, elevated liver enzymes, and low platelet count; PT, prothrombin time; APTT, activated partial thromboplastin time; AST, aspartate aminotransferase; ALT, alanine aminotransferase; BUN, blood urea nitrogen; LN, low normal; ↓, decreased; N, normal; ↑, increased; ↑↑↑, markedly increased; +/–, positive or negative; –, negative.

10% during an uncomplicated pregnancy with the greatest decline occurring during the last trimester.[8] Thrombocytopenia is defined as a platelet count below 150,000/μL.[7] Reasons for thrombocytopenia include increased platelet destruction or decreased platelet production. Thrombocytopenia during pregnancy is most commonly due to increased platelet destruction.[9] Increased platelet destruction can be due to immunologically mediated platelet autoantibody formation, abnormal platelet activation, or platelet consumption. Immune thrombocytopenia during pregnancy is typically caused by ITP.[10] Idiopathic thrombocytopenic purpura is characterized by a decreased platelet count due to the binding of a platelet autoantibody that leads to destruction and clearance of the platelets by cells of the reticuloendothelial system.[5] The majority of these antibodies are of the IgG type, but IgM antibodies also can occur.[11] Antiplatelet antibodies can be identified in 58% to 80% of patients with ITP, and most of these antibodies are directed toward platelet glycoprotein (GP) IIb/IIIa or GPIb/IX.[1,12] The exact reason for the antigenic stimulation and the mode of platelet destruction are unknown at this time. Immunoglobulin G antibody can cross the placenta and lead to transplacental or neonatal

ITP in the newborns of mothers with ITP. It has been estimated that 12% to 65% of newborns of mothers with ITP will have thrombocytopenia at birth.[4,13-15] Moreover, ITP will usually persist in the mother even after delivery.

Antiplatelet antibodies can also occur in gestational thrombocytopenia (GTP), also known as incidental thrombocytopenia. This condition is diagnosed in 74% of women who have thrombocytopenia during pregnancy.[3,9,16] Typically, their platelet counts range between 110,000/μL and 150,000/μL, and rarely do they have platelet counts less than 70,000/μL.[3,16] The thrombocytopenia usually does not develop until the third trimester of pregnancy and does not cause abnormal bleeding in the mother or baby. Moreover, the mother's platelet count usually returns to normal within 2 to 12 weeks following delivery, and thrombocytopenia in the newborn is extremely rare.[3,17]

Other disorders related to thrombocytopenia during pregnancy include thrombotic thrombocytopenic purpura (TTP), hemolytic uremic syndrome (HUS), disseminated intravascular coagulation (DIC), and the syndrome of hemolysis, elevated liver enzymes, and low platelet count (HELLP syndrome).[18]

4. Laboratory tests must be used to differentiate between the various thrombocytopenic disorders associated with pregnancy because many of these disorders can cause harm to the mother or fetus and treatment interventions are necessary to prevent maternal or fetal morbidity or mortality.[6] Idiopathic thrombocytopenic purpura is a diagnosis of exclusion, meaning that no other diagnosis can be determined after evaluating the patient's clinical history, physical examination, peripheral blood counts, and blood smear examination.[1] The platelet count in ITP during pregnancy is generally less than 100,000/μL, and all other laboratory tests used to differentiate the various reasons for thrombocytopenia during pregnancy, such as liver function tests, hemostasis testing, red cell morphology, and kidney function tests are usually normal [**T2**].[7] As mentioned previously, antiplatelet antibodies can be identified in the majority of patients with ITP, although their presence is not required for diagnosis. This is due to the fact that all currently available tests used to identify platelet antibodies suffer from a lack of diagnostic sensitivity, specificity, or both. Platelet antibody detection tests can be divided into 3 chronological groups. Phase I assays use control platelets and the patient's serum. A functional change in the control platelets is measured after they are incubated with the patient's serum. These tests are no longer used to diagnose ITP due to their low diagnostic sensitivity and specificity. Phase II assays measure platelet-specific IgG antibody using various techniques such as immunofluorescence, enzyme-linked immunosorbent assay (ELISA), or flow cytometry. These assays demonstrate high diagnostic sensitivity but low specificity. Phase III assays measure the binding of platelet antibody to specific platelet membrane glycoproteins using immunoblot, immunoprecipitation, and glycoprotein immobilization assays. These tests are highly specific but not very sensitive.[11,19] Platelet antibody tests cannot differentiate ITP from GTP as both conditions can be positive or negative for either platelet-specific or indirect IgG antibodies.[20] A diagnosis of GTP is usually confirmed after delivery by observing no thrombocytopenia in the newborn and a normal platelet count in the mother within 2 to 12 weeks postpartum.

5. The main objective in treating women with ITP during pregnancy is to minimize the risk of bleeding complications that are associated with severe thrombocytopenia. Most therapy is based upon the severity of the maternal ITP. Asymptomatic patients with a platelet count greater than 50,000/μL usually require no treatment.[7] For patients with platelet counts less than 30,000/μL, or for those with active bleeding, the first line of treatment is corticosteroids.[21,22] If the patient does not respond to steroids, or if the platelet count falls below 10,000/μL in the third trimester, high-dose intravenous immune globulin (IVIG) may be administered to raise the platelet count.[2,7] When the platelet count is less than 10,000/μL and both corticosteroids and IVIG are ineffective, a splenectomy is indicated.[22] Platelet transfusions are used only to treat life-threatening bleeding or for patients going to surgery.[7] Traditionally, mothers with ITP delivered their infants by Caesarean section. This mode of delivery was used primarily because of the belief that maternal ITP carried a high risk of neonatal thrombocytopenia and that intracranial hemorrhage in these infants was highly possible if they were delivered vaginally. Several large studies have shown, however, that these beliefs are unfounded.[13,23-25]

Treatment and Follow-up

The patient was treated with varying doses of corticosteroids during the remainder of her pregnancy. Her platelet count during this time ranged from 52,000/μL to 131,000/μL. Seven months after her initial diagnosis, she vaginally delivered a healthy baby girl. The baby was thrombocytopenic at birth, but her platelet count normalized shortly after delivery. The patient is currently maintaining a platelet count of around 90,000/μL and the corticosteroid therapy was stopped.

Keywords

idiopathic thrombocytopenic purpura, gestational thrombocytopenia, thrombotic thrombocytopenic purpura, hemolytic uremic syndrome, disseminated intravascular coagulation, syndrome of hemolysis, elevated liver enzymes, and low platelet count

Acknowledgment

The authors express their appreciation to the patient and her physicians for providing permission to access medical records and to the medical staff at Smoky Hill Family Practice Clinic for their assistance with this case presentation.

References

1. George JN, Raskob GE. Idiopathic thrombocytopenic purpura: Diagnosis and management. *Am J Med Sci.* 1998;36:87-93.

2. Devendra K, Koh LP. Pregnancy in women with idiopathic thrombocytopenic purpura. *Ann Acad Med Singapore.* 2002;31:276-280.

3. Burrows RF, Kelton JG. Fetal thrombocytopenia and its relation to maternal thrombocytopenia. *N Engl J Med.* 1993;329:1463-1466.

4. McCrae KR, Samuels P, Schreiber AD. Pregnancy-associated thrombocytopenia: Pathogenesis and management. *Blood.* 1992;80:2697-2714.

5. Sainio S, Joutsi L, Jarvenpaa AL, et al. Idiopathic thrombocytopenic purpura in pregnancy. *Acta Obstet Gynecol Scand.* 1998;77:272-277.

6. Harmening DM. *Clinical Hematology and Fundamentals of Hemostasis.* Philadelphia: F.A. Davis; 2002:471-480.

7. ACOG practice bulletin. Thrombocytopenia in pregnancy. *Int J Gynaecol Obstet.* 1999;67:117-128.

8. Verdy E, Bessous V, Dreyfus M, et al. Longitudinal analysis of platelet count and volume in normal pregnancy. *Thromb Haemost.* 1997;77:806-807.

9. Burrows RF, Kelton JG. Thrombocytopenia at delivery: A prospective survey of 6,715 deliveries. *Am J Obstet Gynecol.* 1990;162:731-734.

10. Kelton JG. Idiopathic thrombocytopenic purpura complicating pregnancy. *Blood Rev.* 2002;16:43-46.

11. Paidas MJ, Haut MJ, Lockwood CJ. Platelet disorders in pregnancy: Implications for mother and fetus. *Mt Sinai J Med.* 1994;61:389-403.

12. Wang Z-Y, Shen Z-X. Megakaryocytes and platelets in immune thrombocytopenic purpura. *Bailliere's Clin Haematol.* 1997;10:89-107.

13. Payne SD, Resnik R, Moore TR, et al. Maternal characteristics and risk of severe neonatal thrombocytopenia and intracranial hemorrhage in pregnancies complicated by autoimmune thrombocytopenia. *Am J Obstet Gynecol.* 1997;177:149-155.

14. Silver RM, Branch DW, Scott JR. Maternal thrombocytopenia in pregnancy: Time for reassessment. *Am J Obstet Gynecol.* 1995;173:479-482.

15. Takeshi A, Rintaro S, Tsutomu A, et al. Incidence of thrombocytopenia in infants born to mothers with idiopathic thrombocytopenic purpura. *Acta Paediatr Japonica.* 1998;40:112-115.

16. Burrows RF, Kelton JG. Incidentally detected thrombocytopenia in healthy mothers and their infants. *N Engl J Med.* 1988;319:142-145.

17. Samuels P, Bussel JB, Braitman LE, et al. Estimation of the risk of thrombocytopenia in offspring of pregnant women with presumed immune thrombocytopenic purpura. *N Engl J Med.* 1990;323:229-235.

18. Christiaens GC. Immune thrombocytopenic purpura in pregnancy. *Bailliere's Clin Haematol.* 1998;11:373-380.

19. Chong BH, Keng TB. Advances in the diagnosis of idiopathic thrombocytopenic purpura. *Semin Hematol.* 2000;37:249-260.

20. Lescale KB, Eddleman KA, Cines DB, et al. Antiplatelet antibody testing in thrombocytopenic pregnant women. *Am J Obstet Gynecol.* 1996;174:1014-1018.

21. George JN, Raskob GE. Idiopathic thrombocytopenic purpura: A concise summary of pathophysiology and diagnosis in children and adults. *Semin Hemat.* 1998;35:5-8.

22. George JN, Woolf S, Raskob GE. Idiopathic thrombocytopenic purpura: A practice guideline developed by explicit methods for the American Society of Hematology. *Blood.* 1996;88:3-40.

23. Cook RL, Miller RC, Katz, VL, et al. Immune thrombocytopaenic purpura in pregnancy: A reappraisal of management. *Obstet Gynecol.* 1991;78:578-583.

24. Burrows RF, Kelton JG. Pregnancy in patients with idiopathic thrombocytopenic purpura: Assessing the risks for the infant at delivery. *Obstet Gynecol Surv.* 1993;48:781-788.

25. Laros RK, Kagan R. Route of delivery for patients with immune thrombocytopenic purpura. *Am J Obstet Gynecol.* 1984;148:901-908.

A Young Woman With Indurated Skin and Subcutaneous Lesions

Shahnila Latif,[1] Fahim Zaman,[2] Fleurette Abreo,[1] Diana M. Veillon,[1] James D. Cotelingam[1]

[1]*Departments of Pathology and* [2]*Nephrology, Louisiana State University Health Sciences Center, Shreveport, LA*

Patient: 26-year-old African-American woman.

Family History: Non-contributory.

Chief Complaint: Indurated skin and subcutaneous lesions on her abdomen and thighs.

Medical History: End-stage renal disease (ESRD) requiring peritoneal dialysis. History of thrombosis of her subclavian and internal jugular veins and pulmonary embolism after dialysis catheter placement. Coumadin therapy for 6 months with suspected non-compliance as evidenced by significant fluctuation in values for her prothrombin time/International Normalized Ratio (INR) and frequently subtherapeutic coumadin levels. She noticed skin lesions approximately 4 months after beginning coumadin therapy.

Drug History: Coumadin, Nifedipine.

Physical Examination: Indurated skin and subcutaneous lesions on her abdomen and thighs (**Image 1** and **2**).

Additional Diagnostic Studies: A hypercoagulability profile of tests was performed with results shown in **T2**.

Questions

1. What is (are) this patient's most striking clinical and laboratory finding(s)?

2. How do you explain these findings?

3. What is this patient's most likely diagnosis?

4. What is the incidence of this patient's disorder?

5. What is the characteristic clinical presentation of an individual with this patient's condition?

6. What is the etiology of this patient's disorder?

7. What are the typical pathological findings on skin biopsy of an individual with this patient's disorder?

8. What is the differential diagnosis in a patient with signs, symptoms, and laboratory findings similar to those of the patient reported in this case study?

9. What is the treatment for this patient's condition?

T1. Principal Laboratory Findings

Test	Patient's Result	"Normal" Reference Range
Hematology		
Hemoglobin	10.9	11.3-15.4 g/dL
Hematocrit	34.2	34.0-46.0%
Platelet	263	142-405 x10³/µL
MCV	94.1	80.0-99.0 fL
MCH	29.9	26.5-34.0 pg
MCHC	31.8	32.0-35.0 g/dL
Coagulation		
PT	17.0	12.1-14.5 sec
INR	1.38	Therapeutic range: 2.00-3.00
PTT	38.5	24.7-35.5 sec
Mixing studies	No inhibitor detected	Not applicable

MCV, mean corpuscular volume; MCH, mean corpuscular hemoglobin; MCHC, mean corpuscular hemoglobin concentration; PT, prothrombin time; INR, International Normalized Ratio; PTT, activated partial thromboplastin time.

T2. Hypercoagulability Profile

Test	Patient's Result	"Normal" Reference Range
Homocysteine	12.9	5.0-15.0 µmol/L
Anti-thrombin III activity	75	82-125%
Protein C activity	62	74-151%
Protein S activity	65	60-185%
ANA: titer pattern	1:320 Speckled	<1:160
Lupus anticoagulant	Negative	Negative
Anticardiolipin antibodies	Negative	Negative
Factor V Leiden mutation	Negative	Negative
Prothrombin 20210A mutation	Negative	Negative
MTHFR gene mutation	Negative	Negative

ANA, antinuclear antibody; MTHFR, methylenetetrahydrofolate reductase.

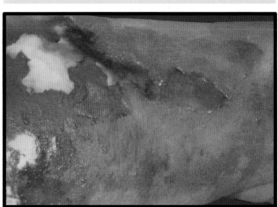

Image 3_Patient's skin biopsy revealing the presence of microthrombi in blood vessels (hematoxylin and eosin stain; 400× magnification).

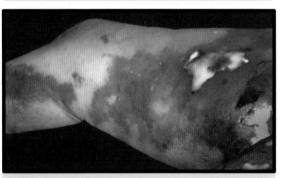

Image 1_Patient's right lower extremity showing areas of coumadin-induced skin necrosis.

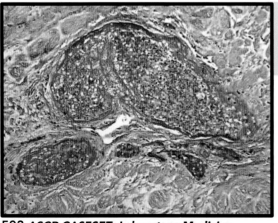

Image 2_Closer view of the same area shown in Image 1 illustrating indurated skin lesions with sloughing.

Possible Answers

1. Indurated skin and subcutaneous lesions on her abdomen and thighs after 4 months of coumadin therapy; mildly prolonged PTT and PT with subtherapeutic INR; mildly decreased antithrombin III and protein C activity; positive ANA titer and speckled ANA staining pattern.

2. Her PT and INR values were consistent with subtherapeutic coumadin levels. Coagulation studies revealed no evidence of an inherited or acquired thrombophilia or a hypercoagulability syndrome. Moreover, molecular studies for Factor V Leiden, Prothrombin 20210A, and MTHFR gene mutations and coagulation studies for lupus anticoagulant and anticardiolipin antibody were not abnormal. Her low protein S and mildly decreased protein C levels were consistent with the subtherapeutic coumadin levels. Her ATIII levels were only mildly decreased, most likely the result of consumption of ATIII due to the ongoing thrombosis that resulted in her skin and subcutaneous lesions. Her positive ANA titer suggested that an autoimmune disorder may have been the primary cause of this patient's renal failure. Because of her rapidly deteriorating clinical condition, additional laboratory studies were not performed.

3. *Most likely diagnosis: coumadin-induced skin necrosis.*

4. The first case report of coumadin-induced necrosis in the United States did not appear in the literature until 1961.[1] The incidence of coumadin-induced skin necrosis is only 0.01% to 0.10% of patients on coumadin.[2] Review of the literature by Cole and colleagues[3] revealed that the most common indication for coumadin therapy in patients who subsequently developed skin lesions was deep vein thrombosis (DVT) and pulmonary embolism (PE). In addition, coumadin-induced skin necrosis occurs more commonly in middle-age women than men.[4]

5. The lesions associated with coumadin-induced skin necrosis are characteristically noted during the first week of therapy, commonly appearing between days 3 and 6 of treatment. However, rare cases in which the skin lesions appeared months after beginning therapy, as in our case, have been reported.[5-8] Interestingly, the majority of patients with coumadin-induced skin necrosis have therapeutic coumadin levels at diagnosis. The most common sites of necrosis are areas of increased subcutaneous fat such as the breasts, thighs, and buttocks. The lesions are usually painful. Petechial hemorrhages are followed by sharply demarcated areas of blue-black ecchymotic discoloration. Hemorrhagic bullae may develop and in many cases progress to gangrenous necrosis. Surgical intervention is required in the most severe cases and lesions may not recur if coumadin therapy is reinitiated. The mortality rate associated with coumadin-induced skin necrosis is approximately 15%.[8]

6. The pathogenesis of coumadin-induced skin necrosis is not well understood. Coumadin produces anticoagulation by inhibiting the activity of the vitamin K-dependent clotting factors (II, VII, IX, and X). Coumadin also inhibits the activity of the anticoagulant proteins, protein C and protein S. Because of the short half-life of these proteins, initiation of coumadin therapy is associated with an imbalance between the anticoagulant and procoagulant proteins. This is the most plausible mechanism of coumadin-induced skin necrosis. Other theories that have been proposed include a localized Shwartzman reaction, an immunologic reaction, and a direct toxic effect of coumadin. Although coumadin-induced skin necrosis occurs in patients with normal coagulation profiles, patients with clotting disorders, including inherited deficiencies in proteins C and S and the Factor V Leiden mutation, are at an increased risk of developing this disorder.[3,4,8] Moreover, delayed appearance of lesions, as occurred in our patient, has been reported. It is suspected that late-onset coumadin-induced necrosis is a result of poor compliance with coumadin dosage schedules, with the patient stopping and subsequently restarting the medication without heparin coverage.[6-8] Laboratory studies to identify any underlying coagulation abnormality in this patient were either normal or non-diagnostic (**T2**).

7. Necrosis and hemorrhage with thrombi in the dermal capillaries and venules of the skin (**Image 3**).

8. The differential diagnosis of lesions arising on the skin of patients receiving coumadin includes: acute necrotizing fasciitis, calciphylaxis (ie, in patients with ESRD), antiphospholipid antibody syndrome, heparin-induced thrombocytopenia, Fournier gangrene, inflammatory breast cancer, decubitus ulcer, and cellulitis.

9. Treatment of coumadin-induced skin necrosis includes discontinuation of coumadin, administration of vitamin K, and institution of heparin therapy in selected cases.[9] Other therapies that have been used include administration of protein C concentrate, infusion of prostacyclin, transfusion with fresh frozen plasma, induction of local hypothermia, administration of systemic vasodilators, induction of sympathetic nerve blockade, and administration of corticosteroids.[4,8] Wound treatment consists of application of topical antibacterial agents and surgical debridement and skin grafting if indicated. In severe cases, amputation of an affected tissue (eg, a breast) may be necessary. Typically, the lesions heal by secondary intention [ie, the lesion heals without the need to bring the opposing margins of the lesion together and the lesion may or may not be sutured; significant scar formation may occur in the absence of primary intention (ie, bringing the opposing margins of the lesion together followed by suturing)]. Early recognition and treatment of coumadin-induced skin necrosis can prevent frank necrosis and gangrene.

Treatment and Course

The patient's condition rapidly deteriorated despite aggressive medical management and she died of septic shock with disseminated intravascular coagulation (DIC).

Keywords

coumadin, skin necrosis, hypercoagulability, International Normalized Ratio, secondary intention

References

1. Kipen CS. Gangrene of the breast–a complication of anticoagulant therapy. Report of 2 cases. *N Engl J Med.* 1961;265:638-640.

2. Koch-Weser J. Coumarin necrosis. *Ann Intern Med.* 1968;68:1365-1367.

3. Cole MS, Minifee PK, Wolma FJ. Coumarin necrosis–a review of the literature. *Surgery.* 1988;103: 271-277.

4. Alves DW, Chen IA. Warfarin-induced skin necrosis. *Hospital Physician.* 2002;38:39-42.

5. Franson TR, Rose HD, Spivey MR, et al. Late-onset, Warfarin-caused necrosis occurring in a patient with infectious mononucleosis. *Arch Dermatol.* 1984;120:927-931.

6. Essex DW, Wynn SS, Jin DK. Late-onset warfarin-induced skin necrosis: case report and review of the literature. *Am J Hematol.* 1998;57:233-237.

7. Koduri PR, Parveez R. Lack of compliance and late-onset warfarin-induced skin necrosis. *Am J Hematol.* 1998;61:218-219.

8. Scarff CE, Baker C, Hill P, et al. Late-onset warfarin necrosis. *Australas J Dermatol.* 2002;43:202-206.

9. Miura Y, Ardenghy M, Ramasastry S, et al. Coumadin necrosis of the skin: report of 4 patients. *Ann Plast Surg.* 1996;37:332-337.

Anemia in a 47-Year-Old Post-Partum Female

Steven H. Kroft, Robert W. McKenna

UT Southwestern Medical School, Dallas, TX

Patient: 47-year-old African American female.

Medical History: None.

Drug History: None.

Chief Complaint: None.

Family History: Unremarkable.

Gynecologic History: Gravida 4/Para 4. Three children by spontaneous vaginal delivery, 1 by Caesarian section. Menorrhagia increasing in severity over past several years.

Physical Examination: Blood pressure 186/90, pulse 88. Bulky, irregular uterus on bimanual examination; pale mucous membranes; otherwise unremarkable.

T1. Principal Laboratory Findings

Test	Abnormal Results	Normal Reference Range
Hemoglobin	7.4	12.0-15.2 g/dL
Hematocrit	22.7	37-46%
MCV1	63	79-101 fL
RDW2	21.2	11.5-14.5%

¹MCV, mean corpuscular volume ²RDW, red blood cell distribution width.

Questions

1. What is the most likely cause of anemia in this patient?

2. What additional laboratory tests would you order to confirm the diagnosis?

3. Why is the patient asymptomatic in the presence of a moderately severe anemia?

4. Why is the MCV low and the RDW high?

5. If this patient were an adult male with no significant medical history, what would be the most important part of his work up?

Results of Additional Laboratory Tests

Uterine ultrasound: discrete masses in the uterus, consistent with leiomyomata.

Serum iron: 11 µg/dL (normal, 48-180 µg/dL).

Total iron binding capacity: 543 µg/dL (normal, 262-474 µg/dL).

Ferritin: 6 ng/mL (normal, 7-282 ng/mL).

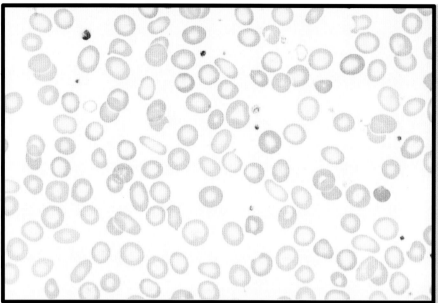

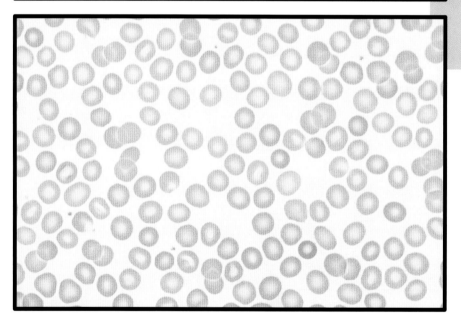

Image 1_Top: Iron deficiency anemia. **Bottom:** Blood smear from a healthy individual. The red blood cells are hypochromic (under-hemoglobinization as evidenced by increased central pallor), and show increased anisocytosis (variability in cell size) and poikilocytosis (variability in cell shape).

Possible Answers _____

1. The most likely diagnosis in this woman with prolonged excessive vaginal bleeding as a result of uterine leiomyomata is iron deficiency anemia. Women have less storage iron than males, and the presence of a negative iron balance induced by chronic blood loss may easily result in an iron deficient state.

2. The laboratory tests that are most commonly utilized in the diagnosis of iron deficiency are serum iron, total iron binding capacity (TIBC), and serum ferritin. Serum iron decreases in iron depleted patients once iron stores are exhausted, so patients with iron deficiency anemia will usually have decreased serum iron. However, serum iron may be normal in iron-deficient patients who have recently received iron supplementation, and it is also usually decreased in the anemia of chronic disease. Therefore, serum iron as an isolated test is essentially useless. The TIBC, which represents the total amount of iron that may be bound by a given volume of patient serum, is essentially a surrogate marker for serum

transferrin. It characteristically increases in iron deficiency and decreases in anemia of chronic disease. However, as a single test it is again of limited utility. Transferrin saturation, the ratio of serum iron to TIBC expressed as a percentage, has been proposed as a useful test for the diagnosis of iron deficiency. In iron deficiency anemia transferrin saturation is almost always less than 15%. However, values less than 15% will sometimes be seen in anemia of chronic disease. The best, commonly available test short of bone marrow examination is measurement of serum ferritin. Serum ferritin levels closely reflect tissue iron stores. In the large majority of cases of iron deficiency anemia, the serum ferritin is low. Low serum ferritin is diagnostic of iron deficiency. While occasionally patients with inflammatory conditions or acute liver disease will have normal levels of serum ferritin, these will generally fall in the low normal range (<50 ng/mL).

3. Iron deficiency anemia develops slowly over prolonged periods of time, thus allowing compensatory mechanisms to develop. In the absence of complicating medical conditions, rather severe degrees of anemia may be surprisingly well tolerated.

4. Iron deficiency anemia represents a cytoplasmic maturation defect in which there is insufficient iron for adequate hemoglobin production. These underhemoglobinized cells are smaller than normal. In very early iron deficiency anemia the red blood cells may be normochromic and normocytic. With increasing severity the cells become microcytic, and eventually hypochromic. The more severe the anemia, the lower the MCV. Maturation defects, whether nuclear or cytoplasmic, tend to result in red blood cells of varying sizes and shapes. The RDW is the coefficient of variation of the red blood cell volume, and thus is a quantitative measure of the variability of red blood cell size in a given patient.

5. Adult males in the United States usually have abundant storage iron because of an iron rich diet and few physiological routes of iron excretion. The presence of iron deficiency in an adult male should prompt investigation for occult blood loss, particularly from the gastrointestinal tract.

Glossary

Bimanual examination: examination of female genital tract performed with 1 hand inside the vagina and 1 on the external abdomen. Allows for palpation of uterus and uterine adnexa.

Menorrhagia: abnormally heavy bleeding during menstrual periods.

Spurious Thrombocytosis in a Burn Patient

Nancy L. Sapanara,[1] Silvio S. Tanev,[1] Vanlila Swami[2]

[1]*Department of Pathology and Laboratory Medicine, Medical College of Pennsylvania and* [2]*Drexel University College of Medicine, Philadelphia, PA*

Patient: 48-year-old woman.

Past Medical History: Not obtainable.

Chief Complaint: The patient was brought to the emergency department (ED) by ambulance after having jumped from a second story window to escape from a burning building. Upon arrival at the ED the patient had no detectable blood pressure or spontaneous respirations.

Family/Social History: Not obtainable.

Physical Examination Findings: Significant findings on physical examination included a 10 cm laceration along the right temporal region with possible skull fracture, blood in the nares and oropharynx, and carbon particles and blood in the sputum. Second-degree burns were found over the trunk and portions of all 4 extremities, comprising approximately 40% of her total body surface area.

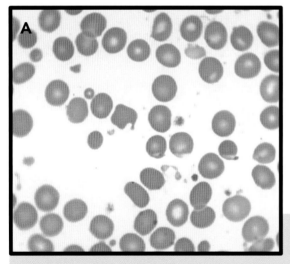 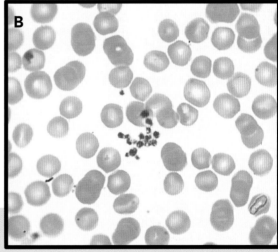

Image 1_A) The patient's peripheral blood smear, illustrating the presence of microcytic RBCs, microspherocytes, schistocytes, and detached pieces of RBC membrane. **B)** An example of platelet clumping. (Wright stain, 100× magnification).

T1. Principal Laboratory Findings

Test	Patient's Result	"Normal" Reference Range
Arterial Blood Gases		
pH	6.97a	7.34-7.44
pO₂	48	74-108 mm Hg
pCO₂	85	32-46
Carboxyhemoglobin	14	0%
Hematology		
WBC count	12.4	4.0-10.8 × 10³/mL
Hemoglobin	12.5	12.0-16.0 g/dL
Hematocrit	36.5	37.0-47.0%
MCV	74.8	81.0-99.0 fL
MCH	25.6	27.0-31.0 pg
MCHC	34.3	31.5-37.0 g/dL
RDW	18.2	11.5-15.5%
Platelet count	728b	150-450 × 10⁹/L
PBS findings:	Numerous microcytic RBCs, microspherocytes, fragmented RBCs (schistocytes), and detached RBC membrane fragments [**Image 1A**]	
Coagulation		
PT	17.3	12.7-14.7 sec
APTT	45.9	24.4-35.5 sec
Chemistry		
Potassium	5.7	3.3-5.1 mmol/L
BUN	14	6-9 mg/dL
Creatinine	0.9	0.4-1.1 mg/dL

aOn 100% O₂ mask. bPlatelet histogram was flagged for "lower and upper region interference" (LURI). WBC, white blood cell; MCV, mean corpuscular volume; MCH, mean corpuscular hemoglobin; MCHC, mean corpuscular hemoglobin concentration; RDW, red blood cell distribution width; PBS, peripheral blood smear; RBCs, red blood cells; PT, prothrombin time; APTT, activated partial thromboplastin time; BUN, blood urea nitrogen.

Questions

1. What is (are) this patient's most striking laboratory result(s)?

2. How do you explain this patient's most striking laboratory result(s)?

3. What does the instrument-generated flag "LURI" indicate?

4. What additional test(s) should be done to confirm your answer to question #3?

5. How do you explain this patient's markedly elevated platelet count?

6. What other conditions are associated with spurious thrombocytosis?

7. What conditions are associated with spurious thrombocytopenia?

Possible Answers

1. Decreased arterial blood pH while the patient was receiving 100% oxygen (O₂), decreased pO₂, and markedly increased pCO₂ and carboxyhemoglobin concentrations; slightly increased

WBC count, decreased MCV, increased RDW, a markedly increased platelet count with the instrument-generated flag of "lower and upper region interference" (LURI), and numerous microcytic RBCs, microspherocytes, fragmented RBCs (schistocytes), and detached RBC membrane fragments upon examination of a peripheral blood smear from this patient [**Image 1A**]; elevated PT and APTT values; and, increased potassium and BUN concentrations.

2. The abnormal arterial blood gas values reflect the patient's near-death condition from inhalation of fumes and then jumping from the second floor of a burning building. Among the other abnormal laboratory findings, the most striking are a markedly increased platelet count with the instrument-generated flag "LURI" and the presence of numerous microcytic RBCs, microspherocytes, fragmented RBCs (schistocytes), and detached RBC membrane fragments on the peripheral blood smear.

3. The platelet histogram flag, LURI, indicates that there are cells slightly smaller than (lower region of the histogram) and slightly larger than (upper region of the histogram) the majority of the patient's platelets. These interfering cells make it impossible for the instrument to determine an accurate range for the size of normal platelets because the interfering cells cause the lower and upper limits of this range and the platelet count to be spuriously elevated.

4. To confirm that the platelet count is spuriously elevated, the platelet count should be estimated from a peripheral blood smear and quantified by an alternate method (eg, manual platelet count). In this case, examination of the patient's peripheral smear revealed that the platelets were quantitatively within the normal range. This finding was confirmed by a manual platelet count of 275×10^9/L.

5. The presence of numerous microcytic and fragmented RBCs caused the "LURI" flag during the automated platelet count giving rise to this patient's falsely elevated platelet count. Interestingly, such changes in RBC morphology have been documented previously in acutely burned patients.[1,2] In 1 report, a burn patient was found to have spurious thrombocytosis due to the presence of numerous microspherocytes that were similar in size to normal platelets.[1] In addition to microspherocytosis, fragmentation and blistering (vesiculation) of RBCs can occur. Careful examination of the background of the peripheral blood smear will often reveal the presence of loose, detached pieces of red cell membrane [**Image 1A**]. These RBC membranes are usually only present in the acute post-burn phase because they are usually cleared from the circulation within 4 hours.[2] It is these fragments which may account in part for the renal failure seen in patients who survive beyond the acute post-burn period.[2] The mechanisms underlying morphologic changes in RBCs following thermal injury have been studied in Sprague-Dawley rats.[3] Rats with 30% full thickness total body surface area burns showed a significant increase in RBC osmotic fragility and decrease in RBC membrane deformability when compared to the control "sham-burn" group.[3] This combination of increased fragility with decreased deformability persisted for 8 hours (the duration of the study) and is the likely cause of RBC loss and fragmentation after acute thermal injury. Numerous fragmented RBCs (schistocytes) may also be seen in the setting of burn-related disseminated intravascular coagulation (DIC). In DIC, the platelet count is usually low; however, when DIC occurs in the post-burn setting the platelet count will be falsely normal, or even elevated, due to the microspherocytes and schistocytes being counted as platelets.

6. Other conditions in which spurious thrombocytosis can occur due to the presence of a large number of small and fragmented RBCs (especially schistocytes) include thrombotic thrombocytopenic purpura (TTP) and hemolytic uremic syndrome (HUS). Both microcytes and schistocytes can be similar in size to platelets and, when present in excessive amounts, can lead to a falsely elevated platelet count using an automated hematology analyzer.

7. Platelet clumps, large and/or giant platelets, and platelet satellitism are the principal causes of spuriously low automated platelet counts. In vitro platelet clumping, or pseudothrombocytopenia (PTCP), is often EDTA-dependent and related to the presence of naturally occurring autoantibodies (predominantly IgM and IgG) with

antiplatelet activity.[4] When platelet clumps are noted on a peripheral smear [I1B] and EDTA-dependent PTCP is suspected, a new sample of blood collected in an alternate anticoagulant, such as sodium-citrate or ammonium oxalate, should be obtained for testing. Large platelets are larger than normal-sized platelets but smaller than a normocytic RBC. Giant platelets are as large as or larger than a RBC, and can be up to 20 μm in diameter. Giant platelets may be seen in a variety of disorders including Bernard-Soulier syndrome, May-Hegglin anomaly, Montreal giant platelet syndrome,[5] and in several autosomal-dominant syndromes including Fechtner syndrome, Sebastian platelet syndrome, and Epstein syndrome.[6] Platelet satellitism, also caused by autoantibodies, is the phenomenon of platelets rosetting around neutrophils or, rarely, around other cells such as neoplastic lymphoid cells. The platelets that are attached as "satellites" to other cells are not detected by automated cell counters and thereby cause spurious thrombocytopenia. Platelet satellitism is caused by EDTA-dependent antiplatelet and antineutrophil IgG antibodies in the patient's serum. Since no clear correlation has been found between these antibodies and any particular disease state or drug, it is thought that they may occur naturally.[7]

Treatment and Outcome

Cardiopulmonary resuscitation and advanced cardiac life support protocols were initiated and performed for more than an hour. Despite these extensive resuscitative measures, the patient could not be revived and was pronounced dead.

Keywords

thermal RBC injury, microspherocyte, schistocyte, spurious thrombocytosis, lower and upper region interference, pseudothrombocytopenia, platelet satellitism

References

1. Akwari AM, Ross DW, Stass SA. Spuriously elevated platelet counts due to microspherocytosis. *Am J Clin Path.* 1982;77:220-221.

2. Lawrence C, Atac B. Hematologic changes in massive burn injury. *Crit Care Med.* 1992; 20:1284-1288.

3. Endoh Y, Kawakami M, Orringer EP, et al. Causes and time course of acute hemolysis after burn injury in the rat. *J Burn Care & Rehab.* 1992;13:203-209.

4. Bizzaro N. EDTA-dependant pseudothrombocytopenia: A clinical and epidemiological study of 112 cases, with 10-year follow-up. *Am J Hematol.* 1995;50:103-109.

5. Becker PS, Clavell LA, Beardsley DS. Giant platelets with abnormal surface glycoproteins: a new familial disorder associated with mitral valve insufficiency. *J Ped Hematol Onc.* 1998;20:69-73.

6. Toren A, Rozenfeld-Granot G, Rocca B, et al. Autosomal-dominant giant platelet syndromes: a hint of the same genetic defect as in Fechtner syndrome owing to a similar genetic linkage to chromosome 22q11-13. *Blood.* 2000;96:3447-3451.

7. Bizzaro N, Goldschmeding R, von dem Borne AE. Platelet satellitism is FC gamma RIII (CD 16) receptor mediated. *Am J Clin Path.* 1995;103:740-744.

Abnormal Red Blood Cell Morphology in an Elderly Male

Naveen Kakkar,[1] Guranjan Deep Singh,[2] Jasbir Dhanoa[2]

Departments of [1]Pathology and [2]Medicine, CMC Hospital, Ludhiana, Punjab, India

Patient: 70-year-old Indian male.

Family History: Unremarkable.

Chief Complaint: Drowsiness after ingestion of a pesticide during a suicide attempt 1 hour prior to presentation.

Medical History: Chronic bronchitis.

Drug History: Unremarkable.

Physical Examination: The patient was drowsy, had an average build, was responsive to painful stimuli, and had no organomegaly.

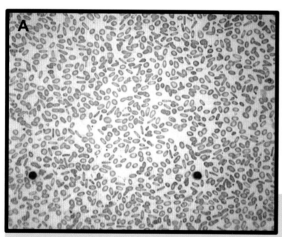 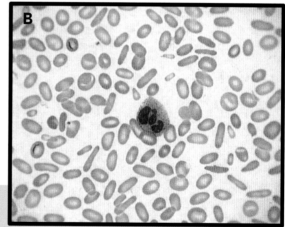

Image 1_Patient's Leishman's stained peripheral blood smear at 400× (**A**) and 1,000× (**B**) magnification showing that ~90% of the red blood cells have oval/elliptical- or rod-shaped morphology.

Questions _____

1. What is (are) this patient's most striking laboratory finding(s)?

2. How do you explain this patient's most striking laboratory finding(s)?

3. What is this patient's most likely diagnosis?

4. What are the incidence, geographical distribution, and inheritance pattern of this patient's condition?

5. What are the principal clinical and hematological features of this patient's condition?

6. What is (are) the defect(s) in the RBCs that cause this patient's RBC abnormality?

T1. Principal Laboratory Findings

Test	Patient's Result	Reference Interval
Hematology		
WBC count	16.5	4.0-11.0 × 10⁶/µL
Hemoglobin	11.7	12.0-16.0 g/dL
Platelet count	300	150-400 × 10⁶/µL
MCV	55	76-96 fL
MCH	16.5	29.5 ± 2.5 pg
MCHC	29.8	33.0 ± 2 g/L
RDW	18.7	11.5-15.0
Differential: Neutrophils	80	40-80%
Lymphocytes	17	20-40%
Metamyelocytes	3	
Peripheral blood smear findings	See [Image 1]	
Reticulocyte count	3.2	0.2-2.0%
Chemistry		
Bilirubin, total	0.8	0.5-1.4 mg/dL
Bilirubin, direct	0.4	0.0-0.4 mg/dL
AST	51	5-50 U/L
ALT	51	5-50 U/L
ALP	136	70-230 U/L
Total protein	6.5	6.0-8.4 g/dL
Albumin	3.6	3.5-5.0 g/dL
BUN	21	15-45 mg/dL
Creatinine	5.4	0.7-1.5 mg/dL

WBC, white blood cell; MCV, mean corpuscular volume; MCH, mean corpuscular hemoglobin; MCHC, mean corpuscular hemoglobin concentration; RDW, red cell distribution width; AST, aspartate aminotransferase; ALT, alanine aminotransferase; ALP, alkaline phosphatase; BUN, blood urea nitrogen.

7. What laboratory investigations can be carried out to diagnose this patient's condition?

8. What other hematological conditions result from RBC membrane abnormalities?

Possible Answers

1. Although this patient's WBC count and creatinine concentration were increased, the most striking laboratory findings were markedly low RBC indices, an increased RDW [**T1**], a modest anemia and reticulocytosis, and the presence of predominantly elliptocytes on his peripheral blood smear (PBS) [**Image 1**].

2. This patient's abnormal RBC indices and increased RDW are most likely due to the large number of elliptocytes observed on this patient's PBS. Elliptocytes can be seen on PBSs from healthy individuals and from individuals with iron deficiency anemia, macrocytic anemia, sickle cell disease, thalassaemia, or hereditary elliptocytosis (HE). In individuals without HE, however, the percentage of elliptocytes on the PBS is typically <25%, while in individuals with HE, this percentage can approach 90% or more.[1]

3. ***Most likely diagnosis:*** *hereditary elliptocytosis as an incidental finding unrelated to the patient's ingestion of a pesticide.* Hereditary elliptocytosis is representative of a family of genetically determined disorders associated with the observation of an excessively large number of elliptically-shaped RBCs on a PBS from individuals with these disorders. Spherocytic elliptocytosis and stomatocytic elliptocytosis are rare variants with more rounded and stomatocytic RBCs, respectively.[2]

4. Hereditary elliptocytosis and its variants occur in the general population with an estimated frequency of 1 in 1,000 to 1 in 5,000. The distribution of HE is worldwide with a much higher frequency (30%) in Malayan aborigines that is related to malarial endemicity in the area where they live. Hereditary elliptocytosis is transmitted as an autosomal dominant trait with the exception of a rare Melanesian variant that has an autosomal recessive mode of inheritance. Homozygous HE, which presents as a transfusion-dependent anemia, is rare, but its existence has been well documented.[3]

5. Hereditary elliptocytosis in its most common form is a mild hemolytic disorder. Most affected patients have a fully compensated hemolytic process with no anemia or splenomegaly. Contrasting with the innocuous clinical picture, however, the PBS of individuals with HE shows 25% to 100% elliptocytes and mild reticulocytosis. In 5% to 20% of individuals with HE, the hemolytic process is incompletely compensated. These patients have mild anemia with a high reticulocyte count and may have splenomegaly,

chronic leg ulcers, or gallstones. As with other hemolytic anemias, abrupt episodes of more severe anemia (crises) may also occur. Such crises are usually precipitated by intercurrent infections or stress. Homozygous HE presents clinically as a chronic transfusion-dependent anemia that responds dramatically to splenectomy. The PBS findings in patients with homozygous HE are characterized by marked poikilocytosis, microelliptocytosis, and RBC fragmentation.

6. The primary defect in HE lies in the protein scaffolding that constitutes the membrane skeleton of RBCs. The quantity of spectrin, the major cytoskeletal protein in the RBC membrane from individuals with HE is normal, but it is structurally abnormal. More than 90% of the spectrin derived from normal RBCs exists in a tetrameric form or as a combination of higher order oligomers. In contrast, the major portion of spectrin molecules extracted from RBCs from individuals with HE exists as dimers. The defect in RBC membrane stability observed in elliptocytes from these individuals is due to the failure of proper spectrin dimer-tetramer association.[4] There are 4 molecular defects that can cause this, each associated with an abnormality or defect in spectrin or proteins required for proper association of spectrin molecules: 1) abnormalities in the α-chain of spectrin; 2) abnormalities in the β-chain of spectrin; 3) a defective protein 4.1; and 4) a defective protein 3. Abnormalities in the α-chain of spectrin occur in 25% to 30% of cases of HE, and several such abnormalities have been identified. In such cases, normal and abnormal spectrins are present in approximately equal amounts in tetrameric and dimeric forms, respectively. Variant spectrins are designated by a superscript identifier that indicates the abnormal domain I of the alpha chain, a region at the head of the spectrin molecule involved in spectrin dimer-dimer interaction (eg, $Sp\alpha^{1/74}$ denotes an abnormal spectrin molecule in which tryptic digestion of domain I of the α-chain of spectrin generates a 74 kilodalton (kD) peptide instead of the normal 80 kD peptide). Other α-chain spectrin variants seen in RBCs from individuals with HE include $Sp\alpha^{1/78}$, $Sp\alpha^{1/65}$, $Sp\alpha^{1/61}$, $Sp\alpha^{1/46}$, and $Sp\alpha^{1/43}$. Two truncated variants of the β-chain of spectrin ($Sp\beta^{220/216}$ and $Sp\beta^{220/214}$) have been described which demonstrate defective dimer self-association. Both of the spectrin variants

fail to undergo enzymatic phosphorylation. Moreover, the structurally alterered β-chain in these spectrin variants is also responsible for defective binding of spectrin to ankyrin, another important component of the RBC cytoskeleton. A defective protein 4.1 is seen in one-third of patients with HE. This defect is seen most commonly in inhabitants of southern France and North Africa. Other abnormalities of the protein 4.1 molecule are associated with abnormally high or low molecular weight. Last, fewer patients exhibit an abnormal protein 3 molecule compared to the other 3 types of cytoskeletal protein abnormalities discussed above.

7. Red blood cell osmotic fragility test, autohemolysis test, and the more complex procedure of isolating and identifying the defect in the spectrin molecule by electrophoretic analysis of the products of enzymatic digestion of spectrin, are useful in the laboratory diagnosis of patients with HE. In individuals with HE, at least 25%, and typically 50% to 90%, of their RBCs are oval-shaped, and 10% occur as elongated, rod-shaped forms. Both the RBC osmotic fragility and autohemolysis tests are normal in individuals with non-hemolytic HE but are increased in patients with spherocytic elliptocytosis or in patients with HE variants and hemolytic disease. Demonstration of the molecular defect in the spectrin molecule confirms the diagnosis; however, the methods (ie, isolation, enzymatic digestion, and electrophoretic analysis) used for this purpose are not routinely available in most clinical laboratories. In addition to the aforementioned laboratory tests, the patient's clinical phenotype, characteristic RBC morphology on a PBS, and family history are of prime importance in the diagnosis of HE.

8. Hereditary spherocytosis, hereditary stomatocytosis, hereditary pyropoikilocytosis, xerocytosis, acanthocytosis (seen in some patients with abetalipoproteinemia), and Rh-Null disease are other disorders associated with RBC membrane defects.

Keywords

hereditary elliptocytosis, spectrin, ankyrin, spherocytosis, osmotic fragility, autohemolysis

References

1. Cutting HO, McHugh WJ, Conrad FG, et al. Autosomal dominant hemolytic anemia characterized by Ovalocytosis. A family study of 7 involved members. *Am J Med.* 1965;39:21-34.

2. Glader BE, Lukens JN. Hereditary spherocytosis and other anemias due to abnormalities of the red cell membrane. In: Lee GR, Foerester J, Lukens J, Paraskevas F, Greer JP, Rodgers GM eds, *Wintrobe's Clinical Hematology,*10th ed. Baltimore: Williams and Wilkins.1999:1133-1159.

3. Palek J, Lux SE. Red cell membrane skeletal defects in hereditary and acquired hemolytic anemias. *Semin Hematol.* 1983;20:189-224.

4. Coetzer T, Zail S. Spectrin tetramer-dimer equilibrium in hereditary elliptocytosis. *Blood.* 1982;59:900-905.

Jaundice and Cola-Colored Urine in a Young Indian Boy

Anureet Kaur,[1] Menka Doomra,[1] Naveen Kakkar,[1] Jasbir Dhanoa[2]

Departments of [1]Pathology and [2]Medicine, Christian Medical College and Hospital, Ludhiana, Punjab, India

Patient: 16-year-old Indian boy.

Medical/Family History: Unremarkable.

Chief Complaint: Fever, jaundice, and passage of cola-colored urine for 1 day. The patient was admitted to the hospital for follow-up.

Physical Examination Findings: The patient was well built and had severe pallor and icterus. There was no organomegaly.

Drug History: Intake of an unbranded white powder given by a non-licensed individual.

Hospital Course: The patient's hematological findings reverted back to normal within 10 days of hospitalization although he developed renal failure consequent to massive hemolysis.

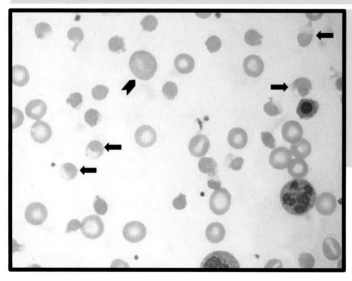

Image 1_Patient's peripheral blood smear showing microspherocytes, bite/blister cells (arrows) with hemoglobin drawn to 1 side of the RBC, irregularly contracted cells, and a polychromatic RBC (arrowhead). A nucleated red blood cell is also present along with a neutrophil. (Leishman stain; 1,000× magnification).

Questions _____

1. What is (are) this patient's most striking clinical and laboratory finding(s)?

2. How do you explain these findings?

3. What is this patient's most likely diagnosis?

4. What is the geographical distribution of this condition?

5. What is the inheritance pattern and the subtypes of this condition?

T1. Principal Laboratory Findings

Test	Patient's Result	Reference Range
Hematology		
WBC count	28.3	4.0-11.0 × 10³/μL
Hemoglobin	3.5	12.0-16.0 g/dL
Hematocrit	11.4	38-47%
Platelet count	211	150-400 × 10³/μL
Reticulocyte count	50.0	0.2-2%
Corrected reticulocyte count	12.6	–
Differential:		
Myelocytes	10	0%
Metamyelocytes	11	0%
Neutrophils	71	40-80%
Lymphocytes	7	20-40%
Eosinophils	1	0-6%
NRBCs	5/100 WBCs	
PBS findings	Anisopoikilocytosis with numerous microspherocytes, bite and blister cells, irregularly contracted cells, few macrocytes and nucleated and polychromatic RBCs; some of the RBCs showed basophilic stippling and Howell-Jolly bodies [**Image 1**]	
Chemistry		
BUN	139	15-45 mg/dL
Creatinine	2.0	0.7-1.5 mg/dL
Bilirubin, total	12.9	0.5-1.4 mg/dL
Bilirubin, direct	1.0	0-0.4 mg/dL
ALT	29	5-50 U/L
AST	244	5-50 U/L
ALP	97	70-230 U/L
LD	5165	230-460 U/L

WBC, white blood cell; NRBCs, nucleated red blood cells; PBS, peripheral blood smear; BUN, blood urea nitrogen; ALT, alanine aminotransferase; AST, aspartate aminotransferase; ALP, alkaline phosphatase; LD, lactate dehydrogenase.

6. What is the pathogenesis of the condition leading to hemolysis in this patient?

7. What are the principal clinical features of this patient's condition?

8. What are the factors which predispose an individual to the clinical manifestations associated with this patient's condition?

9. What are the laboratory investigations which can be carried out to diagnose this patient's condition?

10. What are the other red cell enzymopathies which have hematological manifestations?

Possible Answers

1. Fever, abdominal pain, passage of cola-colored urine, pallor, icterus, severe anemia, leukocytosis, azotemia, hyperbilirubinemia, markedly increased lactate dehydrogenase (LD), and the presence of microspherocytes, bite/blister cells with polychromasia, and nucleated red blood cells in the peripheral blood smear (PBS) (**T1** and **Image 1**).

2. The constellation of this patient's clinical and laboratory findings (eg, markedly decreased hemoglobin and hematocrit levels with a markedly increased serum LD activity), along with the history of intake of an unknown drug and the presence of bite/blister cells and microspherocytes in the PBS, are characteristic of acute oxidant damage to the red blood cells and hemolysis due to glucose-6-phosphate dehydrogenase (G6PD) deficiency.

3. ***Most likely diagnosis:*** *acute hemolysis due to G6PD deficiency.* Deficiency of G6PD is the most common metabolic disorder of red blood cells.

4. The incidence of the deficiency state varies from 20% among African Bantu males to 12% in African-American men and 8% in Brazilian blacks. G6PD deficiency is also prevalent among the Greek population with a maximum incidence of 20% to 32% in the low lands. In Cambodia, South China, and India, the incidence is 14.0%,

5.5%, and 2.6%, respectively. It is rare among Native Americans.

5. G6PD deficiency is a sex-linked trait with the gene for G6PD located on the X-chromosome (band Xq28). It is expressed in males carrying the variant of the gene, whereas heterozygous females are usually clinically normal. Because of inactivation of 1 of the 2 X-chromosomes (Lyon hypothesis), heterozygotes have 2 populations of RBCs—normal and G6PD deficient. The degree of lyonisation and the degree to which the abnormal G6PD variant is expressed decide the enzyme activity in females, which may be normal, moderately reduced, or grossly deficient. More than 400 biochemical variant forms of G6PD are recognized. The normal G6PD enzyme is designated as type G6PD B. The most common variant is G6PD A—encountered primarily in individuals of central African descent. This is followed by G6PD Mediterranean in prevalence. The other commonly occurring variants are G6PD A+ and G6PD Canton. The names for the newer variants are designated according to the location of the individual in whom they were first described.

6. G6PD is an enzyme of the hexose monophosphate (HMP) shunt pathway, which metabolizes 5% to 10% of the glucose used by RBCs. It catalyzes oxidation of glucose-6-phosphate (G6P) to 6-phosphogluconolactone with simultaneous reduction of nicotinamide adenine dinucleotide phosphate (NADP) to reduced NADP (NADPH). The latter is an important reducing compound for conversion of oxidized glutathione (GSSG) to glutathione (GSH) which protects red cells against free radical (eg, superoxide anion) oxidative injury. Individuals with G6PD deficiency, especially when exposed to certain drugs, are unable to maintain adequate levels of reduced glutathione in their RBCs leading to oxidation of hemoglobin sulfhydryl groups. Hemoglobin precipitates within RBCs, forming Heinz bodies. These membrane-bound inclusions lead to mechanical trapping of affected red cells in splenic capillaries resulting in hemolysis. Both intravascular and extravascular hemolysis occurs in these patients.

7. The common clinical features of G6PD deficiency are acute hemolytic anemia, favism,

congenital non-spherocytic hemolytic anemia, and neonatal hyperbilirubinemia. **Acute hemolytic anemia** occurs only after exposure to certain offending agents (drugs, infections, acidosis). After 2 to 4 days of exposure to the offending agent, all signs and symptoms of acute hemolytic anemia are observed which include jaundice, pallor, and dark colored urine, with or without abdominal and back pain. There is an abrupt decrease of 3 to 4 g/dL in hemoglobin concentration. The anemia is self-limited because the older susceptible population of RBCs is replaced by younger RBCs with sufficient G6PD activity. A similar clinical presentation occurs in **favism** on ingestion of fresh fava beans (*Vicia fava*; European broad bean) or inhalation of pollen from the fava plant. In **congenital non-spherocytic hemolytic anemia**, anemia, jaundice, and hyperbilirubinemia occur, along with hemolysis in the absence of a triggering factor. Beyond infancy, signs and symptoms of G6PD deficiency are subtle, and mild to moderate anemia is the rule. **Neonatal hyperbilirubinemia** occurs due to ingestion of drugs, chemicals, and/or fava beans by mothers in late gestation leading to accelerated RBC destruction or impaired liver clearance of bilirubin.

8. Hemolytic crisis occurs only after exposure to certain offending agents, including drugs, infections, exposure to fava beans, and diabetic acidosis. Drugs associated with hemolysis in G6PD deficiency include antimalarials (Primaquine, pamaquine), sulphonamides (Sulphamethoxazole), nitrofurantoin, analgesics (acetaminophen, aspirin, phenacetin), isoniazid (INH), methylene blue, and nalidixic acid. G6PD deficiency due to accidental exposure of children to naphthalene (present in moth balls) has also been reported. The common infectious agents which trigger hemolysis in G6PD deficient individuals are *Salmonella*, *E. coli*, *b-hemolytic streptococci*, and *Rickettsiae*.[1,2]

9. The diagnosis of G6PD deficiency can be made by indirect or direct methods. **Indirect methods** include hematological and biochemical changes. Hematological changes include a fall in hemoglobin concentration by 4 to 8 g/dL and marked anisopoikilocytosis following an acute hemolytic episode. The peripheral blood smear shows microspherocytes, irregularly contracted cells,

and eccentrocytes (blister or bite cells). Blister cells are red blood cells in which the hemoglobin appears to be drawn to 1 side of the cell, leaving an unstained non-hemoglobin containing cell membrane. (**Image 1**). Also seen are red cell fragments, polychromatic RBCs, and basophilic stippling. There is associated moderate leukocytosis and thrombocytosis. Reticulocytosis occurs within 5 days. Heinz bodies can be demonstrated by supravital staining early in the hemolytic episode. Biochemical changes that provide indirect evidence of hemolysis in G6PD deficiency include hyperbilirubinemia, raised plasma hemoglobin, markedly elevated serum lactate dehydrogenase (LD) activity, low serum haptoglobin level, and positive tests for urine hemoglobin and hemosiderin. **Direct methods** involve demonstration of deficient or reduced activity of G6PD. It is important that this testing is not carried out during an acute hemolytic episode as reticulocytosis can give rise to a false negative result, the younger RBCs being rich in G6PD. Accurate estimation of G6PD deficiency is possible if testing is carried out 2 to 3 months following an acute hemolytic episode when reticulocytosis has subsided and steady state hematopoiesis has been restored. The majority of these screening tests demonstrate the presence or absence of G6PD by the ability of the red cells to generate NADPH from NADP with simultaneous oxidation of an appropriate substrate. The laboratory techniques used to demonstrate G6PD deficiency include the brilliant cresyl blue dye test, methemoglobin reduction test, and the fluorescent spot test.[3] An enzyme assay which spectrophotometrically measures the rate of reduction of NADP to NADPH is also available. Common deficient G6PD variants can also be diagnosed by restriction enzyme digestion of the appropriate PCR product.[4] More recently, denaturing high performance liquid chromatography (DHPLC) has been used for rapid detection of G6PD mutations.[5]

10. Other red cell enzymopathies which have hematological manifestations include those associated with enzymes of the Embden-Meyerhof pathway (pyruvate kinase, hexokinase, phosphofructokinase, phosphoglycerate kinase and aldolase), enzymes involved in nucleotide metabolism (adenylate kinase deficiency, pyrimidine 5-nucleotidase), and other enzymes of the HMP shunt pathway (glutathione reductase, glutathione synthetase).

Keywords

G6PD, lyonisation, hemolysis, anisopoikilocytosis, blister cell, glutathione

References

1. Frank JE. Diagnosis and management of G6PD deficiency. *Am Fam Physician.* 2005;72:1277-1282.

2. Glader B. Hereditary hemolytic anemias due to enzyme deficiencies. In: Greer JP, Foerester J, Lukens JN, Rodgers GM, Paraskevas F, Glader B, editors. *Wintrobe's Clinical Hematology,* 11th ed. Philadelphia: Lippincott Williams and Wilkins; 2004: 1115-1140.

3. Jiang J, Ma X, Song C, et al. Using the fluorescence spot test for neonatal screening of G6PD deficiency. *Southeast Asian J Trop Med Public Health.* 2003;34S:140-142.

4. Al-Ali AK, Al-Mustafa ZH, Al-Madan M, et al. Molecular characterization of glucose-6-phosphate dehydrogenase deficiency in the Eastern Province of Saudi Arabia. *Clin Chem Lab Med.* 2002;40:814-816.

5. Tseng CP, Huang CL, Chong KY, et al. Rapid detection of glucose-6-phosphate dehydrogenase gene mutations by denaturing high-performance liquid chromatography. *Clin Biochem.* 2005;38:973-980.

Mild Anemia, Microcytosis, and Target Cells in a Man From Thailand

Jonathan Marotti, Bradley Bryan, Parul Bhargava

Department of Pathology, Beth Israel Deaconess Medical Center, Boston, MA

Patient: 35-year-old man from Thailand.

Chief Complaint: Referred to gastroenterology for further evaluation of mild anemia.

History of Present Illness: This patient was referred to gastroenterology for further evaluation of newly-diagnosed asymptomatic anemia. He reported no chest pain, shortness of breath, weakness, hematochezia, diarrhea, or constipation, and only occasional mild epigastric discomfort after eating spicy foods, but did not report dysphagia. His weight and appetite have been stable.

Past Medical History: The patient has no significant past medical history and was not taking any medications.

Family History: There was no family history of colorectal cancer.

Social History: The patient is a recent immigrant from Thailand who has been in the United States for the past year. He is not married. He does not smoke or drink alcohol. He eats only once a day, but reports a balanced diet of red meat, green, leafy vegetables, and fruit.

Physical Examination Findings: The patient was alert, oriented, and in no apparent distress. The patient's blood pressure was 100/70 mm Hg and his heart rate was 72 beats per minute. He was afebrile. A head-ear-eyes-nose-throat (HEENT) examination was unremarkable. No lymphadenopathy or scleral icterus was noted. The cardiovascular examination was unremarkable. The lungs were clear to auscultation bilaterally. The abdomen was soft, non-tender, and with positive bowel sounds. There was no organomegaly. Edema of the lower extremities was not present. The neurologic examination was grossly normal.

Additional Tests: Based on the findings observed on the patient's peripheral blood smear (**Image 1A**), alkaline (**Image 1B**) and acid (**Image 1C**) hemoglobin electrophoresis was performed.

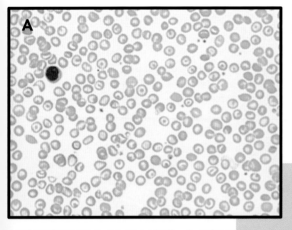

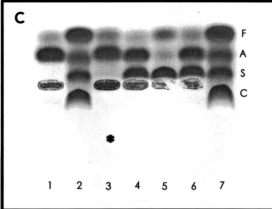

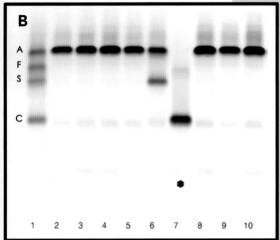

Image 1_The patient's peripheral blood smear, illustrating (**A**) microcytic red blood cells with slight hypochromasia, abundant target cells, an absence of pencil cells or anisopoikilocytosis typically seen in iron deficiency anemia, and no intracellular crystals, coarse basophilic stippling, dacrocytes, or Howell-Jolly bodies (Wright stain, 40× magnification). Alkaline (pH 8.6) (**B**) and acid (pH 6.2) (**C**) hemoglobin (Hb) electrophoresis of a hemolysate prepared from the patient's EDTA whole blood specimen demonstrated, when compared with the Hb standard containing Hb's A, F, S, and C (**B**, lane 1), no band in the HbA position, a band (13.6%) in the HbF position, and a large band (86.3%) in the HbC position (ie, A-, F+, C++) (**B**, lane 7). Acid Hb electrophoresis demonstrated, when compared with the Hb standard (**C**, lane 7), the presence of (**C**, lane 3) a large band in the HbA position, a band in the HbF position, and no band in the HbC position (ie, A+, F+, C-).

Questions _____

1. What is the most striking peripheral blood smear finding?

2. What are the diagnostic possibilities based on peripheral blood smear findings alone?

3. What are the patient's other most striking clinical and laboratory findings?

4. How do you explain this patient's most striking clinical and laboratory findings?

5. What is this patient's most likely diagnosis?

6. What are other possible diagnostic considerations given the available findings?

7. What laboratory methods are available for diagnosing this patient's disease?

8. What is the pathogenesis of this patient's condition?

9. What is the prevalence and geographic distribution of this patient's disease?

10. What treatment and counseling should this patient receive?

Possible Answers _____

1. Abundant target cells (**Image 1A**). Pertinent negative findings include the absence of pencil cells or anisopoikilocytosis pointing against an iron deficiency state. Also, no intracellular

T1. Prinicipal Laboratory Findings

Test	Patient's Result	Reference Interval
Hematology		
WBC count	5.7	$4.0–11.0 \times 10^3/\mu L$
RBC count	6.49	$4.6–6.2 \times 10^6/\mu L$
Hemoglobin	13.6	14.0–18.0 g/dL
Hematocrit	37.6	40–52%
MCV	58	82–98 fL
MCH	20.9	27–32 pg
MCHC	36.0	31–35%
RDW	17.1	10.8–15.5%
Reticulocyte count	1.2	1.2–3.2%
Platelet count	260	$150–440 \times 10^3/\mu L$
Differential count: Neutrophils	54.3	50–70%
Lymphocytes	37.8	18–42%
Monocytes	4.8	2–11%
Basophils	1.2	0–4%
Eosinophils	2.0	0–2%
Coagulation		
PT	13.5	10.4–13.1 sec
INR	1.2	0.9–1.1
PTT	35.8	22.0–35.0 sec
Chemistry		
BUN	12	6–20 mg/dL
Creatinine	0.9	0.5–1.2 mg/dL
Iron	143	45–160 ug/dL
TIBC	224	260–470 ug/dL
Ferritin	460	30–400 ng/mL
Transferrin	172	200–360 mg/dL
Vitamin B_{12}	637	240–900 pg/mL
Folate	7.5	2.0–20 ng/mL

RBC, red blood cell; WBC, white blood cell; MCV, mean corpuscular volume; MCH, mean corpuscular hemoglobin; MHC, mean corpuscular hemoglobin concentration; RDW, red cell distribution width; PT, prothrombin time; INR, International Normalized Ratio; PTT, partial thromboplastin time; BUN, blood urea nitrogen; TIBC, total iron binding capacity.

"crystals," coarse basophilic stippling, Howell-Jolly bodies, or dacrocytes were seen.

2. Target cells, or codocytes, are the result of an increased surface-to-volume ratio and signify either excessive loss of internal content (volume) of the red cell or excessive cell membrane formation.[1] The major causes of decreased hemoglobin (Hb) production, and, thus, decreased internal content, include iron deficiency anemia (IDA), thalassemias, and certain hemoglobinopathies (hemoglobins E, C, SC, and S). An increase in membrane formation results when there is abnormal production of certain cell membrane components, particularly cholesterol. Examples include severe liver disease, especially obstructive jaundice, and lecithin-cholesterol acyltransferase (LCAT) deficiency.[1] The patient had no signs or symptoms of obstructive jaundice. Asplenism can lead to an increase in excess membrane formation because fragments of the membrane are no longer removed. In this case, one would expect to see Howell-Jolly bodies on the peripheral blood smear. It is important to be aware that improper smear preparation can also produce target cells. High humidity and slow air drying during smear preparation can cause hemoglobin to abnormally precipitate centrally and along the rim of the red cell.[1] In addition, HbC disease produces hemoglobin with decreased solubility that abnormally precipitates, forming both target cells and distinctive intracellular crystals.[1] These crystals were not seen in this patient's peripheral blood smear. In thalassemias, the mean corpuscular volume (MCV) is typically low with a preserved or high red blood cell (RBC) count (as seen in this patient); however, a review of the peripheral blood smear often shows, in addition to targets, tear-drop forms (dacrocytes) with or without coarse basophilic stippling. Iron deficiency typically shows anisopoikilocytosis with hypochromasia and pencil forms (thin elliptocytes), features that were notably absent on the patient's peripheral blood smear. In summary, target cells can be found in IDA, thalassemias, hemoglobinopathies, liver disease, LCAT deficiency, post-splenectomy, and after improper smear preparation. Given the patient's relatively unremarkable clinical history, lack of evidence of liver disease, and lack of typical morphologic features of iron deficiency and asplenism, the leading differential diagnostic considerations on morphologic grounds include a hemoglobinopathy or thalassemia. Among the common hemoglobinopathies (ie, HbE,

HbC, HbSC) that lead to the formation of target cells, the lack of C crystals, suggestive of HbC disease, and sickle forms, suggestive of HbSC, makes HbE disease a more likely consideration. Correlation with clinical and additional laboratory data, in particular hemoglobin electrophoresis findings, is needed for further assessment.

3. The patient is clinically asymptomatic. On physical examination, he is anicteric with no organomegaly noted. He has had no prior surgeries or traumas. Specifically, his spleen has not been removed, nor is there evidence of cholecystectomy; the latter, if present, may indicate chronic hemolysis with pigment stones. His complete blood count findings were consistent with marked microcytosis and hypochromasia. Finally, the most striking finding in the alkaline hemoglobin electrophoresis pattern was a major band in the HbC position with no HbA present (**Image 1B**). The acid hemoglobin electrophoresis pattern showed a band in the HbA position along with elevated HbF (**Image 1C**).

4. The most striking initial laboratory finding in this patient was microcytosis (MCV of 58 fL; normal range: 82 to 98 fL). The major differential diagnostic considerations for microcytosis include IDA, thalassemias, certain hemoglobinopathies, red cell fragmentation syndromes, hereditary membrane disorders (eg, hereditary pyropoikilocytosis, homozygous elliptocytosis), hemolytic anemias, and various inflammatory states.[2] The patient's normal iron studies essentially exclude IDA. There was no evidence of hemolysis (normal reticulocyte count and no schistocytes or microspherocytes observed on the peripheral blood smear), which makes red cell fragmentation syndromes and other hereditary and acquired hemolytic anemias unlikely. The normal-to-high RBC count, together with the low MCV, points towards a thalassemic picture. The mean corpuscular hemoglobin (MCH) was decreased, indicating a decreased amount of hemoglobin in the red blood cells. As discussed above, the most striking finding on the peripheral blood smear was abundant target cells. Target cells are especially prominent in hemoglobin E, C, SC, and S diseases.[1] Therefore, hemoglobin electrophoresis is required for further assessment. As seen in the alkaline electrophoresis pattern (**Image 1B**), the patient's sample showed a major band in the HbC position and the absence of HbA. This finding is diagnostic of a hemoglobinopathy, but does not indicate which Hb variant is present since hemoglobins E and O migrate in a similar position to HbC. Acid electrophoresis showed a major band in the A position and an absent band in the HbC position (**Image 1C**). This finding excludes HbC as the cause of this patient's hemoglobinopathy. While HbO-Arab is found primarily in individuals of Bulgarian or African-American descent, HbE is found in individuals from Southeast Asia.[3] Given the ethnic background of the patient (discussed below), along with his microcytosis (O-Arab is typically normocytic), an HbE variant is favored as the cause of his hemoglobinopathy. Clinically, homozygous HbE disease causes an asymptomatic mild microcytic anemia[4]; therefore, the overall clinical and laboratory findings of the patient are most consistent with HbE disease.

5. *Most likely diagnosis: HbE disease.*

6. Hemoglobin E/β-thalassemia is the major alternative diagnostic consideration. Both HbE disease and HbE/β-thalassemia are characterized by anemia, the presence of HbE by hemoglobin electrophoresis, and target cells on the peripheral blood smear. However, there can be significant differences in clinical presentation, peripheral blood smear findings, and other laboratory data that may aid in distinguishing between HbE disease versus HbE/β-thalassemia. Hemoglobin E disease causes only a mild, usually asymptomatic, anemia with microcytosis and erythrocytosis. Since both β genes carry the mutation, no HbA should be seen on hemoglobin electrophoresis. Typically, HbF is only mildly increased in this disorder. In 1 series of 7 patients with HbE disease, the mean HbF level was 3.4 ± 2.4%.[5] In contrast, HbE/β-thalassemia typically has a greater degree of HbF elevation. In the same study,[5] the mean HbF level in 43 patients with HbE/β-thalassemia was 27.3 ± 15.9%, and in a different series of 16 patients HbF levels ranged from 9.0% to 36.6%.[6] Hemoglobin A2 levels are difficult to estimate as this hemoglobin coelutes with HbE. The presence of even a minute quantity of HbA, in the absence of a history of a blood transfusion, would indicate compound heterozygosity for E/β-thalassemia. Clinically, individuals with HbE/β-thalassemia

appear markedly different from individuals with HbE disease and can have a more devastating clinical course. It is often detected in childhood and is characterized by severe anemia with jaundice, marked splenomegaly, growth retardation, and increased risk of infection.[7] The peripheral blood smear can show numerous nucleated red blood cells and anisopoikilocytosis with dacrocytes, elliptocytes, red blood cell fragments, and coarse basophilic stippling.[3] However, it should be noted that there is remarkable variability in the severity of the anemia and subsequent clinical phenotype of HbE/β-thalassemia.[4-10] For example, Premawardhena and colleagues were able to classify 109 patients with HbE/β-thalassemia into 5 groups based largely on transfusion requirements.[10] Group 1 patients required none or only minimal transfusions, while group 5 patients were completely transfusion dependent. This phenotypic diversity was present even though the difference in steady-state hemoglobin levels was small between the various groups (6.3 g/dL in groups 1 and 2, versus 5.5 g/dL in groups 3 to 5).[10] A mechanism to explain this clinical variability remains unclear. Possibilities include the exact nature of the β-thalassemia mutations, coinheritance of α-thalassemia mutations, and factors that lead to an increase in hemoglobin F.[11-13] In the case of this patient, given the complete absence of HbA, only a modestly-elevated HbF (13.7%), and a clinically-benign course, a diagnosis of HbE disease is favored. However, the possibility of a clinically-mild presentation of hemoglobin E/β-thalassemia could not be entirely excluded; family studies, if possible, can be very helpful in this differential.

7. Hemoglobin electrophoresis is the principal laboratory method for diagnosing HbE disease and other hemoglobinopathies.[3,14,15] It is usually performed sequentially in 2 ways using a hemolysate prepared from anticoagulated whole blood. Alkaline electrophoresis at pH 8.6, using cellulose acetate or agar as the support medium, is the initial method, followed by acid electrophoresis at pH 6.2 using an agar medium and a citrate buffer. During alkaline electrophoresis, hemoglobin is negatively charged and migrates toward the positive electrode (anode). The amino acid substitutions that occur in abnormal hemoglobin molecules alter their net charge,

causing an electrophoretic migration pattern that differs from that observed for the normal (non-mutated) hemoglobin molecule. A standard containing 4 known hemoglobins (A, F, S, and C) is used as a reference and results in 4 distinct bands. Following electrophoresis, the hemoglobin pattern observed for the patient's sample can then be compared with the standard. However, interpretation of alkaline electrophoresis patterns is limited because of comigration of various hemoglobin variants. Specifically, hemoglobins C, E, and O-Arab all migrate in the C position, and hemoglobins S, D, G, and Lepore all migrate in the S position; therefore, acid electrophoresis is frequently performed as a complementary test. Agaropectin is a negatively-charged sulfated polysaccharide within the agar medium that binds to hemoglobin amino acids.[3] The degree to which agaropectin binds to hemoglobin depends on the hemoglobin variant. The differential binding of hemoglobin variants to agaropectin during acid electrophoresis results in a migration pattern that differs from alkaline electrophoresis. For example, HbC is now separated from HbE and HbO-Arab; the latter 2 variants comigrate with HbA under these conditions. Alternative methods that can also be used to identify less common hemoglobin variants include isoelectric focusing, high performance liquid chromatography (HPLC), globin electrophoresis, capillary electrophoresis, and amino acid/DNA sequencing.[14]

8. Hemoglobin A is the principal oxygen-transport protein within red blood cells. In humans, HbA consists of a tetramer comprised of 2 α-globin chains and 2 β-globin chains, each associated with an iron-containing heme group. Chromosome 16 contains 2 α-globin chain genes and chromosome 11 contains 1 β-globin gene. Quantitative defects in structurally-normal globin chain production are termed thalassemias, while production of structurally-abnormal globin chains with amino acid substitutions are called hemoglobinopathies. In 1954, 2 independent groups first detected an abnormal hemoglobin variant, which was called hemoglobin E (HbE).[16,17] It is now known that HbE results from the amino acid substitution of lysine (DNA codon, AAG) for glutamic acid (DNA codon, GAG) at the 26th amino acid position of the β-globin chain.[18] This substitution creates

an alternative or "cryptic" splicing site on exon 1 that, when utilized, leads to the production of nonfunctional messenger RNA and a subsequent reduction in the amount of normal β-globin mRNA produced.[19] This results in a thalassemic-like phenotype. In addition, even though HbE has normal oxygen affinity, it is also mildly unstable.[20,21] In the heterozygous state, the relative proportion of HbE is approximately 30%, with the remainder being HbA. In the homozygous state, the proportion of HbE varies from about 85% to 98% with the remainder being HbF.[3]

9. Hemoglobin E is the most common hemoglobinopathy in Southeast Asia. The highest numbers of affected individuals are found in Thailand where the overall prevalence has been estimated to be 13%.[12] In northeast Thailand, the prevalence of HbE reaches 50%.[12] Large numbers of individuals with HbE are also seen in Indonesia, Bangladesh, northeast India, and Sri Lanka. Additionally, it has been reported that up to 3,000 children are born with the more severe hemoglobinopathy, HbE/β-thalassemia, each year in Thailand, and there are approximately 100,000 HbE/β-thalassemia patients in Thailand.[10] These numbers are of particular importance as Southeast Asian immigrant communities continue to increase in Europe and North America.[22,23]

10. As this patient is currently asymptomatic, no treatment is necessary; however, a few critical counseling issues should be addressed. First, since the patient is not iron deficient, both he and his primary care providers should be aware that, despite his marked microcytosis, iron replacement therapy is not warranted. Iron overload due to transfusions and excess gastrointestinal absorption are the major causes of morbidity and mortality in thalassemic patients.[24] Since HbE/β-thalassemia cannot be entirely excluded in this case, genetic counseling to determine inheritance risk for future progeny is important. If his spouse carries the β-thalassemia trait, their children can be at risk for β-thalassemia major. Hence, genetic testing or family studies, if possible, are of particular importance to establish the exact genetic defect causing the abnormal hemoglobin found in the patient's blood.

Keywords

hemoglobin E disease, anemia, microcytosis, target cells

References

1. Glassy EF. *Color Atlas of Hematology: An Illustrated Field Guide Based on Proficiency Testing.* Northfield, IL: College of American Pathologists; 1998.

2. Mach-Pascual S, Darbellay R, Pilotto PA, et al. Investigation of microcytosis: A comprehensive approach. *Eur J Haematol.* 1996;57:54–61.

3. Hoyer JD, Kroft SH. *Color Atlas of Hemoglobin Disorders: A Compendium Based on Proficiency Testing.* Northfield, IL: College of American Pathologists; 2003.

4. Rees DC, Styles L, Vichinsky EP, et al. The hemoglobin E syndromes. *Ann NY Acad Sci.* 1998;850:334–343.

5. Tyagi S, Pati HP, Choudhry VP, et al. Clinico-heamatological profile of HbE syndrome in adults and children. *Hematology.* 2004;9:57–60.

6. Mehta, BC, Agarwal MB, Varandani DG, et al. Hemoglobin E-thalassemia: A study of 16 cases. *Acta Haemat.* 1980;64:201–204.

7. Fucharoen, S, Ketvichit P, Pootrakul P, et al. Clinical manifestations of β-thalassemia/hemoglobin E disease. *J Pediatr Hematol Oncol.* 2000;22:552–557.

8. Fucharoen S, Winichagoon P. Clinical and hematologic aspects of hemoglobin E β-thalassemia. *Curr Opin Hematol.* 2000;7:106–112.

9. Katsanis E, Luke K, Hsu E, et al. Hemoglobin E: A common hemoglobinopathy among children of Southeast Asian origin. *CMAJ.* 1987;137:39–42.

10. Premawardhena A, De Silver S, Arambepola M, et al. Hemoglobin E-β-thalassemia: Progress report from the International Study Group. *Ann NY Acad Sci.* 2005;1054:33–39.

11. Winichagoon P, Fucharoen S, Chen P, et al. Genetic factors that affect clinical severity in β-thalassemia syndromes. *J Pediatr Hematol Oncol.* 2000;22:573–580.

12. Sanchaisuriya K, Fucharoen G, Sae-ung N, et al. Molecular and hematologic features of hemoglobin E heterozygotes with different forms of α-thalassemia in Thailand. *Ann Hematol.* 2003;82:612–616.

13. Rees DC. Hemoglobin F and hemoglobin E/β-thalassemia. *J Pediatr Hematol Oncol.* 2000;22:567–572.

14. Clarke GM, Higgins TN. Laboratory investigation of hemoglobinopathies and thalassemias: Review and update. *Clin Chem.* 2000;46:1284–1290.

15. Bain BJ, Amos RJ, Bareford D, et al. The laboratory diagnosis of haemoglobinopathies. *Br J Haemat.* 1998;101:783–792.

16. Itano HA, Bergren WR, Sturgeon P. Identification of a fourth abnormal human hemoglobin. *J Am Chem Soc*. 1954;76:2278.

17. Chernoff AI, Minnich V, Chongchareonsuk S. Hemoglobin E, a hereditary abnormality of human hemoglobin. *Science*. 1954;120:605–606.

18. Hunt JA, Ingram VM. Abnormal human hemoglobins. VI. The chemical difference between hemoglobins A and E. *Biochim Biophys Acta*. 1961;49:520–536.

19. Traeger J, Wood WG, Clegg JB, et al. Defective synthesis of HbE is due to reduced levels of βE mRNA. *Nature*. 1980;288:497–499.

20. Frischer H, Bowman J. Hemoglobin E, an oxidatively unstable mutation. *J Lab Clin Med*. 1975;85:531.

21. Macdonald VW, Charache S. Differences in the reaction sequences associated with drug-induced oxidation of hemoglobins E, S, A, and F. *J Lab Clin Med*. 1983;102:762–772.

22. Vichinsky EP, MacKlin EA, Waye JS, et al. Changes in the epidemiology of thalassemia in North America: A new minority disease. *Pediatrics*. 2005;116:818–825.

23. Lorey F. Asian immigration and public health in California: Thalassemia in newborns in California. *J Pediatr Hematol Oncol*. 2000;22:564–566.

24. Rund D, Rachmilewitz, E. β-thalassemia. *N Eng J Med*. 2005;353:1135–1146.

Long-Standing Microcytic Anemia in a 29-Year-Old Woman

Peggy Soung Sullivan, Anthony W. Butch

Department of Pathology and Laboratory Medicine, Geffen School of Medicine, University of California at Los Angeles, Los Angeles, CA

Patient: 29-year-old woman of Asian descent.

Chief Complaint: Long-standing microcytic anemia.

History of Present Illness: The patient has been anemic for many years with hemoglobin (Hb) concentrations ranging from 8.9 to 10.5 g/dL. Red blood cells (RBCs) have been microcytic with a mean cell volume (MCV) around 60 fL. She is occasionally fatigued, but is active and runs several miles at a time for exercise. The patient has never received a blood transfusion and has never had hepatomegaly or splenomegaly.

Medical History: Non-contributory. The patient takes vitamin C, iron, folate, vitamin B_{12}, and multi-vitamins. She has never smoked and does not drink alcohol.

Family History: The patient is a single resident physician with 1 sibling and no children. Her mother died in her mid-50s from adenocarcinoma of the esophagus. There is a family history of coronary artery disease, diabetes, hyperlipidemia, and hypertension.

Physical Examination: No abnormal findings were noted. Her vital signs were: temperature, 99.6° F; pulse, 58 beats/minute; blood pressure, 88/56 mm Hg.

Additional Diagnostic Tests: Analysis of Hb variants was performed on the patient's blood using high performance liquid chromatography (HPLC) with results as shown in **Figure 1**.

Questions _____

1. What are this patient's most striking clinical and laboratory findings?

2. How do you explain these findings?

3. What is this patient's differential diagnosis?

4. Which laboratory tests are most useful in distinguishing between the different possible causes of this patient's condition?

5. What other laboratory tests could be performed on this patient?

6. What is this patient's most likely diagnosis?

7. What is the genetic basis of this disease?

8. What additional tests are needed to confirm the diagnosis?

9. What clinical findings are associated with this patient's disease?

T1. Principal Laboratory Findings

Analyte	Patient's Result	Reference Interval
Hematology		
WBC count	8.5	$3.3–9.3 \times 10^3/\mu L$
RBC count	5.56	$3.76–4.93 \times 10^3/\mu L$
Hemoglobin	10.0	11.5–14.6 g/dL
MCV	60.8	79.0–95.0 fL
MCH	18.0	26.0–32.6 pg
MCHC	29.6	31.7–35.5 g/dL
RDW	24.3	10.7–15.5%
Platelet count	202	$143–398 \times 10^3/\mu L$
Reticulocyte count, auto	2.78	0.55–2.08%
Absolute reticulocyte #	0.1546	$0.0216–0.0919 \times 10^6/\mu L$
Immature reticulocyte fraction	20.9	3.4–14.9%
Chemistry		
Sodium	136	136–146 mmol/L
Potassium	3.5	3.6–5.0 mmol/L
Chloride	101	97–110 mmol/L
Total CO_2	26	25–32 mmol/L
Glucose	91	65–110 mg/dL
Urea nitrogen	6	8–20 mg/dL
Total protein	7.6	5.8–8.1 g/dL
Albumin	4.9	3.4–4.7 g/dL
Bilirubin, total	1.5	0.2–1.5 mg/dL
Alkaline phosphatase	39	35–110 U/L
AST	21	15–50 U/L
ALT	14	5–50 U/L
Calcium	9.7	8.6–10.1 mg/dL
Triglycerides	90	<150 mg/dL (desirable)
Cholesterol	161	<200 mg/dL (desirable)
HDL-cholesterol	48	>40 mg/dL (desirable)
LDL-cholesterol (calculated)	95	<130 mg/dL (desirable)
Ferritin	83	8–150 ng/mL
Folate, serum	>40.0	5.6–19.3 ng/mL
Iron	80	17–156 µg/dL
Total iron binding capacity	261	250–450 µg/dL
Iron saturation	31	20–45%

WBC, white blood cell; RBC, red blood cell; MCV, mean cell volume; MCH, mean cell hemoglobin; MCHC, mean cell hemoglobin concentration; RDW, red blood cell distribution width; CO_2, carbon dioxide; AST, aspartate aminotransferase; ALT, alanine aminotransferase, HDL, high density lipoprotein; LDL, low density lipoprotein.

T2. Serum Markers of Iron Status in Microcytic Hypochromic Anemias

Disorder	Iron	TIBC/ Transferrin	% Saturation	Ferritin	Transferrin Receptor
Iron deficiency	↓	↑	↓	↓	↑
Chronic inflammation	↓	N or ↓	N or ↓	N or ↑	N
Thalassemia	N	N	N	N or ↑	N
Sideroblastic anemia	↑	N	↑	↑	N

TIBC, total iron binding capacity; ↓, decreased; ↑, increased; N, normal.

10. What is the most appropriate treatment for this patient's disease?

11. Is screening and/or genetic counseling recommended for this patient's disease?

Possible Answers

1. The most striking clinical finding is the long-standing anemia despite oral intake of iron, folate, vitamin B_{12}, and multi-vitamins. The most striking laboratory findings are the increased red blood cell (RBC) count with a decreased hemoglobin (Hb), mean cell volume (MCV),

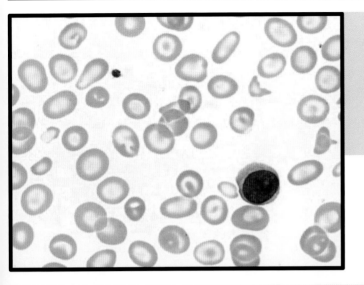

Image 1_Patient's peripheral blood smear illustrating marked hypochromic microcytic red cells, numerous target cells, polychromasia, poikilocytosis, and anisocytosis with numerous small teardrop forms, ovalocytes, and schistocytes (red cell fragments).

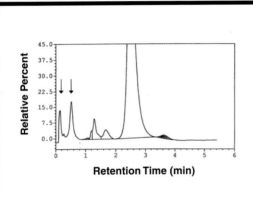

Figure 1_Hb separation by HPLC (Bio-Rad Variant beta-thal short program) revealed a normal Hb F of 0.3% (reference interval, 0-1.8%), a low Hb A2 of 1.6% (reference interval, 2.3-3.5%), and 2 distinct unknown peaks with very short retention times (<0.6 minutes).

mean cell hemoglobin (MCH), and mean cell hemoglobin concentration (MCHC), and the increased RBC distribution width (RDW) and reticulocyte count (**T1**). Other notable findings are numerous target cells, poikilocytes, and anisocytes on the peripheral blood smear (**Image 1**).

2. The patient's laboratory findings confirm a long-standing microcytic, hypochromic anemia. The decreased Hb, MCV, and MCH indicate a quantitative defect in Hb production.

3. The differential diagnosis for microcytic anemia includes iron deficiency, a chronic inflammatory disorder, thalassemia, and sideroblastic anemia. Iron deficiency is the most common cause and can be due to a nutritional deficiency or increased iron requirements due to blood loss or other conditions. Long-standing chronic

inflammation as a result of infection, collagen vascular diseases, and malignancies such as carcinoma and lymphoma, can also produce a microcytic hypochromic anemia. Thalassemias are a heterogeneous group of hereditary disorders resulting in impaired production of either alpha- or beta-globin chains. Sideroblastic anemia is due to defective synthesis of heme and can be inherited (x-linked, autosomal dominant, and autosomal recessive), acquired or secondary to various drugs and toxic agents such as lead or ethanol.[1]

4. The complete blood count and RBC morphology on a peripheral blood smear can be very similar for both iron deficiency anemia and thalassemia. Various RBC indices routinely provided by electronic RBC cell counters can be helpful for differentiating between these 2 conditions. The MCV tends to be lower in thalassemia

compared with iron deficiency, and MCV cutoffs of 72 to 75 fL have been recommended for distinguishing between the 2 disorders.[2] The Hb and RBC count can also be used with the MCV to derive indices to discriminate between iron deficiency and thalassemia.[3,4] Another index often used is the RDW. A normal RDW is commonly found in thalassemia whereas an elevated RDW is common in iron deficiency. However, the RDW can be elevated in some thalassemias, such as hemoglobin H (Hb H) disease and delta beta-thalassemia.[5] Serum markers of iron status are helpful in differentiating between various causes of microcytic hypochromic anemias (**T2**). Since this patient takes iron supplements, and has normal values for serum markers reflective of iron status, it is unlikely she is iron deficient. An MCV of 61 also argues against this diagnosis. Moreover, the patient does not have a history of an underlying chronic inflammatory disorder. Basophilic stippling and 2 distinct RBC populations are not seen in the peripheral blood film, arguing against lead poisoning and sideroblastic anemia. Numerous target cells are present, which is consistent with a thalassemia.

5. Other tests that can be performed include Hb electrophoresis, brilliant cresyl blue staining of peripheral blood films, isoelectric focusing, and Hb fractionation by high-performance liquid chromatography (HPLC). Hemoglobin H migrates rapidly in agarose gel electrophoresis at alkaline pH and appears anodal to Hb A. The distance between Hb H and Hb A is approximately the same as the distance between Hb A_2 and Hb A. If standard alkaline gel electrophoresis times are used, Hb H can be missed since it will migrate off the gel. It is important to be aware of this possibility and to use shorter electrophoresis times (20 minutes using the Beckman Paragon system) when one suspects the presence of Hb H.[6] In addition, a faint band of Bart's Hb (gamma$_4$) is often seen an equal distance between Hb H and Hb A. Hemoglobin A_2 is often decreased and Hb F can be elevated. When using agarose gel electrophoresis at acid pH, a faint band of Hb H can be detected at the point of application.[6] Isoelectric focusing can also be used to detect Hb H; however, this technique is rarely performed by clinical laboratories and is usually only available from reference laboratories. The amount of Hb H detected by any of these methods varies from 1% to 40% of the total Hb.[7] Brilliant cresyl blue staining of peripheral blood films may also be diagnostically helpful in detecting characteristic Hb H inclusions within RBCs.[8,9] Denaturation and precipitation of unstable Hb H results in diffuse stippling of the RBCs (Hb H inclusions). Brilliant cresyl blue staining was performed (1% brilliant cresyl blue in isotonic saline) on a fresh EDTA-anticoagulated blood sample from this patient and peripheral blood films were examined at 1- and 4-hour intervals. Although reticulocytes stained positive, no Hb H inclusions were observed (data not shown). It is noteworthy that brilliant cresyl blue staining has been shown to be an excellent screening test for Hb H, with studies reporting sensitivities as high as 100% in detecting Hb H inclusions.[8,9] However, the performance of the brilliant cresyl blue test can vary widely and has been reported to give false-negative results, depending on the dye manufacturer and dye lot-to-lot variability.[6,8] Hemoglobin fractionation by HPLC of blood from this patient showed the following percentages for each Hb species (reference intervals): Hb A, 97.4% (95% to 98%); Hb A_2, 1.6% (2.3% to 3.5%); Hb F, 0.3% (0.0% to 1.8%) (**Figure 1**). The reduced Hb A_2 (1.6%) suggests alpha-thalassemia or Hb E. Two abnormal peaks with short retention times were noted (arrows in **Figure 1**) and most likely represent Hb H, a tetramer of 4 beta-globin chains.[10] These peaks were not included in the calculation to determine the percentage of each Hb. A peak corresponding to Hb E was not seen.

6. ***Most likely diagnosis:*** *Hb H disease (clinically manifested as thalassemia intermedia).*

7. Hemoglobin molecules are made up of 2 pairs of different globin chains. Each polypeptide chain contains a porphyrin derivative called heme, and polypeptide chains without the heme moiety are called globins. In normal adults, Hb A is the major hemoglobin and is composed of 2 identical alpha-globin chains and 2 identical beta-globin chains. Thalassemias are a group of hereditary disorders caused by mutations or deletions in 1 or more globin genes resulting in decreased or absent globin chain production. Alpha-thalassemia results from diminished alpha-globin chain production and is usually an inherited disorder except in very rare circumstances.[11]

The majority of alpha-thalassemias are caused by a deletion of 1 or more alpha-globin genes; nondeletional (inactivation) mutations are less common.[11] Because there are 4 alpha-globin genes on chromosome 16, there are 5 possible deletional combinations. The severity of the disease is related to the number of affected genes. Deletion of both genes from 1 or both chromosomes is called alpha-thalassemia 1 (the double deletion was identified first), whereas deletion of only 1 gene from 1 or both chromosomes is called alpha-thalassemia 2. Heterozygous and homozygous are used to denote 1 or 2 affected chromosomes, respectively. A single alpha-chain deletion (heterozygous alpha-thalassemia 2), also called alpha-thalassemia trait, is clinically silent and found worldwide. These deletions are very common and are found in 30% of African Americans and more than half the people living in Saudi Arabia, India, Thailand, Papua New Guinea, and Melanesia.[12,13] Deletion of 2 alpha-globin genes (homozygous alpha-thalassemia 2 and heterozygous alpha-thalassemia 1), also called thalassemia minor, is associated with a mild anemia, microcytic RBCs and erythrocytosis. The double gene deletion on 1 chromosome (heterozygous alpha-thalassemia 1) is common in Southeast Asia and the Mediterranean basin, but is rare among African Americans. Thus, ethnic origin should be considered when screening for thalassemia. Deletion of 3 alpha-globin genes (compound heterozygote alpha-thalassemia 1/alpha-thalassemia 2) results in Hb H disease and is clinically classified as thalassemia intermedia. Hemoglobin H disease exhibits marked phenotypic variability and manifests as a moderate to severe hemolytic disease. The excess beta-globin chains are unstable and form tetramers (Hb H) that precipitate slowly within RBCs (Heinz bodies), causing hemolysis or removal from the circulation by the reticuloendothelial system.[11,14] Clinical severity of the disease is related to the amount of Hb H in RBCs. Hemoglobin H disease is usually caused by detection of both alpha-globin genes on 1 chromosome and deletion of a single alpha-globin gene on the other chromosome. Less common is a point mutation or small insertion/deletion of 1 of the alpha-globin chains on the other chromosome (nondeletional Hb H disease). Hemoglobin H disease is particularly common in Southeast Asia and southern China and is also found in Middle Eastern and Mediterranean populations. It is estimated that Hb H disease is present in 420,000 people in Thailand.[15] Hemoglobin H disease is rarely seen in African Americans.[14] Deletion of all 4 alpha-globin genes (homozygous alpha-thalassemia 1) results in the complete absence of alpha-globin chain production and is not compatible with life. It is also called Hb Bart's hydrops fetalis. An affected fetus dies in utero or soon after premature birth and has gamma-globin tetramers (Hb Bart's) with very high oxygen binding capacity in RBCs. Homozygous alpha-thalassemia 1 syndrome is the most common cause of hydrops fetalis in Southeast Asian and southern China, however it is rarely observed in other populations.[8,14]

8. DNA-based genotyping would be needed to confirm the diagnosis of Hb H disease. Southern blot analysis of alpha-globin genes can be performed for diagnosis of the most common deletional mutations.[8] Gap-polymerase chain reaction methods have also been developed for some of the more common Mediterranean and Southeast Asian single- and double-gene mutations.[16] Large deletions encompassing the entire zeta-alpha-globin gene cluster can be difficult to detect, requiring probes distal to the deletional breakpoints.[17] Tests to detect less common non-deletional point mutations are often based on direct nucleotide sequencing of a selectively amplified polymerase chain reaction (PCR) product. Multiplex PCR and reverse dot-blot hybridization with multiple probes have been used to simplify detection of numerous point mutations; however, a simple approach for all alpha-thalassemia point mutations has not been developed.[11] Southern blot analysis using 2 DNA probes (1 directed to the alpha-globin gene and the other to the zeta globin gene) revealed this patient had 3 alpha-globin genes deleted. A single alpha-globin gene deletion (-4.2 kb) on 1 chromosome 16 and 2 alpha-globin gene deletions (Southeast Asian type) on the other chromosome were identified. The -4.2 kb deletion is 1 of the most common single alpha-gene deletions.[18] The Southeast Asian type deletion is 1 of the 3 most common deletions involving both alpha-globin genes; the other 2 (Mediterranean and -20.5 kb) are found in the Mediterranean population.[11,14,19]

9. The clinical findings in Hb H disease can be quite variable. Some patients are asymptomatic and have a mild disorder, while others have severe anemia with in vivo hemolysis, hepatosplenomegaly, and require frequent blood transfusions.[11,14] Infants with Hb H disease can have Hb levels that are near normal in the absence of hepatosplenomegaly.[8] Patients with nondeletional alpha-globin gene mutations typically have a more severe form of the disease than patients with deletional mutations.[11,20-23] Wide variations in clinical severity are observed in patients with the same genotype, suggesting that other poorly defined factors contribute to the severity of the disease.[11] Marked variation in Hb levels has been observed, ranging from 7.0 to 11.4 g/dL among 41 female patients with deletional Hb H disease.[24] The age at diagnosis also varies widely, ranging from birth to 74 years.[8] A study of 114 Chinese patients with Hb H disease found that only 24% presented with clinical symptoms such as jaundice, anemia, and gallstones. Most patients were found to have Hb H disease after routine health evaluations related to work or pregnancy, or after presenting with infection.[20] Other presenting features include mild dysmorphic facial features, scleral icterus, splenomegaly, and hepatomegaly.[8,20] The majority of Hb H patients have a fluctuating anemia throughout life but typically are not transfusion-dependent.[8,11,20] On occasion, Hb levels can fall dramatically, requiring transfusions. These episodes tend to surround pregnancy, infection, or the ingestion of oxidative agents or drugs. Iron overload, based on markedly increased serum ferritin, is present in approximately 70% of adults with Hb H disease.[11,20] Ferritin levels do not appear to be associated with transfusion history and are most likely due to increased iron absorption in the setting of in vivo hemolysis and ineffective erythropoiesis.[20] Imaging studies and liver biopsies have shown that the majority of Hb H patients have iron overload and hepatic fibrosis.[20,25,26] Cardiac echocardiography in 25 asymptomatic patients demonstrated a correlation between abnormal left ventricular diastolic dysfunction and serum ferritin levels. Three patients who were not transfusion-dependent developed heart failure from iron overload,[20] and 1 patient developed hemosiderosis and diabetes mellitus.[27]

10. Treatment of Hb H disease is mainly preventive and supportive. Folic acid supplementation is usually recommended, especially during the periconceptional period and beyond.[8,11] Most patients are asymptomatic despite being moderately anemic. Transfusion therapy may be indicated during severe anemia as a result of infection, fever, hypersplenism, or during pregnancy. Splenectomy may lead to clinical improvement in patients with hypersplenism.[8] Cholecystectomy for symptomatic gallstones may also be beneficial. Because of potential complications from iron overload, patients with Hb H disease should be monitored for tissue damage, and chelation therapy should be initiated when indicated. Although there are no guidelines for starting chelation therapy in Hb H patients not dependent on transfusion therapy, therapeutic intervention may be indicated earlier than in transfusion-dependent patients due to the ferrihydride form of iron that causes more tissue damage.[11,20]

11. Prenatal screening is recommended for Hb H disease. The American College of Obstetrics and Gynecology currently advocates screening high-risk couples for the potential of having offspring with thalassemia or sickle cell disease.[28] High-risk groups for Hb H disease include those of Southeast Asian or Mediterranean descent. Some states with a significant proportion of Southeast Asians (eg, California) have implemented universal newborn screening programs to detect Hb H disease.[29] In California, the prevalence of Hb H disease among all newborns is 1 per 15,000. African Americans are not at high risk for Hb H disease since heterozygous alpha-thalassemia 1 is rare among those of African ancestry.[14] However, it should be noted that in areas where multiracial births are common, offspring of African ancestry have been found to have Hb H disease.[29] Couples at increased risk for beta- or alpha-thalassemia should have an MCV obtained as part of the complete blood count. If the MCV is low and iron deficiency anemia has been excluded, follow-up testing should be performed, such as Hb electrophoresis or fractionation and molecular genetic studies.[28,30] It is strongly recommended that all individuals with Hb H disease near or at reproductive age have his or her partner screened for alpha- and beta-thalassemia carrier status.[11,28,30] If the partner has heterozygous

alpha-thalassemia 2 (a single alpha-globin gene deletion or inactivation), the fetus has a 25% chance of having Hb H disease. If the partner has homozygous alpha-thalassemia 2, the fetus has a 50% risk of having Hb H disease. If the partner has heterozygous alpha-thalassemia 1, the fetus has a 25% chance of having Hb H disease and a 25% chance of having Hb Bart's hydrops fetalis. Lastly, if the partner has Hb H disease, the fetus has a 50% chance of having Hb H disease and a 25% chance of having Hb Bart's hydrops fetalis. Prenatal diagnosis is generally not warranted for fetuses at risk for Hb H disease;[11] however, genetic counseling and prenatal diagnosis should be available for fetuses at risk of Hb Bart's hydrops fetalis.[6,11,28,30] Analysis of fetal DNA may be obtained by chorionic villus sampling or amniocentesis. Ultrasound monitoring may also be offered as an alternative to invasive procedures; however, hydropic changes may not be evident until the second trimester.[11,28,30]

Keywords

alpha-thalassemia, alpha-globin chains, hemoglobin H disease, hemoglobinopathy

References

1. Meredith JL, Rosenthal NS. Differential diagnosis of microcytic anemias. *Lab Med.* 1999;30:538–542.

2. Lafferty JD, Crowther MA, Ali MA, et al. The evaluation of various mathematical RBC indices and their efficacy in discriminating between thalassemic and non-thalassemic microcytosis. *Am J Clin Pathol.* 1996;106:201–205.

3. Mentzer WC. Differentiation of iron deficiency from thalassemia trait. *Lancet.* 1973;1:882.

4. England JM, Fraser PM. Differentiation of iron deficiency from thalassemia trait by routine blood count. *Lancet.* 1973;1:449–452.

5. Bessman JD, Gilmer PR, Gardne FH. Improved classification of anemias by MCV and RDW. *Am J Clin Pathol.* 1983;80:322–326.

6. Hall RB, Haga JA, Guerra CG, et al. Optimizing the detection of hemoglobin H disease. *Lab Med.* 1995;26:736–742.

7. Weatherall DJ, Clegg JB, eds. *The Thalassemia Syndromes*, 4th ed. Oxford, England: Blackwell Science Ltd; 2001:493–507.

8. Pan L, Eng H, Kuo C, et al. Usefulness of brilliant cresyl blue staining as an auxiliary method of screening for alpha-thalassemia. *J Lab Clin Med.* 2005;145:94–97.

9. Skogerboe KJ, West SF, Smith C, et al. Screening for alpha-thalassemia. Correlation of hemoglobin H inclusion bodies with DNA-determined genotype. *Arch Pathol Lab Med.* 1992;116:1012–1018.

10. Joutovsky A, Hadzi-Nesic J, Nardi MA. HPLC retention time as a diagnostic tool for hemoglobin variants and hemoglobinopathies: A study of 60,000 samples in a clinical diagnostic laboratory. *Clin Chem.* 2004;50:1736–1747.

11. Chui DHK, Fucharoen S, Chan V. Hemoglobin H disease: Not necessarily a benign disorder. *Blood.* 2003;101:791–800.

12. Dozy AM, Kan YW, Embury SH, et al. Alpha-globin gene organisation in blacks precludes the severe form of alpha-thalassaemia. *Nature.* 1979;280:605–607.

13. Weatherall DJ, Clegg JB. Inherited haemoglobin disorders: An increasing global health problem. *Bull World Health Organ.* 2001;79:704–712.

14. Hoffman R, Benz E, Shattil S, et al (eds.). *Hematology: Basic Principles and Practice*, 4th ed. Philadelphia: Churchill Livingstone; 2005:578–580.

15. Angastiniotis M, Modell B, Englezos P, et al. Prevention and control of haemoglobinopathies. *Bull World Health Organ.* 1995;73:375–386.

16. Baysal E, Huisman TH. Detection of common deletional alpha-thalassemia-2 determinants by PCR. *Am J Hematol.* 1994;46:208–213.

17. Waye JS, Eng B, Chui DH. Identification of an extensive zeta-alpha-globin gene deletion in a Chinese individual. *Br J Haematol.* 1992;80:378–380.

18. Lau YL, Chan LC, Chan YYA, et al. Prevalence and genotypes of alpha- and beta-thalassemia carriers in Hong Kong—implications for population screening. *N Eng J Med.* 1997;336:1298–1301.

19. Old JM. Screening and genetic diagnosis of haemoglobin disorders. *Blood Reviews.* 2003;17:43–53.

20. Chen FE, Ooi C, Ha SY, et al. Genetic and clinical features of hemoglobin H disease in Chinese patients. *N Engl J Med.* 2000;343:544–50.

21. Charoenkwan P, Taweephon R, Sae-Tung R, et al. Molecular and clinical features of Hb H disease in northern Thailand. *Hemoglobin.* 2005;29:133–40.

22. Li DZ, Liao C, Li J, et al. Hemoglobin H hydrops fetalis syndrome resulting from the association of −SEA deletion and the [alpha]Quong Sze[alpha] mutation in a Chinese woman. *Eur J Haematol.* 2005;75:259–261.

23. Papassotiriou I, Traeger-Synodinos J, Vlachou C, et al. Rapid and accurate quantitation of Hb Bart's and Hb H using weak cation exchange high performance liquid chromatography: Correlation with the alpha-thalassemia genotype. *Hemoglobin.* 1999;23:203–11.

24. Waye JS, Eng B, Patterson M, et al. Hemoglobin H disease in Canada: Molecular diagnosis and review of 116 cases. *Am J Hematol.* 2001;68:11–15.

25. Ooi GC, Chen FE, Chan KN, et al. Qualitative and quantitative magnetic resonance imaging in haemoglobin H disease: Screening for iron overload. *Clin Radiol.* 1999;54:98–102.

26. Hsu HC, Wang CC, Peng HW, et al. Hemoglobin H disease—10 years' experience. *Chin Med J* (Taipei). 1990;45:34–38.

27. Chim CS, Chan V, Todd D. Hemosiderosis with diabetes mellitus in untransfused hemoglobin H disease. *Am J Hematol.* 1998;57:160–163.

28. Rappaport VJ, Velazquez M, Williams K. Hemoglobinopathies in pregnancy. *Obstet Gynecol Clin N Am.* 2004;31:287–317.

29. Lorey F, Cunningham G, Vichinsky EP, et al. Universal newborn screening for Hb H disease in California. *Genetic Testing.* 2001;5:93–100.

30. Leung TN, Lau TK, Chung TKH. Thalassemia screening in pregnancy. *Curr Opin Obstet Gynecol.* 2005;17:129–134.

Anemia and Severe Erythrocytic Morphologic Abnormalities in Two Young Patients

Luis A. Guarda

Department of Pathology, Florida Hospital, Orlando, FL

Patient #1: A 3-year-old Vietnamese girl was admitted complaining of tiredness and pallor for the last 10 days. She had had a febrile illness in the week prior to admission. Physical examination confirmed pallor and disclosed a grade 2/6 left parasternal systolic murmur.

Patient #2: A 19-year-old African-American female was admitted complaining of upper abdominal and rib pain, which began 5 days before seeking medical attention. She admitted to having had similar symptoms 1 year prior to this admission. Physical examination revealed pale conjunctivae and a grade 2/6 systolic murmur.

Questions

1. What are these patients' most striking laboratory results?

2. How do you explain these patients' most striking laboratory results?

3. What conditions should be further investigated and which additional tests should be ordered on these patients?

4. What is the most likely diagnosis for each of these patients?

5. What are the treatment recommendations for these patients?

Possible Answers

1. *Patient #1.* Markedly decreased hemoglobin (Hb) and hematocrit; low MCV and MCH; decreased WBC count with decreased neutrophils and increased lymphocytes; markedly increased nucleated RBCs with marked reticulocytosis; markedly abnormal RBC morphology, including the presence of target cells; decreased RBC osmotic fragility [**T1**] and [**Image 1**];

and, **hypergammaglobulinemia**. *Patient #2.* Markedly decreased hemoglobin and hematocrit; low-normal MCV and MCH; increased WBC count with decreased neutrophils, increased bands; a few nucleated RBCs with marked reticulocytosis; and markedly abnormal RBC findings, including the presence of **sickle** cells [**T2**] and [**Image 2**].

2. Microcytic-hypochromic **anemia** (*Patient #1*; low hemoglobin, hematocrit, MCV, and MCH) and normocytic-normochromic **anemia** (*Patient #2*; low hemoglobin and hematocrit with low-normal MCV and MCH). Moreover, both patients demonstrated pallor and parasternal systolic murmurs, findings consistent with anemia. Nucleated red blood cells (RBCs) were observed on the peripheral blood smear from both of these patients. Circulating nucleated RBCs are abnormal except in the neonatal period and often enter the circulation during periods of bone marrow stress caused by severe hemolysis. Both patients had an elevated reticulocyte count (**reticulocytosis**), which is a reliable indicator of accelerated erythropoiesis, especially when hemolysis is severe enough to produce anemia. **White blood cell abnormalities:** *Patient #1* had leukopenia and neutropenia. Common causes of non-neoplastic neutropenia include therapeutic drugs, such as analgesics and antibiotics, certain

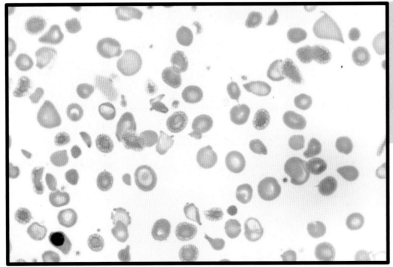

Image 1_Peripheral blood smear of Patient #1, indicating a variety of abnormal RBC morphology findings, including polychromasia, hypochromia, anisocytosis, microcytosis, poikilocytosis, target cells, dacrocytes, and a nucleated RBC.

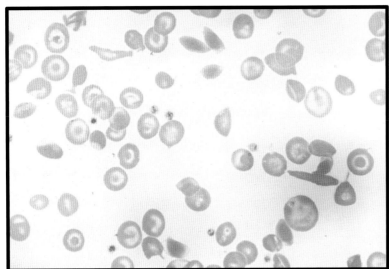

Image 2_Peripheral blood smear of Patient #2, indicating a variety of abnormal RBC morphology findings, including anisocytosis, poikilocytosis, target cells, and sickle cells.

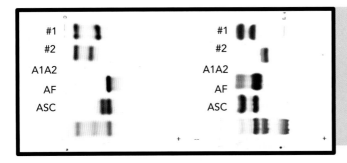

Image 3_Cellulose acetate, pH 8.6 (left) and citrate agar, pH 6.2 (right) hemoglobin electrophoresis patterns for Patients #1 and #2 and for standards containing hemoglobins A1A2, AF, and ASC. Identity of bands from cathode (-) to anode (+) is: (cellulose acetate, left); C, S, F, A(A1A2); (citrate agar, right); F, A(A1A2), S, C.

T1. Principal Laboratory Findings: Patient #1

Test		Patient's Result	"Pediatric" Reference Range
Immunohematology			
WBC count		5.7	6.0-17.0 × 10³/µL
Hemoglobin		5.4	9.7-14.2 g/dL
Hematocrit		17.1	34.0-40.0%
MCV		64.3	70.0-86.0 fL
MCH		20.4	23.0-31.0 pg
Platelet count		245	150-450 × 10³/µL
Differential:	neutrophils	13	35-45%
	lymphocytes	68	40-55%
	monocytes	8	2-6%
	eosinophils	1	0-5%
	basophils	0	0-2%
	bands	9	0-12%
	metamyelocytes	1	0%
	nucleated RBCS	77	0/100 WBCs
	reticulocytes	5.1	0.5-1.5%
	polychromasia	2+	
	hypochromia	2+	
	anisocytosis	3+	
	microcytosis	3+	
	poikilocytosis	3+	
	schistocytosis	Occasional	
	spherocytes	Occasional	
	target cells	1+	
	dacrocytes	1+	
	sickle cells	n.o.	
Osmotic fragility	decreased	normal	
G6PD	normal	normal	
Direct Coombs	negative	negative	
Chemistry			
Iron		79	35-171 µg/dL
TIBC		178	21-481µg/dL
%TS		44	30-44%
Quantitative IgG level		1,700	570-1,280 mg/dL

WBC, white blood cell; MCV, mean corpuscular volume; MCH, mean corpuscular hemoglobin; RBCs, red blood cells; G6PD, glucose-6-phosphate dehydrogenase; TIBC, total iron binding capacity; TS, transferrin saturation = [Iron/TIBC] × 100; n.o., none observed.

infections (our patient had a clinically undefined febrile illness), and autoimmune disease. *Patient #2* had increased neutrophilic bands in the context of an increased WBC count. This is probably a non-specific finding, but it could be an indication of an early left-shift as seen in stress or infection. **Abnormalities in red cell morphology ([Image 1] and [Image 2]). Polychromasia:** Commonly seen when erythrocytes are delivered prematurely to the peripheral circulation and correlate with the presence of reticulocytosis. **Hypochromasia**

T2. Principal Laboratory Findings: Patient #2

Test		Patient's Result	"Adult" Reference Range
Hematology			
WBC count		12.9	$4.3\text{-}10.8 \times 10^3/\mu L$
Hemoglobin		7.1	12.0-16.0 g/dL
Hematocrit		20.5	37.0-47.0%
MCV		80.7	79.0-97.0 fL
MCH		28.2	27.0-32.0 pg
Platelet count		243	$150\text{-}400 \times 10^3/\mu L$
Differential:	neutrophils	37	50-70%
	lymphocytes	39	20.5-45.0%
	monocytes	7	1-15%
	eosinophils	1	0-5%
	basophils	0	0-2%
	bands	15	0-12%
	metamyelocytes	0	0%
	nucleated RBCS	2	0/100 WBCs
	reticulocytes	6.5	0.6-2.8%
	polychromasia	1+	
	hypochromia	n.o.	
	anisocytosis	3+	
	microcytosis	n.o.	
	poikilocytosis	3+	
	schistocytosis	n.o.	
	spherocytes	n.o.	
	target cells	1+	
	dacrocytes	n.o.	
	sickle cells	present	
Chemistry			
Bilirubin, total		2.4	0.1-1.5 mg/dL

WBC, white blood cell; MCV, mean corpuscular volume; MCH, mean corpuscular hemoglobin; RBCs, red blood cells; n.o., none observed.

and microcytosis were observed on the peripheral blood smear from *Patient #1* and are an indicator of impaired hemoglobin synthesis. These findings are important because, in addition to patients with iron deficiency anemia, they are characteristically seen on peripheral blood smears from patients with thalassemia. **Anisocytosis:** A non-specific finding observed on the peripheral blood smears from both patients, which can be seen in a variety of conditions including early iron or vitamin B_{12}/folate deficiency, anemia secondary to systemic disease, bone marrow infiltration, and hemolytic

processes. **Poikilocytosis:** Distortion of red cell shapes was markedly present on the peripheral blood smears from both patients and is of particular diagnostic value because certain poikilocytes suggest only 1 or a few disease entities. **Target and tear drop cells,** also known as codocytes and dacrocytes, respectively, were present on the peripheral blood smears of both patients. These cells can be seen in a variety of conditions, including hemolytic anemias, thalassemias, and various hemoglobinopathies. **Schistocytes and spherocytes:** The presence of only an occasional schistocyte and spherocyte on the peripheral blood smear from *Patient #1* is probably a non-specific finding. Artifactual cells, which appear similar to schistocytes and spherocytes, can sometimes be seen at the feathered edge of peripheral blood smears. **Sickle cells:** Their presence in *Patient #2* is virtually diagnostic for a sickling disorder of which sickle cell disease should be the primary consideration. Moreover, this patient complained of pain in the upper abdomen and ribs and admitted to similar episodes of pain in the past, which is suggestive of sickle cell crisis. In addition, the presence of sickle cells should trigger consideration of a concomitant thalassemia or hemoglobinopathy, due to other abnormal hemoglobins, including Hb C, Hb C$_{Harlem}$, Hb D, Hb O$_{Arab}$. **Other laboratory findings:** Hypergammaglobulinemia in *Patient #1* was probably due to infection or a chronic inflammatory process. This patient's negative direct Coombs test suggests that she did not have an immune hemolytic anemia, while her decreased osmotic fragility test result suggests a thalassemia and/or other hemoglobinopathy. *Patient #2* had an elevated serum total bilirubin concentration, which can best be explained on the basis of significant in vivo hemolysis.

3. Based on the clinical history, ethnic background, and laboratory findings for *Patients #1* and *#2*, particularly the alterations in erythrocyte morphology, a hemoglobinopathy is a likely possibility that should be investigated by hemoglobin (Hb) electrophoresis. This test is based on the different relative mobilities of the various types of hemoglobins in an electric field applied across a solid support medium in a buffer with a specific pH and ionic strength. Electrophoresis on cellulose acetate in an alkaline buffer at pH 8.6 and on citrate-agar at acid pH 6.2 is often adequate for detecting and diagnosing the majority of common hemoglobinopathies. A principal advantage of citrate-agar hemoglobin electrophoresis is that hemoglobins D and G, which co-migrate with Hb S on cellulose acetate, and hemoglobins E and O, which co-migrate with Hb C by cellulose acetate hemoglobin electrophoresis, can be separated by citrate-agar hemoglobin electrophoresis. Cellulose acetate and citrate-agar hemoglobin electrophoresis of a RBC lysate prepared from whole blood obtained from *Patients #1* and *#2* were performed with the results shown in I3. The cellulose acetate hemoglobin electrophoresis

pattern for *Patient #1* demonstrated a complete absence of Hb A, a band with anodal mobility slightly less than that expected for Hb A, and a much slower band in the position of Hb C [**Image 3**]. The citrate-agar gel electrophoresis pattern demonstrated only 2 bands, 1 in the position of Hb A and another in the position of hemoglobin F (Hb F) [**Image 3**]. This hemoglobin electrophoresis pattern is consistent with hemoglobin E-β^0-thalassemia.[1-3] The cellulose acetate hemoglobin electrophoresis pattern for *Patient #2* demonstrated 2 major bands in the positions of Hb S and Hb C, whereas this patient's citrate-age gel electrophoresis pattern demonstrated no Hb A band, a major band in the position of Hb S, and a band cathodal to Hb S [**Image 3**]. This hemoglobin electrophoresis pattern is consistent with Hb S-O$_{Arab}$ hemoglobinopathy.[1,3,5]

4. ***Most likely diagnosis:*** *Patient #1*, hemoglobin E-β^0-thalassemia; *Patient #2*, Hb S-O$_{Arab}$ hemoglobinopathy. Due to its high prevalence in individuals from Southeast Asia, Hb E is 1 of the most common structurally abnormal hemoglobins encountered in the world. It is due to a substitution of lysine for glutamic acid at the 26th amino-acid position of the hemoglobin β-chain. Other major hemoglobin disorders in individuals from Southeast Asia include α- (Hb H disease) and β-thalassemia. The thalassemias are among the most common hemoglobin abnormalities and their geographic distribution follows that of malaria. The majority of affected persons in the United States originate from the Mediterranean basin, Africa, or Southeast Asia. The thalassemias are classified based on the hemoglobin chain affected and thus there are α-, β-, γ-, and δ-thalassemias. The underlying genetic defect is a gene deletion or codon substitution, which causes complete or partial failure to produce the corresponding hemoglobin chain.[1-3] Heterozygosity for these hemoglobin abnormalities ranges from 4% to 20% and, therefore, double heterozygotes are common. Due to the high rate of immigration of people from Southeast Asia to the United States, Hb E is not a rare hemoglobinopathy anymore, thus permanently altering the genetic pool of the United States.[1] Hemoglobin E-β-thalassemia has clinical manifestations of thalassemia major or intermedia, depending on the severity

associated with the coinherited thalassemia gene. Patients with the β^0-gene will tend to have more severe symptoms than a patient with the β^+ form of thalassemia. In spite of being 1 of the most common hemoglobinopathies, if not the most common worldwide, the natural history of β-thalassemia is poorly understood.[4] With regard to *Patient #2*, Hb S disease and trait constitute common abnormalities observed in laboratories that perform hemoglobin electrophoresis. The absence of any Hb A means that this patient has Hb S disease. Hb S has valine substituted for glutamic acid at the sixth amino acid position of the β-chain. The morbidity associated with sickle cell disease is due to the relative increased viscosity, insolubility, and polymerization of Hb S, which distort the membrane of the erythrocyte and produces the characteristic sickle appearance of the sickle cell. The clinical manifestations in individuals with Hb S are largely dependent on the amount of Hb S present, which varies depending on genetic background (eg, sickle cell trait versus sickle cell disease versus combinations of Hb S with other abnormal hemoglobins or with a thalassemia).[1,5] Hemoglobin O-Arab (Hb O_{Arab}) is rarely encountered and is due to lysine substitution for glutamic acid at the 121st amino acid position in the β-chain. It was first described in an Israeli Arab and thus the designation, Hb O_{Arab}. It has been found in blacks of the western hemisphere and in individuals in Bulgaria.[1,3] Heterozygotes for Hb O_{Arab} are clinically silent and do not suffer from anemia or hemolysis. Rare cases of homozygous Hb O_{Arab} hemoglobinopathy have been described and such individuals presented with frontal bossing, splenomegaly, and hemolytic anemia.[1] The heterozygous condition associated with the presence of both Hb S and Hb O_{Arab} causes a slightly milder form of sickle cell disease, intermediate in severity between homozygous sickle cell disease and the disease associated with the presence of both Hb S and Hb C.[1]

5. Careful assessment of a patient's clinical presentation and basic hematological indices, as well as thorough microscopic morphologic examination of an adequately prepared blood smear, are essential to determining the most appropriate treatment modalities in patients with a confirmed hemoglobinopathy. *Patient #1*: If the clinical manifestations of this patient's disease

continue to be severe and recurrent and if failure to thrive or skull deformity due to expansion of the bone marrow in the cranial bones develops, regular blood transfusions may be needed.[4] A program of repeated blood transfusions will often assure normal bone growth and development, but unfortunately, by the age of 12, many patients with hemoglobin E-β^0-thalassemia start to develop growth failure, hypogonadism, cardiac disease, and the complications of iron overload. *Patient #2*: Appropriate treatment of this patient depends on the frequency and severity of the vasoocclusive crises, also known as sickle cell crises or painful crises, which occur in individuals with Hb S disease, which can produce infarctions of various organs, such as spleen, kidneys, retina, brain, bones, and joints.[6] Treatment is directed toward preventing and managing such vasoocclusive crises. In addition, such patients must be monitored for organ damage, to prevent and treat infections (which often are the trigger for more serious complications), and to maintain adequate hydration. Hydroxyurea has been introduced as a mainstay of therapy because it increases fetal hemoglobin (Hb F), but also seems to have an effect on red cell hydration, vascular adherence, granulocytes, and reticulocytes, all of which play a role also in the adverse sequelae associated with sickle cell crisis. There is also a role for transfusions or partial exchange transfusions in patients with life-threatening, prolonged, or frequently recurring crises. Patients who have had recurrent life-threatening episodes of sickle cell crisis may benefit from long-term maintenance blood transfusions. Bone marrow transplantation is an option that could be entertained in very young patients and gene therapy is still under investigation.[6] It must be emphasized, however, that these treatment modalities apply to patients with sickle cell disease and, by analogy, in the treatment of the rare patient with a Hb S-O_{Arab} hemoglobinopathy.

Keywords _____

thalassemia, sickle cell disease, hemoglobinopathy, electrophoresis

References _____

1. Fairbanks VF. *Hemoglobinopathies and Thalassemias. Laboratory Methods and Case Studies.* New York: Brian C Decker Division of Thieme-Stratton. 1980; 164,172

2. Fishdeler AJ, Hoffman GC. A practical approach to the detection of hemoglobinopathies: Part I. The introduction and thalassemia syndromes. *Lab Med.* 1987;18:368-372.

3. Fishdeler AJ, Hoffman GC. A practical approach to the detection of hemoglobinopathies: Part III. Nonsickling disorders and cord blood screening. *Lab Med.* 1987;18:513-518.

4. Oliveri NF. The a-thalassemias. *N Engl J Med.* 1999;341:99-109.

5. Fishdeler AJ, Hoffman GC. A practical approach to the detection of hemoglobinopathies: Part II. The sickle cell disorders. *Lab Med.* 1987;18:441-443.

6. Steinberg MH. Management of sickle cell disease. *N Engl J Med.* 1999;340:1021-1030.

Severe Chronic Neutropenia in a Mother and Her Infant

Steven H. Kroft

Department of Pathology, Medical College of Wisconsin, Milwaukee, WI

Patient: 23-year-old Hispanic woman.

Chief Complaint: Neutropenia with recurrent infections.

History of Present Illness: The patient was presently asymptomatic, despite severe neutropenia.

Past Medical and Surgical History: Previously, the patient had severe, lifelong neutropenia, with multiple episodes of pneumonia during childhood, none of which were life threatening.

Family History: The patient has a 16-month-old son who has been neutropenic since birth.

Physical Examination: Vital signs: temperature, 98.6°F; pulse, 82 beats per minute; respiratory rate, 12 breaths per minute; blood pressure, 111/74 mm Hg. The patient was a well-appearing young woman with unremarkable physical examination findings.

Results of Additional Diagnostic Procedures and Tests: A trephine bone marrow biopsy was performed followed by morphologic review of stained smears prepared from blood and bone marrow (Image 1). A 500-cell bone marrow aspirate differential count revealed the presence of: 0.2% myeloblasts, 6.6% promyelocytes and myelocytes, 52.4% metamyelocytes, bands, and segmented neutrophils, 25% erythroid precursors, 13% lymphocytes, 2% monocytes, 0.8% eosinophils, and 0.2% basophils. The myeloid:erythroid (M:E) ratio was 2.5:1.

Questions

1. What are the patient's most striking clinical and laboratory findings?

2. How do you explain this patient's most striking clinical and laboratory findings?

3. What is this patient's most likely diagnosis?

4. What are the morphologic features of this patient's disorder?

5. What is the mechanism of neutropenia in patients with this disorder?

6. What is the molecular pathogenesis of this disorder?

7. What is the treatment and prognosis of this disorder?

Possible Answers

1. Multiple episodes of non-life-threatening respiratory infection associated with severe, chronic neutropenia (**T1**). Also significant is the fact that

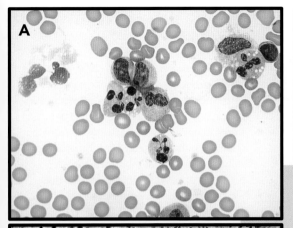

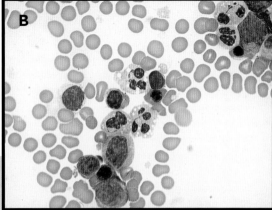

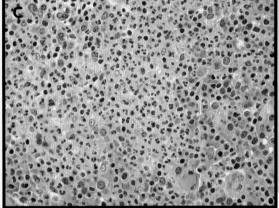

Image 1_The patient's trephine bone marrow biopsy findings, illustrating examples (panels **A** and **B**) of granulocytes, including mature neutrophils that appear pseudohypersegmented but do not contain the 5 or more nuclear lobes of true hypersegmented neutrophils. The nuclear lobes are small and pyknotic-appearing and are separated by abnormally long, often irregular, filaments. There is also distinct cytoplasmic vacuolization in the mature neutrophils. The less mature granuloctypes are morphologically unremarkable. An H&E-stained section (**C**) demonstrated the presence of zones containing sheets of mature neutrophils.

T1. Principal Laboratory Findings

Test	Patient's Result	Reference Interval
WBC count	1.4	4.4–11.0 × 10³/μL
Hemoglobin	13.9	12.3–15.3 g/dL
Platelet count	265	150–450 × 10³/μL
Manual differential: Neutrophils	27	40–62%
Bands	4	1–9%
Lymphocytes	56	27–40%
Monocytes	4	2–8%
Eosinophils	8	0–4.5%
Basophils	1	0–2%
Absolute neutrophil count	0.4	1.8–7.8 × 10³/μL
Absolute lymphocyte count	0.8	1.0–4.8 × 10³/μL

WBC, white blood cell.

the patient's infant child is similarly affected with severe neutropenia. The patient's mature neutrophils show abnormal morphology, including pyknotic nuclei, long, thin, or irregular filaments between nuclear lobes, and cytoplasmic vacuoles (**Image 1**, panels **A** and **B**). The marrow section showed areas consisting of sheets of mature granulocytes (**Image 1C**). To determine the possible causes of neutropenia, it is important to determine whether it represents a congenital or acquired phenomenon. The patient's history of lifelong neutropenia, presumably dating from childhood, strongly supports a congenital condition. Moreover, the fact that the patient's 16-month-old child appears to be similarly affected suggests either an autosomal dominant or X-linked dominant mode of inheritance. A dominant mode of inheritance is unusual for congenital neutropenias and represents an important clue to the correct diagnosis. The only acquired cause of neutropenia that could conceivably be transferred from a mother to an infant would be autoimmune neutropenia, via passive transfer of an antibody directed against neutrophils. The persistence of neutropenia at

16 months in the child, however, rules out this possibility.

2. The causes of neutropenia are myriad, and can be conveniently grouped into 4 major categories of defects: proliferation, survival, maturation, and distribution.[1] **Proliferation defects** are characterized by decreased amounts of marrow granulocytes, often with an arrest of maturation. These can be congenital, as in cyclic neutropenia or Kostmann's syndrome, or acquired, such as occurs with exposure to certain drugs and toxins. The robust granulocytic compartment in the present marrow excludes a proliferation defect. **Survival defects** are typically characterized by a granulocytic hyperplasia with a shift toward immaturity of the granulocytic series. Examples include autoimmune neutropenia and severe bacterial infection. In the present case there is a shift toward more mature granulocytes (**Image 1B**), largely ruling out this mechanism of neutropenia. **Maturation defects** are characterized by bone marrow granulocytic hyperplasia, but abnormal neutrophil maturation and intramedullary cell death (ie, ineffective granulopoiesis). Examples include megaloblastic anemia, myelodysplastic syndromes, and Chediak-Higashi syndrome. Given the morphologic abnormalities in the granulocytes of this patient, this mechanism cannot be excluded. However, the morphologic changes seem to be limited to only the most mature granulocytes, whereas maturation defects typically cause morphologic abnormalities throughout the spectrum of granulocyte maturation. Finally, **distribution defects** are characterized by normal total body granulocytes but reduced circulating granulocytes, either due to defective release from the bone marrow, increased margination (ie, adherence to the endothelium of blood vessels), or pooling in the spleen. This type of defect can be seen as a result of normal physiologic variation (eg, increased margination in people of African descent), complement activation (as may occur with exposure of blood to artificial membranes), or from hypersplenism. This mechanism remains a possibility in this case. Based on the preceding discussion, we may conclude that this patient suffers from a congenital/inherited form of chronic neutropenia that follows either an autosomal or X-linked dominant inheritance pattern that is due to either a maturation or distribution defect in neutrophils.

3. **Most likely diagnosis:** *myelokathexis.* Myelokathexis is a rare form of congenital neutropenia, first described by Zuelzer in 1964.[2] Originally, this disorder was thought to result from failure of release of neutrophils from the marrow (kathexis = retention). Patients typically have baseline absolute neutrophil counts between 0.0 and $0.5 \times 10^3/\mu L$.[3,4] As in this patient, lymphopenia is often present as well. Most patients have a family history, and the inheritance pattern appears most often to be autosomal dominant with variable penetrance.[4-6] This inheritance pattern is unique among the congenital neutropenia syndromes. Patients suffer from recurrent infections, particularly pneumonia, otitis, and sinusitis.[3,5] One-third to one-half of patients have warts, hypogammaglobulinemia, infections, and myelokathexis (WHIM) syndrome.[5] Thus, patients appear to be susceptible to human papillomavirus infections but do not have increased morbidity due to other common viral infections.[3] Opportunistic infections are not seen in this disorder.

4. The morphologic features of the cells observed in the patient's bone marrow are characteristic of myelokathexis, including mature neutrophils with unusual nuclear segmentation, abnormally long or irregular intranuclear filaments, pyknotic-appearing nuclei, and cytoplasmic vacuolization. Curiously, the granulocyte compartment may appear to be "right-shifted," with large numbers of mature forms. Earlier granulocyte precursors were morphologically normal. Notably, an examination of bone marrow from the patient's child revealed identical morphologic findings to those observed in the mother's bone marrow (data not shown).

5. Two primary theories have been proposed for the mechanism of neutropenia in this disorder: increased apoptosis of marrow neutrophils (maturation defect), and abnormal release of neutrophils (distribution defect). Experimental evidence for increased apoptosis exists, with demonstration of increased annexin V binding by flow cytometry.[4] In addition, neutrophils show decreased expression of bcl-x, a protein involved in apoptosis. No direct experimental

evidence exists for abnormal release of neutrophils, although recent studies related to the molecular pathogenesis of myelokathexis shed light on this issue (see below).

6. Most kindreds with myelokathexis/WHIM syndrome have heterozygous mutations in the chemokine receptor 4 (CXCR4) gene on chromsome 2q21.[6-8] Interaction of CXCR4 and its ligand, CXC-chemokine L12 (CXCL12), is important in the homing of hematopoietic cells and in lymphocyte trafficking. The main cellular response to receptor-ligand interaction is chemotaxis and integrin-mediated adhesion. Mutations in CXCR4 result in normal expression of the molecule but with truncation of the cytoplasmic tail. This is a gain of function mutation with enhanced chemotactic response to CXCR4-CXCL12 binding in both neutrophils and lymphocytes.[6] Thus, this molecular defect yields insight into the pathogenesis of this disorder, with an enhanced CXCR4 response possibly resulting in inappropriate retention of neutrophils in the marrow, either due to defective release or reuptake, and impaired lymphocyte trafficking resulting in lymphopenia and hypogammaglobulinemia.[3] Notably, recent data indicates that patients with myelokathexis/ WHIM syndrome who do not have CXCR4 mutations still have altered leukocyte responses to CXCR4/CXCL12 binding, providing a unifying explanation for the molecular pathogenesis of this syndrome.[7]

7. In contrast to other inherited disorders resulting in severe neutropenia, there are no reports of early death in patients with WHIM syndrome.[5] Patients with this syndrome appear to mount an adequate neutrophil response to bacterial infections. Thus, while there is increased susceptibility to bacterial infections, these run a benign course, and treatment with conventional antibiotics is sufficient. Notably, patients respond well and rapidly to therapy with recombinant granulocyte colony-stimulating factor (G-CSF), including sustained neutrophil responses for the duration of therapy.[5] Interestingly, the morphology of bone marrow neutrophils and serum immunoglobulin levels tend to normalize with G-CSF therapy.

Keywords

myelokathexis, WHIM syndrome, neutropenia, granulocyte colony stimulating factor

References

1. Foucar K. Neutropenia. In: Kjeldsberg CR, ed. *Practical Diagnosis of Hematologic Disorders.* Vol. 1. Chicago: ASCP Press; 2006:227–237.

2. Zuelzer WW. "Myelokathexis"—A new form of chronic granulocytopenia. Report of a case. *N Engl J Med.* 1964;270:699–704.

3. Gulino AV. WHIM syndrome: A genetic disorder of leukocyte trafficking. *Curr Opin Allergy Clin Immunol.* 2003;3:443–450.

4. Aprikyan AA, Liles WC, Park JR, et al. Myelokathexis, a congenital disorder of severe neutropenia characterized by accelerated apoptosis and defective expression of bcl-x in neutrophil precursors. *Blood.* 2000;95:320–327.

5. Hord JD, Whitlock JA, Gay JC, et al. Clinical features of myelokathexis and treatment with hematopoietic cytokines: A case report of 2 patients and review of the literature. *J Pediatr Hematol Oncol.* 1997;19:443–448.

6. Gulino AV, Moratto D, Sozzani S, et al. Altered leukocyte response to CXCL12 in patients with warts, hypogammaglobulinemia, infections, myelokathexis (WHIM) syndrome. *Blood.* 2004;104:444–452.

7. Balabanian K, Lagane B, Pablos JL, et al. WHIM syndromes with different genetic anomalies are accounted for by impaired CXCR4 desensitization to CXCL12. *Blood.* 2005;105:2449–2457.

8. Hernandez PA, Gorlin RJ, Lukens JN, et al. Mutations in the chemokine receptor gene CXCR4 are associated with WHIM syndrome, a combined immunodeficiency disease. *Nat Genet.* 2003;34:70–74.

Easy Bruising, Cataracts, and Hearing Loss in a 27-Year-Old Female

Alexandra Harrington, Patrick C. J. Ward, Steven H. Kroft

Department of Pathology, Medical College of Wisconsin, Milwaukee, WI

Patient: 27-year-old female.　　**Chief Complaint:** Easy bruising.

History of Present Illness: The patient presented to the hematology clinic for evaluation of lifelong easy bruising and thrombocytopenia. As a child, she was diagnosed with immune thrombocytopenic purpura (ITP), which was apparently refractory to both medical and surgical interventions. In the past, however, platelet transfusions had successfully raised her platelet counts prior to surgery.

Past Medical and Surgical History: Presumed ITP refractory to corticosteroids, Rituxan, WinRho, plasma exchange, intravenous immunoglobulin (IVIG), and splenectomy; end-stage renal disease secondary to Alport's syndrome, status post related donor kidney transplant; diabetes; hearing loss; cataracts.

Family History: Unknown, as the patient is adopted.

Physical Examination: Vital signs: temperature, 99.6°F; pulse, 94 bpm; respiratory rate, 12 rpm; blood pressure, 137/83 mm Hg. The patient was obese and cushingoid (eg, buffalo hump, obesity, striations). Skin examination revealed a bruise on the right upper extremity and multiple abdominal bruises at insulin injection sites. A left upper quadrant scar, consistent with a splenectomy scar, was present. There was no hepatomegaly, lymphadenopathy, or petechiae.

Questions

1. What are the patient's most striking clinical and laboratory findings?

2. How do you explain this patient's most striking clinical and laboratory findings?

3. What is this patient's most likely diagnosis?

4. How do you best explain the discrepancy between the automated and manual platelet counts?

5. What is the genetic basis of this patient's condition?

6. What additional tests are available to confirm this diagnosis?

7. With which disease is this patient's condition most often misdiagnosed?

8. What is the treatment for individuals with this patient's disease?

Possible Answers

1. The most striking clinical findings are a history of medically- and surgically-refractory thrombocytopenia, presenting as easy bruising during childhood, a history of renal failure secondary to Alport's syndrome requiring a renal transplant, obese and cushingoid body habitus,

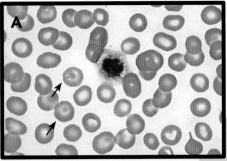

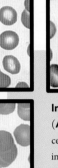

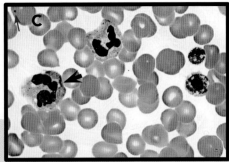

Image 1_The patient's peripheral blood smear revealed (**A**) giant, well-granulated platelets, occasional target cells (black arrows) and (**B**) small, basophilic Döhle-like inclusion bodies within many of the neutrophils (blue arrow). Also seen were rare large Döhle-like inclusion bodies (**C**, arrowhead) and occasional Howell-Jolly bodies within the red blood cells (red arrow). The leukocyte inclusions are, in general, smaller than those seen in May-Hegglin anomaly and are not accompanied by the toxic changes that are typically present in sepsis.

and multiple bruises which could be explained by recent trauma. The most striking laboratory findings include severe thrombocytopenia with an elevated mean platelet volume, giant platelets, small Döhle-like bodies in many neutrophils, target cells, and Howell-Jolly bodies in the red blood cells (**T1** and **Image 1**).

2. The patient's clinical and laboratory findings suggest a congenital macrothrombocytopenia syndrome. This rare inherited group of disorders, including May-Hegglin anomaly, Sebastian syndrome, Fechtner syndrome, Epstein syndrome, Bernard-Soulier syndrome, DiGeorge syndrome, Gray platelet syndrome, and X-linked macrothrombocytopenia with dyserythropoiesis is characterized, as the name implies, by low platelet counts and giant platelets (defined as platelets equal to or greater than the size of a red cell). Congenital macrothrombocytopenias are variable in their clinical presentations, ranging from asymptomatic, incidentally-discovered conditions to severe bleeding disorders.[1,2] A subset of these disorders—May-Hegglin anomaly, Sebastian syndrome, Fechtner syndrome, and Epstein syndrome—are characterized by mutations in the myosin heavy chain 9 (MYH9) gene, and are therefore classified as MYH9-related diseases.[1-3] Despite the genetic commonality and shared macrothrombocytopenia, the individual disorders are distinguished by variable

manifestations of Alport's syndrome, (including nephritis, cataracts, and hearing loss) and variable presence of leukocyte inclusions. For example, patients with May-Hegglin anomaly and Sebastian syndrome do not have clinical signs of Alport's syndrome but do have different types of Döhle-like leukocyte inclusions, which can be discriminated from each other ultrastructurally. Fechtner syndrome patients have the triad of nephritis, cataracts, and hearing impairment, along with Döhle-like bodies within the leukocytes. Finally, patients with Epstein syndrome have hearing impairment and nephritis but do not have identifiable leukocyte inclusions. These 4 macrothrombocytopenia syndromes may represent a single disorder (MYH9-related disease) with variable expression of the discussed clinical and laboratory findings[3] (**T2**).

The red blood cell changes in this case, including Howell-Jolly bodies and increased target cells, can be explained by the prior splenectomy. A normally-functioning spleen will remove red cell inclusions from circulating erythrocytes. The patient's cushingoid body habitus is the result of her chronic corticosteroid use.

3. ***Most likely diagnosis:*** *Fechtner syndrome.* This syndrome was first described in 1985 by Peterson and colleagues in a study of a family with nephritis, cataracts, deafness,

T1. Principal Laboratory Findings

Test	Patient's Result	"Normal" Reference Range
Hematology		
White blood cell count	9.0	4.5–13.0 × 10³/μL
Red blood cell count	5.1	4.4–5.8 × 10⁶/μL
Hemoglobin	15.8	13.0–17.0 g/dL
Hematocrit	47	40–50%
Mean corpuscular volume	92	80–100 fL
Platelet count	10	150–350 × 10³/μL
Mean platelet volume	15.1	7.5–9.5 fL
Manual platelet count	22	150–350 × 10³/μL
Manual		
Differential: Neutrophils	76	40–62%
Lymphocytes	18	27–40%
Monocytes	5	0–8%
Eosinophils	1	0–4%
Basophils	1	0–2%
Peripheral blood smear review	Döhle-like bodies in neutrophils	
	Giant platelets	
	Howell-Jolly bodies	
	Target cells	
Chemistry		
Blood urea nitrogen	15	6–23 mg/dL
Sodium	138	133–145 mmol/L
Potassium	4.3	3.5–5.1 mmol/L
Chloride	103	98–112 mmol/L
Bicarbonate	27	21–32 mmol/L
Creatinine	1.0	0.4–1.2 mg/dL
Glucose	102	70–110 mg/dL
Calcium	9.4	8.4–10.5 mg/dL

T2. Laboratory and Clinical Features of Myosin Heavy Chain 9 (MYH9)-Related Disease

	Giant Platelets	Döhle-Like Inclusions	Hearing Loss	Nephritis	Cataracts
Epstein syndrome	+	-	+	+	-
Fechtner syndrome	+	+	+	+	+
May-Hegglin anomaly	+	+	-	-	-
Sebastian syndrome	+	+	-	-	-

macrothrombocytopenia, and small, pale blue, irregularly-shaped cytoplasmic inclusions resembling Döhle bodies within their leukocytes.[4] In this original report, it was demonstrated that these inclusions are ultrastructurally distinct from the light microscopically-similar inclusions seen in May-Hegglin anomaly and the Döhle bodies seen in toxic neutrophils. On Wright-Giemsa-stained smears, Fechtner inclusions were smaller and paler than May-Hegglin inclusions, and compared with the irregularly-distributed Döhle bodies of sepsis, Fechtner inclusions were present in nearly every cell examined and were present without other toxic changes.[4]

4. A manual platelet count was performed in this case because of the inaccuracy of automated counts in the presence of significant numbers of giant platelets. Most automated analyzers enumerate platelets based on cell size thresholds. When platelets are enlarged, analyzers may count them as red cells or even leukocytes, thus reporting a falsely-low platelet count.

5. In addition to their clinical heterogeneity, the MYH9-related disorders are genetically heterogeneous. The group shares mutations in the MYH9 gene, located on chromosome 22q12-13, which encodes for the heavy chain of the non-muscle myosin IIA (NMMHC-IIA) protein, a cytoskeleton protein in hematopoietic cells.[2] In the literature, 22 different MYH9 gene mutations have been described in 77 unrelated families with disease associated with this genetic locus.[3] The majority of these mutations are transmitted in an autosomal dominant fashion, with a minority (20%) representing sporadic, acquired mutations.[1]

6. Immunofluorescence and immunocytochemical assays for neutrophil NMMHC-IIA protein are available.[1,3,5,6] In MYH9-related disease, this protein abnormally localizes in the cytoplasm of leukocytes. The localization of NMMHC-IIA corresponds to the Döhle-like inclusions seen on Giemsa-stained preparations.[3] These localization assays are performed on peripheral blood and are highly sensitive and specific.[6] Additionally, MYH9 gene mutation analysis can be performed, but these assays are not widely available.[5]

7. Congenital macrothrombocytopenias are often misdiagnosed as immune thrombocytopenic purpura (ITP),[2,7] an acquired autoimmune disorder characterized by peripheral destruction of platelets. Peripheral blood smear examination may provide diagnostic clues in differentiating these 2 entities. Though present in varying proportions, giant platelets may be seen in both conditions, the result of multiple mechanisms in congenital macrothrombocytopenias and accelerated platelet production in ITP.[2] In general, a greater proportion of platelets will be enlarged in the congenital macrothrombocytopenias as compared with ITP.[1] The presence of leukocyte inclusions limits the differential to MYH9-related disorders, as previously discussed. If available, previous platelet counts may also be helpful. Patients with congenital syndromes will have persistently-low platelet counts since birth, while normal platelet counts may have been documented at a previous time in patients with ITP. Finally, obtaining a detailed history and physical examination is important. Of note, because some of the disease manifestations of the congenital syndromes do not present until later in life, such as cataracts, nephritis, and deafness, a detailed family history is essential, especially in the pediatric population.[7]

8. Despite the thrombocytopenia, the majority of patients with MYH9-related disease do not have clinically-significant bleeding problems[1,2] and in general do not require treatment. When serious bleeding does occur, platelet transfusions, recombinant factor VII, and antifibrinolytics may be effective.[1] Patients may require prophylactic platelet transfusions prior to procedures or surgery.[1] As illustrated in this case study, patients are usually unresponsive to the standard ITP therapies of corticosteroids, IVIG, and splenectomy.

Keywords _____

immune thrombocytopenic purpura, macrothrombocytopenias, Fechtner syndrome, MYH9-related disease

References _____

1. Kunishima S, Saito H. Congenital macrothrombocytopenias. *Blood Reviews.* 2006;20:111–121.

2. Beutler E, Coller BS, Lichtman MA, et al, eds. *William's Hematology.* New York, NY: McGraw-Hill; 2005.

3. Seri M, Pecci A, Di Bari F, et al. MYH9-related disease May-Hegglin anomaly, Sebastian syndrome, Fechtner syndrome, and Epstein syndrome are not distinct entities but represent a variable expression of a single illness. *Medicine.* 2003;82:203–215.

4. Peterson LC, Rao KV, Crosson JT, et al. Fechtner syndrome—A variant of Alport's syndrome with leukocyte inclusions and macrothrombocytopenia. *Blood.* 1985;65:397–406.

5. Pecci A, Noris P, Invernizzi R, et al. Immunocytochemistry for the heavy chain of the non-muscle myosin IIA as a diagnostic tool for MYH9-related disorders. *Br J Haematol.* 2002;117:164–167.

6. Balduini CL, Cattaneo M, Fabris F, et al. Inherited thrombocytopenias: A proposed diagnostic algorithm from the Italian Gruppo di Studio dele Plastrine. *Haematologica.* 2003;88:582–592.

7. Young G, Luban N, White JG. Giant platelet disorders in African-American children misdiagnosed as idiopathic thrombocytopenic purpura. *J Pediatr Hematol Oncol.* 1999;21:231–236.

Hyperkalemia in 2 Elderly Men

Naveen Kakkar,[1] Shweta Goyal[2]

Departments of [1]Pathology and [2]Biochemistry, Christian Medical College and Hospital, Ludhiana, Punjab, India

Characteristic	Patient 1	Patient 2
Description	65-year-old man	84-year-old man
Chief Complaint	Cough and fever for 4 days	Asymptomatic. The patient presented in the outpatient service for a routine blood check as a part of an immigration requirement.
Physical Examination Findings	The patient was disoriented and tachypneic. He had bilateral harsh breath sounds, mild hepatomegaly, and no splenomegaly.	Unremarkable, including no organomegaly.
Drug History	Unremarkable	Unremarkable
Medical History	He was a diagnosed case of chronic obstructive airway disease.	He was a diagnosed case of essential hypertension.
Family History	Unremarkable	Unremarkable

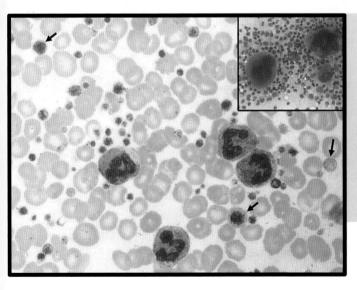

Image 1_Peripheral blood smear findings in Patient 1 illustrating normocytic-normochromic red blood cells, leukocytosis with mild left shift, eosinophilia, basophilia, and marked thrombocytosis with platelet anisocytosis and numerous giant platelets (arrows). The patient's bone marrow aspirate (inset) showed numerous clusters of megakaryocytes (Leishman stain; 1,000× magnification). Similar findings (data not shown) were observed in the peripheral blood smear and bone marrow aspirate from Patient 2.

T1. Principal Laboratory Findings

Test		Results on Patient No.		Reference Range
		1	2	
Hematology				
Hemoglobin		12.8	15.9	12.0-16.0 g/dL
Hematocrit		39.9	47.5	38-47%
WBC count		32.0	20.2	4.0-11.0 × 10³/mL
Platelet count		2,582	2,365	150-400 × 10³/mL
Differential:	Myelocytes	2	2	0%
	Metamyelocytes	3	4	0%
	Neutrophils	89	58	40-80%
	Lymphocytes	2	21	20-40%
	Eosinophils	2	13	0-6%
	Basophils	2	2	0-1%
PBS and bone marrow findings	Normocytic normochromic red blood cells, leukocytosis with mild left shift, eosinophilia, basophilia, and marked thrombocytosis with platelet anisocytosis and numerous giant platelets. The bone marrow aspirate showed numerous clusters of megakaryocytes (**Image 1**, inset)			
Chemistry				
BUN		46.2	22.8	6.0-20.0 mg/dL
Creatinine		2.7	1.4	0.7-1.5 mg/dL
Serum sodium		138	135	137-145 mEq/L
Serum potassium		5.9	10.0	3.5-5.5 mEq/L
Plasma potassium		3.8	n.d.[a]	3.5-5.5 mEq/L
Chloride		100	92	97-107 mEq/L
Bicarbonate		21	16	24-30 mEq/L

[a]*The patient refused blood collection for repeat potassium testing. WBC, white blood cell; PBS, peripheral blood smear; BUN, blood urea nitrogen.*

Questions _____

1. What are the most striking clinical and laboratory findings in these patients?

2. How do you explain these findings?

3. What is the most likely diagnosis in these patients?

4. What is the explanation for the increased *serum*, but normal *plasma*, potassium concentration observed in these patients?

5. What clinical conditions can result in an artefactually increased serum potassium concentration?

6. What pre-analytical conditions can result in an artefactually increased serum potassium concentration?

7. Why is it important to differentiate between the causes of an artefactually increased serum potassium concentration?

8. How can a suspected artefactually increased serum potassium concentration be confirmed?

9. What are the dangers in the clinical management of patients with a confirmed artefactually increased serum potassium concentration?

Possible Answers _____

1. Leukocytosis with mild left shift, eosinophilia, basophilia, marked thrombocytosis with numerous giant forms in the peripheral blood smear and increased megakaryocytes in the bone marrow aspirate (**Image 1**), and hyperkalemia based on *serum* potassium concentration, but normokalemia (Patient 1) based on *plasma* potassium concentration. (**T1**).

2. The constellation of the clinical and laboratory findings in these patients is characteristic of the myeloproliferative disorder, *essential thrombocythemia*, with pseudohyperkalemia secondary to marked thrombocytosis.

3. ***Most likely diagnosis:*** *essential thrombocythemia with pseudohyperkalemia.*

4. The intracellular concentration of potassium is 23 times higher than that of plasma. This concentration gradient is maintained by an active RBC Na-K-ATPase pump which depends on oxidative energy for its function. The difference between serum and plasma potassium values is typically ~0.2 mEq/L.[1] Pseudohyperkalemia is defined as a serum versus plasma potassium difference of >0.4 mEq/L. During the clotting process, platelets release potassium; however, the amount of potassium released during this process in patients without thrombocytosis does not significantly disturb electrolyte homeostasis. On the other hand, in patients with very high platelet counts, the additional potassium released by platelets is significant, leading to a concomitant increase in the *serum* potassium concentration.[2]

5. Pseudohyperkalemia has been reported in patients with myeloproliferative diseases and marked thrombocytosis[3,4] or leukocytosis (eg, in patients with infectious mononucleosis or an acute leukemia).[2,4] This phenomenon has also been reported in patients with Hodgkin's lymphoma or rheumatoid arthritis.

6. Pseudohyperkalemia can also occur due to in vitro hemolysis during a difficult venipuncture, delayed separation of serum, refrigeration of the blood sample, or inadvertent contamination of the blood sample collection container with a potassium-containing anticoagulant [eg, dipotassium ethylenediaminetetraacetic acid (K_2EDTA)].

7. If pseudohyperkalemia is not recognized as a possible cause of an elevated serum potassium concentration, patients with pseudohyperkalemia due to thrombocytosis, leukocytosis, or pre-analytic causes may be inappropriately treated, while those with hyperkalemia due to clinically important causes may not be treated appropriately, especially if a repeat blood specimen is obtained for repeat *serum* potassium testing. The potassium values on the initial and subsequent *serum* samples could be essentially the same and the clinician and the laboratory professional might assume, incorrectly, that the patient's hyperkalemia is real, when, in fact, it could be due to an in vitro artifact.

8. By obtaining another blood specimen from the patient by careful phlebotomy using a collection tube containing an anticoagulant without potassium (eg, sodium heparin). If the hyperkalemia is due to thrombocytosis, leukocytosis, or a pre-analytic cause, the difference in potassium values between the serum and plasma samples will be >0.4 mEq/L, with the lower value obtained on the *plasma* sample. If this difference is only ~0.2 mEq/L, and both values are increased above the upper limit of the reference range for potassium, the hyperkalemia is not due to an in vitro cause, and the clinician can look for and appropriately treat the potential in vivo clinical cause of the patient's hyperkalemia. Other clues consistent with pseudohyperkalemia due to thrombocytosis, leukocytosis, or pre-analytic causes are normal electrocardiogram findings and clinical findings not consistent with the signs and symptoms of hyperkalemia.

9. Hyperkalemia is characterized by confusion, generalized weakness, flaccid paralysis, weakness of the respiratory muscles, bradycardia, cardiac conduction defects, and cardiac arrest. Therefore, hyperkalemia is a life-threatening medical emergency requiring immediate initiation of potassium lowering measures. In patients with pseudohyperkalemia due to unrecognized pre-analytic causes, unnecessary potassium lowering treatment might be initiated which can cause fatal hypokalemia. Thus, ascertaining the cause

of an increased serum potassium concentration is important in avoiding inappropriate treatment decisions that could harm the patient.[5]

Keywords

essential thrombocythemia, potassium, pseudohyperkalemia, thrombocytosis

References

1. Fort JA. Thrombocytosis and hyperkalemia revisited. *Am J Pediatr Hematol Oncol.* 1989;11:334-336.

2. Colussi G, Cipriani D. Pseudohyperkalemia in extreme leukocytosis. *Am J Nephrol.* 1995;15:450-452.

3. Ifudu O, Markell MS, Friedman EA. Unrecognized pseudohyperkalemia as a cause of elevated potassium in patients with renal disease. *Am J Nephrol.* 1992;12:102-104.

4. Ho AM, Woo JC, Kelton JG, et al. Spurious hyperkalemia associated with severe thrombocytosis and leukocytosis. *Can J Anaesth.* 1991;38:613-615.

5. Stankovic AK, Smith S. Elevated serum potassium values: the role of preanalytic variables. *Am J Clin Pathol.* 2004;121:S105-112.

Myeloblastic Proliferation in the Peripheral Blood of a Neonate With Down Syndrome

Rachel B. Flamholz,[1] Diana M. Veillon,[1] Majed Jeroudi,[2] Vishwas S. Sakhalkar,[2] Mary L. Nordberg,[1,3] James D. Cotelingam[1]

[1]*Departments of Pathology and* [2]*Pediatrics, Louisiana State University Health Sciences Center, and the* [3]*Feist-Weiller Cancer Center, Shreveport, LA*

Patient: A male neonate born at 36 weeks gestation, with a prenatal diagnosis of constitutional trisomy 21. Hypoxia developed shortly after birth followed by respiratory distress requiring mechanical ventilation.

Physical Examination Findings: Hepatosplenomegaly, ascites, and a diffuse papular skin rash.

Results of Other Diagnostic Procedures: Ultrasonography revealed bilateral hydronephrosis. Flow cytometry using CD14-fluoroisothiocyanate (FITC) and CD34-phycoerythrin (PE) staining demonstrated the presence of a population of CD14 negative, CD34 positive blast cells [**Image 1B**]. Fluorescence in situ hybridization (FISH) analyses for chromosomes 21 and 13 demonstrated 3 copies of chromosome 21 in all cells evaluated and a normal diploid copy number of chromosome 13 [**Image 1C**], while FISH analysis for rearrangements in the mixed lineage leukemia (MLL) gene on chromosome 11 (11q23) demonstrated that all cells evaluated had an intact, non-rearranged 11q23 locus [**Image 1D**].

Questions

1. What disorders are among the differential diagnosis in this patient? Why?

2. How do you distinguish between the diagnoses constituting the differential diagnosis?

3. What is this patient's most likely diagnosis?

4. What are the genetic characteristics of this patient's hematologic disorder?

5. How should this patient's disorder be treated?

Possible Answers

1. Transient myeloproliferative disorder (TMD) of infancy, acute megakaryoblastic leukemia (AML), and congenital acute leukemia (CAL)

constitute the differential diagnosis because each of these disorders is known to occur in Down syndrome-affected infants.

2. Based on differences in the epidemiologic, clinical, genetic, and laboratory features associated with each of the disorders, TMD, AML, and CAL. Transient myeloproliferative disorder of infancy occurs in approximately 10% of newborns with Down syndrome and is characterized by marked peripheral blood leukocytosis and megakaryoblastic proliferation in the bone marrow and/or peripheral blood. Hemoglobin and platelet counts may be normal or decreased. Splenomegaly and hepatomegaly are variably present. The hepatomegaly is often marked and occasionally results in hepatic fibrosis and insufficiency. By definition, TMD should resolve with supportive care in less than 3 months. However, approximately 30% of these infants will go on to develop AML subtype M7 (AML-M7) within 3 years. These cases may respond to modified

T1. Principal Laboratory Findings

Test	Day After Birth	No Ara-C Treatment			Ara-C Treatment			Reference Range
		1	3	5	20	30	40	
Hematology								
WBC count		129	139	60	2.8	4.8	5.5	9.4-34.0 × 10³/µL
Hematocrit		36.4	30.7	40.0	27.5	24.2	24.2	45-67%
Platelet count		119	150	67	67	813	502	142-405 × 10³/µL
Differential:	%							
	Neutrophils	11						32-62%
	Bands	1						5-9%
	Blasts	68	72	61	0	0	0	0%
	Lymphocytes	12						26-36%
	Monocytes	8						0-12%
NRBCs/100 WBCs	100						0/100 WBCs	
Flow Cytometry								
Positive for antigens	CD: 7, 23, 34, 41, 42b, 56, 61, 71							
Negative for T- and B-cell antigens	CD: 2, 5, 10							
Negative for myelomonocytic and granulocytic antigens	CD: 13, 14, 15, 117, HLA-DR (and cytoplasmic MPO)							

WBC, white blood cell; NRBC, nucleated red blood cell; CD, cluster of differentiation; HLA, human leukocyte antigen; MPO, myeloperoxidase.

T2. Distinguishing Clinical, Morphological, and Molecular Characteristics in Infants With Transient Myeloproliferative Disorder, Acute Megakaryoblastic Leukemia, or Congenital Acute Leukemia

Characteristic	Type of Hematologic Disorder		
	TMD	AML-M7	CAL
Age of onset	Newborn	6 months to 1 year	Newborn
Bone marrow infiltration with blasts	Low	Extensive	Extensive
Common cytogenetic features	Isolated trisomy 21	Trisomy 21 with other clonal cytogenetic abnormalities	11q23 or t(1;22)(p13;q13) translocation
Proposed molecular mechanism	*GATA-1* mutation	*GATA-1* mutation and increased	*MLL* gene rearrangement or fusion of *RBM15* and *MKL1* genes of disease telomerase activity

TMD, transient myeloproliferative disorder; AML-M7, acute megakaryoblastic leukemia-M7 subtype; CAL, congenital acute leukemia; GATA-1, principal portion of the DNA gene motif recognized by the GATA-1 transcription factor; RBM, RNA-binding motif protein-15 gene; MKL1, megakaryoblastic leukemia-1 gene.

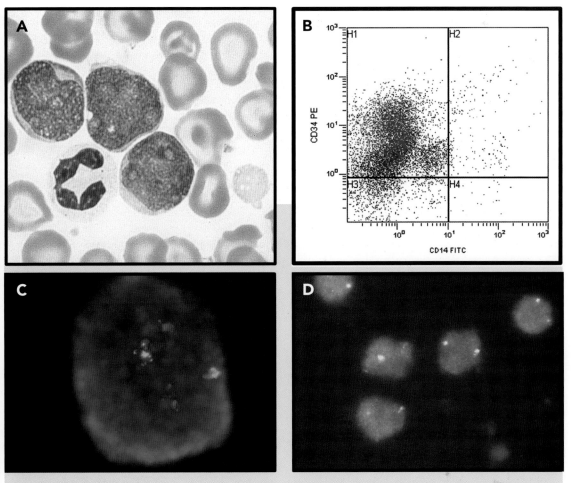

Image 1_A) Patient's peripheral blood smear illustrating the presence of multiple blast forms (Wright-Giemsa stain; 400× magnification); **B**) Flow cytometry dot plot of CD14-fluoroisothiocyanate (FITC) versus CD34-phycoerythrin (PE) staining, using gating parameters based on CD45 identification of blast cells, illustrating a population of blasts (red dots; CD34-positive and CD14-negative) and normal cells (blue dots); **C**) Fluorescence in situ hybridization (FISH) analysis using multicolor probes for specific loci on chromosomes 21 and 13. The cell shown exhibits 3 copies of chromosome 21 (redish signals) and a normal (2) copy number of chromosome 13 (greenish signals). **D**) Fluorescence in situ hybridization analysis for rearrangement of the MLL gene at locus 11q23. FISH photomicrograph demonstrating that all cells contain an intact (non-rearranged) 11q23 locus (normal copy number of 2 yellow signals per cell).

therapy for childhood acute myeloid leukemia, but most relapse and long-term survival is poor.[1-5] Acute megakaryoblastic leukemia may also develop without prior TMD and in the absence of Down syndrome. When TMD develops in the absence of Down syndrome, mosaicism or somatic mutation for trisomy 21 is present.[6] Some differences between TMD and AML-M7 are outlined in **T2**. Age at onset is the most consistent difference between the disorders TMD, AML, and CAL, with both TMD and CAL presenting during the first few days of life and AML after 6 months.[1,2,5] Other differences between these disorders are less specific. In both TMD and AML-M7, blast forms variably express CD33, CD34, CD36, CD38, CD45, and the megakaryocytic antigens, CD41 and CD61. Terminal deoxynucleotidyl transferase (TdT) activity is absent and CD7 and/or CD56 expression may be seen. Although minor differences in immunophenotype have been noted,[5] the morphology and immunophenotypic profile of TMD blasts are essentially indistinguishable from that of AML-M7.[1,7] It is also important to differentiate TMD from CAL. Congenital acute leukemia is defined as a leukemic process presenting between birth and 1 month of age. The incidence of CAL is estimated at 1 in 5 million births.[8]

3. ***Most likely diagnosis:*** *transient myeloproliferative disorder.* In acute myeloproliferative disorders associated with Down syndrome, blast forms are usually 12 to 15 μm in diameter, have round nuclei, and a moderate amount of basophilic cytoplasm with occasional cytoplasmic blebs. Coarse azurophilic granules may be present in the cytoplasm. Promegakaryocytes, micromega-karyocytes, and dyserythropoiesis are commonly observed. Blast forms may reveal scattered granular periodic acid Schiff (PAS) positivity and are negative for myeloperoxidase and Sudan Black B by cytochemistry. Platelet peroxidase is frequently present by electron microscopic cytochemistry. Erythroid differentiation may also be present.[9]

4. Chromosome X inactivation studies have demonstrated that TMD is a clonal disorder. On cytogenetic analysis, TMD blasts usually have only constitutional trisomy 21, while blasts in AML may reveal additional complex cytogenetic abnormalities. However, because complex cytogenetic aberrations are rarely identified in TMD,[10] this is not a reliable distinguishing feature. The most common additional clonal abnormality in TMD is trisomy 8. Cases with 11q23 abnormalities have also been described.[11] Moreover, FISH studies have demonstrated other cytogenetic abnormalities in both megakaryoblasts and erythroid precursors from patients with TMD.[1,3] Transient myelo-proliferative disorder is believed to originate from fetal hematopoietic cells in the liver,[12] a hypothesis supported by the occasional finding of erythroid differentiation in TMD.[13] The DNA binding protein, GATA-1 (GATA binding protein 1 or globin transcription factor 1), is an erythroid transcription factor expressed by megakaryocytes, erythrocytes, and basophils derived from a specific multipotential progenitor cell (CFU-E/B/Meg).[14] The GATA-1 binding protein recognizes the DNA sequence (or motif), WGATAR, where W and R refer to any pyrimidine or purine, respectively, and GATA refers to guanine-adenine-thymine-adenine.[3] Ito and colleagues have documented GATA-1 expression in all 7 of the TMD patients they investigated.[15] More recent studies have shown that both TMD and AML-M7 demonstrate mutations in exon 2 of the *GATA-1* gene on the X chromosome, a finding which was absent in other types of leukemias.[3] Although the exact mutation may vary between individual cases, all relevant mutations lead to expression of a shortened form of the GATA-1 transcription factor, with resultant abnormal megakaryocyte differentiation. One patient in the report by Hitzler and colleague[16] developed AML-M7 1 year following the diagnosis of TMD. In this child, the identical *GATA-1* mutation was found in the TMD blasts and the AML-M7 blasts, suggesting that AML-M7 may evolve directly from TMD. These studies support the concept that *GATA-1* mutations are early developments in TMD.[3,16] In addition, the TMD clone may remain detectable by minimal residual techniques, even when it is undetectable by traditional methods such as routine microscopy of the bone marrow.[17] Currently, there is no reliable way to predict which cases of TMD will reappear or persist as AML-M7. Additional studies to identify reliable predictors of transformation to acute leukemia would be invaluable. Additionally, the *GATA-1* mutation may prove to be a reliable marker of persistent disease, thereby facilitating appropriate therapy for patients with TMD.

5. Typically, TMD resolves without treatment. However, infants born with severe disease may die.[18] These infants may be born with hydrops fetalis due to hepatic or cardiac infiltration. Most investigators recommend supportive care for the treatment of infants with TMD. However, others prefer to use low-dose cytosine arabinoside (Ara-C) in the treatment of the subset of TMD patients with a higher risk of mortality.[19] The ideal dose and timing of Ara-C therapy are currently under investigation.[20] A recent study by the Pediatric Oncology Group recommended chemotherapy under 4 circumstances[19]: 1) leukemic blasts greater than 100,000/μL in the peripheral blood, 2) organ infiltration with impairment, 3) hydrops fetalis at birth, and 4) when disseminated intravascular coagulation (DIC) is present.

Treatment and Course

The patient was extubated on the second postnatal day. Double volume exchange transfusion was performed immediately thereafter. Following 3 days of supportive care, he developed abdominal distention, which resulted in respiratory distress. Therapy with low-dose Ara-C was initiated and was complicated by bone marrow suppression. On the fifth postnatal day, our patient was transferred to another institution. Hepatosplenomegaly resolved 6 days after treatment with Ara-C with marked symptomatic improvement. On postnatal day 30, microscopic examination of a bone marrow aspirate revealed trilineage hematopoiesis with adequate maturation, and no CD34 positive blast population was identified on flow cytometric analysis of the bone marrow. In addition, lymphoid and myeloid markers were appropriate for age. At that time and over the next few months, the leukocyte and differential count normalized [**T1**], indicating resolution of the myeloproliferative disorder and recovery from bone marrow suppression.

Keywords

transient myeloproliferative disorder, Down syndrome, acute megakaryoblastic leukemia, congenital acute leukemia, fluorescence in situ hybridization, flow cytometry

References

1. Jaffe ES, Harris NL, Stein H, Vardiman JW, eds. World Health Organization classification of tumours. Pathology and genetics of tumours of hematopoietic and lymphoid tissues. Lyon, France: IARC Press. 2001:101-102.

2. Collins RD, Swerdlow SH, eds. *Pediatric hematopathology.* Philadelphia: Churchill Livingstone; 2001:178-182.

3. Mundschau G, Gurbuxani S, Gamis AS, et al. Mutagenesis of *GATA-1* is an initiating event in Down syndrome leukemogenesis. *Blood.* 2003;101:4298-4300.

4. Lange B. The management of neoplastic disorders of haematopoiesis in children with Down's syndrome. *Br J Haematol.* 2000;110:512-524.

5. Karandikar NJ, Aquino DB, McKenna RW, et al. Transient myeloproliferative disorder and acute myeloid leukemia in Down syndrome. An immunophenotypic analysis. *Am J Clin Pathol.* 2001;116:204-210.

6. Brissette MD, Duval-Arnould BJ, Gordon B, et al. Acute megakaryoblastic leukemia following transient myeloproliferative disorder in a patient without Down syndrome. *Am J Hematol.* 1994;47:316-319.

7. de Tar MW, Dittman W, Gilbert J. Transient myeloproliferative disease of the newborn: Case report with placental, cytogenetic, and flow cytometric findings. *Hum Pathol.* 2000;31:396-398.

8. Pui C-H, Kane JR, Crist WM. Biology and treatment of infant leukemias. *Leukemia.* 1995;9:762-769.

9. Bozner P. Transient myeloproliferative disorder with erythroid differentiation in Down syndrome. *Arch Pathol Lab Med.* 2002;126:474-477.

10. Kounami S, Aoyagi N, Tsuno H, et al. Additional chromosome abnormalities in transient myelopoiesis in Down syndrome patients. *Acta Haematologica.* 1997;98:109-112.

11. Granzen B, Reinisch I, Skopnik H, et al. Transient myeloproliferative disorder with 11q23 aberration in 2 neonates with Down syndrome. *Ann Hematol.* 1998;77:51-54.

12. Miyauchi J, Ito Y, Kawano T, et al. Unusual diffuse liver fibrosis accompanying transient myeloproliferative disorder in Down syndrome: A report of 4 autopsy cases and proposal of a hypothesis. *Blood.* 1992;80:1521-1527.

13. Zipursky A, Brown E, Christensen H, et al. Leukemia and/or myeloproliferative syndrome in neonates with Down syndrome. *Semin Perinatol.* 1997;21:97-101.

14. Romeo P, Prandini M, Joulin V, et al. Megakaryocytic and erythrocytic lineages share specific transcription factors. *Nature.* 1990;344:447-449.

15. Ito E, Kasai M, Hayashi Y, et al. Expression of erythroid specific genes in acute megakaryoblastic leukemia and transient myeloproliferative disorder in Down syndrome. *Br J Haematol.* 1995;90:607-614.

16. Hitzler JK, Cheung J, Li Y, et al. *GATA-1* mutations in transient leukemia and acute megakaryoblastic leukemia of Down syndrome. *Blood.* 2003;101:4301-4304.

17. Taub JW. Down syndrome and megakaryocytic leukemia/transient myeloproliferative disorder: When does it begin? *Blood.* 2003;101:4228.

18. Hayashi Y, Eguchi M, Sugita K, et al. Cytogenetic findings and clinical features in acute leukemia and transient myeloproliferative disorder in Down's syndrome. *Blood.* 1988;72:15-23.

19. Al-Kasim F, Doyle JJ, Massey GV, et al. Incidence and treatment of potentially lethal diseases in transient leukemia of Down syndrome: Pediatric Oncology Group Study. *Pediatr Hematol Oncol.* 2002;24:9-13.

20. Gamis AS, Hilden JM. Transient myeloproliferative disorder, a disorder with too few data and many unanswered questions: Does it contain an important piece of the puzzle to understanding hematopoiesis and acute myelogenous leukemia. *Pediatr Hematol Oncol.* 2002;24:2-5.

Vulvar and Oral Lesions in a 34-Year-Old Woman

Beverly J. Brent, Meenakshi Nandedkar

Armed Services Blood Bank Center, National Naval Medical Center, Bethesda, MD

Patient: 34-year-old woman.

Chief Complaint: Intermittent fever and vulvar pain.

History of Present Illness: The patient reported that she frequently had re-occurring oral and vulvar lesions.

Physical Examination Findings: Large, erosive, bilateral, necrotic vulvar and oral lesions were found, which were painful on touching. Some necrotic debris at the urethra was noted.

Additional Diagnostic Procedures: A vulvar biopsy revealed marked acute inflammation associated with necrosis and obliterative vasculitis but no epithelioid granulomas were identified. A bone marrow biopsy was performed with results as shown in (**T2**) and (**Image 1B**).

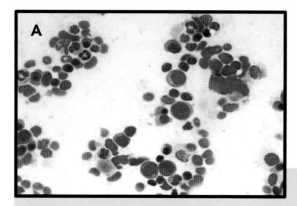
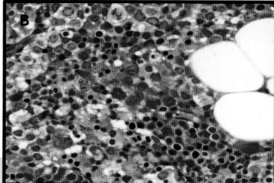

Image 1_Patient's peripheral blood smear (**A**) illustrating leukopenia with blasts and neutrophils with bilobed nuclei (Pelger-Huet anomaly) and bone marrow aspirate (**B**) illustrating a hypercellular bone marrow with an increased number of immature/undifferentiated cells and a decreased number of erythroid cells. Wright-Giemsa stain; 100× magnification.

Questions _____

1. What are this patient's most striking clinical and laboratory findings?

2. How do you explain this patient's most striking clinical and laboratory findings?

3. What is this patient's most likely diagnosis?

4. What additional tests are recommended to confirm this diagnosis?

5. How is this patient's disease subtyped?

6. What is this patient's final diagnosis?

T1. Principal Laboratory Findings

Test	Patient's Result	Reference Interval
Hematology		
WBC count	20.1	$4.0\text{-}11.0 \times 10^3/\mu L$
Corrected WBC count	18.1	$4.0\text{-}11.0 \times 10^3/\mu L$
NRBC count	11/100	1/100 WBC
RBC count	2.77	$4.20\text{-}5.40 \times 10^6/\mu L$
Hemoglobin	8.4	12.0-16.0 g/dL
Hematocrit	24.2	37.0-47.0%
MCV	87.2	81.0-99.0 fL
MCH	30.2	27.0-32.0 pg
MCHC	34.5	31.0-37.0%
RDW	15.8	11.5-14.5%
Blasts	28	<0%
MPV	7.3	7.4-10.4 fL
Platelet count estimate	27	$150\text{-}450 \times 10^3/\mu L$
ESR	111	0-15 mm/h
Manual Differential Count		
Neutrophils	87.3	51.0-67.0%
Lymphocytes	11	21-35%
Monocytes	1.2	4.0-8.0%
PBS Morphology		
WBCs	Leukopenia, many blasts, and neutrophils with bilobed nuclei (Pelger-Huet anomaly) (**Image 1A**)	
RBCs	Normocytic-normochromic	
Platelets	Few hypogranular and agranular platelets	

WBC, white blood cell; NRBC, nucleated red blood cell; MCV, mean corpuscular volume; MCH, mean corpuscular hemoglobin; MCHC, mean corpuscular hemoglobin concentration; RDW, red blood cell distribution width; MPV, mean platelet volume; ESR, erythrocyte sedimentation rate; PBS, peripheral blood smear.

7. What diseases are most often associated with pancytopenia?

8. What is the most common laboratory indicator of erythropoiesis?

9. What is the prognosis for individuals with our patient's disease?

10. What is the most appropriate treatment for this patient?

The views expressed in this article are those of the author(s) and do not necessarily reflect the official policy or position of the Department of the Navy, Department of Defense, or the United States Government.

Possible Answers

1. The most striking clinical findings were fever and recurrent oral/vulvar lesions. The most striking laboratory findings included marked leukopenia, pancytopenia; markedly increased ESR; peripheral blood smear findings of an excessive number of blast cells, thrombocytopenia, some hypogranular and agranular platelets, and normocytic-normochromic anemia (**T1**) (**Image 1A**); and, a hypercellular bone marrow with obliterative vasculitis and an increased number

T2. Principal Bone Marrow Findings

Morphology

Cellularity:	Hypercellular with large aggregates and sheets of immature cells
Granulopoiesis:	Decreased; not all stages of maturation present; polymorphonuclear cells and bands seen; no Auer rods observed
Erythropoiesis:	Markedly decreased with RBCs exhibiting progressive forms of maturation
Megakaryopoiesis:	Mildly increased with micromegakaryocytes and dysmegakaryocytes
Lymphocytes:	Few, scattered
Plasma cells:	Few, mostly mature, some with cytoplasmic Russell bodies

Flow Cytometry

Marker	+/-	Percentage of positive cells in blastregion of dot-plot
CD3	-	
CD4	-	
CD5	-	
CD8	-	
CD13	+ (mod)	81%
CD19	-	
CD20	-	
CD33/CD71	+	40%
CD34	+	1%
CD34/CD117	+	14%
Glycophorin	-	
EMA	-	
Cytokeratin	-	

Cytogenetics (FISH Analysis)

Normal karyotype; negative for CBFB rearrangement [inv(16) or t(16;16)]

RBCs, red blood cells; +/-, positive/negative; CD, cluster of differentiation; mod, moderate; EMA, epithelial membrane antigen; FISH, fluorescence in situ hybridization; CBFB, core binding factor-b; inv, inversion; t, translocation.

of immature/undifferentiated cells and markedly decreased erythroid cells (**T2**) (**Image 1B**).

2. Our patient's clinical and laboratory findings suggest a non-specific necrotizing inflammatory disorder such as Behcet's syndrome or a hematologic disorder such as refractory anemia with excess blasts (RAEB). The patient's peripheral blood smear (eg, pancytopenia) and bone marrow findings, especially obliterative vaculitis, favors a diagnosis of RAEB. Vasculitis may develop before or after a hematologic disorder and its etiology is unknown.[1] One hypothesis on how vaculitis may develop involves activation of B cells and the synthesis of organ-specific and non-organ-specific autoantibodies. Another hypothesis involves severely impaired macrophage function which results in decreased clearance of immune complexes, neutrophil chemotaxis, and organ injury from

increased superoxide anion production. Another hypothesis suggests that changes in the bone marrow play a significant role in the etiology of vasculitis. To distinguish between Behcet's syndrome and RAEB as the cause of our patient's laboratory findings, correlation of laboratory findings with clinical findings was required because pancytopenia is not a typical feature of Behcet's syndrome; however, this syndrome has been associated with clonal myeloid disorders. Behcet's syndrome (or disease) is a rare complication of myelodsyplastic syndrome (MDS) with only 10 cases having been reported up to 1997.[2] Behcet's syndrome is characterized by recurrent oral/genital ulcers and eye/skin lesions. The tissue injury that occurs in patients with this syndrome is caused by excessive production of reactive oxygen species (ROS) by activated neutrophils. On the other hand, patients with MDS are usually characterized by decreased production of ROS. Moreover, when Behcet's disease is associated with MDS, trisomy 8 is the most common karyotypic abnormality observed, involving 8.9% to 18.4% of patients with MDS-associated Behcet's syndrome.[2] Trisomy 8 occurs in MDS patients more frequently than in patients with Behcet's disease. The findings by Ohno and colleagues suggest that this chromosomal abnormality may predispose a subgroup of MDS patients with trisomy 8 to Behcet's disease.[2] In the majority of patients studied by this group of investigators, Behcet's disease occurred after the onset of MDS. In addition, increased concentrations of cytokines and growth factors were found in serum from these patients prior to the onset of Behcet's disease. It has been suggested that trisomy 8 may contribute to the pathogenicity of MDS-associated Behcet's syndrome by producing such serum factors as granulocyte-colony stimulating factor (G-CSF), tumor-necrosis factor-alpha (TNF-a), interleukin-6 (IL-6), and IL-8.[2] Lastly, anemia, thrombocytopenia, and peripheral blood smear findings consistent with excess immature white blood cells rarely occur in patients with Behcet's disease. Therefore, when these findings occur, clinicians should consider MDS with trisomy 8 as a possible diagnosis.

3. **Most likely diagnosis:** *refractory anemia with excess blasts (RAEB)*. Most patients with RAEB are older than 50 years of age and males and females are affected equally. In addition, this

syndrome evolves into AML in about 30% to 50% of cases.

4. Additional testing to confirm the diagnosis of RAEB and identify its subtype should include morphologic analysis of stained bone marrow and reticulum smears, using Wright-Giemsa, hematoxylin-eosin (H&E) and iron stains; flow cytometry using lymphoma/leukemia cell markers; and cytogenetics. In addition, measurement of serum iron, vitamin B_{12}, and folic acid levels is useful in identifying the anemia as refractory, if the patient is not responsive to therapy to reverse the anemia.[1] Our patient's bone marrow demonstrated decreased erythroid cells with scanty, stainable iron content consistent with a normocytic-normochromic anemia (**T2**) (**Image 1B**). Flow cytometry findings were consistent with a clonal proliferation of myeloid cells resulting in impaired hematopoiesis, consistent with acute myeloid leukemia (AML) (**T2**) (P=0.1, log-rank test). Cytogenetic findings, including fluorescence in situ hybridization (FISH) analysis for the core binding factor-b (CBFB) rearrangement, [*inv(16) or t(16;16)*], indicated a normal karyotype and no CBFB rearrangement.

5. Patients with MDS demonstrate significant clinical variability.[3] The French-American-British (FAB) classification criteria for MDS include <30% blasts in the bone marrow and peripheral blood with evidence of ineffective hematopoiesis.[3] The World Health Organization (WHO; 2001 guidelines) classification critiera for MDS indicate 20% blasts in the peripheral blood or bone marrow as consistent with a diagnosis of AML. Moreover, WHO provides criteria for subtyping RAEB based on the percentage of peripheral blood and bone marrow blast cells. Patients with <5% peripheral blood blast cells and 5% to 9% bone marrow blast cells are classified as RAEB-1, while those with 5% to 19% peripheral blast cells and 10% to 19% bone marrow blast cells are classified as RAEB-2.[4] Moreover, Albitar and colleagues reported that the similarity in outcome data for patients with AML and MDS does not necessarily imply that these diseases are biologically similar because there is significant overlap when these 2 diseases are distinguished based on the percentage of peripheral blood and bone marrow blast cells.[3] Their data suggests that

a classification scheme based on the biology of MDS is needed. Strupp and colleagues analyzed the subtypes of RAEB according to the FAB classification criteria: hematological characteristics, karyotype anomalies, and prognosis.[5] Their findings supported the elimination of Auer rods as a criterion for classification of RAEB using the new WHO classification scheme. Lastly, there is concern among hematopathologists that patients classified previously as RAEB-t (refractory anemia with excess blasts in transformation) using the FAB classification scheme based on a peripheral blood blast count of at least 5% are now reclassified as RAEB-2. The concern stems from the fact that this feature predicts a median survival similar to that of patients with AML, it does not reflect their unfavorable prognosis, and it increases the prognostic heterogeneity of the RAEB-2 category.

6. Because of our patient's peripheral blood findings of pancytopenia with leukoerythroblastosis and a blast cell count of 5% and bone marrow hypercellularity (90%), no clonal abnormalities, and trilineal myelodysplasia with 12% blasts, our patient's final diagnosis is RAEB-2. Our patient's normal karotype was not at odds with this interpretation because 52% of patients with MDS lack a karotypic abnormality.

7. Hypersplenism (HS) due to liver cirrhosis or a hepatoma, aplastic anemia (AA), and myelodysplastic syndrome (MDS) are the most common diseases associated with pancytopenia.

8. The reticulocyte count is a common diagnostic indicator of erythropoietic activity. Flow cytometry was applied by Kabutomori and colleagues to examine whether the number of total and immature reticulocytes was decreased in blood from patients with HS, AA, or MDS and pancytopenia.[6] Because MDS involves an intrinsic defect in the maturation of hematopoietic cells in the bone marrow, the number of reticulocytes may not increase when the level of erythropoietin increases. They concluded that the number of total and immature reticulocytes was highly decreased in patients with MDS and pancytopenia.[6]

9. Median survival of patients with RAEB is about 9 months, although there are occasional long-term survivors.[7] Moreover, median survival in patients with RAEB-1 is 18 months and 10 months in patients with RAEB-2. In patients with RAEB, periodic hematologic evaluation of blood and bone marrow is essential to prolonged survival in these patients.

10. In most cases, the treatment of patients with RAEB should be highly individualized. Most patients with RAEB require treatment for weeks to months. Since the response to cytotoxic therapy is poor, a concurrent, symptomatic treatment regimen, including blood transfusion and administration of antibiotics as needed, is required. If the disease progresses to AML and the patient can sustain standard therapy for AML, this therapy is utilized in such patients. Moreover, patients with RAEB who are under 50 years of age and have a histocompatible donor should be considered for stem cell transplantation.[7] Patients with MDS and RAEB are at increased risk for progression to AML. In these patients, treatment options are limited because of the refractory nature of their disorder to conventional cyto-reductive chemotherapy.

Keywords

refractory anemia with excess blasts (RAEB), Behcet's syndrome, myelodysplastic syndrome, acute myeloid leukemia, FAB classification scheme

References

1. Philippe B, Couderc LJ, Droz D, et al. Systemic vasculitis and myelodysplastic syndromes. A report of 2 cases. *Arthritis Rheum.* 1997;40:179-182.

2. Ohno E, Ohtsuka E, Watanabe K, et al. Behcet's disease associated with myelodysplastic syndromes. A case report and a review of the literature. *Cancer.* 1997;79:262-268.

3. Albitar M, Manshouri T, Shen Y, et al. Myelodysplastic syndrome is not merely "preleukemia". *Blood.* 2002;100:791-798.

4. Jaffe EJ, Harris NL, Stein H, Vardiman JW (eds): *World Health Organization Classification of Tumours. Pathology and Genetics of Tumours of Haematopoietic and Lymphoid Tissues.* Lyon, France: IARC Press; 2001.

5. Strupp C, Gattermann N, Giagounidis A, et al. Refractory anemia with excess blasts in transformation: Analysis of reclassification according to the WHO proposals. *Leukemia Res.* 2003;27:397-404.

6. Kabutomori O, Kanakura Y, Iwatani Y. Marked decreases of total and immature reticulocytes in myelodysplastic syndrome among patients with pancytopenia. *Acta Haematologica.* 2003;109:212-213.

7. Beutler E, Lichtman MA, Coller BS, Kupps TJ, Seligjohn U (eds.): *Williams Hematology.* 6th ed. New York: McGraw-Hill Companies; 2001, 1036-1037.

Fatigue and Easy Bruising in a 32-Year-Old Woman With a History of Heart Problems

Diana L. Cochran-Black,[1] Linda K. Burnside[2]

[1]*Department of Medical Technology, Wichita State University, and* [2]*Wichita Clinic, Wichita, KS*

Patient: 32-year-old Hispanic woman.

History of Present Illness: The patient presented to her physician with complaints of extreme fatigue, increasing bruisability, and heavy menstrual bleeding. She had a long history of easy bruising, but the number of bruises had become increasingly more obvious over the last few weeks.

Medical History: The patient denied a history of epistaxis or other sites of bleeding. She also denied any weight loss. Her previous medical history included hypertension, chronic sinusitis, mitral valve prolapse, and Prinzmetal angina. She had undergone 2 heart catheterizations without complications.

Physical Examination: She demonstrated many small ecchymoses over her lower and upper extremities. Splenomegaly and lymphadenopathy were absent.

Questions

1. What are this patient's most striking clinical and laboratory findings?

2. What is this patient's differential diagnosis?

3. What additional laboratory tests are warranted in order to make a definitive diagnosis?

4. What is the most likely diagnosis for this patient?

5. What is the appropriate treatment for this patient's medical condition?

6. What is the prognosis for this patient?

Possible Answers

1. Easy bruising, decreased platelet count and white blood cell count, elevated d-dimer level, and an increased number of immature white blood

cells in the peripheral blood and bone marrow (**T1** and **Images 1** and **2**).

2. The physical examination and initial laboratory features point to a diagnosis of acute leukemia. Based on the morphology of the immature white blood cells, the peripheral blood and bone marrow differentials point to a differential diagnosis of acute myelogenous leukemia (AML) with a French-American-British (FAB) classification of M2.

3. Additional laboratory tests used to differentiate between the various types of acute leukemia include cytochemical stains, immunophenotyping, chromosome analysis, and molecular genetics studies (**T2**).

4. ***Most likely diagnosis:*** *Acute promyelocytic leukemia (APL)*. Based on the flow cytometry, FISH, PCR, and chromosomal analyses, the patient has the microgranular form of acute promyelocytic leukemia with a FAB classification of M3v. It is difficult to differentiate between microgranular promyelocytes and type II myeloblasts seen in

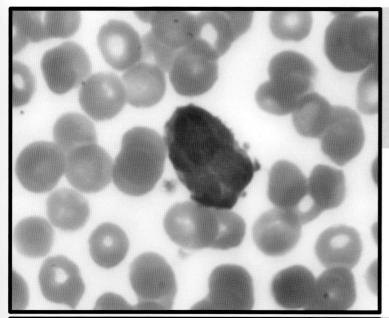

Image 1_Patient's Wright-Giemsa-stained peripheral blood smear illustrating a microgranular promyelocyte with a bilobed nucleus.

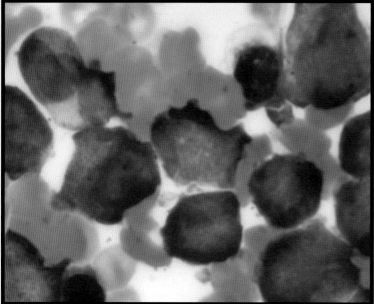

Image 2_Patient's Wright-Giemsa-stained bone marrow aspirate illustrating microgranular promyelocytes with lobulated nuclei.

acute myelogenous leukemia (AML-M2). M3v is also easily confused with acute myelomonocytic (AML-M4) and acute monocytic leukemia (AML-M5) when using morphology alone to differentiate.[1] The blasts reported in the initial differential counts for this patient are most likely microgranular promyelocytes.

Acute promyelocytic leukemia, FAB classification M3, comprises 5% to 15% of all cases of AML2-6 and the microgranular variant (M3v) is seen in approximately 15% to 20% of APL

patients.[7,8] The disease is characterized by the proliferation of abnormal promyelocytes. Additionally, most patients with APL present with a mild to moderate form of disseminated intravascular coagulation (DIC).[4,9,10] The median age of onset for this disease is 30 to 40 years and a higher incidence is seen in Latinos.[11] Those with M3v tend to be female, non-white, and have a higher incidence of infection at the time of presentation.[1]

T1. Initial Laboratory Findings

Test	Patient's Result	"Normal" Reference Range
Hematology		
Peripheral Blood		
White blood cell count	2.0	5.0–10.0 × 10³/µL
Red blood cell count	4.58	3.70–5.20 × 10⁹/µL
Hemoglobin	14.1	12.0–16.0 g/dL
Hematocrit	39.7	37.0–47.0%
MCV	86.7	80.0–96.0 fL
MCH	30.8	26.0–34.0 pg
MCHC	35.5	32.0–36.0%
Platelet count	47.0	150–400 × 10³/µL
RDW	13.0	<14.6%
MPV	9.4	7.4–11.0 fL
Differential:		
Segmented neutrophils	23	50–70%
Lymphocytes	33	20–40%
Monocytes	13	4–8%
Eosinophils	1	0–6%
Blast cells	30	0%
Bone Marrow Differential		
Myeloblasts	53	1–5%
Promyelocytes	16	1–8%
Myelocytes	2	1–20%
Metamyelocytes	1	6–22%
Bands	3	6–36%
Segmented neutrophils	1	9–27%
Lymphocytes	8	3–24%
Monocytes	1	1–3%
Nucleated RBC precursors	14	8–57%
Coagulation		
PT	14.1	9.2–12.6 seconds
D-dimer	6.0	0–2.4 mg/L

MCV, mean corpuscular volume; MCH, mean corpuscular hemoglobin; MCHC, mean corpuscular hemoglobin concentration; RDW, red blood cell distribution width; MPV, mean platelet volume; PT, prothrombin time.

T2. Additional Laboratory Findings

Test	Patient's Result
Flow cytometry	% Positive
CD45	95
CD2	96
CD34	96
CD13	98
CD33	96
CD117	96
Myeloperoxidase	97
HLA-DR	23
FISH analysis	Positive for *PML/RARα* gene rearrangement
Chromosome analysis	46,XX,t(15;17)(q22;q21.1)
PCR analysis	Positive for the short form of the t(15;17) *PML-RARα* translocation

FISH, fluorescence in-situ hybridization; PCR, polymerase chain reaction; PML/RARα, promyelocytic leukemia/retinoic acid receptor alpha.

Acute promyelocytic leukemia and the microgranular variant can be differentiated from other forms of AML through the combination of morphology, cytochemical reactions, immunophenotype, chromosome, and molecular genetic analyses.

Morphologically, the promyelocytes seen in APL can be divided into 1 hypergranular and 4 microgranular subtypes (**T3**).[12]

Cytochemical staining of the neoplastic cells in both M3 and M3v demonstrates a strong positive reaction with myeloperoxidase, Sudan black B, and napthol AS-D chloroacetate esterase.[1,7]

The typical immunophenotype for M3 and M3v is HLA-DR and CD34 negative and CD13, 33, 45, and 117 positive.[13,14] In addition, M3v is usually CD2 positive.[10]

Cytogenetic and molecular genetic studies make an unequivocal diagnosis of APL.[14] Both the classical and variant subtype of APL are associated with the 15;17 chromosome translocation [t(15;17)(q22;21)].[15,16] The translocation links the retinoic acid receptor alpha (*RARα*) gene on chromosome 17 with the *PML* gene on chromosome 15. The formation of this new fusion

T3. Morphology Subtypes of Acute Promyelocytic Leukemia (APL)

Subtype 1: Hypergranular APL	Predominantly hypergranular promyelocytes with multiple auer rods.
Subtype 2: Microgranular APL	Predominantly bilobed promyelocytes with few, fine, or no granules.
Subtype 3: Microgranular APL	Predominantly promyelocytes with non-granular basophilic cytoplasm and cytoplasmic projections.
Subtype 4: Microgranular APL	Predominantly normal-looking promyelocytes without granules and without folding or lobulation of the nucleus.
Subtype 5: Microgranular APL	Predominantly myeloblasts (>60%) with a small proportion of promyelocytes.

protein inhibits the differentiation of myeloid cells and promotes their survival.[17] The *RARα/PML* gene rearrangement is the most common molecular marker for APL[16,18]; however, in recent years several researchers have reported 4 other rearrangements that have been linked with the *RARa* gene. These genes include *PLZF, NPM, NuMA,* and *STAT5b.*[19,20]

5. In adults, APL is now the most curable form of acute myelogenous leukemia.[21] It is imperative that prompt therapy is initiated due to this disorder's association with DIC and the disease's great response with all-trans retinoic acid (ATRA).[9,22] For induction, the therapy of choice for APL is ATRA, either alone or combined with anthracycline-based chemotherapy.[23] All-trans retinoic acid works by inducing the differentiation of leukemic promyelocytes into mature granulocytes. It also leads to rapid resolution of the DIC.[21,24] After complete remission, ATRA is also used for maintenance therapy.[23] A potentially fatal side effect of ATRA is retinoic acid syndrome (RAS). The symptoms of this syndrome include fever, acute renal failure, respiratory distress, pleural and pericardial effusion, interstitial pulmonary infiltrates, hypotension, and weight gain.[25,26] The concurrent use of chemotherapy with ATRA has reduced the likelihood of this syndrome.[21]

6. The prognosis for a patient diagnosed with APL is very good. Complete remission rates of 70% to 90% can be expected when using ATRA combined with chemotherapy.[21,22,27] The overall 5-year disease survival rate is estimated to be between 50% and 70%.[22,23,28] Patients who relapse have been successfully treated with arsenic compounds.[22] Prognostic factors that indicate a low risk for relapse include an initial white count of <10,000/μL and a platelet count of >40,000/μL.[21]

Patient Treatment and Follow-up

The patient received induction treatment with idarubicin, ara-C, and ATRA. She tolerated the treatment very well and is now considered to be in complete remission.

Acknowledgments

The authors express their appreciation to the patient and her physicians for providing permission to access medical records and to the laboratory staff at the Wichita Clinic for their assistance with this case study. We would also like to thank Mouna Todorov, MD, of Heartland Pathology for providing the peripheral blood and bone marrow photos.

Keywords

acute promyelocytic leukemia, microgranular or hypergranular variant, all-trans retinoic acid (ATRA), promyelocytic leukemia/retinoic acid receptor alpha (PML/RARa), disseminated intravascular coagulation

References

1. Davey FR, Davis RB, MacCallum JM, et al. Morphologic and cytochemical characteristics of acute promyelocytic leukemia. *Am J Hematol.* 1989;30:221–227.

2. Bennett JM, Catovsky D, Daniel MT, et al. Proposals for the classification of acute leukemias. *Br J Haematol.* 1976;33:451–461.

3. Groopman J, Ellman L. Acute promyelocytic leukemia. *Am J Hematol.* 1979;7:395–408.

4. McKenna RW, Parkin J, Bloomfield CD, et al. Acute promyelocytic leukaemia: A study of 39 cases with identification of a hyperbasophilic microgranular variant. *Br J Haematol.* 1982;50:201–214.

5. Stone RM, Mayer RJ. The unique aspects of acute promyelocytic leukemia. *J Clin Oncol.* 1990;8:1913–1921.

6. Spell DW, Velagaleti GVN, Jones DV, et al. Translocation (15;17) and trisomy 21 in the microgranular variant of acute promyelocytic leukemia. *Cancer Genet Cytogenet.* 2002;132:74–76.

7. Varghese L, Janckila A, Yam LT. Acute promyelocytic leukemia: New methods in diagnosis and treatment. *J Ky Med Assoc.* 1999;97:61–65.

8. Avvisanti G, LoCoco F, Mandelli F. Acute promyelocytic leukemia: Clinical and morphologic features and prognostic factors. *Semin Hematol.* 2001;38:4–12.

9. Nagendra S, Meyerson H, Skallerud G, et al. Leukemias resembling acute promyelocytic leukemia, microgranular variant. *Am J Clin Pathol.* 2002;117:651–657.

10. Stasi R, Bruno A, Venditti A, et al. A microgranular variant of acute promyelocytic leukemia with atypical morpho-cytochemical features and an early myeloid immunophenotype. *Leuk Res.* 1997;21:575–580.

11. Douer D, Preston-Martin S, Chang E, et al. High frequency of acute promyelocytic leukemia among Latinos with acute myeloid leukemia. *Blood.* 1996;87:308–313.

12. Neame PB, Soamboonsrup P, Leber B, et al. Morphology of acute promyelocytec leukemia with cytogenetic or molecular evidence for the diagnosis: Characterization of additional microgranular variants. *Am J Hematol.* 1997;56:131–142.

13. Exner M, Thalhammer R, Kapiotiss, et al. The "typical" immunophenotype of acute promyelocytic leukemia (APL-M3): Does it prove true for the M3-variant? *Cytometry.* 2000;42:106–109.

14. Rizzatti EG, Portieres FL, Sergio LR, et al. Microgranular and t(11;17)/*PLZF-RAR*a variants of acute promyelocytic leukemia also present the flow cytometric pattern of CD14, CD34, and CD15 expression characteristic of *PML-RAR*a gene rearrangement. *Am J Hematol.* 2004;76:44–51.

15. Bennett JM, Catovsky D, Daniel MT, et al. A variant form of hypergranular promyelocytic leukaemia (M3). *Br J Haematol.* 1980;44:169–170.

16. LoCoco F, Avvisati G, Diverion D, et al. Rearrangement of the *RAR*a gene in acute promyelocytic leukaemia: Correlation with morphology and immunophenotype. *Br J Haematol.* 1991;78:494–499.

17. Grignani F, Testa U, Rogaia D, et al. Acute promyelocytic leukemia: From genetics to treatment. *Blood.* 1994;83:10–25.

18. Redner RL, Rush EA, Faas S, et al. The t(15;17) variant of acute promyelocytic leukemia expresses a nucleophosmin-retinoic acid receptor fusion. *Blood.* 1996;87:882–886.

19. Melnick A, Licht JD. Deconstructing a disease: *RAR*a, its fusion partners and their roles in the pathogenesis of acute promyelocytic leukemia. *Blood.* 1999;93:3167–3215.

20. Dong S, Tweardy DJ. Interactions of *Stat5b-RAR*a, a novel acute promyelocytic leukemia fusion protein, with retinoic acid receptor and *STAT3* signaling pathway. *Blood.* 2002;99:2637–2646.

21. Tallman MS, Nabhan C, Feusner JH. Acute promyelocytic leukemia: Evolving therapeutic strategies. *Blood.* 2002;99:759–767.

22. Chen Z, Chen G-Q, Shen Z-X, et al. Treatment of acute promyelocytic leukemia with arsenic compounds: In vitro and in vivo studies. *Semin Hematol.* 2001;38:26–36.

23. Tallman MS, Andersen JW, Schiffer CA, et al. All-trans retinoic acid in acute promyelocytic leukemia: Long-term outcome and prognostic factor analysis from the North American intergroup protocol. *Blood.* 2002;100:4298–4302.

24. Visani G, Gugliotta L, Tosi P, et al. All-trans retinoic acid significantly reduces the incidence of early hemorrhagic death during induction therapy of acute promyelocytic leukemia. *Eur J Haematol.* 2000;64:139–144.

25. Frankel SR, Eardley A, Heller G, et al. All-trans retinoic acid for acute promyelocytic leukemia results of the New York study. *Ann Intern Med.* 1994;120:278–286.

26. Candoni A, Damiani D, Michelutti A, et al. Clinical characteristics, prognostic factors and multidrug-resistance related protein expression in 36 adult patients with acute promyelocytic leukemia. *Eur J Haematol.* 2003;71:1–8.

27. Fenaux P, Chromienne C, Degos L. Acute promyelocytic leukemia: Biology and treatment. *Semin Oncol.* 1997;24:92–102.

28. Arber DA, Stein AS, Carter NH, et al. Prognostic impact of acute myeloid leukemia classification. *Am J Clin Pathol.* 2003;119:672–680.

Pericardial Effusion in a 29-Year-Old HIV(+) Man

Corey J. Shamah,[1] Judith O. Pretell,[2] Steven H. Kroft[2]

Departments of [1]Internal Medicine, Division of Neoplastic Diseases, and [2]Pathology, Medical College of Wisconsin, Milwaukee, WI

Patient: 29-year-old man.

Chief Complaint: Substernal chest pain for 3 days prior to hospital admission.

Past Medical History: Human immunodeficiency virus (HIV) positive, but not on highly active antiretroviral therapy (HAART); congenital deafness; hepatitis B; syphilis.

Physical Examination Findings: Vital signs: temperature, 99°F; blood pressure, 129/80 mmHg; heart rate, 93 bpm; respiratory rate, 18 rpm; pulse oximetry, 99% on room air. The patient was thin, awake, and alert. Cardiac examination revealed muffled heart sounds and 15 mm Hg pulsus paradoxus. The remainder of the examination was unremarkable.

Results of Additional Diagnostic Procedures: Full body computed tomography (CT) scans revealed a moderately sized pericardial effusion without other lesions (**Image 1A**). Seven hundred milliliters of blood-tinged, turbid pericardial fluid were obtained from a tube pericardiostomy and sent for cytologic analysis (**Image 1B**), a cell block preparation was used for immunohistochemistry for human herpes virus-8 (HHV-8) latent nuclear antigen (**Image 1C**), and flow cytometry was performed on a sample of the pericardial fluid (**Figure 1**).

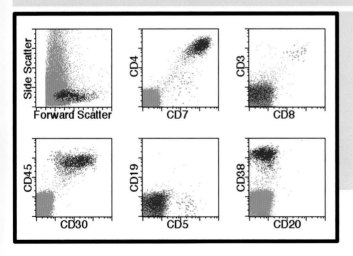

Figure 1_Flow cytometry demonstrates a dominant population of cells (red) with variable forward light scatter properties and moderate to low side scatter. The cells are positive for CD4, CD7, CD45, CD30, and CD38, but are negative for CD3, CD5, CD8, CD19, and CD20. The cells were additionally negative for CD2 and surface immunoglobulin (not shown).

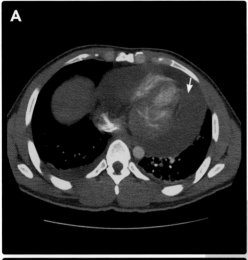

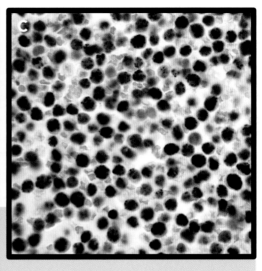

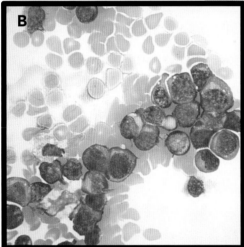

Image 1_(A) CT scan revealing a large pericardial effusion (arrow); (**B**) Wright-stained cytocentrifuge preparation of the pericardial fluid revealed a population of medium to large cells with generally regular nuclei, coarsely-clumped chromatin, 1 to several nucleoli, and small to moderate amounts of deeply-basophilic cytoplasm; (**C**) and immunohistochemistry for HHV-8 latent nuclear antigen on a cell block preparation from pericardial fluid reveals coarse granular nuclear reactivity in the abnormal cells.

Questions _____

1. What are this patient's most striking clinical and laboratory findings?

2. How do you explain this patient's most striking clinical and laboratory findings?

3. What is this patient's likely diagnosis?

4. What is the characteristic clinical presentation of individuals with this disorder?

5. What are the pathologic characteristics of this disorder?

6. What pathologic feature in this case provided the definitive diagnosis?

7. What treatment options are available for this patient's condition?

Possible Answers _____

1. The presence of pulsus paradoxus, muffled heart sounds, and a pericardial effusion on imaging studies; leukopenia (neutropenia), thrombocytopenia, markedly decreased CD4(+) T-cell count, and a prominent increase in leukocytes in the pericardial fluid, consisting of a proliferation of monotonous medium to large cells that express the T-cell-associated antigens CD4 and CD7 and the activation antigens CD30 and CD38, but which lack other T-cell and B-cell antigens (**T1**, **Image 1A,** and **Figure 1**). These cells also show evidence of infection with HHV-8 and Epstein-Barr virus (EBV) by immunohistochemistry and polymerase chain reaction

T1. Principal Laboratory Findings

Test	Patient's Result	"Normal" Reference Range
Hematology		
WBC count	2.5	$4.0–10.0 \times 10^3/mL$
Hemoglobin	14.9	13–17 g/dL
Hematocrit	45	42–52%
Platelet count	85	$150–350 \times 10^3/mL$
Differential: Neutrophils	37	40–70%
Lymphocytes	46	20–45%
Monocytes	15	2–8%
Eosinophils	1	0–4%
Basophils	1	0–2%
CD4(+) T cells	16	467–1,085/mL
Chemistry		
Sodium	135	135–145 mmol/L
Potassium	3.5	3.5–5.1 mmol/L
Chloride	100	98–109 mmol/L
CO_2	29	22–32 mmol/L
BUN	7	6–23 mg/dL
Creatinine	0.8	0.7–1.3 mg/dL
Microbiology		
EBV PCR (pericardial fluid)	Positive	Negative

WBC, white blood cell; CD, cluster of differentiation; BUN, blood urea nitrogen; EBV, Epstein-Barr virus; PCR, polymerase chain reaction.

(PCR) analysis of EBV deoxyribonucleic acid (DNA), respectively.

2. Pulsus paradoxus and muffled heart sounds are physical examination findings associated with a pericardial effusion (accumulation of fluid in the pericardial sack surrounding the heart). Pulsus paradoxus is characterized by an excessive drop (>10 mm Hg) in systolic blood pressure during inspiration. Inspiration causes increased venous return, and thus, an increase in right heart volume. Normally, this volume increase causes the right ventricle to expand in the direction of the free wall. However, when it is unable (as with a pericardial effusion) the enlarged right ventricle can only be accommodated by the interventricular septum bowing to the left. This leads to a decreased left ventricular volume and lower systolic blood pressure during inspiration. Pericardial effusions may be caused by a variety of clinical conditions, including infection, malignancy, radiation, collagen vascular disease, uremia, trauma, and hypothyroidism. In the present case, the effusion is likely the result of the cellular proliferation illustrated in **Image 1B**. We can conclude this is an abnormal (neoplastic) proliferation based on several features. First, the cells in the fluid are generally medium to large in size and show monotonous cytologic features. In reactive effusions, the lymphocytes are typically small and regular, with densely clumped chromatin. Alternatively, in highly-reactive fluids, the lymphocytes may show a spectrum from small to large cells with a full spectrum of reactive cytology, including plasmacytoid lymphocytes, immunoblasts, and plasma cells. Second, the immunophenotype is not that of any normal cell. The expression of CD4 and CD7 suggests T-cell lineage, but the lack of any other T-cell markers indicates this is an aberrant (ie, neoplastic) population. All normal T cells express surface CD3, and the vast majority also express CD2 and CD5. Also, normal T cells do not express the activation antigen CD30. Leukopenia, neutropenia, and thrombocytopenia are common hematological findings associated with HIV infection and have multifactorial etiologies. The low CD4(+) count is a hallmark of acquired immunodeficiency syndrome (AIDS), the pathogenesis of which is viral-mediated destruction of CD4(+) T cells, resulting in diminished cellular immunity.

3. **Most likely diagnosis:** *primary effusion lymphoma (PEL).*

4. Primary effusion lymphoma presents in patients with advanced HIV infection, usually with CD4(+) T-cell counts of less than 100/mL.[1] It is rarely seen in patients who are immunocompromised from organ transplantation.[2] Primary effusion lymphoma presents in a unique fashion, with a proliferation of cells in the fluids of the pleural, pericardial, or peritoneal cavities, resulting in clinically-detectable effusions in these spaces. Rare cases presenting in the cerebrospinal fluid have also been described.[1,2] In distinct contrast to most forms of non-Hodgkin lymphoma, PEL is not associated with any detectable mass lesions in the vast majority of cases.[3] Essentially,

this disorder can be considered a "fluid phase" lymphoma of the serous body cavities.

5. In addition to its unique clinical presentation, PEL is also unique pathologically. Although this is genotypically a B-cell lymphoma (based on the presence of clonal immunoglobulin gene rearrangements in most cases), most often the cells display a "null cell" immunophenotype, with an absence of markers of either B-cell or T-cell lineage. The tumors are identifiable as being of hematolymphoid derivation based on the expression of CD45 (leukocyte common antigen). In addition, the cells express activation antigens such as CD30, CD38, and CD71. Finally, they express markers suggesting differentiation toward the terminally differentiated plasma cell stage of B-cell development, including CD138, VS38c, and MUM-1/IRF4.[1] A small minority of PEL cases express 1 or more B-lineage markers, such as CD19, CD20, or surface immunoglobulin, providing a clue to their derivation. However, they may also aberrantly express T-cell-associated antigens, such as CD2, CD4, or CD7, which may cause diagnostic confusion.[4] The present case was remarkable in that cells from the patient's pericardial fluid brightly co-expressed both CD4 and CD7 (**Figure 1**), strongly suggesting T-cell lineage. CD30 expression, while uniformly present in PEL, is also a hallmark of anaplastic large cell lymphoma, and, in fact, the immunophenotype was entirely compatible with this diagnosis. However, the clinical context (pericardial effusion in an HIV(+) patient) and the cytologic features suggesting plasmacytic differentiation pointed toward the correct diagnosis of PEL. Cytologically, tumor cells from individuals with PEL are typically large, with multiple prominent nucleoli, coarsely-clumped chromatin, and variably-abundant, deeply-basophilic cytoplasm. Some cases are strikingly pleomorphic, with marked anisocytosis, nuclear irregularity, multinucleation, and nuclear lobation. Other cases of PEL show a more monomorphic proliferation of cells with regular nuclei, as in the present case. Corresponding to the immunophenotypic findings, some cases have a distinctly plasmacytic appearance, with eccentrically-placed, round nuclei, deeply-basophilic cytoplasm, and a paranuclear hough. Overall, the cells in fluids from individuals with PEL tend to be described as having cytologic features intermediate between those of immunoblastic lymphoma and anaplastic large cell lymphoma.

6. The most important pathologic feature of PEL, which allowed definitive identification in the present case, is its universal association with HHV-8, also know as Kaposi's sarcoma-associated Herpes virus. This virus, which is assumed to play a causative role in this lymphoma, is also the causative agent of Kaposi's sarcoma and a subset of cases of multicentric Castleman's disease. Demonstration of the presence of this virus is required for a definitive diagnosis of PEL.[5] This can be accomplished with PCR or immunohistochemistry. Detection by PCR of specific HHV-8 DNA sequences has the advantage of extreme sensitivity, but since it will also detect the presence of DNA from a bystander virus not present in the neoplastic cells, it lacks specificity. Immunohistochemistry for HHV-8 latent nuclear antigen will clearly demonstrate the presence of the virus in the nuclei of the neoplastic cells, as in the present case. Another unique feature of PEL is the presence of dual viral infection of the neoplastic cells in most cases. Specifically, the cells in the large majority of PEL cases are latently infected with EBV in addition to HHV-8. This may be detected with either PCR or in-situ hybridization testing for EBV-encoded RNAs (EBER), both of which are highly specific and sensitive tests. The cells do, however, express EBV latent membrane protein-1 (LMP-1).[2] Because EBV is not uniformly present, demonstration of this virus in the neoplastic cells is not a requirement for the diagnosis of PEL.

7. Given the rarity of this neoplasm, there is no consensus treatment. Primary treatment consists of HAART, and case reports exist of complete responses with this as the only treatment.[2] Other treatment modalities are combination chemotherapy and high dose methotrexate.[2] There is generally no role for rituximab (anti-CD20) therapy, given that these tumors are usually CD20 negative. Case reports of treatment of PEL with intracavitary cidofovir and systemic bortezomib are described in the literature; however, outcomes are generally poor, with a median overall survival of approximately 6 months.[6-8]

Keywords

primary effusion lymphoma, non-Hodgkins lymphoma, AIDS

References

1. Boulanger E, Gerard L, Molina J, et al. Prognostic factors and outcome of human herpesvirus 8-associated primary effusion lymphoma in patients with AIDS. *J Clin Oncol.* 2005;23:4372–4380.

2. Dotti G, Fiocchi R, Motta T, et al. Primary effusion lymphoma after heart transplantation: A new entity associated with human herpesvirus-8. *Leukemia.* 1999;13:664.

3. Ely SA, Powers J, Lewis D, et al. Kaposi's sarcoma-associated herpesvirus-positive primary effusion lymphoma arising in the subarachnoid space. *Human Pathol.* 1999;30:981–984.

4. Wilson KS, McKenna RW, Kroft SH, et al. Primary effusion lymphomas exhibit complex and recurrent cytogenetic abnormalities. *Br J Haematol.* 2002;116:113–121.

5. Jaffe ES, Harris NL, Stein H, et al. editors. *World Health Organization Classification of Tumors, Pathology and Genetics, Tumors of the Haematopoietic and Lymphoid Tissues.* Lyon: IARC Press; 2001:179–180.

6. Luppi M, Trovato R, Barozzi P, et al. Treatment of herpesvirus associated primary effusion lymphoma with intracavitary cidofovir. *Leukemia.* 2005;19:473–476.

7. An J, Sun Y, Fisher M, et al. Antitumor effects of bortezomib (PS-341) on primary effusion lymphomas. *Leukemia.* 2004;18:1699.

8. Simonelli C, Spina M, Cinelli R, et al. Clinical features and outcome of primary effusion lymphoma in HIV-infected patients: A single institution study. *J Clin Oncol.* 2003;21:3948–3954.

New-Onset Thrombocytopenia and Anemia in a Patient With a Complex Medical History

Amanda Rivera-Begeman, Wendy Chamberlain, Steven H. Kroft

Department of Pathology, University of Texas Southwestern Medical Center, Dallas, TX

Patient: 52-year-old African-American male.

Chief Complaint and History of Present Illness: New-onset seizure secondary to a chronic subdural hematoma. Patient also complained of abdominal fullness and tenderness of 6 months duration.

Past Medical History: Insulin-dependent diabetes mellitus (diagnosed 20 years ago), end-stage renal disease on dialysis, peripheral neuropathy, hypertension, and cholecystitis status post cholecystotomy tube.

Drug History: Reglan (5 mg PO q.H.S), Digoxin (0.125 mg PO qday), Flagyl (250 mg PO qid), Lortab (PRN), Lactulose (PRN).

Past Family History: His mother died of myocardial infarction at age 62; his father died of myocardial infarction at age 65.

Social History: Married, father of 5, living at a rehabilitation center while recovering from cholecystitis and placement of a cholecystotomy tube. Thirty pack/year smoker.

Physical Examination: He was alert and oriented but somewhat uncooperative. He was tachycardic (90 bpm) and hypothermic (35.6°C) with hepatosplenomegaly and bilateral toe amputations.

Results of Additional Diagnostic Procedures: A bone marrow (BM) aspirate revealed a prominent population of medium-sized mononuclear cells and many large cells scattered throughout the aspirate (**Image 1**). The core biopsy of the BM showed findings as illustrated in **Image 2**. Flow cytometry performed on the BM revealed the findings illustrated in **Image 3**.

T1. Principal Laboratory Findings

Analyte	Patient's Result	"Normal" Reference Range
Hematology		
WBC count	5.6	4.1-10.9 × 10³/μL
RBC count	2.85	4.3-5.7 × 10⁶/L
Hemoglobin	8.7	13.2-16.2 g/dL
Hematocrit	28.1	40.0-52.0%
Platelet count	30	150-450 ×10³/μL
MCV	98.4	80-100 fL
RDW	17.3	10.8-13.8%
Coagulation		
PT	15.0	9.8-11.9 sec
PTT	45.0	24.4-34.5 sec
Fibrinogen	150	190-400 mg/dL
D-dimers	4.5	<0.5 μ/mL
Chemistry		
Triglycerides	151	50-150 mg/dL
ALT	7	10-40 U/L
AST	15	13-40 U/L

WBC, white blood cells; RBC, red blood cells; MCV, mean cell volume; RDW, red cell distribution width; PT, prothrombin time; PTT partial thromboplastin time; ALT, alanine aminotransferase; AST, aspartate aminotransferase.

Questions

1. What are this patient's most striking clinical and laboratory findings?

2. How do you explain this patient's most striking clinical and laboratory findings?

3. What condition(s) is (are) suggested by this patient's most striking clinical and laboratory findings?

4. What is (are) the etiology (etiologies) of this patient's condition(s)?

5. How is (are) this patient's condition(s) typically treated?

Possible Answers

1. Hepatosplenomegaly; normocytic anemia and severe thrombocytopenia; elevated PT, PPT, and D-dimers; hypofibrinogenemia. In addition, the smear of the patient's BM aspirate demonstrated a prominent population of medium-sized lymphoid cells with irregular nuclei, moderately condensed chromatin, and small nucleoli (**Image 1**). In addition, the BM aspirate also demonstrated a prominent population of histiocytes with abundant, vacuolated cytoplasm containing phagocytized cells and debris. The histiocyte illustrated in **Image 1A** contains mainly platelets, whereas the histiocyte illustrated in **Image 1B** contains both platelets and erythrocytes. The BM core biopsy contained infiltrates of medium-sized cells with irregular nuclei and small to moderate amounts of eosinophilic cytoplasm arranged in linear clusters suggesting an intrasinusoidal location (**Image 2A**). A CD3 stain of the patient's core biopsy demonstrated that the infiltrating cells were T cells and highlighted their intrasinusoidal localization (**Image 2B**). Flow cytometry analysis of the patient's BM (**Image 3**) demonstrated a population of T cells (illustrated in red; 19%) that were larger in size (as indicated by high forward light scatter) than other T cells (green; 4.2%) and natural killer (NK) cells (yellow; 0.81%) in the sample. The cells illustrated in red in **Image 3** were positive for: CD2 (*data not shown*), CD3, CD7, CD56, and T-cell receptor (TCR) γδ and negative for: CD4, CD5, CD8, CD57, and TCR.

2. The patient's normocytic anemia and severe thrombocytopenia are attributable to the prominent red blood cell and platelet phagocytosis observed in the BM aspirate (**Image 1**). In addition, given that the patient had splenomegaly, it is likely that hypersplenism contributed to these findings as well. Taken together, the patient's high PT and PTT, low fibrinogen, and elevated D-dimer level suggest the presence of disseminated intravascular coagulation (DIC). The atypical lymphocytes observed in the patient's BM suggested the presence of a lymphoma. This possibility was supported by the flow cytometry findings of an aberrant T-cell population (illustrated in red in **Image 3**). The

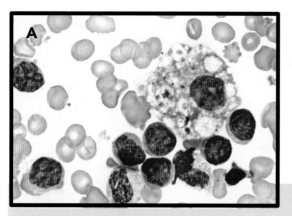
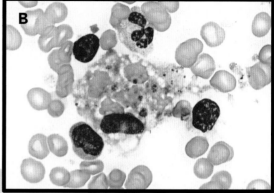

Image 1_Wright-Giemsa stain of the patient's BM aspirate illustrating **A**) a prominent population of medium-sized lymphoid cells with irregular nuclei, moderately condensed chromatin, and small nucleoli and a histiocyte (upper right) containing many platelets and **B**) a histiocyte (center) containing both platelets and red blood cells.

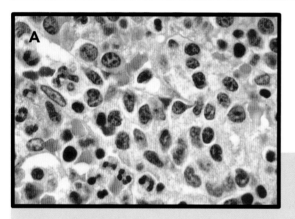
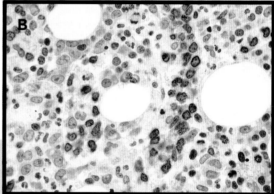

Image 2_Patient's core biopsy illustrating **A**) an infiltrate of medium-sized cells with irregular nuclei, apparently in an intrasinusoidal location (a sinusoidal endothelial cell nucleus is seen on the left side of the field) (H&E stain) and **B**) the identity of the infiltrating cells as T cells (CD3 stain) and the intrasinusoidal localization of these cells.

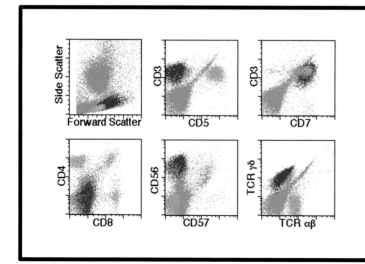

Image 3_Flow cytometry results on the patient's BM indicating a population of T cells (illustrated in red; 19%) that were larger in size [as indicated by higher forward light scatter] than other T cells (green; 4.2%) and natural killer (NK) cells (yellow; 0.81%) in the sample. The cells illustrated in red were positive for: CD3, CD7, CD56, T-cell receptor (TCR) γδ, and CD2 (scattergram not shown above), and negative for: CD4, CD5, CD8, CD57, and TCR αβ.

cells illustrated in red in **Image 3** can be distinguished from normal TCR γδ-expressing T cells on the basis of several features:[1] 1) They are distinctly larger than the other T cells in the sample. Based on forward light scatter characteristics by flow cytometry, the various T-cell subsets in the majority of patients with reactive T-cell proliferations are similar in size; 2) TCR γδ cells are normally a minor T-cell subset; 3) normal TCR γδ cells are CD4(-) and show a spectrum of CD8 expression from negative to dim, rather than the complete absence of CD8 seen in the current case; 4) while normal TCR γδ cells may be CD5(-), usually the majority show CD5 expression that is only slightly dimmer than that of TCR T cells. The patient's hepatosplenomegaly could represent infiltration by lymphoma cells, hemophagocytic histiocytes, or both. In addition, liver infiltration by these cells could also have contributed to the patient's coagulopathy.

3. **Most likely diagnosis:** *hemophagocytic syndrome in association with hepatosplenic T-cell lymphoma.*

Systemic hemophagocytic syndrome (SHS) is characterized by the presence of abundant hemophagocytic histiocytes in BM, cytopenias, consumptive coagulopathy, hypofibrinogenemia, and organomegaly.[2,3] Other commonly associated signs and symptoms of hemophagocytic syndrome are fever, elevated liver enzymes, and hypertriglyceridemia. Although our patient did not have a fever at presentation, he subsequently developed a fever. Lymphadenopathy, skin rashes, and neurologic symptoms can also occur in patients with SHS. The atypical lymphoid cells present in the patient's BM and the aberrant T-cell immunophenotype by flow cytometry indicate the presence of a malignant T-cell process. The presence of hepatosplenomegaly and the distinctly sinusoidal infiltrate of abnormal T-cells in the patient's BM core biopsy are highly characteristic of hepatosplenic T-cell lymphoma (HSTCL).[4-6] HSTCL typically presents as hepatosplenomegaly in young males. Pathologically, in patients with HSTCL, the spleen shows massive red pulp infiltration by aberrant T cells, often with a particular predilection for the splenic red pulp sinuses.[4,6] Moreover, the liver and BM are invariably involved, and each shows a distinctly sinusoidal pattern of infiltration by aberrant T cells.[4-6] Most patients with HSTCL

express TCR γδ on the T-cell surface, as seen in this case, rather than TCR αβ which is expressed on the surface of most normal T cells and the T cells of most patients with a peripheral T-cell lymphoma. Also, T cells from patients with HSTCL characteristically lack expression of CD4, CD8, and CD5 antigens, while CD56 expression is common.[4,6] In addition, HSTCL cells have a cytotoxic T-cell phenotype, with all cases expressing the cytotoxic granule-associated protein TIA-1.[7]

4. Two main forms of SHS are recognized—primary (familial) and secondary—the latter associated with either infection or malignancy.[3,8,9] Both forms are associated with proliferation of benign macrophages that demonstrate avid phagocytosis of hematolymphoid cells in reticuloendothelial organs and BM. Familial hemophagocytic syndrome is an autosomal recessive disorder, usually presenting in infancy, associated with constitutional defects in the cytotoxic function of T cells and NK cells.[8] The defect in cytotoxicity results in uncontrolled T-cell and monocyte activation and hypercytokinemia. Infection-associated hemophagocytic syndrome usually occurs in immunocompromised hosts and can be due to viruses (including Epstein-Barr virus, cytomegalovirus, and herpes viruses), bacteria, fungi, or parasites.[3] Patients with infection-associated hemophagocytic syndrome also have defective cytotoxic function, T-cell and macrophage activation, and hypercytokinemia, but the cytotoxic defect is transient in these patients. Hemophagocytic syndrome may also be seen in association with a variety of malignancies, especially in patients with non-Hodgkin lymphoma derived from an overabundance of cytotoxic T cells or NK cells.[3,10-14] The strongest association between hemophagocytic syndrome and non-Hodgkin lymphoma is seen in patients with extranodal NK/T-cell lymphoma of the nasal type[15,16] and in patients with the gamma/delta TCR-expressing form of subcutaneous panniculitis-like T-cell lymphoma[12,17] (recently re-classified as cutaneous γδ T-cell lymphoma[18]). Hemophagocytic syndrome has been reported uncommonly in association with hepatosplenic T-cell lymphoma.[10,13,14,19] While hemophagocytic syndrome in patients with malignancies may be a result of associated infection, it is thought that hemophagocytic syndrome in patients with

cytotoxic lymphomas are a result of secretion of cytokines by malignant cells.[3] While the etiology of HSTCL is essentially unknown, it occurs with greater frequency in patients who are immunosuppressed following solid organ transplantation.[20] In addition, HSTCL is very strongly associated with isochrome 7q. Trisomy 8 is also seen in the majority of cases.

5. The therapeutic approach to secondary hemophagocytic syndrome is largely supportive care and treatment of the associated infection or malignancy. Hepatosplenic T-cell lymphoma is generally treated with combination chemo-therapy regimens for aggressive non-Hodgkin lymphoma.

Treatment and Course

The patient was started on chemotherapy (cyclophosphamide), but died within a month of diagnosis. Unfortunately, hepatosplenic T-cell lymphomas are extremely aggressive. Patients may initially respond to chemotherapy but frequently relapse. The median survival is only 16 months.[4] In addition, hemophagocytosis is a negative prognostic indicator in patients with non-Hodgkin lymphoma.

Keywords

hemophagocytic syndrome, hepatosplenic T-cell lymphoma, hepatosplenomegaly, flow cytometry

References

1. Jamal S, Picker LJ, Aquino DB, et al. Immunophenotypic analysis of peripheral T-cell neoplasms. A multiparameter flow cytometric approach. *Am J Clin Pathol.* 2001;116:512-526.

2. Risdall RJ, McKenna RW, Nesbit ME, et al. Virus-associated hemophagocytic syndrome: A benign histiocytic proliferation distinct from malignant histiocytosis. *Cancer.* 1979;44:993-1002.

3. Janka G, Imashuku S, Elinder G, et al. Infection- and malignancy-associated hemophagocytic syndromes. Secondary hemophagocytic lymphohistiocytosis. *Hematol Oncol Clin North Am.* 1998;12:435-444.

4. Belhadj K, Reyes F, Farcet JP, et al. Hepatosplenic gammadelta T-cell lymphoma is a rare clinicopathologic entity with poor outcome: Report on a series of 21 patients. *Blood.* 2003;102:4261-4269.

5. Vega F, Medeiros LJ, Bueso-Ramos C, et al. Hepatosplenic gamma/delta T-cell lymphoma in bone marrow. A sinusoidal neoplasm with blastic cytologic features. *Am J Clin Pathol.* 2001;116:410-419.

6. Jaffe ES, Ralfkiaer E. Hepatosplenic T-cell lymphoma. In: Jaffe ES, Harris NL, Vardiman JW, eds. *World Health Organization Classification of Tumours. Pathology and Genetics of Tumours of Haematopoietic and Lymphoid Tissues.* Lyon: IARC Press, 2001:210-211.

7. Cooke CB, Krenacs L, Stetler-Stevenson M, et al. Hepatosplenic T-cell lymphoma: a distinct clinicopathologic entity of cytotoxic gamma delta T-cell origin. *Blood.* 1996;88:4265-4274.

8. Ishii E, Ueda I, Shirakawa R, et al. Genetic subtypes of familial hemophagocytic lymphohistiocytosis: correlations with clinical features and cytotoxic T lymphocyte/natural killer cell functions. *Blood.* 2005;105:3442-3448.

9. Henter JI, Arico M, Elinder G, et al. Familial hemophagocytic lymphohistiocytosis. Primary hemophagocytic lymphohistiocytosis. *Hematol Oncol Clin North Am.* 1998;12:417-433.

10. Falini B, Pileri S, De Solas I, et al. Peripheral T-cell lymphoma associated with hemophagocytic syndrome. *Blood.* 1990;75:434-444.

11. Takahashi N, Miura I, Chubachi A, et al. A clinicopathological study of 20 patients with T/natural killer (NK)-cell lymphoma-associated hemophagocytic syndrome with special reference to nasal and nasal-type NK/T-cell lymphoma. *Int J Hematol.* 2001;74:303-308.

12. Gonzalez CL, Medeiros LJ, Braziel RM, et al. T-cell lymphoma involving subcutaneous tissue. A clinicopathologic entity commonly associated with hemophagocytic syndrome. *Am J Surg Pathol.* 1991;15:17-27.

13. Allory Y, Challine D, Haioun C, et al. Bone marrow involvement in lymphomas with hemophagocytic syndrome at presentation: A clinicopathologic study of 11 patients in a Western institution. *Am J Surg Pathol.* 2001;25:865-874.

14. Chin M, Mugishima H, Takamura M, et al. Hemophagocytic syndrome and hepatosplenic gammadelta T-cell lymphoma with isochromosome 7q and 8 trisomy. *J Pediatr Hematol Oncol.* 2004;26:375-378.

15. Chan DW, Liang R, Kwong YL, et al. Detection of T-cell receptor delta gene rearrangement in T-cell malignancies by clonal specific polymerase chain reaction and its application to detect minimal residual disease. *Am J Hematol.* 1996;52:171-177.

16. Kwong YL, Chan AC, Liang R, et al. CD56+ NK lymphomas: clinicopathological features and prognosis. *Br J Haematol.* 1997;97:821-829.

17. Salhany K, Macon W, Choi J, et al. Subcutaneous panniculitis-like T-cell lymphoma. Clinicopathologic, immunophenotypic, and genotypic analysis of alpha/beta and gamma/delta subtypes. *Am J Surg Pathol.* 1998;22:881-893.

18. Willemze R, Jaffe ES, Burg G, et al. WHO-EORTC classification for cutaneous lymphomas. *Blood.* 2005;105:3768-3785.

19. Nosari A, Oreste PL, Biondi A, et al. Hepato-splenic gammadelta T-cell lymphoma: a rare entity mimicking the hemophagocytic syndrome. *Am J Hematol.* 1999;60:61-5.

20. Khan WA, Yu L, Eisenbrey AB, et al. Hepatosplenic gamma/delta T-cell lymphoma in immunocompromised patients. Report of 2 cases and review of literature. *Am J Clin Pathol.* 2001;116:41-50.

Immunology Overview

Christopher R. McCudden

Immunology is defined as the study of the immune system, which is the source of host defense against infectious diseases or foreign substances. The immune system recognizes these foreign agents through complex innate and adaptive mechanisms involving hematopoietic effector cells, cytokines, and immunoglobulins. Disorders of the immune system include hypersensitivity reactions, autoimmune diseases, and malignancies, and this chapter is divided accordingly. Many of the clinical vignettes cross the boundaries of a given discipline in clinical pathology, underscoring the dynamic interplay of this and other organ systems. The largest subset of cases in this chapter relate to hematologic malignancies, particularly those with associated paraproteinemias. A brief overview follows to provide background for further understanding.

Hematologic Malignancies

Hematologic malignancies represent a heterogeneous group of neoplasms with profoundly diverse clinical presentations and biologic characteristics. Classification of these tumors largely parallels the hematopoietic ontogeny, and provides a framework for diagnosis and treatment. Clonal proliferations of maturing B-lymphocytes comprise malignancies of cells destined for immunoglobulin section. Based on the corresponding normal developmental stage, B-cell neoplasms are classified as precursor B-cell and mature B-cell neoplasms. Mature B-cell neoplasms are further sub-divided into pre-germinal center (eg, mantle cell lymphoma), germinal center (eg, follicular lymphoma), and post-germinal center (eg, multiple myeloma) neoplasms, similarly corresponding to developmental stage. Post-germinal center neoplasms are derived from mature B-cells that typically express or secrete class-switched immunoglobulins, and include marginal zone and mucosa-associated lymphoid tissue (MALT) lymphomas, as well as plasma cell dyscrasias. With the exception of cases I-CS-15 (Leukemia Arthritis) and I-CS-22 (Cryglobulinemia), all of the immune system malignancies cases in this section represent mature B-cell neoplasms. Plasma cell dyscrasias are well represented in this chapter, with cases of light chain deposition disease (LCDD), amyloidosis, multiple myeloma, plasma cell leukemia, and Waldenström macroglobulinemia.

Plasma Cell Dyscrasias

Plasma cell dyscrasias (PCDs) include hematological malignancies that arise from terminally differentiated and antibody-producing B-cells. Plasma cell dyscrasias include multiple myeloma, plasmacytomas, and plasma cell leukemia, as well as diseases resulting from excess immunoglobulin production, such as light chain deposition disease and amyloidosis. Other lymphomas that may demonstrate significant plasma cell differentiation including lymphoplasmacytic lymphoma/Waldenström macroglobulinemia, can also be considered forms of PCD. The diagnostic criteria of various plasma cell dyscrasias are summarized in **Table 1**.

Pathophysiology of Multiple Myeloma

Multiple myeloma represents 1 of the most common clinically encountered hematologic neoplasms. Although the process is not entirely understood, a complex series of genetic 'hits' ultimately promotes clonal expansion of the affected plasma cell. Chromosomal aberrations are identified in the majority of cases by routine karyotype or fluorescence in-situ hybridization (FISH) analysis, and some of the most frequently encountered abnormalities demonstrate relevant prognostic utility. Inappropriate expression and subsequent stimulation of toll-like receptors (TLRs) and interleukin-6 receptors promotes cell division and proliferation. Molecular changes, including mutations in N- and K-Ras along with dysregulation of p16 methylation further promotes survival of the malignant clone. The symptoms of myeloma arise as cytokines are released from malignant plasma cells stimulating bone turnover resulting in the hallmark lytic bone lesions, the bone marrow is progressively overwhelmed by the malignant proliferation, and renal function is impaired by secreted immunoglobulin.

Diagnostic Tools

Plasma cell dyscrasias are diagnosed using a combination of physical findings, radiology reports, patient history, and range of laboratory tests. These tests include serum protein electrophoresis, morphologic and immunohistochemical bone marrow evaluation, cytogenetic studies (including karyotpe and FISH analysis), and flow cytometry. Flow cytometry is 1 of the key immunology tools used for diagnosing hematological malignancies. Immunophenotypic findings that define various B-cell neoplasms are summarized in **Table 2**. For plasma cell dyscrasias, flow cytometry can identify aberrant immunophenotypic features and confirm clonality.

Table 1. Diagnostic Criteria and Clinical Features of Plasma Cell Dyscrasias

Plasma Cell Dyscrasia	Clinical Features	Diagnostic Criteria*
Light chain deposition disease	Symptoms of organ dysfunction (usually renal)	Light chain deposits in tissue biopsy (kappa 80%); do NOT stain with Congo red; elevated serum free light chains; urine free light chains; serum monoclonal immunoglobulin (common, but not universal)
Amyloidosis (AL)	Organomegaly; variable presence of heart failure, renal failure, bleeding, neuropathy, bone pain, purpura	Birefringent light chain deposits in tissue biopsy (usually lambda); binds Congo red dye; serum monoclonal immunoglobulin very common; elevated serum free light chain
Multiple myeloma	Bone pain, fractures, fatigue, weakness, frequency infections	Evidence of end organ damage (CRAB), usually >=10% plasma cells, monoclonal immunoglobulin (usually >=3 g/dL for IgG), abnormal serum free light chains**
Smoldering myeloma	None	Monoclonal immunoglobulin >= 3 g/dL and/or >=10% plasma cells in bone marrow
Plasma cell leukemia	Weakness, fatigue, bone pain	>2 x 10⁹/L plasma cells in peripheral blood (or 20% of leukocyte differential); other findings include plasma cells in extramedullary tissue; monoclonal immunoglobulin
Waldenström macroglobulinemia	Weakness, fatigue, anemia, hyperviscosity syndrome triad (mucosal bleeding, visual disturbance, neurological abnormality)	Monoclonal IgM in serum, coagulopathy, cryoglobulins, >= 10% lymphoplasmacytic infiltrate in bone marrow

*2008 WHO criteria.
** Cases beginning on pages 643 and 649 list older criteria to define multiple myeloma.

Table 2. Immunophenotypes Associated With Plasma Cell Dyscrasias

Plasma Cell Dyscrasia	+ Markers	- Markers	± Markers
Multiple myeloma	CD138, CD38, CD56*, cIg* MUM1/IRF4	CD5, CD19, CD23, CD103	sIg, CD117, CD20, CD52, CD10, cyclin D1
Plasma cell leukemia	CD38, CD138, MUM1/ IRF4	CD19, CD20,	CD45, sIg, cIg, CD56
Waldenström macroglobulinemia	CD19, CD20, CD22, CD38, sIgM*, cIgM* MUM1/IRF4	CD5, CD10, CD23, CD103, cyclin D1	CD43
MALT lymphoma	CD19, CD20, CD22, CD79a, sIg*, MUM1/IRF4, bcl-2	CD5, CD10, CD23*, CD103, bcl-6*, cyclin D1	cIg, CD21, CD35, CD43

*In category >50% of the time; sIg- surface immunoglobulin, IgG, IgA, IgM or uncommonly IgD, or very rarely IgE; cIg-cytoplasmic immunoglobulin; sIg-surface immunoglobulin; MUM1/IRF4 -multiple myelomaoncogene 1)/IRF4 (interferon regulatory factor 4); + indicates present in most cases; - indicates absent in most cases; ± indicates variably present or absent.

Suggested Reading

1. Mais DD. *Quick Compendium of Clinical Pathology.* Chicago: ASCP Press, 2009.

2. *WHO Classification of Tumours of Haematopoietic and Lymphoid Tissues.* 4th edition. Edited by SH Swerdlow et al. WHO Press, 2008.

3. McPherson RA, Pincus MR. *Henry's Clinical Diagnosis and Management by Laboratory Method.* Saunders; 21st edition, 2006.

4. Lin P. Plasma cell myeloma. *Hematol Oncol Clin North Am.* 2009 Aug;23(4):709-27.

Chronic Allergic Rhinitis in an Adult Male

Michael Constantinescu, Diana M. Veillon, Mary Lowery Nordberg, Marjorie R. Fowler, Deepti Shukla, James Cotelingam

Department of Pathology, Louisiana State University Health Sciences Center, Shreveport, LA

Patient: 46-year-old male.

Family History: Unremarkable.

Chief Complaint: Weakness, fatigue, and lymphadenopathy of 4 weeks duration.

Medical History: Allergic rhinitis since age 16 years. Two years previously, he was hospitalized with myocardial infarction. At that time, his absolute eosinophil count (AEC) was $1,200 \times 10^6$/mL.

Drug History: Aspirin daily, a beta-blocker (carvedilol), and an angiotensin converting enzyme inhibitor (lisinopril).

Physical Examination: Significant for hepatosplenomegaly and lymphadenopathy.

Results of Other Diagnostic Procedures: A bone marrow biopsy revealed normal cellularity with increased numbers of maturing eosinophilic forms [**Image 1**]. The blast count was not increased. Fluorescence in situ hybridization (FISH) using locus specific probes for the t(9;22) BCR/ABL translocation showed a normal signal pattern in peripheral blood leukocytes.

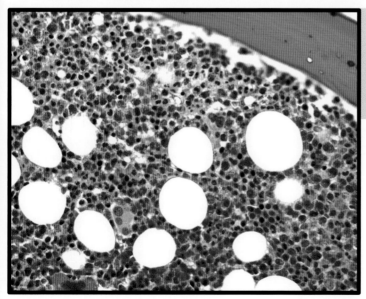

Image 1_Bone marrow biopsy findings illustrating the predominance of eosinophilic myeloid precursors (hematoxylin-eosin stain; magnification, 400×).

T1. Principal Laboratory Findings

Test	Patient's Result	"Normal" Reference Range
Hemoglobin	15.0	12.6-16.6 g/dL
Hematocrit	43.5	39.0-49.0%
WBC count	59.1	3.4-9.2 × 10⁶/μL
RBC count	4.6	4.3-5.6 × 10⁶/μL
MCV	95	81-97 fL
MCH	33	27-33 pg
MCHC	343	2-35 g/dL
RDW	12.1	10.2-13.4%
Segmented neutrophils	4.1	1.5-6.9 × 10⁶/μL
Eosinophils	49	0.00-0.45 × 10⁶/μL
Lymphocytes	4.1	0.5- 4.1 × 10⁶/μL
Monocytes	2.4	0.1-1.1 × 10⁶/μL
Quantitative IgE	1,275	0-158 IU/mL

WBC, white blood cell; RBC, red blood cell; MCV, mean corpuscular volume; MCH, mean corpuscular hemoglobin; MCHC, mean corpuscular hemoglobin concentration; RDW, red cell distribution width; IgE, immunoglobulin E.

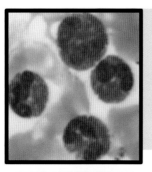

Image 2_Peripheral blood smear findings illustrating the presence of an increased number of eosinophils (Wright's stain; magnification, 600×).

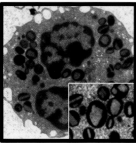

Image 3_Electron microscopic morphology of the eosinophil (magnification, 4,400×). Inset shows the characteristic eosinophil granules (magnification, 30,000×).

Questions

1. What is(are) this patient's most striking clinical and laboratory findings?

2. How do you explain this patient's most striking clinical and laboratory findings?

3. How do you explain this patient's bone marrow findings?

4. How are eosinophils enumerated in peripheral blood?

5. What is the most likely cause of this patient's most striking clinical and laboratory findings?

6. What is the pathophysiology of this patient's most striking clinical and laboratory findings?

7. What other diagnoses should be considered?

8. What are the ultrastructural features of eosinophils?

Possible Answers

1. Markedly elevated whole blood WBC count, eosinophilia (increased AEC) [**Image 2**], markedly increased quantitative serum IgE level, and the presence of increased numbers of maturing eosinophils in the patient's bone marrow.

2. The principal causes of eosinophilia are parasitic infection, atopic/allergic disease, drug-induced, fungal infection, and inflammatory and autoimmune diseases. Worldwide, the most common cause of eosinophilia is **parasitic infection.** The parasites that most commonly cause eosinophilia include *Ascaris lumbricoides, Wuchereria bancrofti, Toxocara canis, Ancylostoma duodenale, Strongyloides stercoralis, Trichinella spiralis, Schistosoma* spp., *Fasciolopsis buski,* and *Echinococcus* spp. A stool examination for ova, cysts, and parasites is essential for the diagnosis of most intestinal causes of eosinophilia.[1,2] In industrialized countries such as the United States, **atopic/allergic diseases** such as seasonal or perennial rhinitis (hay fever), asthma, and drug reactions account most frequently for

eosinophilia. The eosinophil count and the intensity of the symptoms vary in tandem. In the active phase of allergic conditions, nasal secretions reveal an increased number of eosinophils. Atopic asthma, which is associated with an abnormal IgE response to aeroallergens, is also associated with eosinophilia. In the latter, a strong familial predisposition is common. Eosinophils are involved in the pathophysiology of asthma by contributing to airway inflammation. **Drug-induced** eosinophilia has been associated with the use of antibiotic, antifungal, antipsychotic, antiepileptic, anticoagulant, antiglycemic, and antihypertensive drugs. Most drug-related allergic reactions with eosinophilia are associated with systemic manifestations. **Fungal infections** with *Coccidioides immitis* or *Aspergillus* spp. may result in eosinophilia. Some patients with brucellosis, cat scratch disease, *Chlamydia pneumoniae* pneumonia, and mycobacterial diseases may also manifest eosinophilia. Scarlet fever has been associated with an increased number of eosinophils, especially in the second and third weeks of illness. The **inflammatory and autoimmune conditions** most often associated with eosinophilia include rheumatoid arthritis, systemic lupus erythematosus, and inflammatory bowel disease. In addition, other causes of eosinophilia include hyper-IgE syndrome (Job syndrome), IgA deficiency, Wiskott-Aldrich syndrome, certain T-cell neoplasms, Hodgkin lymphoma, and rarely, tumors of the lung, colon, and pancreas. Increased serum IgE levels can occur in patients with allergic disorders, parasitic infections, immune deficiency, and bronchopulmonary aspergillosis.

3. Cytokines and growth factors are involved in the bone marrow eosinophil production. In the normal adult bone marrow, eosinophils represent approximately 3% of hematopoietic cells, with 1% of these being mature forms. Eosinophils originate from bone marrow stem cells and migrate to the blood where their half-life is 18 hours before they enter a tissue phase. There is approximately 1 circulating eosinophil for every 100 eosinophils in tissue. The cytokines, interleukin-3 (IL-3) and interleukin-5 (IL-5), and the growth factor, granulocyte macrophage colony stimulating factor (GM-CSF), regulate the differentiation and growth of eosinophil precursor cells. In the absence of these factors,

eosinophils undergo apoptosis.[3] Interleukin-5 is responsible for terminal differentiation. The migration of these cells from the circulation into tissue is a multi-step process that involves complex interactions between eosinophils and endothelial cells. Integrins, selectins, and other adhesion molecules mediate this process. Eosinophils preferentially bind to P-selectin. The molecules reportedly responsible for initiating the chemoattraction of eosinophils are platelet activating factor (PAF), C5a, and C-C chemokines.

4. The eosinophil count may be obtained by counting cells in a modified Neubauer chamber (wet count), enumeration in peripheral blood (differential count), or using automated cell counting methods. The most accurate automated method for eosinophil enumeration is 1 based on the detection of eosinophil peroxidase. Manual differential counts are less accurate because of aggregation of eosinophils at the feathered edge of the smear. An AEC is preferable to the percentage of eosinophils, as the latter depends on the total white blood cell count. The normal limit of the reference range for eosinophils in adults is 0.45×10^6/mL. Higher counts are normal in newborn infants. Eosinophil counts vary with the patient's age, amount of exercise, and environmental stimuli. Eosinophil counts are slightly higher at night, probably due to diurnal cortisol variation. Eosinophilia is often classified as mild ($0.7\text{-}15 \times 10^6$/mL), moderate ($15\text{-}50 \times 10^6$/mL), or severe (greater than 50×10^6/mL).

5. **Most likely cause of this patient's most striking clinical and laboratory findings:** *allergic rhinitis-induced eosinophilia.*

6. Eosinophilia is a pathophysiologic process mediated by T-lymphocytes that produce IL-5. The production of IL-5 is increased in patients with asthma, parasitic infections, hypereosinophilic syndromes, and following IL-2 therapy. Eosinophilia secondary to allergic or infectious processes is associated with specific T-cell responses. Antigen presenting cells activate Th-2 cells and secrete proinflammatory factors, resulting in eosinophil chemoattraction.[3] Antibodies to IL-5 reportedly diminish eosinophilia in some cases.

7. In the differential diagnosis of eosinophilia, the hypereosinophilic syndromes should be considered. The hypereosinophilic syndromes include **"idiopathic hypereosinophilic syndrome" (IHES), eosinophilia-myalgia syndrome, toxic oil syndrome, eosinophilic fasciitis, and eosinophilic leukemia**. These are rare diseases associated with persistent eosinophilia, organ involvement, and tissue damage. **Idiopathic hypereosinophilic syndrome** has been defined as a persistent unexplained eosinophilia (eosinophil count greater than $1,500/mm^3$) for more than 6 months with signs and symptoms of organ involvement (bone marrow, spleen, liver, heart, or central nervous system). The eosinophils in IHES may be large and dysmorphic with increased nuclear lobation and occasional ring forms. Cytoplasmic vacuoles may be present. The bone marrow is often hypercellular with increased numbers of eosinophils. The major basic protein within the eosinophil granules is responsible for the tissue damage. Involvement of the heart is characterized by an early necrotic stage, followed by mural thrombosis, endocardial fibrosis, and subsequent heart failure. Valvular dysfunction and thromboembolic phenomena may also occur. The cause of IHES is unknown. The proliferation of eosinophils may be polyclonal or monoclonal. In some patients there is a clonal pattern of X-chromosome inactivation, suggesting a neoplastic origin. Most patients have no karyotypic abnormalities. A monoclonal proliferation of T-lymphocytes with overproduction of eosinophil-related cytokines may rarely be the cause of the eosinophilia, and should be excluded. The **eosinophilia-myalgia syndrome** appears to be caused by ingestion of 1,1'-ethylidenebis-contaminated L-tryptophan. A perivascular eosinophilic and lymphocytic infiltrate is identified in fascia, skeletal muscle, skin, and lung. The **toxic oil syndrome** is a hypereosinophilic syndrome with pleural effusion, hypoxia, peripheral neuritis, and vasculitis. A possible association with aniline-denatured rapeseed oil fraudulently marketed as "pure olive oil" has been suggested. **Eosinophilic fasciitis** is characterized by fibrosis of superficial fascia and eosinophilia. **Eosinophilic leukemia** clinically resembles IHES but has evidence of clonal cytogenetic abnormalities. Eosinophilic forms, from the promyelocytes to mature eosinophils, are found in the peripheral blood and bone marrow. Trisomy 8 and isochromosome 17q have been identified in some cases. A t(5;12)(q33;p13) translocation is the most commonly encountered structural chromosome abnormality. In patients with this translocation, eosinophilic forms from promyelocytes to mature eosinophils are found in the peripheral blood and bone marrow. The translocation fuses the ETV/TEL gene at 12p13 to the platelet-derived growth factor receptor-beta (PDGFRb), a receptor for tyrosine kinase that maps to 5q33.[4] Platelet-derived growth factor receptor-beta has attracted considerable attention as it is uniquely inhibited by the new pharmaceutical tyrosine kinase inhibitor, imatinib mesylate (Gleevec, Novartis M).[5-7] Other cytogenetic abnormalities associated with eosinophilic leukemias include t(8;13)(p11;q12) and other FGFR1 gene (8p11) translocations.[8-12]

8. Ultrastructurally, eosinophils have a characteristic appearance.[8,13] They contain primary cytoplasmic granules, specific secondary granules, small granules that contain arylsulfatase and acid phosphatase, tubular vesicular structures (microgranules), and arachidonic acid-containing lipid bodies [**Image 3**]. Specific granules are larger than the primary granules and contain a dense crystalloid core rich in lysophospholipase in a loose matrix. The central core contains a major basic protein. This protein imparts the orange color to the eosinophil granules. The internal dissolution of these crystalline cores results in cytoplasmic vacuoles, and their fusion results in the development of dipyramidal Charcot-Leyden crystals. The less dense matrix contains peroxidases, eosinophil-derived neurotoxin, and eosinophilic cationic protein. The granule content of the eosinophils increases with progressive maturation. Eosinophil granules are hypodense in IHES. Peters and colleagues[14] found that the hypodensity of the granules of IHES was due to smaller and less numerous granules with a decrease in major basic protein.

Keywords

eosinophilia, allergic rhinitis, hypereosinophilic syndromes, translocation, immunoglobulin E

References

1. Brigden ML. A practical workup of eosinophilia. *Postgrad Med.* 1999;105:193-210.

2. Robinson J, Ahmed Z, Siddiqui A, et al. A patient with wheezing, sinusitis, elevated IgE, and eosinophilia. *Ann Allergy Asthma Immunol.* 1999;82:144-149.

3. Rothenberg ME. Eosinophilia. *N Engl J Med.* 1998;338:1592-1600.

4. Golub TR, Barker GF, Lovett M, et al. Fusion of PDGF receptor beta to a novel ets-like gene, tel, in chronic myelomonocytic leukemia with t(5;12) chromosomal translocation. *Cell.* 1994;77:307-316.

5. Cross NC, Reiter A. Tyrosine kinase fusion genes in chronic myeloproliferative diseases. *Leukemia.* 2002;16:1207-1212.

6. Apperley JF, Gardembas M, Melo JV, et al. Response to imatinib mesylate in patients with chronic myeloproliferative diseases with rearrangements of the platelet-derived growth factor receptor beta. *N Engl J Med.* 2002;347:481-487.

7. Pardanani AD, Reeder TL, Porrata LF, et al. Imatinib therapy for hypereosinophilic syndrome and other eosinophilic disorders. *Blood.* 2003;101:3391-3397.

8. Schumacher HR, Cotelingam JD. *Chronic Leukemia: Approach to Diagnosis.* New York: Igaku-Shoin; 1993:245-259.

9. Bain BJ. Eosinophilic leukemias and the idiopathic hypereosinophilic syndrome. *Br J Haematol.* 1996;95:2-9.

10. Bhatnagar S, Patwari AK, Narayan S, et al. Idiopathic hypereosinophilic syndrome. *Indian Pediatr.* 1999;36:824-827.

11. De Vriese AS, Kips JC, Vogelaers DP, et al. Pitfalls in the diagnosis of hypereosinophilic syndrome. A report of 2 cases. *J Intern Med.* 1997;241:165-170.

12. Oliver JW, Deol I, Morgan DL, et al. Chronic eosinophilic leukemia and hypereosinophilic syndromes. Proposal for classification, literature review, and report of a case with a unique chromosomal abnormality. *Cancer Genet Cytogenet.* 1998;107:111-117.

13. Jaffe ES, Harris NL, Stein H. *WHO Classification of Tumours. Pathology and Genetics of Tumours of Hematopoietic and Lymphoid Tissues.* Lyon, France: IARC Press; 2001:32-34.

14. Peters MS, Gleich GJ, Dunnette SL, et al. Ultrastructural study of eosinophils from patients with the hypereosinophilic syndrome: A morphological basis of hypodense eosinophils. *Blood.* 1988;71:780-785.

Diarrhea, Abdominal Pain, Weight Loss, and Malnutrition in an Adult Woman

Qing H. Meng, Stephen Hill, Gillian Luxton

Department of Pathology and Molecular Medicine, McMaster University, Ontario, Canada

Patient: 29-year-old woman.

Chief Complaint: Recurrent vomiting, diarrhea, abdominal pain with muscle weakness, and fatigue for the past 6 months. She described an early satiety and bloating sensation post-prandially. She had recently lost about 30 pounds. She complained of numbness and tingling of her fingers that radiated up to her shoulders and from her feet to her hips, but was more marked distally. She stated that her footdrop condition had worsened. She was experiencing increased muscle wasting, especially in the palmar aspect of her hands.

Medical History: In 1992, she was diagnosed with chronic inflammatory demyelinating polyneuropathy, and in 1994, she was diagnosed with type 1 diabetes mellitus and Hashimoto thyroiditis. In addition, she had gastroparesis, peptic ulcer disease, iron deficiency anemia, and menorrhagia.

Family History: Her mother had breast cancer, and there was no family history of any autoimmune diseases.

Drug History: She was taking several medications, including levothyroxine, daily to relieve the symptoms of her diseases listed above.

Physical Examination: She appeared thin with some edema of the feet and loss of peripheral tone. All of her vital signs were within normal limits; her cardiovascular system was normal; her lungs were clear; her liver was palpable and slightly tender along the edge; there was no evidence of splenomegaly; and bowel sounds were present. Sensation in her arms and hands was generally decreased with no clear nerve pattern involvement. Muscle strength ranged from 4/5 to 5/5. Her glucose levels were monitored closely, and despite adequate glucose control, her symptoms noted above were not eliminated or relieved.

Questions _____

1. What is(are) this patient's most striking laboratory result(s)?

2. How do you explain this patient's most striking laboratory test results?

3. Which additional laboratory test(s) are appropriate to the follow-up of this patient?

T1. Principal Laboratory Findings

Test	Patient's Result	"Normal" Reference Range
Hematology		
WBC count	11.8	$4.0\text{-}11.0 \times 10^3/\mu L$
RBC count	4.25	$3.25\text{-}5.50 \times 10^6/\mu L$
Hemoglobin	10.8	11.5-14.0 g/dL
Hematocrit	35.4	37.0-47.0%
MCV	83.3	82-99 fL
MCHC	33.0	30-35 g/dL
RDW	26.8	11.5-16.0%
Platelet count	426	$150\text{-}400 \times 10^3/\mu L$
Differential: granulocytes	8.2	$2.0\text{-}7.5 \times 10^3/\mu L$
monocytes	0.9	$0.2\text{-}0.8 \times 10^3/\mu L$
eosinophils	0.10	$0.04\text{-}0.40 \times 10^3/\mu L$
basophils	0.00	$0.02\text{-}0.10 \times 10^3/\mu L$
Chemistry		
Glucose (random)	356	50-80 mg/dL
Ketones	Negative	Negative
BUN	5.6	4-12 mg/dL
Creatinine	0.6	0.6-1.1 mg/dL
Sodium	138	135-145 mEq/L
Potassium	4.6	3.5-5.5 mEq/L
Chloride	107	98-107 mEq/L
Calcium	7.5	8.6-10.2 mg/dL
Phosphorus	1.3	2.5-4.5 mg/dL
Magnesium	0.6	0.6-1.1 mEq/L
CK, total	27	38-120 U/L
Total protein	5.5	6.0-8.0 g/dL
Albumin	3.0	3.5-5.5 g/dL
A/G ratio	1.2	1.4-1.6
Bilirubin, total	0.2	0.1-1.1 mg/dL
ALP	140	40-120 U/L
AST	53	<35 U/L
Quantitative Igs: IgG	1170	635-1465 mg/dL
IgA	109	70-352 mg/dL
IgM	235	41-207 mg/dL
TSH	55	0.4-5.0 µU/mL
Free T4	0.8	0.8-2.7 µg/dL
Iron	8	50-167 mg/dL
TIBC	178	223-447 µg/dL
%TS	16	20-50%
Ferritin	9	12-160 ng/mL
CRP	2	<0.8 mg/dL
Vitamin D (25-OH)	7.6	9-38 ng/mL

WBC, white blood cell; RBC, red blood cell; MCV, mean corpuscular volume; MCHC, mean corpuscular hemoglobin concentration; RDW, red cell distribution width; BUN, blood urea nitrogen; CK, creatine kinase; A/G, albumin/globulin; ALP, alkaline phosphatase; AST, aspartate aminotransferase; Igs, immunoglobulins; TSH, thyroid stimulating hormone; T4, thyroxine; TIBC, total iron binding capacity; TS, transferrin saturation; CRP, C-reactive protein.

4. What is the most likely diagnosis relevant to this patient?

5. What is the most appropriate treatment for this patient's current, previously undiagnosed disease?

Possible Answers

1. Low hemoglobin, hematocrit, calcium, phosphorus, total protein, albumin, A/G ratio, iron, TIBC, %TS, ferritin, and vitamin D values; high glucose, ALP, AST, IgM, and CRP values, and a markedly increased TSH value [**T1**]; and, increased IgG and IgA gliadin antibodies, a markedly increased IgA t-Transglutaminase antibody concentration, and positive results for both anti-reticulin and endomysial antibodies [**T2**].

2. This is a complicated case with many abnormal laboratory findings suggestive of multi-organ or -system involvement. Thus, several co-existent diseases or a single disease affecting more than 1 organ or organ system may be present. Combining the information from this patient's history, physical examination findings, and laboratory test results are required to understand this patient's disease(s). Our patient's low hemoglobin, hematocrit, MCV, serum iron, ferritin, %TS, and increased RDW are consistent with microcytic, hypochromic, iron deficiency anemia (IDA), which can be caused by menorrhagia and malabsorption syndrome. The TIBC can be normal or high in patients with IDA and is typically low in patients with anemia of chronic disease (ACD). In patients with IDA, however, %TS is typically <9% and

T2. Immunology Test Results

Test	Patient's Result	"Normal" Reference Range
IgA anti-endomysial Ab	Positive	Negative
Anti-reticulin Ab	Positive	Negative
IgA anti-t-Transglutaminase Ab	100	<20 KEU/mL
Gliadin antibodies: IgG	47	<20 KEU/mL
IgA	47	<20 KEU/mL

Ig, immunoglobulin; Ab, antibody; t-Transglutaminase, tissue transglutaminase.

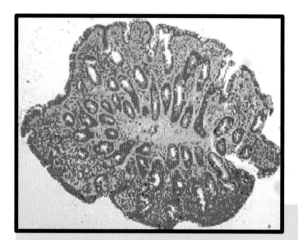 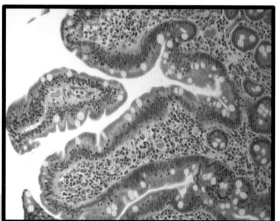

Image 1_Biopsy tissue from the small intestine of the patient presented in this case study revealed (**A**) villous atrophy with deepened crypts and (**B**) irregular epithelium with lymphocyte infiltrates consistent with a diagnosis of celiac disease.

in patients with ACD it is typically >15%. Thus, our patient's %TS value of 16% may indicate presence of ACD.[1] In support of this suggestion, our patient's high glucose, ALP, AST, and low 25-OH-vitamin D values with hepatomegaly; markedly increased TSH and borderline low free T4 concentrations despite levothyroxine replacement therapy; and, low total protein, albumin, and A/G ratio values; and peripheral edema are consistent with her previously established type 1 diabetes mellitus, and the presence of chronic liver disease, uncontrolled hypothyroidism, due possibly to non-compliance with her levothyroxine therapy, and malnutrition (protein depletion). Moreover, our patient's abnormal liver function test results, when coupled with her increased IgM, low-normal BUN, decreased total protein and albumin values, and multiple positive antibody tests suggests chronic liver damage due to an autoimmune disorder, while

her low 25-OH-vitamin D level could be due to liver disease and/or malabsorption syndrome. Her low calcium, phosphorus, and magnesium values can be attributed to her chronic diarrhea. Her decreased BUN, creatinine, and CK values might be due to long-term muscle wasting, and her increased CRP concentration could be due to inflammatory bowel disease or to her chronic inflammatory demyelinating polyneuropathy. Chronic inflammatory demyelinating polyneuropathy, and its symptoms, may explain the patient's muscle weakness; however, it does not explain her other symptoms such as vomiting, diarrhea, and abdominal pain. Diabetes can cause symptoms similar to those observed in patients with a gastroenteropathy or a peripheral neuropathy; however, severe malnutrition and involvement of the kidneys and cardiovascular system usually do not occur until a late stage of this disease in diabetics whose glucose levels are not well controlled. Moreover, our patient's symptoms could not be eliminated or relieved even when her blood glucose levels were well controlled. Thus, our patient's current signs, symptoms, and laboratory findings cannot be explained entirely by her diabetes. Moreover, her medical history, signs, symptoms, and laboratory findings are consistent with an autoimmune disorder affecting multiple organ systems, including the digestive system. The patient's vomiting, diarrhea, abdominal pain, abdominal distension, muscle wasting, peripheral edema, and malnutrition are also consistent with an autoimmune disorder affecting the digestive system. More specifically, our patient's laboratory findings of IDA, hypoalbuminemia, hypocalcemia, and a low serum level of the fat-soluble vitamin, vitamin D, suggest celiac disease.

3. Tests for antibodies, including anti-endomysial (the most diagnostically accurate laboratory test for the diagnosis of celiac disease), anti-reticulin, anti-tissue transglutaminase, and anti-gliadin, are strongly associated with celiac disease. These antibody tests were performed on serum from our patient with the results shown in **T2**. Our patient's positive results for all of these antibody tests prompted additional confirmation using the "gold standard" method for diagnosing celiac disease—biopsy of the small intestine and microscopic analysis of stained tissue specimens for the characteristic histopathological changes associated with celiac disease [**Image 1**].

4. ***Most likely diagnosis:*** *celiac disease*. Celiac disease (ie, celiac sprue, nontropical sprue, or gluten-sensitive enteropathy) is a hereditary, inflammatory condition of the small intestine in which the initiating factor in certain individuals predisposed to this disease is the ingestion of gluten- and prolamin-containing foods such as wheat, rye, and barley.[2] Patients with celiac disease must avoid foods made from cereal grains containing certain alcohol-soluble proteins ("prolamins") that can damage the mucosa of the small intestine. Examples of prolamins include gliadin, secalin, and hordein found in wheat, rye, and barley, respectively. A gluten-free diet is necessary in the treatment of celiac disease.[3] Moreover, screening studies for anti-gliadin and anti-endomysial antibodies, which are associated with celiac disease, have found that

both genetic and environmental factors are important contributors to the development of this disease. Individuals with celiac disease are intolerant to gluten- and prolamin-containing cereal proteins and ingestion of these proteins in such individuals causes small bowel villous atrophy and malabsorption syndrome. Celiac disease demonstrates a strong association with the human leukocyte antigen (HLA) haplotypes, DR3 and DQW2. These haplotypes are also linked to other diseases, including dermatitis herpetiformis, selective IgA deficiency, and Down's syndrome. Antiendomysial antibodies are found in the serum of 70% to 80% of patients with celiac disease or dermatitis herpetiformis. In addition, celiac disease is associated with other autoimmune diseases such as type 1 diabetes mellitus, thyroiditis, and Sjögren's syndrome. Our patient had both type 1 diabetes mellitus and thyroiditis. In the past, celiac disease has been underdiagnosed due, in part, to the lack of awareness and sufficient experience by clinicians with appropriate diagnostic laboratory tests for this disorder. The current availability of diagnostic screening tests (eg, IgA anti-endoymysial and anti-gliadin antibodies) for this disorder has made it clear that celiac disease is more common than was initially thought. Patients with celiac disease usually exhibit fatigue, nausea, vomiting, chronic diarrhea, irritable bowel syndrome, steatorrhea, and abdominal distention. In children, celiac disease can cause failure to thrive, malabsorption of lactose or fructose, and iron and folate deficiency. Because of its varying clinical presentations, celiac disease is often missed in childhood and discovered in adulthood. Our adult patient had multiple immune system disorders linked to her celiac disease. Physical findings in patients with celiac disease include those of chronic disease and muscle wasting, clubbing, and peripheral edema. Laboratory data supportive of the diagnosis of celiac disease include hematologic and iron studies suggestive of IDA, hypoalbuminemia, hypocalcemia, low serum levels of the fat-soluble vitamins (ie, vitamins A, D, E, and K), and positive tests for antibodies associated with the presence of celiac disease (ie, anti-endoymysial, anti-reticulin, anti-tissue transglutaminase, and anti-gliadin antibodies). In addition, quantitative stool findings in such patients include increased fecal fat content (ie, up to 10% of intake). Moreover, bone development is delayed in up to 80% of children with celiac disease. Among the antibody tests for celiac disease, the anti-endomysial and anti-tissue transglutaminase antibody tests have the highest diagnostic sensitivity for celiac disease. Either of these antibody tests can be used for the diagnosis of celiac disease and for monitoring the adherence of patients with celiac disease to a gluten-free diet. In patients with celiac disease who adhere strictly to a gluten-free diet, the level of these antibodies decreases and eventually becomes undetectable. Despite the diagnostic accuracy of the antibody tests for celiac disease, however, biopsy of the small intestine is still recommended to confirm the diagnosis of celiac disease.[2] Molecular genetic analysis is promising and may help to detect celiac disease susceptibility of certain population but more data need to be accumulated for clinical application.[4]

5. Life-long strategy and dietary restriction of all foods containing gluten is essential. Gluten is the protein present in BROW (Barley, Rye, Oats, Wheat). In addition to a gluten-free diet, all patients who have clinically evident malabsorption should receive a multivitamin preparation and appropriate supplements to correct any iron or folate deficiency. In patients that adhere strictly to a gluten-free diet, the serum level of IgA anti-endomysial antibodies will decrease within 6 to 12 months after the onset of dietary therapy. Following the dietary guidelines for celiac disease, our patient's symptoms were improved and immunoserologic markers were disappeared or the titers were reduced. Since our patient had also had type 1 diabetes and other chronic diseases, treatment (especially diet selection) would be more complicated than a simple celiac disease itself.

Keywords

celiac disease, gluten, prolamin, anti-endomysial antibody

References

1. Wians FH Jr, Urban JE, Keffer JH, et al. Discriminating between iron deficiency anemia and anemia of chronic disease using traditional indices of iron status vs transferrin receptor concentration. *Am J Clin Pathol.* 2001;115:112-118.

2. Farrell RJ, Kelley CP. Current concepts: Celiac sprue. *N Engl J Med.* 2002;346:180-188.

3. Semrad CE, Chang EB. Malabsorption Syndromes. In: Cecil RL, ed. *Cecil textbook of medicine.* Philadelphia: W.B. Saunders, 2000:712-722.

4. Popat S, Hearle N, Hogberg L, et al. Variation in the CTLA4/CD28 gene region confers an increased risk of celiac disease. *Ann Hum Genet.* 2002;66:125-137.

Joint Swelling Weakness in a 39-Year-Old African-American Woman

Adam Seegmiller, M. Qasim Ansari

Department of Pathology, University of Texas Southwestern Medical Center and Parkland Memorial Hospital, Dallas, TX

Patient: 39-year-old African-American woman.

Past Surgical History: None.

Drug History: None.

Chief Complaint: Joint swelling, and stiffness in her hands, shoulders, elbows, and knees.

History of Present Illness: The patient presented to the emergency room complaining of increased joint swelling and stiffness in her hands, shoulders, elbows, and knees. She stated that these symptoms were worse in the morning and improved with activity throughout the day. She stated that her joints were not painful per se. She also indicated that she noticed increasing weakness in her arms and legs over the preceding few weeks. She denied any history of recent fevers or illnesses. She had been taking hydroxychloroquine for lupus, but stopped taking it 4 months prior to presentation. She had not seen a doctor in 8 months.

Past Medical History: Systemic lupus erythematosus (SLE) diagnosed 2 years prior to presentation and a history of gastroesophageal reflux disease (GERD).

Family/Social History: The patient has a cousin diagnosed with SLE. Her father died of congestive heart failure at age 68 years, her mother of a myocardial infarction at age 63 years. She has brothers with diabetes and hypertension. The patient drinks socially, but denied any history of tobacco or drug abuse.

Physical Examination: Vital signs: temperature, 37.3°C; pulse, 82 beats per minute; respiratory rate, 16 breaths per minute; blood pressure (systolic/diastolic), 114/75 mm Hg. The patient appeared well nourished and was in no acute distress. Cardiac examintion detected a systolic ejection murmur, loudest at the left sternal border. There was swelling and decreased range of motion in multiple joints, including the wrists, elbows, shoulders, hands, and knees. The elbow joints were warm to the touch. The skin over the fingers was hard (sclerodactyly) and tight, causing abnormal curvature of the fingers. There was a mild, maculopapular rash with excoriation over the chest and abdomen. Neurologic examination was significant for decreased strength in shoulder and hip flexion and extension.

Results of Additional Diagnostic Procedures and Tests: Her electrocardiogram (ECG) showed normal sinus rhythm with no evidence of acute cardiac pathology. Chest x-ray showed an enlarged heart and a reticulonodular infiltrate in the lower lobes of both lungs. Chest computed tomography (CT) scan further delineated these lesions as patchy ground-glass and faint centrilobular lobules in the posterior lower lobes bilaterally. The CT scan also showed an enlarged pulmonary artery. Echocardiography confirmed cardiomegaly and revealed evidence of pulmonary hypertension. Pulmonary function tests (PFTs) were abnormal and indicative of restrictive lung disease.

Questions

1. What are this patient's most striking clinical and laboratory findings?

2. How do you explain this patient's most striking clinical and laboratory findings?

3. What is this patient's most likely diagnosis?

4. What are the criteria for making this diagnosis?

5. What are anti-nuclear antibodies (ANAs), how is their presence in a patient's serum determined, how is the test for ANAs interpreted, what is the clinical significance of a positive ANA test, and how should our patient's ANA test results be interpreted?

6. Is the magnitude of this patient's increase in cardiac enzymes typical of individuals with our patient's diagnosis? Explain your answer.

7. What is the significance of this patient's abnormal pulmonary findings?

8. What is the most appropriate treatment for this patient?

Possible Answers

1. Swelling and stiffness in multiple joints; weakness in the proximal muscles; sclerodactyly; pulmonary infiltrate with abnormal PFTs; an abnormal echocardiogram indicating pulmonary hypertension; and abnormal laboratory findings (**T1**), including markedly elevated CK, CK-MB, cardiac troponin I (cTnI), AST, ALT, and LD levels, elevated serum uric acid and urine

myoglobin concentration, positive ANA titer and speckled immunofluorescence (IF) pattern, positive dsDNA antibody titer, and positive U1-RNP extractable nuclear antigen (ENA) screen.

2. **Joint swelling and stiffness.** These symptoms could be caused by injury, infection, or inflammation of the joints. Injury and infection were unlikely because the patient gave no history of injury and there was no evidence of injury on physical examination, her symptoms were polyarticular (ie, in more than 1 joint), and there were few features present consistent with infection (eg, warmth, redness, fever, leukocytosis). Given her past medical history of SLE, it is reasonable to assume that these symptoms were the result of this condition or some other inflammatory connective tissue disease. **Muscle weakness.** The consistency of her symptoms of lower and upper extremity weakness suggests either a neurologic or muscular origin. The muscular etiology is favored by laboratory data showing elevated serum and urine levels of several enzymes (eg, CK, AST, ALT, and LD) and substances found in skeletal and other types of muscle or released into the serum (eg, uric acid) or urine (eg, myoglobin) following the breakdown of muscle tissue (*see below*). **Sclerodactyly.** This term is used to describe changes in the skin of the fingers. Initially, there is swelling that develops over time into dermal fibrosis and skin atrophy, making the fingers tight and contracted. This finding is characteristic of localized scleroderma. **Pulmonary findings.** This patient's radiographic and PFT findings are consistent with a restrictive lung disease. These disorders are characterized by diffuse and chronic inflammation of pulmonary connective tissue leading to reduced lung expansion and decreased total lung capacity. The most common causes of these findings include environmental

T1. Principal Laboratory Findings

Test		Patient's Result	"Normal" Reference Range
Hematology			
WBC count		3.1	4.1-11.1 ×10³/μL
Hemoglobin		13.8	12.1-16.1 g/dL
Hematocrit		40.9	36.8-48.7%
Platelet count		326	174-404 ×10³/μL
Chemistry			
Sodium		137	135-145 mEq/L
Potassium		5.1	3.6-5.0 mEq/L
Chloride		102	98-109 mEq/L
CO_2		26	22-31 mEq/L
BUN		13	7-21 mg/dL
Creatinine		0.4	0.6-1.2 mg/dL
Glucose		95	65-110 mg/dL
AST		453	13-40 U/L
ALT		186	10-40 U/L
ALP		75	38-126 U/L
GGT		70	8-78 U/L
LD		1,187	100-190 U/L
CK, total		11,143	30-135 U/L
CK-MB		442	0-3 ng/mL
CK index[a]		4	0-3
cTnI		1.5	0.00-0.09 ng/mL
Uric acid		7.8	2.6-6.0 mg/dL
Urine myoglobin		0.367	<0.025 μg/mL
Immunology			
ANA:	Titer	≥1:2560	<1:160
	Pattern	Speckled	
Anti-dsDNA		1:10	Negative
ENA:	Scl-70	Negative	Negative
	Jo-1	Negative	Negative
	Sm	Negative	Negative
	U1-RNP	Positive	Negative
	SS-A	Negative	Negative
	SS-B	Negative	Negative

[a]CK index = [(CK-MB, ng/mL)/(Total CK, U/L)] x 100.

WBC, white blood cell; BUN, blood urea nitrogen; AST, aspartate aminotransferase; ALT, alanine aminotransferase; ALP, alkaline phosphatase; GGT, gamma-glutamyl transferase; LD, lactate dehydrogenase; CK, creatine kinase; cTnI, cardiac troponin I.

exposures (eg, asbestos), drug-induced pulmonary fibrosis, idiopathic pulmonary fibrosis, and inflammatory connective tissue diseases. **Cardiac abnormalities.** The initial indication of cardiac disease in this patient was the finding of cardiomegaly on radiographic studies. An echocardiogram revealed evidence of pulmonary hypertension (ie, elevated blood pressure in the pulmonary arteries). This may be the source of the heart murmur detected on physical examination. Pulmonary hypertension can be idiopathic or caused by chronic lung disease, valvular heart disease, or recurrent thromboembolic disease. Chronic restrictive lung disease compounded by an inflammatory connective tissue disease is a likely cause of pulmonary hypertension and consequent right-sided cardiac muscle hypertrophy. **Abnormal laboratory findings**. Increased levels of enzymes (ie, CK, CK-MB, cTnI, AST, ALT, LD) and substances released into the serum (uric acid) or urine (myoglobin) when muscle cells undergo necrosis, suggest that the patient's muscle weakness could have been caused by the increased breakdown of muscle tissue. Her positive ANA titer, speckled ANA pattern, positive dsDNA antibody titer, and positive U1-RNP ENA screen are consistent with a connective tissue disease.

3. ***Most likely diagnosis:*** *mixed connective tissue disease (MCTD).* MCTD was defined by Sharp[1] in 1972, as a syndrome with overlapping symptoms of SLE, systemic sclerosis, and polymyositis. However, there is considerable debate about whether or not MCTD is an independent pathologic entity.[2] Mixed connective tissue disease is associated with high titers of antibodies to U1-RNP, a 68-kilodalton (kD) constituent of nuclear ribonucleoproteins (RNPs).

4. There are several different diagnostic algorithms that include criteria for the diagnosis of MCTD. Two of these algorithms appear to be the most diagnostically sensitive (**T2**).[3,4] Both include the criterion of a positive U1-RNP screen (ie, the presence of serum antibodies to the U1-RNP ENA)—the defining feature of this disease. Our patient was positive for these antibodies by enzymeimmunoassay (EIA), and her ANA titer (>1:2560) met the minimum cutoff value for ANA titer required by the algorithm of Kahn and Appelboom[4] for the diagnosis of MCTD.

T2. Criteria for the Diagnosis of MCTD According to the Algorithms of Alarcon-Segovia and Villareal and of Kahn and Appelboom[a]

Positive Criterion	Algorithm of[b]	
	Alarcon-Segovia and Villareal[3]	Kahn and Appelboom[4]
Serological test	Anti-(U1-RNP) titer ∃ 1:1600	Anti-(U1-RNP) titer ∃ 1:1200 in a patient with an ANA titer ∃ 1:2560 and a speckled ANA pattern
Clinical features	∃3; 1 of which must be synovitis or myositis, with others to include:	$3; 1 of which must be Raynaud phenomenon, with others to include:
	swollen hands	swollen fingers
	Raynaud phenomenon	synovitis
	Acrosclerosis	myositis

[a]Adapted from Bennett.[8] [b]For a diagnosis of MCTD, both algorithms require that both criteria (ie, serological test and clinical features) be met. MCTD, mixed connective tissue disease; RNP, ribonucleoprotein; ANA, antinuclear antibody.

Additional criteria required by these algorithms for the diagnosis of MCTD, include some combination of Raynaud phenomenon, swollen hands and/or fingers, synovitis, and myositis. The criteria of Alarcon-Segovia and Villareal[3] add acrosclerosis (hardening of the bones of the face and fingers) to the aforementioned list of clinical signs and symptoms. Our patient had no history of Raynaud phenomenon or acrosclerosis, but she did have a history of joint pain, swelling, and stiffness, as well as physical evidence of swelling and stiffness on this admission, consistent with *synovitis*. She had sclerodactyly, the clinical consequence of chronic inflammation and *swelling of the fingers*, and a defining symptom of limited systemic sclerosis. She also had abundant evidence of *myositis*, including neurologic examination findings consistent with proximal muscle weakness–the pattern seen typically in patients with inflammatory myopathies – and abnormal laboratory test findings consistent with increased breakdown of muscle tissue, including increased *serum* levels of the muscle-derived enzymes, CK, AST, ALT, LD, and the muscle breakdown product, uric acid, coupled with an increased *urine* concentration of the muscle breakdown product, myoglobin. Thus, our patient meets the criteria used in the algorithms of Alarcon-Segovia and Villareal[3] and of Kahn and Appelboom[4] for the diagnosis of MCTD (**T2**).

5. Anti-nuclear antibodies (ANAs) are autoantibodies against certain nuclear antigens that can occur in the serum of patients with various rheumatic diseases. The presence of ANAs in serum can be determined by different methods, including indirect immunoflourescence assay (IFA). The IFA test provides information on whether or not the patient's serum contains ANAs at a clinically significant level and if so, the nature of the nuclear staining pattern caused by a specific patient's ANAs. Using the IFA method, a patient's serum is incubated with cells, usually from a human tumor cell line. If the patient's serum contains autoantibodies against nuclear antigens, they will bind to these antigens in the nucleus of the human tumor cells and form an antigen-antibody complex. The presence of these complexes is detected by adding anti-human IgG antibodies linked to molecules of a substance [eg, fluorescein isothiocyanate (FITC)] capable of fluorescence when exposed to the appropriate wavelength of light energy. If ANAs are present in the patient's serum and bound to the tumor cell nuclear antigens, addition of the fluorescently labeled anti-human IgG antibodies will cause the formation of a (nuclear antigen)-(ANA)-(anti-human antibody-fluorescent label) complex in these cells. Subsequent exposure of these cells to the appropriate wavelength of UV light will cause the fluorescent label to emit light of a characteristic wavelength that can be observed using a fluorescent microscope. If the

test is positive, the patient's serum is diluted and re-tested to determine the highest dilution that still yields a positive ANA test. Patients whose serum contains a high concentration of ANAs will require higher and higher dilutions before the highest dilution still yielding a positive ANA test is found. Because positive ANA tests can be obtained using serum from healthy individuals, a positive ANA must be interpreted carefully. It is estimated that the serum from 20% to 30% of all individuals contains ANAs that will yield a titer of >1:40.[5] Moreover, false-positive ANA tests are particularly common among females and older individuals. For these reasons, it is important to establish an appropriate reference titer above which results are likely to be clinically significant. An ANA titer of >1:160 is regarded generally as clinically significant. However, because no autoimmune disease can, or should, be diagnosed on the basis of a positive ANA test alone,[5] it is important that a positive ANA test be interpreted in conjunction with the patient's history and clinical and other laboratory findings. The specific fluorescent staining pattern of the patient's ANAs is determined by viewing the human tumor cells used in the ANA test using a fluorescent microscope. Several characteristic ANA staining patterns have been described (eg, speckled, diffuse, peripheral, nucleolar, centromeric). However, these patterns are not specific for a single disease entity (ie, the same, or a similar, pattern can be seen in more than 1 disease) (*Note:* For a more thorough discussion of ANA staining patterns and their clinical significance, see Greidinger EL, Hoffman RW. Antinuclear antibody testing: Methods, indications, and interpretation. *Lab Med.* 2003;34:113-117). Therefore, it is important that a positive ANA test be followed up by additional testing to define the specific type of ANAs (ie, the antigen(s) against which the patient's autoantibodies are directed) present in the serum of a patient with a positive ANA test. Examples of specific antigens against which ANAs can be directed include double-stranded DNA (dsDNA) and various extractable nuclear antigens (ENAs) (**T1**). The specific autoantibodies seen in our patient were anti-dsDNA and anti-(U1-RNP). As indicated previously, the presence of anti-(U1-RNP) antibodies in a patient's serum is among the diagnostic criteria for MCTD; however, they can also be found in the serum of patients with

SLE. Anti-dsDNA antibodies are found almost exclusively in the serum from patients with SLE; however, they can be found, albeit at low titer, in the serum of patients with MCTD.[1] On the other hand, while the presence of anti-Sm antibodies is a hallmark of the serum from patients with SLE, these antibodies are not found typically in the serum from patients with MCTD.[1] The constellation of these laboratory findings [ie, positive ANA, dsDNA (low titer), U1-RNP antibody tests, and negative anti-Sm antibody test], when coupled with our patient's clinical and other diagnostic findings, provide strong evidence for the diagnosis of MCTD.

6. No. As discussed previously, elevations of CK, AST, ALT, and LD occur commonly in the serum from patients with inflammatory muscle disorders, including polymyositis, dermatomyositis, and MCTD. However, the magnitude of the increase in CK-MB and cTnI in our patient's serum is unusual for a patient with MCTD. CK-MB is considered a marker of cardiac muscle damage when the CK index is greater than 3 (no units). However, CK-MB levels are often high in serum from patients with inflammatory myopathies, because the regenerating muscle in these conditions makes a significant amount of the MB isoform of CK.[6] Consequently, CK-MB is not a reliable marker of cardiac injury in such conditions. Cardiac troponin I (cTnI) is specific for cardiac muscle injury and usually is not elevated as a consequence of the skeletal muscle damage that occurs in patients with inflammatory myopathies.[7] Our patient had a normal ECG, no clinical signs or symptoms of an acute coronary syndrome, a marginally increased CK index, and only a relatively modest increase in cTnI concentration compared to the magnitude of the increase in cTnI concentration (ie, >1.5 ng/mL) that occurs typically in patients with an acute coronary syndrome. These findings suggest that there may be some ongoing sub-acute or chronic myocardial process occurring in our patient. Myocarditis is a known complication of MCTD.[6,8] In some cases, myocardial inflammation may be a primary autoimmune phenomenon. In fact, circulating anti-myocardial antibodies have been detected in serum from some patients with MCTD; however, this finding does not correlate with clinically evident cardiac disease.[9] Myocardial inflammation has also been

attributed to the secondary effects of pulmonary hypertension and cardiomegaly.[8] Both pulmonary hypertension and cardiomegaly were present in our patient.

7. Our patient's restrictive pulmonary disease and pulmonary hypertension are significant in the context of the diagnosis of MCTD because it has been reported that 85% of patients with MCTD demonstrate some evidence of pulmonary disease[8] and pulmonary hypertension appears to be a common feature of MCTD.[10] Pulmonary symptoms in affected individuals can include dyspnea, chest pain, and cough. However, similar to our patient, 73% of patients with MCTD are asymptomatic for these particular pulmonary symptoms. Moreover, in patients with MCTD, PFTs commonly show a restrictive pattern with decreased vital capacity (VC) and reduced carbon monoxide diffusion capacity (DLCO). Pulmonary hypertension can be caused by chronic interstitial lung disease associated with a number of different conditions. However, in patients with MCTD there appears to be an additional primary defect in the pulmonary vasculature. Pulmonary arterioles show intimal proliferation and medial hypertrophy, which are independent of the effects of pulmonary fibrosis.[7] Other features of our patient's disease commonly occur in patients with MCTD, including leukopenia and GERD. Leukopenia, particularly in the lymphocyte lineage, is found in 50% to 75% of patients with MCTD.[1,8] The degree of leukopenia is thought to correlate with disease activity. Our patient was leukopenic (**T1**), with a low percentage of lymphocytes on the differential cell count (17%). In addition, esophageal disturbances are known to occur in both patients with scleroderma and MCTD.[9] Thus, our patient's GERD may be an additional consequence of her MCTD. Lastly, the cardiac, pulmonary, and gastrointestinal manifestations of MCTD may cluster together. Lash[9] reported 5 cases of MCTD with myocarditis. Each of these patients also had pulmonary fibrosis and esophageal dysmotility. This clustering may indicate an interaction between systems, (ie, pulmonary disease leads to pulmonary hypertension, and myocardial damage). Alternatively, it may just reflect multi-system involvement correlating with more severe MCTD.

8. As in most collagen vascular diseases, MCTD is treated with immunosuppression drug therapy.[8] Glucocorticoids are used initially, but may be supplemented with stronger immunosuppressant agents. Anti-malarial drugs or methotrexate can be used in patients susceptible to severe glucocorticoid-related side effects. Pulmonary hypertension requires treatment with calcium channel blockers, angiotensin-converting enzyme (ACE) inhibitors, or intravenous administration of prostacyclin. In patients with MCTD who respond well to steroid therapy, the prognosis is good.[8] Patients with MCTD and pulmonary and cardiac complications, however, do more poorly.[8,9] Pulmonary hypertension, like that seen in our patient, is the most common cause of death in patients with MCTD.

Keywords

mixed connective tissue disease, antinuclear antibodies, restrictive lung disease, pulmonary hypertension

References

1. Sharp GC, Irvin WS, Tan EM, et al. Mixed connective tissue disease – an apparently distinct rheumatic disease syndrome associated with a specific antibody to an extractable nuclear antigen (ENA). *Am J Med.* 1972;52:148-159.

2. Venables PJ. Undifferentiated connective tissue diseases: mixed or muddled? *Lupus.* 1998;7:95-100.

3. Alarcon-Segovia D, Villareal M. Classification and diagnostic criteria for mixed connective tissue disease. In: *Mixed Connective Tissue Disease and Antinuclear Antibodies.* Kasukawa R, Sharp G, eds. Amsterdam: Excerpta Medica. 23.

4. Kahn MF, Appelboom T. Syndrom de Sharp. In: *Les Maladies Systemiques.* Kahn MF, Peltier AP, Meyer O, Piette JC, eds. Paris: Flammarion. 545.

5. Kavanaugh A, Tomar R, Reveille J, et al. Guidelines for clinical use of the antinuclear antibody test and tests for specific autoantibodies to nuclear antigens. *Arch Pathol Lab Med.* 2000;124:71-81.

6. Kiely PDW, Bruckner FE, Nisbit JA, et al. Serum skeletal troponin I in inflammatory muscle disease: relation to creatine kinase, CKMB and cardiac troponin I. *Ann Rheum Dis.* 2000;59:750-751.

7. Erlacher P, Lercher A, Falkensammer J, et al. Cardiac troponin and beta-type myosin heavy chain concentrations in patients with polymyositis or dermatomyositis. *Clin Chim Acta.* 2001;306:27-33.

8. Bennett RM. Mixed connective tissue disease and other overlap syndromes. In: *Kelley's Textbook of Rheumatology,* 6th ed, Ruddy S, Harris ED, Sledge CB, eds. Philadelphia:W.B. Saunders. 1244-1254.

9. Lash AD, Wittman AL, Quismorio FP. Myocarditis in mixed connective tissue disease: clinical and pathologic study of 3 cases and review of the literature. *Semin Arthritis Rheum.* 1986;15:288-296.

10. Oetgen WJ, Mutter ML, Lawless OJ, et al. Cardiac abnormalities in mixed connective tissue disease. *Chest.* 1983;83:185-188.

Muscular Weakness and Respiratory Distress in a Pediatric Patient

Amanda Rivera-Begeman, Ravindra Sarode

Department of Pathology, University of Texas Southwestern Medical Center, Dallas, TX

Patient: 9-year-old Hispanic male.

Past Surgical History: None.

Chief Complaint: Increasing muscular weakness, dysphonia, dysphagia, dyspnea, and abdominal pain.

Past Medical History and History of Present Illness: Patient was diagnosed with myasthenia gravis (MG) 6 months ago, and had a 2.5 year prior history of visual complaints and dysphagia. His last admission for dysphagia was 1 week prior to this presentation. Within 48 hours after being discharged from another hospital, the patient returned to our medical center with the above chief complaint.

Drug History: Pyridostigmine (30 mg PO q8h); Prednisone (75 mg PO qd), increased from qod at last admission; Zantac (75 mg PO bid).

Family History: Unremarkable.

Growth and Development: Unremarkable.

Immunizations: Up to date.

Physical Examination: Afebrile. Used accessory muscles to breathe and had tachypnea. Breath sounds were clear and equal. Patient was awake and alert, but was very anxious and agitated. Motor strength was decreased in the upper extremities to 4/5.

T1. Principal Laboratory Findings

Test	Patient's Result	"Normal" Reference Range
WBC count	14.2	4.1-10.9 × 10³/mL
Hemoglobin	16.6	13.2-16.2 g/dL
Hematocrit	49.1	40-52%
Platelet count	441	140-450 × 10³/mL
PT	11.6	9.8-11.9 sec
aPTT	26.4	24.4-34.5 sec

WBC, white blood cell; PT, prothrombin time; aPTT, activated partial thromboplastin time.

Questions

1. What are this patient's most striking clinical and laboratory findings?

2. How do you explain this patient's most striking clinical and laboratory findings?

3. What condition(s) is (are) suggested by this patient's most striking clinical and laboratory findings?

4. How is (are) this patient's condition(s) typically treated?

Possible Answers

1. Muscular weakness, dysphonia, dysphagia, dyspnea, abdominal pain, and decreased motor strength in an individual recently diagnosed with MG. Except for a modest leukocytosis, the results of all laboratory tests, including hemo-globin and hematocrit (ie, the patient was not anemic), performed on this patient were within normal limits [**T1**].

2. This patient's signs and symptoms were consistent with myasthenic crisis. Potential causes of myasthenic crisis include: drug-induced MG, Lambert-Eaton myasthenic syndrome (LEMS), neurasthenia, hyper- or hypothyroidism, botulism, and intracranial mass lesions. *Drug-induced MG*: Penicillamine (used in treating scleroderma or rheumatoid arthritis) can cause true MG, but the muscle weakness associated with penicillamine treatment is usually mild and disappears after discontinuing its use. In very large doses, aminoglycoside antibiotics can cause muscle weakness in healthy individuals or exacerbation of muscle weakness in MG patients. Procainamide (an anti-dysrhythmic agent) can also cause muscle weakness. *Lambert-Eaton myasthenic syndrome*: a presynaptic disorder of the neuromuscular junction that can cause muscle weakness similar to that seen in patients with MG. Patients with LEMS have depressed or absent reflexes, show autonomic changes such as dry mouth and impotence, and show incremental responses (versus decremental in MG) on repetitive nerve stimulation. These

symptoms are caused by autoantibodies directed against calcium channels at the pre-synapse [versus acetylcholine (ACh) receptors at the post-synapse in MG], impairing release of ACh.[1] Patients with *Neurasthenia* can present with muscle weakness and fatigue, but muscle testing usually reveals the "jerky release" characteristic of nonorganic disorders, and the complaint of fatigue in these patients is related to tiredness or apathy (versus decreasing muscle power on repeated effort as occurs in patients with MG).[1] *Hyper- or hypothyroidism* can increase myasthenic weakness. This can be ruled out by laboratory tests of thyroid function. Patients with *botulism* can present with MG-like muscle weakness; however, these patients often have dilated pupils, and repetitive nerve stimulation provides an incremental response.[1] Patients with *intracranial mass lesions* can present with the diplopia seen often in patients with MG.

3. **Most likely diagnosis:** *myasthenic crisis due to myasthenia gravis (MG).*

   Myasthenia gravis is an autoimmune disease mediated by a competitive blockade of the neurotransmitter, acetylcholine (ACh), by IgG antibodies competing for acetylcholine recep-tors (AChR) at the motor endplate. The IgG antibodies are directed against the alpha-subunit of the AChR. Therefore, patients with these autoantibodies present clinically with muscular weakness and/or fatigue. Most commonly, the eyes, mouth, and throat are affected leading to diplopia, dysphonia, and dysphagia. The diaphragm and intercostal muscles can also be affected, which could lead to respiratory failure. Thymic abnormalities can occur with MG in approximately 75% of patients.[1] A computed tomography (CT) or magnetic resonance imag-ing (MRI) scan of the anterior mediastinum can detect an enlarged thymus or the presence of a thymoma. Hyperthyroidism occurs typically in approximately 3% to 8% of patients with MG. Therefore, once MG is diagnosed, thyroid func-tion tests should be performed.[1] Moreover, other autoimmune disorders can be associated with MG, so blood tests for rheumatoid factor and antinuclear antibodies should also be performed. Myasthenic crisis occurs when an exacerbation of muscle weakness occurs that endangers the patient's life. If the diaphragmatic and intercostal muscles are too weak to function appropriately, respiratory compromise ensues, leading to desaturation and respiratory failure. Also, administration of excessive acetylcholinesterase inhibitors could lead to excessive parasympathetic stimulation and build-up of secretions (ie, cholinergic crisis).[2] An MG patient with dysphagia may aspirate these secretions, leading to respiratory compromise and possibly respiratory failure. In our patient's case, perhaps a combination of both scenarios occurred, leading to respiratory failure.

4. The treatment of patients with MG includes: administration of acetylcholinesterase inhibitors, thymectomy, and plasmapheresis. *Acetylcholinesterase inhibitors* (eg, pyridostigmine) inhibit the degradation of ACh by cholinesterase to override the competitive inhibition of ACh by autoantibodies to the AChR. In patients with myasthenic crisis, use of acetylcholinesterase inhibitors should be temporarily discontinued to avoid uncertainties about overdosage and cholinergic stimulation of pulmonary secretions.[3] Glucocorticoids (eg, prednisone) for immunosuppression are used when ACh inhibitors alone fail. *Thymectomy* decreases the level of circulating autoantibodies, as the thymus is the site of antibody-producing T-cells. However, this operation is not appropriate during myasthenic crisis.[3] In the absense of a thymoma, up to 85% of patients with MG experience improvement after thymectomy, with 35% achieving drug-free remission of their disease.[3] *Plasmapheresis* is used in the treatment of acute exacerbations, crisis, and disabling MG refractory to other therapies. This procedure reduces the plasma level of autoantibodies to levels that will allow improvement in the patient's condition.[4] Ultimately, plasmapheresis can be life-saving. In this procedure, the patient is connected to a pheresis machine via peripheral or central venous access. Whole blood is removed, cellular components are separated from plasma by centrifugation, the plasma is collected, and the cellular components returned to the patient. Usually, the patient's plasma is replaced with 5% albumin alone; however, fresh frozen plasma should be added in a 1:1 ratio if liver function or coagulation tests (ie, PT and aPTT) are abnormal.[4] Also, caution should be taken when performing plasmapheresis on pediatric patients to insure that the amount of blood in the pheresis machine is not less than 15% of the patient's estimated blood volume (EBV). If the EBV is less than 15%, one should consider priming the machine with blood.[4]

Treatment and Course

Plasmapheresis was performed immediately on the patient presented in this case study and he was continued on pyridostigmine and prednisone therapy. Plasmapheresis was continued for 4 days with progressive improvement in the patient's muscle strength and overall neurologic status. The patient was successfully extubated after 2 days and was transferred from a pediatric intensive care unit (PICU) to a general medical unit after 4 days. He received physical and speech therapy and progressed from a liquid to a soft-solid diet. He was scheduled for a thymectomy the following month.

Keywords

myasthenia gravis, acetylcholine

References

1. Drachman DB. Myasthenia gravis and other diseases of the neuromuscular junction. In: *Harrison's Principles of Internal Medicine* (14th ed), Fauci AS, Braunwald E, Isselbacher KJ, et al, eds. New York: McGraw-Hill, 1998,2470-2471.

2. McLeod BC. *Apheresis Principles and Practice*. Bethesda, MD: American Academy of Blood Banks, 1997;294.

3. Yamada KA, Tahseen M, Awadalla S. Neurologic emergencies in internal medicine. In: *The Washington Manual of Medical Therapeutics* (29th ed), Carey CF, Lee HH, Woeltje KF, eds. Philadelphia: Lippincott-Raven Publishers, 1998;490-491.

4. *American Academy of Blood Banks Technical Manual (14th ed)*. Bethesda, MD: AABB, 2002;127-145.

Vision Loss in a 22-Year-Old Woman

Steffini Stalos

Department of Pathology, University of Texas Southwestern Medical Center, Dallas, TX

Patient: 22-year-old African-American woman.

Chief Complaint: Monocular blindness.

History of Present Illness: The patient presented twice to an outside hospital with left-sided weakness. One episode occurred shortly after giving birth. These episodes occurred within 18 months of each other. Her brain and cervical spine magnetic resonance imaging (MRI) scans were negative and the weakness resolved with steroids. Up until this point in time, she was presumably affected by multiple sclerosis. A third episode of weakness prompted a visit to the author's institution, where the patient did not respond to steroids but did respond to a course of plasmapheresis. One month later, she presented to the emergency department with 1 week of complete vision loss in her right eye, and her vision improved significantly after another round of plasmapheresis.

Medical History: She denied smoking, drinking, or intravenous drug use.

Family History: Her mother had an unspecified leukemia.

Physical Examination: She was alert, oriented to time, person, and place, afebrile, and had normal vital signs. Her motor strength, light touch perception, and deep-tendon reflexes were normal. Her gait was slightly affected by past paresis. Extraocular movements were intact. Her right pupil was dilated and fixed and did not respond to light. No lymphadenopathy or rash was present.

Additional Diagnostic Tests: An MRI of her cervical spine revealed T2 hyperintensity from the cervicomedullary junction to C7. An MRI of her thoracic spine revealed T2 hyperintensity from T2 to T7. The brain MRI was negative. Chest x-ray was normal.

Questions

1. What are this patient's most striking clinical and laboratory findings?

2. What is this patient's differential diagnosis?

3. How is this patient's disease differentiated from multiple sclerosis (MS)?

4. Which laboratory tests are most useful in distinguishing between the different possible causes of this patient's condition?

5. What other laboratory tests might be useful in evaluating this patient's condition?

6. What are NMO IgG antibodies and what are their significance?

7. What is this patient's most likely diagnosis?

T1. Principal Laboratory Findings

Test	Patient's Result	Reference Interval
Hematology		
WBC count	9.0	4.0–11.0 × 10³/µL
Hemoglobin	11.2	12.0–15.0 g/dL
Hematocrit	33.7	34–44%
Platelet count	276	170–404 × 10³/µL
ESR	16	0–15 mm/h
Chemistry		
Creatinine	0.6	0.6–1.2 mg/dL
Glucose	116	65–200 mg/dL
AST	49	13–40 U/L
ALT	63	10–40 U/L
Vitamin B₁₂	339	211–911 pg/mL
Folate	10.4	>5.4 ng/mL
CRP	<0.5	0.0–0.9 mg/dL
MBP, CSF	32.5	<1.5 ng/mL
Oligoclonal bands, CSF	Negative	Negative
Drug screenᵃ	Negative	Negative

ᵃAmphetamines, barbiturates, phencyclidine (PCP), cannabinoids, and benzodiazepines. WBC, white blood cell; ESR, erythrocyte sedimentation rate; AST, aspartate aminotransferase; ALT, alanine aminotransferase; CRP, C-reactive protein; MBP, myelin basic protein; CSF, cerebrospinal fluid.

8. How does the pathophysiology of this disease differ from MS?

9. What is the most appropriate treatment for this patient's disease?

Possible Answers

1. Three episodes of transverse myelitis and optic neuritis are striking clinical findings. The most striking laboratory finding is seropositivity for neuromyelitis optica (NMO) IgG antibodies (**T1**).

2. The differential diagnosis of neurologic decline includes central and peripheral neuropathies. Underlying etiologies of neuropathies include nutritional deficiencies, toxins, infections (eg, neuroborreliosis, AIDS, vasculopathy [eg, vasculitis, occlusive stroke secondary to hypercoagulability], metabolic [eg, diabetes], and idiopathic causes [eg, neuromyelitis optica]).[1] Vitamin deficiencies, diabetes, and infectious agents (eg, *Borrelia burgdorferi* and HIV infection) can result in peripheral neuropathies. With vasculitides such as Wegener granulomatosis or Goodpasture syndrome, a neuropathic phenomenon of mononeuritis multiplex may occur. Mononeuritis multiplex may present with nonspecific symptoms and sensory and motor neuropathy. Underlying causes of mononeuritis multiplex may also include Lyme disease, HIV/AIDS, hepatitis, or a systemic inflammatory process.[2]

3. This disease is commonly confused with MS, and the most useful criteria to differentiate this disease from MS are the criteria shown in **T3**. The absolute criteria of myelitis, optic neuritis, and absent brain lesions can be further supported by major or minor criteria for a diagnosis of NMO.[3] The clinical presentation is the strongest indicator for disease. For example, the presence of a longitudinally-extensive cord lesion, together with a brain MRI scan that is normal or demonstrates only nonspecific white matter lesions, is 94% sensitive and 96% specific for NMO.[4]

4. The other diseases of the differential can be worked up by various methods (**T1**). A simple blood glucose measurement, Vitamin B₁₂/folate levels, toxicology screen, and immunologic studies can exclude diabetes, cobalamin/folate deficiencies, commonly-abused medications, and infectious agents as causes of the patient's symptoms. Since NMO is a condition that prompts workup for concomitant autoimmune/vasculitic diseases (eg, lupus, Wegener granulomatosis, and Goodpasture syndrome), appropriate studies for ruling in or out these disorders should be ordered as well. Lupus anticoagulant and other hypercoagulability factors were negative in this patient. Lack of appropriate imaging findings (Wegener tends to have arteriolocentric nodules on chest x-ray), no hemoptysis, normal creatinine, negative c- and p-ANCA, a normal C-reactive protein, and a barely-elevated erythrocyte sedimentation rate tends to exclude Wegener granulomatosis and Goodpasture syndrome as causes of this patient's clinical and laboratory findings.

T2. Principal Immunology Findings

Test		Patient's Result	Reference Interval
NMO Ab, IgG		Positive	Negative
Myelin IgG Ab, IFA		Negative	Negative
HIV Ab		Negative	Negative
ANA screen		Negative	Negative
dsDNA Ab		Negative	Negative
c-ANCA		Negative	Negative
p-ANCA		Negative	Negative
Lyme disease Ab		Negative	Negative
HAV Ab, IgM		Negative	Negative
HBsAg		Negative	Negative
HCV Ab		Negative	Negative
HBcAb, IgM		Negative	Negative
HSV 1 & 2, PCR		Negative	Negative
RPR		Non-reactive	Non-reactive
Lupus anticoagulant:	DRVVT	30.9	26.3–40.2 sec
	PTT La	32.1	29.3–47.7 sec
INR		1.0	0.9–1.3
Protein C activity		92	88–184%
Protein S activity		78	58–138%
Factor V Leiden mutation		Negative	Negative
ACA:	IgG	1.4	<12 GPL
	IgM	0.3	<9 MPL
B2 Glycoprotein I:	IgG	<12	<12 SGU
	IgA	<20	<20 SAU
	IgM	<20	<20 SMU
APA:	IgG	1.2	<10 GPS U/mL
	IgA	<0.1	<20 APS U/mL
	IgM	2.0	<6 MPS U/mL
AT3		99.0	81–33%

NMO, neuromyelitis optica; Ab, antibody; IFA, indirect immunofluorescence assay; HIV, human immunodeficiency virus; ANA, antinuclear antibody antigen; dsDNA, double stranded deoxyribonucleic acid; c-ANCA, cytoplasmic antineutrophil cytoplasmic antibody; p-ANCA, perinuclear antineutrophil cytoplasmic antibody; HAV, hepatitis A virus; HBsAg, hepatitis B surface antigen; HCV, hepatitis C virus; HBcAb, hepatitis B core antibody; HSV, human syncytial virus; PCR, polymerase chain reaction; dRVVT, dilute Russell Viper Venom Time; PTT La, partial thromboplastin time, lupus anticoagulant; INR, international normalized ratio; ACA, anti-cardiolipin antibody; APA, anti-phospholipid antibody; AT3, anti-thrombin 3.

5. Cerebrospinal fluid (CSF) cell count and evaluation for pleocytosis is indicated. In patients with NMO, pleocytosis of >50 × 10³ WBC/L or 5 × 10³ neutrophils/L can be observed. Testing for CSF oligoclonal bands and serum NMO IgG antibodies can also be useful. Currently, the inclusion of NMO IgG antibodies among the criteria for diagnosing NMO has been proposed but not finalized (**T3**). Oligoclonal bands can be found in CSF from individuals with NMO, but less frequently than in those with MS; however, the oligoclonal bands of MS persist, while those of NMO may disappear over time.[5]

T3. Proposed Diagnostic Criteria for Neuromyelitis Optica (NMO)a

Diagnosis of NMO requires:	All "Absolute Criteria" met **AND** 1 "Major Supportive Criteria" **OR** 2 "Minor Supportive Criteria" met.

Absolute Criteria

- Optic neuritis
- Acute myelitis
- No clinical disease outside the optic nerves and spinal cord

Major Supportive Criteria

- Negative[b] brain MRI at disease onset
- Spinal cord MRI with T2-signal abnormality extending over >3 vertebral segments
- CSF pleocytosis[c]

Minor Supportive Criteria

- Bilateral optic neuritis
- Severe optic neuritis with fixed visual acuity worse than 20/200 in at least 1 eye
- Severed, fixed, attack-related weakness[d] (MRC grade 2 or less) in 1 or more limbs

"Potential" Revisions to Diagnostic Criteria for NMO

- Inclusion of extraoptic-spinal clinical symptoms and signs of brain MRI lesions, if other criteria met
- Requirement for >3 segment spinal cord MRI lesion
- Integration of NMO-IgG serologic status into diagnostic schema

[a]Modified from Ref. 3. [b]Normal or not meeting radiological diagnostic criteria for multiple sclerosis (MS). [c]>50 × 103 WBC/L or >5 × 103 neutrophils/L. [d]MRC, Medical Research Council. MRI, magnetic resonance imaging. CSF, cerebrospinal fluid.

6. Neuromyelitis optica can be difficult to distinguish from MS; therefore, using indirect immunofluorescence (IFA) to detect the presence of serum NMO autoantibodies (NMO IgG) may be useful in distinguishing NMO from MS. If it is present, it may serve as a biomarker distinguishing NMO from MS. The NMO IgG antibody test is positive in approximately 60% to 80% of individuals diagnosed with NMO. The IFA for NMO IgG antibodies is 58% to 76% sensitive and 94% to 100% specific, but a newer assay developed by Toshiyuki touts a higher sensitivity.[6,7] Neuromyelitis optica IgG recognizes the aquaporin 4 (AQ4) water channel. This

channel is found on CNS microvessels, pia, sub-pia, and Virchow-Robbin spaces. The presence of NMO IgG antibodies portends a relapsing history of myelitis and optic neuritis.[1,6]

7. ***Most likely diagnosis:*** *neuromyelitis optica (NMO).* Devic syndrome, or NMO, is diagnosed by clinical presentation (**T3**) and is characterized by an inflammation and swelling of the optic nerves, such that orbital pain, decreased visual acuity, decreased color perception, and scotomas (optic neuritis) result. Optic neuritis tends to occur with binocular visual disturbance, as opposed to monocular in patients with MS. Episodes of optic neuritis are accompanied by transverse myelitis after a period of weeks, months, or even years. Moreover, NMO occurs as 1 of 2 subtypes: monophasic or relapsing.

8. Often confused with MS, NMO is similar in that it is also a demyelinating disease of the central nervous system, but there are distinctions between them. Unlike the cell-mediated mechanism that causes MS, NMO is characterized by a humoral mechanism of onset. Specifically, NMO develops as a perivascular deposition of immunoglobulins with concomitant complement activation and eosinophilic infiltrates. In contrast, the plaques of MS begin as perivenularly-distributed macrophages and T lymphocytes. In addition, the lesions found in NMO are absent from the brain but present in at least 3 spinal segments. The lesions of MS tend to occur in the brain matter.[5] Moreover, unlike MS, NMO has a race predilection for non-whites. Lastly, patients with MS often enter a progressive phase of the disease, but attacks can remit. Neurologic damage in individuals with NMO, however, tends to be residual, and thus damage accumulates with each successive attack. It is thought that the attacks are so severe that they preclude appreciation of progressive axonal deterioration. It is uncommon for MS to result in complete blindness. Paraplegia, or severe neurologic deficit, afflicts individuals with MS and affects their quality, but not quantity of life. Neuromyelitis optica affects the mortality rate, with respiratory failure resulting in the death of one-third of patients with this disease.[3]

9. Most treatment regimens rely on steroids. As first line therapy, intravenous administration of

corticosteroids is given for acute attacks of optic neuritis/myelitis. A commonly-used protocol for the administration of steroids involves infusion of methylprednisolone (1,000 mg) for 5 consecutive days. An oral prednisone taper may follow. To prevent future attacks, neurologists employ a regimen of azathioprine (2 to 3 mg/kg/d) in combination with oral prednisone (1 mg/kg/d).[4] Should the patient become steroid resistant, plasmapheresis can be used as an alternative therapy. Other immunosuppressive agents (eg, mitoxantrone, azathioprine, mycophenolate mofetil, and rituximab) have been used as well. A prophylactic regimen has been proposed using immunomodulatory agents. It is recommended that immunomodulatory agents be used even before diagnosis of NMO, as well as in NMO IgG seropositive patients. Because the presence of serum NMO IgG antibodies portends a high risk for relapse, the recommendation is that prophylactic therapy be continued for 5 years.[8] Moreover, the frequency of long-term visual impairment differs in patients affected with monophasic versus relapsing NMO. Regardless of treatment, 60% of patients with relapsing NMO will be blind (ie, less than 20/200 visual acuity) in at least 1 eye, while only 22% of patients with monophasic NMO suffer similar visual disturbances.[3]

Patient Follow-up

The patient continues to suffer from episodic weakness and residual right-sided blurry vision. In lieu of plasmapheresis, she responded well to treatment with oral steroids and rituximab.

Keywords

neuromyelitis optica, optic neuritis, transverse myelitis, multiple sclerosis, corticosteroids

References

1. Friedemann P, Sven J, Orhan A, et al. Antibody to aquaporin 4 in the diagnosis of neuromyelitis optica. *PLoS Med.* 2007;4:133.

2. Gorson KC. Vasculitic neuropathies: Update. *Neurologist.* 2007;13:9–12.

3. Wingerchuk DM, Hogancamp WF, O'Brien PC, et al. The clinical course of neuromyelitis optica (Devic's syndrome). *Neurology.* 1999;53:1107.

4. Wingerchuk DM. Diagnosis and treatment of neuromyelitis optica. *Neurologist.* 2007;13:2–11.

5. Bergamischi R. Importance of cerebrospinal fluid exam in differential diagnosis of Devic's neuromyelitis optica by multiple sclerosis. *Neurol Sci.* 2003;14:95–96.

6. Lennon VA, Wingerchuk DM, Kryzer TJ, et al. A serum autoantibody marker of neuromyelitis optica: Distinction from multiple sclerosis. *Lancet.* 2004;364:2106–2112.

7. Toshiyuki T, Kazuo F, Ichiro N, et al. Establishment of a new sensitive assay for antihuman aquaporin 4 antibody in neuromyelitis optica. *Tohoku J Exp Med.* 2006;210:307–313.

8. Matiello M, Jacob A, Wingerchuk DM, et al. Neuromyelitis optica. *Curr Opin Neurol.* 2007;20:255–260.

Recurrent Sinusitis

Monte S. Willis, M. Jane Latimer

Department of Pathology, University of Texas Southwestern Medical Center, Dallas, TX

Patient: 62-year-old male.

Past Medical History: Hypertension.

Chief Complaint: Recurrent sinusitis.

Past Surgical History: None.

Drug History: Recently on antibiotics (see above). No known drug allergies.

History of Present Illness: The patient reported ongoing upper respiratory and sinus infections since November 2001. In that time, his physician prescribed an unknown antibiotic, oral steroids, and a nasal decongestant for the treatment of his sinusitis. Approximately 7 days later, he developed a waxing and waning low-grade fever (37°C to 38°C). He then went to another physician and was prescribed another unknown antibiotic and steroids, which he took over the next 7 days. During this week, he indicated that his ears began to "tingle" and he started "turning red." He then went to a third physician who prescribed the fluoroquinolone antibiotic, gatifloxicin (Tequin). After taking Tequin, he developed bright red ears, which were painful to the touch. Ear pain and rash are rare (<0.1%) side effects of Tequin. He then went to a fourth physician, who prescribed a second course of Tequin. He subsequently developed a red, swollen ankle and came to the emergency room for assistance.

Family/Social History: The patient's brother has coronary artery disease; his father died of prostate cancer; and his grandmother had diabetes mellitus. He states that he smoked 1 pack of cigarettes a day from approximately 1960 to 1965. The patient denied alcohol and illicit drug use.

Physical Examination: Vital signs: temperature, 37.3°C; heart rate, 123 bpm; respiratory rate, 18/ minute; blood pressure, 108/80 mm Hg. The physical examination was within normal limits. The oropharynx was clear without exudates and sinus tenderness was absent.

Results of Additional Diagnostic Procedures and Laboratory Tests: Computed tomography (CT) scans of the head and sinuses were negative. A renal sonogram revealed enlargement of the right kidney and the presence of fluid in the right pleural space. A renal biopsy demonstrated microscopic findings compatible with an immune-mediated glomerulonephritis with crescent formation and the presence of granulomas. A chest X-ray revealed a peribronchovascular opacity overlying the hilar angle and non-specific pulmonary and pleural abnormalities. A chest CT identified a peribronchovascular ground glass appearance and consolidation not readily apparent on the plain radiographic films in the hilar region. Several bands of subsegmental atelectasis or scarring in the lung base were also identified.

T1. Principal Laboratory Findings

Test		Patient's Result	"Normal" Reference Range
Whole Blood			
WBC count		35.1 × 10³	4.1-11.1 × 10³/μL
Differential:	Neutrophils	93	36-72%
	Bands	2	0-11%
	Lymphocytes	3	20-51%
	Monocytes	1	4-11%
	Eosinophils	1	1-7%
RBC count		3.21 × 10⁶	4.27-5.99/μL
Hemoglobin		9.2	13.2-16.9 g/dL
MCV		88.9	76.2-98.6 fL
Platelet count		682	174-404 × 10³/μL
Aerobic and anaerobic cultures		Neg	Neg
Serum			
Sodium		130	135-145 mmol/L
BUN		79	7-21 mg/dL
Creatinine		2.3	0.6-1.2 mg/dL
Phosphorous		6.0	2.4-4.5 mg/dL
Calcium		8.1	8.4-10.2 mg/dL
CRP		5.9	0.0-0.8 mg/dL
ESR		>130	0-10 mm/h
EPO		17	0-19 mIU/mL
TIBC		125	262-474 μg/dL
TS %		16	20-50 %
Iron		20	60-200 μg/dL
Ferritin		1859	16-323 ng/mL
ANCA:	IFA pattern [**Image 1**]	Cytoplasmic	Negative
	Antibody titer	>1:640	≥1:20
	MPO Ab level	< 3.0	< 9.0 U/mL
	PR3 Ab level	= 100	< 3.5 U/mL
Urine			
Glucose		100	0 mg/dL
Protein		30	0 mg/dL
All other urine dipstick tests		Neg or WNL	Neg or WNL
Microscopy:	RBCs	14	0-3/hpf
	WBCs	None	0-5/hpf
	Casts	0-2 Hyaline	None/hpf

MCV, mean corpuscular volume; BUN, blood urea nitrogen; CRP, C-reactive protein; ESR, erythrocyte sedimentation rate; EPO, erythropoietin; TIBC, total iron-binding capacity; TS, transferring saturation; ANCA, antineutrophil cytoplasmic antibodies; IFA, indirect fluorescence immunoassay; MPO, myeloperoxidase; Ab, antibody; PR3, proteinase 3 (a 29 kilodalton serine protease); WNL, within normal limits; hpf, high power field.

T2. Criteria for Categorizing ANCA Staining Patterns

Pattern	Type of Staining Using Slides Containing Neutrophils[a] Fixed In		Recommended Antibody Confirmatory Test[b]
	Ethanol	Formalin	
cANCA	Cytoplasmic (granular)	Cytoplasmic (granular)	PR3 and MPO
pANCA	Perinuclear[c]	Cytoplasmic (granular)	MPO and PR3
aANCA[d]	Cytoplasmic and perinuclear variants	Cytoplasmic (granular, weakly positive, or negative)	None

[a]And some eosinophils interspersed among the neutrophils.
[b]Quantitative serum test.
[c]If eosinophil nuclei stain positive, antinuclear antibodies (ANA) are present.
[d]Also known as xANCA pattern in older literature.
ANCA, antineutrophil cytoplasmic antibodies; PR3, proteinase 3; MPO, myeloperoxidase.

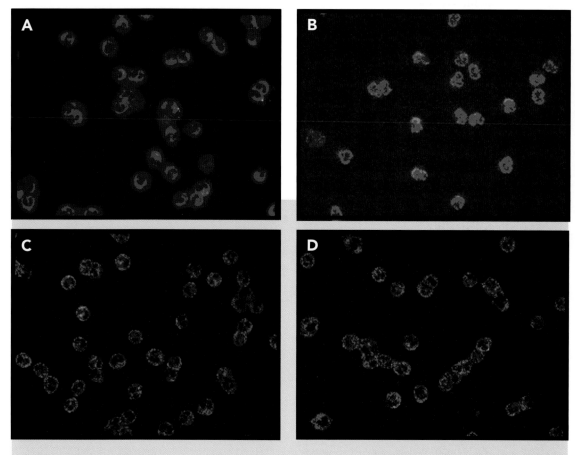

Image 1_ANCA staining patterns by IFA: (**A**) Case study patient's serum demonstrating cANCA pattern on ethanol-fixed neutrophils; (**B**) representative pANCA pattern on ehtanol-fixed neutrophils; (**C**) representative cANCA pattern of formalin-fixed neutrophils from serum that demonstrated a similar cANCA pattern on ethanol-fixed neutrophils; (**D**) representative cANCA pattern of formalin-fixed neutrophils from serum that demonstrated a pANCA pattern on ethanol-fixed neutrophils (ie, normal pANCA staining patterns). Photomicrographs by Monte S. Willis, MD, PhD.

Questions

1. What are this patient's most striking clinical and laboratory findings?

2. How do you explain this patient's most striking clinical and laboratory findings?

3. What condition(s) does this patient's laboratory and other findings suggest?

4. What is the spectrum of clinical and laboratory findings that might be seen in this patient's disease?

5. What is the most appropriate treatment for this patient?

Possible Answers

1. This patient's most striking clinical and laboratory findings are peribronchovascular infiltrations and other abnormal lung findings by CT; fluid in the right pleural space; enlargement of the right kidney; glomerulonephritis with crescent formation; the presence of renal granulomas; markedly increased WBC count (leukocytosis) with increased neutrophils (neutrophilia); a left shift; decreased lymphocytes, RBCs, and hemoglobin; increased platelet count; markedly increased ESR, CRP (C-reactive protein), BUN, creatinine, and ferritin; markedly decreased iron, TIBC, and %TS; decreased serum sodium concentration (hyponatremia); cANCA IFA pattern with strongly positive cANCA and PR3 antibody titers; and, the presence of glucose, protein, RBCs, and hyaline casts in the urine.

2. The most likely explanations for this patient's striking clinical and laboratory findings are:
   cANCA IFA pattern and positive PR3 antibody titer. Antineutrophil cytoplasmic antibodies (ANCA) to neutrophil antigens are mainly of 2 types, cytoplasmic (cANCA) or perinuclear (pANCA), distinguished by their characteristic pattern on indirect fluorescence assay (IFA) staining of human neutrophil substrates [**Image 1**]. Indirect fluorescence assay is performed using glass slides containing ethanol- or formalin-fixed human neutrophils (which have other

granulocytes present such as eosinophils). After adding a patient's serum to these slides, antibodies specific for proteins in the cytoplasm or perinuclear area of the neutrophils bind to these antigens creating a characteristic staining pattern after the addition of fluorescein isothiocyanate (FITC)-labeled anti-human IgG. The pattern of immune complexes formed by (protein antigen)-autoantibody-(anti-human IgG)-FITC are visualized using a fluorescence microscope and categorized as cANCA, pANCA, or atypical (aANCA) according to the criteria indicated in **T2**.[1] The cANCA pattern is characterized by diffuse cytoplasmic staining of neutrophils, the pANCA pattern by perinuclear staining of the neutrophils, and the rarer aANCA pattern by characteristics that neither definitively establish the pattern as cANCA or pANCA. The staining (fluorescence) observed with ethanol-fixed neutrophils using this patient's serum was consistent with a cANCA pattern in which staining predominates in the cytoplasm [**Image 1A**]. Staining of the nuclei of both neutrophils and eosinophils on ethanol-fixed slides is indicative of the presence of antinuclear antibodies (ANAs) and generally rules out the presence of an ANCA. Confirmation of ANAs is provided by the absence of (or markedly reduced) staining of the nuclei of formalin-fixed neutrophils. Rarely, ANA and ANCA autoantibodies may be present simultaneously. The pANCA pattern is associated with staining of the perinuclear region of ethanol-fixed neutrophils [**Image 1B**]. In addition, confirmation of the cANCA pattern using ethanol-fixed neutrophils is provided by the same staining pattern being observed using formalin-fixed neutrophils [**Image 1C**]. A pANCA pattern using alcohol-fixed neutrophils converts to a cANCA pattern when formalin-fixed neutrophils are used [**Image 1D**]. The specificity of the antibodies recognized as cANCA is a 29 kilodalton serine protease, proteinase 3 (PR3) which is found in the cytoplasm of neutrophils 90% of the time. Sometimes other antigens contribute such as myeloperoxidase (MPO). The pANCA is much less closely correlated with myeloperoxidase (MPO) and other antigens capable of producing this reactivity include elastase, cathepsin G, lysozyme, lactoferrin, and others. Cytoplasmic antineutrophil antibodies (cANCA) with PR3 specificity are found characteristically in the sera of patients with the autoimmune disease, Wegener granulomatosis (WG). Perinuclear antineutrophil antibodies (pANCA) are found in 50% to 70% of patients with ulcerative colitis, 80% of patients with chronic active hepatitis, and 20% of patients with SLE.[2,3] When patients have involvement of the respiratory tract and glomerulonephritis in WG, the diagnostic specificity of a cANCA pattern with a positive PR3 antibody titer for WG is 90% to 97%.[4,5] In the absence of renal disease, the specificity is lower (around 70%). Thus, these data and clinical findings from the present case of renal and lung involvement strongly support a diagnosis of WG in this patient. The role of cANCA in the pathogenesis of WG is not clear; however, experimental studies have suggested that the presence of PR3 antibodies is likely an epiphenomenon and not a direct cause of the pulmonary and renal tissue damage that occurs in patients with WG.[3,6] Moreover, these antibodies appear to be produced in pulmonary lymphoid tissue and are present in the serum of patients with active generalized WG, but not in the serum of patients in clinical remission.[7,8] In addition, experimental studies have demonstrated that activation of neutrophils (and monocytes) leads to the translocation of proteinase-3 from intracellular compartments to the cell surface.[7] This normally intracellular component is then available for recognition by the immune system as "non-self." The initiating factors involved in this disease process are currently unknown. The cANCA protein/enzyme enhances the respiratory burst and degranulation effects that occur during neutrophil activation, as well as adherence (inflammation) and results in subsequent damage to pulmonary and renal endothelial cells.[6,10] There is no direct evidence for T-cell involvement in this process; however, there is histological evidence of CD4+ T-cells in areas of infiltrating lesions and increased serum levels of soluble interleukin-2 (IL-2) receptors in patients with WG.[6] Approximately two-thirds of patients with WG present initially with sinusitis and 85% of patients with WG demonstrate sinusitis at some time during the course of their disease.[11,12] A CT scan of the sinuses is more informative than plain radiographs in assessing the presence of sinusitis. The patient presented in this case study, however, had clear sinuses for which there are several possible explanations. He may have had a subclinical sinus infection that

was not detected by CT or his sinusitis may have been adequately treated with antibiotics during the 2 to 3 week period prior to the CT scan. Antibiotic therapy, while treating his sinusitis secondary to WG, would not have an effect on the other manifestations of WG.

Criteria for Categorizing ANCA Staining Patterns

Abnormal x-ray (peribronchovascular opacity) and lung CT findings (peribronchovascular ground glass appearance). The most common pulmonary findings in patients with WG include the presence of pulmonary infiltrates (67%) and nodules (58%).[11] Pulmonary involvement occurs at presentation in up to 45% of patients with WG and in 87% of patients during the course of their disease.[11] The most common radiographic findings are bilateral, multiple, cavitating pulmonary lesions.[6] Computed tomography of the chest, however, commonly detects pulmonary infiltrates and nodules not apparent on conventional radiographs. Pulmonary morbidity in patients with WG is significant and pulmonary function tests may detect obstructive defects secondary to the lung tissue endothelial lesions and scarring that occur in up to 55% of patients with WG.[7]

Leukocytosis with neutrophilia and a left shift. These laboratory findings are commonly found in patients with an infection or inflammatory disease, such as WG.

Normocytic anemia. Generally, the most common cause of anemia is anemia of chronic disease (ACD), which can occur as a normocytic anemia (ie, decreased Hb and normal MCV) as seen in our patient. In patients with ACD, the decreased delivery of iron to new RBCs being produced in the reticuloendothelial system (RES) (ie, bone marrow, liver, and spleen) causes derangements in RBC production. Anemia of chronic disease can develop within weeks of onset of a systemic disease (eg, WG), independent of bone marrow involvement or hematologic complication. Increased breakdown of RBCs, abnormalities in iron mobilization, and the inhibition of erythropoiesis by inhibitory cytokines have all been implicated in the pathogenesis of ACD. In addition, a slight decrease in RBC survival occurs in patients with ACD that probably results from sequestration in the tissues of the RES.[13]

Increased ferritin and decreased iron, TIBC, and %TS. Low serum iron and transferrin saturation in the presence of an increased serum ferritin concentration reflects decreased utilization of iron stores. Low serum iron occurs typically as a generalized response to the presence of infection, as a result of IL-1 release from macrophages, or a malignancy (eg, WG). In such patients, both anabolic and catabolic responses occur, including an increase in the serum concentration of such acute-phase reactants as C-reactive protein (CRP), haptoglobin, ceruloplasm, fibrinogen, and ferritin, and a decrease in serum iron and hematocrit. In addition to the cytokine IL-1, other cytokines such as tumor necrosis factor-alpha (TNF-α) are released by macrophages and inhibit the production of erythroid precursors. The anemia in patients with ACD is generally not severe and medical management of ACD involves treatment of the underlying disorder causing the anemia.[13]

Increased ESR and CRP. An increased erythrocyte sedimentation rate (ESR) is due to alterations in plasma protein levels, especially fibrinogen and CRP. Both fibrinogen and CRP are acute-phase reactants whose concentration increases 12 to 24 hours after the onset of an inflammatory process or tissue damage (eg, the marked inflammation and tissue damage that occurs in patients with autoimmune diseases such as WG).[14] An elevated ESR may be associated with the presence of acute or chronic infection(s), malignancy, collagen vascular disease, abnormal serum proteins, severe anemia, and physiologic stress (such as marked obesity and pregnancy). In addition, the ESR can be increased in disease states such as chronic renal insufficiency and congestive heart disease.[14]

Enlargement of the right kidney, glomerulonephritis, increased serum BUN and creatinine, and the presence of glucose, protein, RBCs, and hyaline casts in the urine. The combination of these clinical and laboratory findings is consistent with significant renal dysfunction. Renal disease, defined by pathologic findings on biopsy or the presence of functional abnormalities, is observed at presentation in 11% to 18% of patients with WG and in 77% to 85% of these patients during the course of their disease.[6] The presence of hematuria in this patient suggests the presence of a vasculitic and/or nephritic process, such as WG. Generally, other manifestations of WG are present before renal disease is apparent. However, once present, renal disease may progress rapidly from a mild disease to a fulminant glomerulonephritis within days to weeks followed by end-stage renal failure. The presence of RBC casts has nearly a 100% positive predictive value for glomerulonephritis; however, the casts observed in our patient's urine were hyaline casts. If the glomerulonephritis in WG is left untreated, the mean survival time is approximately 5 months.[6] Even with treatment, initial and recurrent renal damage can lead to chronic renal insufficiency requiring dialysis and transplantation in some patients.

Hyponatremia. The regulation of plasma sodium and water content are under the control of the renin-angiotensin system and antidiuretic hormone (ADH). Renin is produced in the kidney in response to decreased volume and catalyzes the production of angiotensin I, which is converted to angiotensin II in the lungs. Angiotensin II stimulates aldosterone production (produced in the zona glomerulosa of the adrenal gland), which enhances the reabsorption of sodium and excretion of potassium in the renal distal tubules. Antidiuretic hormone is produced by the posterior pituitary gland in response to increased serum osmolarity or decreased intravascular volume, arterial pressure, and plasma volume, and acts by enhancing the uptake of water by increasing renal tubular permeability to water. Hyponatremia can occur in patients with renal insufficiency as seen in WG by disrupting these physiologic pathways of sodium and water regulation.

3. *Most likely diagnosis: Wegener's granulomatosis.*

4. Wegener granulomatosis can occur in any age group; however, the mean age is approximately 40 years.[7] This disease is characterized by granulomatous vasculitis of the upper and lower airways and the kidney.[7] Involvement of small arteries and veins can occur systemically of variable severity. Typical pulmonary, nasopharyngeal, otologic, ophthalmic, dermatologic (a

hallmark of systemic vascular diseases), musculoskeletal, neurologic, and cardiac manifestations of WG include: cough, hemoptysis, and pleuritis (***pulmonary***); sinusitis, nasopharyngeal obstruction, purulent or bloody discharges, ulcers, septal perforations, external saddle nose deformity (***nasopharyngeal***); serous or suppurative otitis media, conductive or, less commonly, sensorineural hearing loss, vertigo (***otologic***); conjunctivitis, scleritis, iritis, proptosis, retinal or corneal lesions, loss of vision (***ophthalmic***); skin ulcers, palpable purpuric rash, subcutaneous nodules, papules, and vesicles (***dermatologic***); arthralgias, myalgias, synovitis, symmetric arthritis which can mimic rheumatoid arthritis in distribution but is a non-erosive arthritis (***musculoskeletal***); peripheral neuropathy (***neurologic***); pericarditis and symptomatic or asymptomatic pericardial effusions (***cardiac***). Typical laboratory findings in patients with WG include: leukocytosis, elevated ESR, mild anemia, mild hypergammaglobulinemia, and a mildly elevated rheumatoid factor (RF) level.[6] The finding of a swollen ankle in this patient likely represents arthralgias associated with WG.

5. The most effective drug treatment for WG is cyclophosphamide (Cytoxan, 2 mg/kg/day) in conjunction with corticosteroids. The leukocyte count should be monitored and adjusted during therapy to keep the leukocyte count greater than 3,000/μL, which generally maintains the neutrophil count above 1,500/μL. Therapy generally induces a clinical remission without causing severe enough leukopenia to increase the risk of infection. Maintenance of cyclophosphamide treatment should be continued for 1 year following complete remission and tapered to discontinuation. Corticosteroids (prednisone 1 mg/kg/day) should be given daily during the induction of treatment for the first month with conversion to an alternate day dosage (every other day), and subsequently discontinued after 6 months. Greater than 90% of patients with WG demonstrate a marked improvement in their disease and 75% achieve complete remission on this drug regimen.[5] The cANCA titer does not generally decrease with treatment and can remain elevated for years. Thus, therapy should not be governed solely by cANCA titers and should depend more on objective measures of disease progression or remission.

Treatment and Course

The patient described in this case study was started on cyclophosphamide (125 mg orally, once daily) and prednisone (60 mg orally, once daily) therapy; however, his renal function deteriorated (his creatinine level of 2.3 mg/dL at admission rose to 3.8 mg/dL upon discharge from the hospital approximately 1 week later). Because vasculitic granulomas characteristic of WG were observed on his renal biopsy, an open lung biopsy was deemed unnecessary to confirm the diagnosis. The patient's blood pressure was controlled with a combination of a beta blocker (metoprolol tartrate, 25 mg, orally, once daily) and a calcium channel blocker (felodipine, 20 mg, orally, once daily). To treat his hyponatremia, sodium chloride tablets were given. In addition, antibiotic therapy with trimethoprim-sulfamethoxazole (TMP-SMX; 800 mg/160 mg, orally, twice daily) was initiated as this drug combination has been shown to reduce the incidence of relapse in patients with WG.[15] The patient did not experience joint pain or fever for several days before he was discharged. After 1 month of therapy, the patient achieved evidence of clinical remission with a normal chest X-ray and decreased CRP level (2.1 mg/dL compared to 5.9 mg/dL found at his initial admission).

References

1. Hoffman GS, Specks U: Antineutrophil cytoplasmic antibodies (Review). *Arthritis Rheum.* 1998;41:1521-1537.

2. Saxon A, Shanahan F, Landers C, et al. A distinct subset of antineutrophil cytoplasmic antibodies is associated with inflammatory bowel disease. *J Allergy Clin Immunol.* 1990;86:202-210.

3. Savige J, Gillis D, Benson E, et al. International Consensus Statement on testing and reporting of antineutrophil cytoplasmic antibodies (ANCA). *Am J Clin Pathol.* 1999;111:507-513.

4. Van der Woude FJ, Rasmussen N, Lobatto S, et al. Autoantibodies against neutrophil and monocytes: Tool for diagnosis and marker of disease activity in Wegener's granulomatosis. *Lancet.* 1985;1:425-429.

5. Nolle B, Specks U, Ludemann J, et al. Anticytoplasmic autoantibodies: Their immunodiagnostic value. *Ann Intern Med.* 1989;111:28-40.

6. Calabrese LH, Duna G. Vasculitis associated with antineutrophil cytoplasmic antibody. In: *Kelley's Textbook of Rheumatology,* 6th ed. Ruddy S, ed. Philadelphia: W.B. Saunders; 2001:1168-1176.

7. Fauci AS. The vasculitis syndromes. In: *Harrison's Principles of Internal Medicine* 15th ed. Braunwald E, Fauci AS, Kasper DL, et al, eds. New York: McGraw-Hill; 2001:1960-1963.

8. Baltaro RJ, Hoffman GS, Gallin JI, et al. Immunoglobulin G antineutrophil cytoplasmic antibodies are produced in the respiratory tract of patients with Wegener's granulomatosis. *Am Rev Respir Dis.* 1991;143:401-407.

9. Csernok E, Schmitt WH, Ernst M, et al. Membrane surface proteinase 3 expression and intracytoplasmic immunoglobulin on neutrophils from patients with ANCA-associated vasculitides. *Adv Exp Med Biol.* 1993;336:45-50.

10. Mayet WJ, Csernok E, Szymkowia KC, et al. Human endothelial cells express proteinase 3, the target antigen of anticytoplasmic antibodies in Wegener's granulomatosis. *Blood.* 1993;82:1221-1229.

11. Hoffman GS, Kerr GS, Leavitt RY, et al. Wegener's granulomatosis: An analysis of 158 patients. *Ann Intern Med.* 1992;116:488-498.

12. Fauci AS, Haynes BF, Katz P, et al. Wegener's granulomatosis: Prospective clinical and therapeutic experience with 85 patients for 21 years. *Ann Intern Med.* 1983;98:76-85.

13. Duffy TP. Normochromic, normocytic anemias. In: *Cecil Textbook of Medicine* 21st ed. Goldman L, Bennett JC, Drazen JM, eds. Philadelphia: W. B. Saunders; 2000:853-854.

14. Ravel R. *Clinical laboratory medicine: Clinical application of laboratory data.* St. Louis: Mosby; 1995:642.

15. Stegeman CA, Cohen Tervaert JW, de Jong PE, et al. Trimethoprim-sulfamethoxazole (co-trimoxazole) for the prevention of relapses of Wegener's granulomatosis. Dutch Co-Trimoxazole Wegener Study Group. *N Engl J Med.* 1996;335:16-20.

Acute Presentation of an Uncommon Cause of Renal Failure

Saliman A. Karsou,[1] Abeer Alshukhairy,[1] Ibrahim A. Hashim[2]

[1]*Department of Medicine, King Khalid National Guard Hospital, Jeddah, Saudi Arabia, and* [2]*Department of Pathology, University of Texas Southwestern Medical Center, Dallas, TX*

Patient: 60-year-old male.

Chief Complaint: Fever and sore throat followed by anorexia and abdominal pain, 1 week and 3 days prior to admission to our hospital, respectively.

Past Medical History: Poorly controlled diabetes mellitus, ischemic heart disease, and previous coronary artery bypass graft (CABG) surgery.

Drug History: In addition to long-term medications for diabetes mellitus and ischemic heart disease (oral hypoglycemic drugs, aspirin, oral nitrates, and b-blockers), 1 week prior to admission, the patient took a course of antibiotic (Amoxicillin-Clavulanate) treatment for his upper respiratory tract symptoms. There was no history of illicit drugs use.

Physical Examination: The patient was afebrile, normotensive, euvolemic, and not encephalopathic. He had no skin rash, pericardial rub, or cardiac murmurs. The chest was clear and his abdomen was non-tender. There was no diarrhea and no urinary symptoms. He had no dyspnea and no hemoptysis.

Results of Other Diagnostic Procedures: Ultrasound examination of the abdomen showed gallstones with no biliary obstruction, whereas ultrasound examination of the kidneys showed normal-size kidneys with no obstructive uropathy.

Questions

1. What is (are) this patient's most striking laboratory result(s)?

2. How do you explain this patient's most striking laboratory result(s)?

3. What condition(s) does this patient's laboratory and other findings suggest?

4. Which laboratory and non-laboratory test(s) are appropriate to order on this patient and why?

5. What is this patient's most likely diagnosis?

6. What is the pathophysiology of this patient's condition(s)?

7. What are the principal complications, their cause(s), and the prognosis in individuals with this patient's condition?

8. What is the most appropriate treatment for this patient's condition?

Possible Answers

1. Rapid increase of previously (10 days prior to admission) normal serum urea and creatinine levels; markedly elevated blood glucose levels

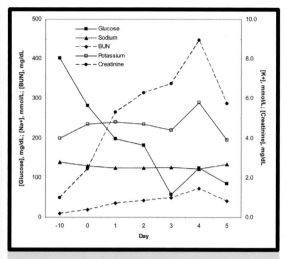

Figure 1_Time course of the patient's results for various laboratory tests 10 days prior (day -10) to hospital admission (day 0) and days 1 through 5 after admission of our patient to the hospital (lower dashed line corresponds to blood urea nitrogen [BUN; primary (left) axis], while upper dashed line corresponds to creatinine [secondary (right) axis]).

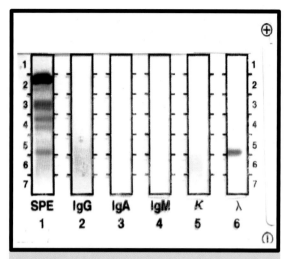

Figure 2_Immunofixation electrophoresis (IFE) pattern of our patient's serum showing a single band of restricted mobility in the gamma region of the serum protein electrophoresis (SPE) lane 1 corresponding to a band in lane 6 to which lambda light chain antiserum was added and no bands in the lanes to which IgG (lane 2), IgA (lane 3), or IgM (lane 4) heavy chain or kappa (6) light chain (lane 5) antiserum was added.

as well as percentage glycated hemoglobin; elevated g-glutamyltransferase (GGT) and β_2-microglobulin levels; decreased serum immunoglobulin levels; and mild thrombocytopenia and anaemia (**T1 and Figure 1**).

2. Increasing serum **urea and creatinine**, that were previously within normal limits, indicates a rapidly deteriorating renal function consistent with acute renal failure (ARF). The differential diagnosis of the ARF in this presentation includes drug therapy (eg, penicillin-induced acute interstitial nephritis,[1] hemolytic uremic syndrome (HUS),[2] post-infectious glomerulonephritis and vasculitis-related rapidly progressive glomerulonephritis,[3] plasma cell dyscrasia [eg, light chain deposition disease (LCDD)]-associated cast nephropathy,[4] or ARF of unknown etiology. The patient is known to have diabetes mellitus, and the markedly elevated blood **glucose** levels as well as percentage **glycated hemoglobin** (13.8%) indicate that his diabetes is not well controlled. However, the rapidly deteriorating renal function cannot be attributed to the poorly controlled diabetes mellitus alone, but it might be a contributing factor. The patient had not been exposed to penicillins or aminoglycosides antibiotics nor to drugs known to cause acute interstitial nephritis. Furthermore, the absence of esinophils in the urine did not support acute interstitial nephritis. Hemolytic uremic syndrome was excluded by the absence of fragmented red blood cells on the peripheral blood smear. Negative **antistreptolysin O**, negative **throat culture**, and normal complement levels (*data not shown*) were not consistent with an acute post-infectious glomerulonephritis. Moreover, negative **anti-neutrophil cytoplasmic antibodies** (ANCA) were not consistent with vasculitis related rapidly progressive glomerulonephritis as the cause of our patient's ARF. Elevated **GGT** [6 × upper limit of normal (ULN)], but normal alkaline phosphatase (**ALP**) levels, and a relatively normal **total bilirubin** indicates mild hepatobiliary dysfunction. These findings are consistent with radiological ultrasound evidence of gallstones but without biliary obstruction. Although GGT is present in high concentration in renal proximal tubules, circulating GGT normally originates primarily from the hepatobiliary system. Elevated GGT levels are usually seen 4 days following acute myocardial infarction suggesting liver injury secondary to cardiac failure,[5] although the patient is known to have ischemic heart disease, there was no clinical or biochemical evidence of

T1. Principal Laboratory Findings

Test		Patient's Result	Reference Range
Hematology			
Hemoglobin		11.8	14.0-17.5 g/dL
Platelet count		69	150-450 × 10³/µL
PBS findings		No fragmented RBCs	
Chemistry			
Albumin		3.5	3.4-4.8 g/dL
Calcium		9.3	8.6-10.2 mg/dL
Bilirubin, total		1.2	<1.1 mg/dL
Uric acid		6.0	3.5-7.2 mg/dL
ALP		226	<270 U/L
GGT		297	11-49 U/L
HbA$_{1c}$		13.8	<7.0%
Immunoglobulins, quant:	IgG	388	650-1,620 mg/dL
	IgA	<25	68-378 mg/dL
	IgM	<25	40-345 mg/dL
Immunology			
β$_2$-Microglobulin		41.7	<1.9 µg/mL
ASO		<80	
ANCA:	MPO	Negative	Negative
	PR3	Negative	Negative
Urinalysis			
Microscopic		Few WBCs and epithelial cells; scant RBCs; moderate number of granular casts; no eosinophils observed	
Microbiology			
Cultures:	Urine	No growth	No growth
	Throat	No β-hemolytic strep	No β-hemolytic strep

PBS, peripheral blood smear; RBCs, red blood cells; ALP, alkaline phosphatase; GGT, gamma-glutamyltransferase; Hb, hemoglobin; SPEP/IFE, serum protein electrophoresis pattern/immunofixation electrophoresis; Ig, immunoglobulin; ASO, anti-streptolysin O; cANCA, cytoplasmic anti-neutrophilic cytoplasmic antibody; MPO, myeloperoxidase antibodies; PR3, autoantibodies to proteinase 3; WBCs, white blood cells; strep, streptococci.

myocardial infarction. Other causes of elevated GGT levels include primary or secondary (metastatic) liver neoplasm, drug therapy, and alcohol intake. Serum **β2-microglobulin** concentration was markedly elevated (>20 × ULN). β$_2$-microglobulin is found on the cell surface of all nucleated cells and is shed into the blood. Elevated levels are seen in conditions (eg, multiple myeloma) associated with an increased number of B-lymphocytes, malignancy, and inflammation. β$_2$-microglobulin is filtered through the glomerulus and catabolized within the renal tubules. Therefore, elevated levels will

be seen in patients with renal insufficiency. Our patient had ARF which makes the interpretation of his β$_2$-microglobulin levels difficult. Circulating immunoglobulins (**IgG, IgA, and IgM**) levels were all decreased with IgA and IgM levels below their assay detection limit and IgG below normal limits. These findings are consistent with secondary immunoglobulin deficiency. Causes of secondary defective immunoglobulin synthesis include: lymphoid malignancy, multiple myeloma, chronic lymphocytic leukaemia, renal failure, diabetes mellitus, and drug therapy.[6] **Albumin** adjusted serum **calcium** levels were within normal limits. The patient had a moderately decreased **hemoglobin** level (anemia) and a mildly decreased **platelet count** (thrombocytopenia), which may be related to impaired renal function and diabetes mellitus. Causes of anaemia include poor nutritional status, blood loss, disseminated intravascular coagulation (DIC), infection, and haematological malignancies.

3. The presence of rapidly deteriorating renal function, anemia, elevated β_2-microglobulin, as well as immunoparesis, suggests a plasma cell dyscrasia as a possible cause of our patient's ARF.

4. A kidney biopsy and serum (SPE) and urine (UPE) protein electrophoresis followed by immunofixation electrophoresis (IFE) if a band of restricted mobility is observed on the SPE and/or UPE gel. In the presence of ARF of unknown aetiology, a kidney biopsy should be performed. The kidney biopsy on our patient showed cast-induced nephropathy consistent with light chain deposition and myeloma kidney. However, renal biopsy findings on their own cannot prove monoclonality. Therefore, a skeletal survey, a bone marrow biopsy, eletrophoretic analysis of serum and urine, and quantitative serum immunoglobulin analysis are indicated to investigate the possibility of multiple myeloma. Our patient's skeletal survey was normal (no evidence of malignancy or lytic lesions), his bone marrow biopsy was consistent with plasmacytosis, the SPE (SPEP) and IFE patterns of our patient's serum were consistent with free lambda light chains and no IgG, IgA, or IgM heavy chains (**Figure 2**), and his serum immunoglobulin (IgG, IgM, and IgA) levels were decreased (**T1**), consistent with immunoparesis. Our patient's urine sample was blood-stained and was not subjected to UPE and IFE. Due to the unavailability of IgD and IgE antisera, IFE with these antisera was not performed.

5. ***Most likely diagnosis:*** *myeloma kidney-induced ARF due to light chain deposition disease (LCDD).*

Light chain deposition disease is a systemic disorder characterized by the deposition of immunoglobulin light chains in various organs.[7] However, since light chains are physiologically filtered through the glomeruli with an elimination rate of 1 to 2 mg/L (lambda light chains),

reabsorbed in the proximal tubules by receptor-mediated endocytosis, and degraded in renal tubular cells by lysosomal enzymes, the kidney is the prominent target for light chain deposition. Moreover, casts composed of monoclonal light chains mixed with Tamm-Horsfall protein (THP) lead to renal tubular changes which are accompanied by interstitial edema and inflammation. The inflammatory infiltrate is typically composed of lymphocytes, monocytes, plasma cells, and rare neutrophils. The intensity of interstitial inflammation may range from minimal to extensive. In time, tubular atrophy and interstitial fibrosis will occur. Most (90%) patients with light chain cast nephropathy will have evidence of multiple myeloma.[8] Light chain deposition disease occurs more frequently among elderly (>50 years) males. It is also facilitated by states of hypovolemia. Our patient was hyperglycemic (serum glucose 401 mg/dL) 10 days prior to admission which may have led to episodes of dehydration facilitating LCDD. Other reported precipitating factors of LCDD include use of radio-iodinated contrast agents,[9] hypercalcaemia, hyperuricemia, acute pyelonephritis, and treatment with non-steroidal anti-inflammatory drugs (NSAIDs).[10-12] Our patient did not receive radio-contrast agents, nor NSAIDs; furthermore, his serum uric acid and calcium levels were within normal limits (**T1**). Although kappa- is more common than lambda-LCDD (68% and 32%, respectively),[13] our patient had lambda-LCDD.

6. It is the tissue affinity of light chains, rather than their circulating levels, that are important in determining their deposition.[14,15] Lambda-LCDD has been reported in a few isolated cases and cohort studies.[8] This may be because of the relative rarity and frequent misdiagnosis of this disease. Renal insufficiency appears in almost all patients with LCDD and rapidly worsens. Although this disease is rarely reported, it should not be rare considering the fact that a necropsy study found LCDD in 5% of multiple myeloma cases.[13] Light chain deposition disease should be suspected in all cases of renal insufficiency of unknown origin. In patients with a plasma cell dyscrasia (eg, multiple myeloma), the abnormal circulating immunoglobulin molecule and subunits (light chains) reach the glomerulus and are associated with various pathologic lesions within the kidney. Free light chains pass through the

glomerular basement membrane and form casts within the cytoplasm of cells of the proximal tubules. Moreover, immunoglobulin molecules or subunits may form paraprotein tissue deposits causing amyloidosis as well as deposition diseases. A number of disease entities are associated with myeloma kidney, including myeloma cast nephropathy, light chain Fanconi syndrome, LCDD, light and heavy chain deposition disease, heavy chain deposition disease, and cryoglobulinemic glomerulonephritis.[8] Light chains may precipitate in various tissues as needle-shaped crystalloid deposits or crystals. When these deposits/crystals are deposited within proximal tubular cells, they lead to disruption of function and in some cases to Fanconi's syndrome with aminoaciduria, glucosuria, and hypophosphaturia.[16] However, if proximal tubular function is severely disrupted, this will lead to renal failure. Although the majority of cases of crystalloid nephropathy have been associated with kappa light chains, there is no association with the type of heavy chain and the development of crystalloid nephropathy.[17,18] Clinical, as well as biochemical and histological investigations, help to distinguish between the different disease entities associated with light and/or heavy chain deposition.

7. Renal insufficiency leading to ARF, volume overload, acidosis, and hyperkalemia. Deposition of light chains leading to cast nephropathy leads in turn to anuric ARF. Full recovery of renal function is unlikely. Anuric acute renal failure has a worse prognosis compared to non-oliguric failure in multiple myeloma.[6,7] About half of all patients with multiple myeloma will develop renal impairment at some stage in their disease and this is usually associated with a poor outcome.[19] By histology, the most common cause of renal impairment is deposition of Bence Jones protein in renal parenchyma leading to cast nephropathy.[20] Other, less common, causes of renal impairment associated with multiple myeloma include amyloidosis and crystalloid deposition.[21,22] Our patient is at risk of poor prognosis due to his age and his poor renal function at presentation. Reduced survival, as well as chronic renal failure, is usually observed in patients with myeloma kidney-induced ARF due to light chain deposition disease (LCDD).[7] Although a markedly elevated β_2-microglobulin

level is a poor prognostic factor in patients with multiple myeloma, its value is limited in assessing prognosis in patients with renal impairment.

8. Therapy for LCDD is aimed at: (1) decreasing the production of light chains, (2) decreasing the concentration of circulating light chains, and (3) disrupting or inhibiting further light chain-Tamm-Horsfall protein interaction. Therapy for our patient included combination chemotherapy with vincristine-adriamycin-methylprednisolone (VAMP), conventional intermittent hemodialysis, as well as 5 sessions of plasma apheresis to reduce the concentration of circulating light chains. The patient had 2 episodes of chest pain and suddenly developed cardiopulmonary arrest. This was attributed to his significant ischemic coronary heart disease.

Keywords

light chain deposition disease, myeloma kidney, acute renal failure, immunoparesis

References

1. Rossert, J. Drug-Induced interstitial nephritis. *Kindney International.* 2001;60:804-817.

2. Caprioli J, Pengb L, Remuzzic G. The hemolytic uremic syndromes. *Curr Opin Crit Care.* 2005;11:487-492.

3. Laube G, Sarkissian A, Hailemariam S, et al. Simultaneous occurrence of the haemolytic uraemic syndrome and acute post-infectious glomerulonephritis. *Eur J Pediatr.* 2001;160:173-176.

4. Markowitz GS. Dysproteinemia and the kidney. *Adv Anat Pathol.* 2004;11:49-63.

5. Burtis CA, Ashwood ER, Bruns DE. *Tietz Textbook of Clinical Chemistry and Molecular Diagnostics.* St. Louis: Elsevier Saunders.

6. Whicher JT, Calvin J, Riches P, et al. The laboratory investigation of paraproteinaemia. *Ann Clin Biochem.* 1987;24:119-132.

7. Pozzi C, D'Amico M, Fogazzi GB, et al. Light chain deposition disease with renal involvement: clinical characteristics and prognostic factors. *Am J Kidney Disease.* 2003;42:1154-1163.

8. Linn J, Markowitz GS, Valeri AM, et al. Renal monoclonal immunoglobulin deposition disease: the disease spectrum. *J Am Soc Nephrol.* 2001;2:1482-1492.

9. Bartels ED, Brun GC, Gammeltoft A, et al. Acute anuria following intravenous pyelography in a patient with myelomatosis. *Acta Med Scand*. 1954;50:296-302.

10. Defrpnzo RA, Humphrey RL, Wright JR, et al. Acute renal failure in multiple myeloma. *Medicine (Baltimore)*. 1975;54:209-223.

11. Cohen DJ, Sherman WH, Osserman EF, et al. Acute renal failure in patients with multiple myeloma. *Am J Med*. 1984;76:247-256.

12. Irish AB, Winearls CG, Littlewood T. Presentation and survival of patients with severe renal failure and myeloma. *Qtrly J Med*. 1997;90:773-780.

13. Ivanyi B. Frequency of light chain deposition nephropathy relative to renal amyloidosis and Bence Jones cast nephropathy in a necropsy study of patients with myeloma. *Arch Pathol Lab Med*. 1990;114:986-987.

14. Ganeval D, Noel LH, Preud'homme JL, et al. Light chain deposition disease: Its relation with AL-type amyloidosis. *Kidney Int*. 1984;26:1-9.

15. Deneroy L, Deret S, Aucouturier P. Overrepresentation of the V_{kIV} subgroup in light chain deposition disease. *Immunol Lett*. 1994;42:63-66.

16. Lajoie G, Leung R, Bargman JM. Clinical, biochemical and pathological features in patients with plasma cell dyscrasia and Fanconi syndrome. *Ultrastruct Pathol*. 2000;24:221-226.

17. Gu X, Barrios R, Cartwright J, et al. Light chain crystal deposition as a manifestation of plasma cell dyscrasias: The role of immunoelectron microscopy. *Hum Pathol*. 2003;34:270-277.

18. Lebeau A, Zeindl-Eberhardt E, Muller EC, et al. Generalised crystal-storing histiocytosis associated with monoclonal gammopathy: Molecular analysis of a disorder with rapid clinical course and review of the literature. *Blood*. 2002;100:1817-1827.

19. Rayner HC, Haynes AP, Thompson, JR, et al. Perspectives in multiple myeloma: Survival, prognostic factors and disease complications in a single center between 1975 and 1988. *Qtrly J Med*. 1991;79:517-525.

20. Kapadia SB. Multiple myeloma: a clinicopathologic study of 62 consecutively autopsied cases. *Medicine (Baltimore)*. 1980;59:380-392.

21. Carstens PHB, Woo D. Crystalline glomerular inclusions in multiple myeloma. *Am J Kidney Dis*. 1989;14:56-60.

22. Keller LS, Faul RJ, Smith P, et al. Crystalloid deposits in the kidney. *Nephrology*. 2005;10: 81-83.

Chest Pain, Dyspnea, and Fatigue in a 57-Year-Old Man

Michael Roth,[1] Julius Aitsebaomo,[2] Monte S. Willis[1]

[1]*Departments of Pathology and Laboratory Medicine and* [2]*Internal Medicine, University of North Carolina, Chapel Hill, NC*

Patient: 57-year-old Caucasian man.

Chief Complaint: Persistent burning chest pain, dyspnea, and fatigue.

History of Present Illness: Symptoms began about 2 years ago but worsened significantly in the past 6 months. Proton pump inhibitor therapy did not alleviate the burning, initially thought to be due to gastroesophageal reflux. The patient's other complaint was increased breathlessness, predominately while in bed, for which diuretic therapy had been instituted. He also admitted to increased urination and a weight loss of 10 pounds, which was attributed to the diuresis.

Past Medical History: The patient is 18 years post aortic valve replacement, has a chronic left bundle branch block (LBBB) on electrocardiogram (ECG), and a history of hepatitis C.

Social History: The patient has a 20 pack/year history of smoking and quit 20 years ago. Currently, he is a painter and has significant occupational chemical and asbestos exposure.

Family History: The patient's mother had kidney cancer, his father had pancreatic cancer, and his sister had breast cancer.

Physical Examination: Vital signs: temperature, 36.2°C; blood pressure, 126/93 mm Hg; heart rate, 70 beats per minute; respiratory rate, 16. Pertinent physical examination findings included a 2/6 holosystolic murmur, identified by cardiac ausculation, along the right sternal border. There was good pulmonary effort with normal respiration. Bibasilar crackles were noted.

Additional Laboratory and Clinical Studies: Chest x-ray: The cardiac silhouette was moderately enlarged when compared with prior studies. There was pulmonary vascular congestion and perihilar edema, as well as some early interstitial edema. There was blunting of the costophrenic angles due to small bilateral pleural effusions.

Electrocardiogram: The QRS voltage was diminished in size, and there was a LBBB and a normal sinus rhythm.

T1. Principal Laboratory Findings

Test	Patient's Result	"Normal" Reference Interval
Hematology		
WBC count	4.6	4.5–11.0 × 109/L
RBC count	4.48	4.50–5.90 × 10^{12}/L
Hemoglobin	12.9	13.5–17.5 g/dL
Hematocrit	38.4	41.0–53.0%
MCV	86	80–100 fL
MCHC	34	31–37 g/dL
RDW	14.5	12.0–15.0%
Platelets	147	150–440 × 10^9/L
Chemistry		
Sodium	139	135–145 mmol/L
Potassium	4.0	3.5–5.0 mmol/L
Chloride	105	98–107 mmol/L
CO_2	25	22–30 mmol/L
BUN	18	7–21 mg/dL
Creatinine	1.3	0.8–1.4 mg/dL
Estimated GFR	>60	> 60 mL/min/1.73m^2
Anion gap	9	9–15 mmol/L
BUN/creatinine ratio	14	Undefined
Glucose, random	89	65–199 mg/dL
Calcium	8.8	8.5–10.2 mg/dL
Magnesium	1.9	1.6–2.2 mg/dL
Phosphorus	3.4	2.4–4.5 mg/dL
CK, total	33	70–85 U/L
CK-MB	3.6	0.0–6.0 ng/mL
Troponin T	0.107	0.0–0.029 ng/mL
NT-proBNP	3,072	0–177 pg/mL
Iron, total	46	35–165 µg/dL
Transferrin	238	200–380 mg/dL
TIBC	300	252–479 µg/dL
% Saturation	15	20–50%
Ferritin	74	0–177 pg/mL
Beta-2-microglobulin	3.55	0.70–1.80 µg/mL

WBC, white blood cell; RBC, red blood cell; MCV, mean corpuscular volume; MCHC, mean corpuscular hemoglobin concentration; RDW, red cell distribution width; BUN, blood urea nitrogen; GFR, glomerular filtration rate; CK, creatine kinase; NT-proBNP, N-terminal propeptide of B-type natriuretic peptide; TIBC, total iron binding capacity.

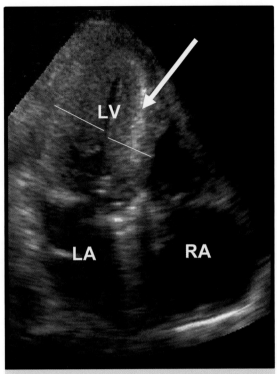

Image 1_The patient's trans-thoracic echocardiographic findings, illustrating left ventricular hypertrophy suggestive of an infiltrative process and left ventricular wall thickening (lines) and the shimmering, or sparkling (arrow), characteristic of amyloid infiltration of the myocardium. Only a minority of patients with cardiac amyloidosis demonstrate this pattern, and newer technology (harmonics) has made this finding less noticeable.[41]

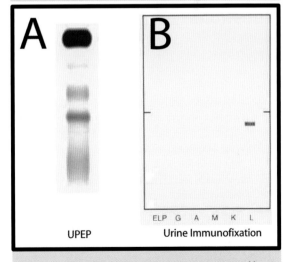

Image 2_The patient's UPE and IFE patterns, illustrating (**A**, UPE) mild selective glomerular proteinuria with excretion of albumin, alpha-, beta-, and gamma-globulins, and (**B**, UIFE) identification of an M-protein consisting of free lambda light chains.

T2. Characterization of Cardiac Involvement in Amyloidosis Classes Based on Underlying Cause of Amyloidosis

Type of Amyloidosis	Underlying Cause	Myofibril Composition	Cardiac Involvement	Tissue Distribution	References
Primary (AL)	Multiple myeloma	Ig light chain	Significant cardiac dysfunction	Kidney	11,22,42,43
		Ig heavy chain		Heart	
				Peripheral nerves	
				Liver	
				Tongue	
Secondary (AA)	Rheumatoid arthritis	SAA	Rare	Kidney	44
				Vascular	
Familial	Familial transthyretin mutation[a]	Transthyretin	Mild clinical cardiac manifestations[b]	Heart[c]	11,42,43
Senile cardiac	Aging	Transthyretin	Yes[d]	Heart	13,42
				Lungs[e]	

[a]Val30Met amino acid substitution. [b]With better outcomes versus AL amyloidosis. [c]Nerve limited. [d]With better outcomes versus AL amyloidosis (mean survival, mo: 11, senile cardiac amyloidosis; 75, AL amyloidosis). [e]To a lesser extent than heart. Ig, immunoglobulin; SAA, serum amyloid A.

Questions

1. What are this patient's most striking clinical and laboratory findings?

2. How do you explain this patient's most striking clinical and laboratory findings?

3. What additional studies would be appropriate to determine the cause of this patient's most striking clinical and laboratory findings?

4. What is this patient's most likely diagnosis?

5. What is the molecular pathogenesis of this patient's disease?

6. How is this patient's condition typically treated?

7. What is this patient's likely clinical course?

Possible Answers

1. Clinically, the most striking findings in this patient were progressive chest pain, intermittent shortness of breath (dyspnea), and reduced ECG voltages with a LBBB. Significant laboratory findings include normocytic anemia, elevated serum levels of N-terminal propeptide of B-type natriuretic peptide (NT-proBNP), cardiac troponin T (cTnT), and β-2-microglobulin (**T1**). Pertinent normal laboratory values include blood urea nitrogen (BUN), creatinine (Creat), ferritin, and transferrin saturation.

2. With a decrease in the ability of the heart to adequately pump out blood, the walls of the heart stretch and release BNP (and its precursor NT-proBNP) in response to the high ventricular filling pressures that are seen in heart failure.[1] In patients with dyspnea, a BNP >100 pg/mL has a sensitivity, specificity, and accuracy of 90%,

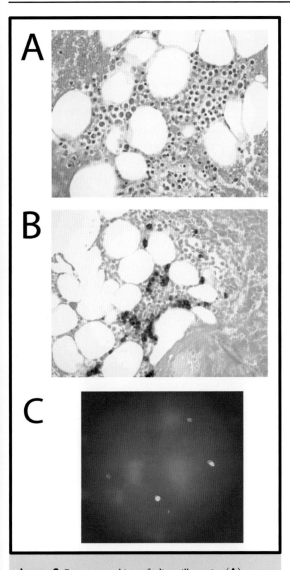

Image 3_Bone marrow biopsy findings, illustrating (**A**) abundant plasma cells with expression of lambda light chain by ISH (**B**) in a blood film made from the patient's clot specimen and (**C**) a cyclin D1:IgH translocation [t(11;14)(q13;q32)] by dual-color FISH, using probes for the cyclin D1 gene (red signal) at 11q13 and the IgH gene (green signal) at 14q32. Single red and green signals and 2 cyclin D1/IgH fusion signals (yellow signals) were observed in 8% of the nuclei containing interphase chromosomes from the patient, consistent with a rearrangement of the primary genes involved in multiple myeloma. ISH, in situ hybridization; FISH, fluorescence in situ hybridization; IgH, immunoglobulin heavy chain.

76%, and 83%, respectively, for diagnosing heart failure.[2] Moreover, serum NT-proBNP levels are typically 4-fold higher than BNP levels, as it is excreted less readily than BNP. This patient's

markedly-increased serum NT-proBNP level (3,072 pg/mL) ruled out a primary lung defect as the cause of his dyspnea and made heart failure the more likely cause.[3] Additionally, the patient had an elevated cTnT level, further indicating that he had cardiac myocyte damage.[4] Elevated cTnT levels are seen in patients with ischemic injury, heart failure, left ventricular hypertrophy, diabetes, and kidney disease.[5,6] During cell turnover, β-2-microglobulin is released into the blood and excreted by the kidneys. The patient's elevated β-2-microglobulin, a constituent of major histocompatibility complex (MHC) class I antigens, likely represents a neoplastic, inflammatory, or an infectious disease process, in lieu of renal disease, as his renal function tests (BUN and Creat) were normal.[7] Low ECG voltages can result from conditions that impede electrical voltage between the heart and the chest wall, such as tamponade, pericardial effusion, emphysema, or infiltrative heart disease. An LBBB is not an uncommon ECG finding, with increasing prevalence with age, and can be associated with progressive infiltrative diseases of the cardiac conduction system. Normocytic anemia results from acute blood loss, anemia of chronic disease (eg, due to infection, inflammation, or malignancy), bone marrow suppression, and chronic renal insufficiency.

3. Echocardiogram (echo), serum and urine protein electrophoresis (SPE and UPE), and an endomyocardial biopsy. An echo is useful in determining the cause of the abnormal laboratory test values and the unexplained ECG abnormalities. An echo performed on the patient revealed substantial symmetric left ventricular wall thickening involving the interventricular septum, thickening of the atrial septum, dilated atria, and diastolic dysfunction (**Image 1**). No evidence of ischemia or vascular occlusion was present, and the patient's prosthetic aortic valve was well seated with normal function. Serum protein electrophoresis and UPE are appropriate to perform in the setting of unexplained anemia, weakness, or fatigue. Additionally, the presence of unexplained heart failure and nephrotic syndrome suggests the possibility of a plasma cell dyscrasia or amyloidosis. Serum protein electrophoresis is usually performed when multiple myeloma, Waldenström macroglobulinemia, primary amyloidosis, or any

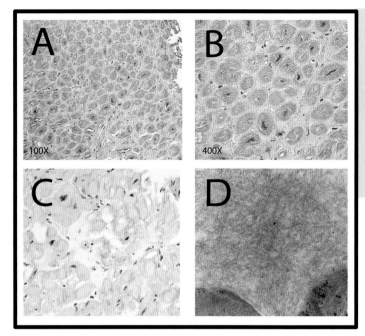

Image 4_Cardiac biopsy findings, illustrating interstitial eosinophilic material with a waxy to fibrillar quality hugging myocytes (H&E stain; 100× [**A**] and 400× magnification [**B**]); an amorphous and homogenous eosinophilic deposit by light microscopy infiltrating the myocardium (Congo red stain) (**C**). Transmission electron microscopy of the biopsy reveals characteristic 8 to 10 nm amyloid fibrils (**D**).

related disorder suggestive of a monoclonal gammopathy is suspected. In these conditions, the SPE pattern (SPEP) demonstrates the presence of a monoclonal protein (M-protein). The monoclonal gammopathies are a group of disorders characterized by the proliferation of a single clone of plasma cells which produce an immunologically-homogeneous protein commonly referred to as an M-protein. This patient's SPEP showed hypoproteinemia and hypoalbuminemia, but no M-protein was observed (not shown). His UPE showed a pattern suggestive of mild selective glomerular proteinuria with excretion of albumin, alpha- and beta-globulins, and the presence of a band of restricted mobility, suggestive of a monoclonal protein (**Image 2A**), which was immunophenotyped subsequently by immunofixation electrophoresis (IFE) as lambda free light chains (FLCs) (**Image 2B**). A bone marrow biopsy is essential in evaluating a patient with an M-protein detected in the serum or urine. A bone marrow biopsy from this patient demonstrated 19% plasma cells (**Image 3A**), many of which were positive for lambda light chain restriction by in situ hybridization (ISH) (**Image 3B**). Moreover, cytogenetic analysis of the bone marrow aspirate revealed a CYCLIN D1/IgH gene fusion product in 8.0% of the interphase nuclei examined (**Image 3C**). An endomyocardial biopsy is useful in classifying the etiology of heart failure. Hematoxylin and eosin (H&E) staining of cardiac tissue from the

patient's biopsy revealed an amorphous to waxy pink infiltrate in the interstitium closely surrounding cardiomyocytes (**Image 4A** and **4B**) and no evidence of granulomatous infiltration suggestive of sarcoidosis. This pattern is classic for cardiac amyloidosis. Moreover, Congo red staining of this tissue, which can be used to differentiate amyloid infiltration from collagen scar, demonstrated dark pink staining deposits that, under polarized light, demonstrated the apple-green birefringence characteristic of amyloid (**Image 4C**). Finally, transmission electron microscopy (TEM) of the cardiac infiltrate demonstrated the presence of rigid fibrils, 8 to 10 nm in diameter, characteristic of amyloid and suggestive of the infiltrative process noted by the echo findings (**Image 4D**) on the patient.

4. ***Most likely diagnosis:*** *cardiac amyloidosis secondary to multiple myeloma.* The diagnostic criteria for multiple myeloma generally requires that 3 criteria are met: (1) the presence of a serum or urinary monoclonal protein; (2) the presence of clonal plasma cells in the bone marrow; and (3) evidence of end-organ damage. In this patient, a urinary monoclonal lambda FLC was identified, a clonal (lambda) plasma cell population (19%) was present in the bone marrow, and the patient had a normocytic anemia. These findings distinguish the monoclonal gammopathies from reactive plasmacytosis due to autoimmune diseases, acquired immunodeficiency syndrome (AIDS),

chronic liver disease, chronic infection, or metastatic carcinoma. In these diseases, the bone marrow plasma cells demonstrate polyclonal light chain restriction. The patient's diagnosis was supported further by the results of the cytogenetic analysis. The most common chromosomal translocations in multiple myeloma involve the immunoglobulin heavy chain (IgH) locus on the long arm of chromosome 14 (14q32). The most common of these translocations, t(11;14)(q13;q32), results in the upregulation of cyclin D1, a finding found in 8% of interphase bone marrow cells from the present patient.[9] The patient's clinical and laboratory evidence of cardiac dysfunction, specifically the combination of left ventricular hypertrophy, dilated atria, and left-sided heart failure with no evidence of cardiac ischemia, strongly supports an infiltrative cardiomyopathy. An infiltrative process produces abnormal cardiac relaxation and the clinical picture of a restrictive cardiomyopathy. This category would include the cardiac involvement observed in patients with hemochromatosis, sarcoidosis, or amyloidosis. A patient with a hemochromotosis-related cardiomyopathy would present with a mildly-enlarged left ventricle and unexplained heart failure. Serum tests would show elevated transferrin saturation and ferritin level. In light of the patient's normal iron indices, iron deposition in the myocardium was considered unlikely. The possibility of sarcoid heart disease in the evaluation of an otherwise-healthy, middle-aged individual with cardiac symptoms must be recognized. Granulomatous infiltration of the atrioventricular node can cause conduction abnormalities and infiltration of the myocardium can result in ventricular arrthymias. When granulomatous infiltration of the myocardium is extensive, heart failure can result. The diagnosis of heart failure due to granulomatous infiltration can be made by endomyocardial biopsy demonstrating granulomatous infiltration. Of the 3 infiltrative processes, hemochromatosis-related cardiomyopathy, sarcoidosis, and amyloidosis, amyloidosis is the only 1 with a link to multiple myeloma because the immunoglobulin light chain is the building block of the amyloid fibril.

5. Amyloidosis refers to the deposition of protein in tissues that has an anti-parallel beta-pleated sheet confirmation by x-ray diffraction, a characteristic fibrillar structure by TEM (**Image 4A**), and the ability to bind Congo red, Thioflavine T, and sulfated Alcian blue stains. It is important to understand that the deposition of proteins that form amyloid is a common final pathway that may have different causes. The characteristics of the different forms of amyloidosis are summarized in **T2**. Immunoglobulin amyloidosis, as in this patient, constitutes about 85% of all newly-diagnosed cases of amyloidosis and results from multiple myeloma and other plasma cell dyscrasias.[10] Secondary amyloidosis refers to reactive amyloid fibrils containing the proteins (acute-phase reactants) produced during the acute phase response in patients with systemic inflammatory diseases such as rheumatoid arthritis, tuberculosis, leprosy, and inflammatory bowel syndrome.[11] Senile systemic amyloidosis occurs due to misfolding of the acute-phase protein, transthyretin (prealbumin), and can be found in 25% of patients older than the age of 80 years. This disease is thought to result from the intrinsic propensity of transthyretin to assume a pathologic conformational structure with age.[12] Although this condition is usually benign, cardiac conduction disturbances can occur.[13] Familial amyloidosis occurs due to a mutation that results in an amino acid substitution, which renders a formerly normal protein as amyloidogenic.[12] Transthyretin and lysozyme are the prototypical culprit proteins.[14] Lastly, hemodialysis-associated amyloidosis can occur in patients with chronic renal failure. In such cases, amyloid protein is deposited primarily in the bone and joints.[10] Moreover, in addition to the typical proteins that constitute amyloid fibrils, co-deposition of other proteins (eg, apolipoproteins, glycoaminoglycans, serum amyloid P) can occur after the initial amyloid product is desposited in the tissue.[15,16] These additional proteins may promote the formation of fibrils, stabilize and prevent their degradation, bind specific extracellular matrix components, or prevent proteolytic events and metabolism of fibrils.[17,18] The biochemical properties of the light chains in immunoglobulin amyloidosis may determine their toxicity in cardiac amyloidosis. In support of this hypothesis, it has been determined that the infusion of light chains from patients with cardiac amyloidosis induces diastolic dysfunction in isolated mouse hearts.[19] Amyloidogenic properties of AL amyloid disease may include the ability of these light chains to aggregate,

which directly correlates with their amino acid composition at specific sites within the FLC molecule.[12,20,21]

6. Both cardiac-related symptoms and the underlying disease should be treated in cardiac amyloidosis. The mainstay of heart failure therapy due to AL amyloidosis is diuretics.[22] Angiotensin converting enzyme (ACE) and angiotensin II inhibitors and calcium channel blockers are poorly tolerated in patients with cardiac amyloidosis.[22] Amyloid fibrils bind digitalis and nifedipine, which may be the reason there is increased toxicity and hemodynamic deterioration with these drugs, respectively, in the treatment of patients with cardiac amyloidosis.[23-25] Because of the high risk of thromboembolic events in patients with cardiac amyloidosis and atrial fibrillation, warfarin anticoagulation, unless major contraindications exist, is strongly indicated in the treatment of such patients.[22] The atria in patients with severe cardiac amyloidosis can be infiltrated, dysfunctional, or occluded by thrombi, even in patients with normal sinus rhythm.[26-28] Therapy for symptomatic cardiac amyloidosis is generally supportive; however, patients with early symptoms may respond to treatment of the underlying disease (ie, their plasma cell dyscrasia). Extended therapy with melphalan and either prednisone or dexamethasone results in a modest improved efficacy compared with other treatment regimens in patients with primary amyloidosis.[29,30] Short courses of high-dose melphalan combined with high-dose dexamethasone results in better outcomes than other combination drug therapies.[31] In a study of 46 patients not eligible for hematopoietic stem cell transplantation, including 32 patients with cardiac involvement, a hematologic response was seen in 67% and a complete hematologic remission in 33% of these patients.[31] Nearly 48% of these patients were found to have a >2 mm reduction in interventricular septal thickness associated with heart failure resolution. However, high-dose dexamethasone is not well tolerated in heart failure patients. Improvement in the survival of patients with AL amyloidosis occurs in patients who undergo autologous hematopoietic stem cell transplantation with high-dose melphalan therapy.[32] Unfortunately, cardiac amyloidosis is associated with increased morbidity and mortality, and reduced survival after therapy compared with patients with amyloidosis without cardiac involvement.[32] Moreover, the majority of patients with cardiac amyloidosis have systemic disease, making them poor candidates for cardiac transplantation. In 1 study, only 4% of symptomatic patients with cardiac amyloidosis were found to have isolated cardiac involvement.[33] The few centers that do accept patients with AL amyloidosis for cardiac transplantation require that patients have: 1) isolated cardiac disease; and 2) unacceptable risk of complications due to hematopoietic stem cell transplantation and chemotherapy.[34] Following cardiac transplantation, high-dose chemotherapy and autologous hematopoietic stem cell transplantation within 12 months is performed, resulting in short-term durable hematopoietic results and improved cardiac performance.[35-37]

7. Among patients with primary amyloidosis, as in this patient, long-term survival is poor. Mean survival is 6 to 9 months in patients with heart failure, and 1.1 years in patients without cardiac involvement.[33] Death in patients with amyloidosis and cardiac involvement is generally attributable to heart failure or arrhythmias; however, renal failure, infection, and gastrointestinal hemorrhage have been reported as other causes of death in such patients.[38,39] Only 7% of patients with primary amyloidossis and symptomatic cardiac involvement survive 10 years.[38] However, a recent report described a patient that survived 20 years after being diagnosed with biopsy-proven amyloidosis,[40] which may indicate improvements in evolving cardiac treatment options for some patients. Nevertheless, the diagnosis of cardiac amyloidosis portends a grave prognosis. In patients with cardiac amyloidosis and clinical manifestations of heart failure, the median survival is 4 months. Most patients die of either heart failure or cardiac arthymia.[38]

Patient Follow-up

After the authors' patient was diagnosed with cardiac amyloidosis secondary to multiple myeloma, the patient was referred to an oncologist and started on high-dose melphalan and dexamethasone therapy. Within 45 days, his cardiac function had improved noticeably. Subsequently, the patient underwent a successful autologous bone marrow transplant. Sixty days post-transplantation, his cardiac function remained stable, although he remained on heart failure medication (Metoprolol, Aldactone, and Lasix), and his serum lambda FLC concentration decreased substantially from the baseline value of >18 mg/dL to 3.5 mg/dL. He has complained of increased constipation, which could be due to gastrointestinal mucosal or neuromuscular infiltration of amyloid.

Keywords

amyloidosis, Congo red, apple-green birefringence, transthyretin, multiple myeloma, free light chain, melphalan, dexamethasone, hematopoietic stem cell transplantation

References

1. Kinnunen P, Vuolteenaho O, Ruskoaho H. Mechanisms of atrial and brain natriuretic peptide release from rat ventricular myocardium: Effect of stretching. *Endocrinology.* 1993;132:1961–1970.

2. Maisel AS, Krishnaswamy P, Nowak RM, et al. Rapid measurement of B-type natriuretic peptide in the emergency diagnosis of heart failure. *N Engl J Med.* 2002;347:161–167.

3. Hunt PJ, Richards AM, Nicholls MG, et al. Immunoreactive amino-terminal pro-brain natriuretic peptide (NT-PROBNP): A new marker of cardiac impairment. *Clin Endocrinol.* 1997;47:287–296.

4. Katus HA, Remppis A, Scheffold T, et al. Intracellular compartmentation of cardiac troponin T and its release kinetics in patients with reperfused and nonreperfused myocardial infarction. *Am J Cardiol.* 1991;67:1360–1367.

5. Wallace TW, Abdullah SM, Drazner MH, et al. Prevalence and determinants of troponin T elevation in the general population. *Circulation.* 2006;113: 1958–1965.

6. Nunes JP, Mota Garcia JM, Farinha RMB, et al. Cardiac troponin I in aortic valve disease. *Int J Cardiol.* 2003;89:281–285.

7. Bethea M, Forman DT. Beta 2-microglobulin: Its significance and clinical usefulness. *Ann Clin Lab Sci.* 1990;20:163–168.

8. Criteria for the classification of monoclonal gammopathies, multiple myeloma and related disorders: A report of the International Myeloma Working Group. *Br J Haematol.* 2003;121:749–757.

9. Chesi M, Bergsagel PL, Brents LA, et al. Dysregulation of cyclin D1 by translocation into an IgH gamma switch region in 2 multiple myeloma cell lines. *Blood.* 1996;88:674–681.

10. Hassan W, Al-Sergani H, Mourad W, et al. Amyloid heart disease. New frontiers and insights in pathophysiology, diagnosis, and management. *Tex Heart Inst J.* 2005;32:178–184.

11. Dubrey SW, Cha K, Skinner M, et al. Familial and primary (AL) cardiac amyloidosis: Echocardiographically similar diseases with distinctly different clinical outcomes. *Heart.* 1997;78:74–82.

12. Merlini G, Bellotti V. Molecular mechanisms of amyloidosis. *N Engl J Med.* 2003;349:583–596.

13. Kyle RA, Spittell PC, Gertz MA, et al. The premortem recognition of systemic senile amyloidosis with cardiac involvement. *Am J Med.* 1996;101:395–400.

14. McCutchen SL, Lai Z, Miroy GJ, et al. Comparison of lethal and nonlethal transthyretin variants and their relationship to amyloid disease. *Biochemistry.* 1995;34:13527–13536.

15. Gallo G, Wisniewski T, Choi-Miura NH, et al. Potential role of apolipoprotein-E in fibrillogenesis. *Am J Pathol.* 1994;145:526–530.

16. Kisilevsky R, Young ID. Pathogenesis of amyloidosis. *Baillieres Clin Rheumatol.* 1994;8:613–626.

17. Husby G, Stenstad T, Magnus JH, et al. Interaction between circulating amyloid fibril protein precursors and extracellular tissue matrix components in the pathogenesis of systemic amyloidosis. *Clin Immunol Immunopathol.* 1994;70:2–9.

18. Tennent GA, Lovat LB, Pepys MB. Serum amyloid P component prevents proteolysis of the amyloid fibrils of Alzheimer disease and systemic amyloidosis. *Proc Natl Acad Sci USA.* 1995;92:4299–4303.

19. Liao R, Jain M, Teller P, et al. Infusion of light chains from patients with cardiac amyloidosis causes diastolic dysfunction in isolated mouse hearts. *Circulation.* 2001;104:1594–1597.

20. Hurle MR, Helms LR, Li L, et al. A role for destabilizing amino acid replacements in light-chain amyloidosis. *Proc Natl Acad Sci USA.* 1994;91: 5446–5450.

21. Myatt EA, Westholm F, Weiss D, et al. Pathogenic potential of human monoclonal immunoglobulin light chains: Relationship of in vitro aggregation to in vivo organ deposition. *Proc Natl Acad Sci USA.* 1994;91:3034–3038.

22. Falk RH. Diagnosis and management of the cardiac amyloidoses. *Circulation.* 2005;112:2047–2060.

23. Gertz MA, Skinner M, Connors LH, et al. Selective binding of nifedipine to amyloid fibrils. *Am J Cardiol.* 1985;55:646.

24. Griffiths BE, Hughes P, Dowdle R, et al. Cardiac amyloidosis with asymmetrical septal hypertrophy and deterioration after nifedipine. *Thorax.* 1982;37:711–712.

25. Rubinow A, Skinner M. Cohen AS. Digoxin sensitivity in amyloid cardiomyopathy. *Circulation.* 1981;63:1285–1288.

26. Dubrey S, Pollak A, Skinner M, et al. Atrial thrombi occurring during sinus rhythm in cardiac amyloidosis: Evidence for atrial electromechanical dissociation. *Br Heart J.* 1995;74:541–544.

27. Modesto KM, Dispenzieri A, Cauduro SA, et al. Left atrial myopathy in cardiac amyloidosis: Implications of novel echocardiographic techniques. *Eur Heart J*. 2005;26;173–179.

28. Santarone M, Corrado G, Tagliagambe LM, et al. Atrial thrombosis in cardiac amyloidosis: Diagnostic contribution of transesophageal echocardiography. *J Am Soc Echocardiogr*. 1999;12:533–536.

29. Grogan M, Gertz MA, Kyle RA, et al. Five or more years of survival in patients with primary systemic amyloidosis and biopsy-proven cardiac involvement. *Am J Cardiol*. 2000;85:664–665,A611.

30. Kyle RA, Gertz MA, Greipp PR, et al. A trial of 3 regimens for primary amyloidosis: Colchicine alone, melphalan and prednisone, and melphalan, prednisone, and colchicine. *N Engl J Med*. 1997;336:1202–1207.

31. Palladini G, Perfetti V, Obici L, et al. Association of melphalan and high-dose dexamethasone is effective and well tolerated in patients with AL (primary) amyloidosis who are ineligible for stem cell transplantation. *Blood*. 2004;103:2936–2938.

32. Skinner M, Anderson J, Simms R, et al. High-dose melphalan and autologous stem-cell transplantation in patients with AL amyloidosis: An 8-year study. *Ann Intern Med*. 2004;140:85–93.

33. Dubrey SW, Cha K, Anderson J, et al. The clinical features of immunoglobulin light-chain (AL) amyloidosis with heart involvement. *QJM*. 1998;91:141–157.

34. Simons M, Rajkumar SV, Falk HF. Amyloid cardiomyopathy. In: Rose B, ed. *UpToDate*. Waltham, MA; 2007.

35. Dubrey SW, Burke MM, Hawkins PN, et al. Cardiac transplantation for amyloid heart disease: The United Kingdom experience. *J Heart Lung Transplant*. 2004;23:1142–1153.

36. Kpodonu J, Massad MG, Caines A, et al. Outcome of heart transplantation in patients with amyloid cardiomyopathy. *J Heart Lung Transplant*. 2005;24:1763–1765.

37. Pelosi F Jr, Capehart J, Roberts WC. Effectiveness of cardiac transplantation for primary (AL) cardiac amyloidosis. *Am J Cardiol*. 1997;79:532–535.

38. Kyle RA, Gertz MA, Greipp PR, et al. Long-term survival (10 years or more) in 30 patients with primary amyloidosis. *Blood*. 1999;93:1062–1066.

39. Kyle RA, Gertz MA. Primary systemic amyloidosis: Clinical and laboratory features in 474 cases. *Semin Hematol*. 1995;32:45–59.

40. Fealey ME, Edwards WD, Grogan M, et al. Primary cardiac amyloidosis with 20-year survival. *Cardiovasc Pathol*. 2006;15:331–335.

41. Rahman JE, Helou EF, Gelzer-Bell R, et al. Noninvasive diagnosis of biopsy-proven cardiac amyloidosis. *J Am Coll Cardiol*. 2004;43:410–415.

42. Ng B, Connors LH, Davidoff R, et al. Senile systemic amyloidosis presenting with heart failure: A comparison with light chain-associated amyloidosis. *Arch Intern Med*. 2005;165:1425–1429.

43. Gertz MA, Kyle RA, Thibodeau SN. Familial amyloidosis: A study of 52 North American-born patients examined during a 30-year period. *Mayo Clin Proc*. 1992;67:428–440.

44. Uda H, Yokota A, Kobayashi K, et al. Two distinct clinical courses of renal involvement in rheumatoid patients with AA amyloidosis. *J Rheumatol*. 2006;33:1482–1487.

Atypical Cells in the Cerebrospinal Fluid of a 43-Year-Old Man With Perioral Parasthesias

Soon Bahrami, John R. Parker, Sandra C. Hollensead

Department of Pathology and Laboratory Medicine, University of Louisville School of Medicine, Louisville, KY

Patient: 43-year-old Caucasian man.

Family History: Unremarkable.

Chief Complaint: Persistent numbness and tingling of the left lower lip and jaw for 2 weeks.

History of Present Illness: In addition to his chief complaint, the patient reported nausea and vomiting every morning. One month prior to the onset of present symptoms, the patient noted a subcutaneous mass on his left leg.

Past Medical History: The patient was diagnosed with multiple myeloma 1 year prior when he presented to his physician with back pain and was found to have renal insufficiency and hypercalcemia. Serum and urine immunofixation electrophoresis identified monoclonal IgG kappa and free lambda light chain M-components, respectively. A bone marrow aspirate and biopsy confirmed the diagnosis of multiple myeloma with 90% replacement of the marrow by plasma cells. Cytogenetic workup of the bone marrow demonstrated several chromosomal abnormalities including deletion of 13q. He had undergone multiple cycles of chemotherapeutic regimens with the most recent treatment administered 4 months prior to current presentation. There is no other significant past medical history.

Results of Additional Diagnostic Procedures: Cerebrospinal fluid (CSF) obtained from a lumbar puncture had a glucose level within normal limits and an elevated protein of 71 mg/dL (reference range: 12-60 mg/dL). Examination of a cytospin preparation for cell count demonstrated 131 total cells with 83% plasma cells, 11.5% lymphocytes, and 5.5% monocytes; 8 red blood cells were present. Morphologic examination revealed numerous atypical plasma cells with conspicuous nucleoli and binucleate forms in a background of a few lymphocytes and monocytes (Image 1). Flow cytometry of the CSF did not reveal any abnormal cell populations. Serum and urine immunofixation electrophoresis confirmed the presence of IgG kappa and lambda free light chain M-components, respectively. A previous fine needle aspiration (FNA) of the subcutaneous leg mass was positive for plasma cells morphologically similar to those seen in the CSF (**Image 2**), establishing the diagnosis of extramedullary plasmacytoma. A magnetic resonance imaging (MRI) scan of the brain was within normal limits.

Questions

1. What is (are) this patient's most striking clinical and laboratory findings?

2. How do you explain the patient's most striking clinical and laboratory findings?

3. What is this patient's most likely diagnosis?

T1. Principal Laboratory Findings

Test		Patient's Result	"Normal" Reference Range
Hematology			
WBC count		3.1	4.8-10.8 × 10^3/μL
Hemoglobin		7.5	14.0-18.0 g/dL
Hematocrit		20.5	42-54%
Platelet count		26	155-367 x 10^3/μL
Differential:	Granulocytes	49	44-78%
	Lymphocytes	34	12-34%
	Monocytes	10.9	3-12%
	Eosinophils	4.6	0-5%
	Basophils	1.5	0-2%
Chemistry			
Sodium		140	138-147 mmol/L
Potassium		3.3	3.5-5.0 mmol/L
Chloride		101	100-108 mmol/L
CO_2		27	22-30 mmol/L
BUN		16	7-20 mg/dL
Creatinine		6.8	0.8-1.5 mg/dL
Calcium		9.3	8.4-10.2 mg/dL
b_2-microglobulin	33.3	1.0-1.7 mg/dL	
IgA		30	80-450 mg/dL
IgG		578	750-1560 mg/dL
IgM		30	46-304 mg/dL

WBC, white blood cell; BUN, blood urea nitrogen; IgA, immunoglobulin A; IgG, immunoglobulin G; IgM, immunoglobulin M.

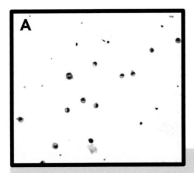 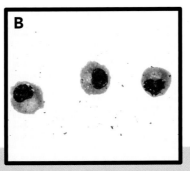 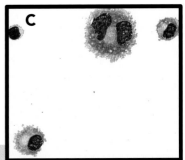

Image 1_Wright-Giemsa stained cells from CSF cytocentrifuge preparation illustrating (**A**) increased cellularity at low power (100×) and (**B**) identification of these cells as plasma cells at higher power (400×), including (**C**) some atypical and binucleate forms (600×).

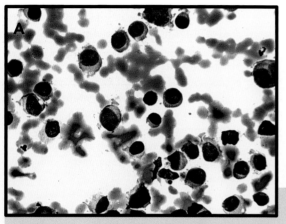
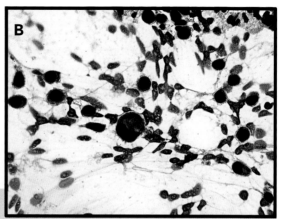

Image 2_Fine needle aspiration (FNA) of the patient's subcutaneous leg mass, using both Diff-quik (**A**) and Papanicolaou (**B**) stains, revealing the presence of numerous atypical plasma cells (600×).

4. What is the characteristic clinical presentation of an individual with this patient's condition?

5. What are the criteria for making this diagnosis?

6. What is the pathogenesis of this patient's disease?

7. What is the prognosis for this patient?

8. What treatment options are available for this patient's condition?

9. How did performing a cell count on the CSF contribute to this case?

Possible Answers

1. Persistent perioral parasthesias; abnormal laboratory findings of elevated creatinine, pancytopenia, elevated β_2-microglobulin and decreased immunoglobulins; identification of M-components in both the serum (IgG kappa) and urine (lambda free light chains); subcutaneous plasmacytoma; and, atypical plasma cells and elevated protein in the CSF.

2. Many of the patient's abnormal laboratory findings can be explained by the patient's previously assigned diagnosis of multiple myeloma. The increased creatinine reflects renal failure secondary to tubular damage resulting from light chain proteinuria. Anemia is a common feature of multiple myeloma and occurs because of bone

marrow replacement by the malignant clone and renal loss of erythropoietin.[1] In this patient's case, previous chemotherapeutic treatments with melphalan, a nitrogen mustard agent, have likely also contributed to the severity of the patient's anemia and to the neutropenia and thrombocytopenia. The electrophoresis results confirm the presence of active plasmacytic disease in this patient, and secondary extramedullary plasmacytomas are a common finding in patients with multiple myeloma. Other typical features of multiple myeloma include a hypogammaglobulinemia of normal (or unaffected) immunoglobulins, and elevated β_2-microglobulin levels may also be present.[2] However, it is important to note that elevation of β_2-microglobulin can also occur in patients with renal failure,[3] which is likely a contributing factor in the current case. The differential diagnosis of parasthesias includes multiple sclerosis, nutritional deficiencies, medications, alcohol, neoplasms, infections (herpes zoster), and various neuropathies.[4] Increased protein in the CSF, often with marked elevation, is commonly seen in infectious conditions of the central nervous system (CNS) including bacterial and tuberculous meningitis and cerebral abscesses. Slight elevations in protein may be seen in sarcoidosis and systemic lupus erythematosus involving the CNS. Neoplastic processes and especially leukemias involving the CSF will also result in an elevated CSF protein level.[4] Plasma cells are an abnormal finding in CSF and may be seen in infectious and noninfectious inflammatory conditions of the CNS including viral and tuberculous meningitis, neurosyphilis, cerebral cysticercosis, multiple sclerosis, and subacute sclerosing panencephalitis.[5] They may also be seen in neoplastic plasma cell processes (ie, meningeal involvement in multiple myeloma or leptomeningeal myelomatosis), in which atypical plasma cells are often found in the CSF.

3. **Most likely diagnosis:** *leptomeningeal myelomatosis.* In light of the patient's active disease course with multiple myeloma, the CSF findings demonstrate multiple myeloma involving the CNS.

4. Neurologic complications in patients with multiple myeloma are not uncommon and include peripheral neuropathies, cranial nerve palsies, spinal cord compression, and various encephalopathies.[6] These complications may be secondary to vertebral compression fractures, base of skull and bony involvement elsewhere, amyloid deposition, hyperviscosity syndrome, metabolic derangements including hypercalcemia and uremia, and toxicity from various treatments. However, invasion of the CNS in the form of leptomeningeal myelomatosis (LMM) is a rare event. The prevalence of LMM in patients with multiple myeloma is estimated to be 1%.[6] A review of 23 patients with LMM established a median age of 54 years at the time multiple myeloma was diagnosed.[6] A median interval of 13 months occurred before LMM was diagnosed. In 1 of the patients, LMM was the presenting feature that led to the diagnosis of multiple myeloma. The majority of patients with LMM have advanced stage multiple myeloma (Salmon-Durie stage III) at the time of diagnosis. Immunologic subtyping revealed IgG-secreting plasma cell dyscrasias to be the most common followed by IgA. However, some early reports have suggested that IgA- and IgD-secreting plasma cells may be disproportionately likely to spread to the leptomeninges.[7] Patients with LMM may present with a broad variety of neurologic signs and symptoms. The characteristic clinical presentations include mental status changes, headaches, seizures, cranial neuropathies, diffuse or localized weakness, diffuse or localized parasthesias, visual changes, and confusion.[6,7] Magnetic resonance imaging may be negative as in our patient or it may demonstrate cranial leptomeningeal contrast enhancement or leptomeningeal-based mass lesions.[6] If these signs or symptoms develop in a patient with

multiple myeloma, a CSF evaluation for the presence of LMM should be performed.

5. The definitive test for diagnosing LMM is examination of the CSF.[6-8] Cytologic examination of CSF from patients with LMM will reveal plasma cells with pleomorphism. High nuclear-cytoplasmic (N/C) ratios, binucleated forms, and conspicuous nucleoli may also be present. Rare mitoses are seen. The number of cells present may vary from 1 to 605 cells/µL.[9] Rarely, a few lymphocytes may be seen in the background. However, the absence of cells in the CSF consistent with an inflammatory response is the more common finding. This has been speculated as facilitating the spread of myeloma cells once they have entered the leptomeninges. It also provides evidence that the neurologic symptoms are directly related to the presence of the malignant cells rather than secondary to an associated inflammatory response.[7] In addition to positive cytologic findings, the CSF often shows elevation in the protein levels which may vary from a slight to marked increase.[9] Glucose levels are typically within normal reference limits. Ancillary tests may be useful if further confirmation of the diagnosis is warranted. These tests include serum, urine, and CSF electrophoresis and immunofixation electrophoresis. The monoclonal protein found in the CSF should match the serum/urine findings. The CSF may be sent for flow cytometry; however, it is important to remember that a negative result does not rule out the presence of LMM, because plasma cell fragility or hemodilution of specimens may lead to negative results.[10] If necessary, immunocytochemical stains can be helpful in identifying cells in the CSF containing cytoplasmic monoclonal immunoglobulins.[8] However, morphologic identification of atypical plasma cells with elevated CSF protein in the setting of a patient with multiple myeloma, demonstrating neurologic signs and symptoms, fulfills the criteria for a diagnosis of LMM.

6. Multiple myeloma, a B cell neoplasm, occurs when the postgerminal center bone marrow plasmablasts or plasma cells become transformed into myeloma cells.[2] The pathogenetic mechanisms of this disease are complex and consist of a multistep process.[11] A precursor lesion, monoclonal gammopathy of undetermined significance (MGUS), has been found to contain

chromosomal abnormalities which lead to karyotypic instability. These MGUS plasma cells are predisposed to have additional genetic events which lead to the evolution of multiple myeloma and advanced progression of the disease. One of the earliest cytogenetic effects identified is a translocation at 14q32 resulting in activation of an oncogene at 1 of numerous translocation partner regions. This process is thought to be the point at which the plasma cell clone is immortalized. The myeloma cells generate a microenvironment in the bone marrow that supports proliferation of the malignant clone via secretion of interleukin 6 (IL-6), tumor necrosis factor a (TNFa), vascular endothelial growth factor (VEGF), and insulin-like growth factor 1 (IGF1), which play important roles in the pathogenesis of this disease. IL-6 is a key growth and survival factor for multiple myeloma cells. It is produced by the bone marrow stromal cells, and it activates signal transduction pathways which induce proliferation and inhibit apoptosis in myeloma cells. TNFa upregulates adhesion molecules which facilitate attachment of the myeloma cells in the bone marrow. VEGF production and secretion is stimulated by IL-6, and an autocrine loop is established as VEGF secreted by the myeloma cells increases IL-6 production by the bone marrow stromal cells. IGF1 acts by inducing proliferation of myeloma cells and improving the effect that IL-6 has on the myeloma cells. Late occurring genetic and molecular events further advance the disease process often resulting in extramedullary manifestations of disease. It is likely at this stage that a patient may develop LMM. However, some research has supported the idea that LMM is just a development in the constellation of extramedullary manifestations of a particularly aggressive multiple myeloma rather than an indicator of disease progression.[6] There is supporting evidence that many of the cases of LMM result from hematogenous spread of abnormal plasma cell clones leading to the initial seeding of the leptomeninges. Moreover, up to one-third of patients with LMM have evidence of circulating plasma cells (plasma cell leukemia) in their peripheral blood, and this may be a risk factor for the development of LMM.[12] In patients with LMM and no apparent evidence of circulating plasma cells, it is hypothesized that their disease arises from lymphocytes that may be progenitors of plasma cells, or the failure to

detect plasma cells in the blood of these patients. Local extension from adjacent bony lesions in the skull may also occur.[9] Other reports support the notion that plasma cells may have entered the leptomeninges earlier in the disease course and then undergone proliferation over time.[13] Most of the chemotherapeutic agents used in the treatment of multiple myeloma cannot cross the blood brain barrier, thus allowing plasma cells that have infiltrated the meninges to survive and proliferate even while the patient's disease is being treated.

7. The development of LMM in patients with multiple myeloma heralds a terminal event in the disease course. The median survival from the time of diagnosis of leptomeningeal involvement is 1.5 months.[7,9,12,13] The patient in this particular case died 5 weeks after the diagnosis of LMM was made. Moreover, there is evidence that particular unfavorable prognostic indicators are associated with the development of LMM.[9] These indicators include deletion of 13q14, high tumor mass, plasmablastic morphology, additional extramedullary manifestations, and the presence of circulating plasma cells. The cytogenetic abnormality, subcutaneous plasmacytoma, and high tumor mass were identified in the present case. Estimation of the degree (%) of marrow replacement by plasma cells (tumor mass) impacts staging of multiple myeloma which helps determine prognosis; <20% (Stage I), 20-50% (Stage II) and >50% (Stage III).[1] Other parameters used in staging are the level of the M-component, renal function, serum calcium levels, lytic bone lesions, hemoglobin levels, and non-M component immunoglobulin levels. Median survival in all patients with multiple myeloma is 3 years with 10% survival at 10 years.[1] Additional poor prognosticators in multiple myeloma include deletion of 17p13, high proliferation index identified by the Ki-67 antigen, and increased levels of M-component β_2-microglobulin.[1]

8. There is no consensus regarding standard therapy for LMM. Treatment modalities include intrathecal chemotherapy with methotrexate, cytarabine, or thiotepa in adjunct with hydrocortisone.[6,13] These agents may or may not be administered concurrently with systemic chemotherapy. Cranial or craniospinal irradiation can

also be performed alone or in combination with chemotherapy. Based on limited information from case reports, the combination of intrathecal chemotherapy and craniospinal irradiation may be the most effective treatment modality for LMM; however, the prognosis still remains very poor.[12] In rare instances, some patients have responded to therapy, including achieving sterilization of their CSF.[7] Thus, despite the poor prognosis in patients with LMM, an attempt at treatment is reasonable.

9. In the present case, only the CSF cell count led to the diagnosis of LMM since MRI of the brain and flow cytometry of the CSF were negative. This case underscores the importance of accurate cell classification when performing cell counts on body fluids such as CSF.

Keywords

leptomeningeal myelomatosis, multiple myeloma, cerebrospinal fluid, cytology

References

1. Grogan TM, Van Camp B, Kyle RA, et al. *Plasma cell neoplasms in the World Health Organization Classification of Tumours: Pathology & Genetics, Tumours of Haematopoietic and Lymphoid Tissues.* Lyon, France: IARC Press; 2001:142-156.

2. Sirohi B, Powles R. Multiple myeloma. *Lancet.* 2004;363:875-887.

3. Perosa F, Luccarelli G, Prete M, et al. Increased serum levels of [beta]2m-free HLA class I heavy chain in multiple myeloma. *Br J Haematol.* 1999;106:987-994.

4. Ferri FF. *Ferri's Clinical Advisor: Instant Diagnosis and Treatment.* Philadelphia, PA: Elsevier Mosby; 2005.

5. Truong LD, Kim HS, Estrada R. Meningeal myeloma. *Am J Clin Pathol.* 1982;78:532-535.

6. Schluterman KO, Fassas A, Van Hemert RL, et al. Multiple myeloma invasion of the central nervous system. *Arch Neurol.* 2004;61:1423-1429.

7. Leifer D, Grabowski T, Simonian N, et al. Leptomeningeal myelomatosis presenting with mental status changes and other neurologic findings. *Cancer.* 1992;70:1899-1904.

8. Cavanna L, Invernizzi R, Berte R, et al. Meningeal involvement in multiple myeloma: Report of a case with cytologic and immunocytochemical diagnosis. *Acta Cytol.* 1996;40:571-575.

9. Fassas A, Muwalla F, Berryman T, et al. Myeloma of the central nervous system: Association with high-risk chromosomal abnormalities, plasmablastic morphology and extramedullary manifestations. *Br J Haematol.* 2002;117:103-108.

10. Braylan RC. Impact of flow cytometry on the diagnosis and characterization of lymphomas, chronic lymphoproliferative disorders and plasma cell neoplasias. *Cytometry.* 2004;58A:57-61.

11. Seidl S, Kaufmann H, Drach J. New insights into the pathophysiology of multiple myeloma. *Lancet Oncol.* 2003;4:557-564.

12. Petersen SL, Wagner A, Gimsing P. Cerebral and meningeal multiple myeloma after autologous stem cell transplantation. A case report and review of the literature. *Am J Hematol.* 1999;62:228-233.

13. Patriarca F, Zaja F, Silvestri F, et al. Meningeal and cerebral involvement in multiple myeloma patients. *Ann Hematol.* 2001;80:758-762.

A Swollen Painful Knee in an Elderly Man With Acute Myelogenous Leukemia

Satish K. Solanki, Shahnila Latif, Diana M. Veillon, Mary L. Nordberg, Steven J. Saccaro,

James D. Cotelingam, Seth M. Berney

Louisiana State University Health Sciences Center, Shreveport, LA

Patient: 60-year-old Caucasian male.

Chief Complaint: Sudden onset of severe pain and swelling in the left knee, right ankle, and right great toe, 1 day after initiation of chemotherapy for recently diagnosed acute myelomonocytic leukemia (AML-M4).

Medical History: This patient had no past history of arthritis. Prophylactic treatment with allopurinol was started prior to initiation of chemotherapy with daunorubicin and cytarabine.

Physical Examination: On examination, the patient was afebrile, normotensive (blood pressure, 120/70 mm Hg); and the left knee, right ankle, and right great toe were warm to the touch, tender to palpation, and had effusions. In addition, the left knee was swollen [**Image 1**].

Gross and Microscopic Histologic Finding: Under aseptic conditions, 18.0 mL of turbid fluid was aspirated from the left knee. Microscopically, no crystals were detected under polarized light. Gram stain and microbial cultures were negative. The WBC and RBC counts were 3,285/mm^3 and 360/mm^3, respectively. However, atypical mononuclear cells were identified on light microscopy [**Image 2**]. Flow cytometric immunophenotyping of synovial fluid cells from our patient was performed with the results shown in **Image 3**.

Questions

1. What is the interpretation of this patient's flow cytometric immunophenotyping results?

2. Based on the constellation of this patient's clinical and laboratory findings, what is the most likely diagnosis?

3. Which age group is most commonly affected by this patient's condition or disorder?

4. What is the usual clinical presentation of this patient's condition?

5. What is the pathogenesis of this patient's condition?

6. What is the preferred diagnostic test for establishing the diagnosis of this patient's condition?

7. What is the best therapy for this patient's disorder?

Possible Answers

1. A predominance of myelomonocytic cells which expressed CD10, CD11b, CD13, CD14, CD15, CD33, CD38, myeloperoxidase, and HLA-DR [**Image 3**]. These results were similar to those

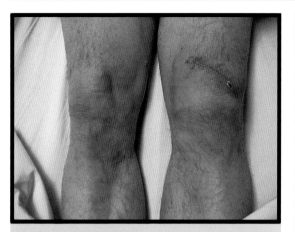

Image 1_Medial aspect of our patient's left knee (note degree of swelling in comparison to his right knee).

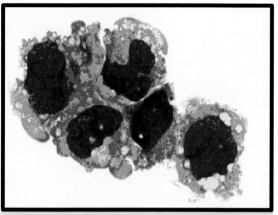

Image 2_Nucleolated leukemic cells with delicate chromatin and cytologicatypia (Wright-Giemsa stain; 1,000× magnification) observed on microscopic examination of our patient's synovial fluid.

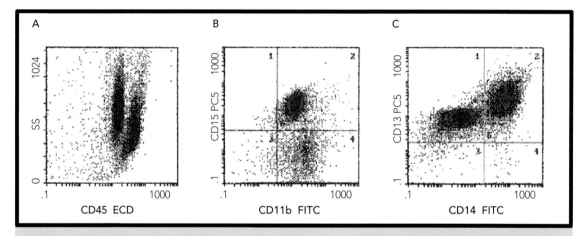

Image 3_Representative flow cytometric dot plots of the cells in synovial fluid from our patient illustrating **A**) CD45 (leukocyte common antigen) versus side scatter showing a predominance of CD45-positive cells; **B**) CD11b (myeloid cells) and CD15 (neutrophils, monocytes) co-expression on the leukemic cells; and, **C**) CD14 (monocytes) and CD13 (monocytes, neutrophils) expression with varying levels of maturation within the hematopoietic cells.

obtained during a prior bone marrow evaluation. The presence of CD13+/CD14- and CD13+/CD14+ cells is a characteristic finding in acute myelomonocytic leukemia.

2. **Most likely diagnosis:** *leukemic arthritis.*

   Any form of arthritis may occur in patients with leukemia. Therefore, the diagnosis of this condition may be difficult, and prior to considering leukemic arthritis as the cause of joint swelling in a patient with leukemia, infectious and crystalline forms of arthritis must be excluded. Moreover, the type and severity of the leukemia,

the therapy, and its effect on the immune system significantly influence the differential diagnosis. In clinical practice, joint infections and crystal-induced arthritis are observed more frequently than leukemic arthritis.[1-4]

3. Arthritis is a well-known complication of leukemia in both children and adults.[5,6] Seward reported the first case in 1930.[7] Since then, many case reports and series have been published. Arthritis is rarely an initial manifestation of acute leukemia in adults. However, in children with arthritis, leukemia is an important consideration and should be excluded since failure to diagnose

leukemic arthritis may be associated with a significant delay in treatment.[5,8] The prevalence of leukemic arthritis in relation to specific types of leukemia is unknown. However, arthritis is more frequently a complication of childhood than adult leukemia, where the incidence varies between 12% to 65% in children versus 4% to 13% in adults.[9,10]

4. One or more painful and swollen joints. Moreover, the signs and symptoms of leukemic arthritis may appear before, after, or concurrent with the diagnosis of leukemia.[5,11,12] Arthritis is commonly asymmetric, pauciarticular, and may be either insidious or of sudden onset. Its manifestations may be additive or migratory and most frequently large joints are involved; however, other joints may also be involved.[9,13] In addition, joint pain may be intermittent or persistent and the severity of the pain is frequently out of proportion to the observed inflammation.[5] Bone pain in leukemia is caused by expansion of the marrow compartment. Since the ends of bones are within joint capsules, such bone pain may not be readily associated with leukemic arthritis. In leukemic arthritis, however, effusion is a frequent accompaniment.

5. Synovial infiltration by leukemic cells is considered the predominant pathogenic mechanism for the occurrence of leukemic arthritis. This mechanism is supported by the observation that leukemic arthritis subsides as the disease remits and reappears as the disease relapses.[10] Other possible mechanisms include a synovial reaction to periosteal or capsular infiltration, hemarthrosis, and immune complex-induced synovitis. Recently, an increased amount of interleukin-1 beta (IL-1β) secreted by an over-expanded B cell clone in the synovium has been reported and may contribute to the resulting joint destruction.[14]

6. The gold standard for the diagnosis of leukemic arthritis is the demonstration of malignant cells in a synovial biopsy.[9,15,16] However, as in this case, joint fluid analysis for leukemic cells is also invaluable.[2,5,17-21] Indirect immunofluorescent assay (IFA) techniques utilizing monoclonal antibodies to leukemia cell antigens have also been used successfully.[5,18-21] In addition, flow cytometry is considered by some to be more

accurate than IFA methods because it provides a specific profile of leukemic cells and false negative synovial biopsies may be observed in cases with a patchy cellular infiltrate.[5,17] Prior to considering leukemic arthritis as the cause of joint swelling in a patient with leukemia, infectious and crystalline forms of arthritis must be excluded. Moreover, serologic tests for antinuclear antibodies and rheumatoid factor are noncontributory and X-ray findings are non-specific.[11]

7. Nonsteroidal anti-inflammatory drugs (NSAIDs) can help alleviate the symptoms of leukemic arthritis.[4,22] Intra-articular steroid injections have also been found to be safe and effective for alleviating symptoms in patients with osteoarthritis of the knee[23]; however, the value of intra-articular steroid injection for the relief of symptoms of leukemic arthritis has not been clearly established.[5] Nevertheless, such treatment may be beneficial, since IL-1β mediated, or other immunologic mechanisms may play a role in the etiology of this disease. In addition, many patients respond to chemotherapy for their underlying disease,[1,19] and radiation therapy has been useful in refractory cases.[5]

Treatment and Course

Treatment of our patient with chemotherapy, intra-articular methylprednisolone acetate (Depo-Medrol) injection, and analgesics resulted in rapid resolution of his symptoms.

Keywords

leukemic arthritis, crystal-induced arthritis, acute myelogenous leukemia, interleukin-1 beta

References

1. Costello PB, Brecher ML, Starr JI, et al. A prospective analysis of the frequency, course, and possible prognostic significance of the joint manifestations of childhood leukemia. *J Rheumatol.* 1983;10:753-757.

2. Luzar MJ, Sharma HM. Leukemia and arthritis: Including reports on light, immunofluorescent and electron microscopy of the synovium. *J Rheumatol.* 1983;10:132-135.

3. Isenberg DA, Shoenfeld Y. The rheumatologic complications of hematologic disorders. *Semi Arth Rheum*. 1983;12:348-358.

4. Silverstein MN, Kelly P. Leukemia with osteoarticular symptoms and signs. *Ann Intern Med*. 1963;59:637-645.

5. Evans TI, Nercessian BM, Sanders KM. Leukemic arthritis. *Semin Arthritis Rheum*. 1994;24:48-56.

6. Seda H, Alarcon GS. Musculoskeletal syndromes associated with malignancies. *Curr Opin Rheumatol*. 1995;7:48-53.

7. Seward BP. Lymphatic leukemia with severe pains in the joints. *Med J Rec*. 1930;131:444-446.

8. Cimaz R, Lippi A, Falcini F. Elbow arthritis: A rare inaugural manifestation of acute leukemia. *Rev Rhum Engl Ed*. 1999;66:520-522.

9. Spilberg I, Meyer GJ. The arthritis of leukemia. *Arthritis Rheum*. 1972;15:630-635.

10. Thomas LB, Forkner CE, Frei E, et al. The skeleton lesions of acute leukemia. *Cancer*. 1961;14:608-621.

11. Cabral DA, Tucker LB. Malignancies in children who initially present with rheumatic complaints. *J Pediatr*. 1999;134:53-57.

12. Taylor HG, Davis MJ, Hothersall TE. Hairy cell leukemia and rheumatoid arthritis. *Br J Rheumatol*. 1991;30:391-392.

13. Gagnerie F, Taillan B, Euller-Ziegler L, et al. Arthritis of the knees in B cell chronic lymphocytic leukemia: A patient with immunologic evidence of B lymphocytic synovial infiltration. *Arthritis Rheum*. 1988;31:815-816.

14. Rudwaleit M, Elias F, Humaljoki T, et al. Overexpanded B-cell clone mediating leukemic arthritis by abundant secretion of interleukin-1 beta: A case report. *Arthritis Rheum*. 1998;41:1695-1700.

15. Fort JG, Fernandez C, Jacobs SR, et al. B cell surface marker analysis of synovial fluid cells in a patient with monoarthritis and chronic lymphocytic leukemia. *J Rheumatol*. 1992;19:481-484.

16. Traycoff RB, Pascual E, Schumacher HR. Mononuclear cells in human synovial fluid. Identification of lymphoblasts in rheumatoid arthritis. *Arthritis Rheum*. 1976;19:743-748.

17. Sanders KM, Nercessian BM, Todd WM, et al. Leukemic arthritis diagnosed by flow cytometry of synovial fluid. *J Rheumatol*. 1993;20:1621.

18. Harden EA, Moore JO, Haynes BF. Leukemia-associated arthritis: Identification of leukemic cells in synovial fluid using monoclonal and polyclonal antibodies. *Arthritis Rheum*. 1984;27:1306-1308.

19. Schaller JG. Arthritis as a presenting manifestation of malignancy in children. *J Pediatr*. 1972;81:793-797.

20. Gramatzki M, Burmester GR, Konig HJ, et al. Synovial fluid involvement in null cell acute lymphoblastic leukemia diagnosed with monoclonal antibodies. *J Rheumatol*. 1988;15:500-504.

21. Fam AG, Voorneveld C, Robinson JB, et al. Synovial fluid immunocytology in the diagnosis of leukemic synovitis. *J Rheumatol*. 1991;18:293-296.

22. Weinberger A, Schumacher HR, Schimmer B, et al. Arthritis in acute leukemia. Clinical and histopathological observations. *Arch Intern Med*. 1981;141:1183-1187.

23. Raynauld JP, Buchland-Wright C, Ward R, et al. Safety and efficacy of long-term intra-articular steroid injection in osteoarthritis of the knee: A randomized double-blind, placebo-controlled trial. *Arthritis Rheum*. 2003;48:370-377.

"CRAB" Findings in a Patient With Fatigue and a History of Poor Appetite

Mandolin Ziadie, Frank H. Wians, Jr.

Department of Pathology, The University of Texas Southwestern Medical Center, Dallas, TX

Patient: 52-year-old African-American female.

Chief Complaint: None; the patient was seen for follow-up of a recent stem cell transplant. The patient denied any major symptoms (eg, bone pain, poor appetite); however, she reported minimal fatigue and poor appetite that had only recently returned to normal.

History of Present Illness: Two years prior to this most recent clinic visit, the patient had presented to the emergency department with flu-like symptoms and was found to have normocytic/normochromic anemia. The work-up that followed included serum (SPE) and urine (UPE) protein electrophoresis, immunofixation electrophoresis (IFE), a bone marrow biopsy and examination, and imaging studies of the axial skeleton. SPE revealed the presence of an M-spike in the gamma-region of the gel at a concentration of 6.4 g/dL. IFE, performed on the patient's serum, demonstrated the presence of an IgG kappa monoclonal immunoglobulin (Figure 1A). SPE of a sample from the patient's 24-hour urine collection demonstrated an M-spike, subsequently identified by IFE as IgG kappa. Microscopic examination of the patient's stained bone marrow biopsy demonstrated the presence of aberrant plasma cells constituting 64% of all cells observed in the bone marrow. Imaging studies of her axial skeleton revealed lytic lesions in both humeri and femurs, and in the skull, a compression fracture of the T12 vertebra, and a plasmacytoma in her left-side sixth rib. Laboratory testing revealed normal serum electrolytes, calcium, and creatinine levels. The patient started a prolonged chemotherapeutic regimen that included 3 cycles of vincristine, adriamycin, and dexamethasone (VAD), combination therapy with Thalidomide and Decadron, and Decadron maintenance therapy. Each regimen provided only a short-term reduction in the size of her serum M-spike and in her urine free light chain excretion rate. As a prelude to an autologous stem cell transplant, the patient underwent a repeat bone marrow biopsy, SPE, and UPE. The bone marrow biopsy demonstrated 27% aberrant plasma cells, while the SPE again showed an M-spike consistent with IgG kappa (0.38 g/dL); however, the UPE of a sample from a 24-hour urine collection was negative for any intact or free light chain immunoglobulins (data not shown). The patient underwent stem cell mobilization followed by bone marrow myeloablation using high-dose melphalan therapy and stem cell transfusion. She tolerated the procedure well, requiring only administration of packed red blood cells and platelets to maintain an adequate cell count of these formed elements while engraftment was occurring.

Past Medical History: Hypertension, community-acquired pneumonia, and hip repair with insertion of bilateral intramedullary nails. The patient had no known drug allergies and was currently taking: Bactrim DS (1 tablet po bid every Saturday and Sunday); Acyclovir (400 mg bid); Protonix (40 mg qd); Norvasc (5 mg qd); potassium chloride (20 mEq qd).

Family/Social History: The patient's father died of colon cancer; she had no family history of any hematologic malignancies. She denied use of alcohol, tobacco, or drugs of abuse.

Physical Examination: The patient appeared comfortable and in no acute distress. No abnormal findings were noted on complete physical examination.

T1. Principal Post-Stem Cell Transplantation Laboratory Findings

Test	Patient's Result	"Normal" Reference Range
Hematology		
WBC count	4.1	4.1-10.9 × 10³/μL
Hemoglobin	11.5	12.0-15.2 g/dL
Hematocrit	35.1	37-46%
Platelet count	38	140-450 × 10³/μL
Bone marrow exam	Occasional (2%) atypical plasma cells of insufficient number to be considered neoplastic	
Chemistry		
Calcium	9.6	8.4-10.2 mg/dL
Creatinine	0.8	0.6-1.2 mg/dL
Special Chemistry		
SPEP	Multiple M-spikes present in gamma-region	
Serum IFE	Consistent with presence of monoclonal IgG kappa (2 distinct subtypes), IgG lambda, and free lambda light chains (Figure 1B)	

WBC, white blood cell; SPEP, serum protein electrophoresis pattern; IFE immunofixation electrophoresis.

T2. Diagnostic Criteria for Diagnosis of Multiple Myeloma[a] (MM)[2]

Criterion	Characteristic
1	BM mPCs ≥10% and/or biopsy-proven plasmacytoma[b]
2	Monoclonal protein (M-protein) in serum and/or urine[c]
3	Myeloma-related organ dysfunction (≥1 "CRAB" finding):
	Serum [Ca²⁺] > 10.5 g/dL or > ULN
	Serum [creatinine] >2 mg/dL
	[Hb] < 10 g/dL or 2 g/dL < LLN
	Lytic bone lesions or osteoporosis without fractures[b]

[a]*All 3 criteria must be met.*
[b]*If sole defining criterion, ≥30% monoclonal plasma cells (mPCs) required in bone marrow (BM).*
[c]*If no M-protein detected (non-secretory MM), ≥30% monoclonal plasma cells (mPCs) required in bone marrow (BM). CRAB, hypercalcemia-renal dysfunction-anemia-lytic bone lesions; ULN, upper limit of normal; Hb, hemoglobin; LLN, lower limit of normal.*

Questions

1. What is this patient's most likely diagnosis?

2. What are the diagnostic criteria associated with this patient's disorder?

3. What other disorders should be included in the differential diagnosis of a patient with an M-spike by SPE?

4. What are the criteria for the clinical and laboratory evaluation of patients with monoclonal gammopathies?

5. What is the most striking finding among this patient's post-stem cell transplant laboratory findings?

T3. Guidelines for the Clinical and Laboratory Evaluation of Monoclonal Gammopathies[a]

Guideline (G) No.	Topic	Recommendation
G1	SPE and UPE	Perform serum and urine HRE[b] for all patients suspected of having a PCD; quantify level of any M-protein by densitometry
G2	IFE	Perform IFE[c] to define abnormal M-protein type
G3	Densitometry	Follow M-protein concentration by densitometry[d]
G4	Nephelometry	Direct measurement of Ig's by nephelometry is indicated at diagnosis of PCD; however, nephelometry should not be used to screen patients for an M-protein
G5	Urine protein excretion rate	Quantify daily urinary excretion of monoclonal free light chains: • In all patients with MM, WG, amyloidosis, and related disorders • Use a ≥100× concentration aliquot from a 24-h urine collection • Type the light chains by IFE
G6	Frequency of SPE/UPE/IFE testing	Monitor changes in serum or urine M-protein levels by HRE at intervals of: • 1-2 months for patients being treated for MM, WM, or amyloidosis • Every year for patient with low level MGUS
G7	Hyperviscosity syndrome	Perform serum viscosity measurement and SPE prior to first plasma exchange to correlate M-protein level with degree of hyperviscosity and clinical symptoms; use the level to anticipate need for repeat plasma exchange
G8	Cryoglobulins	Assess in all patients with an M-protein and specific complications due to cold sensitivity, especially in patients with a monoclonal IgM M-component
G9	Techniques for evaluating M-proteins	To evaluate M-protein, use HRE, IFE, ISELECT,[e] and/or ISUBTRACT

[a]Adapted from Ref 4. [b]HRE, high resolution electrophoresis (gel- or capillary-based). [c]IFE not indicated in obvious cases of polyclonal gammopathy; however, it may be indicated when there is asymmetry of a polyclonal elevation.
[d]And at diagnosis to define the level of "uninvolved" immunoglobulins. [e]For identification of heavy-chain disease.[5]
SPE, serum protein electrophoresis; UPE, urine protein electrophoresis; IFE, immunofixation electrophoresis; Ig's, immunoglobulins; PCD, plasma cell dyscrasia; MM, multiple myeloma; WG, waldenström macroglobulinemia; ISELECT, immunoselection; ISUBTRACT, immunosubtraction.

6. How do you explain this finding?

7. What is the significance of this finding?

8. Does this finding have any impact on the patient's prognosis?

9. What is the standard therapy for this patient's disorder?

Possible Answers _____

1. ***Most likely diagnosis:*** *multiple myeloma.* Multiple myeloma is defined as a clonal proliferation of aberrant bone marrow plasma cells accompanied by monoclonal protein production and destructive bone lesions.[1]

2. The most common clinical manifestations of multiple myeloma are summarized by the acronym, "CRAB": hyper**c**alcemia, **r**enal dysfunction

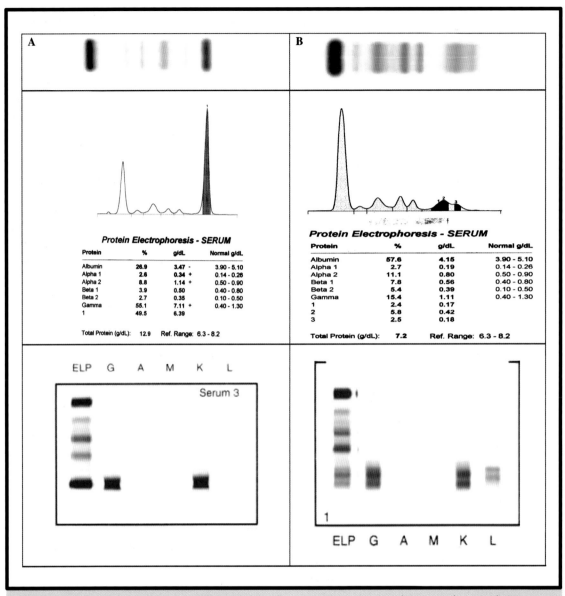

Figure 1_Patient's prior (**A**) and most recent (**B**) SPEP (top panel), densitometric tracing/report (middle panel), and IFE (bottom panel), demonstrating the presence of an M-spike in the gamma-region (**A**; top and middle panels) of the IgG kappa type (**A**; bottom panel), and the presence of M-spikes in the gamma-region (**B**; top and middle panels) consisting of the IgG kappa (2 distinct subtypes), IgG lambda, and free lambda light chain types (**B**, bottom panel). IFE, immunofixation electrophoresis; ELP, electrophoresis lane; G, immunoglobulin G (IgG) antiserum lane; A, immunoglobulin A (IgA) antiserum lane; M, immunoglobulin M (IgM) antiserum lane; k, free kappa light chain antiserum lane; L, free lambda light chain antiserum lane.

(ie, increased serum creatinine concentration), **a**nemia, and lytic **b**one lesions.[2] The most recent diagnostic criteria for multiple myeloma are summarized in **T2**.[2]

3. Although monoclonal protein spikes (M-spikes) are most often seen upon SPE or UPE of serum or urine from patients with a plasma cell dyscrasia, they can also be seen upon SPE of serum and/or urine from patients with lymphoma, carcinoma, chronic infections, solitary and multiple plasmacytomas, plasma cell leukemia, amyloidosis, smoldering (or indolent) myeloma, and monoclonal gammo-pathy of undetermined significance (MGUS).[2,3] Interestingly, non-secretory multiple myeloma is

associated with an absence of an M-spike(s) by SPE, UPE, or IFE.

4. In 1999, a panel of experts published 9 guidelines for the clinical and laboratory evaluation of patients with monoclonal gammopathies[4] that are summarized in **T3**.

5. Despite the fact that the patient had no evidence of residual disease on examination of her bone marrow, she continued to have an abnormal serum protein electrophoresis pattern (SPEP). Moreover, the SPEP originally seen on electrophoresis of her serum had changed significantly from a single IgG kappa M-protein to an oligoclonal pattern consisting of IgG kappa, IgG lambda, and free lambda light chains. It is likely that the patient's markedly decreased platelet count and modestly decreased hemoglobin and hematocrit values (**T1**) were due to continued bone marrow recovery following melphalan therapy and stem cell transplantation.

6. Transient oligoclonal (ie, >2 M-protein bands on SPEP) and monoclonal gammopathies occur in at least 50% of all patients after stem cell transplant and in at least 10% of patients with multiple myeloma treated with stem cell transplant.[3,6] These bands have been shown to appear between 2 to 6 months post-stem cell transplant and persist on SPEPs for an average of 6 months.[3]

7. When oligoclonal bands or a monoclonal band with a different immunophenotype than the band observed initially are observed, the differential diagnosis includes a change in M-protein production by the original plasma cell clone, the emergence of a second malignant clone, or the evidence for immune system regeneration following stem cell transplant therapy. To date, most studies favor the latter hypothesis; the bands represent a benign phenomenon associated with the recovery of immune function in patients who have received a stem cell transplant with or without myeloablative bone marrow therapy prior to stem cell transplantation.[3,6-8]

8. One study of patients with multiple myeloma who were treated with stem cell transplantation, with or without prior myeloablation, revealed a significant relationship between the appearance of abnormal protein bands by SPE and IFE after transplantation and a higher likelihood of positive clinical response, event-free survival, and overall survival.[6]

9. For more than 2 decades, the standard therapy for patients with symptomatic multiple myeloma has included a wide variety of chemotherapeutic regimens. The most commonly used regimens include combined melphalan and prednisone therapy and the combination of vincristine, adriamycin, and dexamethasone (VAD).[1] Such treatments are associated with a median survival of 2 to 3 years. Other chemotherapeutic regimens, which have been used as both frontline and relapse therapies, include pulse dexamethasone and combined therapy with thalidomide and dexamethasone.[1] Unfortunately, almost all patients who initially respond to chemotherapy eventually relapse. In recent years, high-dose chemotherapy followed by autologous stem cell transplantation has become an important alternative frontline treatment for younger patients (<70 years) as well as a rescue therapy for patients who relapse after chemotherapy. This treatment achieves higher complete response rates compared to chemotherapy alone. Prolonged survival (>6 years), however, remains rare.[9]

Keywords

plasma cell dyscrasia, multiple myeloma, M-protein, vincristine-adriamycin-dexamethasone (VAD), stem cell transplant, oligoclonal bands

References

1. Hoffman R, Benz Jr. EJ, Shattil SJ, et al, eds. *Hematology: Basic Principles and Practice.* 4th ed. Philadelphia, PA: Elsevier, Inc. 2005:1398-1410.

2. Durie BGM, Kyle RA, Belch A, Bensinger W, et al. Myeloma management guidelines: A consensus report from the Scientific Advisors of the International Myeloma Foundation. *The Hematology J.* 2003;4:379-398.

3. Alexanian R, Weber D, Liu F. Differential diagnosis of monoclonal gammopathies. *Arch Pathol Lab Med.* 1999;123:108-113.

4. Keren DF, Alexanian R. Goeken JA, et al. Guidelines for clinical and laboratory evaluation of patients with monoclonal gammopathies. *Arch Pathol Lab Med.* 1999;123:106-107.

5. Chan MHM, Cheung RCK, Lam CWK. Test and teach. Laboratory characterisation of paraproteins, Part 1. *Pathology.* 2001;33:379-381.

6. Zent CS, Wilson CS, Tricot G, et al. Oligoclonal bands and Ig isotype switching in multiple myeloma treated with high-dose therapy and hematopoietic cell transplantation. *Blood.* 1998;91:3518-3523.

7. Mitus AJ, Stein R, Rappeport JM, et al. Monoclonal and oligoclonal gammapathy after bone marrow transplantation. *Blood.* 1989;74:2764-2768.

8. Gerritsen EJA, van Tol MJD, Lankester AC, et al. Immunoglobulin levels and monoclonal gammopathies in children after bone marrow transplantation. *Blood.* 1993;82:3493-3502.

9. Abeloff MD, Armitage JO, Niederhuber JE, et al, eds. *Clinical Oncology.* 3rd ed. Philadelphia, PA: Elsevier, Inc. 2004:2968-2969.

A Large Skull Mass in a 67-Year-Old Woman

Cynthia Rutherford[1] Frank H. Wians, Jr.[2]

Departments of [1]Internal Medicine and [2]Pathology, UT Southwestern Medical Center, Dallas, TX

Patient: 67-year-old woman.

Chief Complaint: She noticed a firm mass on the vortex of her scalp that had slowly increased in size for the past 7 to 8 months.

History of Present Illness: She had been well previously with no history of recurrent infections or bone pain.

Past Medical History: She had a 20-year history of hypertension; arteriopathy, having previously undergone a carotid endarterectomy and femoro-popliteal bypass surgery.

Current Medications: Amlodipine, benazepril, and hydrochlorothiazide for hypertension; clopidogrel and aspirin for arterial disease.

Family History: Her mother died at age 78 of a stroke; she also had hypertension. Her father was a smoker and died of lung cancer at age 70. One of her 2 sisters died at age 43 of alcoholic cirrhosis, while the other died at age 78 of diabetes and chronic heart failure. She has 3 children, including 2 daughters–one with hypertension and the other healthy.

Social History: Married, with a very supportive family; moderately heavy (1 pack/day for 40 to 50 years) smoker and drinker (2 glasses of liquor/day).

Physical Examination Findings: All vital signs were within normal limits; her blood pressure was well controlled; no significantly abnormal findings on review of systems; and she had no evidence of bruits or arterial insufficiency.

Results of Additional Diagnostic Procedures: A skull X-ray revealed a large skull defect and a computed tomography (CT) scan of the head demonstrated a 5×7 cm intra- and extra-cranial mass (tumor). The tumor was surgically removed with tumor free margins, examined histologically, and shown to be a monoclonal plasmacytoma with lambda light chain restriction. During her post-surgery hospitalization, she underwent a bone marrow biopsy, a skeletal survey, hematology and chemistry tests (**T1**), and serum (**Figure 1A**) and urine (**Figure 1B**) protein electrophoresis. The skeletal survey demonstrated only the skull lesion with no evidence of additional bone lytic lesions.

She continued to do well following the surgery to remove the plasmacytoma and her follow-up therapy included radiation of the skull and, 6 months later, repair of her skull defect. Six months after this repair, she maintained normal hematocrit, calcium, and creatinine values; however, her β-2-microglobulin (β2-MG) level increased slowly over the 1-year period following her initial presentation. A repeat skeletal survey performed 1-year after her initial presentation demonstrated no lytic bone lesions.

Because the patient complained of aches and pains in her lower back and right hip, a magnetic resonance imaging (MRI) scan of her pelvis and lumbo-sacral spine was performed and demonstrated extensive involvement by tumor, with some bony destruction, despite the unremarkable skeletal survey. Hydrocodone was prescribed for bone pain. She continued to maintain normal hemoglobin, serum calcium, and renal function; however, her β2-MG concentration increased to 3.8 mg/L (reference range: 0.8-2.2 mg/L), serum lambda free light chain (FLC) concentration increased significantly to 772 mg/L from the level measured at diagnosis [43.7 mg/L (reference range: 5.7-26.3 mg/L); kappa:lambda ratio = 0.01 (reference range: 0.26-1.65)], and small monoclonal bands were observed in both her serum and urine (24 h collection) protein electrophoresis patterns [SPEP, **Figure 2A**; UPEP, **Figure 2B**] that were not suitable for monitoring her response to treatment.

T1. Principal Laboratory Findings

Test		Patient's Reference	Result Interval
Hematology			
WBC count		5.7	4.1-11.1 × 10³/µL
Hemoglobin		14.3	13.2-16.9 g/dL
Hematocrit		43	36.8-48.7%
Platelet count		343	174-404 × 10³/µL
Bone marrow biopsy, mPCs		16	1-4%
Chemistry			
Calcium		9.9	8.4-10.2 mg/dL
Uric acid		7.0	2.6-6.0 mg/dL
Creatinine		0.8	0.6-1.2 mg/dL
BUN		14	7-17 mg/dL
Total protein		7.0	6.3-8.2 g/dL
Albumin		4.5	3.5-5.8 g/dL
Special Chemistry			
Protein electrophoresis:	Serum	See **Figure 1A**	No M-component present
			Normal electrophoretic pattern
	Urine	See **Figure 1B**	
Quantitative Ig's:	IgG	533	694-1618 mg/dL
	IgA	165	68-378 mg/dL
	IgM	<25	60-263 mg/dL
Free kappa light chains, serum		0.44	3.3-19.4 mg/L
Free lambda light chains, serum		43.7	5.7-26.3 mg/L
Kappa/lambda ratio		0.01	0.26-1.65
Beta-2-microglobulin		2.2	0.8-2.2 mg/L

WBC, white blood cell; mPCs, monoclonal plasma cells; Ig's, immunoglobulins; UA, urinalysis; M-component, monoclonal component.

T2. Criteria for Classifying Various Plasma Cell Dyscrasias[a]

Criterion	Type of Plasma Cell Dyscrasia				
	MM	NSM	MGUS	SM	SPB
Bone Marrow (BM) Monoclonal Plasma Cells					
Present in BM and/or tissue biopsy at any level				+	
<10%			+		+
≥10%	+	+			
≥30%	+b	+b			
Biopsy-Proven Plasmacytoma					
Present	+	+	+b	+	+b
Present in bone at a single site only				−	+c
Monoclonal Protein in Serum and/or Urine					
Present at any level	+	−	+	+	
Low [M–protein]: [IgG]serum <3.0 g/dL or <3.5 g/dL (SPB only) [IgA]serum <2.0 g/dL [κ or λ]urine <1.0 g/24h			+		±
Myeloma-Related Organ Dysfunction[d]					
BM plasmacytosis and SPB only				−	+
[Calcium]serum, [Creat]serum, and [Hb] all WNL; no bone lesions on full skeletal X-ray survey and/or other imaging studies			+	−	
≥1 "CRAB" Finding: **C**alcium[serum] >10.5 mg/dL or ULN	±	±	−	±	−
Renal insufficiency ([Creat]serum >2 mg/dL)	±	±	−	±	−
Anemia ([Hb]<10 g/dL or 2 g/dL<LLN)	±	±	−	±	−
Lytic **B**one lesions or osteoporosis w/o fractures	±	±	+b	±	+b
Clinical or Laboratory Features of Amyloidosis or Light–Chain Deposition Disease Absent			+		

[a]Adapted from Reference 1. [b]If a solitary, biopsy–proven plasmacytoma or osteoporosis alone without (w/o) fractures is the sole defining criterion, then ≥30% plasma cells are required in the bone marrow. [c]X–rays and MRI and/or FDG PET scans, if performed, must be negative outside the primary site. [d]Other types of end organ dysfunction can support classification as myeloma if proven to be myeloma related.

+, present; −, absent; ±, may be present or absent.

MM, multiple myeloma; NSM, non–secretory myeloma; MGUS, monoclonal gammopathy of undetermined significance; SM, smoldering (or indolent) myeloma; SPB, solitary plasmacytoma of bone; BM, bone marrow; Creat, creatinine; Hb, hemoglobin; M–protein, monoclonal protein; k, kappa free light chains; l, lambda free light chains; WNL, within normal limits; ULN, upper limit of normal; LLN, lower limit of normal; w/o, without; MRI, magnetic resonance imaging; FDG, fluorodeoxyglucose; PET, positron emission tomography.

T3. Staging of Multiple Myeloma According to the IMWG Criteria[a]

Criterion		Stage	Median Survival, Months post-D$_x$
[β2-MG], mg/L	[Albumin], g/dL		
<3.5	>3.5	I	62
Not meeting criteria for Stages I or III		II	44
>5.5	n.a.	III	29

[a]Adapted from Reference 4. IMWG, International Myeloma Working Group; β2-MG, beta-2-microglobulin; Dx, diagnosis; n.a., not applicable.

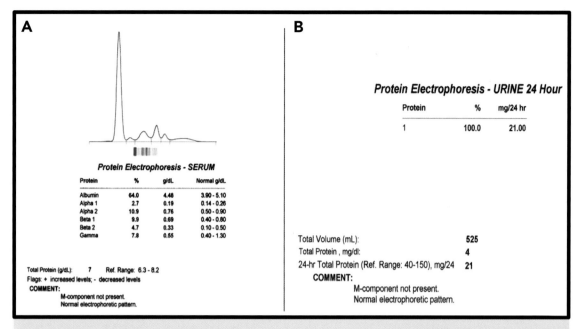

Figure 1_Patient's initial serum (SPEP) and urine (UPEP) protein electrophoretic patterns, illustrating (**A**) a normal total protein concentration (7.0 g/dL) and no visible M-component in the SPEP and (**B**) a normal UPEP from a 24 h urine specimen with a normal total protein concentration (21 mg/24 h) and no visible M-component in the UPEP.

Questions _____

1. What is (are) this patient's most striking *initial* clinical and laboratory finding(s)?

2. How do you explain these findings?

3. What is this patient's most likely diagnosis?

4. What is the stage of this patient's disorder?

5. What are the typical serum and/or urine electrophoretic findings in individuals with this patient's disorder?

6. Are measurements of free light chains (FLCs) in serum and/or urine useful in the diagnosis of individuals with this patient's disorder?

7. Based on her subsequent electrophoretic findings, 1 year after initial diagnosis, why was there no discrete band of restricted mobility observed in the gamma-region of the patient's SPEP (**Figure 2A**), while the patient's UPEP (**Figure 2B**) and serum and urine immunofixation electrophoresis patterns (IFEPs) all demonstrated easily visible discrete bands

in the gamma-region of the UPEP and in the lambda light chain antiserum lanes of the serum (**Figure 2A**) and urine (**Figure 2B**) IFEPs?

8. How should this patient's disorder be treated?

9. How should this patient's response to therapy be monitored?

10. Is this patient a candidate for a peripheral blood stem cell transplant?

Possible Answers _____

1. A large skull tumor with pathology demonstrating a monoclonal plasmacytoma with intracellular lambda-chain staining; a large bony defect in the skull, but no additional lytic bone lesions; bone marrow plasmacytosis; no serum or urine M-component by electrophoresis; no hypercalcemia; no abnormal renal function tests; decreased serum IgG and IgM concentrations; increased β2-microglobulin level.

2. A solitary plasmacytoma of bone and bone marrow plasmacytosis >10% are pathognomonic of a plasma cell dyscrasia (PCD). Recently, Durie

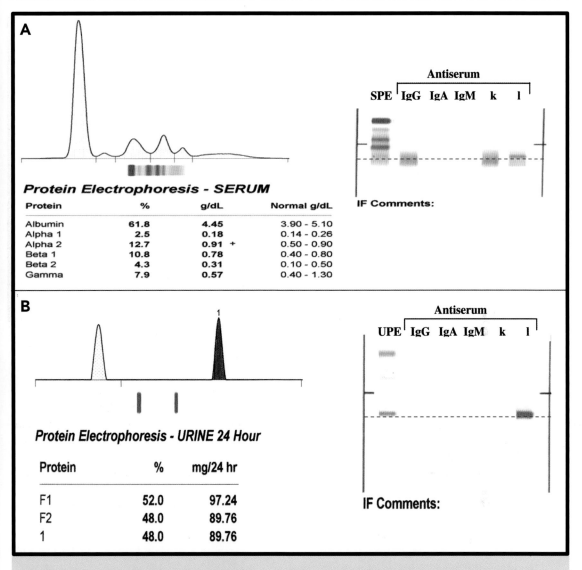

A

Protein Electrophoresis - SERUM

Protein	%	g/dL	Normal g/dL
Albumin	61.8	4.45	3.90 - 5.10
Alpha 1	2.5	0.18	0.14 - 0.26
Alpha 2	12.7	0.91 +	0.50 - 0.90
Beta 1	10.8	0.78	0.40 - 0.80
Beta 2	4.3	0.31	0.10 - 0.50
Gamma	7.9	0.57	0.40 - 1.30

IF Comments:

B

Protein Electrophoresis - URINE 24 Hour

Protein	%	mg/24 hr
F1	52.0	97.24
F2	48.0	89.76
1	48.0	89.76

IF Comments:

Figure 2_Patient's serum (SPEP) and urine (UPEP) protein electrophoretic patterns approximately 1 year after initial presentation, illustrating no visible M-component in the SPEP (**A**) and a single distinct band in the lambda (l) light chain antiserum lane of the immunofixation (IF) electrophoresis pattern (IFEP) (dotted red line), and a discrete band (peak 1) in the UPEP (**B**) from a 24 h urine specimen and a distinct band in the lambda (l) light chain antiserum lane that corresponds with a discrete band in the UPE lane of the IFEP (dotted red line). The lambda free light chain urinary excretion rate is approximately 90 mg/24 h.

and colleagues[1] presented the results of a consensus report on myeloma management, including a standardized approach for classifying various PCDs [ie, multiple myeloma (MM), non-secretory myeloma (NSM), monoclonal gammopathy of undetermined significance (MGUS), smoldering myeloma (SM), and solitary plasmacytoma of bone (SPB)] and for staging myeloma (**T2**). The criteria for classifying PCDs include 1 or more of the following findings: hypercalcemia,

renal dysfunction (based on increased creatinine concentration), anemia (based on decreased hemoglobin concentration), and the presence or absence of lytic bone lesions. The tetrad of findings relevant to these criteria have been summarized by the acronym, "CRAB," (hyper**C**alcemia-**R**enal dysfunction-**A**nemia-Lytic **B**one lesions) (**T2**).[1]

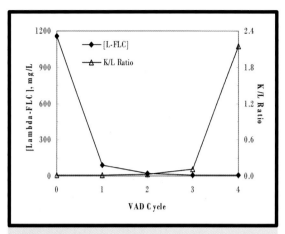

Figure 3_Changes in patient's serum lambda free light chain (L-FLC) concentration and kappa/lambda (K/L) FLC ratio following treatment with vincristine-adriamycin-dexamethasone (VAD).

3. ***Most likely diagnosis:*** *an "apparent" non-secretory myeloma (NSM).* In our patient, all 3 criteria of the current Durie classification scheme for PCDs were met for NSM (**T1**). Our patient had (1) monoclonal plasma cells in the bone marrow[3] 10% and a biopsy-proven plasmacytoma; (2) no monoclonal protein present in the serum and urine, but a biopsy proven plasmactyoma; and (3) myeloma-related organ dysfunction (ie, MRI evidence of pelvic and lumbo-sacral spine tumor involvement with some bony destruction, despite normal skeletal survey findings and normal values for calcium, creatinine, and hemoglobin). Moreover, the plasmacytoma was shown by immunohistochemistry to consist of a population of plasma cells with intracellular staining for only lambda light chains. Monoclonal plasma cells from most patients with NSM are able to synthesize a monoclonal protein, but they are unable to secrete the monoclonal protein into the blood.[2,3] In addition, a small subset of patients (approximately 10% to 15%) with NSM are non-producers of monoclonal protein and their tumor plasma cells contain no detectable immunoglobulins.[3] Non-secretory myeloma accounts for only 1% to 5% of all patients with MM.[2]

4. Although several staging systems for MM have been reported,[1] the simplest of these is the system developed by the International Myeloma Working Group (IMWG)[4] using only serum $\beta2$-MG and albumin levels, to which median

survival data in months post diagnosis have been added (**T3**). Based on our patient's values for $\beta2$-MG (2.2 mg/L) and albumin (3.8 g/dL), and using the IMWG Staging System, our patient's MM stage is Stage 1 with a predicted median survival of 62 months (**T3**).

5. The serum and urine protein electrophoresis patterns in patients with NSM typically demonstrate an absence of monoclonal proteins by standard electrophoretic techniques (ie, SPE and UPE). However, using more analytically sensitive techniques [eg, isoelectric focusing (IEF) and immunofixation electrophoresis (IFE)], monoclonal proteins may be detected in the serum and/or urine from some patients with NSM. This case illustrates the importance of performing IFE on serum and/or urine in patients with a biopsy-proven plasmacytoma and normal SPEP and UPEP findings.

6. Yes. The recent advent of analytically sensitive and specific assays for the direct quantitative nephelometric measurement of kappa- and lambda-FLCs in serum or urine, and the use of the ratio of kappa:lambda FLCs, has reduced the number of patients falsely classified as NSM.[2] Because the peer-reviewed published evidence in support of the clinical utility of serum (and urine) FLC measurements in classifying PCDs has only been emerging recently, FLC criteria are not included in the PCD classification scheme of Durie.[1] Nevertheless, the FLC data [ie, serum positive for lambda-light chains by IFE, urine positive for Bence Jones protein (free lambda light chains), and a markedly reduced kappa/lambda ratio] for the patient presented in this case study are consistent with similar findings in a group of patients with NSM evaluated by Drayson and colleagues[5] using FLC measurements. Recently, Katzmann and colleagues[6] validated the diagnostic performance of nephelometric FLC assays in detecting FLC diseases.

7. Because of significant differences in the analytical sensitivity of SPE and UPE methods in detecting immunoglobulins compared to IFE. The analytical sensitivity of SPE and UPE for FLCs is approximately 500 to 2,000 mg/L and 10 to 20 mg/L, respectively. Urine protein electrophoretic techniques have higher sensitivity to FLCs than SPE because the urine sample is concentrated

25x to 200x, based on the urine total protein concentration. Therefore, SPE is particularly insensitive to the detection of low concentrations of FLCs. The combined (kappa + lambda) FLC concentration in the serum from our patient was approximately 60 mg/L (**T1**). In contrast to SPE, serum and urine IFE has approximately 10-fold higher analytical sensitivity [150 to 500 mg/L (or 200 mg/L by IFE versus 2,000 mg/L by SPE)] to FLCs than SPE. In contrast to SPE, UPE, and IFE methods, the analytical sensitivity of quantitative nephelometric assays for FLCs is 1.5 to 3.0 mg/L (or approximately 1,000- and 10-fold higher analytical sensitivity than SPE and IFE, respectively).[1]

8. Frontline treatment options for patients with multiple myeloma include[1]:

   • Thalidomide + dexamethasone*

   • VAD regimen**

   • Melphalan or other alkylating agents in combination with corticosteroids***

9. *Recently touted as a new standard of care for initial therapy in patients with multiple myeloma.[7] However, unresolved issues with this treatment include: the optimum thalidomide dose, increased risk of venous thromboembolism, necessitating prophylactic anticoagulation, and side effect profile including mental status changes and neuropathy.

   **VAD, vincristine-adriamycin (doxorubicin)- with pulse dexamathasone.

   ***Used in older patients or those who are not candidates for subsequent stem cell transplantation.

   The VAD regimen was selected for this patient, rather than thalidomide-dexamethasone, because of her arteriopathy and the known thrombotic risk with thalidomide-dexamethasone therapy.

   Approaches to monitoring response to therapy in patients with MM typically include following changes in the concentration of the major monoclonal protein in serum and/or urine with a reduction in monoclonal protein of >50%,

when coupled with other laboratory and clinical evidence of favorable response to therapy, regarded generally as the definition of "response" to therapy. It remains to be proven, however, if changes in serum free light chain levels are a similarly reliable measure of response to therapy, although they are quite widely used in clinical practice for this purpose, especially in patients with NSM where conventional paraprotein monitoring is not possible. Radiological studies are generally less helpful in monitoring treatment response. Although skeletal survey is helpful as an initial diagnostic test or to detect disease progression, lytic lesions do not usually show healing. Therefore, skeletal survey is not helpful in following response to therapy in patients with MM. MRI scans are more sensitive in detecting bone marrow infiltration and subtle bone destruction, which may be missed by skeletal survey, as it was in this patient, but MRI is not sufficiently sensitive enough to monitor treatment response. In contrast to MRI, fluoro-deoxyglucose positron emission tomography (FDG-PET) scanning can be very helpful in monitoring response to treatment in patients with MM. However, this imaging modality is expensive and has precluded its widespread use for this purpose. Because FDG-PET scanning measures tissue (tumor) activity, it can be used to monitor response to treatment, with successful response to therapy indicated when initially positive lesions become negative. Moreover, FDG-PET scanning provides a unique tool for evaluating response to therapy and relapse in patients with NSM.[8] The beneficial effects of 4 cycles of VAD chemotherapy in our patient are demonstrated by significant suppression of her serum free lambda light chain level from 1,160 mg/L immediately prior to treatment to approximately 4 mg/L after treatment and normalization of her serum K/L FLC ratio (**Figure 3**).

10. Yes. Autologous peripheral blood stem cell transplantation (PBSCT), while not curative, has been shown to prolong survival in patients with MM and is an integral component of therapy for eligible patients (ie, those with responsive disease who are less than 70 years of age and do not have co-morbid conditions). Because allogeneic bone marrow transplantation has such high morbidity and mortality in patients with MM, this treatment is confined to the research setting.[1]

Keywords

nonsecretory myeloma, plasmacytoma, free light chains, beta-2-microglobulin, fluorodeoxyglucose positron emission tomography, peripheral blood stem cell transplantation

References

1. Durie BGM, Kyle RA, Belch A, et al. Myeloma management guidelines: A consensus report from the Scientific Advisors of the International Myeloma Foundation. *Haematol J.* 2003;4:379-398.

2. Non-secretory myeloma. In: *Serum Free Light Chain Analysis,* Bradwell AR, Mead GP, Carr-Smith HD eds. Birmingham, UK; Drapkins & Co. 2004;79.

3. Raubenheimer EJ, Dauth J, Senekal JC. Non-secretory IgA k myeloma with distended endoplasmic reticulum: A case report. *Histology.* 1991;19:380-382.

4. Greipp RR, San Miguel JF, Fonseca R, et al. Development of an International Prognostic Index (IPI) for myeloma: Report of the International Myeloma Working Group. *Haematol J.* 2003;4(suppl 1);S43-S44.

5. Drayson MT, Tang LX, Drew R, et al. Serum free light-chain measurements for identifying and monitoring patients with nonsecretory multiple myeloma. *Blood.* 2001;97:2900-2902.

6. Katzmann JA, Abraham RS, Dispenzieri A, et al. Diagnostic performance of quantitative 6 and 8 free light chain assays in clinical practice. *Clin Chem.* 2005;51:878-881.

7. Richardson P, Anderson K. Thalidomide and dexamethasone: A new standard of care for initial therapy in multiple myeloma. *J Clin Oncology.* 2006;24:334-336.

8. Durie BGM, Waxman AD, D'Agnolo A, et al. Whole-body ^{18}F-FDG PET identifies high-risk myeloma. *J Nucl Med.* 2002;43:1457-1463.

Why Do I Still Have a Bruise Around My Knee?

Yiqing Chi,[1] Alberto Locante,[1] Valerie Lindgren,[1] Damiano Rondelli[2]
Syed A. Abutalib,[2] Sujata Gaitonde[1]
Departments of [1]Pathology and [2]Medicine, University of Illinois, Chicago

Patient: A 45-year-old African-American female.

Chief Complaint: The patient presented to the emergency department with the chief complaint of a bruise around her right knee, which occurred after a fall approximately 10 days prior to presentation.

History of Present Illness: In addition to her persistent right knee bruise, she reported fatigue and shortness of breath after mild exertion of approximately 3 months' duration.

Past Medical History: Non-smoker with no history of alcohol abuse and no chronic medical conditions.

Physical Examination: Vital signs: temperature, 36.6°C; heart rate, 119 beats /minute; respiratory rate, 19 per minute; blood pressure, 122/66 mm Hg. Pertinent physical examination findings included labile mood, sinus tachycardia, conjunctival pallor, and hepatomegaly (liver span of 10 cm).

Principal Laboratory Findings: See **T1**. The abnormal CBC and coagulopathy were of paramount concern and peripheral blood smear and mixing studies were performed. There was partial correction on mixing studies suggesting the presence of inhibitors.

Peripheral Blood Smear Findings: Anemia, leukocytosis, thrombocytopenia with 28% atypical cells with basophilic cytoplasm and occasional eccentrically-placed nucleus with fine chromatin and nucleoli (**Figure 1**).

Bone Marrow: Bone marrow aspirate and core biopsy demonstrated a hypercellular marrow diffusely infiltrated by blasts with irregular nuclear contour, basophilic cytoplasm, and prominent nucleoli (**Figure 2**). The CD138 immunohistochemical staining of the biopsy specimen highlighted the plasmablasts that are cytoplasmic kappa restricted (**Figure 3A, 3B,** and **3C**). The Ki-67 (proliferation index marker) was approximately 5%.

Flow Cytometry: Immunophenotypic analysis by flow cytometry demonstrated an abnormal plasma cell population expressing CD45 negative/CD19 negative/CD38 positive/CD138 positive/CD56 negative/kappa restricted immunophenotype (**Figure 4**).

Cytogenetic Study: Three (20%) of the cells examined were normal. The remaining 80% exhibited complex aberrations and contained 78 to 90 chromosomes, with most cells in the 78 to 83 (hypertriploid) range. A composite karyotype of 12 cells was generated with the aid of interphase fluorescence in situ hybridization (FISH) studies using probes for IGH (14q32)/CCND1 (11q13), IGH/FGFR3 (4p16), IGH/MAF (16q23), TP53 (17p13.1), D13S319 (13q14.3), CEP 9 (9 centromere), CEP 15 (15 centromere), and D5S23/D5S721 (5p15.2), all from Vysis/Abbott Molecular (Des Plaines, IL).

The karyotype, described with respect to triploidy, was: 78~90<3n>,XXX[12],+X[6], del(1)(p11p31)[12],der(?)t(1;?)(q12;?)[6], +2[5],+3[11],+4[7],+6[2],i(6)(p10)[4], +7[7],+7[4],+add(7)(p12)[4],add(8)(q24.3)[12], +add(8)(q24.3) [11],+9[10],-10[3],+11[12], +11[3],+12[4],-13[12],-14[12],+15[2], -16[12],i(16)(p10)[9],dup(16)(q11.1q21)[8], del(17)(q11.2)[12],+del(17)(q11.2)[11], +der(17)t(1;17)(q21;q25) [3],+der(17)t(1;17)[3], +18[7],+18[3],+19[8],-20[12],+21[7],+?dup(21)(q22q22)[12],+?dup(21)[11],-22[6], +22[2],+1~10mar[cp12] (**Figure 5A**). Salient among the abnormalities were gains of chromosomes 3, 7, 9, 11, and 19; structural abnormalities of chromosome 1; and relative loss of chromosome 13. Notably, FISH analysis using the IGH/MAF probes was positive for translocation (**Figure 5B**).

Additional Diagnostic Procedures: Computed tomography scan showed hepatomegaly and diffusely heterogeneous, moth-eaten appearance of the osseous structures with focal lytic lesions in T7 and L4 vertebral bodies (**Figure 6**). The echocardiogram showed normal cardiac function with an ejection fraction of 56%.

Follow-up of This Patient: The patient was treated with bortezomib, a proteasome inhibitor, liposomal doxorubicin, and steroids. Her renal failure improved in concordance with improvement in primary disease and dialysis was prevented. She developed severe dilated cardiomyopathy (CMP) precluding further treatment with lisosomal doxorubicin. Fortunately, CMP reversed with time. She is currently doing well and awaiting definitive treatment while on a new treatment regimen that includes cyclophosphamide, etoposide, cisplatin, and bortezomib. Thalidomide was held after a single cycle due to grade 3 reversible neuropathy.

Questions _____

1. What is this patient's most likely diagnosis and what are the diagnostic criteria for this disorder?

2. What are the usual clinical and laboratory findings in patients with this disorder?

3. How do you explain her coagulopathy?

4. What are the characteristic pathologic and immunophenotypic findings of this disorder?

5. What are the cytogenetic abnormalities associated with this patient's disorder and what is their prognostic relevance?

6. What is the prognosis of this disorder?

7. What is the treatment for this disorder?

Possible Answers _____

1. ***Most likely diagnosis:*** *primary plasma cell leukemia (PCL).* Plasma cell leukemia is a rare form of plasma cell dyscrasia, accounting for approximately 1% to 2% of all plasma cell neoplasms.[1] According to the World Health Organization (WHO) classification of hematopoietic neoplasms, PCL is diagnosed when circulating peripheral blood plasma cell counts exceed 2×10^9/L or greater than or equal to 20% of total peripheral blood white cells. It may occur at the

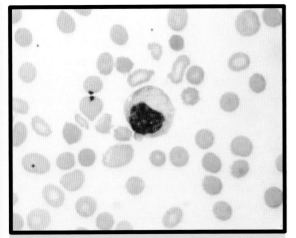

Figure 1_Peripheral blood with circulating atypical cell demonstrating plasmacytoid features (Wright Giemsa stain, original magnification 1000×).

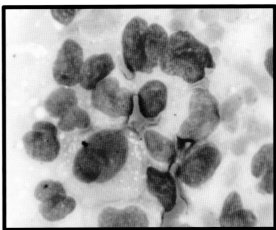

Figure 2_Bone marrow aspirate showing plasmablasts (Wright Giemsa stain, original magnification 1000×).

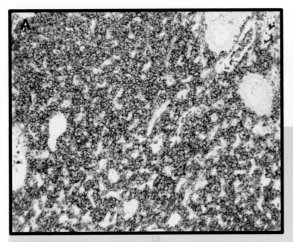

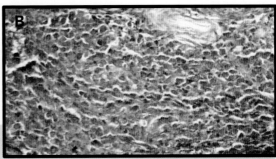

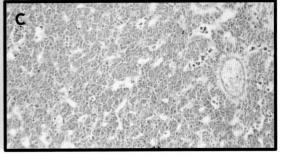

Figure 3_Bone marrow core biopsy showing diffuse CD138 positivity with (**A**) kappa light chain restriction, (**B**) kappa immunohistochemical stain, and (**C**) lambda immunohistochemical stain. Original magnification 400×.

time of diagnosis (primary PCL) or evolve as a leukemic transformation of a previously diagnosed plasma cell myeloma (secondary PCL).[2]

Our patient presented with primary PCL without prior history of plasma cell myeloma (MM); therefore, it was not considered as a secondary PCL.

2. Clinically, patients usually present with weakness, fatigue, and bone pain. Laboratory findings include anemia (80%), leukocytosis (80%), thrombocytopenia (50%), and other laboratory abnormalities, such as renal insufficiency,

hypercalcemia, and elevated lactate dehydrogenase (LDH).[3] They also have elevated monoclonal immunoglobulin in the serum, 50% with IgG, and 15% with IgA, similar to the incidence in MM. IgD and IgE are rare. Bence Jones protein is found in urine in approximately 80% of the patients.[3] Compared with MM, patients with primary PCL usually have more adverse prognostic indicators on initial presentation, such as extramedullary involvement (hepatosplenomegaly), severe anemia, thrombocytopenia, hypercalcemia, renal failure, and higher serum LDH and β_2-microglobulin levels.[3,4] Thus, primary PCL resembles both clinical features of end-stage

T1. Principal Laboratory Findings

Test	Patient's Result	"Normal" Reference Range
Hematology		
WBC count	25.4	3.9–12.0 × 10³/µL
RBC count	1.56	3.8–5.4 × 10⁶/µL
Hemoglobin	4.6	11.7–16.0 g/dL
Hematocrit	15.0	35–49%
MCV	96.0	80–99 fL
MCH	29.4	26–35 pg
MCHC	30.7	32–37 g/dL
RDW	26.5	11.6–15
Platelets	129	150–450 × 10³/µL
MPV	8.3	6.5–11.0 fL
Neutrophils	38	35–75%
Lymphocytes	47	19–56%
Monocytes	9	2–12%
Basophils	0	0–2%
Absolute neutrophils	9.7	1.3–7.5 × 10³/µL
Absolute lymphocytes	7.9	1.3–4.2 × 10³/µL
Absolute monocytes	2.3	0.2–1.0 × 10³/µL
Absolute eosinophils	1.5	0–0.5 × 10³/µL
Absolute basophils	0	0–0.15 × 10³/µL
Nucleated RBC	2/100	
Hematology PB w/ Asp		
WBC count	13.0	3.9–12.0 × 10³/µL
RBC count	2.87	3.8–5.4 × 10⁶/µL
Hemoglobin	8.6	11.7–16.0 g/dL
Hematocrit	25.3	35–49%
MCV	88.4	80–99 fL
MCH	29.9	26–35 pg
MCHC	33.8	32–37 g/dL
RDW	20.5	11.6–15
Platelets	109	150–450 × 10³/µL
MPV	8.7	6.5–11.0 fL
Neutrophils	32	35–75%
Lymphocytes	14	19–56%
Monocytes	3	2–12%
Basophils	0	0–2%
Eosinophils	10	
Promyelocytes	0	
Myelocytes	1	
Metamyelocytes	1	
Bands	1	
Blasts	0	
Plasma cells/ plasmablast	38	
Absolute neutrophils		1.3–7.5 × 10³/µL
Absolute lymphocytes		1.3–4.2 × 10³/µL
Absolute monocytes		0.2–1.0 × 10³/µL
Absolute eosinophils		0–0.5 × 10³/µL
Absolute basophils		0–0.15 × 10³/µL
Nucleated RBC	3/100	

BUN, blood urea nitrogen; WBC, white blood cell; RBC, red blood cell; MCV, mean corpuscular volume; MCH, mean corpuscular hemoglobin; MCHC, mean corpuscular hemoglobin concentration; RDW, red blood cell distribution width; PT, prothrombin time; PTT, partial thromboplastin time; INR, international normalized ratio; MPV, mean platelet volume; LDH, lactate dehydrogenase.

MM and acute leukemia. Although cases have been reported in people as young as 21 years,[5] the median age at presentation is generally above 50 years.[6]

Our patient had severe anemia (hemoglobin, 4.6 mg/dL), mild thrombocytopenia (109 × 10⁹/L), leukocytosis (25.4 × 10⁹/L), and renal failure (Cr 5.5). She also had markedly elevated β_2-microglobulin (49.2 mg/dL) and elevated LDH (518 mg/dL). Her serum total protein, albumin, and immunoglobulin levels were lower than normal. Interestingly, she had unexplained coagulopathy with elevations in all routine coagulation parameters including PT (20 sec), PTT (141 sec), INR (1.6), and TT (>20 sec).

3. The coagulation abnormalities were refractory to fresh frozen plasma (FFP) replacement therapy and no schistocytes were evident on serial phosphate buffered saline (PBS) washes consistent with the presence of inhibitors and absence of thrombotic thrombocytopenic purpura (TTP), respectively. The D-dimer levels were mildly

T1. Principal Laboratory Findings (continued)

Test	Patient's Result	"Normal" Reference Range
Hematology BM Aspirate		
Neutrophils	4	
Lymphocytes	0	
Monocytes	0	
Basophils	0	
Eosinophils	1	
Promyelocytes	0	
Myelocytes	0	
Metamyelocytes	0	
Bands	3	
Plasma cells/ plasmablast	90	
Chemistry		
Sodium	136	135–145 mmol/L
Potassium	5.0	3.5–5.3 mmol/L
Chloride	104	98–108 mmol/L
Bicarbonate	16	24–32 mmol/L
Anion gap	16	3–11
Calcium	10.2	8.6–10.6 mg/dL
BUN	24	6–20 mg/dL
Special Chemistry		
β_2-microglobulin	49.2	1.1–2.4 mg/dL
IgG	344	791–1643 mg/dL
IgA	29	66–436 mg/dL
IgM	<25	43–279 mg/dL
LDH	518	90–180 mg/dL

Serum Protein Electrophoresis		
Total protein	5.6	6–8.3 g/dL
Albumin	3.03	3.75–5.01 g/dL
α1	0.47	0.19 g/dL
α2	0.57	0.48–1.05 g/dL
β	0.93	0.48–1.10 g/dL
γ	0.60	0.62–1.51 g/dL
κ free light chain	2240	0.33–1.94 mg/dL
λ free light chain	0.36	0.57–2.63 mg/dL
κ/λ	6222.22	0.26–1.65
Coagulation Studies		
PT	19.5	11.5–15.6 sec
INR	1.54	0.9–1.2
Urine Protein Electrophoresis		
κ free light chain	2660	0.14–2.42 mg/dL
λ free light chain	0.27	0.02–0.67 mg/dL
κ/λ	9851.85	2.04–10.37

elevated (0.6 µg/mL), implicative of fibrinolytic pathway activation. Combined abnormalities of mixing studies and refractoriness of coagulation parameters to FFP make disseminated intravascular coagulation (DIC) or chronic liver disease less likely. The patient's primary concern was the persistent bruise on her right knee, which can be explained by abnormalities observed in both primary (platelet dysfunction from renal failure and mild thrombocytopenia) and secondary (abnormal coagulation profile) hemostasis. The coagulation parameters improved substantially

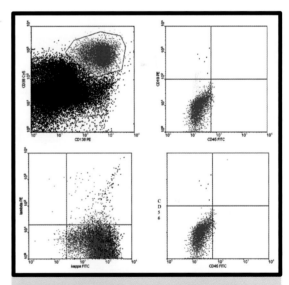

Figure 4_Flow cytometry dot plot identifying plasmablasts as CD45 negative/CD19 negative/CD38 positive/CD138 positive/CD56 negative.

with resolution of the "knee bruise" after treatment of PCL, suggesting that the inhibitor was plasma cell protein being excreted by malignant cells.

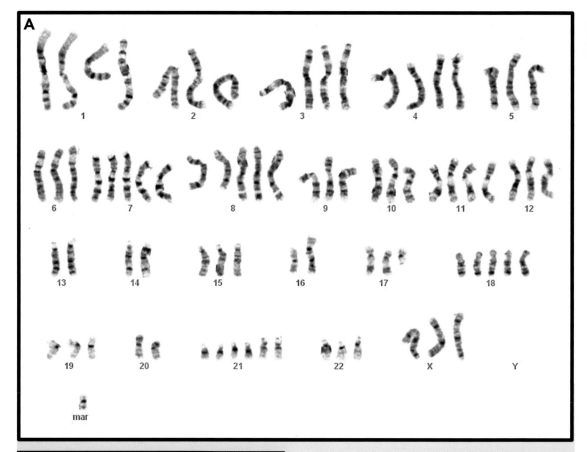

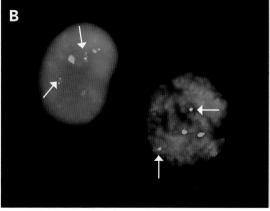

Figure 5_(A) Representative karyotype demonstrating hypertriploidy with 79 chromosomes (see text for details). (**B**) FISH analysis using the dual color, dual fusion IGH (green) and MAF (red) gene probes. Yellow, or green next to red, signals (arrows) indicate that a translocation has occurred.

Patients with plasma cell dyscrasias can manifest a vast array of coagulation abnormalities. Pathophysiologic interactions between monoclonal immunoglobulins and coagulation factors, platelets, and vessels produce these hemostatic abnormalities. Bleeding is the most common finding, although major, spontaneous bleeding is uncommon despite frequent abnormal screening hemostasis tests. The etiology of bleeding in these patients is multifold and includes vascular infiltration by malignant cells, hyperviscosity syndrome, thrombocytopenia secondary to bone marrow infiltration or treatment, uremia, and coagulopathies secondary to liver dysfunction, sepsis, and monoclonal immunoglobulins, which serve as inhibitors of the coagulation factors (antibodies that either inhibit the activity or increase the clearance of a clotting factor).[7] The exact role of paraproteins in many of these conditions has not been completely investigated at this time. Several unique hemostatic derangements are associated with circulating

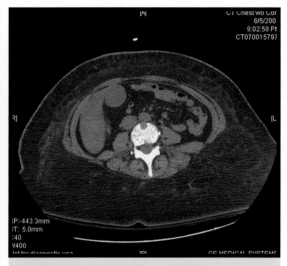

Figure 6_Computed tomography scan showing hepatomegaly and focal lytic lesions in T7 vertebra.

paraproteins/monoclonal immunoglobulins and these include inhibition of fibrin polymerization, qualitative platelet dysfunction, acquired von Willebrand factor deficiency, heparin-like circulating anticoagulants, acquired coagulation factor deficiencies, acquired hypercoagulable state, and acquired inhibitors of coagulation. A normal D-dimer and normal fibrinogen with prolonged partial thromboplastin time not corrected by mixing studies indicates the presence of a circulating inhibitor.[8] We believe our patient had a monoclonal paraprotein that functioned as an inhibitor.

4. Primary PCL usually has a spectrum of morphologically atypical and immature plasma cells in the peripheral blood and bone marrow. The neoplastic cells may occasionally resemble normal plasma cells with basophilic cytoplasm, prominent Golgi zone, and an eccentric nucleus. There may be atypical plasma cells with large size, central nucleus, and inconspicuous Golgi zone. More commonly, the neoplastic plasma cells exhibit a blastic morphology (high nucleus to cytoplasm ratio, open non-clock-face and fine lacy chromatin, prominent nucleolus, and inconspicuous to absent Golgi zone).[6,9] In all 4 cases reported by Johnson and colleagues,[4] the plasma cells vary from small mature plasma cells to large anaplastic blastic cells.

Our patient's marrow and peripheral blood demonstrated a spectrum of plasma cells with a predominance of plasmablasts and fewer atypical plasma cells. Immunophenotypic features of primary PCL are similar to MM. The neoplastic plasma cells are positive for CD38 and CD138. The CD56 (neuronal cell adhesion molecule [NCAM]) marker, which is characteristically expressed on myeloma cells, is typically absent.[10] Expression of CD20 is more frequent in PCL, while in MM the expression of HLA-DR and CD117 is comparatively more common. The CD2, CD3, and CD16 are consistently negative and the expression of CD10, CD13, and CD15 is similar in PCL and MM cells.

Immunophenotypic analysis of our patient's peripheral blood and bone marrow aspirate by flow cytometry revealed an abnormal plasma cell population with CD45 negative/CD19 negative/CD38 positive/CD138 positive/CD56 negative immunophenotype. The neoplastic cells did not express CD2, CD3, CD10, CD13, CD15, CD16, CD20, HLA-DR, or CD117.

5. Because primary PCL is rare, relatively few cases have been studied cytogenetically or with fluorescence in situ hybridization (FISH) analysis. However, cytogenetic analyses, including FISH, play an increasingly important role in determining prognosis in plasma cell dyscrasias. The aberrations in PCL are similar to those in MM but are detected more frequently in PCL with nonrandom abnormalities detectable in the usually complex karyotypes. While hyperdiploidy, with trisomies of 3, 5, 7, 9, 11, 15, 19, and 21, is common in MM, most cases of PCL are pseudodiploid or hypodiploid with recurrent loss of the long arm of chromosome 13 (85% of PCL versus 26% in MM) and translocations involving the immunoglobulin gene (*IGH* at 14q32) and various partner genes.[11-14] The most common partners for *IGH* translocation in both PCL and MM are cyclin D1 (CCND1 at 11q13), *MAF* (musculoaponeurotic fibrosarcoma oncogene at 16q23), and *FGFR3* (fibroblast growth factor receptor 3 at 4p16); the *FGFR3* and *MAF* translocations are cryptic cytogenetically but can be detected by FISH analysis.

Our patient carried the *IGH/MAF* translocation. Both *IGH/MAF* and *IGH/FGFR3* rearrangements are associated with a poor prognosis in MM.[15] Our patient had a hyperdiploid karyotype with extra copies of all the common trisomies in MM except 5 and demonstrated relative loss of chromosome 13, which is a poor prognostic indicator. Loss of the TP53 gene, which has a poor prognosis in MM, was not detected in this patient.

6. Patients with PCL have a poor prognosis. The median survival is 6.8 months for primary PCL and 1.3 months for secondary PCL with conventional chemotherapy.[16] Hematopoietic stem cell transplantation is a definitive treatment strategy; however, the outcome is still poor with a median survival of approximately 28 months.[17]

7. As therapy for PCL evolves, new regimens with novel agents that target specific cellular processes allow a more optimistic prognosis. The more aggressive clinical behavior of PCL has prompted investigators to seek treatment strategies not otherwise amenable to a typical patient with MM. These strategies include the addition of novel agents to induction therapy followed by allogeneic stem-cell transplantation. Bortezomib, a proteasome inhibitor, has emerged as a promising new agent when combined with chemotherapy.[18,19] Further prospective studies are required with integration of novel agents to frontline therapy in improving outcomes for patients with PCL.

Keywords

plasma cell leukemia, multiple myeloma, coagulopathy, FISH analysis, stem cell transplant, bortezomib

References

1. Dimopoulos MA, Palumbo A, Delasalle KB, et al. Primary plasma cell leukaemia. *Br J Haematol*. 1994;88:754–759.

2. Grogan TM, Van Camp B, Kyle RA, et al. Plasma cell neoplasms. In: Jaffe ES, Harris NL, Stein H, et al, eds. *WHO Classification: Pathology and Genetics of Tumors of Haematopoietic and Lymphoid Tissues*. Lyon, France: IARC Press; 2001:144.

3. Kosmo MA, Gale RP. Plasma cell leukemia. *Semin Hematol*. 1987;24: 202–208.

4. Johnson MR, Del Carpio-Jayo D, Lin P, et al. Primary plasma cell leukemia: Morphologic, immunophenotypic, and cytogenetic features of 4 cases treated with chemotherapy and stem cell transplantation. *Ann Diagn Pathol*. 2006;10:263–268.

5. Raj RS, Najeeb S, Aruna R, et al. Primary plasma cell leukemia occurring in the young. *Indian J Cancer*. 2003;40:116–117.

6. Kyle RA, Maldonado JE, Bayrd ED. Plasma cell leukemia. Report on 17 cases. *Arch Intern Med*. 1974;133:813–818.

7. Sallah S, Nguyen N, Abdallah J, et al. Acquired hemophilia in patients with hematologic malignancies. *Arch Pathol Lab Med*. 2000;124:730–734.

8. Eby C. Bleeding and thrombosis risks in plasma cell dyscrasias. *Hematology*. 2007:158–164.

9. Woodruff RK, Malpas JS, Paxton AM, et al. Plasma cell leukemia (PCL): A report on 15 patients. *Blood*. 1978;52:839–845.

10. Pellat-Deceunynck C, Barille S, Jego G, et al. The absence of CD56 on malignant plasma cells is a hallmark of plasma cell leukaemia and of a special subset of multiple myeloma. *Leukemia*. 1998;12:1977–1982.

11. Garcia-Sanz R, Orfao A, Gonzalez M, et al. Primary plasma cell leukemia: Clinical, immunophenotypic, DNA ploidy, and cytogenetic characteristics. *Blood*. 1999;93:1032–1037.

12. Avet-Loiseau H, Daviet A, Brigaudeau C. Cytogenetic, interphase, and multicolor fluorescence in situ hybridization analyses in primary plasma cell leukemia: A study of 40 patients at diagnosis, on behalf of the Intergroupe Francophone du Myelome and the Groupe Français de Cytogénétique Hématologique. *Blood*. 2001;97:822–825.

13. Lloveras E. Cytogenetic and fluorescence in situ hybridization studies in 60 patients with multiple myeloma and plasma cell leukaemia. *Cancer Genet Cytogenet*. 2004;148:71–76.

14. Chang H, Sloan S, Li D, et al. Genomic aberrations in plasma cell leukemia shown by interphase fluorescence in situ hybridization. *Cancer Genet Cytogenet*. 2005;156:150–153.

15. Moreau P, Facon T, Leleu X, et al. Régis Bataille and Hervé Avet-Loiseay for the Intergroupe Francophone du Myélome. Recurrent 14q32 translocations determine the prognosis of multiple myeloma, especially in patients receiving intensive chemotherapy. *Blood*. 2002;100:1579–1583.

16. Noel P, Kyle RA. Plasma cell leukemia: An evaluation of response to therapy. *Am J Med*. 1987;83:1062–1068.

17. Saccaro S, Fonseca R, Veillon DM, et al. Primary plasma cell leukemia: Report of 17 new cases treated with autologous or allogeneic stem-cell transplantation and review of the literature. *Am J Hematol*. 2005;78:288–294.

18. Musto P, Rossini F, Gay F, et al. Efficacy and safety of bortezomib in patients with plasma cell leukemia. *Cancer*. 2007;109:2285–2290.

19. Finnegan DP, Kettle P, Drake M, et al. Bortezomib is effective in primary plasma cell leukemia. *Leuk Lymphoma*. 2006;47:1670–1673.

Markedly Decreased Serum Sodium Concentration in a Patient With Multiple Myeloma

Zhongxin Yu, K. Michael Parker, Kenneth E. Blick
University of Oklahoma Medical Center, Oklahoma City, OK

Patient: 56-year-old male.

Past Medical History: Non-contributory.

Chief Complaint: Low back pain, cough, and altered mental status (confusion and disorientation).

Drug/Family/Social History: Non-contributory.

Results of Additional Diagnostic Procedures: The patient was admitted to the hospital for additional laboratory (**Figure 1**) and diagnostic testing. Bone marrow biopsy showed plasmacytosis >30%; chest X-ray demonstrated right lower lobe pneumonia; additional radiologic studies showed lytic bone lesions of the skull, C-5 cervical spine, and an aged compression fracture at L-1 of the lumbar spine; and computed tomography (CT) and magnetic resonance imaging (MRI) scans of the brain were unremarkable.

Questions

1. What is (are) this patient's most striking laboratory finding(s)?

2. How do you explain this patient's most striking laboratory finding(s)?

3. What is this patient's most likely diagnosis?

4. How is this patient's condition distinguished from other causes of hyponatremia?

5. What are the 2 principal methods for quantifying serum sodium concentration used routinely in most clinical laboratories in the United States and how do they differ?

6. What testing should be performed to confirm pseudohyponatremia as the cause of a markedly decreased serum sodium concentration?

7. Why was this patient's anion gap markedly decreased?

8. In patients with pseudohyponatremia, how should the serum sodium concentration be monitored?

9. How is pseudohyponatremia treated?

Possible Answers

1. This patient has several abnormal test results for a variety of analytes (**T1**); however, the most striking are a peripheral blood smear with 5% plasma cells and marked Rouleaux; markedly decreased serum sodium, calcium, and albumin concentrations; markedly decreased calculated anion gap and albumin/globulin (A/G) ratio; increased IgG and total protein concentrations; and IgG kappa monoclonal gammopathy. In addition, after admission to the hospital, this patient's osmolar gap {ie, measured osmolality – calculated osmolality, where calculated osmolality was determined using the equation: $2[Na] + ([Glucose]/18) + ([BUN]/2.8)$} was large on several days, but narrowed when the calculated osmolality was determined using serum sodium

T1. Principal Laboratory Findings

Test	Patient's Result	"Normal" Reference Range
Hematology		
WBC count	13.0	$4.0\text{-}11.0 \times 10^3/\mu m^3$
RBC count	2.98	$4.70\text{-}6.10 \times 10^6/\mu m^3$
Hemoglobin	10.0	13.0-18.0 g/dL
Hematocrit	28.1	39.0-52.0%
MCV	94.3	82.0-99.0 fL
MCH	33.6	27.0-34.0 pg
MCHC	35.6	32.0-36.0 g/dL
Platelet count	202	$140\text{-}440 \times 10^3/\mu m^3$
Neutrophils	69	39-78%
Bands	2	0-12%
Lymphocytes	19	15-56%
Monocytes	5	2-14%
Plasma cells	5	0-1%
Anisocytosis	Mild	
Rouleaux	Marked	
Chemistry		
Sodium	123	135-145 mmol/L
Potassium	3.6	3.5-5.1 mmol/L
Chloride	102	96-108 mmol/L
Anion gap	2	5-17
BUN	8	7-18 mg/dL
Creatinine	0.7	0.8-1.2 mg/dL
Glucose	130	65-110 mg/dL
Calcium	6.2	8.6-10 mg/dL
Triglycerides	327	40-160 mg/dL
Cholesterol	123	120-200 mg/dL
HDL-cholesterol	<10	35-80 mg/dL
LDL-cholesterol	48	<130 mg/dL
Total protein	9.9	6.4-8.4 mg/dL
Albumin	1.4	3.4-5.0 mg/dL
A/G ratio	0.2	1.0-2.2 mg/dL
Phosphate	1.4	2.5-4.5 mg/dL
Magnesium	1.9	1.6-2.6 mg/dL
Random urine sodium	99	(not established) mmol/L
Random urine osmolality	511	300-900 mOsm/kg
IgG	5530	700-1,600 mg/dL
IgA	58	70-400 mg/dL
IgM	39	40-230 mg/dL
SPE pattern	IgG kappa monoclonal gammopathy	
Arterial Blood Gases		
pH	7.48	7.38-7.42
pCO_2	34	35-45 mm Hg
HCO_3	26	24-26 mmol/L

WBC, white blood cell; RBC, red blood cell; MCV, mean corpuscular volume; MCH, mean corpuscular hemoglobin; MCHC, mean corpuscular hemoglobin concentration; BUN, blood urea nitrogen; HDL, high-density lipoprotein; LDL, low-density lipoprotein; A/G, albumin/globulin; SPE, serum protein electrophoresis.

values obtained by a different method for quantifying the patient's serum sodium concentration than the method used initially (**Figure 1**).

2. All of this patient's abnormal test results are explained, either directly or indirectly, by the large amounts of paraprotein that are present in the serum of patients with multiple myeloma—a condition known to cause falsely decreased serum sodium values (ie, pseudohyponatremia) when sodium concentration is measured using an *indirect* ion-selective electrode (ISE) method.

3. ***Most likely diagnosis:*** *pseudohyponatremia in a patient with multiple myeloma due to measurement of serum sodium concentration using an indirect ISE method.*

4. Whenever a markedly low serum sodium concentration is observed on any patient, the first question to ask is: Is this a true hyponatremia? Sodium is the major cation in the extracellular fluid (ECF) and its concentration in plasma is maintained in healthy individuals within the narrow range of 135 to 145 mmol/L. The plasma sodium concentration reflects the balance between sodium intake and output. *Hyponatremia* is defined as a serum sodium concentration less than 135 mmol/L. The most common causes of true hyponatremia are: 1) depletional due to reduced sodium intake from food; 2) increased sodium loss in urine, feces, or sweat, such as in patients using diuretic agents or with diarrhea or extensive burns; and 3) dilutional, such as in patients with chronic renal insufficiency, nephrotic syndrome, or the

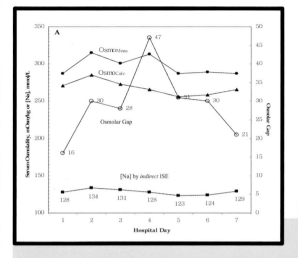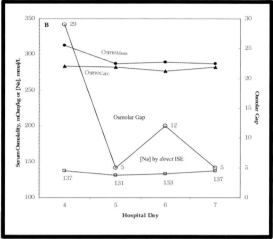

Figure 1_Patient's serum sodium concentration by **A**) indirect (Synchron LX20 instrument, Beckman Coulter, Brea, CA) and B) direct ion-selective electrode (ISE) method (i-STAT instrument, i-STAT Corporation, East Windsor, NJ), calculated (OsmoCalc) and measured (OsmoMeas) osmolality, and osmolar gap on hospital days 1 through 7 (A) or 4 through 7 (**B**). OsmoCalc=2[Na, mmol/L]+[Glucose, mg/dl)/18]+[BUN, mg/dL)/2.8][1]; OsmoMeas was determined using the Advanced™ Micro Osmometer, Model 330 (Advanced Instruments Inc., Norwood, MA); Osmolar gap=OsmoMeas-OsmoCalc. Na, sodium ion concentration; BUN, blood urea nitrogen; Osmo, osmolality; Meas, measured; Calc, calculated.

syndrome of inappropriate anti-diuretic hormone secretion (SIADH) in which an increased ECF volume with a diluted serum sodium concentration. All of these conditions cause true hyponatremia and require immediate medical attention. *Pseudohyponatremia* is an artifactual hyponatremia most commonly caused by severe hypertriglyceridemia (usually, >1,500 mg/dL) or, less often, by severe hyperproteinemia (usually, >10 g/dL). Pseudohyponatremia occurs as a consequence of how serum sodium is measured. The most commonly used method for quantifying serum sodium concentration is ion-selective electrode (ISE) potentiometry. Only a small percentage of clinical laboratories use flame emission spectroscopy; however, this method is considered the reference method for sodium measurement.[2] Spectrophotometric methods for sodium measurement based upon the interaction of sodium with chromogenic macrocyclic ionophores that are capable of selectively complexing sodium have also been described.

5. Indirect and direct ISE potentiometry. Direct ISE methods measure the ion activity in an undiluted sample, whereas indirect ISE methods measure the ion activity in a pre-diluted sample. Sodium is dissolved only in the water portion of serum. In the context of marked hyperparaproteinemia

(as occurs in patients with multiple myeloma) and/or hyperlipidemia, protein and/or lipid occupy more space in a given volume of serum, resulting in a decrease in the percentage of water (with its sodium content). Consequently, an artifactually low serum sodium concentration is obtained due to the fact that less sodium is present in a given volume of serum, even though the concentration of sodium present in the water phase may be unaltered. This phenomenon usually occurs with an indirect ISE method in which a pre-diluted sample is used for testing. For example, in a specimen containing 1 gram of sodium dissolved in 0.8 liters of water and 0.2 liters of an insoluble substance, the sodium concentration should be 1 g/0.8 L (or 1.25 g/L). However, if this specimen is diluted 100-fold with water (eg, by adding 99 liters of water to the 1 liter of specimen), then the total volume of 100 liters of solution consists of 99.8 liters of water and 0.2 liters of insoluble substance. Because the volume (0.2 L) of the insoluble substance is small compared to the 99.8 L of water, the volume contributed by this substance to the total volume (ie, approximately 100 L) is negligible. The sodium concentration measured in this specimen is 1 g/100 L or 0.01 g/L. When this value is multiplied by the dilution factor (ie, 100), the final sodium concentration is 1.00

g/L. Thus, an error has occurred because the true sodium concentration should be 1.25 g/L. The falsely low result of 1.00 g/L is caused by ignoring the volume contributed by the insoluble substance after dilution of the specimen.

6. To confirm pseudohyponatremia, serum osmolality should be measured. Actually, for any hyponatremic patient, the initial approach is to measure the serum osmolality to determine whether the hyponatremia represents a true hypo-osmolar state.[3] Osmolality is a colligative property of solutions that depends only on the number of solute particles present in a given volume of solution. The 3 types of solutes most often encountered in biological fluids are: electrolytes, organic molecules, and colloids. Sodium and its counter ions [eg, chloride (Cl^-)] are the major contributors to serum osmolality. The other 2 principal, active osmolar solutes in serum are urea and glucose. The reference interval for serum osmolality in healthy individuals is typically 282-300 mOsm/kg of water (H_2O). No sex- or age-related differences in serum osmolality values have been reported.[2] To estimate serum (or plasma) osmolality, several formulas have been proposed.[4,5] The most commonly used formula for estimating serum osmolality is: osmolality (mOsm/kg) = 2[Na, mmol/L] + ([Glucose, mg/dL]/18) + ([BUN, mg/dL]/2.8).[1] Under normal physiologic conditions, the calculated osmolality is similar to the measured osmolality so that the difference between them (ie, the osmolar gap) in healthy individuals is approximately 12 (range: 7-19 mOsm/kg H_2O).[6] Thus, in a patient with hyponatremia, an increased osmolar gap suggests the presence of either pseudohyponatremia due to hyper-paraproteinemia or hypertriglyceridemia, or an increased concentration of a solute (eg, ethanol, etc) whose concentration is not included in the formula stated above for calculating serum osmolality. During his hospital stay, our patient's osmolar gap ranged from 16 mOsm/kg H_2O to 47 mOsm/kg H_2O (**Figure 1A**). High osmolar gap values in this range may be seen in patients with pseudohyponatremia. To further support this conclusion, our patient's serum sodium concentration was measured by a direct ISE method (i-STAT instrument, i-STAT Corporation, East Windsor, NJ). Using the i-STAT instrument, the serum sodium values obtained on our patient

were higher than those obtained by an indirect ISE method, resulting in higher values for calculated osmolality and much smaller values for the osmolar gap (**Figure 1B**). These findings support further the conclusion that the low sodium concentration measured initially in our patient's serum was due to pseudohyponatremia and his myeloma-related hyperproteinemia and his hypertriglyceridemia.

7. The anion gap is a calculated measurement representing the balance between the concentration of serum anions and cations. If the sum of the principal anions in serum, Cl^- and HCO_3^-, is subtracted from the Na^+ value (ie, Na^+ - $[Cl^- + HCO_3^-]$), this difference (or "gap") in serum from healthy individuals is usually approximately 12 (range: 7-16). This "gap" is due to the concentration of unmeasured anions (eg, lactate, proteins, SO_4^{2-}, HPO_4^{2-}) in serum.[1] An increased anion gap is often seen in metabolic acidosis and occurs due to a decrease in the HCO_3^- concentration along with a concomitant increase in unmeasured anions such as lactate, and beta-hydroxybuterate. In contrast, a reduced anion gap is observed typically as a consequence of hypergammaglobulinemia (positively charged proteins), hypercalcemia, or hypermagnesemia. Moreover, a consistently low (eg, 1-3) anion gap, signifies the presence of high levels of a basic (or positively-charged) protein (eg, a paraprotein).[7]

8. Because this patient is known to have hyperproteinemia due to multiple myeloma, his serum sodium concentration should be assessed using a direct ISE method.

9. Hyponatremia is a relatively common electrolyte disturbance. Its high prevalence and potential neurologic sequelae make a logical and rigorous differential diagnosis mandatory before any therapeutic intervention.[3] Recognition of pseudohyponatremia as an explanation for a low serum sodium concentration is important because of the nature of the follow-up treatment in patients with pseudohyponatremia versus "true" hyopnatremia. Pseudohyponatremia does not require treatment; however, if misdiagnosed as "true" hyponatremia and unnecessarily treated with fluid restriction—the typical treatment to correct true hyponatremia—dehydration

and impairment of the blood flow in the micro-circulation can occur.

Keywords

hyponatremia, pseudohyponatremia, ion-selective electrode, multiple myeloma, osmolality, osmolar gap

References

1. Burtis CA, Ashwood ER. *Tietz Fundamentals of Clinical Chemistry*, 5th edition. Philadelphia: W.B.Saunders Company; 2001, 740.

2. Kaplan LA, Pesce AJ. *Clinical Chemistry: Theory, Analysis, Correlation*, 3rd edition. St. Louis: Mosby; 1996, 461-446.

3. Milionis HJ, Liamis GL, Elisaf MS. The hyponatremic patient: A systematic approach to laboratory diagnosis. *CMAJ.* 2002;166:1056-1062.

4. Weisberg HF. Osmolality-calculated "delta" and more formulas. *Clin Chem.* 1975;21:1182-1184.

5. Holmes JH. Measurement of osmolality in serum, urine, and other biololgic fluids by the freezing point determination. In: Preworkshop manual on urinalysis of renal function studies, Chicago: ASCP, Commission on Continuing Education, 1962.

6. Garcia-Morales EJ. Osmole gap in neurologic-neurosurgical intensive care unit: its normal value, calculation, and relationship with mannitol serum concentrations. *Crit Care Med.* 2004;32:986-991.

7. Pincus MR. Interpreting laboratory results: reference values and decision making. In: *Henry JB, Clinical Diagnosis and Management by Laboratory Methods*. Philadelphia: WB Saunders Company. 19th edition; 1996, 85.

Biclonal M-Spike in a 7-Year-Old Child

Karen Fritchie, Monte S. Willis

Department of Pathology & Laboratory Medicine, University of North Carolina, Chapel Hill, NC

Patient: 7-year-old previously healthy male.

Chief Complaint: The patient presented with a 2-week history of low-grade intermittent fever and pain in multiple joints including the wrists, shoulders, and ankles.

History of Present Illness: The patient initially developed a fever of 102°F 2 weeks prior to admission accompanied by headache and eye pain. His primary care physician performed a strep test and throat culture, both of which were negative. The patient later developed periumbilical abdominal pain and presented to his local emergency room where a urinalysis was performed and was within normal limits. His fever subsided for 3 days after this visit, subsequently returning to approximately 104°F. He began experiencing wrist pain and shoulder pain and edema of his lower extremities. He was admitted to a local hospital, found to be pancytopenic, and subsequently transferred to our facility for further workup.

Past Medical History: The patient was born at term, demonstrated normal growth and development patterns, and had no history of surgeries or prior hospitalizations.

Social History: The patient lives with his mother (a smoker), 1 sibling, and 2 cats.

Family History: The patient's mother has a history of rheumatoid arthritis and the removal of cervical lymph nodes for unknown reasons. His maternal grandmother had a history of Grave's disease and hepatitis C. His maternal grandfather had a history of diabetes.

Physical Examination Findings: On physical examination, an annular rash of the chest, face, abdomen, and thighs was identified along with mild conjunctivitis and bilateral periorbital and lower extremity edema.

Additional Laboratory and Clinical Studies: An MRI of the abdomen demonstrated hepatosplenomegaly, portal hepatitis lymphadenopathy, periportal edema and gallbladder wall thickening, pulmonary interstitial edema, and small left pleural effusion. Whole body fluorodeoxyglucose positron emission tomography (FDG-PET) scan to look for cancers such as lymphoma using labeled glucose was performed, and no foci suspicious for malignancy were identified suggesting no underlying neoplastic process was present. A bone marrow biopsy identified non-specific changes such as a slightly hypocellular bone marrow (70%), increased megakaryocytes, and a mildly left-shifted granulopoiesis with <5% blasts. Bone marrow cytogenetics were normal. Renal biopsy (after 2 weeks of hospitalization) demonstrated ultrastructural changes consistent with type I membranoglomerulonephritis (**Image 1**). Serum protein electrophoresis (SPE) identified 2 monoclonal proteins that were immunophenotyped by immunofixation electrophoresis (IFE) as IgG lambda (~0.7 g/dL) and IgM lambda (too low to quantify) (**Image 2**). Serum IgM concentration was elevated (701 mg/dL; reference range: 35–290 mg/dL) while the IgG concentration was high, although in the normal range (1,375 mg/dL; reference range: 490–1,400 mg/dL). Urine protein electrophoresis (UPE) on a random urine sample revealed a selective glomerular proteinuria with excretion of moderate amounts of albumin and small amounts of alpha- and beta-globulins (total protein concentration, 184 mg/dL). Urine IFE demonstrated the presence of monoclonal IgG lambda, a kappa free light chain (FLC), and 2 monoclonal bands of lambda FLCs. Cryoglobulin analysis revealed 3 monoclonal components corresponding to IgG lambda, IgM lambda, and kappa FLCs within a polyclonal IgM background (data not shown).

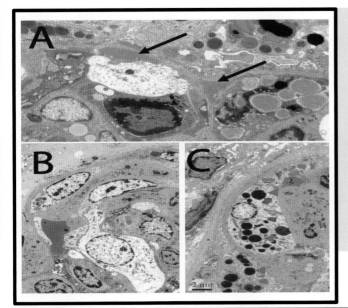

Image 1_Transmission electron microscopy of tissue from the patient's renal biopsy illustrating **A**) electron dense membrane deposits reflecting the deposition of circulating immune complexes (arrows); **B**) endocapillary mononuclear cell hypercellularity indicative of the proliferative aspects of membranoproliferative disease; and, **C**) the presence of large phagolysosomes in many of the mononuclear cell elements containing black, presumably proteinaceous, material indicative of phagocytosed paraproteins (ie, cryoglobulins).

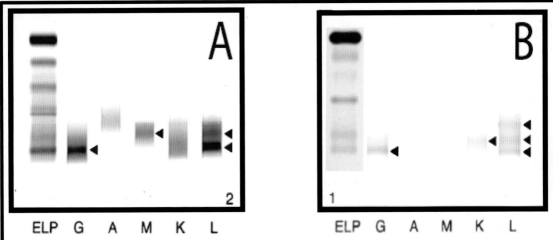

Image 2_Monoclonal antibodies identified in this 7-year-old patient's serum (**A**) by SPE (IgM lambda and IgG lambda monoclonal proteins [arrowheads]) and urine (**B**) by UPE (IgG lambda, as well as kappa and lambda free light chains [arrowheads]).

T1. Principal Laboratory Findings

Test	Patient's Result	"Normal" Reference Range
Hematology		
WBC count	3.5	4.5–13.5 × 10³/μL
RBC count	3.24	4.00–5.20 × 10⁶/μL
Hemoglobin	8.8	11.5–15.5 g/dL
Hematocrit	26.1	35.0–45.0%
MCV	81	77–95 fL
Platelet count	38	150–440 × 10³/μL
ESR	42	0–15 mm/h
PBS examination	Atypical and rare plasmacytoid lymphocytes present; toxic granulation and vacuolation present	
Chemistry		
Sodium	131	135–145 mmol/L
Potassium	4.2	3.4–4.7 mmol/L
CO₂	18	22–30 mmol/L
BUN	26	5–17 mg/dL
Creatinine	1.4	0.4–0.9 mg/dL
Glucose, random	87	65–199 mg/dL
Calcium	8.2	8.8–10.9 mg/dL
Magnesium	1.9	1.6–2.2 mg/dL
Phosphorous	2.7	4.0–5.7 mg/dL
Albumin	1.8	3.5–5.0 g/dL
Bilirubin	0.4	0.0–1.2 mg/dL
AST	58	15–40 U/L
ALT	78	10–35 U/L
ALP	201	175–420 U/L
GGT	29	16–68 U/L
LD	691	420–750 U/L
CRP	4.6	0.0–1.0 mg/dL
C3	<40	88–171 mg/dL
C4	<8	15–48 mg/dL
Haptoglobin	119	37–264 mg/dL

BUN, blood urea nitrogen; AST, aspartate aminotransferase; ALT, alanine aminotransferase; ALP, alkaline phosphatase; GGT, gamma glutamyl transferase; LD, lactate dehydrogenase; CRP, C-reactive protein; C3, complement component-3; C4, complement component-4; WBC, white blood cell; RBC, red blood cell; MCV, mean corpuscular volume; ESR, erythrocyte sedimentation rate; PBS, peripheral blood smear.

T2. Immunology Test Findings

Test	Patient's Result	"Normal" Reference Range
ANA	1:80 (speckled pattern)	Negative
ENA Ab screen	4	<20 ENA U
RF	<6.3	0.0–15.0 U/mL
ANCA IFA	Negative	Negative
MPO ELISA	Negative	Negative
MPO quant	2.5	<=20
PR3 ELISA	Negative	Negative
PR3 quant	3.4	<=20
dsDNA	Negative	Negative
APA panel: DRVTT	34.2	0.0–37.9 sec
Lupus APTT	29.1	28.2–44.7 sec
ACA IgG	5	0–23 GPL
ACA IgM	4	0–11 MPL

ANA, anti-nuclear antibodies; ENA, extractable nuclear antigens; Ab, antibody; RF, rheumatoid factor; ANCA, anti-neutrophilic cytoplasmic antibodies; IFA, immunofluorescence antibody; MPO, myeloperoxidase; Quant, quantitative; PR3, proteinase-3; ELISA, enzyme-linked immunosorbent assay; dsDNA, double-stranded deoxyribosenucleic acid; APA, anti-phospholipid antibody; DRVTT, dilute Russell viper venom time; APTT, activated partial thromboplastin time; ACA, anti-cardiolipin antibody.

Questions

1. What are this patient's most striking clinical and laboratory findings?

2. How do you explain this patient's most striking clinical and laboratory findings?

3. What is this patient's most likely diagnosis?

4. What conditions are most often associated with this patient's diagnosis?

5. What age groups does this disease normally affect?

6. Are urinary M-spikes a common finding in this patient's disease?

T3. Brouet's Modified Classification of Cryoglobulinemia[a]

Cryoglobulin Class	Cryoglobulins Present	Associated Diseases
Type I	Isolated monoclonal Igs	Monoclonal gammopathy Multiple myeloma Waldenström macroglobulinemia
Type II	2 components: 1) a monoclonal component 2) a polyclonal IgG	Hepatitis C virus infection Autoimmune disease Sjögren syndrome Chronic lymphocytic leukemia Non-Hodgkin lymphoma
Type III	Absence of a monoclonal component consisting of 1 or more classes of polyclonal Igs	SLE Biliary cirrhosis Rheumatoid arthritis Viral infections[b] Bacterial infections[c]

[a]Adapted from Shihabi 2006.[21] [b]Cytomegalovirus (CMV), Epstein-Barr virus (EBV), human immunodeficiency virus (HIV), hepatitis B virus (HBV). [c]Leprosy, syphilis (spirochetes).

T4. Summary of Major Studies on Pediatric Cryoglobulinemia

Underlying Disease	Year Reported	No. of Patients (mean age, y; range)	Country	Principal Findings	Reference
Henoch-Schönlein purpura	1977	30 (6.7 y; 2–13)	UK	47% of patients with HSP, 64% with chronic nephritis, and 0% of those who recovered from HSP were CG +	15
Autoimmune disease	1980	250 (n.g.)	US	Patients with SLE, a presumptive AID, or chronic bacterial/viral infection[a] were CG +	16
Schistosomiasis	1983	202 (6–14 y)	Nigeria	33% of patients with schistosomiasis were CG + compared with only 8% of control subjects; No. of children CG + decreased with treatment	14

[a]Subacute bacterial endocarditis and viral or bacterial meningitis when the infectious agent was isolated.
HSP, Henoch-Schönlein purpura, characterized by typical rash and any 2 of 3 major clinical manifestations: 1) joint disease; 2) microscopic hematuria or proteinuria; 3) gastrointestinal disease (abdominal pain, melena); UK, United Kingdom; US, United States; CG +, cryoglobulin positive; SLE, systemic lupus erythematosus; AID, autoimmune disorder; No., number; n.g., not given.

7. What is the composition of cryoglobulins?

8. What is the pathogenesis of this disease?

9. How is this patient's condition typically treated?

Possible Answers

1. The most striking clinical findings include fever, migrating arthralgias, erythematous rash, and periorbital and peripheral edema. The most striking laboratory findings at presentation were

pancyopenia, the presence of monoclonal proteins in serum and urine, subsequently identified as cyroglobulins, elevated liver aminotransferases (AST and ALT), elevated renal function tests (BUN and creatinine), decreased complement components (C3 and C4), low serum phosphorous and albumin concentrations, and elevated erythrocyte sedimentation rate (ESR) and serum C-reactive protein (CRP) concentration.

2. In a patient with pancytopenia, elevated liver aminotransferases, elevated BUN and creatinine, and decreased complement the differential diagnosis includes: 1) a neoplastic process; 2) bacterial or viral infection with bone marrow suppression; 3) post-streptococcal glomerulonephritis or minimal change disease; or 4) a rheumatological disorder. Because of this patient's profound pancytopenia, a series of additional laboratory tests were performed to determine if an underlying neoplastic process was present in the bone marrow. A bone marrow biopsy identified nonspecific changes including a slightly hypocellular bone marrow (70%), increased megakaryocytes, and a mildly left-shifted granulopoiesis with <5% blasts. Bone marrow cytogenetics did not detect any abnormalities. Clinically, a positron emission tomography (PET) scan to look for cancers such as lymphoma was performed, and no foci suspicious for malignancy were identified. Taken together, these findings suggest that an underlying neoplastic process was not responsible for his clinical presentation. To investigate underlying bacterial and viral causes of illness, both serological assays and polymerase chain reaction (PCR) methods were used. Pertinent positive results include the presence of an anti-Epstein-Barr virus (EBV) IgG and a positive IgG anti-EBV viral capsid antigen; however, no IgM anti-EBV viral capsid antigen was detected, indicating that this was not an acute illness. Moreover, EBV viral load by quantitative PCR was performed and revealed a low positive result (<250 copies of EBV genome/mL), consistent with the serological findings. Since quantitative EBV viral load correlates well with severity of illness in pediatric patients,[1] a recent, but non-acute, EBV infection was likely present in this patient. The patient was HIV negative by IFA and pooled PCR. Serologic testing for *Ehrlichia*, *Rickettsia rickettsii*, Parvovirus B19, CMV, Leptospiridia, *Bartonella quintana*, *Francisella tularensis*, *Brucella*, and *Arboviruses* was negative.

Anti-streptolysin O and anti-DNase B were also negative indicating that a recent streptococcal infection was unlikely. Blood, urine, and fecal cultures were negative. These findings suggest that an infectious etiology to his clinical presentation was not likely. Studies were undertaken to determine the underlying cause of this patient's renal disease. Upon admission, urinalysis demonstrated urine sediment including red cell casts and proteinuria (3+). Abnormally-elevated serum creatinine and BUN were identified at admission (1.4 mg/dL and 26 mg/dL, respectively [**T1**]) which spiked sharply at day 12 of hospitalization to 2.6 mg/dL and 34 mg/dL, respectively. A needle biopsy of the kidney was performed during this spike, which detected ultrastructural changes consistent with type I membranoglomerulonephritis and having features suggestive, but not diagnostic, of cryoglobulinemia (**Image 1**). No morphologic evidence of a thrombotic microangiopathy was identified, consistent with the lack of schistocytes on multiple blood smears. This made either hemolytic uremic syndrome (HUS) or thrombotic thrombocytopenic purpura (TTP) an unlikely cause of this patient's renal disease. To evaluate the possibility of an underlying rheumatological disorder, tests to detect autoantibodies were performed. Pertinent positive tests included a positive (1:80) antinuclear antibody (ANA) which had a speckled pattern (**T2**). This ANA was undetectable 6 weeks after admission. Tests for rheumatoid factor, double-stranded deoxyribosenucleic acid (dsDNA), extractable nuclear antigen (ENA), and anti-neutrophilic cytoplasmic antibodies (ANCA) (including myeloperoxidase [MPO] and proteinase-3 [PR3]) were negative during his hospitalization (**T2**).

3. ***Most likely diagnosis:*** *Type II cryoglobulinemia of unknown etiology.*

Cryoglobulinemia indicates the presence of 1 or more immunoglobulin types in the blood that precipitate in serum below 37°C and redissolve upon warming. Cryoglobulins form secondary to the intrinsic characteristics of the immunoglobulins. These characteristics include the subclass of IgG antibody formed and post-translational modification of the antibodies themselves. The underlying pathogenesis of cryoglobulinemia can be classified by characterizing the immunoglobulins in the precipitate according to the Brouet classification

(**T3**). The Brouet classification has been used widely for the past 30 years and subdivides cryoglobulinemia into 3 types: type I, type II, and type III.[2] Type I cryoglobulinemia is associated with lymphoproliferative disorders, while types II and III are associated with infections and autoimmune diseases. The patient in the present case demonstrated a biclonal cryoglobulin, which may be found in both types I and II cryoglobulinemia. The fact that his bone marrow biopsy and PET scan did not reveal a lymphoproliferative disorder, and because his cryoglobulins occurred in a polyclonal background, a diagnosis of type II cryoglobulinemia was made.

4. Type II cryoglobulinemia is primarily associated with viral infections in adults. Up to 90% of patients with type II cryoglobulins have serologic evidence of HCV infection.[3] Epstein-Barr virus, HIV, and HBV infections can result in type II cryoglobulins.[4] While the most common cause of type II cryoglobulinemia is hepatitis C infection, this patient's serology and qualitative PCR for HCV were negative. Similarly, hepatitis B serologic tests (HBsAg, HBsAb, and HBcAb) were negative. Clinical findings of type II cryoglobulinemia include Raynaud phenomenon, arthralgias, lower extremity purpura, liver disease, abdominal pain, and leukocytoclastic vasculitis of the dermis.[5] Renal involvement occurs in up to 50% of cases, and isolated proteinuria or hematuria are the most common presentations.[5] Mesangial expansion and hypercellularity with electron-dense deposits (**Image 1A**) between the basal lamina and endothelial cells were visible on ultrastructural examination of renal biopsy tissue.[5] However, the most common light microscopy finding in renal biopsy tissue from patients with type II cryoglobulinemia is membranoproliferative glomerulonephritis (corresponding to the electron microscopy identified in **Image 1B**).[5] Immunofluorescent staining of this tissue shows glomerular deposits with immunoglobulins and variable amounts of complement.[5] Electron microscopy may show phagocytosed crygloblins in monocytes which appear as dark, membrane-bound bodies in lysosomes (**Image 1C**).[5] While the patient falls well below the median age for type II cryoglobulimia, his clinical presentation is consistent with this diagnosis based on his clinical findings, including arthralgia,

transaminitis, abdominal pain, proteinuria, and the histopathology findings indicated above.

5. Type II cryoglobulinemia usually presents in patients in their 40s and 50s, with a female predominance (2:1).[5] This is consistent with the underlying diseases that are responsible for cryoglobulinemia, such as multiple myeloma (average age of onset, 65 years), mixed connective tissue diseases (systemic lupus erythematosus [SLE], 15 to 40 years; Sjögren's, 30 to 40 years; systemic sclerosis, 30 to 50 years), and hepatitis C (65% of those infected with HCV are between 40 to 49 years).[6-8] These demographics indicate that cryoglobulinemia in a pediatric patient is not common. Cryoglobulins have been sparsely reported in pediatric patients over the past 4 decades. We have been able to identify 5 single case studies of pediatric patients with cryoglobulins and concomitant: 1) pulmonary cirrhosis and psoriasis (1961);[9] 2) Mononucleosis and hepatitis B (1993);[10] 3) streptococcal infection with evidence of a vasculitic process (1978);[11] 4) sickle cell disease with cold agglutinins (1963);[12] and, 5) IgA nephropathy (2003).[13] However, these studies do little to elucidate the associations between various diseases and cryoglobulins. Additionally, we were able to identify 3 larger studies (n = 30 to 250 patients) that shed light on the association between cryoglobulins and pediatric disease processes (**T4**). Specifically, Schistosoma infection, Schölein-Henoch purpura, and autoimmune diseases have been associated with an increased prevalence of cryoglobulins in pediatric patients.[14-16] Schölein-Henoch purpura, *Schistosoma* infections, and autoimmune diseases such as systemic lupus erythematosus are rare in the United States. While no screening tests for SLE to determine its prevalence in pediatric patients have been performed, it is estimated that 5,000 to 10,000 children in the United States are affected.[17] Yang and colleagues investigated 250 patients suspected of having immune complex-mediated disorders and found that 50% of them were positive for cryoglobulins. Significant correlations exist between the presence of cryoglobulins, serum hypocomplementemia, and C1q activity (evidence of immune complexes) in patients with SLE;[16] however, only 60% of patients with cryoglobulins had immune complexes demonstrable by a positive test for C1q activity.[16] The patient in the present case did have a positive

(1:80 titer) ANA antibody with a speckled pattern (**T2**) and hypocomplementemia (decreased C3 and C4), but no other autoantibodies were identified. The possibility of an underlying autoimmune disease with immune complex deposition would explain many of his clinical and laboratory findings; however, no definitive diagnosis can be made at this time.

6. It is rare to identify urinary Bence Jones proteins with cryoglobulin properties. One of the earliest reports was by Alper in 1966 on a patient with multiple myeloma.[18] While we did not test specifically for cryoglobulins in the urine, IFE of the patient's urine detected an IgG lambda monoclonal antibody. This antibody isotype is the same as that in the cryoglobulin fraction of serum (cf, **Image 2A** versus **2B**). Therefore, it is likely that we identified a cryoglobulin in our patient's urine.

7. Cryoglobulins are unique immunoglobulins that precipitate at temperatures <37°C (mostly at 0°C to 4°C) and re-dissolve upon warming. Approximately 95% of cryoglobulins are immune complexes that have a rheumatoid factor (RF) component (anti-IgG). These can be referred to as mixed cryoglobulins, which are differentiated from monoclonal bands without RF or antigen-antibody complexes. The remaining fraction (~5%) comprise the monoclonal proteins observed in patients with monoclonal gammopathies. These proteins have unique amino acid sequences that cause poor solubility at low temperatures (ie, increased precipitation in the cold). Other proteins precipitate in the cold such as fibrinogen in plasma (cryofibrinogen) and fibronectin.[19] Cyroprecipitate is made up of antibodies (including RF), albumin, fibronectin, fibrinogen, viruses, and bacteria.[19,20] In type I cyroglobulinemia, only antibodies are found. In mixed cryoglobulinemias (types II and III), many components are found including RF. The RF-immunoglobulin complex can cause RF and immune-complex vasculitis in skin, nerves, kidney, joints, and liver.[21] This may account for several of the laboratory findings in the present patient, including elevated liver enzymes. Low affinity RFantibodies (anti-IgG) are antibodies that form naturally and likely play a role in clearing immune complexes by activating complement. Rhematoid factor can react with other antigens, such as microorganisms coated with IgG antibodies, leading to complement activation and agglutination. It is hypothesized that HCV stimulates B cells, inducing a polyclonal IgM RF, although other factors play a role in the IgM RF factor found in type II cryoglobulinemia associated with HCV infection.[22]

8. The cryoglobulins in mixed cryoglobulinemias (type II and type III) tend to precipitate in the small vessels of multiple types of tissues due to their decreased solubility in plasma. Histologically, a leukocytoclastic vasculitis is observed which results from immune complex deposition, complement activation, and leukocyte infiltrates. Arterioles, venules, and capillaries are particularly vulnerable to this deposition, and this vasculitis can lead to ischemia, infarction, and purpura. However, not all patients with mixed cryoglobulins develop vasculitis symptoms.[19,20,23]

9. Therapy is based on the underlying cause of the disease, which can be guided by the classification of cryoglobulins. The mainstay of therapy includes immunosuppression and may require plasmapheresis and antiviral therapy depending on the underlying cause of the patient's cryoglobulinemia. Organ failure secondary to vasculitis in HCV warrants plasmapheresis and therapies against B cells (Rituximab) or TNF (Infliximab) and may be applicable to other causes of type II cryoglobulinemia.[24-27]

Patient Follow-up

The patient was treated symptomatically for his edema with lasix. His hypertension was treated using amlodipine (calcium channel blocker), and his elevated phosphate was treated using Renagel, a polymeric phosphate binder. Fresh frozen plasma (FFP), packed red blood cells (RBCs), and platelet concentrates were given periodically as needed for this patient's hypocomplementemia, anemia, and thrombocytopenia, respectively. Serial serum protein electrophoresis patterns (SPEPs) showed a gradual decrease in monoclonal protein, consistent with his gradual clinical improvement. Two weeks after the initial detection of the patient's monoclonal antibodies by SPE, his IgG lambda peaked at 1.0 g/dL (up from 0.7 g/dL), and at 6 weeks after the initial detection his IgG lambda M-protein concentration had decreased to 0.9 g/dL. The patient is currently being followed by the Pediatric Rheumatology and Nephrology Services to monitor his disease progression. Three months after his initial hospitalization he reported occasional bouts of an erythematous/flushing rash of the cheeks, which is also known to occur on other parts of the body. While there has been no fever, the patient remains very susceptible to exercise-induced tachycardia and is still experiencing easy fatigability, although no fever or major intercurrent illness has been experienced. His pancytopenia and hypergammaglobulinemia have improved, although he has a mild anemia and his ESR is still elevated.

Keywords

cryoglobulinemia, pancytopenia, pediatric, renal disease, M-spike, monoclonal antibody

References

1. Pitetti RD, Laus S, Wadowsky RM. Clinical evaluation of a quantitative real time polymerase chain reaction assay for diagnosis of primary Epstein-Barr virus infection in children. *Pediatr Infect Dis J*. 2003;22:736–739.

2. Brouet JC, Clauvel JP, Danon F, et al. Biologic and clinical significance of cryoglobulins. A report of 86 cases. *Am J Med*. 1974;57:775–788.

3. Ferri C, Zignego AL, Pileri SA. Cryoglobulins. *J Clin Pathol*. 2002;55:4–13.

4. Fiorini G, Bernasconi P, Sinico RA, et al. Increased frequency of antibodies to ubiquitous viruses in essential mixed cryoglobulinaemia. *Clin Exp Immunol*. 1986;64:65–70.

5. Schwartz MM. Heptinstall's Pathology of the Kidney. In *Heptinstall's Pathology of the Kidney*, Vol. 2. Philadelphia: Lippincott-Raven Publishers; 1998:1354–1352.

6. Alter MJ, Kruszon-Moran D, Nainan OV, et al. The prevalence of hepatitis C virus infection in the United States, 1988 through 1994. *N Engl J Med*. 1999;341:556–562.

7. Gaubitz, M. Epidemiology of connective tissue disorders. *Rheumatology* (Oxford). 2006;45:iii3–iii4.

8. Samson D, Singer C. Multiple myeloma. *Clin Med*. 2001;1:365–370.

9. Podgorski J, Wolanska A. Cryoglobulinemia, pulmonary cirrhosis and psoriasis in a 7-year-old girl. *Pediatr Pol*. 1961;36:1171–1175.

10. Doutre MS. Urticaria and angioedema associated with cryoglobulinemia in children. *Allerg Immunol* (Paris). 1993;25:343.

11. Hodson AK, Doughty RA, Norman ME. Acute encephalopathy, streptococcal infection, and cryoglobulinemia. *Arch Neurol*. 1978;35:43–44.

12. Charmot G, Reynaud R, Bergot J. Cryoglobulinaemia and cold agglutinins in painful crises of sickle-cell anaemia. *Lancet*. 1963;18:540.

13. Grech V, Vella C, Aquilina A. Type 2 cryoglobulinemia treated with plasmapheresis associated with IgA nephropathy. *Indian J Pediatr*. 2003;70: 999–1000.

14. Adeiga AA, Ade-Serrano MA. Cryoglobulins in Schistosoma haematobium infection. *Acta Trop*. 1983;40:139–146.

15. Garcia-Fuentes M, Chantler C, Williams DG. Cryoglobulinaemia in Henoch-Schönlein purpura. *Br Med J*. 1977;2:163–165.

16. Yang LC, Norman ME, Doughty RA. A micromethod for the analysis of cryoglobulins via laser nephelometry: Evaluation and comparison to C1q binding activity in autoimmune diseases in pediatrics. *Pediatr Res*. 1980;14:858–862.

17. Lehman TJ. Systemic lupus erythematosus in children and adolescents. In *Dubois' Systemic Lupus Erythematosus*. Wallace D, Hahn B, eds. Philadelphia: WB Saunders; 1996.

18. Alper CA. Cryoglobulinuria: Studies of a cryo-Bence Jones protein. *Acta Med Scand Suppl*. 1966;445:200–205.

19. Kallemuchikkal U, Gorevic PD. Evaluation of cryoglobulins. *Arch Pathol Lab Med*. 1999;123:119–125.

20. Dispenzieri A, Gorevic PD. Cryoglobulinemia. *Hematol Oncol Clin North Am*. 1999;13:1315–1349.

21. Shihabi ZK. Cryoglobulins: An important but neglected clinical test. *Ann Clin Lab Sci*. 2006;36:395–408.

22. Trendelenburg M, Schifferli JA. Cryoglobulins in chronic hepatitis C virus infection. *Clin Exp Immunol*. 2003;133:153–155.

23. Dammacco F, Sansonno D, Piccoli C, et al. The cryoglobulins: An overview. *Eur J Clin Invest*. 2001;31:628–638.

24. Chandesris MO, Gayet S, Schleinitz B, et al. Infliximab in the treatment of refractory vasculitis secondary to hepatitis C-associated mixed cryoglobulinaemia. *Rheumatology* (Oxford). 2004;43:532–533.

25. Lamprecht P, Lerin-Lozano C, Merz H, et al. Rituximab induces remission in refractory HCV associated cryoglobulinaemic vasculitis. *Ann Rheum Dis*. 2003;62:1230–1233.

26. Sansonno D, De Re V, Lauletta G, et al. Monoclonal antibody treatment of mixed cryoglobulinemia resistant to interferon alpha with an anti-CD20. *Blood*. 2003;101:3818–3826.

27. Zaja F, De Vita S, Mazzaro C, et al. Efficacy and safety of rituximab in type II mixed cryoglobulinemia. *Blood*. 2003;101:3827–3834.

Immunofixation Electrophoresis Pattern of Serum From a 50-Year-Old Saudi Woman

Yusra Othman

King Khalid National Guard Hospital, Jeddah, Saudi Arabia

Patient: 50-year-old Saudi woman.

Chief Complaint: Hoarseness, weakness, fatigue, and chronic gum bleeding.

History of Present Illness: She was admitted to the hospital previously and diagnosed with lymphadenopathy, MALT (mucosa-associated lymphoid tissue) subtype non-Hodgkin lymphoma, hypothyroidism, and emphysema.

History of Current Medications: L-thyroxin and Zantac.

Physical Examination Findings: Both eyes were congested and her left eye was swollen. Subsequently, she was seen in an opthalmology clinic and diagnosed with periorbital cellulitis. Review of systems indicated intact central nervous system (CNS) and normal cardiovascular system (CVS) findings. Her abdomen was soft with evidence of splenomegaly and no evidence of any other organomegaly or masses.

Questions

1. What is (are) this patient's most striking clinical and laboratory findings?

2. How do you explain these findings?

3. Why did her initial serum immunofixation electrophoresis (IFE) findings demonstrate a single discrete band in all lanes of the IFE gel?

4. How should her serum be treated to resolve the discrepancy of multiple bands in all lanes of the IFE gel?

5. What is this patient's most likely diagnosis?

6. What is the etiology of this patient's condition?

7. How should this patient's condition be treated?

Possible Answers

1. Fatigue, chronic gum bleeding, splenomegaly, congested and swollen eyes, periorbital cellulitis; anemia (decreased hemoglobin level), increased total protein with decreased albumin, markedly increased globulins, an inverted A/G ratio, and markedly increased serum viscosity; serum protein electrophoresis pattern (SPEP) consistent with a tall, dense band in the gamma region of the SPE gel (**Image 1A**) and abnormal IFE

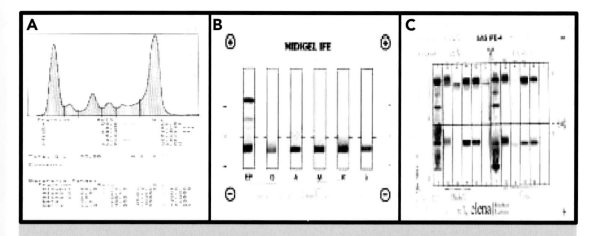

Image 1_Patient's serum protein electrophoresis pattern (SPEP) (**A**), illustrating a tall, dense band in the gamma-region, and immunofixation electrophoresis (IFE) patterns before (**B**) and after (**C**) treatment of the patient's serum with β-mercaptoethanol. In Panel (**C**), the upper left quadrant shows the IFE pattern of the patient's serum pretreated with β-mercaptoethanol for 10 min, while the upper right quadrant shows the IFE pattern of the patient's serum pretreated with β-mercaptoethanol for 30 min. The lower left quadrant shows the IFE pattern of the patient's serum pretreated with β-mercaptoethanol for 60 min. The lower right quadrant shows the IFE pattern of an abnormal control serum of known IgM kappa immunophenotype. Prior to β-mercaptoethanol treatment of the patient's serum, visibly discrete protein bands were observed in all lanes of the IFE gel (**B**), while after treatment of the patient's serum with β-mercaptoethanol, a discrete band of IgM kappa, and some polyclonal IgG, are observed (**C**). Pre-treatment with β-mercaptoethanol for 60 min provided the best resolution of the multiple bands. In all 4 quadrants of panel (**C**), lanes 1-6 represent the lanes to which no antiserum was added (*lane 1*) or to which IgG (*lane 2*), IgA (*lane 3*), IgM (*lane 4*), kappa light chain (*lane 5*), or lambda light chain (*lane 6*) antiserum was added. The horizontal dotted line in panel (**B**) and the solid line in panel (**C**) indicate the point-of-application of serum/antiserum on the IFE gel.

T1. Principal Laboratory Findings

Test	Patient's Result	Reference Interval
Hematology		
WBC count	8.5	4.1-10.9 × 10³/μL
Hemoglobin	9.8	12.0-15.2 g/dL
Platelet count	282	140-450 × 10³/μL
Chemistry[a]		
Total protein	11.2	6.3-8.2 g/dL
Albumin	3.4	3.5-5.2 g/dL
Globulins	7.8	1.3-3.2 g/dL
A/G ratio	0.44	1.5-3.0
IgG	1.72	0.65-1.6 g/dL
IgA	0.11	0.04-0.35 g/dL
IgM	5.84	0.05-0.30 g/dL
Serum viscosity[b]	5.9	1.14-1.34 centipoises

[a]*Liver function tests were normal (data not shown).* [b]*Ordered because her serum appeared highly viscous. WBC, white blood cell; A/G, albumin: globulin ratio.*

findings (ie, protein bands present in all lanes of the IFE gel) (**Image 1B**).

2. Her fatigue is most likely a consequence of her anemia related to chronic gum bleeding, while her congested and swollen eyes with periorbital cellulitis are most likely a consequence of her abnormal protein levels, especially her markedly increased serum globulins and viscosity (hyperviscosity syndrome), and the presence of a large M-protein on SPE. It is not uncommon that opthalmologists order SPE on their patients that present with signs and symptoms of blurred or impaired vision. Moreover, monoclonal proteins are often observed in serum from these patients, which might otherwise go undetected until a later course in their disease. In addition, chronic nasal bleeding and oozing from the gums occur commonly in patients with hyperviscosity syndrome, especially when the serum viscosity is >4 centipoises.[1] Our patient's serum viscosity was 5.9 centipoises (**T1**).

3. Our patient's IFE pattern is classic for the presence of a high concentration of a cryoglobulin that migrates as a single band, precipitates in all lanes of an IFE gel, and is stained with the protein-staining dye used to detect the presence of immunoglobulins in any of the lanes of the SPE gel. This finding, when coupled with her viscous-appearing serum, markedly increased serum viscosity, and presenting symptoms of weakness, fatigue, and bleeding are pathognomonic findings for the large IgM monoclonal protein that is found in the serum of patients with primary (or Waldenström macroglobulinemia. In serum, IgM immunoglobulin monomers combine to form a pentameric molecule that is large in size. An increased concentration of these molecules causes the serum to become viscous. Moreover, other immunoglobulins (eg, IgG and IgA) can bind to the IgM pentameric complex, thus further explaining the presence of discrete immunoglobulin bands in all lanes of the IFE gel, including the lanes to which anti-IgG and anti-IgA antiserum was added.

4. With the disulfide bond reducing agent, β-mercaptoethanol. The use of β-mercaptoethanol to resolve the serum IFE findings observed in our patient, definitively identify the monoclonal protein in the patient's serum, and produce immunoglobulin information consistent with the results obtained from quantitative measurement of serum immunoglobulins by nephelometry has been described previously.[2-4] After pre-treatment of our patient's serum sample with 10% β-mercaptoethanol for 10, 30, or 60 min, followed by repeat IFE of this mixture, the previously observed multiple bands resolved into fewer bands (**Image 1C**). After pre-treatment of our patient's serum with 10% β-mercaptoethanol for 60 min, a single IgM kappa monoclonal protein band was observed that corresponded with the location of the discrete, dense band found in the electrophoresis lane of the IFE gel [**Image 1C**, lower left quadrant].

5. ***Most likely diagnosis:*** *Waldenström macroglobulinemia (IgM M-protein) in a patient with MALT subtype non-Hodgkin lymphoma.* To our knowledge, this patient represents the first reported case of Waldenström macroglobulinemia in Saudi Arabia.

6. Macroglobulinemia results from the uncontrolled proliferation of lymphocytes and plasma cells that secrete large amounts of IgM monoclonal protein; however, the cause of this disease is currently unknown. Waldenström macroglobulinemia is an uncommon B-cell lymphoproliferative disorder (lymphoplasmacytic lymphoma) characterized primarily by bone marrow infiltration with a predominantly intertrabecular pattern and an IgM monoclonal gammopathy.[5,6] However, the concentration of the monoclonal IgM M-protein has little or no prognostic relevance in patients with Waldenström macroglobulinemia.[7] Although Waldenström macroglobulinemia is mainly associated with IgM paraproteinemia, it is occasionally associated with IgG and IgA paraproteins.[5,6,8,9] The high molecular weight IgM molecules contribute to the salient symptoms of this disease, including the serious and potentially fatal complications of hyperviscosity syndrome.[10]

7. The treatment for symptomatic hyperviscosity syndrome is daily plasmapheresis [plasma exchange of 3 to 4 L with albumin (in lieu of plasma) replacement] until the patient is asymptomatic. Our patient underwent plasmapheresis and chemotherapy with cyclophosphamide, vincristine, and prednisone with evidence of clinical improvement; however, a computed tomography (CT) scan of her lungs revealed multiple lesions and she was started on MabThera (antibody specific for the CD20 cell surface marker on B cells) therapy.

Keywords

Waldenström macroglobulinemia, hyperviscosity syndrome, monoclonal gammopathy, immunofixation electrophoresis, β-mercaptoethanol

References

1. Widman, F. *Clinical Interpretation of Laboratory Tests.* 9th ed. Philadelphia: FA Davis, 1983, pp 186-187.

2. Keren DF, Gulbranson, R, Cary JL, et al. 2-Mercaptoethanol treatment improves measurement of an IgM protein by capillary electrophoresis. *Clin Chem.* 2001;47:1326-1327.

3. Doinel C, Ropars C, Salmon C. Agglutination activities of the subunit of one IgM cold agglutinin treated with various reducing agents. *Eur J Immunol.* 1973;9:563-568.

4. Zemmerman B, Grey HM. Non-covalent interaction between immunoglobulin polypeptide chains: stability to dissociation by denaturant. *Biochemistry.* 1972;1:78-84.

5. Dimopoulos MA, Alexanian R. Waldenström's macroglobulinemia. *Blood.* 1994;83:1452-1459.

6. Dimopoulos MA, Panayoitides P, Moulopoulos LA, et al. Waldenström's macroglobulinemia: clinical features, complications and management. *J Clin Oncol.* 2000;18:214-226.

7. Owen RG, Barrans SL, Richards SJ, et al. Waldenström's macroglobulinemia: development of diagnostic criteria and identification of prognostic factors. *Am J Clin Pathol.* 2001;116:420-428.

8. Jandle JH. Mutiple myeloma and related plasma cell dyscrasias. In: *Blood Pathophysiology.* Boston: Blackwell, 1991:349-370.

9. Rolcke D. Cold agglutination, antibodies, and antigens. *Clin Immunol Immunopathol.* 1974;2:266-280.

10. Waldenström J. Incipient myelomatosis or essential hyperglobulinemia with fibronopenia: a new syndrome? *Acta Med Scan.* 1944;117:216.

D

E

I

O

P

R

S